MAGNETIC RESONANCE IMAGING

Second Edition

Volume I

Clinical Principles

C. LEON PARTAIN, M.D., Ph.D.
RONALD R. PRICE, Ph.D.
JAMES A. PATTON, Ph.D.
MADAN V. KULKARNI, M.D.
A. EVERETTE JAMES, JR., Sc.M., J.D., M.D.

Division of Medical Imaging
Department of Radiology and Radiological Sciences
Vanderbilt University Medical Center
Nashville, Tennessee

1988
W.B. SAUNDERS COMPANY
Harcourt Brace Jovanovich, Inc.
Philadelphia   London   Toronto   Montreal   Sydney   Tokyo

W. B. SAUNDERS COMPANY
Harcourt Brace Jovanovich, Inc.

The Curtis Center
Independence Square West
Philadelphia, PA 19106

PHYSICS

LIBRARY OF CONGRESS
Library of Congress Cataloging-in-Publication Data

Magnetic resonance imaging (MRI) / [edited by] C. Leon Partain . . .[et
al.].
    p. cm.
  Includes indexes.
  Contents: v. 1. Clinical applications—v. 2. Physical principles
and instrumentation.
  ISBN 0-7216-1340-3 (set). ISBN 0-7216-2516-9 (v. 1). ISBN
0-7216-2517-7 (v. 2).
  1. Magnetic resonance imaging. I. Partain, C. Leon.
RC78.7.N83M344 1988
616.07'57—dc19

87-26651
CIP

Listed here is the latest translated edition of this book together with the language of the translation and the
publisher.

Japanese (*1st Edition*)—Igaku Shoin/Saunders Ltd., Ichibancho Central Bldg., 22-1 Ichibancho,
        Chiyoda-Ku, Tokyo 102, Japan

Editor: Lisette Bralow
Developmental Editor: Kathleen McCullough
Designer: W. B. Saunders Staff
Production Manager: Bob Butler
Manuscript Editors: Constance Burton/Susan Thomas
Illustration Coordinator: Brett MacNaughton
Indexer: Alexandra Weir

Magnetic Resonance Imaging (MRI)

Volume I ISBN 0–7216–2516–9
Volume II ISBN 0–7216–2517–7
SET ISBN 0–7216–1340–3

Last digit is the print number: 9   8   7   6   5   4   3   2   1

To
David Blane, Teri Ellyn, and Amy Leigh Partain
Amanda Belle Price
James Allen, Jr., and David Lee Patton
Delores J. Kulkarni
Alton Everette and Pattie Royster James

Contributors

W. J. ADAMS, Ph.D.   Software Engineer, Corporate Research and Development Center, General Electric Company, Schenectady, New York
Quantitative NMR Tissue Characterization Using Calculated Images and Automated Image Segmentation

JOSEPH H. ALLEN, M.D.   Professor of Radiology and Radiological Sciences, Vanderbilt University Medical Center, Nashville, Tennessee
Tumor Imaging with Gd-DTPA; Pituitary and Parasellar Region

MARY P. ANDERSON, M.S.   Office of Radiological Health, National Center for Devices and Radiological Health, United States Food and Drug Administration, Rockville, Maryland
Operational Guidelines: United States

WILLIAM H. ANDERSON, M.S.   Research Associate, University of Kansas Medical Center, Kansas City, Kansas
Computer Networks for Medical Image Management

E. R. ANDREW, Ph.D., Sc.D., F.R.S.,   Graduate Research Professor of Physics and Radiology, University of Florida, Gainesville, Florida
NMR in Medicine: A Historical Review

IAN M. ARMITAGE, Ph.D.   Yale University School of Medicine; Yale–New Haven Hospital, New Haven, Connecticut
NMR Evaluation of Tumor Metabolism

TIMOTHY ASHBAUGH, M.S.   Graduate student, Vanderbilt University School of Medicine, Nashville, Tennessee
Dynamic Contrast-Enhanced MRI and Mathematical Modeling

T. WHIT ATHEY   Lecturer, Electical Engineering Department, University of Maryland, Baltimore, Maryland
Operational Guidelines: United States

LEON AXEL, Ph.D., M.D.   Associate Professor, University of Pennsylvania; Department of Radiology, Hospital of the University of Pennsylvania, Philadelphia, Pennsylvania
Future Directions; MRI of Blood Flow

D. R. BAILES, M.Sc.   Department of Medical Physics, University of Manchester, Manchester, United Kingdom
Artifacts in the Measurement of T1 and T2

D. BALERIAUX, M.D.   Professor of Radiology, Université Libre de Bruxelles; Head of the Neuroradiological Clinic in the Department of Radiology, Erasne Hospital, Brussels, Belgium
Surface Coil Imaging of the Spine

P. T. BEALL, Ph.D.   Department of Biology, Texas Woman's University, Houston, Texas
Distinction of the Normal, Preneoplastic, and Neoplastic States by Water Proton NMR Relaxation Times

M. ROBIN BENDALL, B.Sc. (Tasmania), D.Phil. (Oxford), D.Sc. (Griffith)   Senior Lecturer, Griffith University, Brisbane, Australia
Surface Coil Technology

WILFRIED H. BERGMANN, Ph.D.   Senior Research Associate, Department of Physics and Astronomy, Vanderbilt University, Nashville, Tennessee
Hydrodynamic Blood Flow Analysis with Low Temperature NMR Spin Echo Detection

ALBERT H. BETH, Ph.D.   Assistant Professor of Molecular Physiology and Biophysics, Vanderbilt University School of Medicine, Nashville, Tennessee
Advanced Methods for Spin Density, T1, and T2 Calculations in MRI

FELIX BLOCH, Ph.D. (1905–1983)   Max Stein Professor of Physics, Emeritus, Stanford University, Palo Alto, California. Nobel Prize in Physics (for NMR), 1952
Past, Present, and Future of Nuclear Magnetic Resonance

J. L. BLOEM, M.D.   University Hospital, Department of Diagnostic Radiology, Leiden, The Netherlands
Primary Malignant Bone Tumors

R. G. BLUEMM, M.D.   University of Bochum, Marienhospital Herhe, Herhe, German Federal Republic
Primary Malignant Bone Tumors; Fast, Small Flip-Angle Field Echo Imaging

E. BOSKAMP, Ph.D.   Manager, RF Coil Laboratories, Philips Medical Systems, Best, The Netherlands
Surface Coil Imaging of the Spine

PAUL A. BOTTOMLEY, Ph.D.   Physicist, General Electric Research and Development Center, Schenectady, New York
Frequency Dependence of Tissue Relaxation Times

WILLIAM G. BRADLEY, JR., M.D., Ph.D.   Associate Clinical Professor of Radiology, University of California, San Francisco; Director, MR Imaging Laboratory, Huntington Medical Research Institutes and Huntington Memorial Hospital, Pasadena, California
Inflammatory Disease of the Brain; Intracranial Hemorrhage; Future Directions

THOMAS J. BRADY, M.D.   Associate Professor of Radiology, Harvard Medical School; Associate Radiologist and Assistant in Medicine, Massachusetts General Hopital, Boston, Massachusetts
Iron Ethylene bis (2-Hydroxyphenylglycine) as a Hepatobiliary MRI Contrast Agent; Chemical Shift Imaging

ROBERT C. BRASCH, M.D.   Professor of Radiology and Pediatrics; Director, Contrast Media Laboratory, University of California, San Francisco, California
Free Radical Contrast Agents for MRI

H. G. BRITTAIN, Ph.D.   Research Fellow, The Squibb Institute for Medical Research, New Brunswick, New Jersey
Principles of Contrast-Enhanced MRI

RODNEY A. BROOKS, Ph.D.   Neuroimaging Section, NINCDS, National Institutes of Health, Bethesda, Maryland
Image Reconstruction

MARK S. BROWN, Ph.D.   Research Associate, Yale University School of Medicine, New Haven, Connecticut
Pathophysiological Significance of Relaxation

RODNEY D. BROWN, III, Ph.D.   Research Staff Member, IBM, T. J. Watson Research Center, Yorktown Heights, New York
Relaxometry of Solvent and Tissue Protons: Diamagnetic Contributions; Relaxometry of Solvent and Tissue Protons: Paramagnetic Contributions

GORDON L. BROWNELL, Ph.D.   Professor of Radiological Physics, Harvard Medical School; Professor of Nuclear Engineering, Massachusetts Institute of Technology; Radiological Physics, Massachusetts General Hospital, Boston, Massachusetts
Current and Future Frontiers in Medical Imaging

D. J. BRYANT, Ph.D.   GEC Research, Limited, Wembley, Middlesex, United Kingdom
Artifacts in the Measurement of T1 and T2

LAWRENCE J. BUSSE, Ph.D.   Engineering Staff, General Electric—Aircraft Engines; Adjunct Assistant Professor of Radiology, University of Cincinnati, Cincinnati, Ohio
Gradient Coil Technology

RICHARD B. BUXTON, Ph.D.   Instructor, Department of Radiology, Harvard Medical School; Assistant in Applied Physics, Department of Radiology, Massachusetts General Hospital, Boston, Massachusetts
Chemical Shift Imaging

G. M. BYDDER, M.B., Ch.B., F.R.C.R. Senior Lecturer, Royal Postgraduate Medical School, Hammersmith Hospital, London, United Kingdom
Tumors of the Central Nervous System; Artifacts in the Measurement of T1 and T2

ROBERT C. CANBY, M.E.E. Senior Medical Student, University of Texas Southwestern Medical School, Dallas, Texas
Ischemic Heart Disease

GARY R. CAPUTO, M.D. Resident, Department of Radiology, University of California, San Francisco, California
Magnetic Resonance Imaging of the Heart

FRANK E. CARROLL, JR., M.D. Associate Professor of Radiology and Radiological Sciences, Vanderbilt University School of Medicine; Director of Diagnostic Radiology, Vanderbilt University Medical Center, Nashville, Tennessee
Lungs

BRITTON CHANCE, Ph.D. Professor Emeritus, University of Pennsylvania, Philadelphia, Pennsylvania
Phosphorus-31 Spectroscopy and Imaging

JEFFREY A. CLANTON, M.S. Associate in Radiology, Vanderbilt University School of Medicine; Director, Radio and MRI Pharmacy, Vanderbilt University Hospital, Nashville, Tennessee
Oral Contrast Agents; Dynamic Contrast-Enhanced MRI and Mathematical Modeling

HOWARD T. COFFEY, Ph.D. (Physics) Sub-Sea Systems, Inc., Escondido, California
Principles of Superconducting Magnets

SHEILA M. COHEN, Ph.D. Senior Research Fellow, Merck Institute for Therapeutic Research, Merck, Sharp & Dohme Research Laboratories, Rahway, New Jersey
Carbon-13: NMR Spectroscopy

JANET D. COIL, Ph.D. Philips Medical Systems, Inc., Shelton, Connecticut
Planning and Preparation

THOMAS E. CONTURO, B.A. Graduate Student and Medical Student (M.D., Ph.D.) Medical Scientist, Training Program of the National Institutes of Health, Vanderbilt University School of Medicine, Nashville, Tennessee
MRI Optimization Strategies; Understanding Basic MR Pulse Sequences; Advanced Methods for Spin Density, T1, and T2 Calculations in MRI

LARRY T. COOK, Ph.D. Associate Professor of Diagnostic Radiology, University of Kansas; University of Kansas Medical Center, Kansas City, Kansas
Breast; Computer Networks for Medical Image Management

GLENDON G. COX, M.D. Associate Professor, University of Kansas; University of Kansas Medical Center (Bell Memorial Hospital), Kansas City, Kansas
Computer Networks for Medical Image Management

F. C. CREZEE, M.D. Academisch Ziekenhuis van de Vrije Universiteit, Department of Radiology, Amsterdam, The Netherlands
Malignant Lesions of the Paranasal Sinuses

LAWRENCE E. CROOKS, Ph.D. Professor of Electrical Engineering, Department of Radiology, University of California, San Francisco, California
Fundamental Limitations

J. CUPPEN, Ph.D. Department of MRI, Philips Medical Systems Division, Best, The Netherlands
Fast, Small Flip-Angle Field Echo Imaging

RAYMOND DAMADIAN, M.D. President, FONAR Corporation, Melville, New York
NMR Scanning

JOHN L. DELAYRE, Ph.D. Department of Radiology, University of Texas Medical School, Houston, Texas
Localization Methods in NMR

J. DEN BOER, Ph.D. Department of MRI, Philips Medical Systems Division, Best, The Netherlands
Fast, Small Flip-Angle Field Echo Imaging

R. G. M. DE SLEGTE, M.D. Academisch Ziekenhuis van de Vrije Universiteit, Department of Radiology, Amsterdam, The Netherlands
Malignant Lesions of the Paranasal Sinuses

TIMOTHY M. DEVINNEY, M.B.A. Assistant Professor, Owen Graduate School of Management, Vanderbilt University, Nashville, Tennessee
Legal Aspects of MRI

L. S. DE VRIES, M.D. Senior Research Fellow, Hammersmith Hospital, Royal Postgraduate Medical School, London, United Kingdom
Tumors of the Central Nervous System

J. DOORNBOS, Ph.D. University Hospital, Department of Diagnostic Radiology, Leiden, The Netherlands
Primary Malignant Bone Tumors; Fast, Small Flip-Angle Field Echo Imaging

LEO F. DROLSHAGEN, III, M.D.   MRI Fellow, Department of Radiology and Radiological Sciences, Vanderbilt University Medical Center, Nashville, Tennessee
Female Pelvis

EDWARD J. DUDEWICZ, Ph.D.   Professor and Chairman, University Statistics Council, Department of Mathematics, Syracuse University, Syracuse, New York
Advanced Statistical Methods for Tissue Characteristics

SAMUEL J. DWYER, III, Ph.D.   Professor of Diagnostic Radiology, University of Kansas Medical Center, Kansas City, Kansas
Breast; Computer Networks for Medical Image Management

WILLIAM C. ECKELMAN, Ph.D.   Vice-President of Research and Development, The Squibb Institute for Medical Research, New Brunswick, New Jersey
Principles of Contrast-Enhanced MRI

WILLIAM A. EDELSTEIN, Ph.D.   Physicist, Corporate Research and Development Center, General Electric Company, Schenectady, New York
Radio Frequency Resonators

KENNETH R. EFFERSON, Ph.D.   President, American Magnetics, Inc., Oak Ridge, Tennessee
Principles of Superconducting Magnets

STEPHEN G. EINSTEIN   Philips Medical Systems, Inc., Shelton, Connecticut
Planning and Preparation

ALAN EISENBERG, M.D.   Resident, Department of Radiology and Radiological Sciences, Vanderbilt University Medical Center, Nashville, Tennessee
MRI Optimization Strategies

JANE E. ERICKSON, M.H.S.   Research Associate, Center for Hospital Finance and Management, Johns Hopkins University, Baltimore, Maryland
The Economics and Regulation of MRI

JON J. ERICKSON, Ph.D.   Associate Professor of Radiology and Radiological Sciences, Vanderbilt University Medical Center, Nashville, Tennessee
Image Production and Display

RICHARD R. ERNST, DR. PROF.   Full Professor, Laboratorium Für Physikalische Chemie, Technische Hochschule, Zürich, Switzerland
A Survey of MRI Techniques

WILLIAM T. EVANOCHKO, Ph.D.   Assistant Professor of Medicine, University of Alabama, Birmingham, Alabama
Ischemic Heart Disease

THEODORE H. M. FALKE, M.D.   Department of Diagnostic Radiology, University Hospital, Leiden, The Netherlands
MRI Optimization Strategies; Adrenal Glands; Blood Flow in MR Imaging; Primary Malignant Bone Tumors; Sonography and MRI

BRIAN D. FELLMETH, M.D., Ph.D.   Resident in Radiology, Vanderbilt University Medical Center, Nashville, Tennessee; Fellow, Vascular Radiology, University of California, San Diego, California
Practical Pediatric MRI

HARVEY V. FINEBERG, M.D., Ph.D.   Dean, Harvard School of Public Health, Cambridge, Massachusetts
Clinical Efficacy: 5000 MRI Cases Between 0.15 and 0.6 Tesla

JAMES J. FISCHER, M.D., Ph.D.   Professor and Chairman, Department of Therapeutic Radiology, Yale University School of Medicine; Chief, Department of Therapeutic Radiology, Yale–New Haven Hospital, New Haven, Connecticut
NMR Evaluation of Tumor Metabolism

MADELEINE R. FISHER, M.D.   Assistant Professor, Department of Radiology, Northwestern University; Medical Director, MRI, Northwestern Memorial Hospital, Chicago, Illinois
Neck; Prostate and Urinary Bladder

ARTHUR C. FLEISCHER, M.D.   Professor of Radiology and Radiological Sciences, Associate Professor of Obstetrics and Gynecology, Vanderbilt University School of Medicine; Director, Ultrasound Section, Department of Radiology and Radiological Sciences, Vanderbilt University Hospital, Nashville, Tennessee
Breast; Sonography and MRI

MARK P. FREEMAN, M.D.   Clinical Assistant Professor, Department of Radiology, Vanderbilt University Medical Center and Baptist Hospital, Nashville, Tennessee
Ischemic Cerebrovascular Disease

G. T. GAUGHAN, Ph.D.   Group Leader, The Squibb Institute for Medical Research, New Brunswick, New Jersey
Principles of Contrast-Enhanced MRI

HARRY K. GENANT, M.D.   Professor of Radiology, Medicine and Orthopaedic Surgery; Chief of Skeletal Radiology, Department of Radiology, University of California, San Francisco, School of Medicine, San Francisco, California
The Spine

G. J. GERRITSEN, M.D.   Academische Ziekenhuis van de Vrije, Universiteit Department of Otolaryngology, Head and Neck Surgery, Amsterdam, The Netherlands
Malignant Lesions of the Paranasal Sinuses

ANTHONY GIAMBALVO, Ph.D.   Vice-President, FONAR Corporation, Melville, New York
NMR Scanning

S. JULIAN GIBBS, D.D.S., Ph.D.   Associate Professor of Radiology and Assistant Professor of Dentistry, Vanderbilt University; Adjunct Professor, University of Tennessee Space Institute; Radiology Service, Vanderbilt University Hospital, Nashville, Tennessee
Bioeffects

EDWARD J. GOLDSTEIN, Ph.D., M.D.   Assistant Professor of Radiology, Hospital of the University of Pennsylvania, Philadelphia, Pennsylvania; Chairman, Department of Radiology, Los Alamitos Medical Center, Los Alamitos, California
Free Radical Contrast Agents for MRI; Hepatobiliary Contrast Agents

J. C. GORE, Ph.D.   Associate Professor of Radiology, Yale University School of Medicine, New Haven, Connecticut
Quantitative NMR Tissue Characterization Using Calculated Images and Automated Image Segmentation; Legal Aspects of MRI; Pathophysiological Significance of Relaxation; NMR Evaluation of Tumor Metabolism

THOMAS P. GRAHAM, JR., M.D.   Professor of Pediatrics, Director of Pediatric Cardiology, Vanderbilt University Medical Center, Nashville, Tennessee
Gated MRI in Congenital Cardiac Malformations

TOM GREESON, J.D., L.L.D.   Professor of Law, Vanderbilt University, Nashville, Tennessee
Legal Aspects of MRI

J. J. HAGAN, Ph.D.   Senior Research Investigator, The Squibb Institute for Medical Research, New Brunswick, New Jersey
Principles of Contrast-Enhanced MRI

A. S. HALL, Ph.D.   GEC Research, Limited, Wembley, Middlesex, United Kingdom
Artifacts in the Measurement of T1 and T2

STEVEN E. HARMS, M.D.   Director of Magnetic Resonance, Department of Medical Imaging, Baylor University Medical Center, Dallas, Texas
Face, Orbit, and Temporomandibular Joint

JOHN H. HARRIS, JR., M.D., D.Sc.   Professor and Chairman, Department of Radiology, University of Texas Medical School; Chairman, Department of Radiology, Hermann Hospital, Houston, Texas
Musculoskeletal System

CECIL E. HAYES, Ph.D.   Senior Physicist, Applied Science Laboratory, GE Medical Systems, Milwaukee, Wisconsin
Radio Frequency Resonators

C. F. HAZLEWOOD, Ph.D.   Professor, Department of Physiology, Baylor College of Medicine, Houston, Texas
Distinction of the Normal, Preneoplastic, and Neoplastic States by Water Proton NMR Relaxation Times

RICHARD M. HELLER, M.D.   Professor of Radiology and Radiological Sciences, Vanderbilt University Medical Center; Chief, Pediatric Radiology, Vanderbilt University Hospital, Nashville, Tennessee
Practical Pediatric MRI

KENNETH S. HENSLEY, M.S.   Research Associate, University of Kansas Medical Center, Kansas City, Kansas
Computer Networks for Medical Image Management

ROBERT J. HERFKENS, M.D.   Associate Professor of Radiology, Director of Magnetic Resonance Imaging Section, Duke University Medical Center, Durham, North Carolina
High Field MRI

CHARLES B. HIGGINS, M.D.   Professor and Vice-Chairman, Department of Radiology, University of California, San Francisco, School of Medicine; Chief, Magnetic Resonance Imaging, University of California, San Francisco, Medical Center, San Francisco, California
Neck; Magnetic Resonance Imaging of the Heart

G. NEIL HOLLAND, M.Phil.   Picker International, Highland Heights, Ohio
Systems Engineering

MYRON HOLSCHER, D.V.M., Ph.D.   Associate Professor of Pathology, Vanderbilt University School of Medicine; Associate Director, Animal Care, Vanderbilt University Medical Center, Nashville, Tennessee
Dynamic Contrast-Enhanced MRI and Mathematical Modeling

HEDVIG HRICAK, M.D.   Professor of Radiology and Urology, University of California, San Francisco; Chief of Uroradiology Section, Department of Urology, University of California, San Francisco, Medical Center, San Francisco, California
Clinical Potential of MRI; Prostate and Urinary Bladder

NOLA M. HYLTON, Ph.D.   Assistant Professor of Physics, Department of Radiology, Radiologic Imaging Laboratory, University of California, San Francisco, California
MRI Parameter Selection Techniques

MASAHIRO IIO, M.D.   Professor and Chairman, Department of Radiology, University of Tokyo, Tokyo, Japan
Current and Future Frontiers in Medical Imaging

JOANNE S. INGWALL, Ph.D.   Associate Professor of Physiology and Biophysics, Department of Medicine, Harvard Medical School; Biochemist, Brigham and Women's Hospital, Boston, Massachusetts
The Physiological Chemistry of Creatine Kinase in the Heart: Phosphorus-31 Magnetization Transfer Studies

A. EVERETTE JAMES, JR., Sc.M., J.D., M.D.   Professor and Chairman, Department of Radiology and Radiological Sciences, Vanderbilt University School of Medicine; Vanderbilt University Hospital, Nashville, Tennessee
Sonography and MRI; Legal Aspects of MRI; Bioeffects

A. EVERETTE JAMES, III, B.A.   Law Student, University of Illinois, Chicago, Illinois
Legal Aspects of MRI

JEANNETTE CROSS JAMES, B.A.   Student, The Washington College of Law at the American University, Washington, D.C.
Legal Aspects of MRI

JEROME P. JONES, Ph.D.   Diagnostic Physicist, Department of Radiology, Alton Ochsner Medical Foundation, New Orleans, Louisiana
Physics of the MR Image: From the Basic Principles to Image Intensity and Contrast; T1 and T2 Measurement

M. C. KAISER, M.D.   Academisch Ziekenhuis van de Vrije Universiteit, Department of Radiology, Amsterdam, The Netherlands
Malignant Lesions of the Paranasal Sinuses

ALAN J. KAUFMAN, M.D.   Assistant Professor of Radiology and Radiological Sciences, Vanderbilt University Medical Center; Co-Director, Abdominal Imaging, Vanderbilt University Hospital, Nashville, Tennessee
Gastrointestinal Tract

ROBERT M. KESSLER, M.D.   Associate Professor of Radiology, Vanderbilt University School of Medicine; Chief, Neuroradiology, Vanderbilt University Medical Center, Nashville, Tennessee
Ischemic Cerebrovascular Disease

SEYMOUR H. KOENIG, Ph.D.   Research Staff Member, IBM, T. J. Watson Research Center, Yorktown Heights, New York; Adjunct Professor of Physics, University of Illinois, Urbana, Illinois
Relaxometry of Solvent and Tissue Protons: Diamagnetic Contributions; Relaxometry of Solvent and Tissue Protons: Paramagnetic Contributions

W. KOOPS, M.D.   Department of Diagnostic Radiology, University Hospital, Rotterdam, The Netherlands
Fast, Small Flip-Angle Field Echo Imaging

KEITH E. KORTMAN, M.D.   Assistant Clinical Profesor of Radiology, University of California, San Diego; Research Radiologist, Huntington Medical Research Institute; Huntington Memorial Hospital, Pasadena; Sharp Memorial Hospital, San Diego, California
Inflammatory Disease of the Brain

MADAN V. KULKARNI, M.D. Assistant Professor and Clinical Director, Magnetic Resonance Imaging, Vanderbilt University Medical Center, Nashville, Tennessee
Spinal Cord; Gated MRI in Congenital Cardiac Malformations; Breast; Kidneys and Retroperitoneum; Female Pelvis; Musculoskeletal System; Sonography and MRI Correlation; Pitfalls and Artifacts in Clinical MRI; NMR of ^{23}Na in Biological Systems

RANDALL B. LAUFFER, Ph.D. Assistant Professor, Department of Radiology, Harvard Medical School; Director, NMR Contrast Media Laboratory, Massachusetts General Hospital, Boston, Massachusetts
Iron Ethylene bis (2-Hydroxyphenylglycine) as a Hepatobiliary MRI Contrast Agent

RICHARD L. LAWS, B.S. Research Associate, University of Kansas Medical Center, Kansas City, Kansas
Computer Networks for Medical Image Management

JOHN S. LEIGH, JR., Ph.D. Professor of Biochemistry and Biophysics, University of Pennsylvania, Philadelphia, Pennsylvania
Phosphorus-31 Spectroscopy and Imaging

GEORGE C. LEVY, Ph.D. Professor of Science and Technology, Syracuse University; Adjunct Professor of Radiology, S.U.N.Y. Health Sciences Center at Syracuse; Adjunct Professor of Radiology, State University of New York, Health Sciences Center at Syracuse, New York
Advanced Statistical Methods for Tissue Characteristics

OTHA W. LINTON, M.S.J. Associate Executive Director, American College of Radiology, Chevy Chase, Maryland
The Economics and Regulation of MRI

WILFRIED LOEFFLER, Ph.D. Siemens A.G. Medical Engineering Group, Erlangen, German Federal Republic
Systems Optimization

MARK A. LUTHE, B.A. Diasonics, Inc., San Francisco, California
Chemical Efficacy: 5000 MRI Cases Between 0.15 and 0.6 Tesla; Clinical Efficacy: Analysis of 300 MRI Cases at 1.5 Tesla

JAMES R. MacFALL, Ph.D. General Electric Company, Medical Systems Group, Milwaukee, Wisconsin
Impact of the Choice of Operating Parameters on MR Images

S. MAJUMDAR, Ph.D. Associate Research Scientist, Department of Diagnostic Radiology, Yale University School of Medicine, New Haven, Connecticut
Quantitative NMR Tissue Characterization Using Calculated Images and Automated Image Segmentation

ALEXANDER R. MARGULIS, M.D.   Professor and Chairman, Department of Radiology, University of California, San Francisco, School of Medicine, San Francisco, California
Clinical Potential of MRI

R. MATHUR-DE VRÉ, Ph.D   Research Associate, Institut d'Hygiène et d'Epidémiologie, Brussels, Belgium
Biomedical Implications of Relaxation Times of Tissue Water

A. A. MAUDSLEY, Ph.D.   Associate Professor, University of California, San Francisco; Veterans Administration Medical Center, San Francisco, California
Technical Demands of Multiple Nuclei

MURRAY J. MAZER, M.D.   Associate Professor of Radiology and Radiological Sciences; Chief, Angiography Section, Vanderbilt University Medical Center, Nashville, Tennessee
Gated MRI in Congenital Cardiac Malformations

MICHAEL McCURDY, B.S.E.E.   Student, Master of Science in Electrical Engineering, Vanderbilt University, Nashville, Tennessee
Dynamic Contrast-Enhanced MRI and Mathematical Modeling

ALAN C. McLAUGHLIN, Ph.D.   University of Pennsylvania, Philadelphia, Pennsylvania
Phosphorus-31 Spectroscopy and Imaging

SNEHAL D. MEHTA, M.D.   Assistant Professor, University of Texas Health Science Center; Staff, Hermann Hospital, Houston, Texas
Kidneys and Retroperitoneum; NMR of ^{23}Na in Biological Systems

MARK R. MITCHELL, M.D.   Assistant Professor, Department of Radiology and Radiological Sciences, Vanderbilt University Medical Center, Nashville, Tennessee; Simi Valley Adventist Hospital Staff, Simi Valley, California
MRI Tissue Characterization; MRI Optimization Strategies; Understanding Basic MR Pulse Sequences; Advanced Methods for Spin Density, T1, and T2 Calculations in MRI

E. PAUL NANCE, JR., M.D.   Associate Professor of Radiology; Assistant Professor of Orthopaedics and Rehabilitation; Chief, Section of Bone and Joint Radiology, Vanderbilt University School of Medicine; Department of Radiology, Vanderbilt University Hospital, Nashville, Tennessee
Musculoskeletal System

PONNADA A. NARAYANA, Ph.D.   Assistant Professor, The University of Texas Medical School, Houston, Texas
Kidneys and Retroperitoneum; NMR of ^{23}Na in Biological Systems; Localization Methods in NMR

M. O'DONNELL, Ph.D.   Physicist, Corporate Research and Development Center, General Electric Company, Schenectady, New York
Quantitative NMR Tissue Characterization Using Calculated Images and Automated Image Segmentation

WILLIAM H. OLDENDORF, M.D., D.Sc. Professor of Neurology and of Psychiatry, University of California, Los Angeles, School of Medicine; Senior Medical Investigator, VA Brentwood, Veterans Administration, Los Angeles, California
A Comparison of Resistive, Superconductive, and Permanent Magnets

ARNULF OPPELT, Ph.D. Siemens A.G. Medical Engineering Group, Erlangen, German Federal Republic
Systems Optimization

DOUGLAS A. ORTENDAHL, Ph.D. Associate Profesor of Physics, Department of Radiology and Radiologic Imaging Laboratory, University of California, San Francisco, California
MRI Parameter Selection Techniques

C. LEON PARTAIN, M.D., Ph.D. Professor of Radiology, Radiological Sciences, and Biomedical Engineering, Vanderbilt University School of Medicine; Director, Division of Medical Imaging, Vanderbilt University Hospital, Nashville, Tennessee
Breast; Gastrointestinal Tract; Kidneys and Retroperitoneum; Practical Pediatric MRI; Dynamic Contrast-Enhanced MRI and Mathematical Modeling; Legal Aspects of MRI; Future Directions; NMR Physical Principles; Current and Future Frontiers in Medical Imaging

JAMES A. PATTON, Ph.D. Professor of Radiology and Radiological Sciences, Administrative Officer for Radiology, Vanderbilt University Medical Center, Nashville, Tennessee
Thyroid and Parathyroid Glands; Pitfalls and Artifacts in Clinical MRI; Future Directions; Quality Assurance

J. A. PAYNE, B.Sc. GEC-Research, Limited, Wembley, Middlesex, United Kingdom
Artifacts in the Measurement of T1 and T2

ROBERT A. PHILLIPS, Ph.D. Office of Radiological Health, National Center for Devices and Radiological Health, United States Food and Drug Administration, Rockville, Maryland
Operational Guidelines: United States

DAVID R. PICKENS, Ph.D. Assistant Professor of Radiology and Radiological Sciences, Vanderbilt University Medical Center, Nashville, Tennessee
Blood Flow in MR Imaging; Image Production and Display; Gating: Cardiac and Respiratory; Fast Scanning Methods in MRI

GERALD M. POHOST, M.D. Professor of Medicine, Professor of Radiology, University of Alabama School of Medicine; Director, Division of Cardiovascular Disease; Director, Center for NMR Research and Development, University of Alabama Hospitals, University of Alabama at Birmingham, Alabama
Ischemic Heart Disease

C. F. POPE, M.D.   Assistant Professor of Radiology, Yale University School of Medicine, New Haven, Connecticut
Quantitative NMR Tissue Characterization Using Calculated Images and Automated Image Segmentation

ANN C. PRICE, M.D.   Associate Professor of Radiology, Medical College of Virginia, Richmond, Virginia
White Matter/Multiple Sclerosis; Tumor Imaging with Gd-DTPA; Pituitary and Parasellar Region

RONALD R. PRICE, Ph.D.   Professor of Radiology and Radiological Sciences, Associate Professor of Physics and Astronomy, Vanderbilt University; Director, Division of Radiological Sciences, Vanderbilt University Medical Center, Nashville, Tennessee
Blood Flow in MR Imaging; NMR Physical Principles; Quality Assurance; Fast Scanning Methods in MRI; Advanced Methods for Spin Density, T1, and T2 Calculations in MRI; Current and Future Frontiers in Medical Imaging

JAMIE H. PROST, M.S.   General Electric Medical Systems, Waukesha, Wisconsin
Impact of the Choice of Operating Parameters on MR Images

EDWARD M. PURCELL, Ph.D.   Professor Emeritus, Department of Physics, Harvard University, Cambridge, Massachusetts. Nobel Prize in Physics (for NMR), 1952
Foreword

S. S. RANADE, M.Sc., Ph.D.   Member, Ad Hoc Committee in Biophysics, Bombay University; Research Guide Faculty of Biophysics; Officer-In-Charge, Radiobiology Unit, Cancer Research Institute, Bombay, India
Histopathological Correlation

MRUTYUNJAYA J. RAO, M.S.   Digital Equipment Corporation, Marlborogh, Massachusetts
Advanced Statistical Methods for Tissue Characteristics

RUSSELL C. REEVES, M.D.   Assistant Professor of Medicine, University of Alabama School of Medicine, University of Alabama Hospitals and Clinics, Birmingham, Alabama
Ischemic Heart Disease

BRADFORD J. RICHMOND, M.D.   Radiology Staff, Section of Bone and Joint Radiology, Cleveland Clinic Foundation, Cleveland, Ohio
The Spine

STEPHEN J. RIEDERER, Ph.D.   Associate Professor of Radiology and Biomedical Engineering, Duke University Medical Center, Durham, North Carolina
MRI Synthesis

F. DAVID ROLLO, M.D., Ph.D.   Visiting Professor of Radiology and Radiological Sciences, Vanderbilt University School of Medicine, Nashville, Tennessee; Executive Vice-President, Humana, Inc., Louisville, Kentucky
Legal Aspects of MRI

CHARLES E. ROOS, Ph.D.   Professor of Physics, Vanderbilt University, Nashville, Tennessee
Principles of Superconducting Magnets

BRUCE R. ROSEN, M.D., Ph.D.   Lecturer, Harvard/MIT Division of Health Sciences and Technology, Cambridge; Instructor in Radiology, Harvard Medical School; Director of Clinical NMR, Massachusetts General Hospital, Boston, Massachusetts
Chemical Shift Imaging

VAL M. RUNGE, M.D.   Assistant Professor, Tufts University–New England Medical Center Hospitals; Chief of Service, Magnetic Resonance, Department of Radiology, New England Medical Center Hospitals, Boston, Massachusetts
White Matter/Multiple Sclerosis; Tumor Imaging with Gd-DTPA; Pituitary and Parasellar Region; Principles of Contrast-Enhanced MRI; Intravenous Contrast Media

GLYNIS A. SACKS, M.D.   Assistant Professor of Radiology and Radiological Sciences (Ultrasound Section), Vanderbilt University Medical Center, Nashville, Tennessee
Thyroid and Parathyroid Glands

BERNIE J. SAKS, M.D.   Department of Radiology, University of California, San Francisco, School of Medicine, San Francisco, California
Prostate and Urinary Bladder

MARTIN P. SANDLER, M.D., F.C.P. (S.A.)   Associate Professor of Radiology and Medicine; Chief, Nuclear Medicine, Vanderbilt University Medical Center, Nashville, Tennessee
Thyroid and Parathyroid Glands; Gated MRI in Congenital Cardiac Malformations; Adrenal Glands

JOHN F. SCHENCK, M.D., Ph.D.   Adjunct Assistant Professor of Radiology, University of Pennsylvania, Philadelphia; Medical Dental Staff, Ellis Hospital, Schenectady, New York; Technical Staff, Corporate Research and Development Center, General Electric Company, Schenectady, New York
Gradient Coil Technology; Radio Frequency Resonators

MITCH SCHNALL, M.D., Ph.D.   Instructor, Department of Radiology, University of Pennsylvania School of Medicine, Philadelphia, Pennsylvania
Phosphorus-31 Spectroscopy and Imaging

ROGER H. SCHNEIDER, M.Sc.   Director of the Division of Electrical Products, Office of Radiological Health, National Center for Devices and Radiological Health, United States Food and Drug Administration, Rockville, Maryland
Operational Guidelines: United States

C. SEGEBARTH, Ph.D.   Scientific Director of the Department for Magnetic Resonance, Erasme Hospital, Brussels, Belgium
Surface Coil Imaging of the Spine

MAX SHAFF, M.D., F.R.C.R.   Associate Professor, Vanderbilt University Medical Center; Chief, Section of Computed Tomography, Department of Radiology and Radiological Sciences, Vanderbilt University Medical Center, Nashville, Tennessee
Adrenal Glands

TERESA SINNWELL, Ph.D.   Department of Radiology, University of Pennsylvania, Philadelphia, Pennsylvania
Phosphorus-31 Spectroscopy and Imaging

FRANCIS W. SMITH, M.D.   Clinical Senior Lecturer in Medicine, University of Aberdeen; Consultant Radiologist, Specialist in Nuclear Medicine, Aberdeen Royal Infirmary, Aberdeen, Scotland
MRI at Low Field Strength

GREG D. SMITH, M.D.   Resident, Department of Radiology and Radiological Sciences, Vanderbilt University Medical Center, Nashville, Tennessee
MRI Tissue Characterization

HYLTON SMITH, Ph.D., F.I.Biol.   Secretary of International Commission on Radiological Protection, Surrey, United Kingdom
On the Safety of Nuclear Magnetic Resonance Imaging and Spectroscopy Systems

H. D. SOSTMAN, M.D.   Professor of Radiology, Duke University; Attending Radiologist, Duke University Medical Center, Durham, North Carolina
NMR Evaluation of Tumor Metabolism

M. SPERBER, M.D.   Formerly, Academisch Ziekenhuis van de Vrije Universiteit, Department of Radiology, Amsterdam, The Netherlands
Malignant Lesions of the Paranasal Sinuses

DAVID D. STARK, M.D.   Assistant Professor of Radiology, Harvard Medical School; Assistant in Radiology, Massachusetts General Hospital, Boston, Massachusetts
Liver and Spleen

JOHN W. STEIDLEY, Ph.D.   Philips Medical Systems, Inc., Shelton, Connecticut
Planning and Preparation

ALAN A. STEIN, Ph.D., M.B.A.   Diasonics, Inc., San Francisco, California
Clinical Efficacy: Analysis of 300 MRI Cases at 1.5 Tesla; Thin-Slice MRI

EARL P. STEINBERG, M.D., M.P.P. Henry J. Kaiser Foundation Faculty Scholar in General Internal Medicine, Assistant Professor of Medicine and of Health Policy and Management, The Johns Hopkins Medical Institutions; Director, The Johns Hopkins Program for Medical Technology and Practice Assessment, Full-Time Active Staff, The Johns Hopkins Hospital, Baltimore, Maryland
The Economics and Regulation of MRI

R. E. STEINER, M.D., F.R.C.R., F.R.C.P. Emeritus Professor of Diagnostic Radiology, University of London Royal Postgraduate Medical School; NMR Unit, Hammersmith Hospital, London, United Kingdom
Role and Scope of MRI in Diagnostic Medicine

W. HOYT STEPHENS, M.S. Senior Associate in Radiology and Radiological Sciences; Director, Center for Medical Imaging Research, Vanderbilt University Medical Center, Nashville, Tennessee
NMR Physical Principles

BERT TE STRAKE, M.D. Department of Radiology, University Hospital, Groningen, The Netherlands; Consulting Radiologist, MRI, King Faisal Specialist Hospital and Research Centre, Riyadh, Kingdom of Saudi Arabia
Adrenal Glands

A. H. M. TAMINIAU, M.D., Ph.D. Department of Orthopaedic Surgery, University Hospital, Leiden, The Netherlands
Primary Malignant Bone Tumors

ROBERT W. TARR, M.D. Chief Resident in Radiology, Vanderbilt University Medical Center, Nashville, Tennessee
MRI Optimization Strategies; Gastrointestinal Tract; Understanding Basic MR Pulse Sequences

ALBERT TEDESCHI, M.D. Riverview Medical Center; Fellow, Magnetic Resonance Imaging, Vanderbilt University Medical Center, Nashville, Tennessee
Gastrointestinal Tract

ARCH W. TEMPLETON, M.D. Professor and Chairman, Department of Radiology, University of Kansas Medical Center, Kansas City, Kansas
Computer Networks for Medical Image Management

STEPHEN R. THOMAS, Ph.D. Professor of Radiology, University of Cincinnati College of Medicine, Cincinnati, Ohio
Gradient Coil Technology; The Biomedical Applications of Fluorine-19 NMR

JACK TISHLER, M.D. Professor of Radiology, University of Alabama Medical School; University of Alabama Hospitals, Birmingham, Alabama
Gated MRI in Congenital Cardiac Malformations

M. F. TWEEDLE, Ph.D. Director of Research, The Squibb Institute for Medical Research, New Brunswick, New Jersey
Principles of Contrast-Enhanced MRI

B. G. TWEEDY, Ph.D.   Chairman, Chemistry Department, Agriculture Division, Ciba-Giegy Company, Greensboro, North Carolina
Dynamic Contrast-Enhanced MRI and Mathematical Modeling

J. VALK, M.D.   Professor of Radiology, Academische Ziekenhuis van de Vrije Universiteit, Department of Radiology, Amsterdam, The Netherlands
Malignant Lesions of the Paranasal Sinuses

P. VAN DER MEULEN, M.Sc.   Department of MRI, Philips Medical Systems Division, Best, The Netherlands
Fast, Small Flip-Angle Field Echo Imaging

P. VAN DIJK, M.Sc.   Department of MRI, Philips Medical Systems Division, Best, The Netherlands
Fast, Small Flip-Angle Field Echo Imaging

A. T. VAN OOSTEROM, M.D.   Department of Oncology, University Hospital, Antwerpe, Belgium
Primary Malignant Bone Tumors

ARNOUD P. VAN SETERS, Ph.D.   Teacher in Endocrinology, University Medical Center; Staff Member, Department of Endocrinology, University Hospital, Leiden, The Netherlands
Adrenal Glands

W. RICHARD WEBB, M.D.   Professor of Radiology, University of California, San Francisco, California
Mediastinum and Hila

P. W. WEDEKING, Ph.D.   Research Investigator, The Squibb Institute for Medical Research, New Brunswick, New Jersey
Principles of Contrast-Enhanced MRI

FELIX W. WEHRLI, Ph.D.   General Electric Medical Systems, Waukesha, Wisconsin
Impact of the Choice of Operating Parameters on MR Images; Advanced Statistical Methods for Tissue Characteristics

JEFFREY C. WEINREB, M.D.   Associate Professor of Radiology, Columbia University College of Physicians and Surgeons; Director of MRI, St. Luke's/ Roosevelt Hospital Center, New York, New York
Obstetric Problems

JOSEPH D. WEISSMAN, M.D., Ph.D.   Technicare Corporation, Solon, Ohio
Thin-Slice MRI

M. ROBERT WILLCOTT, Ph.D.   President, NMR Imaging, Inc., Houston, Texas
NMR Chemical Principles

ALAN C. WINFIELD, M.D. Professor of Radiology, Vanderbilt University School of Medicine; Director, Abdominal Imaging Section, Vanderbilt University Hospital, Nashville, Tennessee
Breast

GARY L. WISMER, M.D. Clinical Fellow, Neuroradiology, Massachusetts General Hospital, Boston; Staff Radiologist, Nemours Magnetic Resonance Facility, Jacksonville, Florida
Chemical Shift Imaging

GERALD L. WOLF, Ph.D., M.D. Professor of Radiology, University of Pittsburgh; President and Medical Director, Pittsburgh NMR Institute, Pittsburgh, Pennsylvania
Free Radical Contrast Agents for MRI; Hepatobiliary Contrast Agents

I. R. YOUNG, Ph.D. GEC Research, Limited, Wembley, Middlesex, United Kingdom
Artifacts in the Measurement of T1 and T2

EBERHARD ZEITLER, M.D. Professor at the University of Erlangen—Nürnberg; Head of the Diagnostic Department, Radiological Center, General Hospital, Nuremberg, German Federal Republic
Overview of MRI Clinical Applications in Germany

B. G. ZIEDSES DES PLANTES, JR., M.D. Stichting Deventer Ziekenhuizen, Deventer, The Netherlands
Malignant Lesions of the Paranasal Sinuses

Foreword

It is nearly 400 years since the practice of medicine and the study of magnetism were combined in the career of Sir William Gilbert, physician to Queen Elizabeth I, president of the Royal College of Physicians, and author of *De Magnete*, one of the great scientific treatises our civilization has produced. Gilbert studied the magnetic field of the Earth, as revealed by the behavior of compasses, and the interaction of small magnets of lodestone (magnetite: Fe_3O_4) or iron. A tireless experimenter and acute observer, Gilbert was an early practitioner of the scientific method. The lore of the lodestone had become encrusted with myths—such as the efficacy of garlic as a demagnetizing agent. Much worse, the essential difference between *electric* attraction (of rubbed amber for bits of straw) and *magnetic* attraction (of a lodestone for pieces of iron) was not recognized. All of this Gilbert straightened out. He showed that magnetically the Earth resembles a giant lodestone sphere. He had an idea of a magnetic field, which he called an *orb of virtue* in the space surrounding a lodestone, and he emphasized the virtue's extraordinary penetrating power. "No hindrance," Gilbert wrote, "is offered by thick boards, or by walls of pottery or marble, or even metals; there is naught so solid as to do away with this force, or check it, save a plate of iron."

Gilbert made other discoveries in what we now call the physics of ferromagnetism. Magnetic effects *not* enhanced by the peculiar properties of iron were far beyond the reach of his experiments, even if he had known what to look for. *De Magnete* was published in 1600. The next significant advance in our understanding of magnetism did not come until 220 years later, with Oersted's discovery that an electric current in a wire can influence a nearby compass needle.

As a physician, Gilbert recorded no notable discoveries. However, Sir William Harvey, whose revolutionary book on the circulation of blood was published in 1628, was an enthusiastic admirer of Gilbert's scientific investigations and may have derived some inspiration from them. Perhaps that should count as Gilbert's most valuable contribution to medical science. In any case, if one indulges in the familiar fantasy of summoning a figure from the past to witness a scientific advance of the present, one would like to tell *both* William Gilbert and William Harvey about the medical uses of magnetism—not omitting observation of the flow of blood, which is described in Chapters 36 and 98 of this book. Dr. Gilbert himself might be more astonished by the total dependence on ferromagnetism of a society that now stores most of its information, whether on tape or disk, in powdered lodestone!

Even physicists of today, accustomed as they have become to rapid growth in the range and power of their instruments, are awed by the resolution of detail that has been achieved in the NMR image. As for those of us who were exploring the physics of NMR 40 years ago, I believe that few could comment on the pictures in this book without using the word *marvelous*. Yet in retrospect one can trace, as Professor Bloch has done in Chapter 1, a path leading, step by logical step, from I. I. Rabi's molecular beam to today's sagittal section. That seems to be the way science, in our century, produces a genuine marvel.

The development of imaging by nuclear magnetic resonance presents a striking contrast to the beginning of roentgenography. When Roentgen discovered x-rays in November 1895, physics could not even explain, let alone predict, the penetrating power of the mysterious radiation. The electron itself was unknown; the structure of atoms would remain a puzzle for the next 20 years. Nevertheless, within weeks of Roentgen's discovery, eager experimenters on both sides of the Atlantic were displaying pictures of bones and medical applications were already being reported. By June 1896 there existed a journal devoted to x-ray shadowgraphs, termed *skiagraphy*.* From discovery to world-wide medical use: less than one year!

The history of nuclear magnetic resonance was quite different. A long sequence of developments, with branches and several turning points, preceded its eventual use in medicine. That an atomic nucleus can have a magnetic moment was deduced around 1925 from certain features in atomic spectra. The magnetic moment of the proton was measured by Otto Stern in 1933 using a beam of hydrogen molecules. Further developments by I. I. Rabi at Columbia, reviewed in the first chapter by Professor Bloch, led to the molecular beam resonance method. In the thirties, nuclear magnetic moments were interesting mainly as clues to nuclear structure. The collective behavior of the nuclear magnets in condensed matter, properly called *nuclear magnetism*, concerned only a few physicists—notably C. J. Gorter in Leiden, and B. Lazarev and L. Schubnikov in Moscow. In 1937 the Russian physicists were able to demonstrate the magnetization of solid hydrogen in a strong field at low temperature, the protonic analogue of electronic paramagnetism. Gorter actually tried a resonance experiment, but without success, in 1942. So matters stood at the end of World War II, when the experiments at Stanford and at Harvard were conceived, and the proton magnetic resonance was observed in ordinary matter.

By 1950, plus or minus a year or two, the basic physics that underlies NMR imaging was for practical purposes completely understood. That includes: the magnetic dipole moments and electric quadrupole moments of relevant nuclei; the relaxation times $T1$ and $T2$ and their dependence on molecular viscosity; the dynamical behavior of spins of all sorts in oscillating fields, both continuous and pulsed; the chemical shifts that were soon to open up an immense field of application in organic chemistry. No physicist working with NMR at that time would have been surprised to see a proton resonance with a mouse, or a human finger, in the coil. Its amplitude, as in the case of any other largely aqueous substance, would have been quite predictable. Yet with all this knowledge ready to apply, the realization of medically useful NMR images lay more than 20 years in the future. What essential ingredients were lacking?

For one thing, sensitivity. In our first proton resonance in 1945, the sample was nearly 1 kilogram of paraffin. Recalling that, as I look at the image in Figure 2–7, I realize that one millionth of our sample, a 1-milligram lump of paraffin, would shine out in that image as a conspicuous anomaly, possibly identifiable through paraffin's exceptionally short $T1$. Of course, that kilogram of paraffin was an absurdly large sample by our later standards. The real advance in sensitivity in the decades after 1950, although difficult to define neatly, was more like 10^3 than 10^6, still a spectacular gain.

---

* Encyclopedia Brit. *23*:845, 1942. "Archives of Skiagraphy" (see O.E.D. for skiagraph).

The key was computer power and the great advance in sophisticated signal-processing techniques that became feasible as computer speed and memory grew by their own powers of ten. Through that period the active frontiers in NMR were expanding from physics to chemistry and biochemistry. Several ingenious and powerful techniques were developed by chemists using NMR to study molecular structure. In addition to increasing sensitivity by one form or another of signal averaging, computer power is, of course, essential for tomographic reconstruction of the NMR image. In short, NMR imaging could hardly have been developed to its present state, no matter how well established its base in physics, without the modern computer.

But something even more essential was lacking in 1950: the *idea* that a useful interior image was in principle obtainable, and was a goal worth pursuing. For that P. C. Lauterbur, P. Mansfield, and R. Damadian deserve enormous credit. Several more ideas that were needed to accelerate developments were forthcoming, when the time was ripe, from other NMR practitioners.

NMR imaging is so powerful, so general, and at the same time so gentle a diagnostic procedure that it is likely to become part of most people's experience. That seems obvious now, even to an antiquated NMR expert like myself who did *not* foresee it. The prospect must be exhilarating for the scientists involved, from physicists to physicians, very well represented by the contributors to this book. It is challenging to me as a teacher of physics, for I feel that some general public understanding of the essential facts is both desirable and attainable.

How fortunate we are that most ordinary matter, as Gilbert observed, is freely penetrated by a magnetic field. To that we owe both the power and the safety of NMR imaging of today. But the layman undergoing this rather mysterious procedure may ask how one can be so confident that magnetic fields are benign. Weren't x-rays considered harmless at first? The concern is understandable. There is a good answer, an answer based solidly on the fundamental physics and chemistry we have learned in this century: *The interaction of a magnetic field with a molecule is so very slight that neither can seriously perturb the other.*

The explanation is simple. It begins with another fact first recognized by Gilbert: Electricity and magnetism are essentially different. We know now that matter, including living tissue of every sort, is at the molecular level an *electrical* structure. Within it electrons are held in atoms, atoms are bound into molecules, and molecules are linked with one another by the forces of attraction and repulsion between *electric charges*. Magnetism is not directly involved. Nothing like a *magnetic charge* has been found in nature. Physicists have searched assiduously, but in vain, for a magnetic monopole, as it would be called. There is not even one such particle among all the electrically charged particles in the human body—some 10^{28} protons and electrons. Magnetic effects in matter arise exclusively from the *motion* of electric charge—an electron orbiting in an atom or spinning around an axis, a proton orbiting or spinning in an atomic nucleus. Magnetism in matter is a by-product, a side effect, so to speak, of the electrical structure of the atom, and as such it is intrinsically feeble.

To emphasize the point with one important example, consider the water molecule

$$\text{H} \diagdown \quad \diagup \text{H.}$$
$$\text{O}$$

Its "boomerang" shape gives the molecule an electric dipole moment, thereby making liquid water a powerful solvent. That shape represents an equilibrium of *electrical* attractions and repulsions within the molecule, with quantum mechanics governing the motions of all the protons and electrons. The structure is stiff. To bend the molecule straight (H—O—H) by brute force would cost in energy about 50 kcal/mole, roughly five times as much energy as it would take to vaporize the water. Now there is also in this molecule a magnetic interaction, of central importance in NMR, between the two hydrogen nuclei. It is the interaction of each nuclear magnet with the magnetic field of the other. Expressing it in the same units, the energy of this magnetic dipole-dipole interaction is about 10^{-9} kcal/mole, less than one ten-billionth of the energy involved in any major alteration of the molecule's shape. The interaction of one nuclear magnetic dipole with the strong field of an NMR imaging coil can be a few thousand times larger (as in a field of 1 tesla) but is still less than one millionth of the energy exchanged in a typical biochemical reaction. The largest increment of energy associated with the effect of a steady magnetic field on a molecule is the energy required to reverse an electron's spin. In a field of 1 tesla that is 0.003 kcal/mole.

The various oscillating magnetic fields used in NMR imaging, with frequencies up to a few hundred megacyles/second, are generally stronger than, but not different in character from, the alternating magnetic fields in radio waves and around a-c wiring, which imperceptibly pervade our bodies much of the time. As for possible physiological effects of such low-frequency magnetic fields, the ultimate guarantor of safety is the quantum law, $E = h\nu$, which governs the absorption of energy by an individual atom or molecule. If the frequency of alternation ν is lower than 1000 megacycles/second, the quantum energy is less than one-millionth that of a quantum of ultraviolet light. An atom absorbs one quantum at a time. One "x-ray" quantum absorbed by an atom can blow it apart. The disturbance one "radio" quantum can make is so slight that it would be swamped merely by the ever-present thermal agitation of the molecular surroundings.

This assurance that the quantum law gives us is important, for it holds whether the oscillating field is magnetic or electric. As remarked earlier, magnetic interactions with an electrical structure like a molecule are intrinsically weak. No physiological observation I can imagine will tell me whether my hand is penetrated by the Earth's magnetic field (as it has been all my life) or by a steady field ten thousand times stronger. An *oscillating* magnetic field, on the other hand, is necessarily accompanied by an oscillating electric field, induced in accordance with Faraday's law. An oscillating electric field can deposit energy, in the form of heat, in bulk matter and does so readily in a material whose dielectric properties are dominated by the presence of polar molecules, such as water. The result, when it occurs in tissue, is literally nothing but smoothly distributed heat. It is not necessarily negligible, but the precautions called for are the same as in any form of diathermy. I believe that in routine NMR imaging as currently practiced, the amplitudes of alternating electric fields can be kept well below the level at which warming of tissue might be a concern. This question and others related to safety will be thoroughly discussed in Chapters 84 to 86. The point I want to emphasize here is the fundamental difference between the alteration of a specific biochemical structure or process by a low-frequency oscillating field—which appears to me, in view of the quantum law, nearly impossible—and the general warming of a mass of tissue, no more mysterious than if the heat were generated by internal friction.

I write as a physicist, not a biochemist, which is one reason for the qualifying word *nearly* in the preceding sentence. Arguments based on such immutable facts as the electrical nature of matter and the quantum law are compelling, but it would surely be foolish to claim that every potential physiological effect has been thought of and can be categorically ruled out. Nothing can substitute completely for observation over a long period of time of living organisms in a magnetic field. For such empirical testing physics can offer some guidance. Suppose there is some relatively small but definite effect of a magnetic field on a molecular process, unforeseen and awaiting discovery. Imagine, for instance, that the rate of a certain biochemical reaction is changed in the presence of the field. An argument based on a general principle of symmetry in electromagnetism (which I shall not develop here) leads directly to the prediction that the effect of a constant magnetic field upon an electrical structure must be proportional to the *square* of the magnetic field strength, if not to an even higher power. Therefore, a search for new effects should be carried out at the highest possible field strength, in the expectation that a 5-tesla field will be 25 times as effective as a 1-tesla field in evoking a response. Conversely, if a biological system behaves quite normally in a 5-tesla field, confidence that fields of 0.5T or less will not perturb it is greatly strengthened.

My own confident expectation is that clinical experience (accumulating at a rate that may for a while seem exponential) and empirical testing in the 10-tesla range (which ought to be part of a systematic long-term program) will eventually prove beyond question that the extension of William Gilbert's "orb of virtue" into the human body is in the deepest sense benign.

EDWARD M. PURCELL, PH.D.
Gerhardt Gabe University Professor Emeritus
Harvard University

Preface

The continuing developments in MRI techniques and applications following publication of the first edition of Nuclear Magnetic Resonance (NMR) Imaging have been both dramatic and significant. It appears that MRI rapidly is becoming the most comprehensive and efficacious diagnostic imaging modality in medical history. Therefore, we felt the need to initiate a second edition almost immediately after the publication of our first text owing to the rapidity, significance, and number of new developments. It has been a challenge to find a stop frame in the motion picture of innovation in which the current capabilities of MRI techniques will be documented and described most successfully. The refinement of MRI fluoroscopy, MRI angiography, flow measurement, fast scan, cine-mode, and three-dimensional imaging, to name a few areas of research and innovation, continues to revolutionize clinical applications of this discipline. Further, the organ substrate metabolism capability of nuclear magnetic resonance spectroscopy (NMRS) is so important an area that it must be given proper emphasis. This text, then, is an effort by the five editors to summarize the collective experience of many leading scientists and clinical investigators in a comprehensive overview of the field of magnetic resonance diagnostic inquiry.

In order to retain the comprehensive nature of the text and to expand the coverage of research to include more from international laboratories, a two-volume set became a necessity. From a first edition of 40 chapters, this second edition has expanded in size and content to 107 chapters. The group of 90 contributors to the 1983 edition, almost all of whom are represented once again, are joined by 80 additional clinicians and investigators. A second reason for a two-volume set is that even the most diligent will not utilize a cover-to-cover analysis in attempting to master this often complex, and sometimes overwhelming, material. Therefore, the two volumes have been organized as a Clinical Volume I and a Basic Sciences Volume II. This is intended to simplify for the reader the location of that information which is deemed most relevant and timely.

Volume I is composed of 11 subdivisions. Following a historical overview and basic sciences introduction, there are sections on clinical imaging experience in various parts of the body, special applications including contrast media, and a concluding section that forecasts and analyzes future expectations. New to this edition are the four chapters on tissue characterization and the five chapters on the use of contrast enhancement in MRI. Six primary subdivisions appear in Volume II, exploring physics and chemistry, relaxation/relaxometry, instrumentation, MRI site planning, NMR spectroscopy, and new areas of research and development. It is evident that many of the exciting advances found in the research section were in their infancy at the time of the first edition. These include relaxation measurement, flow and organ perfusion measurement, medical imaging networks, contrast agents, in vivo NMRS, and thin-section and fast-scan MRI. Many have been or are about to be introduced clinically.

One often has a sense of inadequacy when charged with the responsibility of recognizing the multiple talents involved with such a monumental project as this. We are deeply indebted to our contributors and hope that they will rejoin us when the need arises to update this text in the future. The editors are especially grateful to the Vanderbilt University Medical Center administration for their enthusiastic interest and support, to our colleagues in Radiology and Radiological Sciences, to the Center for Medical Imaging Research, to our residents and students who stimulate our most creative productivity, and to the publication staff at W. B. Saunders. Finally, the responsibility for the reality of any text often rests with the dedicated efforts and editorial skills of a few significant and special people. For this text, our three very special people are Margaret W. Moore and Pamela S. Moore at Vanderbilt and Kathleen McCullough at Saunders, and to them we express our deepest appreciation.

Participation in the evolution of magnetic resonance imaging and the generation of this book represents opportunities that are tremendously exciting and fulfilling for each of us personally and professionally. It is our hope that a portion of that excitement and satisfaction will be transmitted to the reader as he identifies his areas of interest within these volumes.

C. LEON PARTAIN, M.D., PH.D.
A. EVERETTE JAMES, JR., SC.M., J.D., M.D.

Contents for Volume 1

Contents for Volume 2

I

INTRODUCTION

1

Past, Present, and Future of
Nuclear Magnetic Resonance*

FELIX BLOCH

Like almost every advance in physics, nuclear magnetic resonance (NMR) owes its origin to a chain of preceding developments. An important link in this chain was forged 50 years ago by Otto Stern. Many nuclei had already been understood, from the hyperfine structure of spectral lines, to possess a characteristic electric and magnetic moment. However, the magnetic moments of the proton and the deuteron were not known until their magnitude was determined by Stern and I. Estermann from the deflection of a molecular beam of hydrogen in its passage through an inhomogeneous magnetic field.[1] The study of nuclear moments in molecular and atomic beams was subsequently taken up by I. I. Rabi and his collaborators at Columbia University.[2] During the following years they were able gradually to extend the power of the method by a series of innovations that culminated in the introduction of nuclear magnetic resonance.

This decisive step forward was based on a paper by Rabi, published in 1937, in which he treated the transition between the Zeeman levels of a magnetic moment μ in a constant magnetic field H under the influence of a field rotating at right angles to the constant field. The transition probability was shown to reach its maximum under the resonance condition

$$H\mu = s\hbar\omega \tag{1}$$

where ω is the circular frequency of the rotating field, typically in the range of radio frequencies, and s the spin associated with the magnetic moment. The requirement of a rotating field can be bypassed, since the simpler application of an alternating field calls for only a minor and calculable correction. To observe the effect in a molecular beam, the molecules pass from a region of the homogeneous field H into a region with a strongly inhomogeneous field so that the occurrence of transitions in the former is detected by a change of deflection in the latter. With the condition for resonance thus established and given the spin of a nucleus, the magnetic moment is obtained from Equation (1) by the strength H and the frequency ω of the constant and of the alternating perpendicular field, respectively. The accuracy is limited in principle only by the flight time Δt of the molecule through the transition region, leading to an indeterminancy

$$\Delta\omega \cong 1/\Delta t \tag{2}$$

of the resonance frequency but still allowing a far more precise determination of nuclear moments than had been possible by the earlier methods.

This manuscript was originally prepared by Felix Bloch (1905–1983) for presentation at the 40th Anniversary Symposium, Los Alamos Scientific Laboratory, New Mexico, and is printed here with the permission and assistance of Dr. Bloch's family and with the permission of Dr. Ann Metropolis, Editor, New Directions in Physics. The Los Alamos 40th Anniversary Volume. Orlando, Academic Press, 1988.[9]

3

A second use of magnetic resonance was made shortly before World War II in an experiment by L. W. Alvarez and the author to measure the magnetic moment of the neutron.[3] As an essential difference from the application to molecular beams, however, the scattering of slow neutrons in magnetized iron, rather than the deflection in an inhomogeneous field, was observed to ascertain the establishment of resonance conditions.

The preceding account may seem to deal merely with the prehistory of nuclear magnetic resonance, since the abbreviation NMR is now customarily used in connection with the method introduced after the end of the war by E. M. Purcell and the author.[4,5] Although the observation of resonance is still essential in some of the most important applications, it is not this feature that characterizes the method. There are, in fact, other relevant instances in which resonance is of secondary significance or even entirely absent. The real distinction from earlier methods has to be seen in the novel principle of detection, based upon purely electromagnetic effects, which allows the investigation of nuclear magnetic phenomena in bulk matter and under many different aspects.

It is indicated, under these circumstances, to describe the principle in terms of the macroscopic polarization resulting from the magnetic moments of the nuclei in a sample. Whereas the vector of polarization at thermal equilibrium in a constant magnetic field is static and parallel to that field, its essential dynamic manifestations appear under conditions chosen to result in deviations from parallelity. The polarization is seen, thereupon, to undergo a precession around the direction of the constant field H with the Larmor frequency

$$\omega_L = \gamma H \tag{3}$$

where

$$\gamma = \mu/s\hbar \tag{4}$$

is the gyromagnetic ratio of the nucleus. An alternating voltage of the same frequency is thus induced in an external circuit. It is the signal due to this voltage, combined with the normal methods of amplification, that lends itself to direct observation. To emphasize this truly distinctive feature, the term "nuclear induction" originally was proposed but now is used only in reference to free precession, observed under nonresonant conditions.

As in the earlier applications, an alternating field, perpendicular to the constant field, can lead to resonance. In regard to the polarization, the resulting action is related to free precession in a manner analogous to that of the forced to the free oscillation of the harmonic oscillator, with the resonance condition of Equation (1) seen to be satisfied when the frequency ω of the alternating field equals the Larmor frequency ω_L of Equation (3). The angle of the vector of polarization against the constant field here reaches its maximum, indicated by a maximum of the observed signal. In contrast to the situation in a molecular beam, the accuracy is not limited by the flight time since the nuclei remain in the sample under investigation, but there are other causes of error, comparable to the linewidth $\Delta\omega$ of the resonance.

An obvious cause concerns the homogeneity of the constant field; if H varies by an amount ΔH over the extension of the sample, the resonance frequency of a nucleus, depending on its location, will vary in view of Equation (1) by the corresponding amount

$$(\Delta\omega)_H \cong \gamma\Delta H \tag{5}$$

with γ from Equation (4). Another more fundamental cause arises from the random processes that establish the thermal equilibrium of nuclear moments in the constant magnetic field through interaction with their environment. It is necessary for the effect of these processes upon the vector of polarization to distinguish between the approach toward the equilibrium value of the component parallel to the field and the disappearance of an initial perpendicular component. Depending on the specific properties of the interaction, the two components are found, in general, to change at a different rate, with the inverse characterized by a "longitudinal relaxation time" $T1$ for the parallel component and by a separately observable "transverse relaxation time $T2 \leq T1$ for the perpendicular component. In the observation of resonance this leads to a natural linewidth

$$(\Delta\omega)_n \cong 1/T2. \tag{6}$$

The basic facts, outlined above, already were well understood in the first demonstrations of NMR carried out on the protons in paraffin and water.[4,5] While they merely confirmed with comparable accuracy the value of the magnetic moment, known from magnetic resonance in a molecular beam, not even the order of magnitude of the relaxation time had been surmised until $T1$ was found to be about 3 seconds in water. This result was of particular relevance since there were good reasons to expect, in a liquid of low viscosity, the equality of $T1$ and $T2$ and, hence, from Equation (6) to envisage a natural linewidth of no more than a fraction of a cycle per second. Although the first experiments were carried out in a relatively weak field H, corresponding to a resonance frequency of only a few megacycles per second, such a small linewidth, in principle, would have allowed the determination of the magnetic moment with an accuracy of about one part in 10 millions. The width of the observed resonance, however, was much larger and entirely due to the inhomogeneity of the field according to Equation (5). It became clear, therefore, that greater homogeneity should be attempted, even without realizing at the time that this would lead to further developments of major significance.

The rather primitive instrumentation of the original experiments was soon replaced by better equipment. Besides improvements in the circuits and electronics, the stronger and more homogeneous fields obtained by specially designed magnets were found to greatly enhance the quality of the observed signals. Among the immediate benefits of higher sensitivity and resolution thus achieved, it was possible to determine the magnetic moment of many nuclei either with greater accuracy than had been previously attained or in cases in which it had not been known before. Most of the measurements were carried out on samples in which the molecules containing the nuclei under investigation were dissolved in a liquid in order to obtain resonances of sufficiently small linewidth. Another early application of NMR concerned the structure of crystals. One observes here, in contrast to a liquid, broad resonances due to the fact that the effective field H, acting upon a nucleus, varies over a range determined by the different orientations of neighboring nuclear moments. From the magnitude of the broadening it is possible, therefore, to base conclusions on the distance between neighbors. The rapid change of relative positions in liquids causes such broadening to be averaged out. It is because of this motional narrowing that liquid samples offer distinct advantages when high resolution is important.

The usefulness of NMR had already been widely recognized, and it was actively pursued in many laboratories within a few years after the announcement of the first results.[6,7] It would be impossible, even in bare outline, to describe the great variety of investigations in which NMR was fruitfully applied, first in physics but soon in other branches of science as well. Instead, a few examples will be chosen to indicate at least some of the lines along which the developments have moved and are still in progress.

Once the magnetic moment of the proton had been identified with considerable accuracy, NMR was used conversely as a convenient method for the measurement of magnetic fields. In an interesting version put into practice, the protons in a hydrogeneous liquid are first allowed to reach the equilibrium polarization in a relatively strong field at right angles to the earth's field to be measured. Upon quick removal of this field, the polarization, still perpendicular to the earth's field, begins its free precession around the direction of the latter and induces an alternating voltage in a coil surrounding the sample. Owing to a long relaxation time, the slow exponential decrease of the amplitude allows the timing of several thousand cycles, equivalent to a correspondingly accurate determination of the Larmor frequency ω_L, with the result for the magnitude H of the earth's field obtained from Equation (3) and the known value of γ.

For the measurement of stronger fields, the observation of resonance at a frequency ω for protons similarly yields the value of H from Equation (1). Irrespective of this value, however, one obtains the magnetic moment of a nucleus with known spin s in units of that of the proton moment from the ratio of their respective resonance frequencies, observed in the same field. The magnetic moment of the proton has thus served as a standard and has been calibrated for the conversion of the data into conventional units.

In the course of measuring the magnetic moment of different nuclei, the discovery of the chemical shift came as a by-product. It manifests itself in a slight dependence of the resonance frequency on the compound in which a given nucleus is observed and is due to a shielding of the external magnetic field by the electrons of the molecule. Actually, it is only the relatively small contribution to the shielding by the valency electrons that varies with the compound, but the resulting shifts are sufficiently pronounced and characteristic that they have become an important indicator in chemical analysis. A chemical shift was found not only between different compounds but also between different bonds within the same molecule, a fact that has led to the extended use of NMR for the investigation of molecular structures.

The first evidence of this fact appeared on the introduction of pulse methods for the observation of NMR signals. Instead of the steady state under resonance conditions, one deals here with the transient response of the polarization to an intermittent action of the alternating field. For a pulse of a given short duration the action can be seen to consist in a rotation of the vector of polarization against the direction of the constant field by an angle proportional to the amplitude of the alternating field. In particular, the application of a 90 degree pulse to a sample in an inhomogeneous field, followed by a delayed 180 degree pulse, results after the same further delay in the appearance of a signal called a spin echo. The magnitude of the echo was found for some substances to vary with a change of the delay time in a manner that could be related to internal properties of the molecule. It suggested the possibility of reaching equivalent conclusions more directly from data to be obtained with sufficiently high resolution from the observation of resonances.

The need for high resolution became evident in the studies on ethyl alcohol, which provided the basis for all later research directed at the structure of molecules by means of NMR. In fact, it required very great homogeneity of the magnetic field, as indicated by Equation (5), to reduce the linewidth to about 100 cycles per second, comparable to the chemical shift of three different groups of protons in the molecule. A further reduction, down to the natural linewidth of no more than one cycle per second, was achieved by rapid rotation of the sample, which effectively suppresses the broadening by the remaining inhomogeneity. At this point, a large number of closely spaced resonances, which arise from a very slight coupling between the magnetic moment of protons in neighboring groups, could be resolved.

This type of spin-spin splitting is found for a great variety of compounds in patterns that are highly characteristic of the molecule and occur in the resonances both of protons and of other nuclei typically present in organic molecules. Combined with the chemical shift, these patterns convey a good deal of essential information, such as the spatial arrangement of different radicals within the molecule. For this reason as well as for its nondestructive character and other advantages, the application of high-resolution NMR has been extended to almost the entire field of organic chemistry. In a further natural extension, NMR has become increasingly important to biochemistry and biology, in which it has the special merit of allowing investigations in vivo without interfering with the function of the organism.

The significance of NMR as a valuable tool for research continues to grow both in scope and in quality. There are two particular innovations that contribute to a considerable improvement in the performance of the equipment. The first is due to the attainment of magnetic fields, both more stable and considerably stronger than those obtained from electromagnets, by means of the persistent current in a superconducting coil. Since the signal greatly increases with increasing field and correspondingly increasing frequency, this allows observation even in cases in which only small amounts of the sample substance are available. In addition, the chemical shift is proportional to the field so that a greater spread of the resonances can be achieved.

A second important contribution is made by computers through their extensive use in the processing of data. In a frequent procedure, the alternating field operates in a series of widely spaced 90 degree pulses, and the computer is programmed to produce the Fourier transform of the transient signal that follows each pulse as a result of the free precession of the polarization. By this process the time-dependence of the signal is converted into signal strength versus frequency so that even the result, derived from a single pulse, is the same as that otherwise obtained by scanning through the entire sequence of resonance frequencies. The signal-to-noise ratio is improved, however, by accumulation and averaging over a number of pulses. Besides furnishing a display of the transformed signal, the computer can be further programmed to extract relevant numerical values, such as those of chemical shifts and spin-spin coupling constants, characteristic of an organic molecule.

The applications of NMR in physics, chemistry, and biology have been newly expanded to provide diagnostic information in the field of medicine. Through the introduction of sufficiently large magnets it is now possible, in particular, to investigate specific metabolic processes in the human body by means of high-resolution NMR. The chemical shift between the phosphorus metabolites, observed in the so-called topical magnetic resonance of the isotope ^{31}P, makes it possible to determine their relative concentration and hence to obtain a nonintrusive test for the muscle function in the arm or leg.

One of the most promising clinical applications of NMR, however, is due to the remarkable progress of NMR imaging, or zeugmatography (from the Greek *zeugma*, that which joins together).[8] (The process of imaging using NMR techniques will be referred to throughout this text as magnetic resonance imaging [MRI], a result of common usage also reflected in the title change for the second edition of this text.) What is being joined is the frequency of the signal and the location of the nuclei from which it originates. The principle is a direct consequence of Equation (3), with the difference that H now refers to an inhomogeneous field that has a known dependence of its magnitude on the space variables. Considering particular protons, all those observed to have a given Larmor frequency ω_L are therefore known from their value of γ to be located on a surface

$$H(x,\ y,\ z)\ =\ \omega_L/\gamma\ =\ \text{constant.} \tag{7}$$

There are several schemes, based upon this principle, for arriving at the spatial distribution of protons and thereby at an image representing the shape and location of the tissues within which they are contained. In one of the procedures, the method described above is applied to obtain the frequency distribution from the Fourier transform of the transient signal following a 90 degree pulse. For a constant gradient of H

with the surfaces of given frequency thus being parallel planes, this constitutes a one-dimensional projection of NMR responses along the direction of the field gradient. By rotating the direction, data of different projections can then be processed to give a two-dimensional image analogous to the processing used in x-ray tomography (CT).

NMR imaging can at present resolve details at the submillimeter level of resolution and is in this respect comparable to x-ray CT scanning, avoiding the damage to cells caused by x-rays. As another distinguishing feature of considerable importance, it allows the discrimination between different tissues, such as the gray and the white matter in the brain, or the recognition of a tumor through the difference not only in the density but also in the relaxation time $T1$ as well as $T2$ of their protons. It was found that malignant tissues generally have a longer relaxation time than does normal tissue; although there is some overlap, this difference may prove to be of significance in the detection of cancer.

The fact that NMR has long been firmly established in many fields of endeavor leaves little doubt that its use, aided by the availability of specially designed instrumentation, will be extended in the near future. Nor are there reasons to believe that all potentialities of the method have been exhausted and that major new advances are no longer possible. Given the wide interest in the application to medicine, for example, much progress can be expected as more experience is gained to correlate clinical evidence with the acquisition of NMR data.

Further developments largely depend on success in the attainment of stronger NMR signals. This is of special importance for elements other than hydrogen, since both the abundance of suitable isotopes and the magnitudes of their magnetic moments compare unfavorably with those of the proton. Besides operating at the highest magnetic fields and the lowest feasible temperatures, it is possible in some instances to increase the signal by applying simultaneously with the alternating field for NMR a field at a higher frequency chosen to cause transitions between certain states that are coupled to the Zeeman states of the observed isotope. The effect is the more pronounced the higher the frequency, and it can lead to an increment of the signal by several orders of magnitude where transitions between electronic states are involved. In order to fully exploit such opportunities, the combination of NMR not only with microwave but also with laser techniques may thus become an important auxiliary device.

It is difficult to anticipate the directions in which NMR is going to develop, and there is no assurance that the previous expansion will continue at the same rate. The prospects are not to be underestimated, however. If experience offers any guidance as to the future of NMR, all expectations at the time of its modest beginnings were so far surpassed during the following decades that one should be prepared for more surprises to come.

References

1. Stern O, Estermann I: Magnetic moment of the deuteron. Phys Rev 45:761, 1934.
2. Rabi II, Millman S, Kusch P, Zacharias JR: The molecular beam resonance method for measuring nuclear magnetic moments. Phys Rev 55:526, 1939.
3. Alvarez LW, Bloch F: Quantitative determination of the neutron moment in absolute nuclear magnetons. Phys Rev 57:111, 1940.
4. Bloch F, Hansen WW, Packard ME: Nuclear induction. Phys Rev 69:127, 1946.
5. Purcell EM, Torrey HC, Pound CV: Resonance absorption by nuclear magnetic moments in a solid. Phys Rev 64:37, 1946.
6. Hahn EL: Spin echoes. Phys Rev 80:580, 1950.
7. Gibillard R: A steady state transient technique in nuclear resonance. Phys Rev 85:694, 1952.
8. Lauterbur PC: Image formation by induced local interactions: Examples employing nuclear magnetic resonance. Nature 242:190, 1973.
9. Metropolis A, et al (eds): New Directions in Physics: The Los Alamos 40th Anniversary Volume. Orlando, Academic Press, 1988.

2

NMR in Medicine: A Historical Review

E. R. ANDREW

This chapter gives an account of the historical background of nuclear magnetic resonance (NMR) and its clinical applications. It deals with the discovery of NMR, its applications in physics and chemistry, and its later developments in biology and medicine.[1]

DISCOVERY

The first successful demonstrations of NMR in bulk matter were published in 1946. It is remarkable that two independent groups, quite unknown to each other, working in physics laboratories on opposite coasts of the United States, discovered NMR almost simultaneously. Bloch, Hansen, and Packard,[2] working at Stanford University, and Purcell, Torrey, and Pound,[3] working at Harvard University, published their results in consecutive issues of *Physical Review*. The impact of their work was immediate, and the applications of NMR have widened steadily from physics and chemistry to a surprising range of disciplines from archeology to medicine. The importance of the discovery was recognized by the joint award of the 1952 Nobel Prize for Physics to the two leaders, Professor Felix Bloch and Professor Edward Purcell (Fig. 2–1). Professor Bloch died in 1983; Professor Purcell is an Emeritus Professor at Harvard University.

These early experiments were described in quite different physical terms, and only after discussions between the two groups was it realized that their discoveries were essentially identical. At Harvard the emphasis was on transitions of magnetic nuclei between quantized states in a magnetic field, and on resonance absorption of radiofrequency (rf) energy. At Stanford experiments were focused on the precession of nuclear magnetization in a magnetic field, inducing an electromotive force (EMF) in the surrounding radiofrequency coil. The first description led to the name "nuclear magnetic resonance" for the phenomenon, and the second to the name "nuclear induction." These two descriptions, which can be shown to be quantitatively equivalent,[4] still provide complementary views of the basic phenomenon that are mutually illuminating. Today everyone refers to "nuclear magnetic resonance," but the alternative "nuclear induction" often still is used by physicists and particularly survives in the term "free induction decay" for the NMR signal following an exciting pulse.

Although NMR was first discovered and experimentally demonstrated in ordinary materials in 1946, the phenomenon did have what might be called a prehistory. In 1936 Gorter[5] looked for the resonance of ^7Li nuclei in crystalline lithium fluoride and of protons in crystalline potassium alum, but without success. The failure of these ex-

9

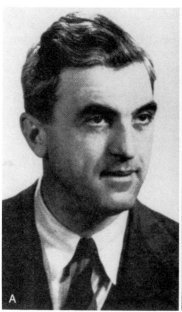
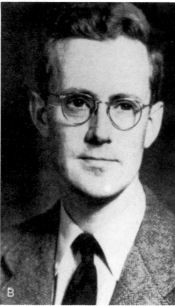

Figure 2–1. *A*, Professor Felix Bloch. *B*, Professor Edward Purcell. (Courtesy of the Nobel Foundation, Stockholm, Sweden.)

periments and of some later attempts[6] subsequently was attributed to the use of unfavorable materials.[7] Meantime, nuclear magnetic resonance first was demonstrated in molecular beams by Rabi and coworkers[8] at Columbia University in 1939. These elegant experiments furnished the first successful example of NMR. While the applications of NMR principles to matter in the tenuous form of molecular beams are similar to applications in ordinary materials, it is the latter that will be the focus of this book.

Now that hospitals are spending large sums on magnetic resonance imaging (MRI) clinical equipment it is sobering to recall that the first NMR experiments were done at almost no cost at all. The Harvard group borrowed a large electromagnet previously used by Professor J. C. Street for his pioneer cosmic ray experiments on the muon which, in turn, had been converted from a discarded generator from the Boston elevated railway. In Stanford an electromagnet was borrowed from the physics lecture theater and only a few hundred dollars was spent, mainly on an oscilloscope. Bloch has recalled[9] how his calibration of the magnet was slightly in error and the field set too high, so that at first the investigators failed to see the NMR signal. As they turned off the magnet their despondence was quickly transformed to elation as the NMR signal drifted across the oscilloscope screen. I have recently learned [9a] that the Harvard group had a similar experience; in their case the magnetic field initially was set too low.

PHYSICS

Over the next few years many workers joined this exciting new field of research, and NMR was detected for almost all magnetic nuclei in the periodic table of the elements. NMR was detected in solids, liquids, and gases; in insulators, semiconductors, and metals; in crystalline, polycrystalline, and amorphous materials; in diamagnetics, paramagnetics, ferromagnetics, and antiferromagnetics; in polymers, membranes, adsorbed and occluded phases; and indeed in matter in all its forms. Resonances in liquids and gases were remarkably sharp, those from solids somewhat broader. By exploiting the sharpness of the resonances from fluids, extremely precise measurements were made of nuclear magnetic moments; nuclear spins were determined or confirmed, and other nuclear parameters obtained.

The resonance frequency and the magnetic field are directly proportional to each other, the constant of proportionality being determined by the gyromagnetic ratio of the nucleus of interest. Consequently, once the NMR frequency had been determined in an accurately known magnetic field, any other unknown magnetic field could be measured with high precision by simply measuring the NMR frequency in that field. NMR thus presented the physicist with an excellent magnetometer for magnetic field measurement in the laboratory. The method was readily extended to the earth's magnetic field, and portable NMR magnetometers became useful in civil engineering projects, in archeologic surveys for buried magnetic artifacts, for aerial geomagnetic surveys, for oceanographic surveys, and for magnetic field measurements in satellites and space vehicles. The high precision of magnetic field measurement enabled more precise measurements to be made of some of the fundamental constants of physics.

From the beginning the importance of relaxation times in NMR had been realized. At Stanford the proton NMR was first found in water, and a paramagnetic salt was dissolved in the water in some experiments with a view to shortening the relaxation time.[2] At Harvard the proton NMR was first found in solid paraffin,[3] and great pains were taken to use an extremely low radiofrequency power level to avoid saturation. The relaxation times $T1$ and $T2$ were introduced from the outset, and the foundations for understanding these basic quantities were laid in famous pioneering papers by Bloch[10,11] and Purcell[12] and their colleagues; to all NMR practitioners interested in relaxation processes, Reference 12 is known simply as BPP. Fundamental studies of relaxation behavior in solids and liquids gave great insight into molecular dynamics in a wide range of materials.

In the early years NMR was detected using a steady source of resonant rf radiation, often referred to as continuous wave (CW) detection. The spectacular discovery of spin echoes by Hahn[13] in 1950 stimulated the widespread use of pulsed NMR. The NMR spectrum could be obtained by Fourier transformation of the free induction decay with tremendous savings of time, and relaxation times could be determined with greater simplicity.

In the first decade of its activity NMR was largely the province of the physicist and the physical chemist. By 1954 some 400 NMR papers had been published and the first book on NMR[4] was able to make reference to all of them. Two later books[14,15] devoted to the fundamental physical principles of NMR have become landmarks in the development of the subject.

CHEMISTRY

Quite early it had been noted by several workers[16–18] that the NMR frequency of a given nucleus was to a small degree dependent on the chemical form in which the element was present. The molecular electrons slightly shielded the nucleus and shifted the resonance; the effect was appropriately called the chemical shift. Consequently, a molecule with nuclei in several environments generated a spectrum with several distinct NMR responses, and the subject of NMR spectroscopy had begun. A very early example[19] of the proton NMR spectrum from ethyl alcohol is shown in Figure 2–2. Spin couplings provided finer features in the NMR spectrum.[20,21] The NMR spectrum was thus a fingerprint of the chemical compound and enabled NMR spectroscopy to become one of the chemist's most valuable structural and analytic tools.

The NMR spectral lines are close together; consequently, the development of high-

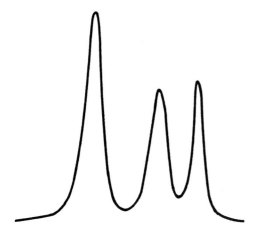

Figure 2–2. Proton NMR spectrum from ethyl alcohol.[19] Reading from left to right the three peaks correspond to CH_3, CH_2, and OH groups. (From Andrew ER: Nuclear Magnetic Resonance. Cambridge, Cambridge University Press, 1955. Used by permission.)

resolution NMR spectroscopy called for extremely uniform magnetic fields, uniform to a part in 10^8 over a 1 ml sample. Varian Associates in California can be credited fairly with opening this field to chemists generally in the late 1950s, by responding to the challenge posed by small proton chemical shift differences and by providing NMR spectrometers with magnets having the requisite uniformity of field. In the quest for improved resolution and sensitivity the proton NMR frequency was steadily advanced from 40 to 60 to 100 MHz, this last frequency corresponding to a magnetic field of 2.3 tesla. Many other nuclei, especially ^{13}C, ^{19}F, and ^{31}P, were exploited under high-resolution conditions. Pulse methods replaced CW, and a dedicated computer became an integral part of the spectrometer system, controlling the pulse sequences, gathering the data, performing the Fourier transforms, and displaying the spectra.

The pursuit of higher and higher resolution and sensitivity has called for still higher magnetic fields, which, in turn, has required a change of magnet technology from the iron electromagnets used hitherto. Using superconducting magnets, proton NMR spectra are recorded now at frequencies up to 600 MHz in fields up to 14 tesla.

Currently no chemistry research laboratory is properly equipped without its high-resolution NMR spectrometer. The widespread use of NMR spectrometers in chemical laboratories has led to the growth of a substantial NMR instrument industry. The principles and practice of NMR are now a feature of chemistry courses at quite elementary levels. The use of high-resolution NMR spectroscopy has spread from chemistry to biochemistry, microbiology, pharmacy, agricultural chemistry, polymer science, and, as we shall see, biology and medicine. Its widespread use in the context of chemistry and biochemistry has brought NMR to the notice of a very wide range of scientists in all disciplines.

We shall note in passing that specimens investigated by chemists and physicists are usually homogeneous and rather less than 1 ml in volume. Consequently, the bore of a superconducting NMR magnet for such work is usually about 5 cm in diameter and the gap between the polefaces of an iron electromagnet is of similar dimensions. This provides just sufficient access for the specimen, its surrounding rf probe, and other accessories.

BIOLOGY

The earliest biologic NMR experiments take us back to the discovery of the phenomenon. Soon after the first successful NMR experiments at Stanford,[2] Bloch obtained a strong proton NMR signal when he inserted his finger into the rf coil of his spectrometer. In 1948 Purcell and Ramsey, in turn, inserted their heads into the 2 tesla field of the Harvard cyclotron; around their heads was a coil connected to a powerful rf generator tuned to the proton NMR frequency. The only sensation recorded was that of the EMFs generated in the metal fillings of their teeth as their heads were moved into and out of the magnet, and detected by their tongues. It is noteworthy that 40 years later there is no evidence of injury or damage arising from this magnetic adventure by these distinguished physicists.

Occasional NMR experiments subsequently were reported on materials of biologic interest.[22,23] A pioneering series of investigations was carried out by Odeblad and his colleagues in Stockholm on tissues and fluids from animals and humans, starting in 1955 and continuing over the next decade. These studies included blood cells,[24,25] cervical mucus,[26] tissues and fluids of the eye[27] and the eye lens,[28] saliva,[29] and muscle.[30] However, substantial advances in the application of NMR in biology awaited the development of high-field, high-resolution, Fourier-transform spectrometers in the late 1960s. In one type of application, high-resolution NMR spectra have been obtained from enzymes and from other proteins and biomolecules in solution, yielding structural and dynamic information of importance in biochemistry and biology. This NMR contribution to molecular biology continues to be an active area at the frontier of research.

In a second type of application, high-resolution NMR spectroscopy has been applied to living systems. First, Moon and Richards[31] reported high-resolution ^{31}P NMR studies of intact red blood cells in which they could assign lines to individual metabolites. This was followed by the recording of a ^{31}P NMR spectrum from an intact freshly excised muscle from a rat's leg by Hoult et al.[32] (Fig. 2–3). It was found possible to maintain muscles in good physiologic condition in the spectrometer and to record the effects of electrical stimulation. The 5 cm diameter bore of a conventional NMR superconducting magnet was nevertheless a severe restriction. Soon magnets with a 10 cm diameter bore were provided, and a wide range of studies on perfused animal hearts,

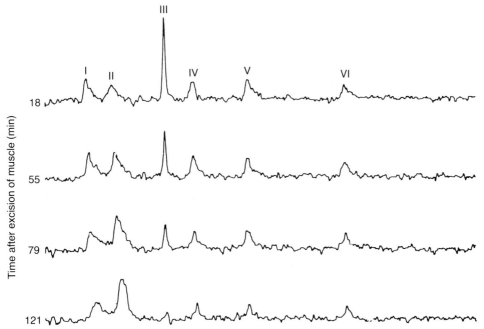

Figure 2–3. ^{31}P NMR spectra from an intact freshly excised rat leg muscle. I, Sugar phosphate and phospholipid; II, inorganic phosphate; III, creatine phosphate; IV, γ ATP; V, α ATP; VI, β ATP. (From Hoult DI et al: Nature *252*:285, 1974. Used by permission.)

kidneys, livers, and other organs were pursued, using mainly ^{31}P NMR but also ^{1}H and ^{13}C NMR spectroscopy.

It was then a natural step to examine whole intact living organisms from bacteria to mice, rats, and rabbits. With animals it is, of course, important to know from what anatomic part or organ the NMR spectrum originates. In some cases this could be achieved by winding the rf coil around the part concerned; in other cases a small rf coil was placed on the surface of the animal to record the NMR signal from the region immediately below.

From animals it is just a further step to man; this stage in the evolution of high-resolution NMR spectroscopy is discussed next. Meantime, in 1973 a rather different application of NMR to living systems appeared in the form of NMR imaging. Here too, before moving on to human beings, the initial applications included intact biologic systems in the form of fruit, vegetables, and small animals. However, it is more convenient to discuss this development as a whole under Medicine: Imaging.

MEDICINE: SPECTROSCOPY

A prerequisite to high-resolution NMR spectroscopy of human beings was the provision of magnets with a very much larger access than those used to date. In 1980 the Oxford Instrument Company in England, a pioneer of many NMR magnet developments, provided superconducting magnets with a field of 2 tesla, a 30 cm diameter horizontal bore, and a high-resolution capability over a region 2 to 4 cm in extent.

It was possible to insert the human hand and arm, foot and leg into such a magnet, and many high-resolution NMR spectra have been recorded of ^{31}P and also of ^{13}C and ^{1}H nuclei. In this way it was possible to monitor the metabolism of both normal and diseased human limbs. The effects of exercise and of a tourniquet could be followed; diseased muscles could be diagnosed and their treatment and course followed in biochemical detail. Magnets of this size have also been used to study clinical problems in the heads of babies.[33]

It is, of course, important to gather the NMR spectra from a clearly defined region in the human anatomy. Several methods have been developed for this. One is by the use of surface coils described previously, but this method is clearly limited to anatomic parts near the surface of the body. The spatial selectivity of surface coils has been improved by combining their use with depth-resolved pulses and selective excitation. An early method of localizing the NMR spectrum from a region well inside the body consists of carefully profiling the magnetic field so that only a small, well-defined volume has the necessary uniformity to yield a high-resolution spectrum. This technique has been termed topical magnetic resonance (from the Greek *topos,* a place). The well-defined volume is at a fixed place in the magnet bore; to change its location in the human subject, the patient must be moved, and this is a distinct inconvenience. A number of ingenious techniques are therefore under current development, using three-dimensional selective excitation to move the region of interest electronically without disturbing the patient.

Later, 2 tesla superconducting magnets with a 100 cm diameter bore and a high-resolution capability have become available. With access of this size the whole human body can be inserted and the high-resolution NMR spectrum obtained from any desired part of the anatomy. A ^{31}P NMR spectrum of the right side of the brain (Fig. 2–4) displays the customary characteristic metabolic spectral lines. Figures 2–2 to 2–4 together demonstrate in a graphic manner the historical progress of NMR spectroscopy from molecules to man.

As may be expected, high-resolution NMR spectroscopy of almost every part of

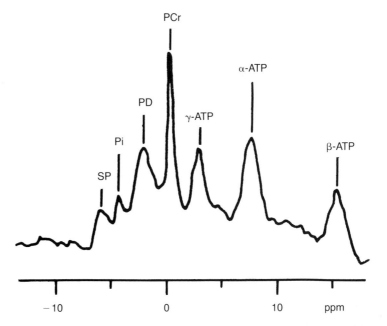

Figure 2–4. ³¹P NMR spectra from a live human head in a field of 1.5 tesla using a surface coil placed over the temple.[54] (Courtesy of Dr. P.A. Bottomley, General Electric Company.)

the human body is now yielding valuable clinical information, especially from organs such as the brain, heart, kidney, and liver, and is contributing to the understanding of cancer, stroke, and heart disease. The technique also is providing information on the metabolic state of kidneys prior to transplantation. While there is no doubt of the value of high-resolution NMR spectroscopy as a research instrument in medicine, its use as a regular diagnostic modality in hospitals is not yet established, and the next few years will be a critical time of clinical evaluation.

As in conventional high-resolution NMR spectroscopy as used in chemistry, the pursuit of higher resolution and sensitivity is leading to the introduction of still higher magnetic fields. Although FDA guidelines in the United States at present limit the application of magnetic fields in human subjects to 2 tesla, wide-bore magnets for NMR imaging and spectroscopy of animals in the range of 4 to 5 tesla are now available, and a feasibility study for a whole-body 10 tesla magnet is in progress. Such a decatesla magnet undoubtedly will be expensive.

Further information on the developments outlined in this section may be found in a book by Gadian[34] and in Chapters 88 to 95.

MEDICINE: IMAGING

In contrast with the steady onward march of NMR spectroscopy from physics through chemistry and biology to medicine, the second strand of clinical applications, namely NMR imaging, represents a distinctly different approach. In 1973, Lauterbur[35] published the first NMR image of a heterogeneous object: two tubes of water. He pointed out the simple fact that if a field gradient is applied to a structured object each nucleus responds with its own NMR frequency determined by its position; the NMR spectrum is the one-dimensional (1D) projection of nuclear density along the gradient direction. Applying the gradient in a series of directions and so obtaining a series of projections, he devised an algorithm to generate a two-dimensional (2D) proton NMR image of the object from its projections, in just the same way as it is done in x-ray CT scanning. This first image is reproduced in Figure 2–5.

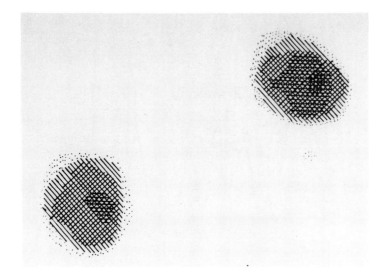

Figure 2–5. The first NMR image. The image is of two tubes of water. (From Lauterbur PC: Nature *242*:190, 1973. Used by permission.)

The impact of this first image and the work that followed has been tremendous. Within a decade of its publication, manufacturers worldwide were producing NMR scanners that generated high-quality images of all parts of the human body, challenging traditional modalities of imaging in clinical practice. It is likely that before long all major hospitals will be equipped with NMR scanners and that the total expenditure for this equipment will overshadow that for all previous uses of NMR. It is, moreover, likely to bring NMR for the first time to the notice of the man in the street and to enter our everyday vocabulary.

Just as in NMR itself there was a prehistory before the final successful breakthrough, so in NMR imaging there was a prehistory in the use of magnetic field gradients. NMR 1D projections were first investigated quite early with simple glass and liquid structures by Gabillard[36–38] in France, who studied their dynamic response as well. Field gradients are an essential feature of the study of molecular diffusion in liquids by the NMR spin-echo method[13,39] and also have been used in the study of phase separation in ^{3}He-^{4}He solutions,[40] in methods of information storage,[41,42] and in the investigation of periodic structures by the NMR diffraction method.[43] In a prophetic patent, filed in 1972, Damadian[44] proposed without detail that the human body might be scanned for clinical purposes by NMR. This proposition was based on his important observation[45] that relaxation times $T1$ and $T2$ were significantly higher in cancerous tissue than in corresponding normal tissue.

In its short life, a variety of terms have been used in the literature to describe this subject, for example, NMR imaging, spin imaging, spin mapping, NMR tomography, and NMR zeugmatography. The first four of these names are rather straightforward and self-explanatory and are clearly equivalent; the last name is intriguingly different and calls for further explanation. Lauterbur in his original article[35] recognized that unlike traditional microscopy, the resolution of detail in NMR images is not related to the wavelength of the illuminating radiation. The resolution and spatial discrimination are determined by the magnetic field and its gradient, while the rf electromagnetic field serves to detect the NMR phenomenon. So both fields must be conjoined in the object, which led Lauterbur to coin the term "zeugmatography" (from the Greek *zeugma*, that which joins together). This name is currently fighting for survival. The most common term today is NMR imaging, although in a medical context this is often abbreviated to MR imaging or MRI.

A field gradient is an essentially 1D probe, and a dozen or more techniques have been advanced for manipulating the gradient to secure 2D or 3D information. In most investigations the 2D projection-reconstruction method originally used by Lauterbur[35] has been replaced by the 2D Fourier imaging method,[46] which generates a 2D image of a selected slice. Both methods may be extended to 3D, but 3D images take a longer time and usually give more information than is needed.

The first NMR imaging experiments were carried out in physics and chemistry laboratories using conventional NMR spectrometers with their limited access. As work progressed, larger magnets became available. For whole-body imaging, air-core resistive magnets up to 0.15 tesla and superconducting magnets up to 2 tesla have been provided; permanent magnets and iron electromagnets are also in use. The specification for field uniformity for NMR imaging is less demanding than for high-resolution NMR spectroscopy; large magnets for whole-body imaging therefore became available several years earlier and at lower cost than for whole-body NMR spectroscopy.

Since hydrogen is the most abundant element in all living organisms, proton NMR lends itself particularly well as a method of imaging in biology and medicine; some work has also been done with ^7Li, ^{13}C, ^{19}F, ^{23}Na, and ^{31}P. As a method of medical imaging, NMR imaging offers some special advantages, namely that it does not use ionizing radiation, is noninvasive, and if properly used is without known hazard. It is therefore a much safer means of imaging than modalities using x-rays, γ-rays, positrons, or heavy ions. In contrast with ultrasound, the radiation penetrates bony structures without attenuation. Besides giving morphologic information, NMR imaging yields additional diagnostic insights through relaxation parameters that are not available from other imaging modalities. Finally, in contrast with x-ray CT scanning, NMR imaging can directly provide images of transverse, coronal, or sagittal slices or of slices of arbitrary orientation.

The first human image, reported in 1976, was of a live finger,[47] followed by the hand[48] and the thorax[49] in 1977, and the head[50] and the abdomen[51] in 1978. Since then, NMR images have improved immensely in quality, both in resolution and in tissue discrimination. Figure 2–6 is a sagittal image of the spine[52] showing the spinal cord, Figure 2–7 is an excellent early sagittal image[53] of the head (1982), and Figure 2–8 is a transverse image of the head[54] taken in a field of 1.5 tesla. The special feature of this last image is that it was taken in the same magnet and of the same normal head as the ^{31}P NMR spectrum shown in Figure 2–4, and demonstrates a potential marriage of the two strands of NMR applied to medicine.

A single NMR image of a defined slice in the body takes about 2 minutes. However, by more economical use of time one may typically obtain ten adjacent slices, each with

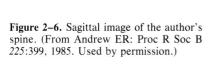

Figure 2–6. Sagittal image of the author's spine. (From Andrew ER: Proc R Soc B *225*:399, 1985. Used by permission.)

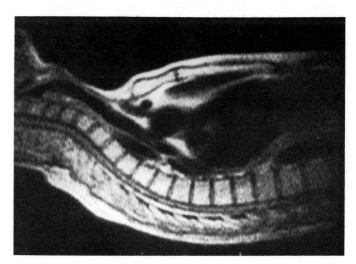

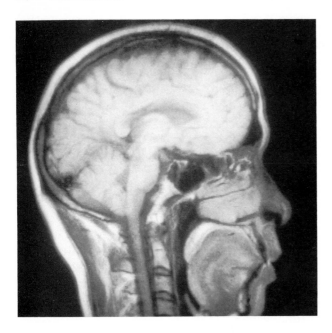

Figure 2–7. Sagittal image of the human head.[53] (Courtesy of Technicare Corporation.)

four spin-echo delay times giving *T2* weighting, a total of 40 images, in 4 minutes, or 6 seconds per slice, which is competitive with x-ray CT scanning; this is the multislice/multiecho technique.[53] Faster images may be obtained by the FLASH technique[54a] and still faster images may be obtained by the echo-planar technique, which enables real-time movie NMR images to be recorded.[55]

Recent advances include the use of paramagnetic contrast agents, such as solutions of gadolinium chelates, to enhance pathologic tissue discrimination (see Chapters 12 and 46 to 52); the measurement of fluid flow in the body (see Chapters 36 and 98); and the development of microimaging techniques (see Chapters 99 and 104).

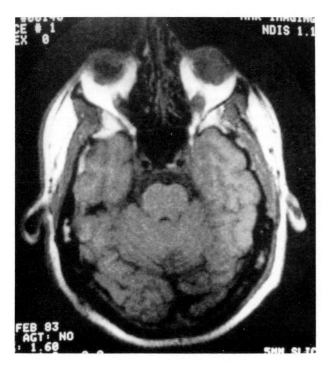

Figure 2–8. Transverse image of the human head in a magnetic field of 1.5 tesla.[54] This image was obtained of the same head and in the same magnet as the ^{31}P spectrum in Figure 2–4. (Courtesy of Dr. P.A. Bottomley, General Electric Company.)

Further information on the developments outlined in this chapter may be found in articles by the author,[53,56] in a book by Morris,[57] and in later chapters.

Physicians have found magnetic resonance imaging to be a valuable addition to their armory of diagnostic techniques. Approaching one thousand whole-body MRI scanners have currently been installed in hospitals worldwide and about one million patients have been examined. We can predict with confidence a further substantial expansion in its use in the years ahead.

References

1. Andrew, ER: A historical review of NMR and its clinical applications. Br Med Bull *40*:115, 1984.
2. Bloch F, Hansen WW, Packard ME: Nuclear induction. Phys Rev *69*:127, 1946.
3. Purcell EM, Torrey HC, Pound RV: Resonance absorption by nuclear magnetic moments in a solid. Phys Rev *69*:37, 1946.
4. Andrew ER: Nuclear Magnetic Resonance. Cambridge, Cambridge University Press, 1955.
5. Gorter CJ: Negative result of an attempt to detect nuclear magnetic spins. Physica *3*:995, 1936.
6. Gorter CJ, Broer LFJ: Negative result of an attempt to observe nuclear magnetic resonance in solids. Physica *9*:591, 1942.
7. Gorter CJ: Spectroscopy at radio frequencies. Physica *17*:169, 1951.
8. Rabi II, Millman S, Kusch P, Zacharias JR: The molecular beam resonance method for measuring nuclear magnetic moments. Phys Rev *55*:526, 1939.
9. Andrew ER: Magnetic resonance discovery celebrated. Nature *233*:374, 1971.
9a. Pound RU: Personal communication, 1985.
10. Bloch F: Nuclear induction. Phys Rev *70*:460, 1946.
11. Bloch F, Hansen WW, Packard ME: The nuclear induction experiment. Phys Rev *70*:474, 1946.
12. Bloembergen N, Purcell EM, Pound RV: Relaxation effects in nuclear magnetic resonance absorption. Phys Rev *73*:679, 1948.
13. Hahn EL: Spin echoes. Phys Rev *80*:580, 1950.
14. Abragam A: The Principles of Nuclear Magnetism. Oxford, Clarendon Press, 1961.
15. Slichter CP: Principles of Magnetic Resonance, 2nd ed. Berlin, Springer-Verlag, 1978.
16. Knight, WD: Nuclear magnetic resonance shift in metals. Phys Rev *76*:1259, 1949.
17. Dickinson WC: Dependence of the F^{19} nuclear resonance position on chemical compound. Phys Rev *77*:736, 1950.
18. Proctor WG, Yu FC: The dependence of a nuclear magnetic resonance frequency upon chemical compound. Phys Rev *77*:717, 1950.
19. Arnold JT, Dharmatti SS, Packard ME: Chemical effects on nuclear induction signals from organic compounds. J Chem Phys *19*:507, 1951.
20. Gutowsky HS, McCall DW, Slichter CP: Coupling among nuclear magnetic dipoles in molecules. Phys Rev *84*:589, 1951.
21. Hahn EL, Maxwell DE: Chemical shift and field independent frequency modulation of the spin echo envelope. Phys Rev *84*:1246, 1951.
22. Shaw TM, Elsken RH: Nuclear magnetic resonance absorption in hygroscopic materials. J Chem Phys *18*:1113, 1950.
23. Jacobsohn B, Anderson WA, Arnold JT: A proton magnetic resonance study of the hydration of deoxyribonucleic acid. Nature *173*:772, 1954.
24. Odeblad E, Lindstrom G: Some preliminary observations on the proton magnetic resonance in biologic samples. Acta Radiol *43*:469, 1955.
25. Odeblad E, Bhar BN, Lindstrom G: Proton magnetic resonance of human blood cells. Arch Biochem Biophys *63*:221, 1956.
26. Odeblad E, Bryhu V: Proton magnetic resonance of human cervical mucus during the menstrual cycle. Acta Radiol *47*:315, 1957.
27. Huggert A, Odeblad E: Proton magnetic resonance studies of some tissues and fluids of the eye. Acta Radiol *51*:385, 1959.
28. Huggert A, Odeblad E: Water of the crystalline lens III proton magnetic resonance studies. Acta Ophthalmol *37*:26, 1959.
29. Odeblad E, Soremark R: Nuclear magnetic resonance of human saliva. Acta Odontol Scand *20*:23, 1962.
30. Odeblad E, Ingelman-Sundberg A: Proton magnetic resonance studies on the structure of water in the myometrium. Acta Obstet Gynecol Scand *44*:117, 1965.
31. Moon RB, Richards JH: Determination of intracellular pH by ^{31}P magnetic resonance. J Biol Chem *248*:7276, 1973.
32. Hoult DI, Busby SJW, Gadian DG, Radda GK, Richards RE, Seeley PJ: Observation of tissue metabolites using ^{31}P nuclear magnetic resonance. Nature *252*:285, 1974.
33. Cady EB, Costello AM deL, Dawson MJ, Delpy DT, Hope PL, Reynolds EOR, Tofts PS, Wilkie DR: Non-invasive investigation of cerebral metabolism in newborn infants by phosphorus nuclear magnetic resonance spectroscopy. Lancet *1*:1059, 1983.

34. Gadian DG: Nuclear Magnetic Resonance and Its Application to Living Systems. Oxford, Clarendon Press, 1980.
35. Lauterbur PC: Image formation by induced local interactions: examples employing nuclear magnetic resonance. Nature *242*:190, 1973.
36. Gabillard R. Mesure du temps de relaxation T_2 en présence d'une inhomogenéité de champ magnétique supérieure à la largeur de raie. C R Acad Sci Paris *232*:1551, 1951.
37. Gabillard R: A steady state transient technique in nuclear resonance. Phys Rev *85*:694, 1952.
38. Andrew ER: Nuclear Magnetic Resonance. Cambridge, Cambridge University Press, 1955, pp 134–136.
39. Carr HY, Purcell EM: Effects of diffusion on free precession in nuclear magnetic resonance experiments. Phys Rev *96*:630, 1954.
40. Walters GK, Fairbank WM: Phase separation in He^3-He^4 solutions. Phys Rev *103*:262, 1956.
41. Anderson AG, Garvin RL, Hahn EL, Horton JW, Tucker GL, Walker RM: Spin echo serial storage memory. Phys Rev *26*:1324, 1955.
42. Andrew ER, Finney A, Mansfield P: Information storage by NMR. Royal Radar Establishment Research Report PD/24/026/AT, 1970.
43. Mansfield P, Grannell PK: NMR "diffraction" in solids? J Phys C: Solid State Phys *6*:L422, 1973.
44. Damadian R: Apparatus and method for detecting cancer in tissue. US patent 3789832, filed 17 March 1972.
45. Damadian R: Tumor detection by nuclear magnetic resonance. Science *171*:1151, 1971.
46. Kumar A, Welti D, Ernst RR: NMR Fourier zeugmatography. J Magn Reson *18*:69, 1975.
47. Mansfield P, Maudsley AA: Planar and line-scan spin imaging by NMR. Proc XIXth Congress Ampere, Heidelberg, 1976, pp 247–252.
48. Andrew ER, Bottomley PA, Hinshaw WS, Holland GN, Moore WS, Simaroj C: NMR images by the multiple sensitive point method: application to larger biological specimens. Phys Med Biol *22*:971, 1977.
49. Damadian R, Goldsmith M, Minkoff L: NMR in cancer: Fonar image of the live human body. Physiol Chem Phys 1977: 97–108.
50. Clow H, Young IR: Britain's brains produce first NMR scans. New Scientist *80*:588, 1978.
51. Mansfield P, Pykett IL, Morris PG, Coupland RE: Human whole body line-scan imaging by NMR. Br J Radiol *51*:921, 1978.
52. Andrew ER: Nuclear magnetic resonance imaging in medicine: physical principles. Proc R Soc [Biol] *225*:399, 1985.
53. Alfidi RJ, Haaga JR, El Yousef SJ, et al: Preliminary experimental results in humans and animals with a superconducting, whole body, nuclear magnetic resonance scanner. Radiology *143*:175, 1982.
54. Bottomley PA, Hart HR, Edelstein WA, et al: NMR imaging/spectroscopy system to study both anatomy and metabolism. Lancet *2*:273, 1983.
54a. Haase A, Frahm J, Matthaei D, Hanicke W, Merboldt J: FLASH imaging. Rapid NMR imaging using low flip-angle pulses. J Magn Reson *67*:258, 1986.
55. Rzedzian R, Mansfield P, et al: Real-time NMR clinical imaging in paediatrics. Lancet *2*:1281, 1983.
56. Andrew ER: NMR imaging. Acc Chem Res *16*:114, 1983.
57. Morris PG: NMR Imaging in Medicine and Biology. Oxford, Clarendon Press, 1986.

3

A Survey of MRI Techniques

RICHARD R. ERNST

The casual observer may be overwhelmed by the multitude of medical imaging techniques using nuclear magnetic resonance (NMR) principles in MRI. It parallels the even greater richness of NMR methods developed in the past 40 years for conventional spectroscopic investigations in physics, chemistry, and biology.[1] There is hardly another technique capable of matching NMR in versatility and potential. The explanation is found in the easy realization of time-domain experiments with an arbitrarily large number of radio frequency pulses of freely selected shape, frequency, and phase, and in the exploitation of time-dependent magnetic fields and magnetic field gradients.

This chapter presents an incomplete but representative survey of the available imaging techniques. It attempts to demonstrate the diversity of approaches by including some examples that appear at present to be of primarily historical interest (although it is hard to predict the trend of future developments).

At first sight, it may not be obvious why macroscopic imaging should employ the phenomenon of nuclear magnetic resonance or how such an imaging concept could be realized. Consider the attenuation of radiation by human tissue, schematically represented in Figure 3–1 for electromagnetic and acoustical radiation. It is apparent that nature provides three windows that permit us to look inside the human body. The x-ray window has been exploited for more than 90 years, starting with the basic experiments by Roentgen in 1895, and has completely revolutionized medical diagnosis. In recent years, computed tomography has had a significant impact on medicine. Despite the potential danger of the sizable radiation dose, x-ray imaging is still one of the most important diagnostic tools.

The second window is the low-frequency ultrasonic window. It led to the development of ultrasonic scanners that produce images of acceptable quality in very fast sequence.

The radio frequency window was not exploited until 1972. This is not surprising, considering the achievable resolution, which is usually limited by the wavelength of the applied radiation through the uncertainty relation. The maximum useful frequency for NMR imaging is in the order of 100 MHz, limiting resolution to about 3 m, which is insufficient even for the imaging of full-grown elephants (Fig. 3–2). On the other hand, the quantum energy involved in radio frequency radiation is extremely low in comparison to typical chemical bonding energies—this in contrast to x-rays, which can easily break bonds and may induce destructive chemical processes (Fig. 3–3).

The potential value of NMR for in vivo studies was recognized in 1971 by Damadian.[2,3] The basic idea of NMR imaging, however, was proposed in 1972 by Lauterbur,[4,5] who suggested the use of magnetic field gradients to distinguish between the signal contributions originating from various volume elements. Since 1972 many techniques of NMR imaging have been proposed. The most successful technique for medical

ELECTROMAGNETIC RADIATION

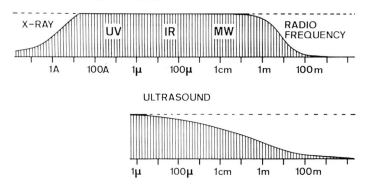

ULTRASOUND

Figure 3–1. Attenuation of radiation by human tissue. Electromagnetic radiation is strongly absorbed except in the x-ray and radio frequency ranges. Acoustical radiation is absorbed except for the low-frequency range, which is suitable for ultrasonic imaging. (Adapted from Ernst RR et al: Principles of Nuclear Magnetic Resonance in One and Two Dimensions. London, Oxford University Press, 1986.)

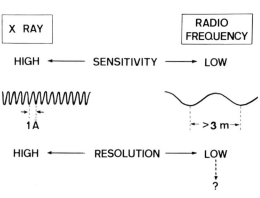

Figure 3–2. Radio frequency irradiation in NMR uses much longer wavelengths than do x-rays. This leads to low sensitivity and, in direct imaging procedures, to extremely low resolution. The sensitivity can be improved by optimized techniques, whereas the attainment of adequate resolution calls for a new imaging principle.

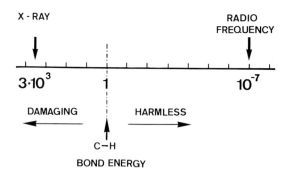

Figure 3–3. The very low quantum energy of radio frequency irradiation precludes adverse chemical effects in tissue. This is in contrast to energetic x-rays, which can easily break chemical bonds and induce damaging chemical processes.

imaging, spin-warp imaging, introduced in 1980 by Edelstein and coworkers,[6,7] is a variant of Fourier imaging suggested in 1975 by Kumar et al.[8,9]

MR IMAGING

MR imaging takes advantage of the magnetic moments of nuclei associated with their spin. The force acting on a nuclear moment μ placed in a magnetic field $\overline{B}$ is the basic interaction that leads to nuclear magnetic resonance. In addition to the magnetic moment, the nuclei possess an angular moment. They can be visualized as gyroscopes that precess under the influence of the applied magnetic field with the angular velocity[1,10]

$$\omega = -\gamma B \qquad (1)$$

about the magnetic field direction (see Chapter 1). The gyromagnetic ratio γ is a measure for the size of the magnetic moment characteristic for a nuclear species.

The precession of a magnetic moment μ or of the magnetization $M = 1/\text{vol} \sum_k \mu_k$ of a volume element does not last indefinitely but is damped exponentially with the transverse relaxation time $T2$. At the same time the equilibrium magnetization M_0 recovers exponentially with the longitudinal relaxation time $T1$ and aligns along the static magnetic field (z-axis). Normally $T2$ is much shorter than $T1$.

By the application of radio frequency pulses it is possible to rotate the magnetization vector about selected axes. For example, a radio frequency field B_1 applied for the time τ along the x-axis rotates the magnetization vector by the angle $\beta = -\gamma B_1 \tau$ about the x-axis. In many experiments $\pi/2$ and π pulses with $\beta = 90$ degrees and 180 degrees, respectively, are used. Pi/2 pulses are useful for rotating the equilibrium magnetization M_0 from the position along the static field (z-axis) into the transverse (x, y) plane for initiating free precession. Pi pulses, on the other hand, are needed for the inversion of the magnetization in order to exploit $T1$ effects or to refocus transverse magnetization.

MR imaging relies on the use of magnetic field gradients to disperse the MR frequencies of the various volume elements of a medical object. The basic idea of MR imaging is illustrated in Figure 3–4. A linear magnetic field gradient applied along an axis of the object leads to resonance frequencies characteristic of the position along this axis. All volume elements in a plane perpendicular to this axis exhibit the same resonance frequency and contribute to the same signal amplitude. The MR spectrum can thus be considered as a one-dimensional projection of the three-dimensional density of the observed nuclear spin species (normally ^{1}H) onto the direction of the field gradient.

Additional experiments are required for the distinction of the volume elements within one of these planes. In effect, a three-dimensional frequency space is required, in which each volume element of the object has its correspondence. Numerous experimental techniques have been proposed for establishing this correspondence.

A general imaging experiment consists of two phases that are often clearly separated in time (Fig. 3–5). The *preconditioning or preparation period* prepares the spins in an initial state for obtaining maximum information on the question to be answered by the MR image. The second phase is the *imaging period*, which serves to differentiate the various volume elements. The preconditioning period is primarily responsible for the image contrast, which is of central importance for the image quality. The imaging period, on the other hand, determines the spatial resolution. Both periods affect sen-

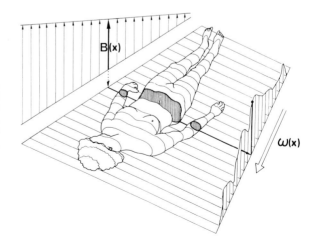

Figure 3–4. Basic idea of NMR imaging: The NMR signal is recorded in the presence of a linear magnetic field gradient $\bar{B}(x)$ such that the resonance frequency ω is a linear function of the spatial coordinate x. (Adapted from Ernst RR et al: Principles of Nuclear Magnetic Resonance in One and Two Dimensions. London, Oxford University Press, 1986.)

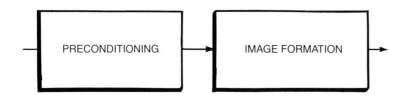

PRECONDITIONING → IMAGE FORMATION →

Figure 3–5. The two phases of an imaging experiment. Preconditioning is responsible for the image contrast, while the image formation process determines the spatial resolution.

CONTRAST   RESOLUTION

sitivity, although the selection of the imaging process is normally decisive in this respect.

Numerous imaging techniques will be discussed in some detail in the following sections. At first a few comments concerning the preconditioning period are in order.

The image contrast can be influenced by various parameters of the object. The most important ones are the spin density $\rho(r)$, the longitudinal relaxation time $T1(r)$, and the transverse relaxation time $T2(r)$. In many cases, all these parameters simultaneously contribute in a nontransparent manner to the image contrast. It is, however, also possible to specifically design the preconditioning process in order to favor the influence of one parameter. Figure 3–6 shows some commonly used preconditioning processes.

In the simplest case, preconditioning consists of a single preparation pulse, usually of rotation angle $\beta = \pi/2$ (Fig. 3–6A). The magnetization is rotated into the xy plane and starts to precess under the influence of magnetic field gradients applied for the imaging process. When a sufficiently long waiting time is inserted between different experiments in order to let the system fully relax, the image contrast will be given primarily by $\rho(r)$. However, for an insufficient waiting time, there is an additional influence of $T1(r)$.

In order to favor the influence of $T1(r)$ on the image contrast, it is possible simply

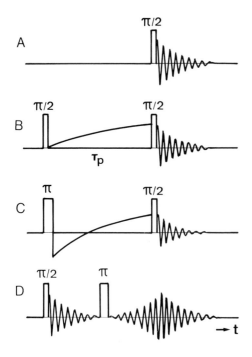

Figure 3–6. Processes of preconditioning or preparation for manipulating the image contrast. *A*, Single pulse creating transverse magnetization, which leads to a free induction decay. *B*, Saturation recovery experiment exploiting *T1* differences. *C*, Inversion-recovery experiment, also sensitive to *T1* variations. *D*, Spin-echo experiment for obtaining *T2* weighted images.

to use a very fast repetition of the experiment shown in Figure 3–6A. To ensure a well-defined initial state for longitudinal relaxation, one may apply a $\pi/2$ prepulse, leading to the "saturation recovery experiment" of Figure 3–6B. Here exclusively, the magnetization recovered during the time τ_p by *T1* processes is imaged. Another *T1* experiment is the inversion recovery sequence of (Fig. 3–6C), in which a π prepulse initially inverts the magnetization. Its recovery proceeds through an intermediate zero value, which can be exploited to suppress undesired components with a characteristic *T1* value.

Spin-echo experiments of the type shown in Figure 3–6D are sensitive to differences in the transverse relaxation *T2*. The free precession is initiated by a $\pi/2$ pulse. At $\tau_p/2$, a π pulse is applied, which refocuses the effects of magnetic field inhomogeneities and possible chemical shift effects. An echo is formed at $t = \tau_p$, at which time all magnetization vectors are again in phase. *T2* relaxation, however, will lead to an irreversible decay of the magnetization, which attenuates the echo amplitude. This can be exploited for *T2*-enhanced imaging.

The refocusing of magnetization by the application of π pulses is a general means for keeping the magnetization under control.

Another type of refocusing is of practical importance in the context of frequency-selective pulses applied in the presence of a magnetic field gradient. In the course of a long selective pulse, some defocusing of magnetization components cannot be avoided. By applying a reversed magnetic field gradient shortly after the pulse, it is possible to refocus the magnetization and generate an echo (see under Line Scan Technique).

CLASSIFICATION OF IMAGING TECHNIQUES

The smallness of the nuclear magnetic moments and the low-resonance frequencies lead to inherently low sensitivity of NMR. Apart from considerations of image contrast, limited sensitivity represents the major obstacle to more imaging experiments, for example, the observation of nuclei different from protons. It is known that sensitivity can always be increased when even more time is available for the measurement. In fact, the available signal-to-noise ratio (S/N) increases with the square root of the total performance time T[11]

$$S/N \propto \sqrt{T} \qquad (2)$$

Of course, in clinical applications, the maximum permissible performance time T is determined by patient-related considerations.

To be of practical use, imaging experiments must be designed with a view to maximizing sensitivity or minimizing performance time.[12,13] The most successful concept in this context is the *multiplex principle*: It is possible to reduce the performance time by a factor N by recording simultaneously N channels of information. This leads to the so-called multiplex advantage, which is the secret of success of many imaging techniques.

It seems sensible to classify imaging techniques according to their inherent sensitivity, measured by the number of parallel recorded channels. Four possible types of experiments are illustrated in Figure 3–7.

Point Measurement Techniques. A single volume element of the object is excited selectively and observed at a time.[14–18] For the construction of a complete image, one volume element after the other must be scanned through sequentially. Point measurement techniques produce a direct image without any intermediate image processing. However, the sensitivity will if necessity be low and the measurement time corre-

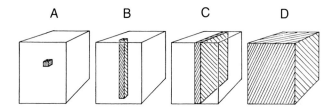

Figure 3–7. Four types of imaging experiments. *A*, Point measurement techniques. *B*, Line measurement techniques. *C*, Plane measurement techniques. *D*, Simultaneous techniques. (From Brunner P, Ernst RR: J Magn Reson *33*:83, 1979. Used by permission.)

spondingly long. Point measurement techniques are of particular merit when a localized area of the object must be investigated in great detail.

Line Measurement Techniques. To increase sensitivity, an entire line of volume elements is excited and observed simultaneously.[19-38] A static magnetic field gradient is applied along this line to obtain the required frequency dispersion for distinguishing the volume elements that are simultaneously observed. Line measurement techniques utilize normally a one-dimensional (1D) pulse-Fourier experiment for simultaneous excitation and observation of the entire line. The reconstruction of the line image requires merely a one-dimensional Fourier transformation.

Plane Measurement Techniques. The sensitivity can be further increased when an entire plane of volume elements is excited and observed at once.[4-9,39-48] Two-dimensional (2D) image reconstruction can, in some procedures, be achieved by a 2D Fourier transformation.[8,9] In other cases, more elaborate reconstruction procedures, for example, filtered back-projection, are required.[49]

Simultaneous Techniques. The most sensitive techniques involve simultaneous excitation and observation of the entire three-dimensional medical object.[9,12,50] Such an experiment, however, can be quite demanding with regard to the amount of data to be acquired and the necessary performance and data processing time.

We shall describe next the most prominent techniques for NMR imaging, classified according to the classification discussed above.

POINT MEASUREMENT TECHNIQUES

The selection of a single volume element in an extended object can be achieved by three different approaches, which may also be used in conjunction: (1) selective excitation of a single volume element; (2) nonselective excitation and selective destruction of unwanted magnetization; and (3) selective observation of a single volume element.

Sensitive Point Technique

The sensitive point technique proposed by Hinshaw[14-16] is a particularly successful member of the class of point measurement techniques. It utilizes nonselective excitation pulses and defocuses all unwanted magnetization originating from volume elements outside the one selected by means of time-dependent field gradients.

The principle of the sensitive point technique is explained in Figure 3–8. A continuous string of strong rf pulses of alternating phase is applied to the sample to create a steady-state transverse magnetization of all volume elements.[51,52] At maximum, half the equilibrium magnetization can be maintained in the steady state.

For the selection of the sensitive point at coordinates (x_0, y_0, z_0), three time-dependent gradients are necessary. A sinusoidally modulated magnetic field gradient $g_x(t)$ is applied along the x-axis such that its nodal plane passes through the point at

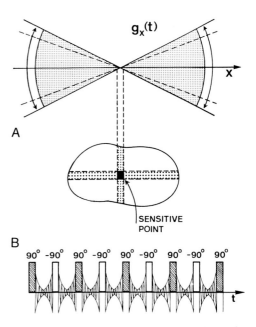

Figure 3–8. Sensitive point technique: A sequence of rf pulses with alternating phases (*B*) generates a steady-state magnetization. Three time-dependent gradients (one of which is shown in *A*) modulate the resonance frequencies of all volume elements except for the sensitive point (intersection of the nodal planes of the alternating gradients). The modulation interferes with the formation of a steady-state magnetization, which is destroyed except for the sensitive point. (Adapted from Ernst RR et al: Principles of Nuclear Magnetic Resonance in One and Two Dimensions. London, Oxford University Press, 1986.)

$x = x_0$ (Fig. 3–8). This gradient modulates the resonance frequencies of all volume elements lying outside the nodal plane. The modulation inhibits the formation of a steady-state transverse magnetization and leads to destruction of the magnetization outside the plane $x = x_0$. Two additional time-varying gradients $g_y(t)$ and $g_z(t)$ are applied simultaneously along the other two axes with nodal planes at $y = y_0$ and $z = z_0$, respectively. When three incommensurate modulation frequencies are used, only the steady-state transverse magnetization of the sensitive point remains and determines the observed signal.

By moving the three nodal planes, it is possible to move the sensitive point systematically through the object. A point-by-point image is then obtained. This simple technique can produce good image quality. However, it is slow. In particular, it should be noticed that after each measured point the magnetization purposely destroyed must be allowed to recover before the next point can be measured. The data acquisition rate is limited to about 1 point per *T1* relaxation time.

Field Focusing NMR (FONAR) and Topical NMR

Another scheme for selecting a "sensitive point" has been suggested by Damadian.[17] In this technique, called FONAR, the static magnetic field is shaped in such a way that good homogeneity is obtained only in one single small volume. The homogeneous region is normally near a saddle point of the field (Fig. 3–9). Most of the object will give rise to a broad background signal, while the region around the saddle point gives a dominant contribution at one frequency. Additional contributions to the same frequency coming from the extended but narrow regions for $\Delta B_0 = 0$ may be negligible under suitable circumstances. The sensitive point is fixed in space, and it is necessary to move the object to record a full image.

This scheme often does not lead to adequate spatial resolution for a high-resolution image, and it may be necessary to enhance selectivity by suitably shaped radio frequency fields. It is a useful method, however, for in vivo spectroscopy to acquire spectral information (chemical shifts) of a localized area within an object. This approach, known as topical NMR,[53] was the first technique for recording resolved NMR

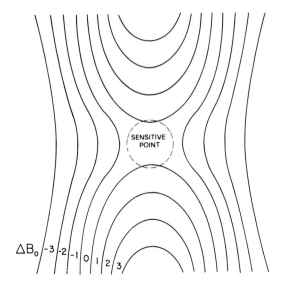

Figure 3–9. Shaping of the static magnetic field used in FONAR and topical NMR. Only the region near the saddle point is sufficiently homogeneous to give rise to strong narrow signals; the remainder of the object contributes only weak broad resonances. (Adapted from Ernst RR et al: Principles of Nuclear Magnetic Resonance in One and Two Dimensions. London, Oxford University Press, 1986.)

spectra of a localized organ in a living being. It allows the study of physiologic processes in a nondestructive and noninvasive manner. Particularly, ^{31}P NMR proved revealing for the measurement of metabolite concentrations and pH in living tissue.[53-56]

Although the requirements for spatial resolution are less severe for in vivo spectroscopy than for imaging, such a simple field-focusing technique is often inadequate for investigating smaller organs, and alternative approaches have been proposed for better localizing the area of observation.

Volume-Selective Pulse Sequences

The selective excitation of a specific volume element within an object is highly desirable in the context of in vivo spectroscopy. Although it is easy to selectively excite a single plane, the selection of a single volume element is more elaborate. It normally involves a three-step process whereby a point in the object is defined by the crossing of three orthogonal planes. This requires the intelligent combination of three "plane-selective" pulses.

Aue et al.[57,58] have described a clever technique for "volume-selective excitation" (Fig. 3–10). By the simultaneous application of a selective $-\pi/2$ and a nonselective $\pi/$

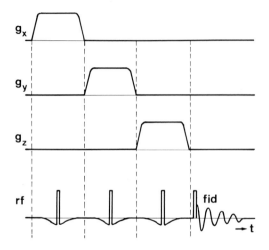

Figure 3–10. Sequence for volume-selective excitation.[57] Each of the three phases destroys the magnetization except within a single plane. In effect, all magnetization, except for the selected plane, is rotated into the xy plane by the combination of a selective and a nonselective $\pi/2$ pulse. $T2$ processes lead to the decay of transverse magnetization. At the end, magnetization in a single volume element remains exclusively. It can be used for local spectroscopy by applying a last pulse.

2 pulse in the presence of a linear field gradient, it is possible to rotate the entire magnetization outside the selected plane into the *x-y* plane, where it decays by *T2* processes. The magnetization in the selected plane remains unperturbed. After three pairs of such pulses in the presence of three field gradients, only the magnetization in a single volume element remains. A final nonselective pulse in the absence of magnetic field gradients then allows volume-selective excitation and the observation of a local NMR spectrum for the distinction of chemical components. Subsequently, many further approaches with the same goal have been described. More advanced techniques no longer require nonselective pulses to be applied in the presence of magnetic field gradients.

Volume-selective pulse sequences can be used for local spectroscopy anywhere within a medical object. However, sensitivity will be relatively low because a large receiver coil must be used and the filling factor with regard to the selected volume element is small.

Surface Coils

Some localization of the observation can also be obtained by properly shaping the receiver and/or transmitter coils. In particular, if observation of a volume element at or near the surface of the object is required, it is possible to employ surface coils.[59-61] A circular coil has a receptive volume approximately equal to a sphere, with a diameter equal to that of the coil. Surface coils allow local spectroscopy without the need of applying magnetic field gradients. They lead to high sensitivity, as the receptive volume fills the entire coil.

In a further refinement, it is possible to exploit the inhomogeneous radio frequency field for further spatial selectivity. An rf pulse of given duration and amplitude acts as a $\pi/2$ pulse only on a two-dimensional surface of constant radio frequency field strength. By properly shaping the pulses or using composite pulse sequences, it is feasible to selectively excite spherical calottes or differently shaped restricted areas of the object.[61-63]

LINE MEASUREMENT TECHNIQUES

In line measurement techniques, a column of volume elements is selected. By means of a linear field gradient applied along this line, the necessary frequency dispersion for distinguishing the volume elements within the line can be obtained. A single-pulse Fourier experiment delivers simultaneously information on the entire line. In comparison with sensitive point methods, substantial time savings can be achieved this way, exploiting the multiplex advantage of Fourier spectroscopy.[1,11,64] The various sequential line techniques differ in the schemes used for selective excitation or detection of the "sensitive line."

Sensitive Line or Multiple Sensitive Point Method

The sensitive line or multiple sensitive point (MSP) technique, suggested by Hinshaw,[16,24] is a straightforward extension of the sensitive point method. Instead of three time-varying gradients, only two time-varying gradients are used, and a static field gradient is applied along the *z*-axis (Fig. 3–11). Again, steady-state free precession is generated by a repetitive pulse sequence. The frequencies of precession between two

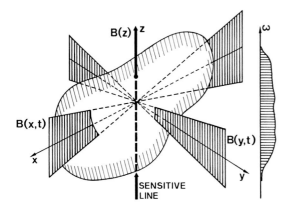

Figure 3–11. The sensitive line technique applies only two time-dependent gradients, while a static gradient is applied along the z-axis. The steady-state magnetization, generated by a sequence of pulses is destroyed by the modulation, except for volume elements in one column. (Adapted from Ernst RR et al: Principles of Nuclear Magnetic Resonance in One and Two Dimensions. London, Oxford University Press, 1986.)

successive pulses are analyzed in order to determine the spin density along the selected line.

The sensitive line technique is simple and leads to fair sensitivity. A few high-quality images have been obtained by the Andrew group using this technique.[19,25]

Line Scan Technique

An inherent disadvantage of the sensitive line technique is the complete saturation of all volume elements outside the investigated sensitive line. Therefore, after each measured line, a waiting time has to be inserted before the next line can be excited. This disadvantage is shared with the sensitive point technique.

The line scan technique, proposed by Mansfield,[29,31] overcomes this deficiency (Fig. 3–12). At first, a single plane of volume elements perpendicular to the x-axis is selected by applying a magnetic field gradient along the x-axis and selectively saturating all volume elements outside this plane by means of tailored excitation.[65] A wide spectrum of frequencies is applied for saturation while the frequency of the selected plane

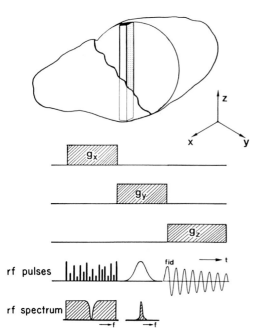

Figure 3–12. The line scan technique[29] selects a plane by saturating all volume elements except for those in a plane perpendicular to the x-axis by tailored excitation (the rf spectrum should be white except for a "dip"). A selective π/2 pulse in the presence of a y-gradient excites the magnetization associated with a column of volume elements, and the signals originating from the entire column are recorded in the presence of a z-gradient. (Adapted from Ernst RR et al: Principles of Nuclear Magnetic Resonance in One and Two Dimensions. London, Oxford University Press, 1986.)

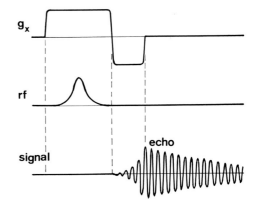

Figure 3–13. In order to refocus the transverse magnetization components after application of a selective pulse, a reversed field gradient is applied after the pulse. The resulting signal shows an echo where all magnetization components are again in phase.

is purposely suppressed to avoid saturation within this plane. A line perpendicular to the y-axis is then selected by a selective rf pulse in the presence of a y-gradient. Finally, the free induction decay of this line is observed in the presence of a z-gradient to disperse the responses of the volume elements along this line. Because a selective pulse has been used for excitation, it is possible to repeat the experiment without delay on another line within the same plane without suffering from saturation effects.

It should be noted that after a selective pulse the various excited magnetization components show significant phase dispersion, which may lead to mutual cancellation. The dispersion can be eliminated by the application of a reversed field gradient for a short time following the pulse.[37,38,66,67] This allows the formation of an echo where all magnetization components are again in phase (Fig. 3–13).

Echo Line Imaging

A modified procedure that also leads to the selection of a single line has been suggested by Hutchison et al.[36–38] Figure 3–14 indicates that by means of a selective 180 degree pulse in the presence of a g_x gradient, an entire plane of spins is inverted.

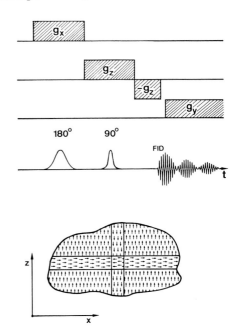

Figure 3–14. Echo line imaging: Transverse magnetization is excited by a $90°_y$ pulse in the presence of a z-gradient, which selects a slice perpendicular to the z-axis. In alternate scans, a 180° pulse applied in the presence of an x-gradient inverts the magnetization in a slice perpendicular to the x-axis. The difference of the free induction decays obtained in the two experiments yields a signal stemming from a column parallel to the y-axis. The arrows (lower left) indicate the distribution of the spin orientation after the $180°–90°_y$ sequence. (Adapted from Ernst RR et al: Principles of Nuclear Magnetic Resonance in One and Two Dimensions. London, Oxford University Press, 1986.)

A subsequent selective 90 degree y-pulse applied in the presence of a g_z gradient rotates the spins of the selected plane perpendicular to the z-axis. Thus, the selected line parallel to the y-axis produces a negative signal, while the remaining plane perpendicular to the z-axis generates a positive signal. The difference of two free induction signals, one obtained with and one without 180 degree pulse, yields a signal that originates exclusively from the selected line. In this scheme, a refocusing gradient has been included to produce an echo before the free induction decay (FID) is sampled in the presence of a g_y gradient.

With this technique, it is possible to repeat the experiment without delay on another line as no saturation has been employed.

PLANE MEASUREMENT TECHNIQUES

Medical imaging normally calls for planar sections through the object to be investigated. From the sensitivity standpoint, it is best to excite simultaneously an entire plane of volume elements, leading to the planar techniques to be discussed. This can be achieved either by a plane measurement or by a fully 3D excitation technique. We will not devote a separate section to 3D techniques but will include in this discussion a few remarks on extensions of 2D techniques to three dimensions.

Projection-Reconstruction Technique

The projection-reconstruction technique was first proposed and used by Lauterbur.[4,5,39–44] The inspiration may have come from x-ray tomography, in which this type of imaging is routinely used. A signal measured in the presence of a strong linear field gradient corresponds to a one-dimensional projection of the object onto the axis of the gradient (Fig. 3–4). It is well known that it is not sufficient to obtain three orthogonal projections in order to reconstruct an image of the object. In fact, a great many projections are needed to acquire sufficient information for a well-resolved image (Fig. 3–15). The number of projections recorded should match the number of resolution elements to be distinguished in one dimension (in the case of 2D imaging), or the number of resolution elements in two dimensions (for 3D imaging).

Let us restrict the discussion to imaging in two dimensions. By means of a selective pulse applied in the presence of a magnetic field gradient, e.g., along the z-axis, one entire plane perpendicular to the z-axis is excited. The FID is then observed in the presence of a magnetic field gradient applied along a line in the xy plane subtending an angle φ with the x-axis. A whole set of FIDs for different angles φ covering the range from $\varphi = 0$ degrees to $\varphi = 180$ degrees is recorded. The signals are Fourier-transformed and yield the required projections. These are then subjected to one of the reconstruction procedures described below.

RECONSTRUCTION PROCEDURES

A number of reconstruction techniques have been developed for x-ray tomography.[49] The same procedures can be used equally well for the reconstruction of NMR images.

A simple method of reconstruction is the back-projection technique. The intensity of each projection is back-projected into the image plane along the direction of projection. If the untreated projections are used for this purpose, a blurred image will be

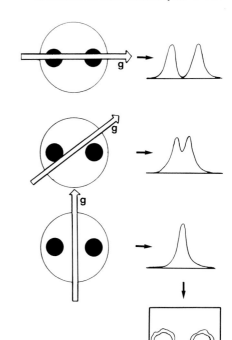

Figure 3–15. Projection-reconstruction technique: By applying gradients with a variable orientation to an object (in this case a phantom with two water-filled cylindrical volumes), a set of spectra is obtained. These spectra correspond to projections of the object (like shadows cast by a distant light source), from which the image of the object is reconstructed. (Adapted from Ernst RR et al: Principles of Nuclear Magnetic Resonance in One and Two Dimensions. London, Oxford University Press, 1986.)

obtained. However, by suitable prefiltering of the projections, it is possible to obtain a faithful image. This is the basic principle of *filtered back-projection*.

Another possibility is *iterative reconstruction*, which also employs the procedure of back-projection. However, after each cycle, new projections of the obtained image are computed and compared with the real projections of the object. The differences are again back-projected in order to improve the image iteratively. The recursive procedure leads to a faithful image without requiring prefiltering of the data.

The *Fourier reconstruction technique* reveals some basic features important in the context of Fourier imaging. It exploits the projection cross-section theorem. Let $S(\omega_1, \omega_2)$ be the desired image of an object in two dimensions and $P(\omega, \phi)$ be a projection of the image obtained by applying a static gradient in the direction at angle ϕ. The *projection cross-section theorem* then states that the 1D Fourier transform $c(t, \phi)$ of the projection $P(\omega, \phi)$ represents a central cross section through the 2D Fourier transform $s(t_1, t_2)$ of the image $S(\omega_1, \omega_2)$. The measured frequencies ω_1 and ω_2 are related to the spatial coordinates x_1 and x_2 through the relations

$$x_i = -\omega_i/(\gamma g), \ i = 1, 2 \tag{3}$$

where g is the magnetic field gradient applied to obtain the projections. The projection cross-section theorem is presented in Figure 3–16.

We can use the theorem to reconstruct an image from projections (Fig. 3–17):

(a) The measured projections $P(\omega, \phi)$ for different directions ϕ of projection are individually Fourier-transformed.

(b) The Fourier transforms represent central cross sections $c(t, \phi)$ through the Fourier-transformed object $s(t_1, t_2)$. By means of an interpolation procedure, a regular grid of sample points is computed in the (t_1, t_2) plane.

(c) A two-dimensional reverse Fourier transformation of $s(t_1, t_2)$ produces the desired image $S(\omega_1, \omega_2)$.

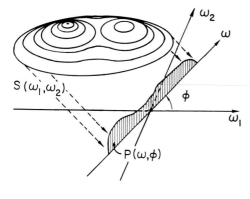

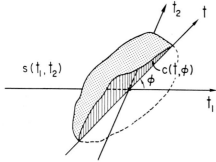

Figure 3–16. Fourier reconstruction: The projection $P(\omega, \phi)$ of the image $S(\omega_1, \omega_2) = S(-\gamma g x_1, -\gamma g x_2)$ onto an axis that subtends an angle ϕ with respect to the ω_1 axis is obtained by applying a gradient in the direction ϕ. The 1D Fourier transform of $P(\omega, \phi)$ is equal to a cross section $c(t, \phi)$ through the origin $t_1 = t_2 = 0$ (central cross section) of the Fourier transform $s(t_1, t_2)$ of the image.

It should be noted that a pulse Fourier experiment permits a direct measurement of the central cross sections $c(t, \phi)$, and the step (a) in the reconstruction sequence can be omitted. The only approximation involved in this image reconstruction procedure is in the interpolation procedure required to obtain a regular grid of sample points. It can be appreciated from Figure 3–17 that the measured sampling points are more densely distributed around the central point, $t_1 = t_2 = 0$, than in the outer parts of the (t_1, t_2) plane. This implies that the "low-frequency components" or the coarse

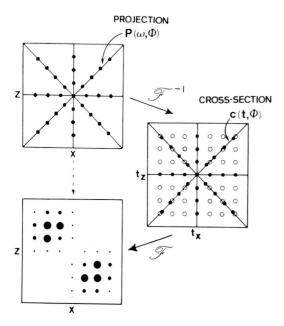

Figure 3–17. Fourier reconstruction technique: The spectra are observed in the presence of gradients with different directions ϕ, (as in Fig. 3–15). These signals correspond to projections $P(\omega, \phi)$ (top left), which can be Fourier-transformed to give cross sections $c(t, \phi)$, with grid points indicated by filled circles (right). These sampling points correspond to time-domain signals (free induction decays) obtained in the presence of gradients applied along the direction ϕ. A regular grid (open circles) is obtained by interpolation, and a two-dimensional reverse Fourier transformation leads to the desired image (lower left). Adapted from Ernst RR et al: Principles of Nuclear Magnetic Resonance in One and Two Dimensions. London, Oxford University Press, 1986.)

features of the image are better represented than the finer details contained in the high-frequency components.

It appears desirable to modify the measurement such that an equally spaced grid of sampling points $s(t_1, t_2)$ is obtained without a need for interpolation. This is indeed possible by Fourier imaging.

Fourier Imaging

Fourier imaging,[8,9] remarkable for its conceptual simplicity, became the most frequently used class of techniques for obtaining NMR images. The various volume elements are localized by three sequential measurements of their frequency coordinates ω_1, ω_2, and ω_3 in gradient fields applied along three orthogonal directions. By exploiting the multiplex concept it is possible to treat all volume elements at the same time and to achieve maximum sensitivity. The technique is loosely related to two-dimensional spectroscopy used in analytic NMR, particularly for the analysis of the structure of biomolecules.[1]

Fourier imaging allows full 3D imaging but also can be reduced to a 2D (planar) version. In the 3D scheme (Fig. 3–18), at first a nonselective pulse excites transverse magnetization in the entire object. In a first, so-called evolution period of length t_1, the magnetization precesses in the presence of a gradient g_x. During the second evolution period t_2, a gradient g_y is applied. Finally, the precessing signal $s(t_1, t_2, t_3)$ is observed during the detection period as a function of t_3 in the presence of a gradient t_3. The precession frequencies during the three periods measure the displacement of the volume element along the three orthogonal directions. Having the three frequency coordinates together with the corresponding signal intensity allows a direct construction of the image. However, a separate measurement of the frequencies under the three gradients would not serve the purpose, as it would be impossible to identify the frequencies belonging to the same volume element.

In Fourier imaging, the signal is observed exclusively during the detection period t_3. The two evolution periods (containing the information for the x- and y-directions) influence the observed signal through the initial phase. The information for the x- and y-directions is phase-encoded in the observed signal. By a systematic variation of the durations of the evolution periods t_1 and t_2 it is possible to retrieve the full signal $s(t_1, t_2, t_3)$, which contains for each volume element a contribution of the form

$$s(t_1, t_2, t_3) = s(x, y, z)\exp\{-i\gamma xg_xt_1 - i\gamma yg_yt_2 - i\gamma zg_zt_3\}, \qquad (4)$$

x, y, z being the coordinates of the volume element.

Figure 3–18. Fourier imaging: In the course of three consecutive phases, gradients are applied along the x, y, and z directions, respectively. The local frequencies during the first two periods, which determine the x and y coordinates of the volume elements, are phase-encoded in the signal, which is observed in the third period in the presence of a z gradient. The parameters t_1 and t_2 are systematically incremented in a series of experiments. A three-dimensional Fourier transformation of the acquired data produces the image.

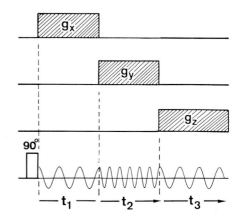

By means of a three-dimensional Fourier transformation it is possible to separate the contributions of the various volume elements

$$S(x, y, z) = \frac{\gamma^3 g_x g_y g_z}{(2\pi)^3} \iiint_0^\infty s(t_1, t_2, t_3) \exp\{i\gamma x g_x t_1 + i\gamma y g_y t_2 + i\gamma z g_z t_3\} \, dt_1 \, dt_2 \, dt_3$$

(5)

In the 2D form of Fourier imaging, the first evolution period t_1 is replaced by a selective pulse applied in the presence of a gradient g_x to select a plane parallel to the y- and z-axes. Again, refocusing of the magnetization after the selective pulse is necessary by applying a reverse g_x gradient during the phase-encoding period.

An example of the recorded signals together with the results after the two successive stages of Fourier transformation is shown in Figure 3–19.

Fourier imaging and the Fourier projection-reconstruction technique are related. The two techniques differ merely in the distribution of the sampling points in the 2D or 3D time domain. Fourier imaging yields an equally spaced grid of sampling points and leads therefore to equal accuracy of high and low image frequency components. Thus the finer details will be better represented by Fourier imaging than in an image obtained with a projection-reconstruction technique. Fourier imaging is less susceptible to artifacts than is the projection-reconstruction technique.

Spin-Warp Imaging

Spin-warp imaging, proposed by Hutchison et al.,[6,7] represents a variant of Fourier imaging that turned out to be particularly easy to implement and has been very successful in commercial instruments.

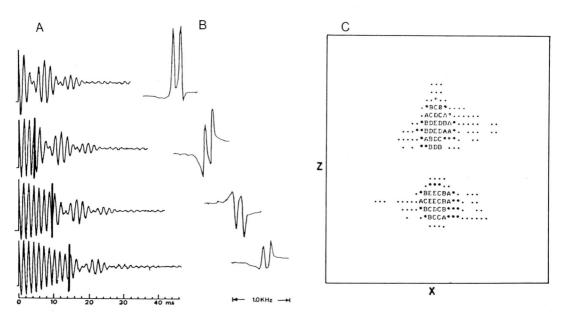

Figure 3–19. Fourier imaging of a phantom consisting of two water-filled capillaries with an inner diameter of 1 mm and a center-to-center separation of 2.2 mm, immersed in D_2O. The tubes are oriented parallel to the y-axis and aligned in the y–z plane. *A*, Time-domain signals: Four typical free induction decays were recorded throughout evolution and detection periods. Normally, observation is restricted to the detection period. In the t_1 and t_2 periods, gradients were applied along the x- and z-axes, respectively (in the t_1 period, the signals from both tubes have the same frequency). *B*, Signals $S(t_1, \omega_2)$ obtained by 1D Fourier transformation with respect to the t_2 time variable. *C*, Signal $S(\omega_1, \omega_2)$ obtained after the second Fourier transformation (absolute-value display). (Adapted from Kumar A et al: J Magn Reson *18*:69, 1975.)

Spin-warp imaging differs from conventional Fourier imaging in that the evolution period is fixed in length and the amplitude of the applied magnetic field gradient(s) is incremented from experiment to experiment. This has the advantage that relaxation effects during the evolution time τ remain the same through all experiments. Because the evolution time τ is kept constant, the resolution in the phase-encoded direction is independent of relaxation and exclusively limited by technical aspects and by a compromise between resolution and sensitivity.

The experimental scheme of spin-warp imaging is shown in Figure 3–20. The excitation is effected by a selective rf pulse in the presence of a g_x gradient. During the evolution period a reversed gradient $-g_x$ is applied to refocus the excited magnetization. At the same time, a gradient g_y, which is incremented systematically from experiment to experiment, serves to obtain the differentiation of the volume elements in the y-direction. Finally, during observation a g_z gradient is used to disperse the volume elements in the z-direction. The gradients may be turned on and off smoothly without adverse effects, provided that the gradient shape is the same in all experiments of a series.

Spin-warp imaging can be extended easily to three dimensions.[7] It also can be combined with measurements of chemical shifts.

Rotating Frame Imaging

Another variant of Fourier imaging, proposed by Hoult,[48] combines the preparation and evolution periods into one single interval. The transverse magnetization is excited by a linearly inhomogeneous rf field, e.g., by an rf field with gradient g_x. Different planes in the medical object will experience different pulse rotation angles $\beta(x)$ (Fig. 3–21). A systematic variation of the pulse length (or amplitude) from experiment to experiment creates a characteristic amplitude modulation of the resulting signal, which carries the x-coordinate information. Detection takes place in the presence of a static g_y field gradient.

Except for the replacement of a static field gradient by an rf field gradient, rotating frame imaging is equivalent to Fourier imaging. The same data processing is required. The major advantage of rotating frame imaging is the absence of switched static field gradients. This takes into account some concern about possible adverse effects of

Figure 3–20. Experimental scheme for spin-warp imaging. In contrast to Fourier imaging (Fig. 3–18), the phase encoding is obtained by increasing from experiment to experiment the amplitude of the gradient g_y, rather than varying the duration of the evolution period τ.

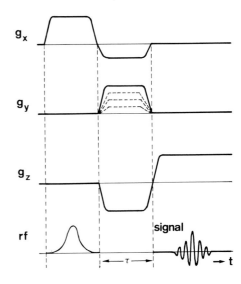

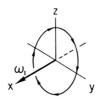

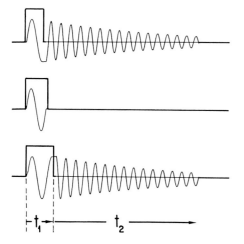

Figure 3–21. Rotating frame imaging: The evolution period consists of a pulse with an inhomogeneous rf field with a gradient g_x. The pulse width t_1 is incremented systematically, leading to an amplitude modulation of the signal as a function of t_1, which depends on the x-coordinate of the volume element. (Adapted from Ernst RR et al: Principles of Nuclear Magnetic Resonance in One and Two Dimensions. London, Oxford University Press, 1986.)

rapidly switched field gradients on human beings. On the other hand, it is much more difficult to create a clean linear rf field gradient. An extension to three dimensions without using switched static field gradients is also more complex.

Planar and Multiplanar Imaging

Two further plane measurement techniques have been proposed by Mansfield.[45] Both are extensions of the line scan technique described earlier. The principle of planar imaging is visualized in Figure 3–22. At first, all parts of the object, except for one single plane, are saturated by the applications of tailored excitation in the presence of a g_x gradient. In contrast to line scanning, a set of parallel columns of volume elements are then simultaneously excited by a suitably shaped multifrequency pulse in the presence of a g_y gradient. Finally, the FID is observed in the simultaneous presence of two properly weighted gradients g_y and g_z, leading to an inclined gradient in the yz plane.

If sufficiently narrow strips of the selected plane are excited (Fig. 3–23), it is possible to project the spin density on a single axis by the application of an inclined gradient such that the contributions of different columns do not overlap. Each column is then separately represented on the same axis.

Thus, a single experiment allows one to image an entire plane (or at least a family of narrow strips of this plane). Planar imaging is an exceptionally fast technique. The inherent trick is the *reduction of the dimension* by the mapping of an entire plane onto a single straight line.

Although the idea behind this technique is quite ingenious, the method has drawbacks. Sensitivity will be rather low, since very narrow strips of the plane have to be selected. In addition, resolution is severely restricted because of the elongated shape of the distinct volume elements (Fig. 3–23).

In a further extension of this technique, Mansfield[45] proposes to image simul-

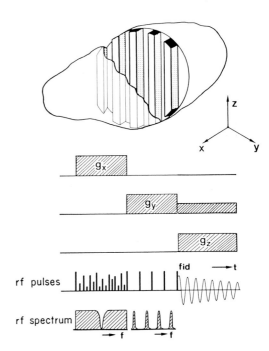

Figure 3–22. In planar imaging, a tailored excitation sequence is applied in the presence of an *x*-gradient, such that the rf spectrum is esentially white with the exception of a dip (compare Fig. 3–12). Except for a plane perpendicular to the *x*-axis, all volume elements are therefore saturated. A different tailored excitation sequence (e.g., a sequence of regularly spaced pulses) with a spectrum consisting of discrete sidebands is then applied in the presence of a *y*-gradient for the excitation of narrow strips in the unsaturated plane. Finally, the signal is observed in the presence of two weighted gradients applied along the *y*- and *z*-axes. (Adapted from Ernst RR et al: Principles of Nuclear Magnetic Resonance in One and Two Dimensions. London, Oxford University Press, 1986.)

taneously an entire 3D object by suitable selective excitation of narrow columns evenly distributed throughout the object. A twofold reduction of dimension can be achieved in this manner. This technique, known as *multiplanar imaging*, has the same advantages and disadvantages as planar imaging but in an even more pronounced form.

Echo Planar Imaging

Echo planar imaging, also proposed by Mansfield,[47] can be considered as another modification of Fourier imaging in which all experiments necessary to reconstruct the image of an entire plane are performed sequentially within a single FID. It is also related to planar imaging but does not require selective excitation of narrow strips.

At first, transverse magnetization of an entire plane of volume elements is excited, e.g., by a selective pulse in the presence of a magnetic field gradient g_z. The signal is observed in the presence of a weak static field gradient g_x and a strong switched gradient

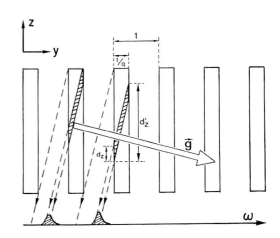

Figure 3–23. The *y*- and *z*-gradients applied in the detection period of the planar imaging method (see Fig. 3–19) must be adjusted in such a way that the skew projections of the individual columns do not overlap. Good spatial resolution in the *z*-direction can be obtained only if the columns are narrow ($1/q \ll 1$). (From Johnson G et al: J Magn Reson *54*:374, 1983. Used by permission.)

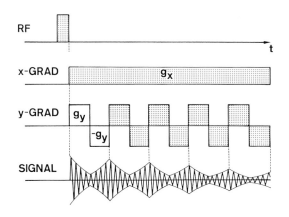

RF

t

x-GRAD g_x

y-GRAD g_y

$-g_y$

SIGNAL

Figure 3–24. Echo planar imaging: The magnetization of a planar section is selectively excited in the presence of a z-gradient (not shown), and observed in the presence of a weak static x-gradient with a switched y-gradient. (Adapted from Ernst RR et al: Principles of Nuclear Magnetic Resonance in One and Two Dimensions. London, Oxford University Press, 1986.)

g_y (Fig. 3–24). This leads to a sequence of echoes owing to the refocusing effect of the reversal of the field gradient.

To understand the principle and to grasp the relationship to Fourier imaging, we can consider this procedure as a sequence of experiments, each lasting from one echo peak to the next. The signal originating from the volume element at coordinates (x, y) in the nth experiment (following the nth echo) is then given by

$$s(nT, t_2) = s(x, y) \exp\{-i\gamma g_x nT - i\gamma g_y t_2\} \qquad (6)$$

where $t_2 = 0$ at the top of the nth echo. The effects caused by g_y in the previous periods have all been refocused, and the phase at the time of the nth echo is entirely determined by the local field yg_x. The signal $s(nT, t_2)$ is exactly the same as the signal $s(t_1, t_2)$ in a 2D Fourier imaging experiment.

The reconstruction in echo planar imaging also requires a 2D Fourier transformation of the signal $s(nT, t_2)$. The method is one of the fastest and most sensitive techniques known today, as sufficient information about an entire plane is acquired during a single FID.

The techniques described in this chapter represent only a small subset of the numerous techniques proposed so far. Additional information can be gained from several monographs written on magnetic resonance imaging.[68–74]

ACKNOWLEDGMENTS

The author is indebted to G. Bodenhausen, A. Wokaun, and Oxford University Press for permission to adapt some of the material contained in Chapter 10 of the monograph Principles of Nuclear Magnetic Resonance in One and Two Dimensions *by R. R. Ernst, G. Bodenhausen, and A. Wokaun (Clarendon Press, 1987). The manuscript has been edited by Mrs. I. Müller.*

References

1. Ernst RR, Bodenhausen G, Wokaun A: Principles of nuclear magnetic resonance in one and two dimensions. Oxford, Clarendon Press, 1987.
2. Damadian R: Tumor detection by nuclear magnetic resonance. Science *171*:1151, 1971.
3. Damadian R: U.S. patent 3.789.832, filed March 17, 1972.
4. Lauterbur PC: Measurements of local nuclear magnetic resonance relaxation times. Bull Am Phys Soc *18*:86, 1972.
5. Lauterbur PC: Image formation by induced local interactions: Examples employing nuclear magnetic resonance. Nature *242*:190, 1973.
6. Edelstein WA, Hutchison, JMS, Johnson G, Redpath TW: Spin warp NMR imaging and applications to human whole-body imaging. Phys Med Biol *25*:751, 1980.
7. Johnson G, Hutchison JMS, Redpath TW, Eastwood LM: Improvements in performance time for simultaneous three-dimensional NMR imaging. J Magn Reson *54*:374, 1983.

8. Kumar A, Welti D, Ernst RR: Imaging of macroscopic objects by NMR Fourier zeugmatography. Naturwissenschaften *62*:34, 1975.
9. Kumar A, Welti D, Ernst RR: NMR Fourier zeugmatography. J Magn Reson *18*:69, 1975.
10. Abragam A: Principles of nuclear magnetism. Oxford, Oxford University Press, 1961.
11. Ernst RR: Sensitivity enhancement in magnetic resonance. Adv Magn Reson *2*:1, 1966.
12. Brunner P, Ernst RR: Sensitivity and performance time in NMR imaging. J Magn Reson *33*:83, 1979.
13. Hoult DI, Lauterbur PC: The sensitivity of the zeugmatographic experiment involving human samples. J Magn Reson *34*:425, 1979.
14. Hinshaw WS: Spin mapping: The application of moving gradients to NMR. Phys Lett *A48*:87, 1974.
15. Hinshaw WS: The application of time dependent field gradients to NMR spin mapping. Proc 18th Ampere Congress, Nottingham, 1974, p 433.
16. Hinshaw WS: Image formation by nuclear magnetic resonance: The sensitive point method. J Appl Phys *47*:3709, 1976.
17. Damadian R, Goldsmith M, Minkoff L: NMR in cancer: FONAR image of the live human body. Physiol Chem Phys *8*:97, 1977.
18. Damadian R, Minkoff L, Goldsmith M, Koutcher JA: Field focusing nuclear magnetic resonance (FONAR) and the formation of chemical scans in man. Naturwissenschaften *65*:250, 1978.
19. Hinshaw WS, Bottomley PA, Holland GN: Radiographic thin-section image of the human wrist by nuclear magnetic resonance. Nature *270*:722, 1977.
20. Hinshaw WS, Andrew ER, Bottomley PA, Holland GN, Moore WS, Worthington BS: Display of cross-sectional anatomy by nuclear magnetic resonance imaging. Br J Radiol *51*:273, 1978.
21. Holland GN, Bottomley PA, Hinshaw WS: ^{19}F magnetic resonance imaging. J Magn Reson *28*:133, 1977.
22. Brooker HR, Hinshaw WS: Thin-section NMR imaging. J Magn Reson *30*:239, 1978.
23. Hinshaw WS: An introduction to NMR imaging: from Bloch equation to the imaging equation. Proc IEEE *71*:338, 1983.
24. Andrew ER, Bottomley PA, Hinshaw WS, Holland GN, Moore WS, Simaroj C: NMR images by the multiple sensitive point method: Application to larger biological systems. Phys Med Biol *22*:971, 1977.
25. Andrew ER, Bottomley PA, Hinshaw WS, Holland GN, Moore WS, Simaroj C: NMR imaging in medicine and biology. Proc 20th Ampere Congress, Tallinn, 1978.
26. Mansfield P, Grannell PK: NMR diffraction in solids. J Phys *C6*:L422, 1973.
27. Mansfield P, Grannell PK: "Diffraction" and microscopy in solids and liquids by NMR. Phys Rev *B12*:3618, 1975.
28. Mansfield P, Grannell PK, Maudsley AA: Diffraction and microscopy in solids and liquids by NMR. Proc 18th Ampere Congress, Nottingham, 1974, p 431.
29. Mansfield P, Maudsley AA, Baines T: Fast scan proton density imaging by NMR. J Phys *E9*:271, 1976.
30. Mansfield P, Maudsley AA: Planar and line-scan spin imaging by NMR. Proc 19th Ampere Congress, Heidelberg, 1976, p 247.
31. Garroway AN, Grannell PK, Mansfield P: Image formation by a selective irradiative process. J Phys C: Solid State Phys *7*:L457, 1974.
32. Mansfield P, Maudsley AA: Line scan proton spin imaging in biological structures by NMR. Phys Med Biol *21*:847, 1976.
33. Mansfield P, Maudsley AA: Medical imaging by NMR. Br J Radiol *50*:188, 1977.
34. Mansfield P: Proton spin imaging by NMR. Contemp Phys *17*:553, 1976.
35. Mansfield P, Pykett IL: Biological and medical imaging by NMR. J Magn Reson *29*:355, 1978.
36. Hutchison JMS, Goll CC, Mallard JR: In-vivo imaging of body structures using proton resonance. Proc 18th Ampere Congress, Nottingham, 1974, p 283.
37. Sutherland RJ, Hutchison JMS: Three-dimensional NMR imaging using selective excitation. J Phys E: Sci Instrum *11*:79, 1978.
38. Hutchison JMS, Sutherland RJ, Mallard JR: NMR imaging: Image recovery under magnetic fields with large non-uniformities. J Phys E: Sci Instrum *11*:217, 1978.
39. Lauterbur PC: Stable isotope distributions by NMR zeumatography. Proc 1st Int Conference on Stable Isotopes in Chemistry, Biology and Medicine, May 1973.
40. Lauterbur PC: Magnetic resonance zeugmatography. Pure Appl Chem *40*:149, 1974.
41. Lauterbur PC: Magnetic resonance zeugmatography. Proc 18th Ampere Congress, Nottingham, 1974, p 27.
42. Lauterbur PC: *In* Dewk RA, Campbell ID, Richards RE, Williams RJP (eds): NMR in Biology. London, Academic Press, 1977, p 323.
43. Lauterbur PC, Kramer DM, House WV, Chen C-N: Zeugmatographic high resolution NMR spectroscopy: Images of chemical inhomogeneity within macroscopic objects. J Am Chem Soc *97*:6866, 1975.
44. Lauterbur PC: Medical imaging by nuclear magnetic resonance zeugmatography. IEEE Trans Nucl Sci *NS26*:2808, 1979.
45. Mansfield P, Maudsley AA: Planar spin imaging by NMR. J Phys C: Solid State Phys *9*:L409, 1976.
46. Mansfield P, Maudsley AA: Planar spin imaging by NMR. J Magn Reson *27*:101, 1977.
47. Mansfield P: Multi-planar image formation using NMR spin echoes. J Phys C: Solid State Phys *10*:L55, 1977.
48. Hoult DI: Rotating frame zeugmatography. J Magn Reson *33*:183, 1979.
49. Brooks RA, Di Chiro G: Principles of computer assisted tomography (CAT) in radiographic and radioisotopic imaging. Phys Med Biol *21*:689, 1976.

50. Bernardo ML, Lauterbur PC: Rapid medium-resolution 3D NMR zeugmatographic imaging of the head. Eur J Radiol *3*:257, 1983.
51. Bradford R, Clay C, Strick E: A steady-state transient technique in nuclear induction. Phys Rev *84*:157, 1951.
52. Carr HY: Steady-state free precession in nuclear magnetic resonance. Phys Rev *112*:1693, 1958.
53. Gordon RE, Hanley PE, Shaw D: Topical magnetic resonance. Progr NMR Spectrosc *15*:1, 1982.
54. Ackerman JJH, Grove TH, Wond GG, Gadian DG, Radda GK: Mapping of metabolites in whole animals by ^{31}P NMR using surface coils. Nature *283*:167, 1980.
55. Gordon RE, Hanley PE, Shaw D, Gadian DG, Radda GK, Styles P, Bore PJ, Chan L: Localization of metabolites in animals using ^{31}P topical magnetic resonance. Nature *287*:736, 1980.
56. Gadian DG: Nuclear Magnetic Resonance and Its Applications to Living Systems. Oxford, Clarendon Press, 1982.
57. Aue WP, Muller S, Cross TA, Seelig J: Volume selective excitation: A novel approach to topical NMR. J Magn Reson *56*:350, 1984.
58. Aue WP, Muller S, Seelig J: Localized ^{13}C NMR spectra with enhanced sensitivity obtained by volume-selective excitation. J Magn Reson *61*:392, 1985.
59. Taylor DJ, Bore PJ, Styles, P, Gadian DG, Radda GK: Bioenergetics of intact human muscle: A ^{31}P nuclear magnetic resonance study. Mol Biol Med *1*:77, 1983.
60. Bendall MR, Gordon RE: Depth and refocusing pulses designed for multipulse NMR with surface coils. J Magn Reson *53*:365, 1983.
61. Shaka AJ, Freeman R: Spatially selective radiofrequency pulses. J Magn Reson *59*:169, 1984.
62. Tycko R, Pines A: Spatial localization of NMR signals by narrow-band inversion. J Magn Reson *60*:156, 1984.
63. Ernst RR, Anderson WA: Sensitivity in magnetic resonance II. Investigation of intermediate passage conditions. Rev Sci Instrum *36*:1696, 1965.
64. Tomlinson BL, Hill HDW: Fourier synthesized excitation of nuclear magnetic resonance with application to homonuclear decoupling and solvent line suppression. J Chem Phys *59*:1775, 1973.
65. Hoult DI: Zeugmatography: A criticism of the concept of a selective pulse in the presence of a field gradient. J Magn Reson *26*:165, 1977.
66. Mansfield P, Maudsley AA, Morris PG, Pykett IL: Selective pulses in NMR imaging: A reply to criticism. J Magn Reson *33*:261, 1979.
67. Mansfield P, Morris PG: NMR imaging in biomedicine. Adv Magn Reson, Suppl 2, 1982.
68. Jaklovsky J: NMR imaging, a comprehensive bibliography. Reading, Mass, Addison Wesley, 1983.
69. Kaufman L, Crooks LE, Margulis AR: Nuclear magnetic resonance imaging in medicine. Tokyo, Igaku Shoin, 1981.
70. Wende S, Thelen M (eds): Kernresonanz-Tomographie in der Medizin. Berlin, Springer, 1983.
71. Roth K: NMR-Tomographie und Spektroskopie in der Medizin. Berlin, Springer, 1984.
72. Petersen SB, Muller RN, Rinck PA: An Introduction to Biomedical Nuclear Magnetic Resonance. New York, G. Thieme Verlag, 1985.
73. Morris PG: Nuclear Magnetic Resonance Imaging in Medicine and Biology. Oxford, Clarendon Press, 1986.

4

NMR Scanning

RAYMOND DAMADIAN
ANTHONY GIAMBALVO

THE DEVELOPMENT OF NMR SCANNING

Converting medicine from a descriptive art to a quantitative science is an objective worthy of the space age. In the late 1960s, ideas for bringing about this transformation were constantly being spawned by the modern view of salt and water biophysics, expressed in the ion exchanger resin theory of the living cell of Damadian.[1-3] A method and apparatus to implement such a change awaited a new technology—nuclear magnetic resonance.

The actual invention, first manifested in a grant application to the Health Research Council of New York City in 1969, occurred during a series of experiments in Pittsburgh aimed at trying to see for the first time a potassium NMR signal from a living cell.[4] The object of the studies was to use the potassium NMR signal as a means of investigating the extent to which a freely movable positive ion, such as potassium, is coupled to the immovable negative ions of the cellular matrix rather than to free-moving cellular anions. The question was a key issue in the ion exchanger resin theory. The opportunity to test the idea came in the summer of 1970. The first experiments were aimed at answering the question, ''Can the NMR signal detect disease?,'' and were performed on the premises of NMR Specialities Corporation in New Kensington, Pennsylvania.

Two groups of rats with malignant tumors were studied. The tumors were surgically removed and put in NMR tubes. Spin-lattice and spin-spin constants of hydrogen for the tumors and a range of normal rat tissues were measured. The results are shown in Table 4–1.

The two malignancies, a Novikoff hepatoma and a Walker sarcoma, had $T1$ values that fell entirely outside the range of normal tissues. No instances of overlap were encountered. The study was also the first determination of $T1$ in normal tissues. A second result from the study was the observation that each soft tissue organ had its own characteristic $T1$ value and that organs could differ in $T1$ by as much as 100 percent. The observation gave rise to the possibility that body-scanning images made by NMR might exhibit much more contrast between organs than could be achieved by conventional x-ray methods. This set of experiments established that the NMR signal could detect disease, and the NMR body-scanning idea came to life.[5]

Apparatus to achieve the body-scanning objective had to satisfy a new condition not required in the measurements on excised tissues and not provided by state-of-the-art NMR instruments. An NMR method was required for ''in-sample'' focusing that could spatially locate the tumor within the body and provide a means for directing the NMR beam to specific sites within the anatomy for a locus-by-locus examination of tissue chemistry.

The focusing NMR (FONAR) concept arises from the implicit constraints on the

Table 4–1. RODENT T_1 RELAXATIONS (HYDROGEN)

	Muscle	Liver	Stomach	Small Intestine	Kidney	Brain
Normal	0.538 ± 0.015	0.293 ± 0.010	0.270 ± 0.016	0.257 ± 0.030	0.480 ± 0.026	0.595 ± 0.007
Tumor	0.736 ± 0.002	0.826 ± 0.013				
	(Walker sarcoma)	(Novikoff hepatoma)				

From Damadian R: Science *171*:1151, 1971. Used by permission.

forced precessions of a nuclear magnetization in an rf driving field. These constraints provide the basis for obtaining spatial resolution of the signal-producing domains of a nuclear resonance sample. Sufficient coupling of the nuclear spins to the radiation field to produce a signal detectable by rf spectroscopy requires that the stringent Bohr frequency condition, $h\upsilon = \mu H_0/I$, be met. It is thus possible to develop a small volume in the working field of the static magnet that contains the correct values of H_0 to bracket the band of the rf pulse.

The principle of the FONAR method (Fig. 4–1) exploits the same property of standard NMR machines that trips up beginners using the apparatus for the first time. Novices discover early that failure to place the NMR probe and sample carefully at the center of the magnetic field produces poor signal or none at all. Centering it produces good signal (shown above the centered sample in Fig. 4–1). Moving the sample too far off center causes it to vanish. Application of this principle in human body scanning requires that the sample (body) be moved with respect to the magnet so as to move the signal-generating volume of the magnet through different regions and organs of the body. Figure 4–2 shows the final form of the apparatus for body scanning by this invention.

A plot of field intensity in the mapping plane of the FONAR NMR scan (Fig. 4–3) shows the field to be approximately saddle-shaped. Vertical height is field intensity, while the z axis is the horizontal and x is into the plane of the paper. When the NMR pickup coil is tuned for resonance at the field value of the saddle point, all parts of the sample lying outside the saddle point either will be immersed in a field of different intensity and not give resonance or will be in a region of the field that is too steeply graded to generate signal. The loci of all points in the field mesh isomagnetic with the

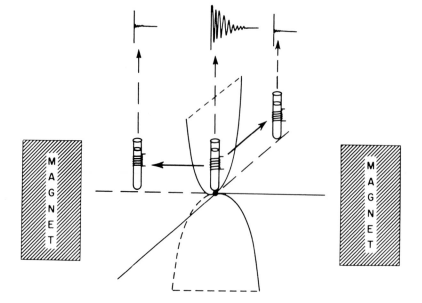

Figure 4–1. Principle of the FONAR method. Centering the NMR sample in the magnet produces good signal (shown above the centered sample). Moving the sample too far off center causes it to vanish.

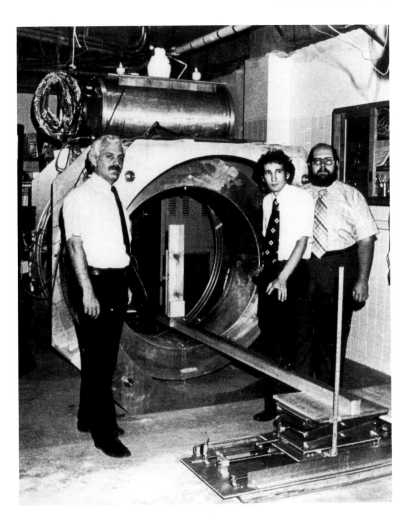

Figure 4–2. World's first NMR scanner for humans. Left to right, Drs. R. Damadian, L. Minkoff, and M. Goldsmith.

saddle point are drawn as dotted lines. These are obtained by cutting across the surface with a plane parallel to the base and passing through the saddle point. The plane is the locus of all points at the same altitude as the saddle point and therefore represents the plane containing all points of magnetic intensity equal to the saddle point. The locus of all points on the saddle surface isomagnetic with the center point is the intersection of this plane with the surface and represents all the off-center elements that could satisfy

Figure 4–3. A field plot of the FONAR magnet and coils on the first NMR scanner for humans.

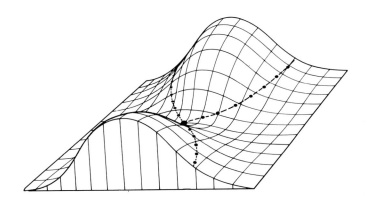

resonance. It can be seen by examining the figure that the off-center elements fall on curvatures of the field that are too steeply graded to give resonance.

A pair of these contour lines, orthogonal to each other and passing through the origin, illustrates the principle (Fig. 4–1).

As shown in Figure 4–1, when the exploring NMR sample is at the plateau of the conic section, a signal is produced both because the resonant frequency is tuned to H_0 and because there is sufficient H_0 uniformity to produce it. The signal vanishes when moved off center along either axis because H_0 departs from the field value of resonance and because the field is too steeply graded to generate signal. The principle shown in Figure 4–4 illustrates the process as it operates during a FONAR body scan.

A description of the invention of human NMR scanning was filed for United States patent in 1972.[6] Scientists generally objected vigorously to the idea of NMR body scanning, claiming that it had no possibility of success. The objections were as follows:

1. A magnet this large, which would have a region of sufficient uniformity to span the human body, could never be built.

2. Major filling factor difficulties would be encountered in the body pickup coil, with a resulting loss in detector signal/noise that would destroy any prospect of a successful medical NMR machine.

3. Tissue penetrability of radiated rf would be insufficient to permit rf to reach the deep interior of the human body and return with an atomic signal.

4. The large sample and its conductivity would so load the Q of the coil as to dampen its signal/noise mercilessly.

Despite the discouraging forecast, we proceeded. The prospect of a machine that could do chemical scans anywhere in the body was irresistible. A machine that could eventually convert the medical discipline from the practice of anatomy to the practice of chemistry was worth the toil and risk of failure.

Further explorations in tissue for elements other than hydrogen that would be useful nuclear probes of disease demonstrated the utility of the sodium nucleus. The amplitude of the tumor sodium signal substantially exceeded the amplitude of the normal signal. The result for phosphorus was similar to that for water. The *T1* relaxations were greater in tumors than in normal tissues. Hoult's 1975 paper,[7] which worked out the ^{31}P spectrum of normal muscle and identified the molecular origin of the spectral lines in the muscle spectrum, provided us with the opportunity to examine the ^{31}P spectrum of malignant muscle for comparison. The ^{31}P spectra obtained by Koutcher from normal and malignant muscle showed differences.[8] The tumor lacked the ATP and phosphocreatine resonances, while the inorganic and sugar phosphate peaks were shifted upfield by 70 Hz.

In a large investigation of human tissues, *T1, T2,* and *T1*ρ were measured in 1000 biopsy specimens taken at surgery. The same general results were obtained in these relaxation determinations of human tissue as in rodent tissue, but with more variation.

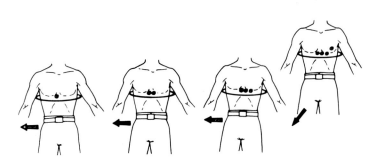

Figure 4–4. First, the torso of the human sample is centered on the resonance aperture. Data are recorded on the NMR signal at the start location, the coordinates stored, and the sample translated to the next location. The data collection process is then repeated with the resonance aperture at the new location. At the end of a scanning line, the resonance aperture is positioned at the start of a new line by a right-angle translation. The process is repeated until a rectangular grid of scanning elements has been completely traversed.

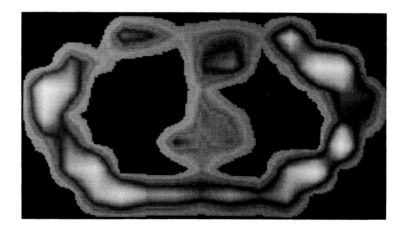

Figure 4–5. First human scan, a cross section through the chest at the level of the eighth thoracic vertebra. The image shows the body wall; the right and left lung fields; the heart encroaching on the left lung field; the cardiac chambers, right atrium, and a ventricle; and a section across the descending aorta.

The increased variance presumably is due to the marked variance in the clinical state of patients ill with cancer as compared with laboratory animal populations. The latter are as near to a homogeneous experimental population as possible. In a typical laboratory animal study, experimental rodents are littermates of the same age and strain, share the same food and water, are inoculated with cancer on the same day, and are commonly tested for disease on the same day after inoculation.

In 1973 Lauterbur suggested an alternative to the FONAR method for NMR scanning analogous to the CT method for x-ray scanning.[9] This was quickly followed by Mansfield's invention of NMR diffraction[10] and Hinshaw's development of sensitive-point imaging[11] employing the method originated by Abe.[12]

Lauterbur's picture of the mouse lent further support to the idea of human body scanning but failed to answer the basic objections of the critics, which centered around the practicability of body-sized uniform magnetic fields, tissue penetrability of rf, and the diminished signal/noise characteristics of large probe coils.

Once the scanner was completed, a trial scan of a phantom chest settled the questions of rf penetrability of large samples. Visible proton signal was obtained from all phantom locations. There was no significant attenuation of signal from the interior of the sample relative to sample nearest the antenna.

Damadian was the subject for the first attempt at a live human scan on May 11, 1977. Baseline blood pressure, respiratory rate, pulse rate, and electrocardiographic determinations exhibited no significant changes. The scan, however, failed owing to excessive loading of the antenna by a sample too large for the dimensions of the rf coil.

A second and successful attempt at the world's first live human scan through the chest of Lawrence Minkoff occurred on July 3, 1977 (Fig. 4–5). The scan time was 4.5 hours, with resolution elements of 4 to 6 mm. The scans were performed at an operating frequency of 2.18 MHz and a magnetic field of 508 gauss.[13] This first scan clearly showed the body wall, the right and left lungs, the heart and its chambers (right atrium and one of its ventricles), and a cut through the descending aorta.

PERMANENT MAGNETS IN NMR SCANNING

Since the inception of the idea to use the principle of nuclear magnetic resonance as a means of scanning the body to obtain diagnostically useful chemical information,[5] the development of NMR scanning has progressed rapidly. Developments have occurred in areas of spectral analysis of tissue and the quantitative measurements of various tissue parameters, such as relaxation times $T1$ and $T2$ and proton density. However, by far the major thrust has come in the area of imaging technology, which represents chemical information as two-dimensional arrays of intensity that portray the details of the human anatomy rather precisely. Whereas the first live human torso image took 4.5 hours and had a data matrix of 1500 points, improvements in technology and technique over the past nine years have led to imaging times on the order of a few minutes and data densities routinely 256×256 (65,536 points). In addition, the amount of detail that can now be exhibited in NMR images is striking and in many instances superior to modern CT scanners.

One of the major areas of intense development and interest has been magnet design. A wide range of magnetic field strength has been used, from approximately 400 gauss to 15,000 gauss. Magnet uniformity has been constantly improving, as this has been recognized to be a key factor in the accurate replication of spatial detail in images. Also, imaging has been performed on all three types of magnets—permanent, resistive, and superconducting.

It has been clear from the start that in order for the NMR scanning technique to reach its full potential, widespread use of the technique was essential. This necessitated a strategy that would make NMR scanners practical for the majority of physicians to have, or have easy access to, thus not restricting their use to research-oriented institutions; NMR scanning also needed to be as inexpensive a diagnostic technique as possible to encourage widespread use. Performance, however, could not be sacrificed in order to achieve the goal of a practical, cost-effective scanner. This is the rationale that provided the impetus for development of a permanent magnet-based NMR scanner.

We have often heard that permanent magnets are inherently inferior to superconducting magnets for any number of reasons. However, all magnets, regardless of the energy source used to produce the magnetic flux, are subject to the same laws of physics. Thus, the fundamental factors that affect scanner performance are the same for permanent, resistive, and superconducting magnets, namely magnetic field strength, magnetic field uniformity, and stability of the magnetic field. How well these factors are controlled determines the level of scanner performance that can be expected, and this fact is independent of the type of magnet one is considering.

Static Magnetic Field Strength

The static magnetic field strength at which an NMR scanning device operates determines a number of important features about the system. First, it dictates the resonant frequency of operation according to the well-known equation $\omega = \gamma H$, where ω = angular frequency, γ = gyromagnetic ratio for the particular nuclei being studied, and H = magnetic field strength. This frequency will be an important determinant in the design of the antenna that is used to transmit and receive the rf energy to and from the subject and will affect other electronic components in the rf portion of the NMR spectrometer. Second, assuming that the remainder of the scanning system has been optimally designed and tuned, the static magnetic field strength has a strong bearing on the signal-to-noise (S/N) performance of the scanner. The S/N is extremely important, since this affects the amount of time that must be spent to obtain high-quality scans. Increased in-plane resolution and thinner slices are current objectives of NMR imaging, in an attempt to improve the anatomic detail. In both cases there is a loss in S/N due to the reduction in the number of nuclei contributing signal per image voxel.

Many have chosen to increase magnetic field strength in order to obtain higher levels of S/N. Indeed, this may be the correct approach in situations in which the rf bandwidth can remain constant and characteristics of the sample under investigation are constant with changing magnetic field strength. But these situations do not exist in NMR scanning. In the case of biologic systems, it is necessary to consider the effect of magnetic field strength on the inherent NMR properties of tissue, such as $T1$ and $T2$, and the influence of $T1$, $T2$, and the chemical shift properties of tissue on the imaging parameters that are chosen.

In general, as magnetic field strength increases, the $T1$ relaxation time also increases, whereas $T2$, which is rather frequency-insensitive, tends to remain the same. In order to achieve the full benefit of increased S/N, which comes with higher field strength magnets, the increase in $T1$ makes it necessary to spend more time between rf pulses to allow for relaxation of the nuclear spin system. In going from 3 kilogauss to 15 kilogauss, the $T1$ relaxation times are approximately doubled. Therefore, in order to take full advantage of the S/N increase that could be generated at this higher magnetic field strength, scan time would also have to double because of the necessity of doubling the repetition time of the scan. As scan times are reduced at the higher field strength, there is a progressive loss of S/N benefit.

Let us consider chemical shift. In hydrogen imaging there are two main contributors to the signal, namely, lipid protons and water protons. These are chemically shifted from each other by approximately 3 ppm, meaning that the frequencies of the signal returning from the sample for lipid protons and water protons are different and that the magnitude of the difference will vary with magnetic field strength or operating frequency. At 3 kilogauss, the chemical shift results in a difference of 38 Hz between returns for lipid and water protons, whereas at 15 kilogauss, the difference is 190 Hz. This is significant because the magnitude of the chemical shift places lower limits on the frequency size of the image pixel. For example, if signal returns from water and lipid are to be represented as coming from a single spatial location in an image, then the pixel size in frequency units must be greater than the chemical shift. Otherwise, two chemically shifted returns that emanate from a single anatomic location will be represented at different spatial locations in the image. In comparing 3 kilogauss with 15 kilogauss, the total bandwidth required to spatially encode the same object will be five times greater at 15 kilogauss than at 3 kilogauss owing to the chemical shift. The factor of 5 increase in bandwidth reduces S/N by 2.2-fold, further diminishing the anticipated gains in S/N from increasing magnetic field strength. To completely offset the loss in S/N due to this increase in bandwidth, scan time would have to increase fivefold.

Thus it can be seen that given a constant scan time, increasing magnetic field strength does not have the purported advantages in S/N that might be expected by the proportional increase in resonant frequency, since other factors that influence S/N also are affected.

A discussion of high field strength versus low field strength is difficult to avoid given the evolution of NMR scanning technology to its current state. Various manufacturers have concentrated their efforts, generally speaking, into the areas of "low" magnetic field strength (3 to 5 kilogauss) or "high" magnetic field strength (10 to 15 kilogauss). More importantly, however, the physics of NMR scanning must allow for high-quality imaging to be performed at magnetic field strengths that are achievable using permanent magnet technology. This has proved to be the case. Information gathered from our NMR scanners over the past several years indicates that a field strength of 3 kilogauss as generated by permanent magnet material provides all that is required for high-quality diagnostic images and efficient scanner operation.

Once one settles on the optimal field strength for a permanent magnet scanning system, the next major question is the design of the magnet. The design determines the size of the magnet; the potential for achieving adequate field uniformity over distances that cover the human torso; cost of the unit; ease with which a particular design can be manufactured, quality-controlled, and installed; and the extent to which the magnet has a fringe field, which impacts siting requirements of the scanner as well as consistent scanner operation.

Magnet Uniformity

The uniformity or homogeneity of the magnetic field is important to NMR imaging, since this factor plays a key role in the accurate spatial localization and replication of anatomy in an NMR image. All imaging techniques make use of a set of three orthogonal magnetic field gradients to spatially encode the information received from the subject being scanned. These gradients are superimposed on the static magnetic field; thus, any nonuniformities in the static field will add to the deliberately imposed magnetic field gradients and distort the linearity of the gradients. As a result, information will be placed in an inappropriate place in the image relative to its actual source point in the body. This leads to image distortion, blurring, and a loss of proper intensity distribution. The effects of magnetic field nonuniformities can be overcome by increasing the magnitude of the imposed gradient so that the inherent uniformities in the magnet represent a smaller portion of the gradient sum that will encode the information. In effect, this increases the pixel bandwidth in the image and concomitantly the overall image bandwidth. Such an approach has proved to be an effective way to reduce the effect of magnet nonuniformities in an image, but as described earlier, the increased bandwidth results in a loss in S/N. Therefore, achieving a high level of uniformity is desirable.

The static magnetic field in the volume of interest can be expressed analytically in the form of a three-dimensional magnetic potential. This can be separated into a polynomial series that describes symmetric terms (i.e., perfect construction) and asymmetric terms (practical errors). The magnitude of these terms, which represent a particular nonuniformity, can be ascertained from field measurements, and this information forms the basis of the magnet correction procedure. The objective in "shimming" then becomes to reduce the magnitude of the coefficients of each polynomial term as much as possible (ideally to zero) such that the equation representing the magnetic field approaches the form:

$$B_z = a_o$$

This equation represents a perfectly uniform magnetic field. Although this is impossible to achieve in practice, it is quite possible to reduce the magnitude of the terms of the polynomial expansion to a few milligauss.

This system of analysis lends itself to treating each term in the expansion separately during the shimming process. One can then predict a shim coil current that will generate a magnetic field specifically designed to cancel the nonuniformity described by that term. If this is done for a series of different terms of the polynomial expansion, the system of shim coils will significantly increase the uniformity of the bare magnet. The actual design of the shim coils may vary depending on the basic geometry of the magnet chosen.

For NMR imaging, magnet uniformities are typically of the order of 10 to 100 ppm over the region of interest. Using a system of shim coils plus the three orthogonal linear gradients that also may be used to shim the static magnetic field, we have achieved a uniformity of 6 ppm over a 30 cm diameter sphere of interest. This has proved quite adequate to obtain high-quality images on our 3000 gauss permanent magnet scanner (FONAR's Beta 3000 Whole Body Imaging System, FONAR Corporation, Melville, New York). With this universal approach to shimming, it is quite possible to achieve a desired level of uniformity, whether the magnet be permanent, resistive, or superconducting.

One point worth noting is that as magnetic field strength increases, the percentage variation in magnetic field strength over a given volume must decrease in order to maintain a constant imaging bandwidth. For example, a magnet at 3 kilogauss with a uniformity specification of 10 ppm has a variation of 0.03 gauss (127 Hz) over the volume of interest; a system operating at twice the field strength (or 6 kilogauss), which has the same uniformity specification of 10 ppm, will vary 0.06 gauss (254 Hz), or twice as much over this same area of interest. As in the case of the chemical shift described earlier, it is the absolute magnitude of the variation that is the important factor in NMR imaging, not the percentage variation that is described in terms of ppm. The absolute magnitude of the nonuniformities will set lower limits on the gradient strength needed and consequently on the bandwidth and S/N performance of the scanner.

Magnet Stability

Magnetic field stability often is purported to be a shortcoming of permanent magnets. In fact, each of three types of magnets has difficulties in terms of stability. Resistive magnets require extremely well regulated current sources in order to maintain a constant magnetic field. This can be very difficult to achieve at the levels of sensitivity that are perceptible by NMR. With superconducting magnets used in NMR imaging, a steady downward drift of magnetic field on the order of 25 to 100 Hz per hour is not uncommon and results from the slow loss of current in the superconducting coils due to some resistive flaw in the system. In addition, superconducting magnets are subject to a potentially "catastrophic instability" in that within some fraction of a second, they can suddenly dump their entire magnetic field, or quench.

In dealing with permanent magnets, the major factor with respect to stability is temperature. The different types of permanent magnet material have temperature coefficients that cover a range of -0.0008 percent change/$^{\circ}$C to -0.2 percent change/$^{\circ}$C. However, the changes in magnetic energy due to changes in temperature of the permanent magnet material are totally reversible over the range of temperature used for scanner operation; thus, the average performance of the magnet material over any cyclical temperature variation will be quite constant.

Importantly, although the magnet material itself may have a certain temperature coefficient, we have found that the dependence of the magnetic field on temperature, as measured in the gap of the magnet, is much less than for the material itself. For example, the permanent magnet that is part of the Beta 3000 scanning system, when placed in a room where ambient temperature is controlled to $70^{\circ} \pm 5^{\circ}$ F, generally exhibits a cyclical variation of ± 5 ppm over a 24-hour period. The lack of sensitivity of the main magnetic field to temperature, as compared with the magnetic material of which it is composed, can be attributed to the fact that the mass of the magnet represents an enormous thermal reservoir that will allow the magnet to change temperature only very slowly. Hence, even with moderately good ambient temperature control the magnetic field is very stable.

In order to compensate for any short-term field changes, as small as they may be, the scanning system employs an automatic compensation that is used prior to each scan. This compensation keeps the system fine-tuned and assures that the spatial location of the slices in multiple-slice acquisition mode remains constant.

We have found that permanent magnets routinely perform in a highly stable fashion, making magnetic field stability a major asset of the permanent magnet NMR scanning system.

Benefits of Permanent Magnet Scanners

Permanent magnets are, quite simply, permanent. Once energized the magnetic material will retain its properties essentially forever; thus, following construction, no additional attention or maintenance is required, and one can basically forget that the magnet is part of the system.

In contrast, superconducting magnets require constant replenishing of liquid helium and liquid nitrogen to be kept operational as well as personnel specially trained in cryogenics to maintain the system. Furthermore, the potential for considerable downtime always exists owing to the unavailability of cryogens or, even worse, a catastrophic quenching of the magnet. In the case of resistive magnets, the ongoing cost of electrical power and the requirement for a substantial water cooling system must be considered. Both the electrical system and the water-cooling system are subject to failure, which may result in system downtime. Not only does the permanent magnet have a clear advantage in operational costs of an NMR scanner when compared with superconducting and resistive magnets, but the potential for downtime due to magnet failure does not exist. Furthermore, since superconducting and resistive magnets can fail, maintenance contracts for scanning systems that employ them cost more than for systems that use permanent magnets.

Superconducting magnets have a solenoidal geometry that can project a 1 gauss fringe field as far as 37 ft at 0.3 tesla, and 67 ft at 1.5 tesla. However, owing to the design of the FONAR permanent magnet, the fringe field is quite small, so that outside the shielded room that houses the magnet there is virtually no remaining fringe field. The advantage of a scanning system with no fringe field is that it may be placed quite easily into pre-existing facilities. Moving elevators, parking lot traffic, and structural steel in the building, for example, are of no consequence to the operation of the scanner. Similarly, the absence of fringe field ensures that there will be no interference with the operation of gamma cameras, CRTs, and the like, which may be in close proximity to the NMR scanner. Obviating the need to reorganize or renovate existing facilities in order to place an NMR scanner results in savings that are often substantial.

Finally, let us consider the 100 ton weight of the permanent magnet. While at first glance this weight may appear to be excessive and restrictive in terms of siting, this has not been the case thus far. It is possible to simply distribute the weight of the magnet over sufficient floor area so that the load-bearing specifications of the floor are not exceeded. For example, if the 100 tons (200,000 lb) were distributed over the recommended floor area of the scanner room, which is 625 sq ft, the floor loading would be 320 lb/sq ft. This is only about twice as much as the weight of an average person. Indeed, the 100 ton magnet already has been installed in a second-floor facility.

FONAR's Beta 3000 Scanner in 1986

Much of the development of the Beta 3000 permanent magnet NMR scanner was based on exploiting the flexibility of designed-into-the-systems electronic configuration. This effort has generated a series of software releases that have made improvements in the ease and speed of operation of the scanner, which translates into increased patient throughput and cost-effectiveness. For example, the latest generation of software employs a totally automatic tuning feature that tunes the rf coil, adjusts receiver gain settings, and centers the transmitter frequency in approximately 30 to 45 seconds. In addition, there is the capability to vary continuously in-plane pixel resolution to values as low as 250 μ per pixel as well as continuous variability of slice thickness to values as low as 2 mm. Importantly, these are user-selectable, and choices can be made at the time of the scan.

The software/hardware configuration of the scanner is such that multiple processes, such as scanning, image review, photography, archiving, and entering of patient information, can be accomplished simultaneously, greatly aiding throughput and operator efficiency.

Another feature of the system is its oblique scanning capability (Fig. 4–6). Operationally, a scan is performed in the axial, sagittal, or coronal plane and is displayed. A multislice cursor is then overlaid, consisting of a number of line cursors representing the slices that the operator chooses to acquire on the next scan. At this point, under trackball control, the operator is free to rotate the line cursors to any angle, to translate the slice positioning to any offset, and to change the slice spacing, all as desired by the operator in real time. Once this selection is made, a single key stroke enters the information and the scan can proceed, yielding images positioned precisely as chosen. This has proved to be a powerful capability in many clinical situations.

A variation of this oblique angle scanning capability has been developed, which enables the operator to position individual slices of a multislice oblique angle scan at different angles relative to each other (Fig. 4–7). This feature is particularly useful in imaging the lumbar spine, where succeeding intervertebral discs are at different angles. With the multiangle oblique (MAO) capability, a single multislice scan can produce slices at the appropriate angles coincident with the disc angles, thereby eliminating the need for additional scans.

The advent of surface coils is a major advance in NMR scanning technology. Surface coils produce exquisite images. They enhance the signal-to-noise performance of the scanner for anatomic structures close to the surface as well as for body limbs. This is accomplished at the expense of the ability to probe deeper-lying structures. Thus, structures such as the knee, ankle, shoulder, elbow, wrist, foot, neck, spine, and temporomandibular joint (TMJ) are particularly well suited for studies using surface coils.

FONAR has undertaken a very active surface coil development program, which has produced thus far 20 surface coils for specific applications (Table 4–2). These coils fall into two basic designs, planar or ring and solenoidal. Ring coils consist of a loop

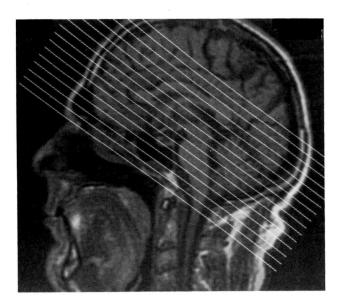

Figure 4–6. Oblique scanning cursor. The angulated lines that overlie a sagittal scout scan of the head indicate position and angle of slices to be obtained on subsequent scan. Line cursors are under trackball control and may be translated, rotated, and spaced as operator wishes.

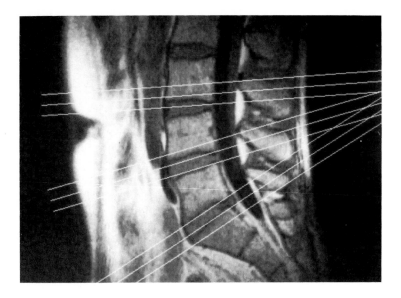

Figure 4–7. Multiangle oblique cursor allows nonparallel positioning of slices, as shown by line cursor overlays, to obtain multiple angle slices in a single scan.

of wire that is applied in planar fashion to the surface of the body; the primary use is for TMJ and breast imaging. The solenoidal surface coils are actually belts that wrap completely around the specific body part, such as the knee or neck. These vary in size or diameter from the smallest, which is designed for the ankle and elbow, to the largest, which is designed for the torso. The ability to use a surface coil with a solenoidal geometry results from the fact that the permanent magnet has a vertically oriented magnetic field (i.e., orientation perpendicular to the long axis of the human body), as opposed to the horizontal magnetic field orientation of the superconducting magnet. The solenoidal type surface coil has the advantage of providing even image illumination across the entire field of view, as opposed to the planar surface coil, with which illumination falls off rapidly as distance from the receiving antenna increases (Figs. 4–8 and 4–9).

The discovery of Damadian in 1971[5] that diseased tissue exhibits elevated $T1$ and $T2$ relaxation times relative to healthy tissue provided the impetus for development of the modern NMR scanner. In fact, the soft tissue contrast and the ability to visualize pathology in an image are the direct result of the inherent differences and changes in normal tissue values for $T1$ and $T2$ relaxation. Whereas accentuating the relative differences in $T1$ and $T2$ by appropriately weighting pulse sequences for $T1$ and $T2$ contrast enhancement may be sufficient for performing clinical evaluation via images, the potential for corroborating or elucidating such findings may be provided through a quan-

Table 4–2. FONAR SURFACE CELLS

Solenoidal Coils	Ring Coils
Ankle/Elbow	Large ring (shoulder)
Ankle/Neck	Small ring (TMJ, orbit)
Neck/Knee	Breast
Neck/Head	Double orbit
Head/Hip	Double ear
Head/Torso	Spine
Small torso	Pediatric head
Large torso	Pediatric body
Wrist	Pediatric spine
Whiplash neck coil	Larynx

Adopted from Damadian R: Science *171*: 1151, 1971.

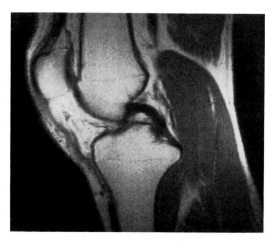

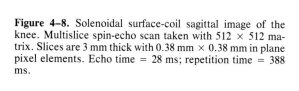

Figure 4–8. Solenoidal surface-coil sagittal image of the knee. Multislice spin-echo scan taken with 512 × 512 matrix. Slices are 3 mm thick with 0.38 mm × 0.38 mm in plane pixel elements. Echo time = 28 ms; repetition time = 388 ms.

titative measure of *T1* and *T2*. Such a measure bridges the gap between the diagnostic image and the biochemistry of the tissue. Furthermore, the potential exists for development of screening procedures on the basis of quantitatively accurate relaxation time measurements. An effort to provide quantitative measurements for *T1* and *T2* and evolve clinical correlations to them is a valuable effort whose importance should not be underestimated.

The method currently employed for measurement of *T1* on the FONAR scanner involves selecting a location in an image (using a cursor) where *T1* is to be measured. Once this point is chosen, a key stroke begins the measurement. Data are collected along a line that includes the point of interest, using a Freeman-Hill partial saturation technique[14] employing 14 different repetition times. Data collection time is 2.5 minutes, and *T1* is computed from a semilogarithmic plot and signal amplitude versus repetition time. The value of computing *T1* from so many measurements is that accuracy is improved; concurrently, there is the possibility of detecting multiple relaxation time fractions, which are not uncommon in biologic tissue. This cannot be done with the more ubiquitous approach to *T1* quantitation, which calculates a value from two points obtained from images acquired at different repetition times.

T1 information is displayed in profile, providing accurate information along an entire line through the image (Fig. 4–10). The *T1* at any point along the line can be read automatically by moving a cursor to that point. It is expected that profiling tumors

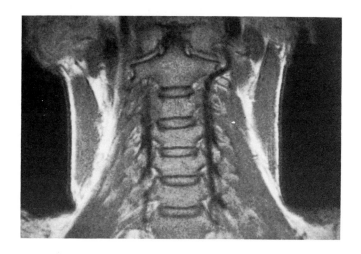

Figure 4–9. Solenoidal surface-coil coronal image of the neck. Same scan parameters as in Figure 4–8.

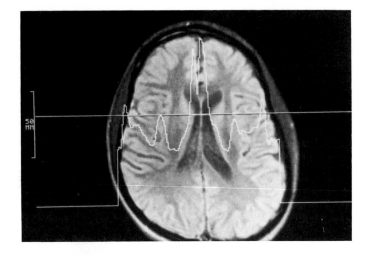

Figure 4–10. Axial head scan on which *T1* measurements were made along the horizontal line as indicated. *T1* profile shows changes in *T1* corresponding to changing anatomic structure in the head. Note the two central peaks corresponding to the ventricles. Movement of point cursor along the line gives read-out of *T1* value at a particular position (not shown). Measurement time for this experiment is 2.5 min.

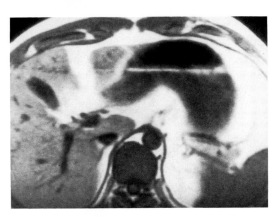

Figure 4–11. Respiratory compensated axial abdomen scan. Slice thickness 7 mm with 1 mm × 1 mm pixels. Echo time = 14 ms; repetition time = 300 ms.

in this fashion will provide additional information regarding possible infiltration into surrounding tissue, which may not be obvious from the image alone.

In addition to these unique features, the Beta 3000 permanent magnet scanner's capabilities include: acquisition matrices of 128 × 128, 256 × 256, or 512 × 512; spin-echo pulse sequences with echo times covering the range from 14 ms to 112 ms; cardiac gating; respiratory compensated scanning, which eliminates respiratory artifacts with no additional hardware or extra scan time (Fig. 4–11); and multislice multiecho scanning.

References

1. Damadian R: Biological ion exchanger resins. III. Molecular interpretation of cellular ion exchange. Biophys J *11*:773, 1971.
2. Damadian R, Goldsmith M, Zaner KS: Biological ion exchanger resin. I. Quantitative electrostatic correspondence of fixed charge and mobile counter ion. Biophys J *11*:739, 1971.
3. Damadian R: Cation transport in bacteria. *In* Critical Review in Microbiology. Cleveland, CRC Press, 1973, pp 377–422.
4. Cope F, Damadian R: Cell potassium by ^{39}K spin echo nuclear magnetic resonance. Nature *228*:76, 1970.
5. Damadian R: Tumor detection by nuclear magnetic resonance. Science *171*:1151, 1971.
6. Damadian R: Apparatus and method for detecting cancer in tissue. U.S. patent 3,789,832, filed 17 March 1972.
7. Hoult DI, Busby SJ, Gadian DG, et al: Observation of tissue metabolites using ^{31}P nuclear magnetic resonance. Nature *252*:285, 1975.

8. Koutcher JA, Damadian R: Four spectral differences in the ^{31}P NMR of normal and malignant tissue. Physiol Chem Phys 9:181, 1977.
9. Lauterbur PC: Image formation by induced local interactions: examples employing nuclear magnetic resonance. Nature *242*:190, 1973.
10. Mansfield P, Grannell PK: NMR 'diffraction' in solids? J Phys C: Solid State Phys 6:L422, 1973.
11. Hinshaw WS: Spin mapping: the application of moving gradients to NMR. Phys Lett *48A*:84, 1974.
12. Abe Z, Tanaka K: U.S. patent 3,932,805, filed 9 August 1973.
13. Damadian R, Goldsmith M, Minkoff L: NMR in cancer, FONAR image of the live human body. Physiol Chem Phys 9:97, 1977.
14. Freeman R, Hill HDW: Fourier Transform study of NMR spin-lattice relaxation by "progressive saturation." J Chem Phys *54*:3367, 1971.

5

Clinical Potential of MRI

ALEXANDER R. MARGULIS
HEDVIG HRICAK

Magnetic resonance imaging (MRI), although introduced by Lauterbur in 1973[1] and subsequently investigated in multiple centers,[2-6] did not become a clinical reality until 1981.[7-10] Since then MRI has advanced at an ever increasing pace, capturing the medical imagination to the extent that there is hardly a medical community in the western world not having magnetic resonance imagers in practice or planning to install one or several of them. Often, even untried devices are ordered from a proliferation of manufacturers in the United States, Europe, and Japan. It is remarkable that this is occurring in spite of fiscal restraints and critical self-examinations that are occurring in these same countries. All this is due to the fact that magnetic resonance imaging is the most revolutionary and significant innovation in diagnostic medicine since the introduction of x-rays by Roentgen in 1896.

MRI has become the accepted modality for the examination of the brain, spinal cord, spine, cancellous bone, and joints.[7-17] It is increasingly used for the staging of neoplasms, particularly in the neck, mediastinum, retroperitoneum, and pelvis.[8,18-38] With ECG gating, it is very useful in the examination of the heart.[39-43] The large blood vessels are also an ideal area for investigation, promising significant future clinical applications. MRI of the upper abdominal organs, the liver, spleen and pancreas, awaits more practical respiratory gating techniques before it can authoritatively challenge high-resolution computed tomography.[8,44,45]

UNIQUE QUALITIES OF MRI

Magnetic resonance imaging is non-ionizing, has produced no harmful biologic effects in the diagnostic range currently utilized, has soft tissue contrast that is 70 to 80 times better than that of the best x-ray CT, and is capable of direct imaging in any plane without reformatting. In addition, it is possible to obtain multiple slices simultaneously, thus providing the performance of MR imaging within the practical limits of reimbursement. MRI also offers a multitude of techniques that can be individualized for the clinical condition investigated, making it possible to greatly increase the diagnostic sensitivity and improve specificity. The current research in paramagnetic contrast media promises even further increased sensitivity and specificity, opening wide areas of research in normal and abnormal physiology.

These unique qualities of MRI are based on the fact that unlike other imaging modalities, which rely on a single physical parameter, MRI depends on at least seven such parameters, which can be selectively enhanced in order to obtain the greatest difference between normal and abnormal tissues. These parameters are (1) proton density; (2) $T1$, the spin-lattice tissue relaxation parameter; (3) $T2$, the spin-spin parameter;

(4) bulk proton motion, the parameter permitting the study of blood flow; (5) chemical shift, which can be used to further differentiate between tissues; (6) diffusion, which can be applied to sizing tissue compartments; and (7) magnetic susceptibility. Techniques are continuously being designed for enhancing individually or in groups the various tissue parameters, and they promise significant increase in pathologic specificity. An example is the Ortendahl "liquefaction imaging," in which areas with increased proton density, $T1$, and $T2$ are selected by computer and imaged, depicting only areas with high water content.[46] Computer-calculated $T1$ or $T2$ images have been available for several years, expanding the differences between various tissues as, for instance, between normal bone marrow and that of acute leukemia in children. The enhancement of parameter differences is generating multiple, new, highly informative techniques.

DISADVANTAGES OF MRI

The medical disadvantages of MRI are predominately related to the length of scanning, which degrades the image of the parts of the body involved in breathing and peristalsis. With multiple sequences the scanning and calibration time often amounts to one hour or more, thus precluding this examination for the critically ill, for those in continuous need of life support, for patients with multiple stabilizing devices, and for the severely claustrophobic. Patients with cardiac pacemakers currently are not admitted for this type of examination, and neither are patients with metallic intracranial clips.

Further medical disadvantages are the presence of many tissue or disease-specific techniques. Unfortunately, there are even more suboptimal techniques. Early papers comparing CT, a mature modality, with MRI in its early development were of low value, as the use of the wrong technique did not reflect the limitations of MRI. Finally, with high magnetic field strengths requiring high RI or with multiple fast repeated 180 degree pulses, heat will build up in the tissues, limiting the application of these potentially useful techniques.

PRESENT CLINICAL STATUS

Brain

Magnetic resonance imaging is at present the imaging modality of choice for almost all indications in the examination of the brain, except when the presence of calcifications is the critical factor (Fig. 5–1).[8,11–15,47] With the use of spin-echo techniques with long pulse intervals (TR) and long echo times (TE) and, if necessary, with the use of two sequences modifying these parameters, MRI surpasses CT or any other modality in demonstrating tumors, vascular lesions, ischemia, edema, trauma, and intracerebral hemorrhage. Although imaging can be done in any plane, in order to save time, most sequences performed by neuroradiologists are in the axial plane.[14] Gadolinium DTPA has been applied to the study of the brain and is particularly valuable in examinations for tumors.[48]

Spinal Cord

MRI is the modality of choice for virtually every affliction involving the spinal cord.[11,12] By changing TR and TE with spin-echo technique, the spinal fluid surrounding

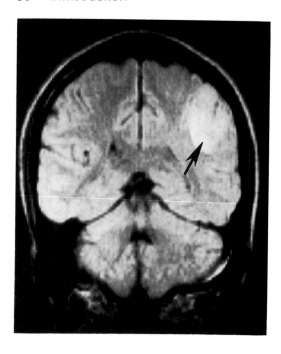

Figure 5–1. A 25-year-old man with seizures. SE (*TR* = 2 sec; *TE* = 28 ms). An ill-defined high-intensity mass (arrow) in the left parietal lobe represents a low-grade astrocytoma.

the cord is well outlined as is the cord itself. Abnormalities in the cord are precisely demonstrated (Fig. 5–2).

Spine

The bony cortex of vertebrae, containing very few free protons, is demonstrated as a black line. The vertebral bone marrow, containing fat and some cellular elements, is studied to great advantage, particularly with the use of surface coils. Trauma, infiltrative and degenerative disease, and tumors are all shown better with MRI than with any other modality. The intervertebral discs are also well demonstrated with MRI. Differentiation between degenerated and normal discs is easily made (Fig. 5–3). Whether MRI is going to replace x-ray CT in the study of herniated discs is not yet clearly established but appears likely.[49,50]

Pelvis

Male Pelvis. The prostate, urinary bladder, seminal vesicles, corpora cavernosa, corpus spongiosum, and ductus deferens are all well demonstrated. Although neoplastic disease contained within the capsule of the prostate cannot be differentiated with certainty from inflammatory disease, the staging of carcinoma of the prostate is done better with MRI than with any other imaging modality.[51] The same is true for tumors of the urethra, seminal vesicles, and urinary bladder.[52–54] Tumors of the urinary bladder are demonstrated with excellent detail (Fig. 5–4), and MRI staging of bladder tumors surpasses that of CT.[52,53]

Female Pelvis. It is in the female pelvis that MRI excels. It is possible to differentiate between endometrium, myometrium, and cervix. An intermediate zone demonstrated with a low-intensity signal using a spin echo (SE) pulse sequence with a long TR is shown located between the high-intensity endometrium and the intermediate-density myometrium. Similarly, anatomy of the cervix is well demonstrated. Benign and ma-

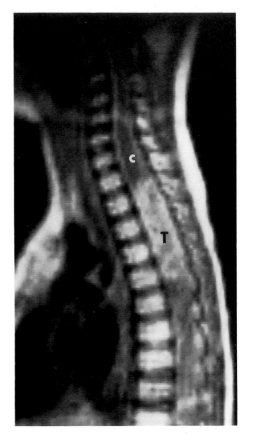

Figure 5–2. On this *T2* weighted image, a solid tumor (T) is seen with high signal intensity (owing to the prolongation of the *T2* parameter). Superior extent of the tumor has a cystic (c) component. The low intensity of this cystic component reflects a long *T1* value. (Courtesy of Dr. M. Brant-Zawadzki.)

lignant corpus tumors are easily displayed (Fig. 5–5). MRI further provides information in the staging of carcinoma of the endometrium.[55] The ovaries and adnexal tissues are seen with less detail because of their proximity to the moving intestines.[56]

Lymph Nodes

By using sequences with short *TR* to differentiate fat from lymph nodes and long *TR* to differentiate nodes from muscle, lymph nodes larger than 1 cm are well delineated

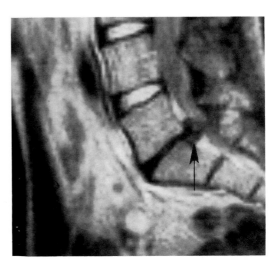

Figure 5–3. A 54-year-old male with sciatica. SE (*TR* = 2 sec; *TE* = 56 ms). There is degenerative disc disease (demonstrated by loss of height and signal intensity) with the extension of the nucleus pulposus (arrow) at the level L5–S1. (Courtesy of Dr. H.K. Genant.)

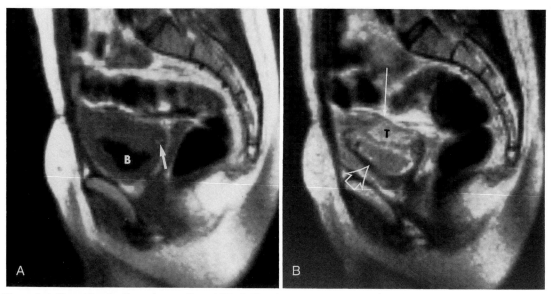

Figure 5–4. Transitional cell carcinoma, Stage T3B. Infiltrating type tumor growth. *A*, SE (*TR* = 0.5 sec; *TE* = 28 ms). Urine in the urinary bladder (B) is imaged with low signal intensity. There is asymmetric bladder wall thickening. In this imaging sequence the bladder wall hypertrophy and tumor cannot be differentiated. There is hemorrhage at the site of recent biopsy (arrow). *B*, *TR* = 2 sec; *TE* = 56 ms. On a *T2* contrast image the hypertrophic normal bladder wall (open arrow) is markedly decreased in intensity. It can be clearly differentiated from the high signal intensity tumor (T). Peritoneal reflection (long arrow).

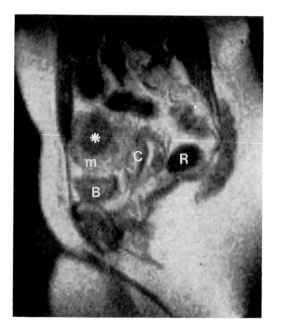

Figure 5–5. Sagittal femal pelvis. SE (*TR* = 1.5 sec; *TE* = 28–56 ms). The uterus is enlarged. The myometrium (*) is imaged with homogenous low signal intensity and is clearly separated from the myometrium (m). Cervix (C); rectum (R); urinary bladder (B).

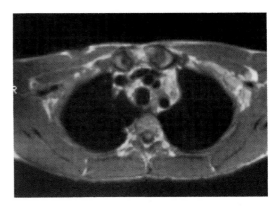

Figure 5–6. Mediastinal adenopathy. ECG-gated axial image. SE (*TE* = 30 ms). Numerous small lymph nodes are imaged with medium signal intensity and are clearly differentiated from the surrounding high-intensity adipose tissue and blood vessels, which exhibit a void of signal.

by MRI.[37,38] Unfortunately, MRI differentiation between benign and malignant nodes is not currently possible.[57] Differentiation of nodes from patent blood vessels by MRI is excellent and sometimes even better than by contrast-enhanced CT (Fig. 5–6). Obtaining MRI views in a sagittal or coronal plane also is frequently of great help.

Heart

With ECG gating and the ability to obtain sagittal, coronal, axial, and oblique views, MRI promises to be the modality of choice in the study of myocardial infarcts.[58–60] Fresh myocardial infarcts show up as areas of acute edema, while chronic infarcts show thinning of the myocardium. Congenital heart disease can also be studied because of the availability of multiple planes of imaging (Fig. 5–7).[42] The thickened pericardium and the effects of constrictive pericarditis are studied with better detail than with any other modality.[41]

Large Vessels

MRI is rapidly becoming the modality of choice for the demonstration of details of dissecting aneurysms.[61,62] Atherosclerotic disease of large vessels and aneurysms are also well studied by this method.[63] With further refinements in technique, it is expected that this modality will replace angiography.

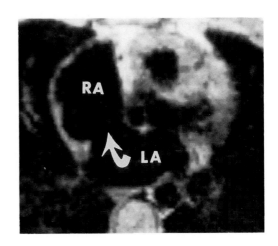

Figure 5–7. Atrial septal defect. Right atrium (RA) is enlarged. A large atrial septal defect (curved arrow) is seen. Left atrium (LA). (Courtesy of Dr. Charles Higgins.)

Lungs and Hila

In the imaging of lungs, MRI is inferior to CT, particularly to high-resolution, thin-slice, and rapid cine CT. Respiratory gating is not yet sufficiently developed for it to be a usable clinical technique. It is surprising, however, that occasionally even small lesions can be demonstrated by this method, particularly in slowly breathing patients. In contrast, lung hila and the mediastinum are often seen better with MRI than with CT, as blood vessels can easily be differentiated from hilar nodes. ECG-gated images are recommended for imaging the mediastinum (Fig. 5–6).

Liver

The liver is one of the most promising areas for MRI studies. Often, MR images demonstrate anatomic detail not obtainable by CT. Although bile ducts, except when very dilated, are not seen as well as with CT, the portal and hepatic veins are seen extremely well without contrast medium injection, thus providing information about anatomic location as well as about the presence of space-occupying lesions. The contributions of fat and water can be separated with chemical shift imaging, thus demonstrating fat infiltration of the liver.[7,64,65] By using multiple spin-echo sequences and inversion recovery technique, metastases and primary tumors of the liver can be seen with great accuracy, matching and sometimes surpassing that of x-ray CT (Fig. 5–8).[65–67] Hemangiomas are also seen and apparently can be identified without the injection of contrast medium.[68,69] Cholangiocarcinoma of the scirrhous type can uniquely be demonstrated by this method.[70]

Spleen

The spleen is an area in which there is very little clinical experience at present. Many studies are under way. While it is proven that tumor invasion and metastases

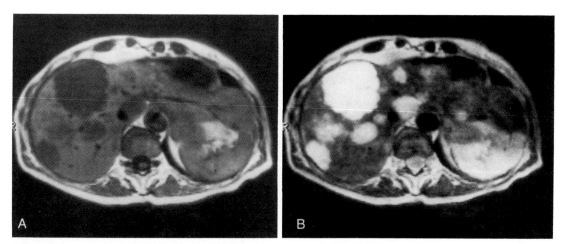

Figure 5–8. Liver metastases. *A*, SE (*TR* = 5 sec; *TE* = 30 ms). Numerous various-sized low-intensity lesions are seen throughout the liver. *B*, SE (*TR* = 2 sec; *TE* = 60 ms). Liver metastases on the *T2* weighted image show high signal intensity in contrast to the lower signal intensity of the remaining liver parenchyma.

can be demonstrated by MRI, the crucial question of whether involvement by lymphoma can be diagnosed has not been answered to date.

Pancreas

The pancreas is an area of disappointment for MRI investigations. It is hoped that MRI may yet justify expectations with improvements in respiratory gating techniques and with the development of new approaches.

Kidneys and Adrenals

The adrenal gland is easily depicted by magnetic resonance. The best imaging sequences are *T1* weighted, offering excellent contrast between the adrenal glands and the surrounding adipose tissue. MRI demonstration of a normal adrenal gland is comparable to that of x-ray CT. Adrenal hyperplasia and adrenal tumors are also easily depicted with MRI. The advantage of MRI over CT in evaluating adrenal pathology is in the patient with previous abdominal surgery, in whom surgical clips in the retroperitoneum preclude diagnostic CT studies.

In the evaluation of the kidneys, magnetic resonance intrinsic contrast permits a clear separation of the cortex (C) and medulla (M) on the *T1* weighted image. While CM differentiation is a sensitive predictor of renal disease, the findings are nonspecific, being seen in a variety of conditions, including inflammatory, obstructive, and even neoplastic renal pathology. In the evaluation of renal tumors, MRI affords improved tumor staging. Staging by MRI has a 92 percent accuracy rate and surpasses that of CT. The advantages lie in the ability of MRI to evaluate tumor extension to the renal vein and inferior vena cava (Fig. 5–9); owing to clear depiction of the blood vessels, the demonstration of perihilar or retrocaval adenopathy by MRI is better than by CT.

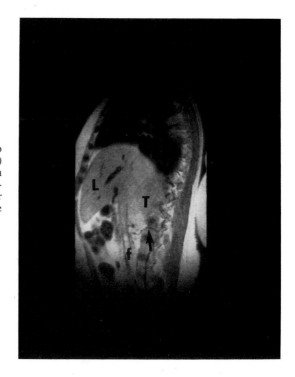

Figure 5–9. Renal cell carcinoma with tumor extension to the inferior vena cava. The large retroperitoneal tumor (T) is a renal cell carcinoma. There is direct tumor extension to the inferior vena cava. The tumor thrombus shows a signal intensity similar to that of the original tumor. Lumbar collateral vessels (arrow). The slow flow proximal to the tumor thrombus (f) is depicted. Liver (L).

Joints

Many investigations are being conducted for the applications of MRI to the study of joint disease, traumatic, degenerative, and neoplastic.[71] The use of surface coils has provided superbly detailed images particularly in the knee.[72,73]

THE FUTURE OF MRI

Certain Directions of Development

MR is a rapidly advancing imaging modality. While some directions of its development are clear, others are still uncertain. The certain directions are as follows.

Improvement in Respiratory Gating. The present types of respiratory gating prolong the examination, sometimes even doubling the examination time and making the entire advantage questionable.[74] It is likely that respiratory gating in the future will be heavily computer-assisted, with the selection of scans that fit each other best. It is also likely that in the not too distant future computers will achieve excellent rearrangements of pixels, even in patients with irregular respiratory motion.

Development of Artificial Intelligence. The development of artificial intelligence, allowing an unerring selection of optimal sequences for the given clinical problem, is a direction promising consistently high-quality studies.

Development of Coils. Further development of optimal coils (surface, elliptical, or special procedure–targeted) will improve spatial resolution. High-resolution small coils may make magnetic resonance imaging microscopy a future clinical reality.

Increased Scanning Speed. Multiple centers currently are engaged in projects aimed at increasing scanning speed. Different approaches are being pursued, from the Mansfield echo planar method to stimulated spin-echo, rapidly repeating, 90 degree pulses and gradient reversal reduced flip angle technique. Reducing scanning time to a few seconds would open the upper abdomen as well as the peritoneal cavity to examinations of better quality.

Spectroscopy. The increasing value of the metabolic and clinical information obtained by spectroscopy is encouraging the pursuit of the exact localization of spectra by imaging. With the reduction of volume of tissue from which the spectrum is obtained, MR imaging spectroscopy may become the ideal diagnostic technique. It is extremely likely that, at least in large medical centers, magnetic resonance imaging and spectroscopy will become inseparable. It should be easily possible to accumulate simultaneously imaging and spectroscopy data from several elements.

Development of Contrast Media. Although there is some controversy about the need for contrast media, with the availability of techniques for enhancing information from the multiple physical MR parameters, the development of paramagnetic contrast media is advancing along several lines.[59,60,75,76] Nitroxides, organic compounds with chelated paramagnetic metals such as gadolinium DTPA, promise to provide more information about the nature of tissue, to more easily separate normal from abnormal, and to narrow the margin of error in the selection of the proper technique. Work on contrast media that are based on monoclonal antibodies is progressing in multiple centers and promises to provide specificity of information.[77]

Integration With Other Modalities. Although magnetic resonance imaging provides information that other imaging modalities cannot, particularly by significantly improving soft tissue contrast resolution, calcifications are not seen, and neither can the bony cortex be evaluated by this method. It is likely that in the future images from x-ray CT and MRI will be compatibly superimposed by computers programmed to accurately superimpose pixels adjusted to the same matrix.

Uncertain Directions of Development

It is by no means established yet which field strength is optimal for imaging. It appears that field strengths anywhere from 0.15 to 1.5 are capable of providing excellent imaging results. As the image quality is the product not only of the magnetic field strength but also of other multiple components composing the system, the controversy appears illogical except for being fueled by commercial interests. Many other considerations come into play, such as the nature of the company providing the magnet, the extent of the service contract, and the cost of the device itself as well as its siting. Both are higher for magnets with a field strength of over 1 tesla.

The nature of the medical institution and the purpose of applications for the instrument are important factors. Higher fields have the advantage of emission of stronger signals and better signal-to-noise ratios, but they have longer $T1$ and motion artifacts are enhanced.

At present, there are also uncertainties about the type of magnet optimal for future developments. While at this stage, cryogenic magnets provide the best images for the investment of time, effort, and funds, it is possible that methods will be developed to improve resistive magnets and make their magnetic fields as homogenous as those of superconducting magnets. As research into the improvement of permanent magnets is advancing and new permanent magnetic materials are developed, it is conceivable that these will also play an important role. Hybrid magnets, combining the best features of permanent, resistive, and cryogenic magnets, may also be developed once MRI becomes the omnipresent diagnostic imaging tool.

MRI is an established clinical imaging modality for almost all conditions involving the brain, spinal cord, bone marrow, and the male and female pelvis. It is undoubtedly going to advance in other areas, for instance, in the mediastinum, in the staging of retroperitoneal tumors, and, with ECG gating, in almost all conditions involving the heart. With surface coils, examination of all the joints, the spine, and the intervertebral discs will be performed preferentially with MRI. With respiratory gating or breathholding techniques in fast-scan methods, MRI will be the preferred modality for the investigation of the liver, spleen, and pancreas. As faster scanning techniques are developed it is possible that even the peritoneal cavity will enter the domain of magnetic resonance imaging. Because of financial considerations and the cost of the MR installations, it will be necessary to develop algorithms favoring the use of less expensive and more accessible modalities for most conditions for which they are adequate. MRI will then be reserved for the conditions in which other modalities would fail.

References

1. Lauterbur PC: Image formation by induced local interactions: examples employing nuclear magnetic resonance. Nature *242*:190, 1973.
2. Hutchinson JMS, Mallard RJ, Goll C: In vivo imaging of body structures using proton resonance. *In* Allen PS, Andre ER, Bates CA (eds): Proc 18th Ampere Congress, Nottingham, 1974. Amsterdam, Elsevier/North Holland, 1975, pp 283–284.
3. Mansfield P, Grannell PK, Maudsley AA: Diffraction and microscopy in solids and liquids by NMR. *In* Allen PS, Andre ER, Bates CA (eds): Proc 18th Ampere Congress, Nottingham, 1974. Amsterdam, Elsevier/North Holland, 1975, pp 431–432.
4. Hinshaw WS: The application of time dependent field gradients to NMR spin mapping. *In* Allen PS, Andre ER, Bates CA (eds): Proc 18th Ampere Congress, Nottingham, 1974. Amsterdam, Elsevier/North Holland, 1975, pp 433–434.
5. Mansfield P, Maudsley AA: Medical imaging by NMR. Br J Radiol *60*:188, 1977.
6. EMI Press Release (''Britain's Brains Produce First NMR Scan''). New Scientist *80*:588, 1978.
7. Pykett IL, Newhouse JH, Buonanno FS, Brady TJ, Goldman MR, Kistler JP, Pohost GM: Principles of nuclear magnetic resonance imaging. Radiology *143*:157, 1982.
8. Margulis AR, Higgins CB, Kaufman L, Crooks LE (eds): Clinical MR Imaging. San Francisco, Radiology Research and Education Foundation, 1983.

9. Pykett IL: MR imaging in medicine. Sci Am *246*:78, 1982.
10. Young IR, Bailes DR, Burl M, et al: Initial clinical evaluation of a whole body nuclear magnetic resonance (NMR) tomograph. J Comput Assist Tomogr *6*:1, 1982.
11. Bradley WJ, Waluch V, Yadley RA, et al: Comparison of CT and MR in 400 patients with disease of the brain and cervical spinal cord. Radiology *152*:695, 1984.
12. Norman D, Mills CM, Brant-Zawadzki M, et al: Magnetic resonance imaging of the spinal cord and canal: potentials and limitations. AJR *141*:1147, 1983.
13. Brant-Zawadzki M, Badami JP, Mills CM, et al: Primary intracranial tumor imaging. A comparison of magnetic resonance and CT. Radiology *150*:435, 1984.
14. Brant-Zawadzki M, Norman D, Newton TH, et al: Magnetic resonance of the brain: the optimal screening technique. Radiology *152*:71, 1984.
15. Young IR, Randell CP, Kaplan PW, et al: Nuclear magnetic resonance (NMR) imaging in white matter disease of the brain using spin-echo sequence. J Comput Assist Tomogr *7*:290, 1983.
16. Moon KL, Genant HK, Helms CA, et al: Musculoskeletal applications of nuclear magnetic resonance imaging. Radiology *147*:161, 1983.
17. Totty WG, Murphy WA, Ganz WI, et al: Magnetic resonance imaging of the normal and ischemic femoral head. AJR *143*:1273, 1984.
18. Dillon WP, Mills C, Kjos B, et al: Magnetic resonance imaging of the nasopharynx. Radiology *152*:731, 1984.
19. Stark DD, Moss AA, Gamsu G, Clark OH, et al: Magnetic resonance imaging of the neck. Part I. Normal anatomy. Radiology *150*:443, 1984.
20. Stark DD, Moss AA, Gamsu G, et al: Magnetic resonance imaging of the neck. Part II. Pathologic findings. Radiology *150*:448, 1984.
21. Webb WR, Gensen BJ, Gamsu G, Sollitto R, Moore EH: Coronary magnetic resonance of the chest: Normal and abnormal. Radiology *153*:729, 1984.
22. Webb WR, Gensen BJ, Sollitto R, Gamsu G, Moore EH: Sagittal MR imaging of the chest. J Comput Assist Tomogr *9*(3):471, 1985.
23. Gamsu G, Stark DD, Webb WR, Moore EH: MRI of benign mediastinal masses. Radiology *151*:709, 1984.
24. Hricak H, Crooks L, Sheldon P: NMR imaging of the kidney. Radiology *146*:425, 1983.
25. Hricak H, Williams RD, Moon KL, et al: NMR imaging of the kidney. Part II. Renal masses. Radiology *147*:765, 1983.
26. Moon KL, Hricak H, Crooks LE, et al: Nuclear magnetic resonance imaging of the adrenal gland: a preliminary report. Radiology *147*:155, 1983.
27. Hricak H, Demas BE, Williams RD, et al: Magnetic resonance imaging in the diagnosis and staging of renal and perirenal neoplasms. Radiology *154*:709, 1985.
28. Hricak H, Higgins CB, Williams RD: NMR imaging in retroperitoneal fibrosis. AJR *141*:35, 1983.
29. Hricak H, Alpers CA, Crooks LE, et al: Magnetic resonance imaging of the female pelvis: initial experience. AJR *141*:1119, 1983.
30. Hricak H, Williams RD, Spring DB, et al: Anatomy and pathology of the male pelvis by magnetic resonance imaging. AJR *141*:1101, 1983.
31. Bies JR, Ellis JH, Kopecky KK, Sutton GP, et al: Assessment of primary gynecologic malignancies: comparison of 0.15T resistive MR with CT. AJR *143*:1249, 1984.
32. Butler H, Bryan PJ, LiPuma JP, Cohen AM, El Yousef S, et al: Magnetic resonance imaging of the abnormal female pelvis. AJR *143*:1259, 1984.
33. Bryan PJ, Butler HE, Lipuma JP, Haagas JR, El Yousef S, Resnick MI, Cohen AM, Malviya VK, Nelson AI, Clampitt M, Alfidi RJ, Cohen J, Morrison SC: NMR scanning of the pelvis: initial experience with a 0.3T system. AJR *141*:1111, 1983.
34. Hricak H, Williams RD: Magnetic resonance imaging and its application in urology. Urology *23*(5):442, 1984.
35. Poon P, McCallum RW, Henkelman MM, et al: Magnetic resonance imaging of the prostate. Radiology *154*:143, 1985.
36. Buonocore E, Hesemann C, Pavlicek W, Montie JE: Clinical and in vitro magnetic resonance imaging of prostate carcinoma. AJR *143*:1267, 1984.
37. Dooms GC, Hricak H, Crooks LE, et al: Magnetic resonance imaging (MRI) of the lymph nodes: Comparison with CT. Radiology *153*:719, 1984.
38. Lee JKT, Heeken JP, Ling D, et al: Magnetic resonance imaging of abdominal and pelvic lymphadenopathy. Radiology *153*:187, 1984.
39. Higgins CB, Stark DD, McNamara M, et al: Multiplane magnetic resonance imaging of the heart and major vessels. Studies in normal volunteers. AJR *142*:661, 1984.
40. Herfkens RJ, Higgins CB, Hricak H, et al: Nuclear magnetic resonance imaging of the cardiovascular system. Normal and pathologic findings. Radiology *147*:761, 1983.
41. Stark DD, Higgins CB, Lanzer P, Lipton MJ, et al: Magnetic resonance imaging of the pericardium. Normal and pathologic findings. Radiology *150*:469, 1984.
42. Fisher MR, Higgins CB: Magnetic resonance and computerized tomography in congenital heart disease. Semin Roentgenol *20*:272, 1985.
43. Pavlicek W, Geisinger M, Castle L, et al: Effects of nuclear magnetic resonance on patients with cardiac pacemakers. Radiology *147*:149, 1983.
44. Moon KL, Hricak H, Margulis AR, et al: Nuclear magnetic resonance imaging characteristics of gallstones in vitro. Radiology *148*:753, 1983.

45. Fisher MR, Wall S, Hricak H, McCarthy S, Kerlan R: Hepatic vascular anatomy on magnetic resonance imaging. AJR *144*:739, 1985.
46. Ortendahl D. Liquefaction imaging. Personal communication, 1986.
47. Young IR, Burl M, Clarke GJ, et al: Magnetic resonance properties of hydrogen: imaging of the posterior fossa. AJR *137*:895, 1981.
48. Wesbey GE, Engelstad BL, Brasch RC: Paramagnetic pharmaceuticals for magnetic resonance imaging. Physiol Chem Phys Med NMR *16*:145, 1984.
49. Chafetz NI, Genant HK, Moon KL, Helms CA, Morris JM: Recognition of lumbar disc herniation with MRI. AJR *141*:1143, 1983.
50. Modic MT, Pavlicek W, Weinstein MA, et al: Magnetic resonance imaging of intervertebral disc disease. Radiology *152*:103, 1984.
51. Hricak H, Dooms GC, Jeffrey RB, et al: Prostatic carcinoma: staging by clinical assessment, CT, and MR imaging. Radiology *162*:331, 1987.
52. Fisher MR, Hricak H: MR of the urinary bladder: normal and benign pathology. Radiology *157*:467, 1985.
53. Fisher MR, Hricak H, Tanagho EA: Urinary bladder MR imaging. Part II. Neoplasm. Radiology *157*:471, 1985.
54. McClure RD, Hricak H: MRI: Its application to male infertility. Radiology *160*:285, 1986.
55. Fisher MR, Hricak H, Lacey CG: MRI evaluation of endometrial carcinoma. Radiological Society of North America, 1984. Work in progress.
56. Dooms GC, Hricak H, Tscholakoff D: Adnexal structures: MR imaging. Radiology *158*:639, 1986.
57. Dooms GC, Hricak H, Crooks LE, Higgins CB: Magnetic resonance imaging of lymph nodes: comparison with CT. Radiology *153*:719, 1984.
58. McNamara MT, Higgins CB, Schechtmann N, Botvinick E, Amparo EG, Cattergee K: Detection and characterization of acute myocardial infarctions in man using gated magnetic resonance imaging. Circulation *71*(4):717, 1985.
59. Wesbey GE, Higgins CB, McNamara MT, et al: Effect of gadolinium DTPA on the magnetic relaxation times of normal and infarcted myocardium. Radiology *153*:165, 1984.
60. McNamara MT, Higgins CB, Ehman RL, et al: Acute myocardial ischemia: magnetic resonance contrast enhancement with gadolinium DTPA. Radiology *153*:157, 1984.
61. Amparo EG, Higgins CB, Hricak H, Sollitto R: Aortic dissection: Magnetic resonance imaging. Radiology *155*:399, 1985.
62. Geisinger MA, Risius B, O'Donnell JA, Zelch MG, Moodie DS, Graor RA, George CR: Thoracic aortic dissections: Magnetic resonance imaging. Radiology *155*:407, 1985.
63. Amparo EG, Hoddick WK, Hricak H, Sollitto R, Justich E, Filly RA, Higgins CB: Comparison of magnetic resonance imaging and ultrasonography in the evaluation of abdominal aortic aneurysms. Radiology *154*:451, 1985.
64. Dixon WT: Simple proton spectroscopic imaging. Radiology *153*:189, 1984.
65. Lee JKT, Dixon WT, Ling D: Fatty infiltration of the liver: demonstration by proton spectroscopic imaging. Radiology *153*:195, 1984.
66. Demas B, Hricak H, Goldberg HI, Margulis AR: Magnetic resonance imaging diagnosis of hepatic metastases in the presence of negative CT studies. J Clin Gastroenterol *7*(6):553, 1985.
67. Stark DD, Felder RC, Wittenberg J, et al: Magnetic resonance imaging of cavernous hemangioma of the liver: Tissue-specific characterization. AJR *145*:213, 1985.
68. Glazer GM, Aisen AM, Francis IR, Gyves JW, Lande I, Adler DD: Hepatic cavernous hemangioma: Magnetic resonance imaging. Work in Progress. Radiology *155*:417, 1985.
69. Ohtomo K, Itai J, Furui S, Yashiro N, Yoshikawa K, Iio M: Hepatic tumors: Differentiation by transverse relaxation time (T2) of magnetic resonance imaging. Radiology *155*:421, 1985.
70. Dooms GC, Kerlan R, Hricak H, Wall S, Margulis AR: MR imaging of cholangiocarcinomas. Radiological Society of North America, 1985 (abstract).
71. Turner DA, Prodromos CC, Petasnick JP, Clark JW: Acute injury of the ligaments of the knee. Magnetic resonance evaluation. Radiology *154*:717, 1985.
72. Fisher MR, Barker B, Amparo EG, Brandt G, Brant-Zawadzki M, Hricak H, Higgins CB: Magnetic resonance imaging using specialized coils. Radiology *157*:443, 1985.
73. Axel L: Surface coils magnetic resonance imaging. J Comput Assist Tomogr *8*:831, 1984.
74. Ehman RL, McNamara MT, Pallack M, Hricak H, Higgins CB: Magnetic resonance imaging with respiratory gating: techniques and advantages. AJR *143*:1175, 1984.
75. Brasch RC, Wesbey GE, Doemeny J, McHamara M, Ehman R: Contrast media for NMR imaging. Invest Radiol *19*:148, 1984.
76. Brasch RC, Ogan MD, Englestad BL: Paramagnetic contrast agents and their application in NMR imaging. *In* Parvez Z (ed): Contrast Media: Biologic Effects in Clinical Application. Vol 3. Boca Raton; CRC Press; 1987.

II

TISSUE
CHARACTERIZATION

6

Impact of the Choice of Operating Parameters on MR Images

FELIX W. WEHRLI
JAMES R. MACFALL
JAMIE H. PROST

Compared with x-ray–based modalities and optical spectroscopy, nuclear magnetic resonance (MR) is a relatively insensitive technique. There are two phenomena that severely limit the achievable signal-to-noise ratio (SNR). The virtual absence of spontaneous emission is a mechanism for re-establishment of thermal equilibrium following excitation of spins from their ground to the excited state.[1] The only available mechanism for dissipation of the excess energy to the environment, spin-lattice relaxation, is a highly inefficient process because of the insulation of the spin system from the lattice.[1] For protons in biologic tissue the time constant for this process (spin-lattice relaxation time $T1$) is of the order of hundreds of milliseconds or seconds.[2] The selection of the imaging strategy is, therefore, paramount to achievement of adequate image quality.

This section discusses the interdependence of the principal operator-selectable parameters, such as matrix size, field of view, slice thickness, number of excitations, and pulse repetition time, on the achievable SNR and scan time. These all affect image quality in one manner or another. It is, therefore, essential that the user develop a good grasp of the interrelationship of these parameters so as to become adept in optimizing image quality within the constraints of the available scan time.

SIGNAL-TO-NOISE MEASUREMENT

Although an unbiased measurement of SNR for the purpose of comparing performance of different imagers is a complicated normalization task,[3] the user is more often concerned with relative SNR measurements.

The SNR in an image can be measured in various ways. A simple measurement on an unprocessed image involves computing the pixel mean and standard deviation in a region of interest (ROI). The SNR is then computed as the ratio of the ROI mean value (with all known constant offsets subtracted) to the standard deviation. This approach includes low spatial frequency variation that can be due to actual object structure or rf field nonuniformity that would not ordinarily be considered "noise." A better approach is to first subtract a low-pass filtered version of the image from the original image before computing the pixel standard deviation. While this is an improvement, the result depends, to some extent, on the filter characteristics.

More often, two images acquired successively or in an interleaved fashion can be subtracted to remove the structure dependence. The so-obtained difference representing the noise should then be reduced by $\sqrt{2}$ to compensate for the noise multiplication of the subtraction process. Alternatively, one can place an ROI box outside the object boundary and calculate the standard deviation for this pixel matrix. This method is hampered by the fact that most MR images are formed from the magnitude of the Fourier transform used in the image reconstruction process. Thus the noise in the object exterior is unipolar, while the noise in the interior is bipolar. The visual effect is that the interior noise is higher than its exterior counterpart. Hence, an underestimate of the true noise results. As long as the noise is consistently measured this way, however, this algorithm is legitimate for comparison purposes. Figure 6–1 compares two of the methods of SNR measurement discussed for a region of interest in a brain image.

Dependence of Signal-to-Noise Ratio on Operating Parameters

The major source of noise in MR images is the electronic noise generated in the receiver circuit and the patient.[4] While with today's technology, the noise of the receiver coil circuit (preamplifier, coil, and so forth) can be reduced to well below 1 dB, noise generated by the patient, resulting from Brownian motion of the ions in the body fluids, can be controlled only to a limited extent, for example, by confining the detection volume using local coils.[5,6]

In addition, the instrument designer is faced with a variety of extraneous signal sources, generating noise that is not statistical in nature. This includes FM radio frequency transmitters and digital systems radiating at frequencies within the bandwidth of the receiver. MR imaging systems, therefore, are typically enclosed by an rf shield to minimize reception of such extraneous signals. We will not dwell on this subject, and henceforth it will be assumed that such coherent noise sources are effectively suppressed.

The electronic noise N_R is given by[4]

$$N_R = \xi\,\Delta v^{1/2}(aR_c \cdot v^{1/2} + bR_p \cdot v^2)^{1/2} \tag{1}$$

In Equation (1) ξ is the coil filling factor, v is the resonance frequency in Hertz, and Δv is the bandwidth of the receiver. R_c and R_p represent the resistances of the coil and patient, respectively, and a and b are constants. Assuming a field of view of D_x

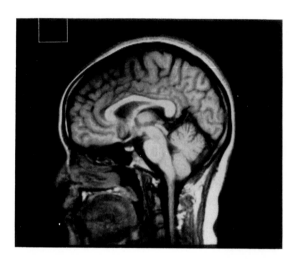

Figure 6–1. The SNR in this sagittal image was calculated from an ROI in the pons by two of the methods described in the text, yielding 40 and 45 for the blurred mask subtraction method vs. noise measurement outside the object boundary, respectively.

cm in frequency-encoding direction and an amplitude of G_x of the read-out gradient, then according to the Larmor relationship, we can write for the receiver bandwidth

$$\Delta v = (\gamma/2\pi)G_x D_x \tag{2}$$

where γ is the magnetogyric ratio.

In abbreviated form we may write for the signal S per pixel

$$S \sim N(X) \cdot \Delta x \cdot \Delta y \cdot d \cdot v^2 \cdot f(TR, TE, T1, T2) \tag{3}$$

In Equation (1) ξ is the coil filling factor, v is the resonance frequency in Hertz, and Δy are the pixel dimensions, and d is the slice thickness. The product $N \cdot \Delta x \cdot \Delta y \cdot d$ thus corresponds to the number of nuclei per voxel that contribute to the signal. $f(TR, TE, T1, T2)$ represents the dependence of the transverse magnetization that induces the signal voltage in the receiver coil on the pulse recycle time (TR), echo delay (TE), and spin relaxation times ($T1$, $T2$), assuming that a spin echo is detected, as is common in MR imaging.

The quantity $f(TR, TE, T1, T2)$ will be addressed in Chapters 7 and 8 discussing the pulse sequence dependence of contrast. It is the principal determinant of contrast between two anatomic regions.

In two-dimensional Fourier transform (2DFT) imaging,[7] we collect a free induction decay (FID) or echo, which is sampled N_x times during the frequency-encoding (detection) period. Each of these signals yields, upon Fourier transformation, a projection or view of the object. In total, N_y projections are collected to create, following a second Fourier transform, an image consisting of $N_x \cdot N_y$ pixels. If we consider further that each projection may result from averaging of n identical FIDs, we obtain for the SNR (Equations [1] to [3])

$$SNR \sim \Delta x \cdot \Delta y \cdot d \cdot \sqrt{N_x} \cdot \sqrt{N_y} \cdot \sqrt{n} \cdot N(X) \cdot f(TR, TE, T1, T2) \cdot 1/\sqrt{\Delta v} \cdot v^2/\sqrt{aR_c v^{1/2} + bR_p v^2} \tag{4}$$

The term $\sqrt{N_x}\sqrt{N_y}$ in Equation (4) results from statistical reduction of noise during data collection. If we consider, in addition, that for the x and y dimension of the field of view (FOV), $D_x = N_x \cdot \Delta x$ and $D_y = N_y \cdot \Delta y$ holds, we can write for the SNR

$$SNR \sim \frac{D_x}{\sqrt{N_x}} \cdot \frac{D_y}{\sqrt{N_y}} \cdot d \cdot \sqrt{n} \cdot N(H) \cdot f(TR, TE, T1, T2) \cdot 1/\sqrt{\Delta v} \cdot f(v) \tag{5}$$

where $f(v) = v^2/\sqrt{aR_c v^{1/2} + bR_p v^2}$.

If we further take into account that the bandwidth Δv is proportional to the number of samples N_x (Equations 2 and 3) and consider only the operator-selectable imaging parameters (excluding pulse-timing parameters), we obtain

$$SNR \sim \frac{D_x}{N_x} \cdot \frac{D_y}{\sqrt{N_y}} \cdot d \cdot \sqrt{n} \tag{6}$$

By denoting the time between consecutive excitations TR and the total scan time T_s,

$$n = T_s/(TR \cdot N_y) \tag{7}$$

follows. Holding SNR constant, we obtain, from rearrangement of Equation (6)

$$T_s \sim TR \left\{ \frac{N_x \cdot N_y}{d \cdot D_x \cdot D_y} \right\}^2 \tag{8}$$

From Equation (8) we recognize the time penalties paid for magnification, increase in matrix size, and decrease in slice thickness when it is desired to keep SNR constant. A simultaneous reduction, for example, by a factor of 2 each in field of view and slice thickness, would require a 64-fold increase in scan time to maintain SNR! Since this is totally impractical, it is important that the imager's intrinsic SNR be high enough so that upon increasing spatial resolution the SNR in the image does not degrade excessively.

While Equations (4) to (8) assume excitation of a single slice only, it is readily recognized that by multiplexing data acquisition for a multitude of slices, utilizing the dead time between data acquisition and the next following excitation pulse, the scan efficiency can be greatly improved.[8] Although this mode of acquisition, which is now standard practice in the large majority of MR scans, does not affect the signal-to-noise ratio in each of the individual slices, it obviously shortens the scan time per slice. Assuming, for example, the time between initial excitation pulse and end of data collection (including computer overhead) to be of the order of t ms, we recognize that TR/t slices can be excited during one pulse repetition. This reduces the scan time per plane by a factor TR/t. In the case of collection of a single echo, typically 20 slices can be excited during a 1 sec TR period.

For the sake of completeness we may further consider volume acquisition techniques such as 3DFT.[9] In this case, the field of view has a third dimension D_z, in addition to previously defined D_x and D_y. We therefore need to phase-encode in z direction by incrementing the phase-encoding gradient $G_z N_z$ times. From Equation (6) it therefore follows for the SNR

$$SNR \sim \frac{D_x}{N_x} \frac{D_y}{\sqrt{N_y}} \frac{D_z}{\sqrt{N_z}} \sqrt{n} \tag{9}$$

Analogously, for constant SNR we may write for the scan time

$$T_s \sim TR \left\{ \frac{N_x \cdot N_y \cdot N_z}{D_x \cdot D_y \cdot D_z} \right\} \tag{10}$$

Note, for example, from Equation (9) that a reduction in the field of view by a factor of 2 in all three linear dimensions reduces the signal-to-noise ratio eightfold. However, the intrinsically high SNR of 3D imaging makes a reduction in voxel size more easily tolerable. Let us assume, for example, $D_z/N_z = d$, i.e., equal slice thickness for the two methods. We then realize that the SNR in the corresponding 3D images, with all other scan parameters held constant, is superior by a factor of $\sqrt{N_z}$. The price for this superior signal-to-noise ratio, of course, is increased scan time. This becomes evident by comparing the minimum scan times for the two techniques.

$$2D: \quad T_{s,min} \sim N_y \cdot n \cdot TR \tag{11}$$

$$3D: \quad T_{s,min} \sim N_y \cdot N_z \cdot n \cdot TR \tag{12}$$

It is, therefore, evident that for a limited number of slices and on the assumption that a single excitation provides adequate signal-to-noise, 2D acquisition is the method of choice. However, if multiple excitations are needed (such as in the case of very small voxels, i.e., very high spatial resolution), 3D may be more appropriate.[10] It is evident from Equation (12) that in order to be competitive with 2D multislice techniques, 3DFT require very short repetition times. While this results in a loss in SNR (SNR is proportional to $[1 - \exp(-TR/T1)]$), the latter is usually tolerable because of the very high intrinsic signal-to-noise afforded by 3DFT.

SLICE THICKNESS

In theory, a true cross-sectional view of the body requires an infinitely thin slice. The thicker the slice, the more closely we approach a projection image. The effect of partial voluming is shown with two images obtained in the coronal plane across the

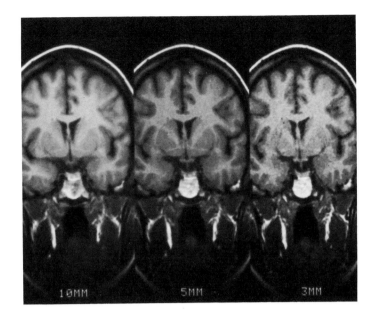

Figure 6–2. Coronal images across the pituitary gland showing the effect of partial voluming. Note that in the thick-slice image (10 mm) the stalk of the pituitary gland is not as well visualized as in the images obtained from thinner slices.

pituitary gland (Fig. 6–2). Note that the 3 mm image enables clear visualization of the stalk of the pituitary gland, whereas this structure is not visible in the 10 mm image, in spite of the fact that the scan coordinates were identical in both images.

In 2DFT the slice thickness is controlled by the magnitude of the slice-selection gradient and the bandwidth of the rf pulse (not to be confused with the sampling frequency bandwidth):

$$\Delta z = 2\pi\delta\nu/\gamma G_z \tag{13}$$

where Δz is the slice thickness and $\delta\nu$ is the bandwidth of the rf pulse in hertz. Hence the slice thickness can be reduced in either of two ways: (a) by narrowing the width of the rf pulse, or (b) by increasing the amplitude of the slice-selection gradient. In practice, $\delta\nu$ is held constant while the slice-selection gradient amplitude is varied. The practical lower limit of slice thickness achievable in this manner in 2DFT imaging is of the order of 2 to 3 mm.

In 3DFT the slice thickness is controlled by the amplitude of the phase-encoding gradient G_z and the duration of the phase-encoding gradient Δt as follows:

$$\gamma G_z \cdot \Delta z \cdot \Delta t = 2\pi \tag{14}$$

FIELD OF VIEW AND PIXEL SIZE

The size of individual pixels is determined by the number of sampling points in x and $y(N_x, N_y)$ and the field of view $D_x D_y$. The field of view is further related to the sampling frequency bandwidth $\Delta\nu$ and the read-out gradient G_x (Equation [2]). By substituting $D_x = N_x \cdot \Delta x$ into Equation (2), we obtain

$$\Delta\nu = (\gamma/2\pi)G_x \cdot N_x \cdot \Delta x \tag{15}$$

For a sampling frequency $\Delta\nu = 32{,}000$ Hz, $N_x = 256$, and a field of view $D_x = 24$ cm, Equation (2) demands for the gradient amplitude $G_x = 0.314$ gauss. The resulting pixel size is $D_x/N_x = 0.094$ cm. The standard procedure for lowering pixel size (i.e., increasing spatial resolution) consists of reducing the field of view. According to Equation (2), a decrease in field of view by a factor of 2 demands a commensurate increase in gradient amplitude. In our example, this would increase the read-out gradient strength to 0.628 gauss/cm.

The effect of reduction in field of view by a factor of 2 in either dimension on spatial resolution is illustrated in Figure 6–3. Note the much improved definition of anatomic detail in the higher-resolution image (Fig. 6–3B). Figure 6–4 shows the effect on SNR as FOV and pixel size are reduced. The two curves were obtained from Equation (6), fitting the three points corresponding to region-of-interest SNR values in muscle and bone from three scans in which the field of view was reduced from 16 to 8 cm.

The second alternative, according to Equation (15), is to lower the bandwidth by a factor of 2. Remembering further that the bandwidth is also the rate at which the free induction decay or spin-echo signal is sampled, it is readily recognized that

$$N_x = \Delta v \cdot t_s \tag{16}$$

holds, where t_s represents the sampling time. From Equation (16) we see that at a bandwidth of 32,000 Hz and 256 samplings, a sampling time $t_s = 8$ ms follows. Hence, by decreasing the bandwidth by a factor of 2, the sampling time would have to be increased to 16 ms. While the user often does not have this option available to increase spatial resolution, it is nevertheless of relevance that the consequences of decreased bandwidth be understood. We have seen earlier (Equation [1]) that the noise is proportional to the square root of the bandwidth. Hence, decreasing the bandwidth by a factor of 2 results in a $\sqrt{2}$ improvement in signal-to-noise. In practice, this may not always be achievable to the full extent, since the increased sampling time may require an adjustment of the echo delay toward longer values. For example, if $T2 = 60$ ms, then an increase of TE from 20 ms to 24 ms results in a signal loss of 6 percent. Thus the potential SNR improvement of 40 percent is reduced to 34 percent.

The third alternative for increasing spatial resolution consists of increasing the number of sampling points, in our example from 256 to 512. This will also increase the sampling time while holding the field of view constant (since the product $N_x \cdot \Delta x$ remains unaltered). Equation (15) indicates that this method does not require an adjustment of either bandwidth or read-out gradient strength. However, since twice as many samples have to be taken, the sampling time in our example increases from 8 to 16 ms.

While an increase in sampling points in frequency-encoding direction does not affect scan time, an increase in the number of points in y does (Equation [11]). In our example, an increase by a factor of 2 in both linear dimensions increases the minimum scan time by a factor of 2.

Typically, the matrix size is held constant and the field of view is decreased whenever operation at higher spatial resolution is required. This approach is favored over an increase in matrix size, since the need for visualization of smaller structures is like a magnification of a portion of the object, i.e., does not require the full field of view.

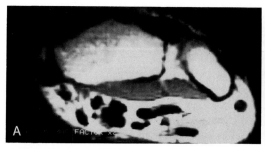 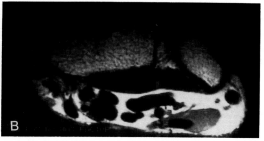

Figure 6–3. Sixty-three MHz transverse images of the wrist obtained at FOVs of 16 cm (*A*) and 8 cm (*B*), corresponding to pixel sizes of 0.62 and 0.31 mm, respectively.

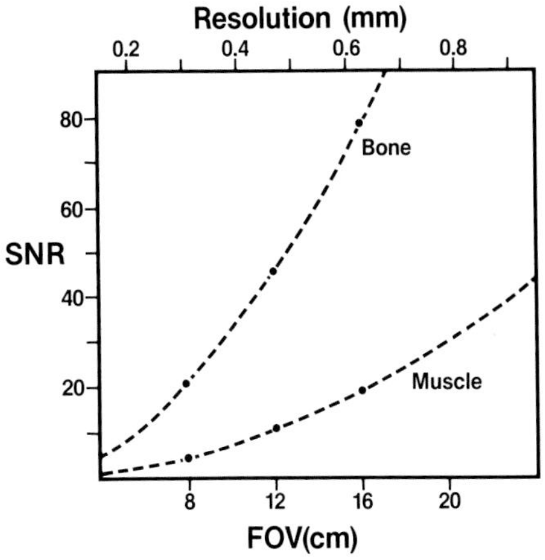

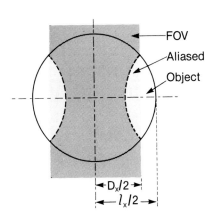

Figure 6–4. Plot of SNR vs. FOV and pixel size. Dots pertain to ROI measurements taken at different FOVs in images recorded under otherwise identical conditions.

SCAN PARAMETER–DEPENDENT ARTIFACTS

Aliasing

The Nyquist theorem[11] demands that in order to unambiguously digitize a frequency, at least two samples per cycle must be taken. In a quadrature receiver, the carrier frequency is set to the center of the band of frequencies $\Delta \nu$ to be digitized, i.e., after conversion to audio frequency in the receiver, a band of frequencies $\pm \Delta \nu/2$ is obtained. Hence, the largest frequency to be digitized is $\Delta \nu/2$. In our situation the Nyquist theorem, therefore, may be stated as follows:

$$2 \cdot \Delta \nu/2 \cdot t_s = N_x \qquad (17)$$

Any frequency exceeding Nyquist's frequency by an amount $\Delta \Delta \nu$ will be converted to a frequency $(\Delta \nu - \Delta \Delta \nu)$. In practice, this may occur whenever the object extends beyond the boundaries of the field of view (Fig. 6–5). Let us assume that the object has a width ℓ_x and the FOV in frequency-encoding direction is D_x such that $\ell_x > D_x$. Whereas $D_x = \Delta \nu/[(\gamma/2\pi)G_x]$ satisfies the Nyquist condition, it is obvious that ℓ_x translates into a frequency greater than $\Delta \nu$. Those portions of the object that lie outside the field of view will also be excited and will emit a signal at a frequency greater than $\Delta \nu/2$. It therefore appears as though the images were folded or wrapped around an axis determined by the boundary of the field of view (Fig. 6–5). This phenomenon, termed aliasing, is rather common. It can be minimized by use of suitable low-pass filters. The

Figure 6–5. Aliasing in frequency-encoding direction. Portions of the object extending beyond the boundaries given by the field of view, thus corresponding to higher than the Nyquist frequency, are folded around the FOV boundaries, back into the image.

images in Figure 6–6, in which a FOV was chosen that does not fully encompass the object, illustrate the relative effect of the filters on the aliasing artifact. Note that the eight-pole Butterworth filter with a steeper roll-off (and thus better attenuation of frequencies above its cutoff point) provides slightly better suppression of the foldover artifact than the corresponding four-pole filter.

Aliasing also occurs in the phase-encoding dimension. One way to suppress the artifact is to avoid excitation of those portions extending beyond the FOV. This can be achieved by using a selective 180 degree pulse with the rf bandwidth and amplitude of the gradient adjusted such that $(\gamma/2\pi)G_yD_y = \delta\nu$, where $\delta\nu$ is the bandwidth of the 180 degree refocusing pulse.[12] The other symbols have been defined earlier. While this method is effective in single-slice acquisition, it is inapplicable to 2DFT multislice operation, since the latter demands selectivity of the 180 degree pulse in z (i.e., perpendicular to the scan plane). Presence and absence of the phase-encoding aliasing artifact for the two modes of operation are shown in Figure 6–7.

Another approach to eliminate or at least minimize aliasing artifacts is the use of surface coils.[13] In this case, signals are typically received only from the region encompassed by the surface coil conductor.

Chemical Shift Phenomenon

Besides the strength of the external magnetic field, it is the intrinsic magnetic fields generated by the surrounding electrons that determine the exact resonance frequency of a nucleus. The most common situation in proton imaging is the chemical shift between water protons and the protons of the CH_2 moiety in long-chain fatty acids as they occur in adipose tissue. The difference in the magnetic field experienced by the two types of protons is of the order of 3.5 ppm of the static magnetic field. This difference δB translates into a frequency difference $\gamma\delta B$, which causes a positional displacement,[14] given as

$$x_0^{\mathrm{w}} - x_0^{\mathrm{f}} = \delta B/G_{\mathrm{x}} \qquad (18)$$

Hence, if a tissue contains both water and fat, we will, in fact, obtain two images that are shifted relative to each other by an amount that is proportional to the ratio of static

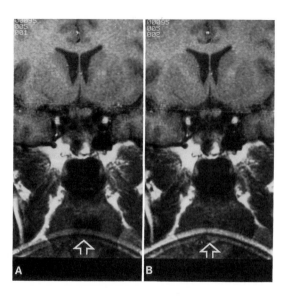

Figure 6–6. Effect of filter attenuation characteristics on aliasing artifact. The images in *A* and *B* were taken with eight-pole and four-pole Butterworth filters, respectively, under otherwise identical conditions, showing aliasing artifact (arrows). Note the somewhat improved suppression of the aliasing artifact in *A*.

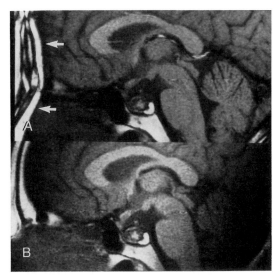

Figure 6–7. Aliasing in the phase-encoding dimension can be minimized by shaping the 180 degree spin-echo pulse in such a manner that spins outside the FOV are not refocused. For this purpose a gradient G_y is applied in the presence of the 180 degree pulse (B). In normal multislice operation, however, the 180 degree pulse is slice-selective, and thus phase-encoding aliasing cannot be prevented (A, arrows).

magnetic field to read-out gradient strength. The effect is illustrated schematically in Figure 6–8 for two tissue species labeled F and W. Note that nuclei W are less shielded by an amount δB. Therefore a frequency ν translates into spatial locations x_F and x_W that differ by an amount $\delta B/G_x$. For the fractional displacement of the two images, we readily see that by dividing Equation (18) by the field of view D_x, we obtain

$$\frac{x_0^w - x_0^f}{D_x} = \frac{\delta B}{G_x D_x} = \frac{\delta \nu}{(\gamma/2\pi)G_x D_x} \tag{19}$$

Hence, the fractional shift is given by the ratio of frequency shift over bandwidth. At a constant bandwidth of 32 kHz, this ratio is 6.98×10^{-3}, or in the case of 256 pixels in frequency-encoding direction 1.79 pixel. Therefore, the displacement in millimeters decreases with decreasing field of view. It is 3.4 mm at 48 cm but only 1.7 mm at 24 cm FOV. Figure 6–9 illustrates the dependence of the chemical shift effect on the choice of FOV, quantitatively confirming these predictions.

From Equation (19) we further note that the relative displacement is inversely proportional to bandwidth. Therefore, if we halve the bandwidth, for example, the chemical shift effect increases twofold.

Techniques have recently been devised that enable correction of the chemical shift effect. Whereas a standard acquisition provides an image that consists of the sum of fat and water images (F + W), it is possible to obtain a difference image (F − W).[15] The two sets of images then can be used to derive a pure fat and a pure water image,

Figure 6–8. Origin of chemical shift effect. Spins labeled F and W differ in their resonance frequency by an amount $\gamma\delta B$, which upon frequency decoding, translates into a pixel displacement $\Delta x = \delta B/G_x$.

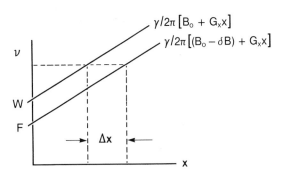

respectively, from which, by applying a 1.8 pixel shift of one of the images in frequency-encoding direction, a chemical shift–corrected image is obtained. Alternatively, one can eliminate the undesired component, for example, by saturating its resonance by means of a frequency-selective pulse prior to slice selection.[16]

Gibbs Phenomenon

Another common effect that is artifactual has its cause in the algorithm used for reconstruction. It typically occurs at boundaries characterized by large signal intensity gradients, such as adipose/muscle, brain/cortical bone, and so forth. Such a nearly vertical signal step cannot faithfully be reproduced by the Fourier transform. Instead, the discontinuity is accompanied by a damped oscillation in either direction (Figs. 6–10 and 6–11). The Gibbs phenomenon, as it is sometimes referred to,[17] results in lines of increased (or decreased) intensity parallel to boundaries separating structures of largely differing signal intensities. Such oscillations are most commonly seen in images in which the Fourier transform resolution is higher than the sampling resolution. Figure 6–10A shows a step function profile after sampling and reconstruction via Fourier transform, both at a resolution of 256 data points. An expanded view is shown in Figure 6–10B. As expected, the Gibbs oscillation is at one half of the pixel frequency. Figure 6–11A shows the same step function sampled at a resolution of 128 and Fourier transformed at the resolution of 256. Again, an expanded view is given in Figure 6–11B. Note that the oscillation frequency is one-half that of the previous case. Also, the spatial distance for damping has increased; thus the artifact is more apparent since it extends farther. Because it has a length of 4 pixels per cycle rather than 2 pixels, it is less obscured by noise.

Thus the Gibbs phenomenon is the result of the particular choice of sampling and transform resolution. More samples will tend to suppress its visibility, while filtration of the Fourier amplitudes can also hide it if resolution is sacrificed.

Figure 6–12 illustrates the Gibbs artifact in a head image obtained from 128 views, reconstructed from a 256 point Fourier transform. Note the distinct lines parallel to

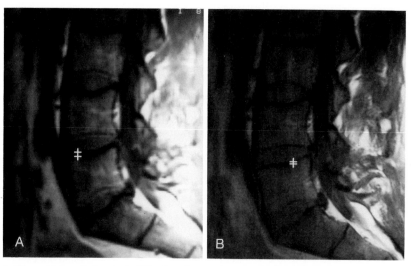

Figure 6–9. Dependence of chemical-shift effect in two images obtained from the same anatomy (sagittal lumbar spine with a FOV of 32 cm [A] and 16 cm [B]). Note the dark lines appearing at the inferior aspect of the vertebral body–disc interface. Measured thickness of the signal void is 2.6 and 1.3 mm, respectively, in good agreement with predictions (2.24 and 1.12 mm).

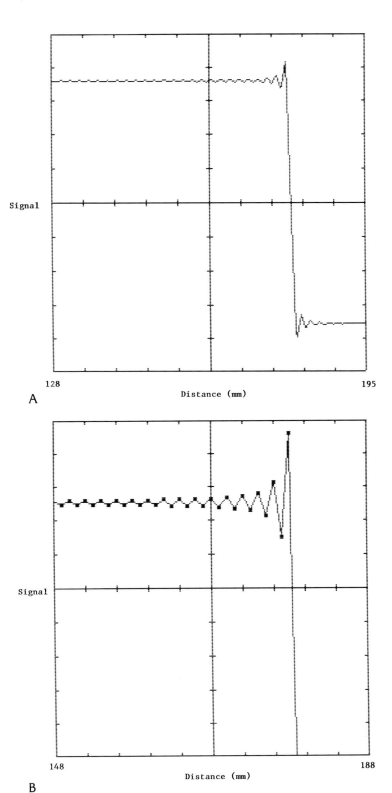

Figure 6–10. *A*, Step function after sampling its Fourier amplitudes with 256 samples and performing a 256 FFT to recover the distorted step function. Continuous curve is from linear interpolation between points. Step amplitude is 10 units, and calculations were scaled for a 100 mm length step in a 256 mm field of view. *B*, Expanded view of *A*, also showing the sample positions resulting from the FFT.

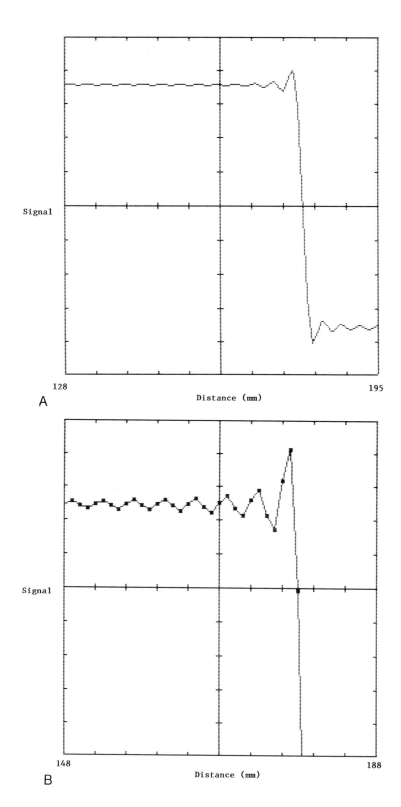

Signal

128   195

A   Distance (mm)

Signal

148   188

B   Distance (mm)

Figure 6–11. *A*, Step function resulting from processing similar to that of Figure 6–10*A* except that the signal amplitudes were sampled at 128 locations only. *B*, Expanded view of *A*, showing the sample locations in the Fourier-transformed signal.

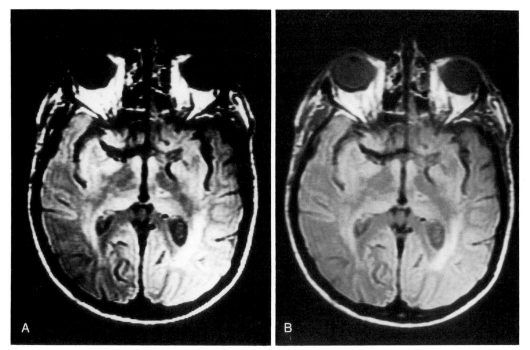

Figure 6–12. Gibbs artifact. Note that the banding at the boundaries of sharp signal drops becomes particularly prominent at narrow window settings. The two images are displayed with window settings of 50(A) and 150(B).

the brain-skull interface, perpendicular to the phase-encoding direction. This artifact is particularly prominent at small window settings (Fig. 6–12A).

ACKNOWLEDGMENTS

The authors are indebted to Ann Shimakawa, General Electric Company, Medical Systems Group, for collecting and analyzing some of the image data, and to Drs. J. Hyde and B. Kneeland for the surface coil images in Figure 6–3. Sue Hallchurch is thanked for the preparation of the manuscript.

References

1. Abragam A: The Principles of Nuclear Magnetism. Oxford, Clarendon Press, 1961.
2. Beall PT, Amtey SR, Kasturi SR: NMR Data Handbook for Biomedical Applications. New York, Pergamon Press, 1984.
3. Edelstein WA, Pfeifer LM, Bottomley PA: A signal-to-noise calibration method for NMR imaging machines. Med Phys *11*:180, 1984.
4. Hoult DI, Lauterbur PC: The sensitivity of the zeugmatographic experiment involving human samples. J Magn Res *34*:425, 1979.
5. Schenck JF, Hart HR Jr, Foster TH, Edelstein WA, Hussain MA: High resolution magnetic resonance imaging using surface coils. *In* Kressel HY (ed): Magnetic Resonance Annual. New York, Raven Press, 1986.
6. Hayes CE, Axel L: Noise performance of surface coils for magnetic resonance imaging at 1.5T. Med Phys *12*:604, 1985.
7. Bottomley PA: NMR imaging techniques and applications: a review. Rev Sci Instr *53*:1319, 1982.
8. Crooks LE, Ortendahl DA, Kaufman L, Hoenninger JC, Arakawa M, Watts J, Cannon CN, Brant-Zawadzki M, Davis PL, Margulis AR: Clinical efficiency of nuclear magnetic resonance imaging. Radiology *146*:123, 1983.
9. Buonanno FS, Pykett IL, Brady TJ, Black P, New PFJ, Richardson EP, Jr., Hinshaw WS, et al: Clinical relevance of two different nuclear magnetic resonance (NMR) approaches to imaging of a low grade astrocytoma. J Comput Assist Tomogr 6:529, 1982.

10. Johnson GA, Thompson MB, Gewalt SL, Hayes CE: Nuclear magnetic resonance at microscopic resolution. J Magn Res 68:129, 1986.
11. Farrar TC, Becker ED: Pulse and Fourier Transform NMR. New York, Academic Press, 1971, Chapter 5.
12. Glover GH: Unpublished work, 1983. See also Bilaniuk LT, Zimmerman RA, Wehrli FW, et al: Cerebral magnetic resonance: A comparison of high and low field strength imaging. Radiology 153:409, 1984.
13. Schenck JR, Foster TH, Henkes JL, Adams WJ, Hayes C, Hart HR, Edelstein WA, Bottomley PA, Wehrli FW: High-field surface coil MR imaging of localized anatomy. Am J Neuroradiol 6:181, 1985.
14. Babcock EE, Brateman L, Weinreb JC, Horner SD, Nunnally RL: Edge artifacts in MR images: chemical shift effect. J Comput Assist Tomogr 9:252, 1985.
15. Dixon WT: Simple proton spectroscopic imaging. Radiology 153:189, 1984.
16. Bottomley PA, Foster TH, Leue WM: In-vivo magnetic resonance chemical shift imaging by selective irradiation. Proc Natl Acad Sci USA 81:6856, 1984.
17. Bracewell RN: The Fourier Transform and Its Applications. New York, McGraw-Hill, 1978.

7

MRI Tissue Characterization

MARK R. MITCHELL
GREG D. SMITH

Although in its infancy, MRI tissue characterization has already demonstrated a potential for improving the accuracy of in vivo tissue typing that is unparalleled in medical imaging. Because MR images are dependent upon a large number of tissue characteristics, including spin density (N), $T1$ and $T2$ relaxation times, flow, diffusion,[1] magnetic susceptibility effects, chemical shift,[2] and a wide variety of contrast agents, the possibility of successful tissue identification with MRI is quite good. Someday it may even provide the long sought "noninvasive biopsy."

This chapter will review the use of $T1$ and $T2$ for in vitro and in vivo tissue identification and introduce the concept of image intensity analysis as an approach to tissue characterization. Tissue maps, called classified images, will also be presented, which demonstrate the use of computer pattern recognition techniques to analyze image intensity characteristics on a set of images created with varying tissue parameter dependence. Computer analysis of image intensity characteristics will be emphasized, as it represents one of the most promising directions for MRI tissue characterization in imaging. Nonimaging MRI techniques for tissue identification will not be discussed.

IN VITRO T1 AND T2 MEASUREMENTS

Since Odeblad started evaluating complex tissues with NMR in the 1950s,[3-8] numerous investigators have tried to determine the relationship between normal and pathologic tissues using a variety of NMR tissue parameters. Damadian and Goldsmith tried to identify neoplastic states for in vitro tissue samples using a "malignancy index" that was based on $T1$ and $T2$ relaxation times.[9-13] A high degree of accuracy was predicted for this approach, but subsequent investigators found that many pathologic processes have overlapping $T1$ and $T2$ characteristics.[14-25] Although these results dampened hopes for using $T1$ and $T2$ as tumor-specific markers, they correctly predicted the high degree of pathologic sensitivity in MR imaging. Bottomley and Beall have written excellent reviews of in vitro $T1$ and $T2$ measurements in normal and pathologic tissues.[26-28] Examples of typical relaxation times for a variety of normal and pathologic tissues of the brain are listed in Table 7–1,[29-32] which illustrates the overlap between different disease states.

The apparent nonspecificity of $T1$ and $T2$ relaxation times is partly due to the fact that many pathologic processes produce edema or an increase in tissue water. The relationship between water content and relaxation times is not simple, however, as evidenced by the inconsistent results in a number of studies comparing water content and relaxation times.[33-38] Koenig demonstrated the effects of complex proteins on the relaxation-enhancing characteristics of a number of paramagnetic agents, postulating

Table 7–1. REPRESENTATIVE *T*1 AND *T*2 VALUES FOR NORMAL AND PATHOLOGIC TISSUES OF THE BRAIN*

Brain Tissue	Frequency (MHz)	*T*1 (ms)	*T*2 (ms)	Reference
In Vitro				
White matter	20	687 ± 95	107 ± 26	28
Gray matter	20	825 ± 59	110 ± 19	28
Tumors				
Glioblastoma	100	1100–1700	90–200	29
Astrocytoma	100	1300–1400	90–130	29
Meningioma	100	1000–1600	70–170	29
Metastasis	100	1300–1500	100–150	29
In Vivo				
White matter	6.3	290 ± 22		30
Gray matter	6.3	365 ± 40		30
Astrocytoma	6.3	546 ± 1048		30
Meningioma	6.3	360 ± 472		30
Neurinoma	6.3	690–785		30
Lipoma	6.3	235–290		30
Ependymoma	6.3	645 ± 70		30
Pituitary				
Adenocarcinoma	6.3	764 ± 180		30
Metastasis				
Renal carcinoma	6.3	605–696		30
White matter	20.9	486 ± 22	69.8 ± 2.1	31
Gray matter	20.9	756 ± 57	82.8 ± 3.2	31
CSF	20.9	2564 ± 349	1996 ± 931	31

* Note the fact that most normal and pathologic states can be differentiated on the basis of their *T*1 and *T*2 values, although there is considerable overlap in the values obtained in different pathologic states. *T*1 and *T*2 values therefore should be sensitive for pathology but rather nonspecific.

that these proteins provide a framework for the agents' interactions with water.[39] Consequently, tissue relaxation times are a function of both the quantity and the state of tissue water. If *T1* and *T2* were dependent only on the quantity of water present in a tissue, they would probably have little value as tissue markers. Their dependence on other tissue characteristics, including the type of proteins present, should increase their potential as tissue-specific markers.

Although in vitro *T1* and *T2* measurements are usually quite precise owing to the number of measurements and signal averages used, the results have still been inconsistent. There are a number of possible reasons for this inconsistency, including variations in hydration, temperature, age of the sample, and field strength.[27,40] Dead tissues also have different *T1*'s than living tissues.[41,42] In addition, some tissues demonstrate nonexponential relaxation curves owing to *T1* and *T2* values in different components of the tissue.[43] These problems make prediction of in vivo imaging results from in vitro *T1* and *T2* measurements extremely difficult and frustrate their use as tissue-specific markers.

IN VIVO EVALUATION OF T1 AND T2

Significant differences between in vitro and in vivo *T1* and *T2* measurements were noted as soon as in vivo evaluation began. *T2* values measured in an imaging system were significantly shorter than those measured in a spectrometer. Differences between spectroscopic and imaging equipment that influence *T1* and *T2* measurements include the size and uniformity of the magnets, inhomogeneities produced by spatially encoding imaging gradients,[1,27,39,44] inaccurate tip angles[45,46] and motion artifacts.[47] The limited

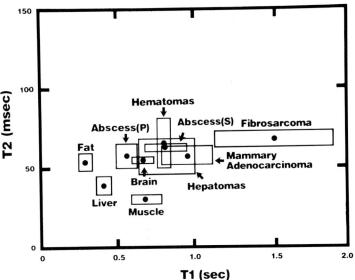

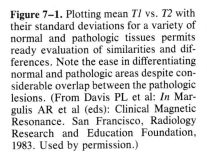

Figure 7–1. Plotting mean *T1* vs. *T2* with their standard deviations for a variety of normal and pathologic tissues permits ready evaluation of similarities and differences. Note the ease in differentiating normal and pathologic areas despite considerable overlap between the pathologic lesions. (From Davis PL et al: *In* Margulis AR et al (eds): Clinical Magnetic Resonance. San Francisco, Radiology Research and Education Foundation, 1983. Used by permission.)

number of measurements and signal averages used for measuring relaxation times in imaging systems also decrease the precision of these measurements.[48–54]

The differences between in vivo and in vitro measurements made acquisition of a good *T1* and *T2* database on an imaging system a necessity before the potential for in vivo tissue characterization could be evaluated. Working toward this goal, Davis evaluated in vivo relaxation measurements by plotting normal and pathologic relaxation times on a graph of *T1* vs *T2* (Fig. 7–1). He concluded that many normal and pathologic processes could be differentiated on the basis of *T1* and *T2* values, but that overlap between many of the lesions studied precluded accurate identification of the pathology on that basis alone. *T1* and *T2* seem to provide sensitivity but to lack the desired specificity.[28–31,55–60]

Although improved methods for measuring in vivo *T1* and *T2* values[61–64] may solve some of these problems, current information suggests that *T1* and *T2* measurements alone will not provide the necessary specificity for tissue characterization. Fortunately, images can be created with information that can be added to basic relaxation data to improve MRI's ability to differentiate tissues.

IMAGE INTENSITY ANALYSIS

MR images can be created so that their intensity is dependent on one or more tissue parameters. Generally, an image has a mixture of *N*, *T1*, and *T2* weighting as described in Chapters 3, 6, and 74. Images can also be generated with a dependence on flow, chemical shift, and possibly diffusion.

Direct analysis of relative image intensity on a variety of images with differing tissue parameter dependence offers an approach to tissue characterization that takes into account the influence of all contributing tissue parameters; it also avoids some of the technical difficulties involved in measuring actual tissue parameters. Image intensity analysis can be performed subjectively or with the aid of a computer. In its simplest form, the MRI practitioner compares the intensity characteristics of suspected pathologic areas with known normal and pathologic tissues within the images; tissues with similar intensities on a variety of images are assumed to represent similar normal or pathologic tissue, whereas those that vary are considered different.

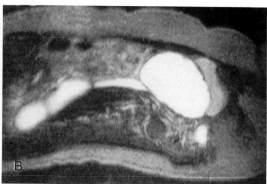

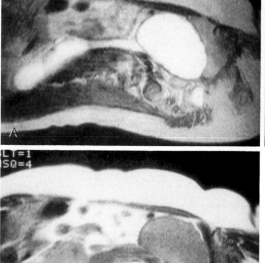

Figure 7–2. Sagittal spin-echo pulse sequences (*A*, 60/2000, *B*, 120/2000, *C*, 30/500) obtained in a patient with a pelvic mass. A communication between the mass and a hydronephrotic ureter can be diagnosed using subjective image-intensity analysis by noting the similarity in intensity between the mass and the dilated ureter in all the images. Note also the difference in intensity between the fluid in the dilated ureter and the bladder.

In a patient with a known pelvic mass (Fig. 7–2), subjective image intensity analysis made it possible to diagnose an unsuspected communication between the cystic mass and a dilated left ureter. On ultrasound examination the dilated ureter was thought to be due to compression of the ureter by the mass because of the clear sonolucent character of the fluid in the collecting system. Careful examination of the MR images disproved this impression by demonstrating that the mass and the ureter had identical image intensity characteristics on images created with a variety of pulse sequences; the fluid in the ureter was also dissimilar when compared with the urine in the opposite collecting system and the bladder. From this, it was concluded that there must be a communication between the mass and ureter; this was confirmed at surgery.

An additional example of this kind of analysis can be seen in Figure 7–3, in a patient with a mucinous cystadenocarcinoma in the pelvis. On some of the images it is impossible to differentiate the uterus from cystic components in the tumor; in other images the uterus and tumor can be easily separated. On all the images the uterus retains an intensity similar to normal muscle, indicating its lack of gross invasion. An endocervical polyp can also be differentiated from the normal uterine cervix by its dissimilar intensity on some of the images. In contrast, note the involvement of the uterine fundus (Fig. 7–4) in a patient with invasion of the uterus by an ovarian cystadenocarcinoma. Although the intensity of the invaded uterus is not the same as the main tumor mass on all the images, it is obviously different from the normal skeletal muscle, which is more typical of normal uterine muscle. The invaded uterus also has pockets of involvement with characteristics very similar to parts of the pelvic mass.

A final example of subjective intensity analysis is shown in Figure 7–5. A glioma had been removed from this patient's left frontal cortex four years previously. On a set of eight multiecho images and a single short *TR* spin-echo image, recurrence of the tumor can be excluded by noting that the intensity in the surgical site is consistently

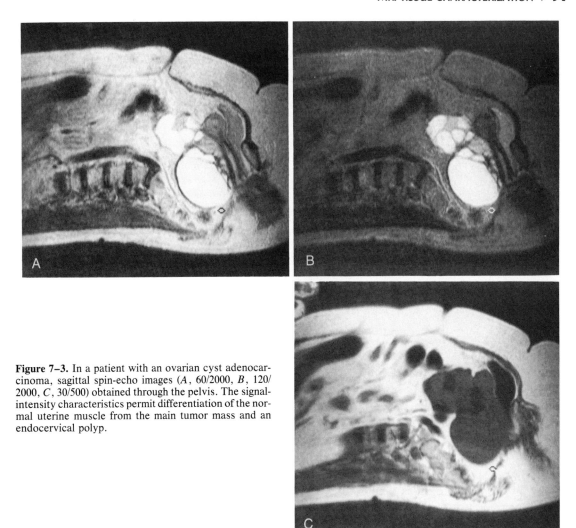

Figure 7-3. In a patient with an ovarian cyst adenocarcinoma, sagittal spin-echo images (*A*, 60/2000, *B*, 120/2000, *C*, 30/500) obtained through the pelvis. The signal-intensity characteristics permit differentiation of the normal uterine muscle from the main tumor mass and an endocervical polyp.

the same as that of ventricular or subarachnoid CSF; this identifies the area as a region of postoperative porencephaly. On some images, periventricular white-matter disease can be identified around the anterior horn of the right lateral ventricle by its unique intensity characteristics. It should be noted that each image in this set permits different comparisons and that many of the images fail to differentiate some of the normal and pathologic tissues; the proper diagnostic conclusion can be drawn only after integrating the findings on all the images.

The process of creating a database of relative image intensity characteristics for particular lesions is just beginning. Only two pulse sequences are generally used, usually designated *T1* or *T2* weighted. Unfortunately, there is little or no standardization in this nomenclature; sequences as diverse as SE 40/1500 and SE 150/3000 have been called *T2* weighted, while *T1* weighted sequences could be PS 200, IR 700/1500, or anything from ISE 200/30/1500 to ISE 700/15/3000, or from SE 15/250 to SE 40/700. In spite of these limitations, several examples of this work will be cited, as it demonstrates the value of MR image intensity analysis.

Using an eight echo volume acquisition with a *TR* of 800 ms, Harms attempts differentiation of high- and low-grade gliomas and edema based on how early the process shows up on the increasingly *T2* weighted images as the *TE* is lengthened from 30 ms

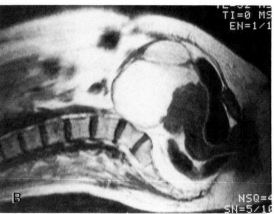

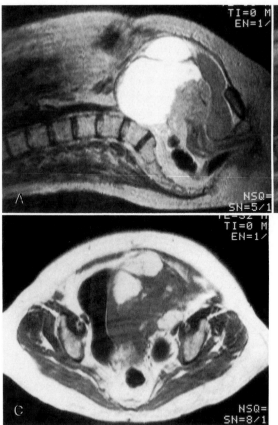

Figure 7–4. In another patient with cystic ovarian adenocarcinoma, a set of spin-echo images (*A*, sagittal 60/2000, *B*, sagittal 32/500, *C*, transverse 32/500) obtained through the pelvis. The image-intensity characteristics indicate invasion of the uterus by the tumor. Note that this is demonstrated only on some of the images.

to 240 ms. It was observed that low-grade tumors and edema become intense with shorter echo times than do the high-grade tumors. The explanation given is that high-grade tumors have a longer *T1* that suppresses the effects of a long *T2* on the images with shorter echo times and therefore less *T2* weighting.[65]

Louis evaluated the image intensity characteristics of lesions producing leukokoria. He differentiates retinoblastoma, Coats' disease, *Toxocara* endophthalmitis, and subretinal hemorrhage on the basis of their intensity, using characteristics on SE 30/500 and SE 90/2000 images without *N, T1,* or *T2* measurements. Retinoblastoma has low intensity on both images. Coats' disease and *Toxocara* endophthalmitis appear moderately intense on the SE 30/500 image, but Coats' disease is "bright" and *Toxocara* endophthalmitis is "very bright" on the SE 90/2000 image. Although subretinal hemorrhage is also "very bright" on the SE 90/2000 image, it can be differentiated from the other entities by the fact that it is also "bright" on the SE 30/500 image.[66]

Subjective tissue characterization based on clinical experience with image intensity variations will continue to develop slowly and methodically, but it will be difficult for the practicing radiologist to acquire this skill because of the diversity of imaging sequences and instrumentation reported in the literature. Fortunately, quantitative evaluation of image intensity can be performed easily using computer techniques originally developed for satellite image processing.

AUTOMATED MRI TISSUE CHARACTERIZATION

The use of sophisticated computing routines for evaluation of MR image intensity characteristics was first demonstrated by Vannier, who formatted MR images so that

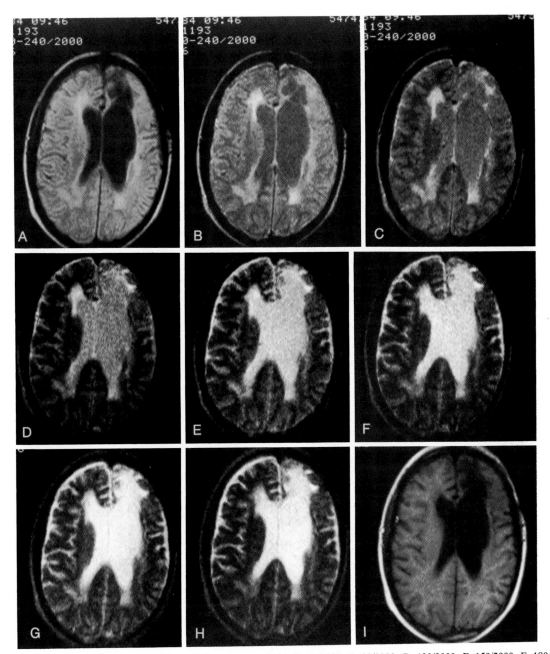

Figure 7–5. Nine transverse spin-echo MR images (*A*, 30/2000, *B*, 60/2000, *C*, 90/2000, *D*, 120/2000, *E*, 150/2000, *F*, 180/2000, *G*, 210/2000, *H*, 240/2000, *I*, 30/300) in a patient four years after removal of a left frontal glioma demonstrate the varied image-intensity characteristics that can be obtained using single spin-echo and multiecho techniques. By visually analyzing the image intensities in all nine images one can exclude tumor recurrence and diagnose porencephaly in the region of the previous tumor by noting that the intensity in the surgical site is always similar to the ventricular or subarachnoid CSF.

they could be analyzed on the NASA LANDSAT satellite image processing system.[67] This work demonstrated that the varied tissue parameter dependence in MR images can be used to identify tissues, with multispectral image processing techniques.[68–71]

The authors have written highly specialized computer programs designed specifically for analysis of MR image intensity data. The programs, based on pattern recognition techniques, have been used to generate the "classified" images presented here. Tissue "signatures" are developed in an interactive fashion from a group of images called a training set. Following training, the computer compares each pixel in similar sets of images with unknown pathology with the "signatures" to determine the identity of each pixel. Each pixel is assigned a gray-scale level or color that has been selected by the operator to indicate a specific tissue or lesion. By assigning an identity to each pixel in the image, the computer generates a "classified" image that combines the discriminatory information on all the images into a single synthetic image.

Determining the optimal input images is critical. An ideal set of images should sample all the desired tissue parameters in a clinically reasonable amount of time. Criteria for selecting the input images are currently being developed. The input images used to create the classified images presented here include an SE 30/300 image and eight multiecho images with TE's from 30 to 240 ms and a TR of 2000 ms. These images were selected because of the speed with which they could be acquired in a clinical setting and because of their diversity of tissue parameter dependence. They are used only for illustration of the technique and not to represent the ideal set of input images.

Graphing the mean image intensity and standard deviation (Fig. 7–6) for the normal and pathologic tissues seen in Figure 7–5 demonstrates the overlap between tissues on many of the images. Each image permits discrimination of different tissues; none of the original images provides enough information to identify all the tissues. Therefore,

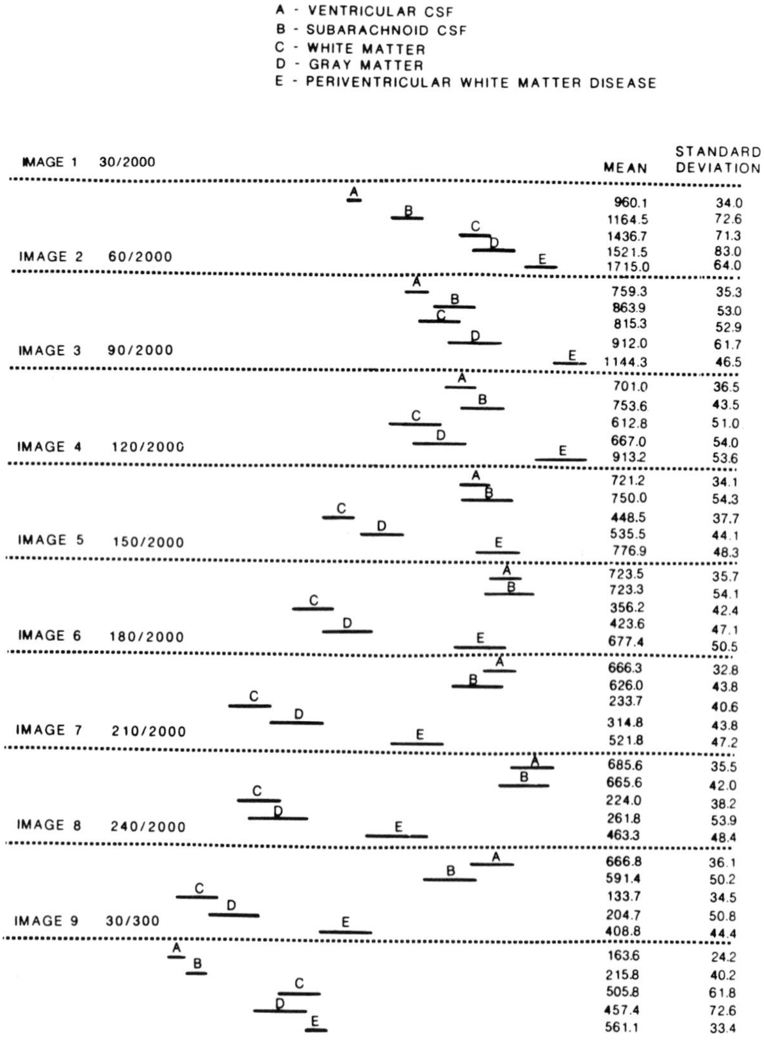

A - VENTRICULAR CSF
B - SUBARACHNOID CSF
C - WHITE MATTER
D - GRAY MATTER
E - PERIVENTRICULAR WHITE MATTER DISEASE

	MEAN	STANDARD DEVIATION
IMAGE 1 30/2000		
A	960.1	34.0
B	1164.5	72.6
C	1436.7	71.3
D	1521.5	83.0
E	1715.0	64.0
IMAGE 2 60/2000		
A	759.3	35.3
B	863.9	53.0
C	815.3	52.9
D	912.0	61.7
E	1144.3	46.5
IMAGE 3 90/2000		
A	701.0	36.5
B	753.6	43.5
C	612.8	51.0
D	667.0	54.0
E	913.2	53.6
IMAGE 4 120/2000		
A	721.2	34.1
B	750.0	54.3
C	448.5	37.7
D	535.5	44.1
E	776.9	48.3
IMAGE 5 150/2000		
A	723.5	35.7
B	723.3	54.1
C	356.2	42.4
D	423.6	47.1
E	677.4	50.5
IMAGE 6 180/2000		
A	666.3	32.8
B	626.0	43.8
C	233.7	40.6
D	314.8	43.8
E	521.8	47.2
IMAGE 7 210/2000		
A	685.6	35.5
B	665.6	42.0
C	224.0	38.2
D	261.8	53.9
E	463.3	48.4
IMAGE 8 240/2000		
A	666.8	36.1
B	591.4	50.2
C	133.7	34.5
D	204.7	50.8
E	408.8	44.4
IMAGE 9 30/300		
A	163.6	24.2
B	215.8	40.2
C	505.8	61.8
D	457.4	72.6
E	561.1	33.4

Figure 7–6. Plotting the mean image intensity and standard deviations for the normal and pathologic tissues seen in Figure 7–5 demonstrates the fact that some of the images readily differentiate some tissues whereas others do not. One must therefore integrate the findings on all the images to get the best idea about the identity of each tissue.

maximum tissue discrimination is possible only when multiple images with varied tissue parameter dependence are used in a synergistic fashion to develop a visual or mathematical identity for each tissue.

By using a computer to analyze these relationships, the information on multiple images can be condensed into a single image, freeing the radiologist from the arduous task of analyzing and comparing intensity changes on numerous images. Thus, the physician can concentrate on correlating anatomic and clinical information with the summated intensity data to arrive at a clinical assessment.

Looking into the future, the computer's job could be broken down into two parts. First, it should determine which pixels have "abnormal" signal intensity characteristics, i.e., those that do not match any of the normal tissues in the computer's data bank. Next the computer could compare the "abnormal" areas with the signatures developed in a group of patients with pathologically proven lesions to determine whether the "lesion" is similar to any of the pathologic entities previously presented to the computer. A list of possible matches could be generated in the order of their likelihood, based on how closely the intensity characteristics in the unknown match the known lesions. The radiologist could then compare this list with the clinical history and anatomic location of the lesion to determine the most likely diagnosis.

Although the full capabilities described above have not been realized, they are not unrealistic. Several examples of classified images have been included here to demonstrate the remarkable ability of the computer to recognize tissues on the basis of their intensity characteristics without the aid of the anatomic information on which the radiologist must rely. Unlike the ideal situation described above, the computer was trained for these examples on parts of the same images used for classification.

The images in Figure 7–5 were used to create a single classified image that combines the intensity information on all the images into a single synthetic image (Fig. 7–7). In this classified image the computer has identified ventricular and subarachnoid CSF in the region of the previous surgery, indicating the presence of postoperative

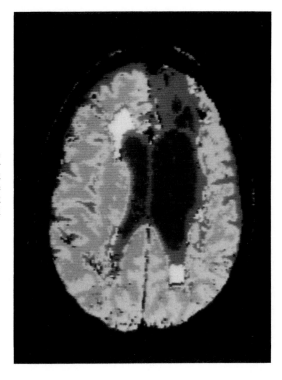

Figure 7–7. Using computer pattern-recognition techniques, all the information in the images in Figure 7–5 can be compressed into a single classified image. On this image one can diagnose the presence of postsurgical porencephaly and the absence of tumor recurrence with considerably less effort than that required to examine and compare all the original images.

porencephaly. Examination of a single classified image therefore permits the same conclusion as visual analysis of all nine original images.

In a classified image the operator can chose the signatures used and the gray level assigned to each tissue. In the images presented here, black was used to indicate the absence of a signature match; therefore, black pixels had intensity characteristics that were unlike any of the tissue signatures being used for classification. Air was given a gray-scale level slightly higher than that of the nonclassified pixels. In general, it is difficult to discriminate between more than five to seven discrete gray levels on a single image; therefore, muscle, scalp, and marrow signatures were not used, leaving these regions unmatched and black, so that the usable gray levels could be assigned to the intracranial structures that were of primary interest.

Since the assignment of a gray level for a particular tissue or pathology is under complete user control, the gray scale can be selected to highlight any features desired. One can produce an image in which all the normal tissues are represented by varying shades of gray, while all pathologic processes or unidentified areas are indicated by white; this highlights the pathology without distinguishing different types of lesions. A complementary image can be created using different gray levels for different pathologic entities to provide further discrimination.

In Figure 7–8 the left half of the image is one of the original source images, and the right half is a classified image with the intensity of each pixel assigned by the computer on the basis of the information in all nine original images. Note the excellent differentiation of normal tissues in this normal volunteer.

In a patient with a cystic brain tumor with surrounding edema (Fig. 7–9), one can again appreciate the superb differentiation of tissues in the classified image. A thin rim of tumor, the cystic center of the tumor, and the surrounding edema can all be easily distinguished from each other and from the surrounding normal tissues. On this classified image a small area of edema was identified in the occipital white matter of the opposite hemisphere that was not appreciated on the original images except in retrospect.

The marriage of computer and practitioner described here promises to be a highly effective means for improving tissue specificity in MRI. The image intensity charac-

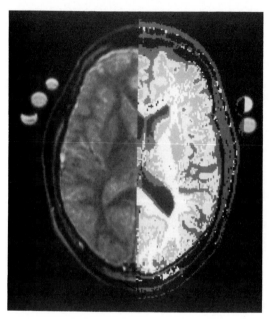

Figure 7–8. An image in a normal volunteer demonstrates the difference between one of the nine original images on the left and the computer-generated classified image on the right.

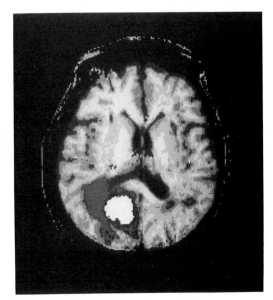

Figure 7–9. A classified image in a patient with a cystic tumor and edema differentiates the cystic portion of the lesion and edema from all the normal tissues.

teristics that are intuitively difficult for the radiologist are the natural domain of the computer, while the anatomic and pathologic knowledge of the radiologist is extremely difficult to model in a computer. Although clinical history, laboratory data, physical findings, and even spacial analysis could be incorporated into the computer analysis, the database and computing power needed to do this will probably be years in coming.

Some of the advantages of direct image intensity analysis are as follows. (1) It can be performed subjectively or by a computer. (2) It avoids some of the problems associated with calculating $T1$ and $T2$ by taking systematic errors into account, since the same systematic inaccuracies should exist in the training set and the unknowns. (3) It includes all tissue parameters that contribute to differences in intensity, both known and unknown. This includes N, flow, diffusion, magnetic susceptibility, and organ perfusion, since anything that causes a consistent difference in intensity will be used in developing the tissue signatures. (4) Computer classification permits the addition of information to the database from any new development in MRI that can be used to produce images; such sources include diffusion images,[72] selective saturation images,[73] chemical shift images, phosphorus or sodium images, spectroscopic images,[2] and images created after injection of contrast agents. The computer simply categorizes the patterns presented to it and looks for them in the future.

Although the computer programs for classification are quite sophisticated, they can never be any better than the database on which the predictions are made. This database must be developed on an appropriate set of images that adequately sample the full range of tissue characteristics in a large number of normal and pathologic cases. The database must also take into account the normal variation in tissues from patient to patient, including such factors as age. Fetal tissue, for instance, has longer relaxation times than adult tissue[43]; body water content also decreases by approximately 2.5 percent per decade from age 40 to 70 years.[74]

There are a number of problems that must be overcome before signatures developed on training sets can be applied in a general fashion to unknown cases. Although the relative intensity between tissues remains the same, actual image intensity varies from day to day and scan to scan even in the same patient.[75] This is only a minor problem for subjective image intensity analysis, since "windowing" can be used to compensate for most of this variation. It is a major problem for computer analysis, since the computer uses measured image intensity for one of its identification parameters and a correction must be made for this variation. The use of internal reference standards is one approach to this problem that is currently being studied by the authors. Inhomogeneity within the images is another problem that must be solved, since variations in intensity in the same tissue located in a different part of the image will decrease the likelihood of correct classification.

In conclusion, although the sensitivity of magnetic resonance imaging is well recognized, its potential tissue characterization is still being explored.

Work using in vitro and in vivo *T1* and *T2* measurements has generally supported the idea that MRI is sensitive to pathology but rather nonspecific. Fortunately, other tissue characteristics are available that can be used to add specificity to the characterization process; these include spin density, diffusion, selective saturation, simple spectroscopic imaging techniques, contrast agents, and evaluation of other nuclei. The use of images with dependence on these tissue characteristics in MRI tissue characterization should dramatically increase MRI's specificity.

Direct visual analysis of image intensity information on a variety of MR images avoids some of the methodological difficulties associated with *T1* and *T2* calculations and utilizes all the parameters that influence the image. Unfortunately, this kind of subjective analysis is difficult and time-consuming and requires a great deal of experience.

Fortunately, however, there is an alternative to subjective intensity analysis. Computer pattern recognition techniques can be used to perform the intensity analysis, compressing the unique characteristics in multiple images into a single "classified" image, with discrete gray levels used to represent recognized normal and pathologic regions. This frees the MRI practitioner to integrate the clinical history and anatomy into the final impression. As mentioned earlier, this form of computer analysis may even provide the "noninvasive biopsy" of the future.

References

1. Wesby GE, Moseley MRE, Ehman RL: Translational molecular self-diffusion in magnetic imaging. I. Effects on observed spin-spin relaxation. Invest Radiol *19*:484, 1984.
2. Dixon WT: Simple proton spectroscopic imaging. Radiology *153*:189, 1984.
3. Huggert A, Odeblad E: Proton magnetic resonance studies of some tissues and fluids of the eye. Acta Radiol *51*:385, 1958.
4. Odeblad E: Studies on vaginal contents and cells with proton magnetic resonance. Ann NY Acad Sci *82*:189, 1959.
5. Odeblad E, Bahr BN, Lindstrom G: Proton magnetic resonance of human red blood cells in heavy-water exchange experiments. Arch Biochem Biophys *63*:221, 1956.
6. Odeblad E, Ryhn U: Proton magnetic resonance of human cervical mucus during the menstrual cycle. Acta Radiol *47*:315, 1957.
7. Odeblad E, Westin B: Some preliminary observances on the PMR in biologic samples. Acta Radiol *43*:469, 1955.
8. Odeblad E, Westin B: Proton magnetic resonance of human milk. Acta Radiol *49*:389, 1958.
9. Damadian R, Zaner K, Hor D, et al: Human tumors detected by NMR. Proc Natl Acad Sci USA *71*:1471, 1974.
10. Damadian R, Zaner K, Hor D: Human tumors by NMR. Physiol Chem Phys *5*:381, 1973.
11. Goldsmith M, Koutcher JA, Damadian R: NMR in cancer. XIII. Application of the NMR malignancy index to human mammary tumours. Br J Cancer *38*:547, 1978.
12. Goldsmith M, Koutcher J, Damadian R: Application of the NMR malignancy index to human gastrointestinal tumors. Cancer *41*:183, 1978.
13. Goldsmith M, Koutcher JA, Damadian R: Nuclear magnetic resonance in cancer. XII. Application of NMR malignancy index to human lung tumours. Br J Cancer *36*:235, 1977.
14. Medina D, Hazlewood CF, Cleveland G, et al: NMR studies on human breast dysplasias and neoplasms. J Natl Cancer Inst *54*:813, 1975.
15. Eggleston JC, Saryan LA, Czeisler JL, et al: NMR studies of several experimental and human malignant tumors. Cancer Res *33*:2156, 1973.

16. Weisman ID, Bennett LH, Maxwell LR, et al: Recognition of cancer in vitro by NMR. Science *178*:1288, 1972.
17. Hollis DP, Saryan LA, Eggleston JC, et al: NMR studies of cancer. J. Natl Cancer Inst *54*:1469, 1975.
18. Barriolhet LE, Moran PR: NMR relaxation spectroscopy in tissues. Med Phys *2*:191, 1975.
19. Hollis DP, Economou JS, Parks LC, et al: Nuclear magnetic resonance studies of several experimental human malignant tumors. Cancer Res *33*:2156, 1973.
20. Hazlewood CF, Chang DC, Medina D, Cleveland G, Nichols BL: Distinction between the preneoplastic and neoplastic state of murine mammary glands. Proc Natl Acad Sci *69*(6):1478, 1972.
21. Hazlewood CF, Cleveland G, Medina D: Relationship between hydration and proton nuclear magnetic resonance relaxation times in tissues of tumor-bearing and non–tumor-bearing mice: Implications for cancer detection. J Natl Cancer Inst *52*(6):1849, 1974.
22. Hollis DP, Economou JS, Parks LC, Eggleston JD, Saryan LA, Czeisler JL: Nuclear magnetic resonance studies of several experimental and human malignant tumors. Cancer Res *33*:2156, 1973.
23. Parrish RG, Kurland RJ, Janese WW, Bakay L: Proton relaxation rates of water in brain and brain tumors. Science *183*:438, 1974.
24. Beall PT, Asch BB, Chang DC, Medina D, Hazlewood CF: Distinction of normal, preneoplastic, and neoplastic mouse mammary primary cell cultures by water nuclear magnetic resonance relaxation times. J Natl Cancer Inst *64*(2):335, 1980.
25. Beall PT, Asch BB, Medina C, Hazlewood C: Distinction of normal, preneoplastic, and neoplastic mouse mammary cells and tissues by nuclear magnetic resonance techniques. Cameron IL, Pool TB (eds): The Transformed Cell. New York, Academic Press, 1981, pp 293–325.
26. Beall PT, Hazlewood CF: Distinction of normal, preneoplastic, and neoplastic states by water proton NMR relaxation times. *In* Partain CL, James AE Jr, Rollo FD, Price RR (eds): Nuclear Magnetic Resonance (NMR) Imaging. Philadelphia, WB Saunders, 1983, pp 312–338.
27. Bottomley PA, Foster TH, Argersinger RE, Pfeifer LM: A Review of Normal Tissue Hydrogen NMR Relaxation Times and Relaxation Mechanisms From 1–100 MHz: Dependence on Tissue Type, NMR Frequency, Temperature, Species, Excision, and Age. Report No. 84CRD072. Schenectady, New York, General Electric Company, 1984.
28. Beall PT, Amtey SR, Kasturi SR: Data Handbook for Biomedical Applications. New York, Pergamon Press, 1984.
29. Ngo FQH, Glassner BJ, Bay JW, Dudley AW, Neaney TF: T1 and T2 relaxation measurements of human brain tissues and NMR imaging optimizations. Proc SMRM, San Francisco, 1983, p 264.
30. Naruse S, Horikawa Y, Tanaka C, Hirakawa K, Nishikawa H, Shimizu K, Kiri M: Fundamental interpretation of NMR-CT image: Comparison of relaxation time in-vitro and NMR-CT image. Proc SMRM, San Francisco, 1983, p 252.
31. Araki T, Inouye T, Matozaki T, Iio M: In vivo T1 measurement of brain tumors by NMR-CT. Proc SMRM, San Francisco, 1983, p 3.
32. Conturo TE, Mitchell MR, Price RR, Beth AH, Partain CL, James AE Jr: Improved determination of spin density, T1, and T2 from three-parameter fit to multiple delay–multiple echo (MDME) NMR images. Phys Med Biol *31*(12):1361, 1986.
33. Hazlewood CF, Cleveland G, Medina D: Relationship between hydration and proton NMR relaxation times in tissues of tumor bearing and non–tumor bearing mice. J Natl Cancer Inst *52*:1844, 1974.
34. Inch WR, McCredie JA, Knispel RR, et al: Water content and proton spin relaxation times for malignant and non-malignant tissues from mice and humans. J Natl Cancer Inst *52*:353, 1974.
35. Ranade SS, Sha S, Korgaonkar KS, et al: Absence of correlation between spin-lattice relaxation times and water content in human tumor tissues. Physiol Chem Phys *8*:131, 1976.
36. Ling GN, Tucker M: Nuclear magnetic resonance relaxation and water contents in normal mouse and rat tissues and in cancer cells. J Natl Cancer Inst *64*:1199, 1980.
37. Hazlewood CF: Water content and proton spin relaxation time for malignant and nonmalignant tissues from mice and humans. J Natl Cancer Inst *52*:625, 1974.
38. Ranade SS, Shah S, Korgaonkar KS, Kasturi SR, Chaughule RS, Vijayaraghavan R: Absence of correlation between spin-lattice relaxation times and water content in human tumor tissues. Physiol Chem Phys *8*:313, 1976.
39. Koenig SH, Brown RD, Adams D, Emerson D, Harrison CG: Magnetic field dependence of 1/T1 of protons in tissue. Invest Radiol *19*(2):76, 1984.
40. Thickman DI, Kundel HL, Wolf G: Nuclear magnetic resonance characteristics of fresh and fixed tissue: The effect of elapsed time. Radiology *148*(1):183, 1983.
41. Gore JC, Doyle FH, Pennock JM: Relaxation rate enhancement observed in vivo by NMR imaging. *In* Partain CL, James AE Jr, Rollo FD, Price RR (eds): Nuclear Magnetic Resonance (NMR) Imaging. Philadelphia, WB Saunders, 1983, pp 94–106.
42. Ling CR, Foster MA: Changes in NMR relaxation time associated with local inflammatory response. Phys Med Biol *27*(6):853, 1982.
43. Kasturi SR, Ranade SS, Shah SS: Tissue hydration of malignant and uninvolved human tissues and its relevance to proton spin-lattice relaxation mechanism. Proc Indian Acad Sci *84B*(2):60, 1976.
44. Hart HR, Bottomley PA, Edelstein WA, et al: Nuclear magnetic resonance imaging: Contrast to noise ratio as a function of strength of magnetic field. Am J Roentgenol *141*:1195, 1983.
45. Joseph PM, Axel L, O'Donnell M: Potential problems with selective pulses in NMR imaging systems. Med Phys *11*(6):772, 1984.
46. Rosen BR, Pykett IL, Brady TJ: Spin lattice relaxation time measurements in two-dimensional nuclear

magnetic resonance imaging: Corrections for plane selection and pulse sequence. J Comput Assist Tomogr 8:195, 1984.

47. Ehman RL, McNamara MT, Brasch RC, Hricak H, Higgins CB: Effect of motion on relaxation times in magnetic resonance imaging. Third Annual Meeting of Society of Magnetic Resonance, New York, August 1984, pp 208–209.

48. Davis PL, Kaufman L, Crooks LE: Tissue characterization. In Margulis AR, Higgins CB, Kaufman L, et al (eds): Clinical Magnetic Resonance. Chapter 6. San Francisco, Radiology Research and Education Foundation, 1983.

49. Ortendahl DA, Hylton N, Kaufman L, Watts JC, Crooks LE, Mills CM, Stark DD: Analytical tools for magnetic resonance imaging. Radiology 153:479, 1984.

50. Diegel JG, Pintar MM: Origin of the nonexponentiality of the water proton spin relaxations in tissues. Biophys J 15:855, 1975.

51. Pykett IL, Rosen BR, Buonanno FS, Brady TJ: Measurement of spin-lattice relaxation times in nuclear magnetic resonance imaging. Phys Med Biol 28:723, 1983.

52. Redpath TW: Calibration of the Aberdeen NMR imager for proton spin-lattice relaxation time measurements in-vivo. Phys Med Biol 27:1057, 1982.

53. Vold RL, Waugh JS, Klein MP, Phelps DE: Measurement of spin relaxation in complex systems. J Chem Phys 48:3831, 1968.

54. Freeman R, Hill HDW: Fourier transform study of NMR spin-lattice relaxation by progressive saturation. J Chem Phys 54:3367, 1971.

55. Araki T, Inouye T, Matozaki T, Iio M: In vivo T1 measurement of brain tumors by NMR-CT. Second Annual Meeting of Society of Magnetic Resonance in Medicine, San Francisco, August 1983, pp 3–4.

56. Davis PL, Kaufman L, Crooks LE, Margulis AR: NMR characteristics of normal and abnormal rats. In Kaufman L, Crooks LE, Margulis AR (eds): Nuclear Magnetic Resonance Imaging in Medicine. New York, Igaku-Shoin, 1981, pp 71–100.

57. Davis PL, Sheldon P, Kaufman L, Crooks LE, Margulis AR, Miller J, Watts J, Arakawa M, Hoenninger J: Nuclear magnetic resonance imaging of mammary adenocarcinomas in the rat. Cancer 51:433, 1983.

58. Herfkens RJ, Davis PL, Crooks LE, Kaufman L, Price D, Miller T, Margulis AR, Watts J, Hoenninger J, Arakawa M, McRee R: Nuclear magnetic resonance imaging of the abnormal live rat and correlations with tissue characteristics. Radiology 141:211, 1981.

59. Herfkens RJ, Sievers R, Kaufman L, Sheldon PE, Ortendahl DA, Lipton MJ, Crooks LE, Higgens CB: Nuclear magnetic resonance imaging of the infarcted muscle: a rat model. Radiology 147:749, 1983.

60. Hutchison JMS, Smith FW: NMR clinical results: Aberdeen. In Partain CL, James AE Jr, Rollo FD, Price RR (eds): Nuclear Magnetic Resonance (NMR) Imaging. Philadelphia, WB Saunders, 1983, pp 231–249.

61. Conturo TC, Mitchell MR, Price RR, Partain CL, James AE: Simultaneous calculation of spin density, T1 and T2 from multiecho MRI data. Paper presented at 33rd Annual Meeting of Association of University Radiologists, Nashville, May 1985.

62. Conturo TC, Mitchell MR, Partain CL, James AE: Dependence of signal intensity on T1 and T2 in the multiecho MRI pulse sequence. Exhibit at 33rd Annual Meeting of Association of University Radiologists, May 1985.

63. Conturo TE, Price RR, Beth AH, Mitchell MR, Partain CL, James AE: Improved determination of spin density, T1 and T2 from a three-parameter fit to multiple delay–multiple echo (MDME) NMR images. Physics Med Biol 31(12):1361, 1986.

64. Schneiders NJ, Ford JJ, Bryan RN: Accurate T1 and spin density NMR images. Med Phys 12(1):71, 1985.

65. Harms SE: Three-dimensional multiple spin-echo MR imaging of intracranial tumors. Radiology 153(P):86, 1984.

66. Louis LS, Haik BG, Albert AB, Cahill P, Zimmerman RD, Lee BCP, Deck MDF: Magnetic resonance imaging in leukocoria. Exhibit at 1984 RSNA, Washington, DC, Nov 1984.

67. Vannier MW, Butterfield RL, Jordan D, Murphy WA, Levitt RG, Gado M: Technical developments and instrument: multispectral analysis of magnetic resonance images. Radiology 154:221, 1985.

68. Anderberg MR: Cluster Analysis for Applications. New York, Academic Press, 1973.

69. Tou JT, Gonzalez RC: Pattern Recognition Principles. Reading, Mass, Addison-Wesley Publishing Co, 1974.

70. Lillesand TM, Keifer RW: Remote Sensing and Image Interpretation. New York, John Wiley & Sons, 1979.

71. Duda RO, Hart PE: Pattern Classification and Scene Analysis. New York, John Wiley & Sons, 1973.

72. Wesby G, Mosely M, Hrovat M, Ehman R: Measurement of translational molecular self-diffusion in proton magnetic resonance imaging (MRI). Third Annual Meeting of Society of Magnetic Resonance in Medicine, New York, August 1984, pp 751–752.

73. Rosen BR, Wedeen VJ, Brady TJ: Selective saturation NMR imaging. J Comput Assist Tomogr 8(5):813, 1984.

74. Mansfield P, Morris PG: NMR Imaging in Biomedicine. New York, Academic Press, 1982, pp 10–32.

75. Ehman RL, Kjos BO, Hricak H, Brasch RC, Higgins CB: Relative intensity of abdominal organs in MR images. J Comput Assist Tomogr 9(2):315, 1985.

8

MRI Optimization Strategies

MARK R. MITCHELL
ALAN EISENBERG
THOMAS E. CONTURO
ROBERT W. TARR
THEODORE FALKE

Selecting the best MRI pulse sequence and timing intervals in a clinical setting is by no means a trivial task. The large number of MRI pulse sequences available, e.g., inversion recovery, spin echo, and partial saturation, each with a large number of possible timing interval combinations, has created a situation in which the options seem overwhelming. Consequently, a variety of computer modeling techniques have been developed to help the MRI practitioner choose appropriate pulse sequences and timing intervals for the problem at hand. This chapter will review several of the optimization strategies that have been proposed, examining their strengths and weaknesses and summarizing their recommendations. Guidelines for implementing these strategies will then be presented.

All of the optimization strategies presented are based on predictions made using mathematical models that describe image pixel intensity (I) as a function of the MRI tissue parameters N (spin density), $T1$, and $T2$, and the pulse sequence timing intervals TI, TE, and TR. Each model generates performance criteria that can be used to compare different pulse sequences and predict the "best" combinations of timing intervals for examining or differentiating specific tissues of clinical interest.

The emphasis in these models has been on developing techniques with maximal sensitivity to subtle pathology. These models do not attempt or claim to optimize the technique for maximal tissue specificity; Chapters 6 to 9 and 63 to 68 on MRI tissue characterization address the quest for increased specificity in MRI.

PULSE SEQUENCE MODELS

Seven models for MRI pulse sequence optimization have been reviewed, including (1) difference plots, (2) contrast-to-noise plots, (3) isointensity curves, (4) modeling of multiple hypothetical lesions, (5) parameter sensitivity, (6) figure of merit, and (7) synthetic image generation. Each discussion will define the performance criterion developed in the model, describe the assumptions used, and evaluate strengths and limitations.

The analysis presented here assumes that the general goal of pulse sequence modeling is selection of screening techniques that will produce images with reasonable anatomic detail and enough contrast between the pathologic and normal tissues to make lesions easily discernible.

General Limitations of the Models

Although the models are based on similar mathematical constructs, the assumptions used in deriving the performance criteria vary. All the models take into account the effects of *T1*, and most consider the effects of *T2*. Although a few include *N* effects, none of the models contains a mathematical expression for molecular self-diffusion, flow, physiologic motion (such as respiratory motion), or magnetic susceptibility effects.

All the models assume single-slice acquisition without considering the time savings available through multislice or multiecho acquisition. Therefore, the predicted optima must be considered in light of the number of slices that can be obtained using these newer techniques; some of the models predict shorter optimal *TR* intervals that may not be long enough for acquisition of more than a few images. The background noise level has also been assumed to be independent of the timing intervals chosen.

Subjective factors have been excluded in all the models; in a clinical setting it becomes immediately apparent that individual preferences have a significant effect on the type of images considered adequate for general examination. Financial constraints and overall patient scanning time also weigh heavily on the choices made when implementing these models.

Most of the models require a database of normal *N*, *T1*, and *T2* values. For the purposes of this discussion, it is assumed that such a database is available or can be generated by a motivated clinician on his own instrumentation. Ideally, this database should be developed on the machine being used for imaging, since relaxation times may vary between manufacturers because of differences in field strength, rf pulse shape, and so forth. It should be noted that the *N*, *T1*, and *T2* values of interest for modeling are not the absolute or "true" values but the values perceived by the imaging device. For instance, if gaussian-shaped rf pulses are used for imaging, *T1* and *T2* measurements should be performed with gaussian-shaped rf pulses even though they introduce a known systematic error. Although "square" rf pulses should yield more accurate relaxation, the results would not be particularly helpful in setting up an imaging technique that "sees" different relaxation properties owing to the differences in the rf pulse shape.

DIFFERENCE PLOTS

The difference in *I* (DI) between two tissues was one of the earliest performance criteria used to model MRI technique selection.[1,2] The *N*, *T1*, and *T2* values of the two tissues to be differentiated must be known and entered into a computer program that produces a graph of predicted *I* and/or DI as the timing intervals are varied. The "optimal" imaging technique is then selected by noting which combination of timing intervals results in the largest DI, on the assumption that larger DI values make tissue differentiation easier.

Simple line graphs, such as those in Figure 8–1, can be used to demonstrate the effects of changing a single timing interval. Visualizing the interrelationship between multiple timing intervals requires a more complex graphic method. A pseudo–three-dimensional "isometric" plot, displaying DI as a function of all possible combinations of two timing intervals, was developed to solve this problem.[2–4] In these plots (Fig. 8–2), the magnitude of DI is represented as a surface on a graph, with the timing intervals varied along the *x*- and *y*-axes. In the plots, peaks represent large DI values, while valleys indicate smaller DI values. Using the timing intervals that correspond to the peaks should produce images with the largest difference in intensity between the tissues.

The peaks and valleys described above can also be displayed with a gray scale or

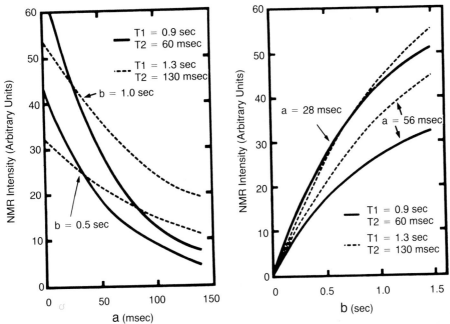

Figure 8–1. The effect on signal intensity of varying *TE* (*a*) and *TR* (*b*) in the spin-echo sequence is demonstrated for two sets of *T1* and *T2* values. (From Crooks LE et al: Radiology *144*:843, 1982. Used by permission.)

with isocontour lines. On the gray-scale display (Fig. 8–3), darker shades of gray indicate larger DI values and therefore more favorable timing interval combinations. The isocontour plots use contour lines similar to those used on topographic maps to represent the peaks and valleys. Figure 8–4 demonstrates such a plot for the predicted DI between gray and white brain matter (GM, WM) using the SE sequence. DI has been scaled so that the maximum value on the plot is 100. Isocontour plots are easier to read and permit negative values for DI, indicating a reversal in the relative intensity of the tissues.

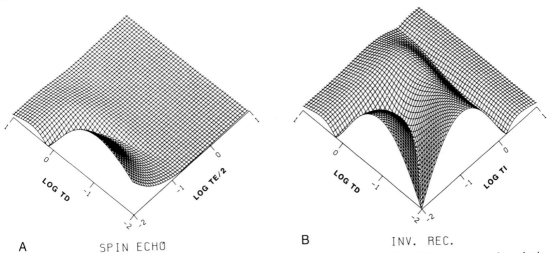

Figure 8–2. Pseudo–three-dimensional plots of calculated difference in signal intensity (DI) between two hypothetical tissues for the spin-echo and inversion-recovery sequences. The peaks on the graph represent areas of maximal DI. Tissue parameter values for the hypothetical tissues modeled were: *A*, N = 1.5, *T1* = 1500 ms, *T2* = 150 ms, *B*, N = 1.0, *T1* = 1000 ms, *T2* = 100 ms. (From Mitchell MR et al: Paper presented at Association of University Radiologists Annual Meeting, Mobile, AL, 1983.)

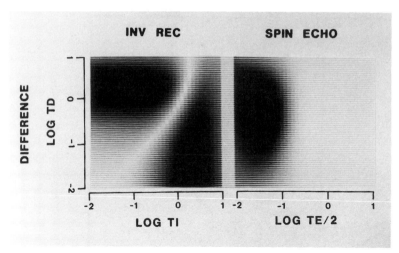

DIFFERENCE

Figure 8–3. The plot of DI in Figure 8–2 can also be presented using a gray-scale display, with black representing a large DI and lighter shades of gray indicating progressively smaller DI values. (From Mitchell MR et al: Paper presented at Association of University Radiologists Annual Meeting, Mobile, AL, 1983.)

A matrix of images created with the multiecho technique demonstrates the correlation between the graphic predictions (Fig. 8–4) and the imaging results (Fig. 8–5). Note that a larger difference between GM and WM is predicted for and seen in the images with long *TR* and short-to-intermediate *TE* values. Also note that the relative intensity of GM and WM is reversed in the images with short *TE* and *TR* intervals, as predicted by a change in sign on the graph. In between these extremes, GM and WM have similar intensity, as predicted on the DI plot by values near zero.

The difference model is simple, incorporates the effects of all three tissue parameters, and permits selection of a single imaging sequence that should provide excellent results. Unfortunately, the use of this model is limited by the fact that it requires a prospective knowledge of the *N*, *T1*, and *T2* values for both tissues of interest. When attempting to maximize the difference between a normal tissue and a lesion, it is unlikely that the tissue parameter values for the lesion will be known in advance, particularly if the nature of the lesion is uncertain, as in most screening situations. The model can be used when two normal tissues need to be differentiated; separating GM and CSF to produce a noninvasive cisternogram, for instance. It is also suitable for follow-up examinations and in screening for a specific lesion, such as multiple sclerosis, in which the probable lesion characteristics are known in advance.

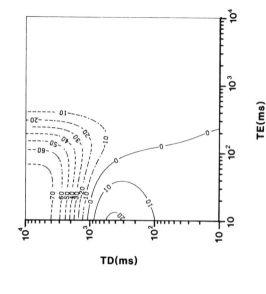

SE

Figure 8–4. Isocontour plot of difference in signal intensity between gray and white matter for all combinations of *TE* and *TR* using the spin-echo sequence. Note the presence of two peaks, one in the lower left where *TE* and *TR* are short, and another in the upper middle portion of the plot where *TE* is intermediate and *TR* is long.

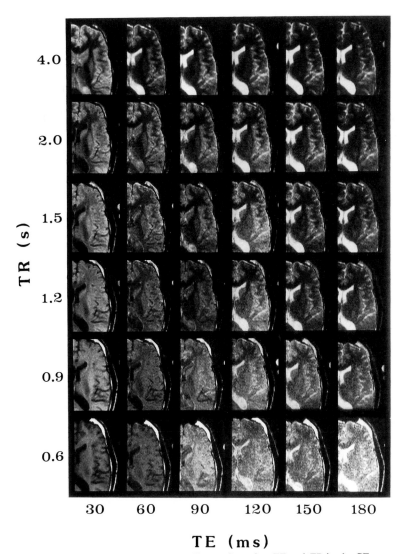

TR (s)

4.0 2.0 1.5 1.2 0.9 0.6

30   60   90   120 150 180

TE (ms)

Figure 8–5. A matrix of images demonstrates the effects of varying *TE* and *TR* in the SE sequence. (From Mitchell MR et al: RadioGraphics 6(2):245, 1985. Used by permission.)

Predicted optimal techniques using the difference model usually have long *TR* intervals that are quite advantageous for multislice-multiecho techniques, since the long *TR* intervals permit acquisition of a large number of slices and echoes simultaneously. This keeps scanning time within reasonable limits.[5] Long *TR* intervals also produce good signal-to-noise levels by providing extra time for longitudinal relaxation, which re-establishes the net magnetization vector.

CONTRAST-TO-NOISE

Contrast-to-noise (C/N) plots are essentially difference plots that have been modified to compare different timing interval combinations while holding total imaging time constant. This is accomplished by multiplying DI by the square root of the number of signal averages that can be performed during a constant acquisition time, or by dividing DI by the square root of *TR*.[6] Since noise is assumed to be constant, the relative signal-to-noise between different techniques is assumed to improve by the square root of the number of signal averages that can be performed during any given total scanning time.

Initial predictions using this model were imprecise because N was assumed to be the same for all tissues; including N dramatically improved the accuracy of the C/N calculations.[7] This is an important point to remember, since a number of the early optimization models used this incorrect assumption about N.

Simple line graphs or isocontour plots can be used with the C/N model. Isocontour plots for optimizing differentiation between GM and WM for the SE and ISE sequences are presented in Figure 8–6.[7] The images in Figures 8–7 and 8–8 have been located

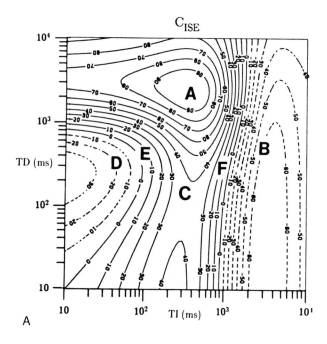

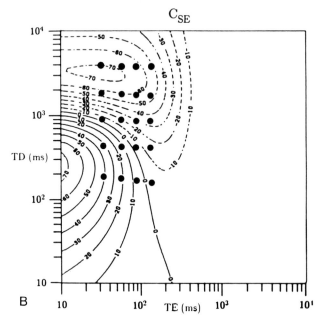

Figure 8–6. Contrast to noise (C/N) plots for GM and WM for all combinations of *TE* vs. *TR* for spin echo (right) and *TI* vs. *TD* (*TD* = *TR* − *TI* − *TE*/2) for inverted spin echo (left). (From Mitchell MR et al: Invest Radiol *19*:350, 1984. Used by permission.)

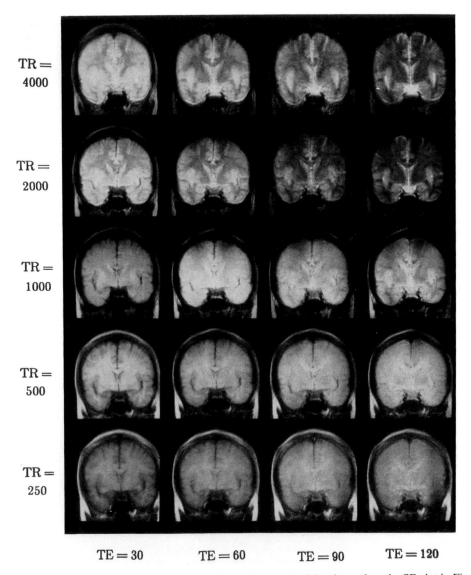

TR = 4000

TR = 2000

TR = 1000

TR = 500

TR = 250

TE = 30   TE = 60   TE = 90   TE = 120

Figure 8–7. SE image timing intervals corresponding to the matrix of dots located on the SE plot in Figure 8–6. (From Mitchell MR et al: Invest Radiol *19*:350, 1984. Used by permission.)

on these plots using their timing intervals; they are identified on the SE plot by a matrix of dots and on the ISE plot with the letters *A* through *F*.

The C/N model shares some of the advantages and disadvantages of the DI model. This includes the significant disadvantage of requiring prospective knowledge of the N, T1, and T2 for the tissues to be differentiated, severely limiting its clinical application for screening.

The major theoretical advantage of this model is that it takes into account the overall scanning time and tries to predict the "best" possible DI in the allotted time. Consequently, the C/N model predicts optimal scanning with shorter *TR* intervals than the difference model because shorter *TR* intervals permit more signal-averaging during a fixed total scanning time. But short *TR* intervals can also limit the number of slices that can be acquired using the multislice-multiecho technique. If the shorter *TR* interval necessitates more than one acquisition to obtain the desired slices, it may take con-

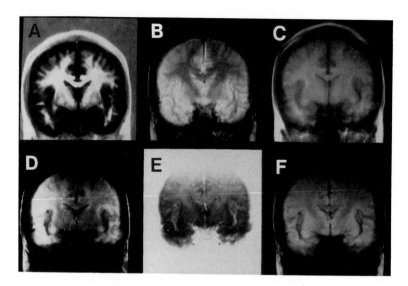

Figure 8–8. ISE images with timing intervals corresponding to the location indicated by the letters on the ISE C/N plot in Figure 8–6 and ISE *T1* sensitivity plot in Figure 8–11. (From Mitchell MR et al: Invest Radiol *19*:350, 1984. Used by permission.)

siderably longer than the optimal sequence predicted with the difference model. Even though a shorter *TR* is used, the short *TR* scan requires the same amount of time as the long *TR* sequence to achieve the predicted improvement in "contrast-to-noise" by using signal averaging. Therefore, C/N comparisons are valid only for sequences with *TR* intervals long enough to acquire all the desired slices in a single acquisition.

To illustrate the problem, consider an SE sequence with a *TR* of 250 ms. This short *TR* permits only five multislice images to be acquired on a Teslacon (TM) 0.5 tesla system, since 44 ms (the minimum *TE* of 30 ms plus 14 ms for the acquisition gate to close) are required for each slice. Although a decrease in the time required for each slice may increase the number of slices that can be acquired, it is unlikely that this time will be shortened sufficiently in the SE sequence to permit a substantial increase in the number of slices that can be acquired during this short *TR*. If a true partial saturation sequence were used instead of SE, the *TE* time could be eliminated and more slices could be acquired. On the other hand, if multiple echoes are used, the *TE* becomes longer and the number of slices that can be obtained in a single acquisition decreases.

Radio frequency heat deposition can also be a problem when short *TR* sequences are used with multiple signal averages in a multislice acquisition owing to the rapidity of rf pulsing, especially at high field strengths.[8]

ISOINTENSITY CURVES

Isointensity curves have been used to indicate the predicted image intensity (*I*) for all combinations of *T1* and *T2* for a specific set of pulse sequence timing intervals.[9,10] On these plots, *T1* and *T2* vary along the *x*- and *y*-axes with isocontour lines indicating *T1-T2* combinations with the same predicted *I*. By following the lines, one can rapidly identify all the combinations of *T1* and *T2* that produce the same image intensity.

Isointensity plots for the SE 50/500, SE 50/1000, and SE 50/2000 techniques are illustrated in Figure 8–9. Normal and pathologic tissues are located on the plot by their *T1* and *T2* values; *N* is assumed to be the same for all tissues. If the tissues fall on the same isointensity line, the model predicts that they will not be differentiated. The ability to differentiate two tissues is assessed by observing the number of isointensity lines

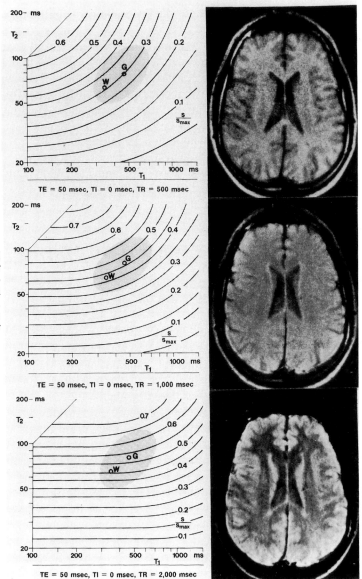

Figure 8–9. Fraction of maximum signal I for gray and white matter is illustrated for graphs of *T1* vs. *T2* for each of three spin-echo sequences. To the right of each graph can be found the corresponding image. (From Zeidses des Plantes BG et al: RadioGraphics *4*:869, 1984. Used by permission.)

separating them. Those that are separated by several lines should have significantly different intensities, and should therefore be easily distinguished.

This model is quite instructive when used to compare the *T1* and *T2* sensitivity of various sequences, providing one of the most effective methods for demonstrating the interaction of *T1* and *T2*.[10] It illustrates that tissues with vastly different *T1* and *T2* values can have identical image intensities because of the competitive effects of *T1* and *T2*. This model also permits simultaneous evaluation of multiple tissues; as many tissues as necessary can be located on the plots.

The model is limited by the number of graphs required to evaluate a wide variety of pulse sequence timing interval combinations; each set of timing intervals requires a different isointensity plot. To select optimal timing parameters, the user must determine which plot separates the tissues under evaluation by the maximum number of isocontour lines. Isointensity plots also require a prospective knowledge of the *T1* and *T2* values to be encountered; in most situations the pathology is not known, and this requirement cannot be met.

The assumption that N is the same for all tissues, although useful for instruction and simplicity, is incorrect; it is now well documented that differences in N contribute significantly to the contrast between different normal tissues and pathologic tissues.[7] Consequently, real tissues cannot be localized on the plots, since differences in N change tissue intensity, and the tissues no longer have a unique intensity that can be plotted as a function of $T1$ and $T2$. This makes the model less suitable for prediction of image contrast in a clinical setting.

Carried to its logical conclusion, the model could be expanded to a three-dimensional plot with axes for N, $T1$, and $T2$. Visual analysis of the plots would be extremely difficult, since one is actually viewing a four-dimensional space, with intensity as the fourth dimension.

MODELING OF MULTIPLE HYPOTHETICAL LESIONS

Droege suggested optimizing for lesion detection by computing the difference in signal intensity between all normal intracranial structures and a set of hypothetical lesions with a wide range of N, $T1$, and $T2$ values.[11,12] If the difference between all the normal tissues and the hypothetical lesion exceeded a predicted noise level by a factor of 4, the lesion was considered identifiable. Calculations were performed for a variety of timing interval combinations for the SE and IR sequences. The results were tabulated, and the pulse sequence techniques that differentiated the largest percentage of lesions were considered optimal.

For CNS screening, good detection rates were noted with the SE 100/2000 and IR 200/1800 sequences. These two sequences tend to work well together because they evaluate different tissue parameters; the SE sequence is more $T2$ weighted, while the IR sequence is relatively $T1$ weighted. Therefore, lesions that are missed by one sequence have a high probability of being detected by the other. The $T1$ and $T2$ combinations that should be detected by each of the recommended sequences are graphically depicted in Figure 8–10. The authors referred to these two techniques as a diagonal set of images.[11,12]

The sequences selected with this model tend to produce images with white lesions on a gray background of normal tissue. Although the uniform intensity of the normal tissues decreases visualization of the anatomic details, it highlights the pathology in a highly desirable manner.

This model has the advantages of predicting a single set of sequences that can be used for general screening without requiring selection of a particular tissue of interest or a guess about which tissues are likely to be involved by pathology. This makes it simple to implement once a normal database has been collected and the appropriate calculations have been performed.

The predictions made with this model are limited by the fact that phase-reconstructed inversion recovery was not included in the analysis. As Chapter 24 explains, magnitude reconstruction discards the negative sign in IR images, significantly decreasing the sequence's potential $T1$ weighting. This skews the results toward short $T1$ intervals, since moderate to long $T1$ intervals produce a "bounce point" artifact that decreases the lesion detection rate. Comparing the phase and magnitude reconstructed IR techniques with this model would be very informative.

One disadvantage of this model is the limited contrast between normal tissues on the suggested sequences; WM, GM, and CSF tend to blend, resulting in loss of familiar

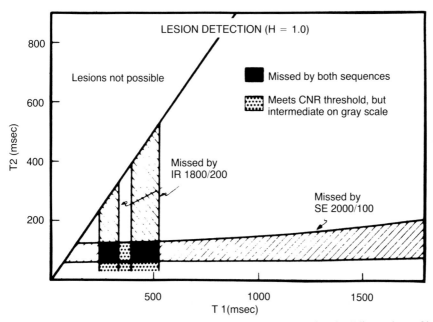

Figure 8–10. *T1* and *T2* values of lesions that will or will not be detected using the "diagonal set of images" suggested by Droege et al. (From Droege RT et al: Radiology *153*:419, 1984. Used by permission.)

landmarks and anatomy. Using the same sequences for every screening examination also eliminates the potential for tailoring the examination to the particular clinical situation by using a technique that would permit even better detection of subtle lesions within a tissue of interest.

PARAMETER SENSITIVITY

Calculating the partial derivative of *I* with respect to specific tissue parameters produces a set of performance criteria called parameter sensitivities.[4] These criteria can be used to predict maximal sensitivity to subtle changes in *N*, *T1*, and *T2* for a wide variety of pulse sequence timing intervals. Each tissue parameter has its own sensitivity parameter; *SN*, *ST1*, and *ST2* (defined in Chapter 21) are used to predict the relative rate of change in intensity due to subtle changes in *N*, *T1*, and *T2*, respectively.

Plots for each of these sensitivities can be created with isocontour lines indicating the magnitude of the sensitivity parameter for all combinations of two timing intervals. The plots indicate the relative sensitivity of the different timing interval combinations for a particular tissue of interest. Only one tissue can be graphed at a time. Therefore, one must determine on a clinical basis the most likely normal tissue to be involved by pathology and then optimize the imaging for that tissue. The sensitivities are scaled so that the maximum value obtained on the plot is 100. High sensitivity values indicate a large change in intensity for a small change in the tissue parameter being evaluated.

Figure 8–11 contains sensitivity plots of *ST1* for the ISE sequence and *ST2* for the SE sequence. Both plots were produced using normal white matter tissue parameter values. ISE images in a normal volunteer and SE images in a patient with multiple sclerosis have been included for comparison with the predictions on the plots in Figures 8–8 and 8–12.

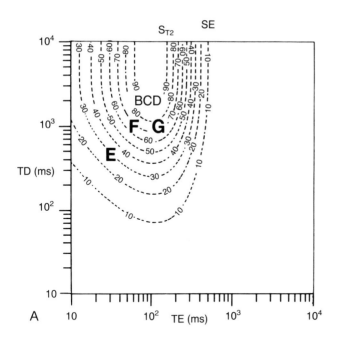

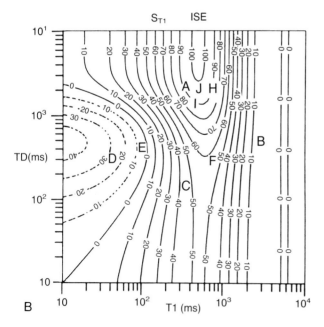

Figure 8–11. Relative sensitivity to changes in *T2* for SE (*A*) and to *T1* for ISE (*B*) predicted by the parameter sensitivity model. Corresponding images can be found in Figures 8–8 and 8–12. (From Mitchell MR et al: Invest Radiol *19*:350, 1984. Used by permission.)

The parameter sensitivity model permits a number of rules of thumb to be deduced that can be used without the aid of computer modeling. These rules of thumb are developed in detail in Chapter 21 and summarized in Table 8–1.

The parameter sensitivity model is limited by the fact that it can evaluate only the potential for signal intensity change in a single normal tissue. Each tissue has its own graphic predictions, making it difficult to select a sequence that will be optimal for a variety of tissues. It is also limited by the fact that it predicts the effects of small changes in individual tissue parameters, with the assumption that the other tissue parameters are not changing enough to alter *I* significantly. Therefore, one must look at all three sensitivity plots and make sure that the techniques selected are not only sensitive to

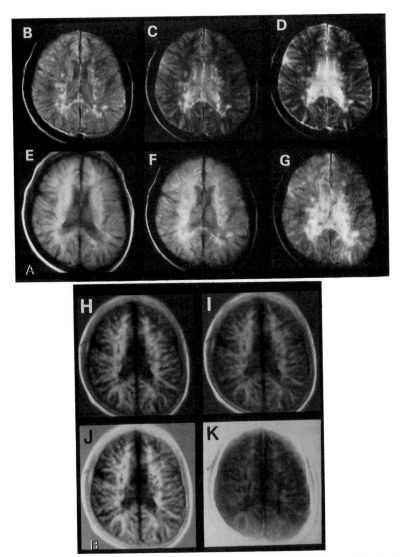

Figure 8–12. Spin-echo and multiecho images in a patient with multiple sclerosis match the timing intervals indicated in Figure 8–11 for the sensitivity to *T2*. (From Mitchell MR et al: Invest Radiol *19*:350, 1984. Used by permission.)

Table 8–1. GUIDELINES FOR SELECTING MRI SCREENING TECHNIQUES

For Sensitivity To:	Pulse Sequences:*	Timing Intervals†		
		TI	*TE*	*TR*
N	PS	—	—	$TR \gg TI$
	SE	—	$TE \ll T2$	$TR \gg TI$
TI	IR (Phase Recon)	$TI = TI$	—	$TR \gg TI$
	ISE (Phase Recon)	$TI = TI$	$TE \ll T2$	$TR \gg TI$
	PS	—	—	$TR = TI$
	PSSE (SE)	—	$TE \ll T2$	$TR = TI$
T2	SE	—	$TE = T2$	$TR \gg TI$

* Pulse sequences have been listed in the order of their potential for tissue parameter weighting; therefore, select the highest sequence possible on each list.
† *TI* and *T2* values are the relaxation times of the normal tissue suspected of harboring the pathology.

the desired parameter but also insensitive to competing parameters. Another limitation is the fact that this model optimizes tissue differentiation for subtle lesions; if the tissue parameter changes in the lesion are large, the sequences selected will not necessarily be those that maximize differentiation of normal and pathologic tissues. It is most useful for selecting screening techniques when subtle changes in a particular normal tissue are being sought.

FIGURE OF MERIT

"Figure of merit" is a performance criterion similar to parameter sensitivity, which uses the partial derivative of the intensity equation but includes a term to account for signal averaging. This is done by multiplying the predicted intensity for a single pulse sequence repetition by the square root of the number of pulse sequence repetitions that can be performed during a constant total scanning time, as in the C/N model.[6] This permits comparison of different scanning techniques on the basis of a constant total scanning time. Figure 8–13 is an isocontour plot of the figure of merit for inversion recovery *T1* discrimination.

The figure of merit model has many of the advantages and limitations of the parameter sensitivity model. In addition, because it optimizes for overall scanning efficiency in a single-slice mode, it may predict an optimal *TR* that severely restricts the number of slices that can be used with the multislice-multiecho technique. If one can perform the number of slices desired, however, using the figure of merit for optimization should be helpful.

SYNTHETIC IMAGES

The difficulty of acquiring images with a wide variety of timing intervals and contrast characteristics has produced considerable interest in the idea of creating synthetic images from *N*, *T1*, and *T2* information calculated from a rapidly acquired set of images. This permits the MRI physician to retrospectively change the timing intervals at will

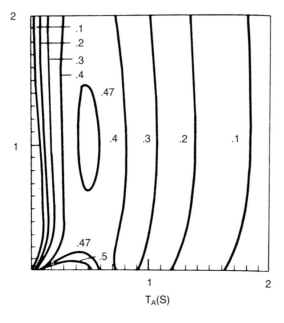

Figure 8–13. *T1* discrimination for IR, as a function of the timing intervals *T1* (*TA*) and *TD* (*TB*) for a tissue with a *T1* of 0.5 sec. (From Edelstein WA et al: J Comput Assist Tomogr *1*:391, 1983. Used by permission.)

in order to produce the desired images without rescanning the patient. The results have demonstrated very good agreement with real images acquired with the same timing intervals.[13]

Accurate synthesis of images obviously requires the accurate N, $T1$, and $T2$ information and correct mathematical models for creating the images. The N, $T1$, and $T2$ images must also be acquired in a reasonable total scan time. If these criteria are met, retrospective image synthesis can save time and increase the number of imaging sequences viewed without increasing total scanning time. These are obviously significant advantages.

One difficulty in using this model is in knowing how to select the kind of image that should be synthesized. Although one could simply generate synthetic images using the "optimal" techniques predicted by the models in this chapter, the value of producing images that include competitive tissue parameter effects is questionable. Once the calculated N, $T1$, and $T2$ images are available, it seems counterproductive to create images using the normal signal intensity equations with $T1$ and $T2$ effects that tend to cancel each other, thus diminishing contrast. Creating images that cannot be acquired directly ($TE = 0$, for instance) may be very helpful.[14] Since the principal object of optimization is the addition of complementary tissue parameter effects and the elimination of competitive effects, it makes more sense to create images using some relationship other than the normal signal intensity equations for the synthesis. Simply adding the N, $T1$, and $T2$ images would produce better contrast in most situations.

GENERAL GUIDELINES

All the optimization strategies described were produced with the aid of computers and require computer hardware and software for full implementation. Nevertheless, several rules of thumb can be developed from the parameter sensitivity model and can be used by the practicing MRI physician without computer assistance. These rules of thumb (Table 8–1)[15–20] allow one to select MRI techniques to screen for subtle pathology in a normal tissue of clinical interest if its N, $T1$, and $T2$ are known. If normal values are not available, the clinician can generate them by scanning a few normal volunteers, provided that the software for measuring tissue parameters is available. Otherwise, literature values obtained at the same field strength can be used as a first approximation.

The MRI user must first select the pulse sequences that provide the best sensitivity to changes in each of the three tissue parameters on the instrumentation being used. True partial saturation and phase-reconstructed inversion recovery or inverted spin echo are good for detecting $T1$ changes. Spin echo is best for $T2$ weighting. N can be evaluated with partial saturation or a spin-echo sequence with a short TE. The timing intervals for each sequence should be selected according to the recommendations in Table 8–1. One of the sequences (usually the $T2$ weighted scan) can be used for screening, with additional sequences performed as needed. The N sensitive sequence provides the greatest signal-to-noise, and therefore optimal anatomic detail, but not the best tissue differentiation. It is probably better to perform all three sequences (one for each tissue parameter) if it can be done in an efficient manner. N and $T2$ weighted scans can usually be acquired at the same time using a multiecho-multislice sequence with asymmetric echoes; adding good $T1$ weighted technique completes the screening. Additional sequences can be added as needed to increase tissue specificity.

Since the final sequences selected are usually a compromise between predicted optima, personal preference, and instrumental limitations, one can use these guidelines to establish a starting technique that can be modified as the user's experience grows.

In conclusion, the wide variety of techniques developed to predict optimal imaging sequences should indicate that the problem of optimization is neither simple nor solved. Further work is needed to include the effects of multislice acquisition, additional tissue parameters, patient throughput, cost, and subjective judgments about what kind of images the MRI practitioners will find most useful.

Although each of the models reviewed has different strengths and weaknesses, they all teach principles about selection of optimal pulse sequences for MRI screening that can be used in both selection and interpretation of different types of MR images. Studying these models and the principles presented throughout this text should assist the MRI practitioner through the maze of different pulse sequences and timing interval combinations that provide the challenge and potential of MRI.

Until the ideal model is developed, the reader is encouraged to select one of the models discussed that can be implemented on the instrumentation being used. From this starting point, the sequences can be adjusted and tailored to fit the needs and preferences of the individual user.

References

1. Crooks LE, Mills CM, Davis PL, et al: Visualization of cerebral and vascular abnormalities by NMR imaging. The effects of imaging parameters on contrast. Radiology *144*:843, 1982.
2. Mitchell MR, Gibbs SJ, Partain CL, James AE: NMR imaging: Optimization of tissue discrimination through manipulation of pulse parameters. Paper presented at Association of University Radiologists Annual Meeting, Mobile, Alabama, March 1983.
3. Mitchell MR, Gibbs SJ, Partain CL, James AE: Computer modeling of NMR pulse sequences. Category I Continuing Education Exhibit, Radiological Society of North America 69th Annual Scientific Meeting, Chicago, November 1984.
4. Mitchell MR, Conturo TE, Gruber TJ, Jones JP: Two computer models for selection of optimal magnetic resonance imaging (MRI) pulse sequence timing. Invest Radiol *19*(5):350, 1984.
5. Crooks LE, Hoenninger J, Arakawa M, Watts J, McCarten B, Sheldon P, Kaufman L, Mills CM, Davis PL, Margulis AR: High-resolution magnetic resonance imaging. Radiology *150*:163, 1984.
6. Edelstein WA, Bottomley PA, Hart HR, Smith LS: Signal, noise, and contrast in nuclear magnetic resonance (NMR) imaging. J Comput Assist Tomogr *7*(3):391, 1983.
7. Wehrli FW, MacFall JR, Shutts D, Breger R, Herfkens RJ: Mechanisms of contrast in NMR imaging. J Comput Assist Tomogr *8*(3):369, 1984.
8. Budinger T: Workshop on RF heating thermophysiology. Soc Magn Reson Med Newslett *5*:2, 1985.
9. Kurtz D, Dwyer A: Isosignal contours and signal gradients as an aid to choosing MR imaging techniques. J Comput Assist Tomogr *8*(5):819, 1984.
10. Zeidses des Plantes, BG Jr, Falke THM, den Boer JA: Pulse sequences and contrast in magnetic resonance imaging. RadioGraphics *4*(6):869, 1984.
11. Droege RT, Wiener SN, Rzeszotarski MS: A strategy for magnetic resonance imaging of the head: results of a semi-empirical model. Part I. Radiology *153*:419, 1984.
12. Droege RT, Wiener SN, Rzeszotarski MS: A strategy for magnetic resonance imaging of the head: results of a semi-empirical model. Part II. Radiology *153*:425, 1984.
13. Bobman SA, Riederer SJ, Lee JN, Suddarth SA, et al: Synthesized MR images: comparison with acquired images. Radiology *155*:731, 1985.
14. Riederer SJ, Suddarth SA, Bobman SA, Lee JN, Wang HZ, MacFall JR: Automated MR image synthesis: feasibility studies. Radiology *153*:203, 1984.
15. Mitchell MR: Optimization of magnetic resonance imaging techniques. Association of University Radiologists Research Symposium 1984—Research in Magnetic Resonance Imaging. Nashville, May 1984.
16. Mitchell MR, Conturo TE, Jones JP, Partain CL, James AE Jr: Understanding MR pulse sequence timing. Annual Meeting of the American Roentgen Ray Society. Las Vegas, April 1984.
17. Mitchell MR, Conturo TE, Gruber TJ, Jones JP, Price RR, Partain CL, James AE Jr: Prospective selection of optimal magnetic resonance imaging (MRI) pulse sequence timing. Society of Magnetic Resonance in Medicine, Third Annual Scientific Meeting, Abstract 19, New York, August 17, 1984.
18. Mitchell MR, Jones JP, Conturo TE, Partain CL, James AE Jr: Basic principles underlying selection of optimal MR imaging pulse sequence timing intervals. 70th Scientific Assembly of the Radiological Society of North America, Paper 598, November 28, 1984.
19. Mitchell MR, Tarr RW, Conturo TE, Partain CL, James AE: Spin echo technique selection: basic principles for choosing MRI pulse sequence timing intervals. RadioGraphics *6*(2): 245, 1986.
20. Mitchell MR, Tarr RW, Conturo TE, Partain CL, James AE: Inverted spin echo (ISE) technique selection: guidelines for optimizing pulse sequence timing intervals. Submitted for publication.

9

Quantitative NMR Tissue Characterization Using Calculated Images and Automated Image Segmentation

J. C. GORE
M. O'DONNELL
C. F. POPE
S. MAJUMDAR
W. J. ADAMS

An important potential advantage of MR imaging is its ability to derive quantitative indices of the intrinsic characteristics of tissues. In this chapter we report our experience in implementing self-normalizing multiple-echo pulse sequences for efficiently producing calculated *T1*, *T2*, and proton density images simultaneously from a single scan. We have analyzed theoretically the performance of such sequences and have investigated their immunity to artifacts arising from imperfections in the rf pulses or main field. The successful implementation of these methods demands gradients and pulses in addition to normal imaging, and these are described. We also summarize our preliminary attempts to automatically analyze these quantitative images to classify tissue regions according to their relaxation characteristics. The feasibility of such quantitative MR images for automated image segmentation in specific clinical applications is demonstrated.

MRI systems generate images sensitive to several intrinsic nuclear magnetic properties of tissue, but conventional proton images represent a complicated convolution of these intrinsic parameters with instrumental and technique features such as receiver coil geometry and pulse sequence timing. Even using several conventional scan sequences in series, there are inherent difficulties in obtaining reliable in vivo measurements of tissue properties. This may account, in part, for the apparently disappointing reliability of in vivo MR measurements in characterizing pathology. Furthermore, because of the fundamental link between image presentation (and consequently image perception) and extrinsic parameters, the design of a general automated analysis system for MRI is very difficult. In particular, a new analysis system may have to be designed for each coil geometry and pulse sequence. Here we explore the use of efficient self-normalizing pulse sequences for direct imaging of the *T1* and *T2* relaxation times of tissue and attempt to use these for automated image quantitation.

Conventional proton MR images are obtained using one of several different pulse sequences. Inversion recovery and partial saturation sequences are used to generate images exhibiting primarily *T1* contrast. Spin-echo sequences are used to generate images exhibiting primarily *T2* contrast. However, the image brightness in all images obtained with these methods is determined by the choice of timing parameters and is also linearly related to both spin-density and receiver-coil sensitivity. Self-normalizing sequences and analysis methods can be used to produce quantitative images, where the image brightness is simply proportional to either *T1* or *T2*. Quantitative *T1* images can be generated by combining two conventional inversion recovery or partial saturation sequences. Quantitative *T2* images can be produced by incorporating more than one echo into a spin-echo sequence (i.e., a multiple-echo sequence). Although conceptually attractive, self-normalizing sequences often are far less efficient than simple sequences, where efficiency is described in terms of the contrast to noise per unit imaging time. We first demonstrate that it is possible to derive sequences that provide simultaneous *T1* and *T2* imaging with efficiencies approaching those of simple sequences.

COMBINED T1-T2 PULSE SEQUENCES

A useful measure for comparing pulse sequences is the contrast to noise ratio achievable per unit time, which quantitatively indicates the discriminant ability of the resultant image to distinguish subtle changes in the MR signal. For example, Edelstein et al.[1] discuss the efficiency of several different pulse sequences sensitive to *T1* contrast, and conclude that the most efficient sequence for *T1* discrimination is the simple saturation recovery method running at a repetition time one-half the average *T1* in the object of interest. This sequence is also more efficient than inversion recovery if *T1* is the only varying quantity. For our purpose, two self-normalizing sequences can be used to generate quantitative *T1* images and can be analyzed in similar fashion. The first sequence, referred to as the inversion-saturation recovery method, consists of an inversion recovery measurement followed after a short delay time (in comparison with *T1*) by a saturation recovery measurement. The second sequence, referred to as the double saturation recovery method, consists of a measurement of a partially saturated spin system followed by another saturation recovery measurement at a different *TR*. For a *T1* of 400 ms, the maximum contrast to noise for the simple saturation recovery method is 0.68; for the inversion-saturation recovery method, it is 0.44; and for the double saturation recovery method, it is 0.20. Consequently, the inversion-saturation recovery method is best for quantitative *T1* imaging but has a reduced efficiency compared with the simple saturation recovery method. However, as we show below, this efficiency may be increased by the use of multiple echoes.

In order to image both *T1* and *T2* simultaneously, the self-normalizing *T1* sequences can be combined with a multiple-echo sequence. Figure 9–1 presents a *T1-T2* sequence based on the inversion saturation recovery method. We have previously shown[2] that the first signal in the first echo train for the inversion-saturation recovery sequence is

$$S_1 = M_0 e^{-TE/T2}\{1 - e^{-TI/T1} - e^{-TI/T1}[1 - e^{-TR'/T1} + \eta(TE, TI)e^{-TR'/T1}]\} \tag{1}$$

and the first signal in the second echo train is

$$S_1' = M_0 e^{-TE/T2}[1 - e^{-TI/T1} + \eta(TE, TI)e^{-TI/T1}], \tag{2}$$

where

$$\eta(TE, TI) = (-1)^N (1 - e^{-TE/2TI}) e^{-(N-1)TE/TI} + (1 - e^{-TE/TI}) \sum_{n=2}^{N} (-1)^n e^{(n-N)TE/TI}$$

and there are *N* echoes.

T₁–T₂ Sequences

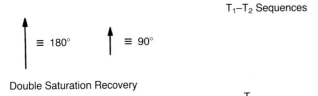

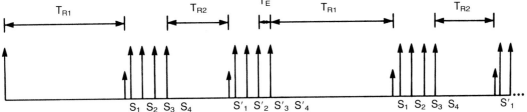

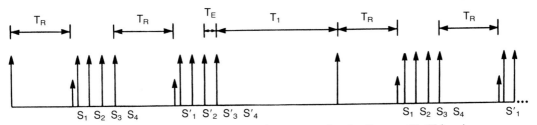

Figure 9–1. Inversion-saturation recovery pulse sequence for simultaneous *T1–T2* imaging.

A self-normalized signal dependent only on *T1* can be obtained from the following expression

$$S(T1) = (S_1 - S'_1)/S'_1 \tag{3}$$

This equation can be used to obtain an estimate of *T1*; by analyzing the propagation of noise through the fit we can also derive the standard deviation of the calculated numbers[2]. We can denote the resultant expression for the signal-to-noise ratio in a quantitative *T1* image as $\Gamma_1(T1)$. The remaining signals in the multiple echo trains for the sequence presented in Figure 9–1 are described by the expressions

$$S_n = S_1 e^{-(n-1)TE/T2} \tag{4}$$

for the first echo train, and

$$S'_n = S'_1 e^{-(n-1)TE/T2} \tag{5}$$

for the second echo train. Consequently, the self-normalized signal, $S(T1)$ for the *n*th echo is the same as for the first echo; this is

$$S(T1) = (S_n - S'_n)/S'_n \tag{6}$$
$$= (S_1 - S'_1)/S'_1.$$

Of course, the signal-to-noise in the estimate of *T1* from the *n*th echo is decreased by the exponential factor related to the echo time. Nevertheless, by simply computing the average of $S(T1)$ over all echoes, the accuracy of the *T1* estimate can be greatly improved. In particular, the *T1* contrast-to-noise from a sequence of *N* echoes is

$$\Gamma_N(TI) = \Gamma_1(TI)N \left(\sum_{n=1}^{N} e^{2nTE/T2} \right)^{-1/2} \tag{7}$$

In the limit that *TE* ≪ *T2*, this reduces to

$$\Gamma_N(TI) = \Gamma_1(TI)N^{1/2} \tag{8}$$

Thus, for a four-echo sequence the *T1* contrast-to-noise can be improved by as much as a factor of 2 compared with the contrast-to-noise for the single-pulse, self-normalizing *T1* sequence. This means that the maximum *T1* contrast-to-noise for a *T1* of 400 ms can be as high as 0.88 for the inversion-saturation recovery sequence.

In Figure 9–2 we present contour plots of the *T1* contrast-to-noise as a function of *T1* and *T2* for a four-echo inversion-saturation recovery sequence. Timing parameters, *TI*, *TR*, *TR1*, and *TR2*, were chosen for maximal contrast-to-noise at a *T1* between 350 and 400 ms, a value appropriate at 0.15 *T* for soft tissues, such as brain. The echo time *TE* was chosen for maximal contrast-to-noise for the *T2* fit at a *T2* between 60 and 70 ms, a value close to the *T2* of white matter. The multiple-echo inversion-saturation recovery sequence exhibits excellent contrast-to-noise over a wide range of *T1* and *T2* (Fig. 9–2). Indeed, the contrast-to-noise for this sequence is comparable to the *T1* contrast-to-noise for the optimized simple saturation recovery sequence.

We should note that multiple echoes can also be used for the simple partial saturation sequence, where addition of echoes will increase the absolute signal-to-noise. However, the sum of a number of echoes for this sequence does not necessarily increase the contrast-to-noise, since *T2* effects can modify *T1* effects. The net result will depend on the sense of *T1* and *T2* variations and on the relative magnitudes of δ*T2*/*TE* and δ*T1*/

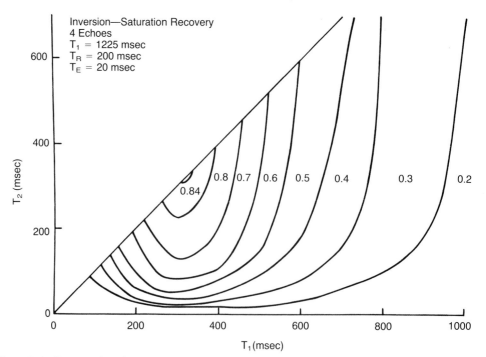

Figure 9–2. Contour plot of *T1* contrast to noise as a function of *T2* and *T1* for the inversion-saturation recovery sequence.

TR, where $\delta T2$ and $\delta T1$ are the variations in relaxation times between two tissues that present different signals. For example, assume that we are trying to differentiate between two tissues, one with $T1 = 350$ ms and $T2 = 70$ ms, the second with $T1 = 500$ ms and $T2 = 80$ ms, using a four-echo sequence with $TE = 20$ ms and $TR = 200$ ms. The contrast-to-noise ratio for the sum of four echoes is only 15 percent better than that for the first echo alone. In such a circumstance, the contrast-to-noise decreases with each successive echo. When $T1$ effects give rise to the contrast, multiple echoes can be used to enhance the contrast-to-noise of saturation recovery sequences only if the $T2$ variations are negligible, or if the echo times for all echoes are significantly less than the $T2$ of all tissues considered. If $T1$ varies in the opposite sense to $T2$ variations, then adding echoes reinforces $T1$ effects. In contradistinction, multiple echoes with echo times comparable to and greater than $T2$ of all tissues may actually be used to *increase* $T1$ contrast-to-noise for self-normalizing sequences. This feature of self-normalizing sequences is very attractive, since it results in quantitative $T1$ images with contrast-to-noise comparable to, or even greater than, the maximum $T1$ contrast-to-noise achievable with more simple pulse sequences.

As noted earlier, the sequence of Figure 9–1 can also be used for simultaneous $T2$ imaging. Each multiple-echo sequence can be used to estimate $T2$, and a combined estimate can be obtained from a weighted sum of the estimates from the two echo trains. We have used the magnitude of the signal from the first echo of each train as the weighting coefficient. That is, the estimated $T2$ can be written as

$$T2 = (S_1 T2 + S_1' T2')/(S_1 + S_1') \qquad (9)$$

In Figure 9–3 the contrast-to-noise for the $T2$ image generated by our self-normalizing sequence is presented as a function of $T1$ and $T2$. There is poor $T2$ contrast-to-noise

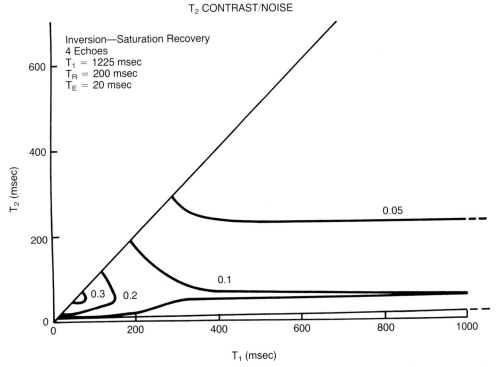

Figure 9–3. Contour plot of $T2$ contrast to noise as a function of $T2$ and $T1$ for the inversion-saturation recovery sequence.

as compared with a simple multiple-echo sequence. The inversion-saturation recovery sequence is thus very efficient for *T1* imaging but is inefficient for *T2* imaging.

Figure 9–4 displays a set of images acquired with this sequence in an adult volunteer. The first and fourth echo images (*A* and *B*) are from the first set of echoes, whereas *C* and *D* are the first and fourth echo images from the second set of echoes. Figure 9–4*A* is much like an inversion recovery image, and Figure 9–4*C* is much like a saturation recovery image. These images were obtained in 15 minutes at a field strength of 0.15 tesla. The timing parameters for the sequence are *TI* = 1225 ms, *TR* = 200 ms, *TE* = 20 ms, and total repetition time *T* = 1.765 s. Four acquisitions of each of 128 projections were taken. Using the analysis method presented previously, images of this type can be used to generate quantitative *T1* images (Fig. 9–5). Each pixel displayed in the image represents a 1.95 × 10.95 × 8 mm voxel. We note that there is a 1:1 correspondence between gray-scale value and the estimated value of *T1* in this image.

The *T2* image generated from the same data used to generate Figure 9–5 is presented in Figure 9–6. As expected, the signal-to-noise in this image is greatly reduced compared with the *T1* image. However, this image also represents a quantitative image of an intrinsic property of tissue. The data sampling time for these images was approximately 6 ms, and the echo time was 20 ms. Thus the data acquisition efficiency was only about 30 percent. This number can be increased by a factor of 2 or more. Consequently, self-normalizing sequences with eight echoes operating at 60 percent efficiency or more, optimized for maximum contrast-to-noise at a *T2* between 50 and 100 ms, should be readily achievable. Once a high efficiency has been obtained, additional echoes will not improve the contrast-to-noise, since the data acquisition time must be correspondingly reduced. In any event, multiple-echo sequences of 60 percent efficiency result in *T1* and *T2* images with contrast-to-noise approximately a factor of 2 better than the images presented in this chapter and represent extremely attractive sequences for simultaneous *T1-T2* imaging.

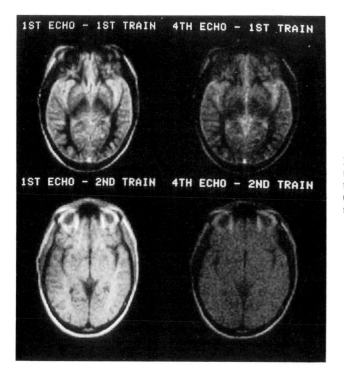

Figure 9–4. Magnitude images of an adult volunteer for the first (*A*) and fourth (*B*) echoes of the first echo train, and the first (*C*) and fourth (*D*) echoes of the second echo train of an inversion-saturation recovery sequence.

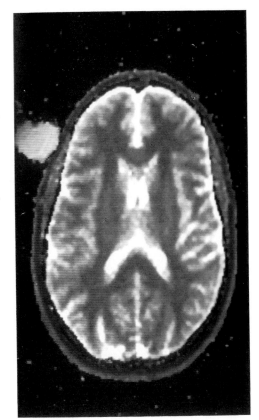

Figure 9–5. *T1* image of adult volunteer generated from inversion-saturation echo sequence of Figure 9–1.

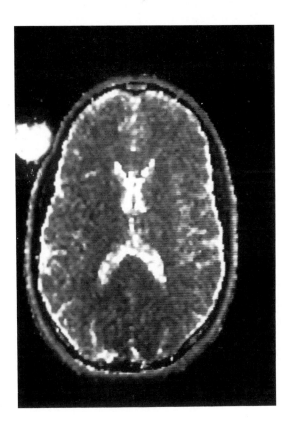

Figure 9–6. *T2* image of adult volunteer generated from same data used to form image in Figure 9–5.

INFLUENCE OF SYSTEM IMPERFECTIONS

The derivation of quantitative estimates of *T1* or *T2* usually assumes a particular analytic relationship between successive echoes. The validity of this assumption depends on the behavior of the rf pulses used to rotate the magnetization. The influence of imperfect inverting pulses in inversion-recovery is well documented and accommodated relatively easily by using a 3- (rather than 2-) parameter fit to the resultant recovery curve. However, the propagation of errors in multiple-echo sequences is more complex and can introduce a variety of effects. In particular, if each refocusing pulse produces a nutation of less than 180 degrees, the subsequent echo is reduced in amplitude and a longitudinal component of magnetization is created. Some of this longitudinal component subsequently is returned to the transverse plane (by later imperfect 180 degree pulses), where it may refocus with later echoes. However, because of its different history, it may be phase-shifted from the "true" echo (i.e., the component that has been always in the transverse plane) and thus give rise to artifactual "ghost" images shifted in the direction of the phase-encoding gradient.[3] We have previously analyzed such effects[3,4] and shown how the error in the estimate of *T2* depends on the magnitude of imperfections in both H_1 and H_0, the rf and static fields, respectively. Errors in H_1 arise from coil inhomogeneity or inappropriate selection of pulse amplitude or duration. Off-resonance effects arise from main-field inhomogeneities or inappro-

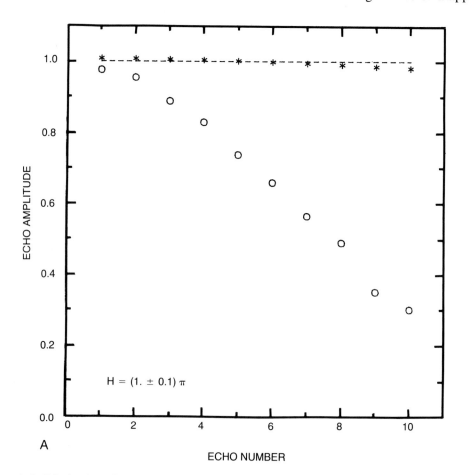

Figure 9–7. Calculated amplitudes of successive echoes in a multiple-echo sequence. The dashed lines represent the ideal situations for a material with infinitely long *T2*. The asterisks (*) denote the result of using composite refocusing pulses. *A* shows the effects of using pulses that are 10 percent incorrect.

priate selection of the transmitter frequency. In effect, H_1 and H_0 imperfections are similar in their consequences and are exacerbated in multiple-slice imaging by the use of spatially selective refocusing pulses. Selective 180 degree pulses are notorious for the fact that they produce complete 180 degree nutations over only a fraction of the total slice affected, so that regions toward the edge experience pulses that are substantially weaker than a 180 degree pulse in their effect. Consequently, selective 180 degree pulses produce echo trains that contain many of the features of rf pulse and main-field imperfections.[5]

The qualitative features of such imperfections are illustrated in Figure 9–7, which shows how the amplitudes of echoes in a 10-echo sequence oscillate and reduce in amplitude with an apparent $T2$ much different from the actual value when the refocusing rf pulses are 10 to 50 percent from being true 180 degree pulses. Such effects may well have been the origin of errors in some previous attempts to estimate $T2$ in imaging systems. In order to optimize our particular approach, three modifications are implemented that are crucial for its success. First, all 180 degree pulses are nonselective, and only one slice is imaged at a time. Second, each 180 degree pulse is actually a composite pulse, i.e., $90_x - 180_y - 90_{-x}$, which partially compensates for deviations in the H_1 inhomogeneity. Third, additional dephasing gradients in the z (slice selection) direction are pulsed on before and after each 180 degree pulse to attenuate the ghost artifacts that arise from field imperfections. These balanced dephasing gradients have no effect on stationary true signals but affect moving spins and artifactual echo com-

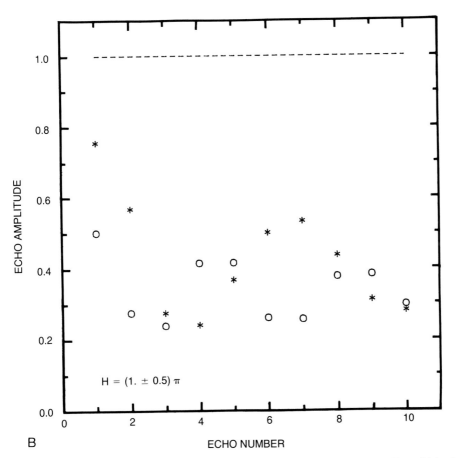

B

Figure 9–7 (*Continued*) B shows the effect of using pulses that are 50 percent incorrect. (From Majundar S, et al: Magn Reson Med *3*:397, 1986. Used by permission.)

Effect of frequency

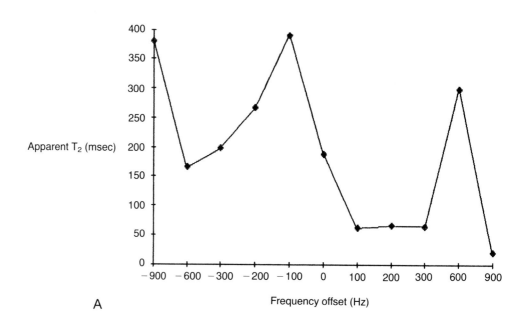

A

Effect of transmitter power

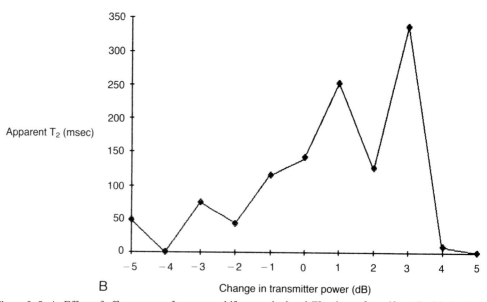

B

Figure 9–8. A, Effect of off-resonance frequency shifts on calculated *T2* values of a uniform liquid phantom. B, Effect of variations in the 180 degree pulse amplitude (measured in dB rf power relative to the ideal case) on calculated *T2* values of a uniform liquid phantom.

ponents. The resultant sequence is then much less susceptible to artifacts even in the relatively nonuniform field of our resistive magnet.[3]

Experiments have been performed explicitly to measure the magnitudes of errors that may nonetheless arise. In particular, we have attempted to estimate the errors in reconstructed *T1* and *T2* calculated images of uniform liquid samples arising from (1)

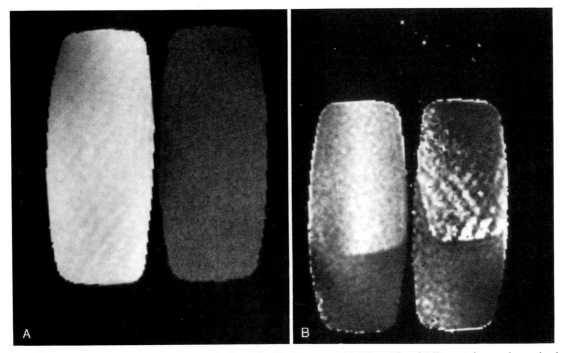

Figure 9–9. *A*, Calculated *T2* image of two uniform liquid phantoms with *T2* = 65 and 160 ms, taken under optimal conditions. *B*, Calculated *T2* image as in (*A*) but with rf transmitter 2 dB incorrect and no ghost-removing additional gradients. A "ghost" artifact is superimposed on the true object.

off-resonance effects (achieved by changing the transmission frequency), (2) rf pulse errors (achieved by altering the transmitted pulse amplitude), and (3) ghost artifacts in the absence of our "ghostbusting" dephasing gradients. Figure 9–8 shows that alterations in the transmitter frequency of as little as 100 Hz cause the echo amplitudes to alter in such a way that the apparent *T2* of a material with *T2* = 160 ms shifts by 60 percent. Similarly, altering rf transmitted power by 1 dB causes a change in the calculated *T2* of almost 50 percent. Figure 9–9 shows the effects of removing the ghost-dephasing gradients on a calculated image in our sequence when the transmitted power is 2 dB incorrect. The ghost artifact adds image intensity to some regions, which apparently compensates for the reduction in intensity that might otherwise arise. However, the estimated *T2* would be incorrect for any nonuniform object because the calculation would include contributions from material displaced in the phase-encoding direction.

These results indicate that without proper precaution the accuracy of *T2* and *T1* estimates using these sequences may be substantially impaired. They indicate that careful adjustment of the rf power and MR frequency is essential even with the use of nonselective composite pulses and additional dephasing gradients.

AUTOMATED IMAGE SEGMENTATION OF CALCULATED IMAGES

Image segmentation may be defined as the problem of decomposing an image into regions of common characteristics. In any automated image-analysis system, segmentation is a necessary first step and is usually a precursor to the process of description, in which measurements of properties within regions of an image are correlated with knowledge about relationships between objects in the scene.

Quantitative MR images of the type described earlier present a unique opportunity for image analysis, since there is a 1:1 correspondence between image brightness and a well-defined intrinsic tissue property. This means that brightness histograms can be used to identify "natural clusters" of indistinguishable volume elements in the image. The method of hierarchical clustering based on histogram analysis of both *T1* and *T2* images is one approach to segmentation of quantitative MR images. The key features of the method presented here are that segmented regions are identified using *both T1* and *T2* information, and that these regions exhibit the same resolution as the original images.

The basic segmentation algorithm is based on a hierarchical approach, in which image decomposition is obtained in multiple steps according to a tree structure (Fig. 9–10), commonly referred to as a dendrogram. Level 1 represents the original *T1* and *T2* images. Using a histogram analysis method described later, the *T1* and *T2* images are parsed into three new subimages, designated at Level 2. The same analysis is then applied to the subimages of Level 2, resulting in new progeny shown on Level 3. This process is continued until one of a set of parsing rules is violated. We note that the parsing from one level to the next is not always even. For example, subimage 21 may not be able to be separated further, yet subimage 22 may go on for several more generations. The parsing stops when all current subimages can no longer be divided (i.e., further separation of any image violates one of the parsing rules). The image is now considered segmented into *N* subimages generated according to the dendrogram (Fig. 9–10). The average values of *T1* and *T2* are then computed in each of the regions. In addition, other features of the region, such as local spatial variations in *T1* and *T2*, can be derived to help classify the properties of the region.

The basic principle of the histogram analysis method is presented in Figure 9–11. The histogram of *T1* values is illustrated for a particular subimage. The histogram is first fit to a double gaussian model

$$p(T1) = P_1 e^{-(T1-\mu_1)^2/2\sigma_1^2} + P_2 e^{-(T1-\mu_2)^2/2\sigma_2^2} \tag{10}$$

using a steepest descent method. Henceforth, we assume that P_1, μ_1, and σ_1 are associated with the most probable element (i.e., $P_1 > P_2$). Using a maximum likelihood criterion, namely that

$$P_1 e^{-(T1^0-\mu_1)^2/2\sigma_1^2} = P_2 e^{-(T1^0-\mu_2)^2/2\sigma_2^2} \tag{11}$$

a threshold, $T1^0$, between the two distributions is generated. In addition, a second threshold is generated using the 2σ point of the most probable distribution on the opposite side of the first threshold (i.e., $T1^1 = \mu_1 \pm 2\sigma_1$). The two thresholds computed

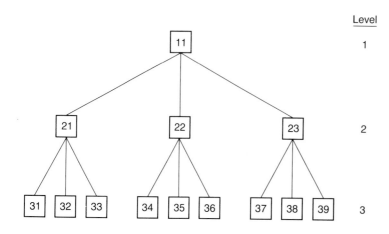

Level

1

2

3

Figure 9–10. Dendrogram, or true structure, for the decomposition of an image using a hierarchical approach.

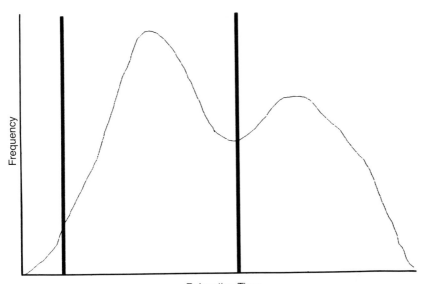

Figure 9–11. Histogram segmentation method, where dark solid lines represent thresholds computed for the histogram for this case.

in this way, represented by the thick solid lines in Figure 9–11, give rise to the following parsing rules:

A. $\mu_1 > \mu_2$

Region I $T1 < T1^0$

Region II $T1^0 \leq T1 \leq \mu_1 + 2\sigma_1$

Region III $T1 > \mu_1 + 2\sigma_1$

B.

Region I $T1 < \mu_1 - 2\sigma_1$

Region II $\mu_1 - 2\sigma_1 \leq T1 \leq T1^0$

Region III $T1 > T1^0$

Accordingly, the image is parsed into three subimages using these rules. Initial parsing is based on $T1$ data and stops only if one of the following four rules is violated:

1. $|\mu_1 - \mu_2| < \delta$
2. σ_1 or $\sigma_2 < \delta$
3. $|\mu_1 - T1^0| + |\mu_2 - T2^0| < |\mu_1 - \mu_2|$
(i.e., the threshold is not between the two means)
4. $(RMSD_1 - RMSD_2)/(RMSD_2) < \epsilon$.

In Rules 1 and 2, the term δ represents the basic histogram interval, which was 10 ms for $T1$ images and 5 ms for $T2$ images. In Rule 4, $RMSD_1$ is the root mean square deviation for fitting the histogram to a single gaussian distribution; similarly, $RMSD_2$ is the root mean square deviation for the double gaussian fit. The term ϵ in Rule 4 is a constant chosen to equal 0.10 in our studies. These four stopping rules are related to the accuracy of modeling the histogram of any subimage as a double gaussian distribution. If the double gaussian model is not valid, then the parsing algorithm assumes that the subimage represents a single gaussian distribution and cannot be subdivided further.

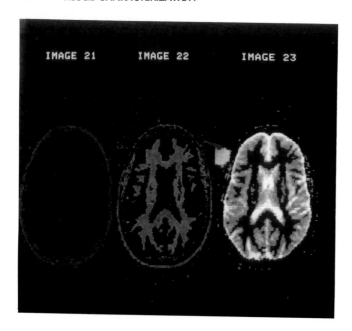

Figure 9–12. First level of segmentation of *T1* image from Figure 9–5.

Once additional *T1* parsing is no longer allowed by these rules, the method switches to *T2* data. The same analysis and stopping rules used for *T1* image parsing are applied to *T2* data. We note that the switch from *T1* to *T2* data does not necessarily occur at the same level for every subimage. For example, subimage 21 may be subdivided into subimages 31, 32, and 33 based on *T2* data, whereas subimage 22 may be subdivided into subimages 34, 35, and 36 based on *T1* data. However, for all images, *T2* parsing is used only after *T1* parsing is no longer valid for a particular subimage.

The segmentation algorithm described has been applied to a number of simultaneous *T1-T2* images obtained with the inversion-saturation recovery sequence. Figures 9–5 and 9–6 present *T1* and *T2* images of a healthy adult volunteer. Using these images as image 11 in the dendrogram of Figure 9–10, the first level of segmentation computed solely with *T1* data is presented in Figure 9–12. Subimage 21 shows the outline of the head, presumably associated with the short *T1* of skin and subcutaneous tissue, while subimage 22 contains primarily gray matter but also a subcutaneous boundary layer of tissue indistinguishable in terms of *T1*. Subimage 23 contains primarily brain gray matter and cerebrospinal fluid (CSF). It is interesting to note that the initial parsing distinguishes two categories of material in the peripheral border of the head. On anatomic grounds we suppose that this distinction represents concentric layers of skin, connective tissue, loose areolar tissue, and fat. Image brightness is proportional to *T1*. We have chosen a convention for image display in which the brightness for each pixel of a subimage is proportional to the *T1* of that pixel, *even if* the parsing to that subimage uses *T2* data. In reality, each pixel in each subimage has both a *T1* and a *T2* value.

Further parsing of the images presented in Figure 9–12 generates 12 independent regions. Several of these regions contain very few pixels, generally representing points along the edge between well-defined regions. However, several of the regions can be associated with the predominate tissue types in the head. In particular, from anatomic considerations it appears that subimage 22 (Fig. 9–12) can be associated with brain white matter. The average *T1* and *T2* in this subimage are 345 ± 30 ms and 72 ± 28 ms, respectively, values well within the range for white matter at this field strength, even though this image may be slightly biased by the inclusion of the subcutaneous region. Similarly, it appears that subimage 45, obtained using both *T1* and *T2* segmen-

Table 9–1. STATISTICAL PROPERTIES OF EIGHT DOMINANT PIXEL SUBGROUPS IN HUMAN BRAIN SCAN THROUGH LATERAL VENTRICLES

% Area	T1 Range	T1 Mean	Standard Deviation
1·4	1–280	66	96
4·6	281–343	330	81
26·1	344–435	394	27
25·0	436–507	471	21
18·1	508–587	543	23
7·6	588–650	618	18
4·0	651–694	670	114
13·0	695–2040	1062	287

tation, can be anatomically associated with gray matter. This image has averaged $T1$ and $T2$ times of 549 ± 130 ms and 82 ± 15 ms, respectively, values well within the range for gray matter at this field strength. Consequently, the segmentation approach appears to parse the $T1$ and $T2$ images into reasonable clusters without using specific templates. From an initial histogram of the type shown in Figure 9–11 we derive eight significant subdistributions, each characterized by a mean, standard deviation, and pixel count. Table 9–1 lists details of the subpopulations discriminated by this method. For quantitative tissue characterization, it is possible that regional variations of one or more such subgroups indicates a deviation from norm; or, we may look for alterations in the subgroup parameters themselves as alternative strategies to more traditional region-of-interest statistical parameters.

Starting with quantitative $T1$ and $T2$ images obtained with an efficient multiple-echo, inversion-saturation recovery pulse sequence, we have begun to investigate the possibility of an automated image-analysis system for tissue characterization. Hierarchical processing of brightness histograms has been used to parse $T1$ and $T2$ images into natural clusters that presumably represent distinct tissue types. Initial parsing is performed according to $T1$. Once parsing is no longer valid for $T1$ data, further parsing is attempted with $T2$ data. Partially reconstructed images, representing the sum of several subimages, can be used to highlight image features at high resolution and with high contrast-to-noise. Our preliminary results using this technique in clinical studies of radiation-treated tumors and for regional gray–white matter ratio measurements suggest that quantitative analysis of such $T1$ and $T2$ images may be useful for tissue characterization and accurate planimetry of tissue types.

References

1. Edelstein WA, Bottomley PA, Hart HR, Smith LS: Signal, noise and contrast in nuclear magnetic resonance imaging. J Comput Assist Tomogr 7:391, 1983.
2. O'Donnell M, Gore JC, Adams WJ: Toward an automated analysis system for nuclear magnetic resonance imaging. 1. Efficient pulse sequences for simultaneous $T1$-$T2$ imaging. Med Physics 13:182, 1986.
3. Majumdar S, Orphanoudakis S, Gmitro A, O'Donnell M, Gore JC: Errors in the measurements of $T2$ using multiple echo MRI techniques. I. Effects of radiofrequency pulse imperfections. Magn Reson Med 3:397, 1986.
4. Majumdar S, Orphanoudakis S, Gmitro A, O'Donnell M, Gore JC: Errors in the measurements of $T2$ using multiple echo MRI techniques. II. Effects of static field inhomogeneity. Magn Reson Med 3:562, 1986.
5. Majumdar S, Gore JC: Effects of selective pulses on the measurements of $T2$ and apparent diffusion in multiecho MRI. Magn Reson Med 4:120, 1987.

III

CLINICAL EXPERIENCE: MRI OF THE BRAIN

10

White Matter/Multiple Sclerosis

VAL M. RUNGE
ANN C. PRICE

The sensitivity of magnetic resonance imaging to intracerebral disease in multiple sclerosis (MS) became apparent immediately following its clinical introduction.[1,2] Both *T1* and *T2* weighted techniques have been utilized to detect plaques, which are usually seen as low signal intensity areas on *T1* images and high signal intensity areas on *T2*. This appearance is due to the prolongation of both transverse and longitudinal relaxation times in the area of abnormality. Although both gliosis and edema presumably play a role in increased relaxation times, the pathologic processes responsible for this change have not been well studied. Not all plaques (even within a single patient) demonstrate the same prolongation of *T1* and *T2*; however, these differences are not thought to accurately reflect disease activity or stage.

In multiple sclerosis, lesions occur in a typical distribution.[3–5] Plaques are seen primarily in the white matter, with periventricular and supraventricular locations being most common. MRI studies (Fig. 10–1) have confirmed this distribution.[6] Lesions commonly are noted in the internal capsule, with the posterior limb seemingly favored. In one early study, brainstem plaques were noted in approximately 25 percent of cases. Gray matter lesions also may be encountered, although these are uncommon. The advent of surface coils has markedly improved the ability of MRI to detect spinal cord lesions, which prior to this time usually were confirmed only at autopsy.[7]

As shown in Figure 10–1, areas of abnormality demonstrate high signal intensity on *T2* weighted images and low signal intensity on *T1*. The use of very long *TR*'s and *TE*'s (classically more "heavily *T2* weighted" images) can be counterproductive, however, for maximum detection of lesions. In these scans, the long *T2* of cerebrospinal fluid is emphasized, making the identification of periventricular lesions difficult, and on occasion decreasing the contrast between white matter plaques and normal surrounding brain. Along the ventricles, the high-intensity lesions are easily lost in the intense signal from CSF. *T1* weighted spin-echo images are not efficacious for lesion detection, even with the use of relatively short *TE*'s and *TR*'s, owing to the low sensitivity of these techniques to *T1* contrast. Indeed, lesions may not be visualized on these short spin-echo techniques (Fig. 10–2), emphasizing the need for *T2* weighted scans.

Inversion recovery sequences are much more heavily *T1* weighted and can detect multiple sclerosis plaques with high sensitivity (Figs. 10–3 and 10–4). These are particularly efficacious for the identification of lesions situated deep within white matter. Because of the low signal intensity of CSF and the broad range of contrast present on these scans, they may be more difficult to interpret. In particular, periventricular abnormalities as well as those near cortical sulci may be difficult to identify.

Field strength as well as imaging technique may have substantial impact upon visualization of lesions. *T1*'s of most tissues increase with field strength; for example,

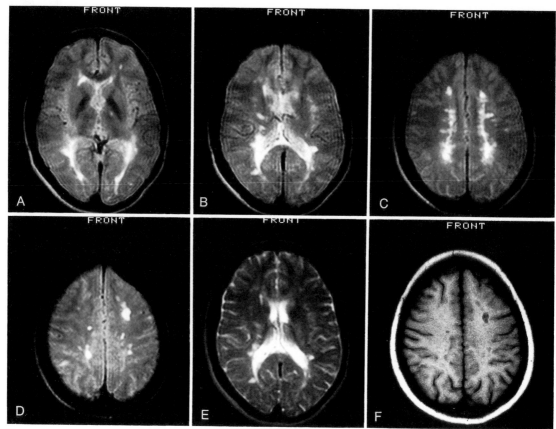

Figure 10–1. *A–D,* Four contiguous axial sections in a patient with multiple sclerosis. *TR/TE* = 2500/70, 1 cm slice thickness, 128 acquisition matrix, 1 tesla field strength. Multiple discrete punctate areas of high signal intensity (long *T2*), becoming almost confluent in the periventricular region, are noted in a classic distribution for the disease. Plaques are observed most commonly in the immediate periventricular region (frontal horns and atria), supraventricular white matter, and internal capsule. *E,* On a more heavily *T2* weighted image (SE 2500/240) some lesions immediately adjacent to the ventricles become less apparent owing to the high signal intensity of CSF (compare with *B*). The ability to identify abnormal areas as contrasted with surrounding normal white matter also may prove to be poorer on these longer *TE* images. To some extent this reflects the lower signal to noise ratios achieved with long *TE*'s. *F,* On a mildly *T1* weighted spin-echo image (SE 800/17) a few lesions may be identified (in this example, in the supraventricular region). However, the intermediate *T2* weighted image (*D*) remains significantly more efficacious. On the *T2* weighted images, lesions typically are of high signal intensity, whereas they are of low signal intensity on *T1* weighted images. This reflects the long *T1* and *T2* of multiple sclerosis plaques when contrasted with normal brain matter.

T1's from 0.5 to 1.0 tesla typically increase by 30 percent. Some tissues, however, may be anomalous. Field strength therefore may affect one's ability to detect lesions, in addition to requiring changes in pulse technique to achieve the same mix of *T1* and *T2* weighting. Combating potential negative aspects to imaging at higher field strengths is the significant advantage of increased signal-to-noise.

With a given imaging technique and field strength, the radiologist must be familiar with the normal appearance of the intracranial contents on MRI. In particular, an area of high signal intensity is normally demonstrated on *T2* weighted images in the distal portion of the posterior limb of the internal capsule (Fig. 10–5). Symmetry in the axial plane aids in recognition of such normal structures. High signal intensity on *T2* weighted techniques adjacent to the frontal horns ("capping") may also be a variant of normal. This finding appears commonly in the elderly and is of unknown etiology and significance.

The ability to achieve high-resolution direct sagittal and coronal images constitutes

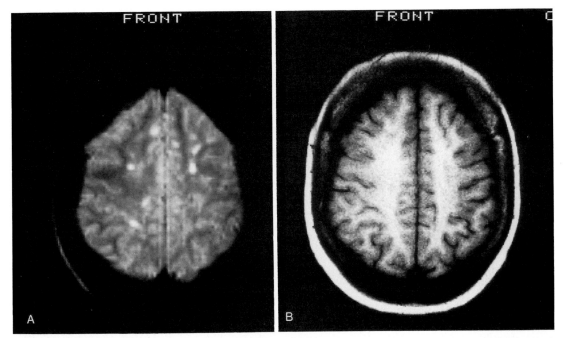

Figure 10–2. A second multiple sclerosis patient with more than seven lesions identified on a SE 2500/70 technique in the supraventricular white matter (*A*). However, the mild *T1* weight (SE 800/17) fails to identify any abnormality (*B*). Short spin-echo techniques, with only mild *T1* weighting, prove to be significantly less efficacious for detection of disease when compared with *T2* weighted images.

a significant advantage of MRI over x-ray CT (Figs. 10–6 and 10–7). This capability is important in the study of multiple sclerosis, particularly in examination of the brainstem and spinal cord, where sagittal images generally are diagnostically superior. For examination of the cord itself, specially designed surface coils provide the most diagnostic images. The true clinical potential of this technique is just now being explored.

The superiority of MRI over x-ray CT for the detection of multiple sclerosis plaques rapidly became readily apparent. Despite the use of thin sections and double-dose delayed scanning, two techniques that improve the "harvest" of lesions,[8-11] MRI remains pre-eminent (Fig. 10–8). Indeed, the use of contrast media and thin sections may further increase the sensitivity of MRI. Preliminary trials[12] indicate that Gd-DTPA (Berlex Laboratories, Cedar Knolls, New Jersey) enhanced MRI can distinguish between active and quiescent lesions in multiple sclerosis. If substantiated in continued clinical trials, this finding would improve substantially our ability to assess activity of disease and effectiveness of treatment regimens. Reliable quantitation of these two parameters has so far eluded physicians to some extent. In the same initial research at the University of Pennsylvania, no new lesions were demonstrated following Gd-DTPA administration (all the enhancing lesions had been previously noted on *T2* weighted images without Gd-DTPA).

By the comparison of CT and MRI, we have been able to improve our criteria for the recognition of MS on x-ray CT, leading to increased awareness of the potential pattern of distribution of lesions and improved film diagnoses.[13]

Progression of disease in multiple sclerosis and a change in the distribution of plaques has been noted temporally in clinical studies with MRI as well as CT.[14-16] In some series, the changes on MRI have corresponded with clinical neurologic findings. However, this issue is complicated by the presence of lesions in clinically "silent" areas of the brain. The use of contrast enhancement should provide a more accurate assessment of disease activity.

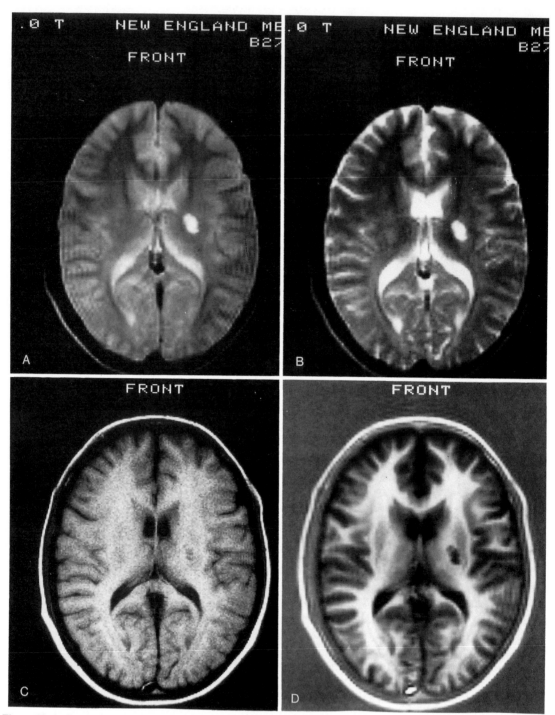

Figure 10–3. A comparison of four imaging techniques in a patient with multiple sclerosis. SE (*A*) 2500/70, (*B*) 2500/140, (*C*) 800/17, IR (*D*) 1500/400/30 (*TR/TI/TE*). A solitary large lesion is identified at this level in the posterior limb of the left internal capsule. The SE 2500/70 *T2* weighted image and the IR (heavy *T1* weight) are equally efficacious for visualization of the lesion. This plaque is poorly seen on the mildly *T1* weighted SE sequence (*C*, SE 800/17). The inversion recovery image demonstrates superior gray–white matter differentiation (compared with the other three imaging techniques), enabling identification of the head of the caudate, the lenticular nucleus, and the thalami. Without the identification of other abnormalities at different brain levels (present in this case but not shown here), a definitive diagnosis of multiple sclerosis could not be made.

Figure 10–4. A comparison of inversion-recovery technique (*A*, 1500/400/30) and *T2* weighted spin-echo imaging (*B*, 1500/70) in the detection of supraventricular abnormalities in a patient with multiple sclerosis. Several discrete areas of abnormal low signal intensity (long *T1*) are more easily identified on the IR sequence, thus proving the superior efficacy of heavily *T1* weighted techniques in certain restricted applications. This is most true for white-matter lesions deep within the corona radiata or centrum semiovale (i.e., lesions deep within white-matter tracts).

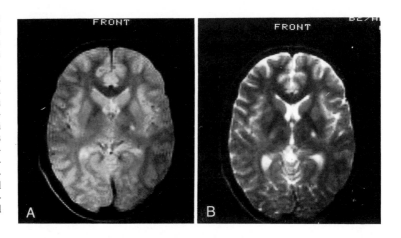

Figure 10–5. Lesions adjacent to the posterior limb of the internal capsule are commonly identified in multiple sclerosis. In this patient, a single plaque is seen on the left: *A*, 2500/70. *B*, 2500/140. Images obtained from a multiecho-multislice acquisition. A subtle increase in signal intensity on heavily *T2* weighted images can, however, be demonstrated in this region in normal subjects (best seen in this case on the second echo, right posterior internal capsule). The radiologist interpreting scans must be familiar with the normal patterns of signal intensity experienced, given the imaging technique and magnetic field strength employed.

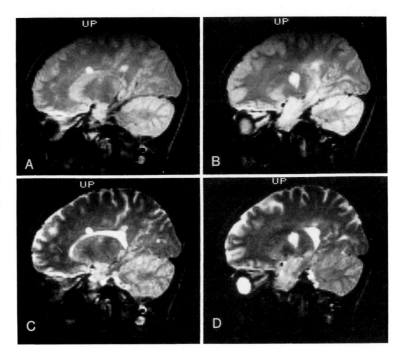

Figure 10–6. Several MS plaques are identified in this individual (same patient as in Figure 10–3) on contiguous 5 mm sagittal sections. *A–B*, SE 2500/70; *C–D*, SE 2500/140. Images from a multiecho-multislice acquisition technique. On the longer *TE* images, the high signal intensity from CSF in the lateral ventricles aids in orientation.

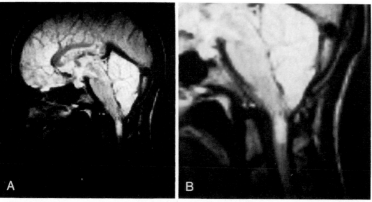

Figure 10–7. A high cervical cord plaque (*A*) on 5 mm sagittal imaging (SE 2500/60). Without the identification of other lesions (which were observed in this patient), a definitive diagnosis of multiple sclerosis cannot be made. Given this image alone for interpretation, ischemic and neoplastic lesions also would need to be included in differential diagnosis. Postacquisition magnification (*B*) improves visualization of the lesion.

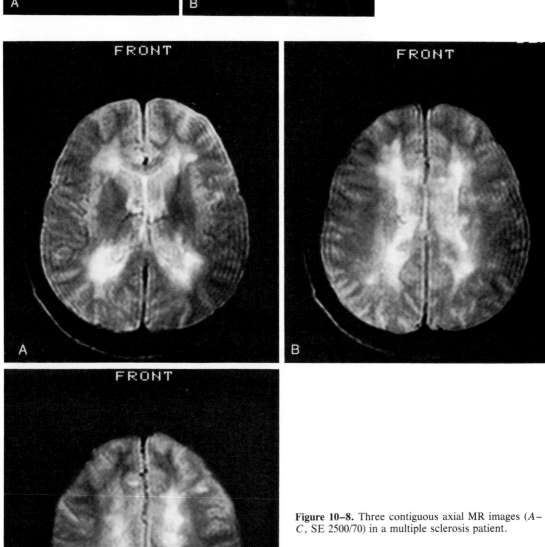

Figure 10–8. Three contiguous axial MR images (*A–C*, SE 2500/70) in a multiple sclerosis patient.

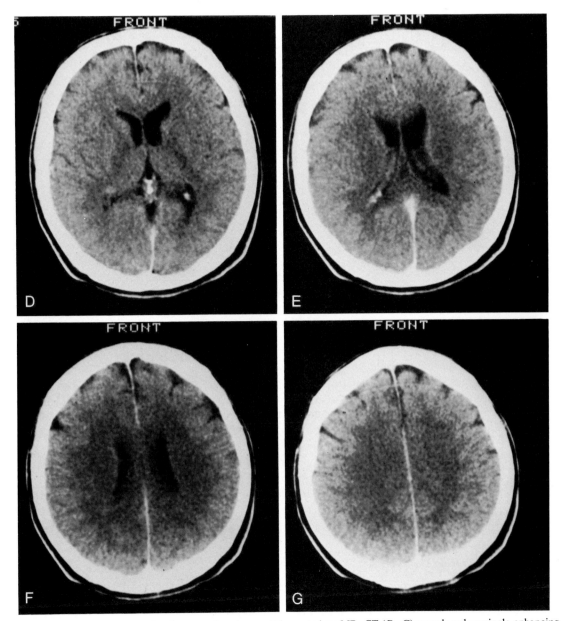

Figure 10–8 (*Continued*) Despite the extensive abnormalities noted on MR, CT (*D–G*) reveals only a single enhancing lesion (immediately anterior to the right ventricular trigone). The x-ray CT was performed with double-dose delayed IV contrast administration and 8 mm sections. The slice thickness on MR was 10 mm.

Figure 10–9 illustrates the MRI findings in a cadaver brain (from a patient with multiple sclerosis). This represents the first reported case correlating MRI and gross pathology. Although this analysis is still ongoing, much is to be learned from such an approach about the true sensitivity of MRI to disease states.

Multiple sclerosis must be differentiated on MRI from other disease entities that cause prolongation of *T1* and *T2*.[17] The presence of a lesion in a known arterial distribution with involvement of both gray and white matter leads to a diagnosis of stroke, not multiple sclerosis, despite any similarity in signal intensity of the lesion. Deep white matter ischemia (DWMI), a common entity in the elderly population, must also be differentiated from multiple sclerosis. This distinction may be difficult, particularly if the clinical question is between advanced disease (in MS), in which plaques may become

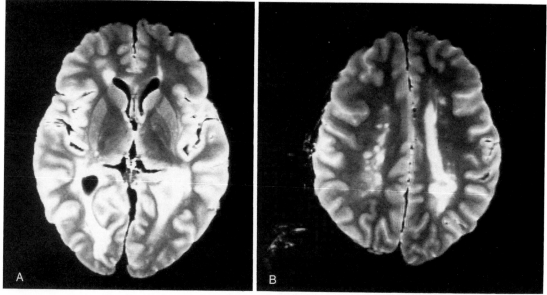

Figure 10–9. Two 3 mm MR axial sections through an autopsy specimen from a multiple sclerosis patient. *TR/TE* = 2.5/35. Greater than 20 discrete well-defined plaques are identified in the millimeter size range.

almost confluent, and DWMI. However, the presence of subcortical infarcts, confluence and symmetry of disease, and extension of white matter involvement to the gray–white matter junction all favor a diagnosis of DWMI.

Magnetic resonance imaging is without question the imaging modality of choice for the diagnosis of multiple sclerosis. Surface coils and high-field imaging have improved spatial resolution and made possible high-quality imaging of the spinal cord and cerebral hemispheres. The use of thin sections (down to 2 mm with our current instrumentation) should further improve lesion detection if clinical questions persist. The administration of an intravenous contrast agent, such as Gd-DTPA, adds the potential for evaluation of blood-brain barrier integrity and thereby improved assessment of disease activity and possible treatment regimens.

ACKNOWLEDGMENTS

With appreciation of the contribution of the MRI Division staff at the New England Medical Center—and in particular Dr. Michael Wood, Dr. John Kirsch, Janis Breslin, Joanne Incerpi, Donna Desmond, Nancy Wysocki, Michele Cochrane, and Noralene Slash.

References

1. Lukes SA, Crooks LE, Aminoff MJ, et al: Nuclear magnetic resonance imaging in multiple sclerosis. Ann Neurol *13*:592, 1983.
2. Young IR, Hall AS, Pallis CA, et al: Nuclear magnetic resonance imaging of the brain in multiple sclerosis. Lancet *2*:1063, 1981.
3. McFarlin DE, McFarland HF: Multiple sclerosis. Part I. N Engl J Med *307*:1183, 1982.
4. McFarlin DE, McFarland HF: Multiple sclerosis. Part II. N Engl J Med *307*:1246, 1982.
5. Brownell B, Hughes JT: The distribution of plaques in the cerebrum in multiple sclerosis. J Neurol Neurosurg Psychiatr *25*:315, 1962.
6. Runge VM, Price AC, Kirshner HS, et al: Magnetic resonance imaging of multiple sclerosis: a study of pulse technique efficacy. AJR *143*:1015, 1984.
7. Maravilla KR, Weinreb JC, Suss R, Nunnally RL: Magnetic resonance demonstration of multiple sclerosis plaques in the cervical cord. AJNR *5*:658, 1985.

8. Reisner T, Maida E: Computerized tomography in multiple sclerosis. Arch Neurol *37*:475, 1980.
9. Haughton VM, Ho KC, Williams AJ, Eldevik DP: CT detection of demyelinated plaques in multiple sclerosis. AJR *132*:213, 1979.
10. Hershey LA, Gado MH, Trotter JL: Computerized tomography in the diagnostic evaluation of multiple sclerosis. Ann Neurol *5*:32, 1979.
11. Sears ES, McCammon A, Bigelow R, Hayman LA: Maximizing the harvest of contrast enhancing lesions in multiple sclerosis. Neurology *32*:815, 1982.
12. Grossman RI, Gonzales-Scarano F, Atlas SW, Galetta S, Silberberg DH: Gd DTPA enhancement in magnetic resonance imaging of multiple sclerosis: a preliminary report. *In* Runge VM, Claussen C, Felix R, James AE Jr (eds): Contrast Agents in Magnetic Resonance Imaging. New York, Excerpta Medica, 1986, pp 121–123.
13. Price AC, Runge VM, Kirshner HS, Allen JH, Partain CL, James AE: Improved diagnosis of multiple sclerosis on CT examination after magnetic resonance image evaluation. 22nd Annual Meeting of the American Society of Neuroradiology, June 1984. Am J Neuroradiol *5*:678, 1984. (Abstract.)
14. Johnson MA, Li DKB, Bryant DJ, et al: Magnetic resonance imaging: serial observations in multiple sclerosis. AJNR *5*:495, 1984.
15. Kirshner HS, Tsai SI, Runge VM, Price AC: Magnetic resonance imaging and other techniques in the diagnosis of multiple sclerosis. Arch Neurol *42*:859, 1985.
16. Weinstein MA, Lederman RJ, Rothner AD, et al: Interval computed tomography in multiple sclerosis. Radiology *129*:689, 1978.
17. Bradley WG Jr, Waluch V, Brant-Zawadski M, Yadley RA, Wycoff RR: Patchy, periventricular white matter lesions in the elderly: a common observation during MR imaging. Noninvas Med Imag *1*:35, 1984.

11

Tumors of the Central Nervous System

L. S. DE VRIES
G. M. BYDDER

In the time between the first and second editions of this textbook, magnetic resonance imaging (MRI) of tumors in the central nervous system (CNS) has come of age. In the previous edition, several cases of tumor were illustrated but the total experience was quite small. Now reports on CNS tumors appear regularly in the world radiologic literature, and the field has rapidly become specialized. There is a wide recognition of the common features of tumors as well as an appreciation of the specific appearances of certain uncommon tumors. Whereas the potential of MRI for CNS tumors was first appreciated for imaging in the posterior fossa, major applications now include the supratentorial compartment and spinal cord. The early results were obtained on a few clinical research prototype machines, but several technical developments have had a major bearing on the improved clinical performance now being achieved. These include surface and closely coupled coils, new pulse sequences, and the paramagnetic contrast agent gadolinium-DTPA (see Chapters 12 and 46 to 52).

In this chapter some of the technical advances of particular relevance to tumor imaging are outlined, and results in the categories of CNS tumor are reviewed.

TECHNICAL FEATURES

High-Resolution Imaging

Initial MR images were produced with a matrix of 64×64 or 128×128; this has been increased so that most manufacturers provide 256×256 resolution. Many technical factors have contributed to this development, including specific features such as better magnetic field homogeneity and longer data collections with pulse sequences as well as less specific features associated with better design and greater experience. The use of closely coupled coils of the spherical type has been the single most important factor in improving machine performance in our experience.[1,2] These coils are simple to produce, being made of children's play helmets with copper tubing wound around them in a spherical configuration (Fig. 11–1). They are available in a range of sizes, and patients are measured in order to ensure that the coil is a satisfactory fit. The level of patient acceptance has been high. The coils are regarded as articles of clothing, which by definition are not claustrophobic. Wearing some sort of helmet as protection when entering the strange environment of an MRI machine has also seemed logical to some patients. Measured improvement in signal-to-noise ratio with these coils has been 2.5 to 3, and the principle is now being applied to orthogonal coils of the same design.

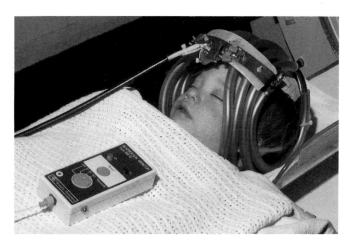

Figure 11–1. Closely coupled spherical receiver head coil in position on a child.

These "generalized" coils have a broader application than local surface coils, since multislice imaging can be performed in any plane without penalty.

Surface Coils

For localized areas within the central nervous system, small surface coils can provide a considerable improvement in image quality.[3] The principal area of application to date has been the spinal cord and spinal column. Small coils have been designed to examine just the cervical, thoracic, or lumbar region, and the results have been useful, although, if more than one region is required, examination time is increased. Less frequent uses include the internal auditory meatus as well as the temporal lobe and superficial tumors such as meningiomas, in which features such as the dural attachment may be demonstrated in detail. Considerable ingenuity has gone into the design of coils, but there is still a range of possible improvements to be made.

Outside of the brain and spinal cord, the orbit has been the principal area of use of surface coils and the improvements in image quality have been notable. There is also scope for detecting nasopharyngeal tumors, and applications in nonmalignant disease such as temporomandibular joint derangements have been successful.

Pulse Sequences

Significant advances have been made in extending the scope and range of application of the three common pulse sequences, and a variety of new pulse sequences have been developed over the last four years. Each of these pulse sequences will be discussed.

Partial Saturation (PS) and Saturation Recovery (SR) Sequences. In this context, partial saturation (PS) is used to indicate a sequence with a 90 degree pulse followed by data collection without a refocusing 180 degree pulse. The term "partial saturation" has also been applied to *T1* dependent (short *TE*, short *TR*) spin-echo sequences, but this usage can be confusing. In keeping with the American College of Radiology convention on nomenclature, we use the term "saturation recovery" (SR) only to describe the situation in which tissues have been saturated or very nearly saturated. In practice this is difficult to achieve, and to do so, we use a 90 degree pulse followed by a spoiler pulse. Following this "dephasing," an additional 90 degree pulse is performed, followed by a data collection. Details of these sequences are presented elsewhere.[4]

Initially it was recognized that the PS sequence with a long *TR* value and a short *TE* value was useful in identifying differences in proton density. Since changes in proton density were usually much less than changes in *T1* and *T2* demonstrated by inversion recovery (IR) or spin-echo (SE) sequences, it was thought that the clinical applications of the PS sequence would remain limited. However, changes in *T1* and *T2* are only one mechanism for the formation of image contrast; PS sequences may be useful in a variety of situations in which image contrast can be generated by flow effects, chemical shift effects, and detection of short *T2* components.[4] In addition, there has been a revival of interest in this sequence as a fast imaging technique with or without the use of contrast-enhancing agents.

Blood flowing into the slice may be highlighted with a PS sequence, since unsaturated blood is fully relaxed and may give a higher signal than tissue within the slice that has been saturated with previous 90 degree pulses. When *TR* of the pulse sequence is decreased, this effect may be increased—a feature that is specific for flowing blood and that may be useful in identification of arteriovenous malformations.

Increased proton density produces an increased signal intensity with this sequence and this may be observed with some tumors but not all. In fact, there may be a striking decrease in proton density in some tumors, particularly if they are calcified.

Recent developments of the PS and SR sequences have included the use of chemical shift effects. By choosing *TE* such that phase contrast between lipid and water components within tissues is developed in opposite directions, a cancellation effect can be obtained, with tissues having roughly equal proportions of lipid and water. This is important in the identification of lipid-containing tumors. It can also be of value in canceling the signal from red marrow, enabling lesions within the spinal column to be seen with greater contrast. The lipids in brain (phospholipids, syringomyelins, and so forth) are tightly bound and do not give a significant signal. The cancellation effect is of importance with triglycerides, in which significant signal is produced by protons within lipid.

Another notable feature of the PS sequence is the fact that it can be used to detect the short *T2* components in tissues, such as the anulus fibrosus and articular cartilage. The earlier data collection provides a higher signal intensity, which may be of value in obtaining thin slices. More recently, attention has been directed toward using reduced flip angles and low values of *TR* to achieve fast scanning. These techniques are generally low in soft tissue contrast, but this problem may be solved to some extent by the use of contrast agents such as intravenous gadolinium-DTPA (Gd-DTPA).

The saturation recovery sequence does not display the flow effects seen with the PS sequence and may be used in conjunction with the PS sequence to identify flow effects both in blood and in CSF.

Spin-Echo Sequence. This is the most common pulse sequence in MRI and is generally used in three forms: the largely *T1* dependent version, the largely *T2* dependent version, and the asymmetric spin echo.[5] The *T1* dependent version (short *TE*, short *TR*) provides useful anatomic detail, whereas the highly *T2* dependent version generally highlights pathologic change. With the trend to higher field systems, it has become clear that the increased *T1* of brain makes it more difficult to achieve high *T2* dependent contrast with spin-echo sequences while keeping the signal from CSF less than that from brain. When the CSF signal is higher than brain, partial volume effect between brain and CSF may simulate periventricular lesions. The asymmetric echo sequence has been used in a manner analogous to that of the PS sequence for identification of chemical shift effects.

The multiecho, multislice, highly *T2* dependent spin-echo sequence is probably the most useful single sequence in MRI of the brain, although it has a number of limitations.

Inversion Recovery Sequence. This sequence can be used in three different forms, a short *TI* version, a medium *TI* version, and a long *TI* version.[6] The short *TI* version shows high sensitivity as well as a greater degree of gray–white matter contrast than does the corresponding spin-echo sequence. The medium *TI* version shows a high level of anatomic detail. It is less sensitive in detection of most malignant tumors than a highly *T2* dependent spin-echo sequence but is more sensitive in some benign tumors, such as meningioma. The medium *TI* sequence is highly sensitive to contrast enhancement, unlike the heavily *T2* weighted spin-echo sequences. The long *TI* inversion recovery sequence is useful in pediatric practice, where the *TI* of infant brain is prolonged.

The IR sequence may be used with a spin echo or a field echo; the latter system makes available the chemical shift features associated with the PS sequence.

Other Sequences. Many other sequences have been developed over the last three years; one (steady state–free precession) has fallen into disuse. With this sequence, contrast was dependent on the parameter *T2/T1*. In many diseases, both *T1* and *T2* are increased so that the ratio changes relatively little, and contrast between normal and abnormal tissues is modest. An exception to this is subacute hemorrhage, in which *T1* is shortened and *T2* may be prolonged.

Echo-planar imaging (EPI) has now been used in the brain, where the long *T2* of brain provides sufficient time to obtain a 64×64 matrix (L. Crooks, personal communication). When used with a short *TI* inversion recovery, the chemical shift artifact from fat can be eliminated. $T1\rho$ imaging has been used in hematomas.[7]

Susceptibility changes may be more important than originally thought, in relation to both iron compounds in the brain and organic paramagnetic ions. Diffusion imaging so far appears to have a limited clinical application.

Derived images have received considerable attention. These include single parameter maps of proton density, and *T1* and *T2*, as well as phase maps. They are computed from two or more images of the three common types: PS and SR, IR, and SE. They permit direct measurement of proton density, *T1*, or *T2*, using a region-of-interest facility.

Synthetic imaging enables an image to be computed with any chosen value of *TR* or *TE* once proton density, *T1*, and *T2* maps have been constructed. So far the technique has been used mainly for teaching purposes.

The relative merits of different pulse sequences for different clinical conditions has been a major field of investigation. Although there is much work still to be done, common patterns of practice have emerged, and any new sequences will have established patterns for comparison.

Intravenous Gadolinium-DTPA

Gadolinium-DTPA (Gd-DTPA) is the first parenteral contrast agent approved for clinical use. It was developed by Schering[8] and was initially used in humans by Felix et al.[9] Clinical trials soon showed a level of contrast enhancement equal to or greater than that available with iodinated contrast agents in x-ray CT.[10,11] The agent is now being used at over 30 different sites in Europe and the United States, although FDA approval for general use is not thought likely until early 1988.

Gadolinium-DTPA has a similar molecular weight to iodinated agents and is distributed within the vascular compartment and extracellular space following intravenous injection. It does not cross the intact blood-brain barrier and is excreted unchanged through the kidneys. It accumulates in tumors in a manner analogous to that of iodinated contrast agents in CT.

Its effect on tissues is to shorten *T1* and *T2*. The effect is complicated by the fact

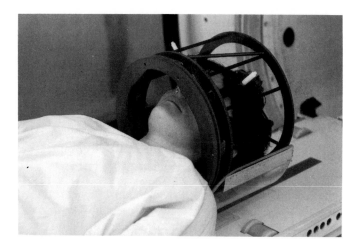

Figure 11–2. Subject shown with an MRI stereotactic frame in position.

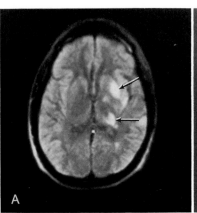
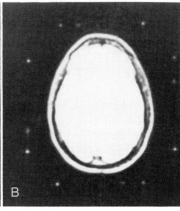

Figure 11–3. Abnormal regions on SE 1500/80, scan (*A*), with image windowed to show coordinate markers (*B*).

that the relaxation *rate* (the reciprocal of the relaxation time) is proportional to concentration so that there is a reciprocal relationship between *T1* and *T2* and gadolinium concentration. In addition, the absolute decrease in *T1* is greater than the absolute decrease in *T2*, since *T1* is always greater than *T2*. In the brain, *T1* is three to six times greater than *T2* at the fields commonly used for imaging so that the absolute changes in *T1* are more significant.

The choice of pulse sequence has a major bearing on whether or not contrast enhancement will be detected. The most sensitive sequences are highly *T1* dependent (such as medium *TI* inversion recovery), and the least sensitive are highly *T2* dependent. In general, decreasing *T1* increases signal intensity of the commonly used pulse sequences, whereas decreasing *T2* decreases signal intensity. The latter effect becomes dominant at high concentrations of Gd-DTPA, but at low concentrations the *T1* dependent increase in signal intensity is more important.

The properties of Gd-DTPA have been reviewed by Weinmann et al.[8] and its mechanism of action by Gadian et al.[12]

Stereotactic Biopsy

Stereotactic biopsy is now an established technique in x-ray CT, so it is not surprising that similar techniques have been developed for use with MRI. There are several practical problems that need to be overcome. The stereotactic frame must not contain ferromagnetic components, nor must there be a conducting pathway in which eddy currents may be induced. Coordinate markers have to be made of MRI-sensitive materials, such as lipids or solutions containing paramagnetic agents. Once these problems have been solved it is possible to use stereotactic biopsy systems in a manner essentially similar to that used in CT (Fig. 11–2). The main clinical application has been in lesions poorly visualized with CT,[13] but the technique is also of value in understanding the appearances of various tissues on MR images (Fig. 11–3).

GENERAL FEATURES OF CNS TUMORS

The first description of CNS tumors visualized with MRI was published in 1980,[14] and since then several reviews of clinical results containing general descriptions of CNS tumors have been published.[15-22] With more experience, variants and exceptions to the general pattern have been increasingly recognized. Nevertheless, the "typical" features of MRI tumors provide a useful clinical starting point.

The proton density of tumors may be increased or decreased; generally there is some increase with malignant tumors, although a decrease is seen with some benign tumors and in regions of dense calcification. The fact that the $T1$ and $T2$ of tumors is usually increased was recognized first by Damadian et al. in the early 1970s,[23] but exceptions to this pattern were seen even at this early stage. With increasing experience it became clear that there may be a wide spread of $T1$ and $T2$ values even within a single histologic classification and that there is overlap between different pathologic groupings. Since the tumor mass may contain calcification and cysts as well as hemorrhagic and necrotic areas, it is not surprising that it has not been possible to find single characteristic values of $T1$ and $T2$. In addition, some gliomas show areas of differing malignancy, and there may be differences within a tumor between viable, well-vascularized, well-oxygenated cells at the rim and cells at the center with inadequate blood supply.

Peritumoral edema produces an increase in $T1$ and $T2$; since this is the same basic change as that usually produced by the tumor mass, there may be difficulties in detecting the margin between the two pathologic processes. It is known from x-ray CT stereotactic biopsy studies that tumor often extends beyond the apparent rim of tumor; similar difficulties in defining the margin between tumor and edema might be expected with MRI. With use of a wider variety of sequences and intravenous Gd-DTPA, definition of the margin between the bulk of the tumor and surrounding edema has improved (Fig. 11–4).

Mass effects are generally better displayed with IR sequences than with SE sequences. This advantage may be particularly marked in comparison with x-ray CT in regions where the CT is obscured by the presence of artifact or by partial volume effect from bone. This includes the apex of the skull, the posterior fossa, and the skull base. In addition, mass effects may be better demonstrated in particular cases by direct sagittal or coronal imaging.

Hydrocephalus is well demonstrated with MRI. The sagittal plane is useful to show the region of the aqueduct. Periventricular edema can be demonstrated without confusion with partial volume effects between brain and CSF using appropriate spin-echo sequences. There are often some remote effects associated with tumors, including periventricular changes unrelated to hydrocephalus as well as changes in the properties of CSF (decreased $T1$ and $T2$) attributable to increased protein content. Ready visualization of the cervical spinal cord is another factor of importance with MRI. Determination of the extent of posterior fossa tumors into the cervical cord is relatively

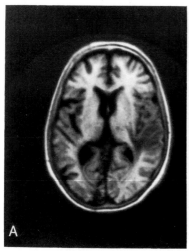 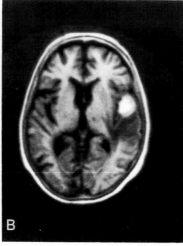

Figure 11–4. Metastasis from carcinoma of the breast: IR 1500/500/44, scans before (A) and after (B) Gd-DTPA. Definition between tumor and edema is improved in B.

straightforward. With the use of Gd-DTPA, dural and meningeal enhancement may be observed. These features may also be present with x-ray CT but are easily obscured by the presence of the adjacent skull.

Acoustic Neuromas

Soon after the first prototype MR images were introduced it was apparent that acoustic neuromas could be visualized on essentially the same basis as on x-ray CT; i.e., tumors down to about 1 cm could be visualized, but resolution was insufficient to demonstrate small tumors within the cerebellopontine angle (CPA) and internal auditory meatus (IAM).[24] With improvements in image quality it became possible to visualize the IAM in normal subjects and to demonstrate small tumors (Fig. 11–5). This extended the range of application of MRI to include acoustic neuromas previously recognizable only by CT cisternography with air or iodinated contrast media.[25-27] With further advances it has been possible to visualize the normal seventh and eighth cranial nerves. Gd-DTPA promises to be useful in doubtful cases involving very small tumors as well as postoperatively, when anatomical planes are lost or distorted.[28]

Care must be taken with the choice of sequence in the examination for acoustic neuromas. There are three sites to consider: intracanalicular, cerebellopontine angle, and posterior fossa. There are also two types of acoustic neuromas: first, those with a long $T1$ and $T2$; and second, those with a normal or only slightly prolonged $T1$ and $T2$. There are also three types of sequence in use: $T1$ and $T2$ dependent forms of spin echo and medium TI inversion recovery. The important normal tissues to consider are CSF, dense bone, fatty marrow, brain, and nerve roots. Essentially, the $T2$ dependent SE sequence is of value in demonstrating the canal and cochlear and vestibular system but may obscure small intracanalicular tumors that have normal values of $T1$ and $T2$. Within the cerebellopontine angle, distinction between tumor and adjacent cerebellum is important. If the tumor has a prolonged $T1$ and $T2$, this may be straightforward (Fig. 11–6); however, with tumors that do not display increased $T1$ and $T2$ values, diagnosis may be difficult (Fig. 11–7). With posterior fossa tumors (larger tumors) there may be difficulties in defining the margin between the tumor and surrounding brain edema. The use of Gd-DTPA provides an additional approach to this problem. The inversion recovery sequence, which is of limited value in demonstrating the IAM, is the sequence most sensitive to contrast enhancement; hence if it is intended to diagnose an acoustic

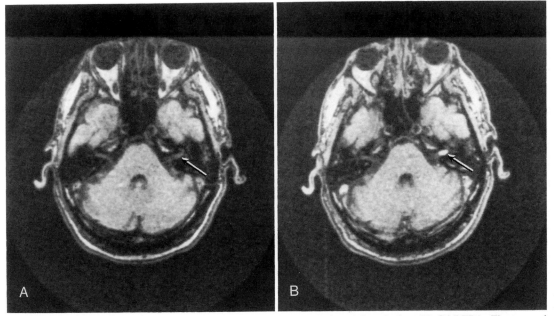

Figure 11–5. Intracanalicular acoustic neuroma: SR 300/22, scans before (*A*) and after (*B*) Gd-DTPA. The tumor is highlighted in *B* (arrows).

neuroma on IR sequence, before-and-after Gd-DTPA scans are both required. Some problems remain. The CSF within the IAM frequently appears to have a shorter *T1* than CSF elsewhere in the subarachnoid space. Occasionally, "flow effects" may be seen within the canal. Use of the short *TE*–short *TR* sequence to distinguish soft tissue of tumor from CSF and use of Gd-DTPA may be helpful in this situation.

MRI offers the potential to visualize acoustic neuromas as small as a few millimeters in diameter regardless of site. It avoids the need for contrast enhancement in most cases and the need for air CT cisternography in small tumors. Broader questions

Figure 11–6. Bilateral acoustic neuromas: SE 1500/80, scan. The tumors are highlighted (arrows).

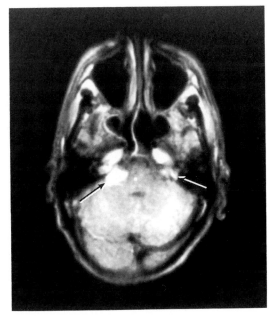

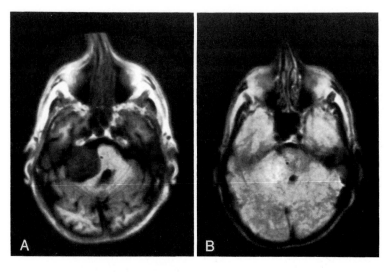

Figure 11–7. Acoustic neuroma: IR 1500/500/44, (*A*) and SE 1500/80, (*B*) scans. The tumor is well seen in *A* and poorly defined in *B*.

about the use of MRI as the general screening examination for all patients with unilateral nerve deafness remain.

Meningioma

The diagnosis of meningioma with MRI has been a matter of considerable interest over the last three years. Two reports have appeared in which the results of unenhanced MRI examinations were inferior to those obtained with contrast-enhanced CT.[28,29] Since meningiomas are important and generally curable lesions that are diagnosed with high accuracy by CT, this represents a major disadvantage for MRI. Since these earlier studies, improved results based on more recent MRI machines and Gd-DTPA contrast enhancement have appeared. There has also been wider appreciation of the fact that highly *T2* dependent sequences may not be the best technique for the diagnosis of meningioma.

A significant proportion of meningiomas show only a slight increase in *T1* over white matter and a *T2* within the normal range for brain. The use of highly *T2* dependent sequences therefore produces little soft tissue contrast. With medium *T1* inversion recovery sequences the slight difference between tumor and white matter may be sufficient to define the lesion (Fig. 11–8). In addition, the greater anatomic detail available

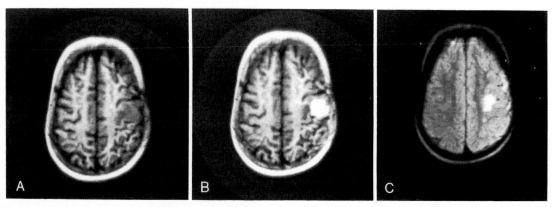

Figure 11–8. Meningioma: IR 1500/500/44, before (*A*) and after (*B*) Gd-DTPA with SE 1500/80, (*C*) scans. The tumor has a normal *T2* and is poorly seen on *C*. Definition and enhancement are better in *A* and *B*.

with IR images helps in identification of lesions. Meningiomas usually enhance with Gd-DTPA, and this enhancement is maximal with the medium *TI* IR sequence (Fig. 11–9). Since highly *T2* dependent sequences normally are used for detecting pathology in the brain (IR sequences are used much less frequently), there is a possibility of missing meningiomas. On the other hand, if IR sequences were used routinely for screening purposes the examination time would be increased. Questions about the use of Gd-DTPA in screening examinations also emerge. Gd-DTPA has been used only in

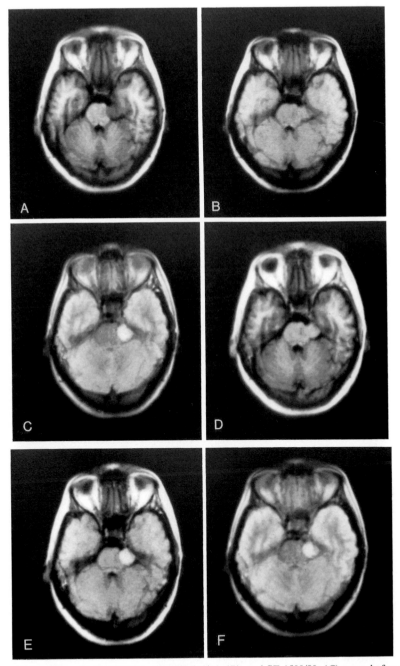

Figure 11–9. Meningioma: IR 1500/500/44, (*A*), SE 544/44, (*B*), and SE 1500/80, (*C*) scans before Gd-DTPA compared with IR 1500/500/44 (*D*), SE 544/44 (*E*), and SE 1500/80, (*F*) scans after Gd-DTPA. Greatest enhancement is seen between *A* and *D*.

a research context to date, but it could possibly be used routinely in the same way as iodinated contrast agents are now used with x-ray CT in order to exclude meningioma.

MRI has potential advantages over CT in demonstrating lesions adjacent to the convexity of the skull at the base of the brain and in the posterior fossa. Meningioma-en-plaque (Fig. 11–10) and dural involvement may be better demonstrated, although calcification is not. It is also possible that measurements of *T1* and *T2* may provide a guide to consistency and therefore surgical approach. Softer tumors may well have a longer *T1* and *T2* than harder tumors. Surface coils have been of value in demonstrating dural attachment adjacent to the skull.

Although results obtained with MRI in meningioma have improved, doubts remain about how an examination sensitive for meningioma can be integrated into routine practice. Since the symptoms of meningioma are not specific, there is often no particular indication to perform an examination specifically designed to detect this tumor. Missing a meningioma may not be important if it is a small incidental finding in the region of the falx, but the same-sized tumor in the optic canal or the foramen magnum may be highly significant. These issues have yet to be resolved, but the need to detect meningiomas in screening examinations may profoundly affect the choice of sequences, the length of time of screening examinations, and the extent to which Gd-DTPA is used in routine practice.

Other Benign Tumors

"Benign" is used in its traditional sense to indicate nonmalignant tumors, excluding, for example, Grades I and II astrocytomas. The common clinical entities include lipoma, epidermoid tumors, craniopharyngiomas, glomus tumors, chordomas, and, for convenience, colloid cysts and arachnoid cysts.

The lipid-containing tumors are of particular interest.[30] If triglyceride can be identified by use of a cancellation technique (PS) or the Dixon asymmetrical echo technique, the diagnosis can be quite specific (Fig. 11–11). The position of germinal layer neoplasms in the midline and the specific sites of predilection of various tumors provide additional information (Fig. 11–12).[31] For example, lipomas may display a cancellation effect. These tumors are also well demonstrated with x-ray CT; in fact, the calcification sometimes seen with them is better visualized with this modality. The appearance of epidermoid tumors is more variable. Craniopharyngiomas are well demonstrated, although specific identification of a lipid-containing cyst has not yet been described.

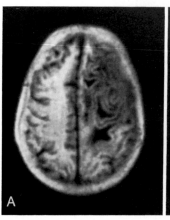
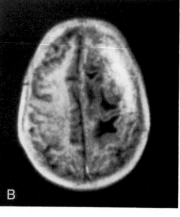

Figure 11–10. Meningioma-en-plaque: IR 1500/500/44, scans before (*A*) and after (*B*) Gd-DTPA. Definition of the tumor is best seen in *B*.

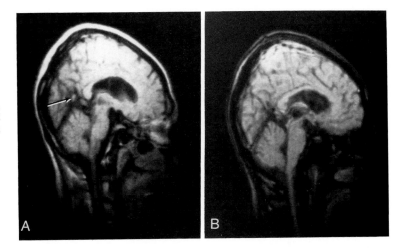

Figure 11–11. Lipoma: SE 544/44, (*A*) and PS 500/22, (*B*) scans. Part of the tumor (arrow) is not seen in *B* owing to cancellation effect.

Pinealomas and other tumors of the posterior end of the third ventricle are well demonstrated, particularly in the sagittal plane, although care must be taken not to mistake the choroid plexus within the third ventricle for tumor.

Similarly, chordomas can be well demonstrated in the sagittal and transverse planes. It is important to note that tumors of soft tissues, apart from brain, generally have a *T2* about half that of normal brain. A 100 percent increase in *T2* may therefore result in signal intensity similar to that of brain, with poor definition of the interface between tumor and brain. Tumors in the base of the skull can be well visualized (Fig. 11–13). Arachnoid cysts may display very long *T1* and *T2* values, but cysts with an increased proton content may display a shorter *T1* and *T2*. Distinction from solid lesions may then be difficult. The sharp margins and absence of edema are helpful signs. Colloid cysts are well seen (Fig. 11–14).

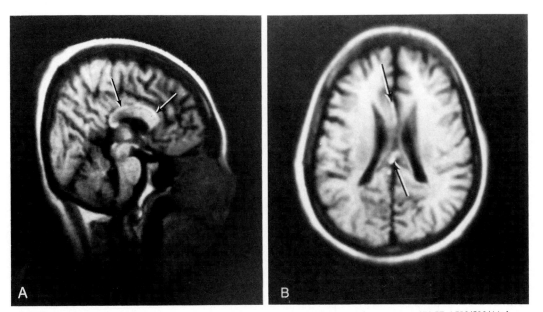

Figure 11–12. Lipoma with partial agenesis of the corpus callosum: sagittal (*A*) and transverse (*B*) IR 1500/500/44, images. The lipoma (arrows) has a high signal.

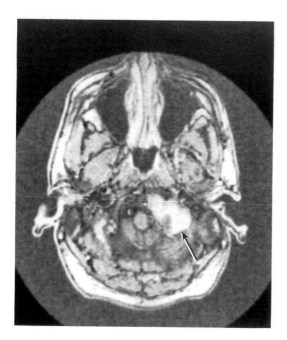

Figure 11–13. Glomus jugulare tumor: IR 1500/500/44, scan. The tumor is well displayed (arrows).

Pituitary Tumors

Some of the same features described for benign tumors of the brain also apply to pituitary tumors.[32–34] In general, the *T1* and *T2* of lesions are similar to those of brain, and calcification is poorly demonstrated. The pituitary stalk is well demonstrated as a high-signal area in normal subjects, and the inferior aspect of the pituitary fossa may contain fat. Extension of tumors outside the pituitary fossa is usually well shown (Fig. 11–15). However, sensitivity in detection of small tumors within the pituitary fossa is

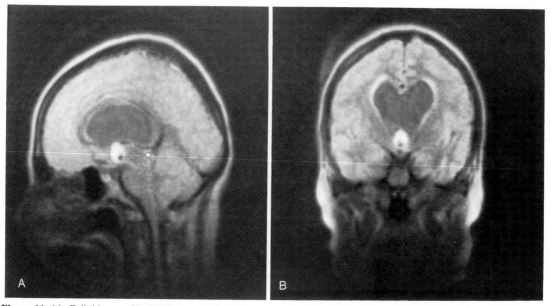

Figure 11–14. Colloid cyst: SE 1500/80, scans in sagittal (*A*) and coronal (*B*) planes. The cyst is seen associated with periventricular edema.

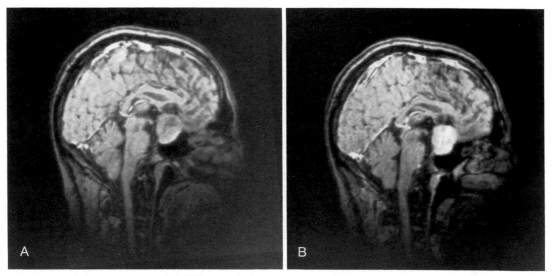

Figure 11–15. Pituitary adenoma: PS 500/22, scans before (*A*) and after (*B*) Gd-DTPA. The extent of the tumor is well defined.

less impressive. It is possible that volume screening of the restricted pituitary region may result in improved image quality in acceptable imaging times.

Contrast enhancement with Gd-DTPA has yet to be systematically evaluated with pituitary tumors, but improvement in existing results may well be possible.

MRI has the advantage that no ionizing radiation is used in the region of the lens of the eye. This may be important, especially as many patients with pituitary lesions are young, with a long life expectancy and high likelihood of requiring follow-up examinations in checking for recurrence or assessing the response to bromocriptine therapy. Recognition of parasellar lesions and their differential diagnosis can also be facilitated with MRI.

Malignant Tumors

For the purposes of this discussion, metastatic lesions are not specifically differentiated from primary tumors, although (as with CT) there are some differences, especially between Grades I and II gliomas and metastases.

In general, malignant tumors display a longer $T1$ and $T2$ than do benign tumors, such as meningiomas, but there is evidence that $T1$ and $T2$ do not necessarily increase with increasing malignancy and that necrotic areas may have shorter values of $T1$ and $T2$ than do surrounding tumor.

The increased relaxation within the tumor is frequently heterogeneous with higher grade tumors (Fig. 11–16), although some lower grade tumors within the brain may be quite uniform (Fig. 11–17). There are a number of circumstances in which areas within tumors with normal values of $T1$ and $T2$ may be seen.[35] These include malignant melanoma metastases, in which the normal or decreased $T1$ and $T2$ may be due to hemorrhage or paramagnetic melanins (Fig. 11–18). In patients who have hemorrhage with tumors, the same feature may be observed (Fig. 11–19). Following radiotherapy, some tumors also display a relatively short $T1$ and short $T2$. On spin-echo images, low signal areas may be seen (Fig. 11–20). These may be due to calcification, hemorrhage, accumulation of paramagnetics (e.g., Fe^{+++}, from hemorrhage), or membranes or capsules within the tumor, but the precise explanation may not be clear in any given case.

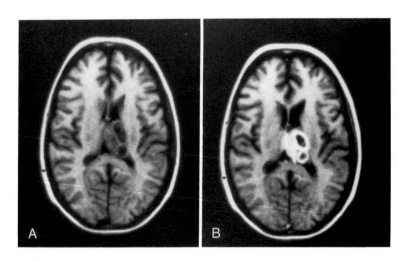

Figure 11-16. Astrocytoma, Grade III: IR 1500/500/44, before (A) and after (B) Gd-DTPA. Heterogeneous tumor showing enhancement.

Cyst formation usually appears as high *T1* and *T2* areas, and a fluid-fluid level may sometimes be observed, possibly as a result of accumulated debris within the tumor.

Patterns of edema vary, although there is a general tendency toward a perifocal pattern with more distinct spread along white matter pathways. Demarcation between tumor and edema can be quite difficult, but varying the *T1* and *T2* dependence of pulse sequence can improve the distinction considerably. Gd-DTPA is also of value, since it may reveal contrast enhancement in areas of apparent edema, indicating that these regions are likely to be tumor rather than edema. Similar difficulties may arise with periventricular changes in distinguishing direct or metastatic spread from edema (Fig. 11-21).[36]

A mass effect is a very important aspect of tumor diagnosis, although it is not invariably present. In addition to ventricular size and shape and the appearance of the basal cisterns, MRI provides a series of gray-white interfaces that are valuable reference points in assessing the presence of a mass effect. The fact that the surface of the brain is readily seen and that it can be visualized in any plane is also useful in assessing mass effects.

Hydrocephalus without localizing features can be a presentation of tumor in colloid cysts as well as in a variety of malignant third ventricular and brainstem lesions.

Studies have been presented detailing the time course of contrast enhancement with malignant tumors, and it is clear that enhancement may persist or even increase

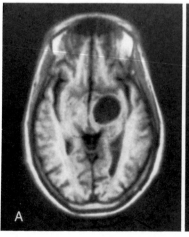
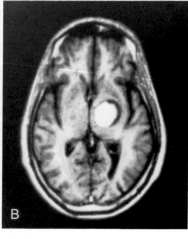

Figure 11-17. Thalamic glioma: IR 1500/500/44, scans before (A) and after (B) Gd-DTPA. The tumor appears more uniform.

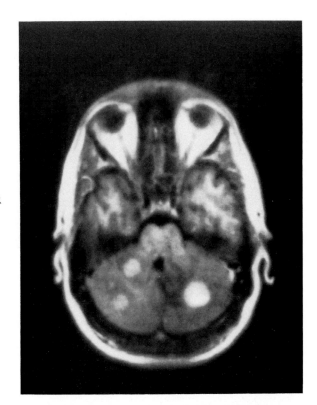

Figure 11–18. Malignant melanoma metastasis: IR 1500/500/44,. The tumors have high signal intensity.

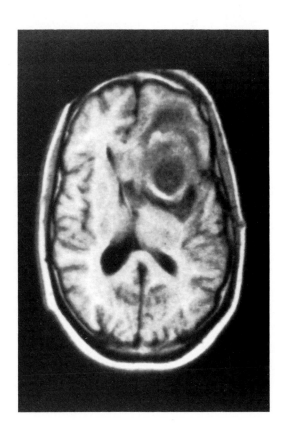

Figure 11–19. Astrocytoma, Grade IV: IR 1500/500/44, scan. There is a ring of high signal intensity due to hemorrhage.

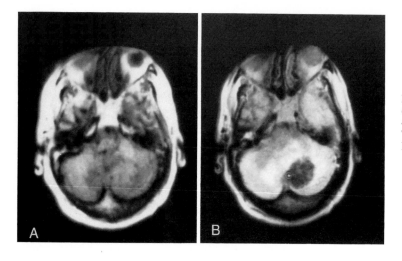

Figure 11–20. Metastasis from carcinoma of the rectum: IR 1500/500/44, (*A*) and SE 1500/80, (*B*) scans. The signal intensity of the mass is low in *B*.

for at least 40 minutes after injection of Gd-DTPA.[31] As with benign tumors, contrast enhancement is almost always maximal with highly *T1* dependent sequences. As with CT, Gd-DTPA may enter cystic areas within tumors.

Infiltrating tumors without obvious mass effect, such as primary lymphoma, may present a problem in diagnosis, since the most striking feature is widespread involve-

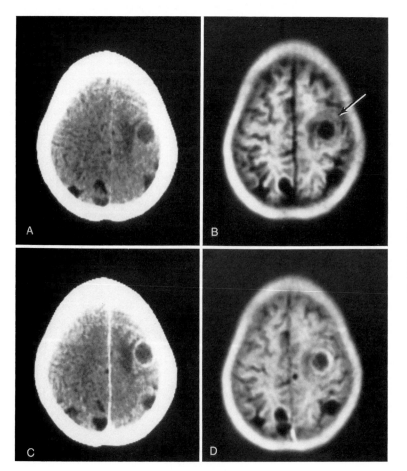

Figure 11–21. Metastasis: CT (*A*) and IR 1500/500/44, (*B*) scans before contrast enhancement compared with CT (*C*) and IR 1500/500/44, (*D*) scans after enhancement. A region of apparent edema in *B* shows enhancement (*D*) and therefore probably represents tumor.

ment of white matter. Although these tumors may display marked enhancement with CT, this has been present in only a minority of our cases.

The advantages of MRI over CT in visualizing the posterior fossa were documented early in the clinical development of the technique,[37,38] but with more experience, advantages are now being recognized in imaging the supratentorial compartment. For example, patients are frequently referred with mass effects apparent on the CT scan but the extent of tumor not demonstrated. In these cases, MRI frequently displays the full extent of the tumor. Uncontrolled epilepsy or the display of delta-wave foci on EEG has been another indication for MRI, because lesions not seen by CT may be apparent.[39] Stereotactic biopsy has been of value in individual cases when the lesion has been incompletely visualized on CT but has been better demonstrated with MRI.

Metastatic lesions display the same general features (Fig. 11–22). They are more frequently multiple, edema is readily apparent, and a high level of contrast enhancement is often seen (Fig. 11–23). Meningeal spread may be apparent with secondary tumors, but there are no specific features distinguishing metastases from high-grade malignant primary tumors. Malignant melanomas are of interest as secondary tumors that frequently display short *T1* and *T2*, probably as a result of hemorrhage within the tumor.

Pediatric Tumors

Among the more common reasons for referral of children are diagnosis of tumors and assessment of shunt problems. The technique for children differs from that for adults. Sedation is necessary for younger children. Smaller spherical coils are used to improve image signal-to-noise ratio. In addition, the sequences used must be adjusted in order to accommodate the increased *T1* and *T2* of the normal pediatric brain. The normal brain changes in size and shape with age, but also *T1* and *T2* decrease, particularly in the first two years of life. The process of myelination can also be visualized during the first two years of life.

The types of tumor observed in children differ from those in adults both in the

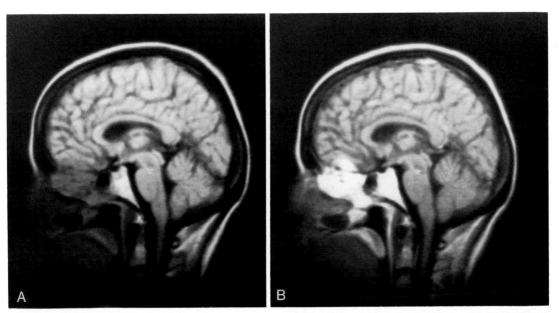

Figure 11–22. Metastasis from carcinoma of the nasopharynx: SE 544/44, scans before (*A*) and after (*B*) Gd-DTPA. The extension of the tumor into the anterior fossa is best seen in *B*.

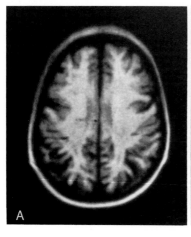 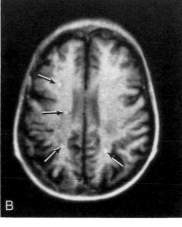

Figure 11–23. Metastases from carcinoma of the breast: IR 1500/500/44, scans before (*A*) and after (*B*) Gd-DTPA. The metastases (arrows) are better defined in *B*.

increased incidence of posterior fossa tumors and in the distribution of histologic types.[40–42] Since many of these tumors occur in the midline, the sagittal plane is of particular value (Fig. 11–24). Because of the longer *T1* and *T2* of normal pediatric brain the contrast between brain and tumor may be reduced; when myelin is relatively sparse, identification of a tumor may be difficult. Some embryonic lesions, such as hamartoma, may display little or no increase in *T1* and *T2* (Fig. 11–25).

Tumor Follow-Up

One of the ongoing problems in follow-up examination is technical change in the machine, making images difficult to compare. The decision of how much change to attribute to the basic pathologic process and how much to attribute to technical change can be very difficult (Fig. 11–26). There are also difficulties in obtaining the same slice level and angulation used in the earlier examination to obtain strict geometric com-

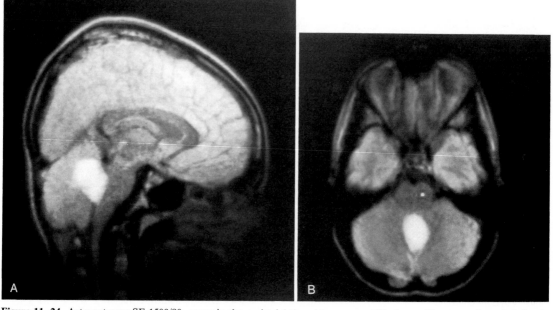

Figure 11–24. Astrocytoma: SE 1500/80, scans in the sagittal (*A*) and transverse (*B*) planes. The tumor is well defined.

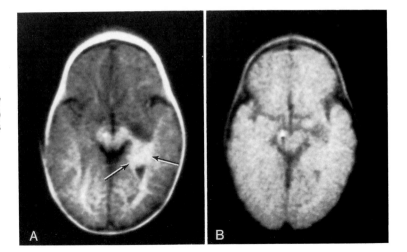

Figure 11–25. Hamartoma: IR 1500/500/44, (*A*) and SE 1500/80, (*B*) scans. The tumor is seen in *A* but is poorly defined in *B*.

parisons. At the present time, Gd-DTPA is available only for single usage in any given patient. As a result, follow-up examinations are generally obtained without contrast enhancement. This too may make it difficult to compare images.

The use of a shunt may produce a radical change in appearance of the brain so that unless a baseline scan is performed at a suitable time following therapy, no adequate reference may be available. After surgery, clips may be inserted. While these do not generally carry the risks that aneurysm clips do, care is necessary to ascertain that they are not ferromagnetic. Frequently, subdural blood accumulation is seen after surgery. The membrane usually displays contrast enhancement, and the meninges elsewhere may display a decreased *T1* or *T2* on contrast enhancement following surgery. The margin of resection is usually associated with an increase in *T2*.

Radiation effects are a further source of confusion. They may be apparent as areas of increased *T2* in a periventricular or peritumoral distribution. In a few high-dose

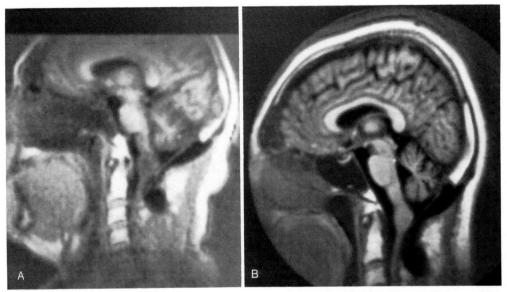

Figure 11–26. Astrocytoma, Grade I, at foramen magnum level: IR 1400/400/13f, scan (*A*) before and IR 1500/500/44, scan (*B*) after radiotherapy. The change in image quality makes assessment of tumor change difficult.

cases, changes are seen within the radiation fields. Distribution within white matter is also seen.

Diagnosis of recurrence is difficult. Changes in size are valuable diagnostically, but increases in *T1* and *T2* have also been seen in cases of recurrence. Secondary effects, including periventricular changes, may also be prominent (Fig. 11–27).

The Spinal Cord

Although the MRI technique for examination of the spinal cord has much more in common with that of the brain than does metrizamide CT or myelography, there are a number of important differences.[43] Surface coils are usually employed for the spinal cord. There is a distinct preference for the sagittal plane, although transverse images are also important (Fig. 11–28). Demonstrating the actual size of the cord is a major feature in diagnosis. CSF signal control, making its signal intensity either distinctly less than that of cord or distinctly greater, is essential in order to accurately determine cord size. Flow effects are frequently seen at the C1–C2 level anterior to the spinal cord.

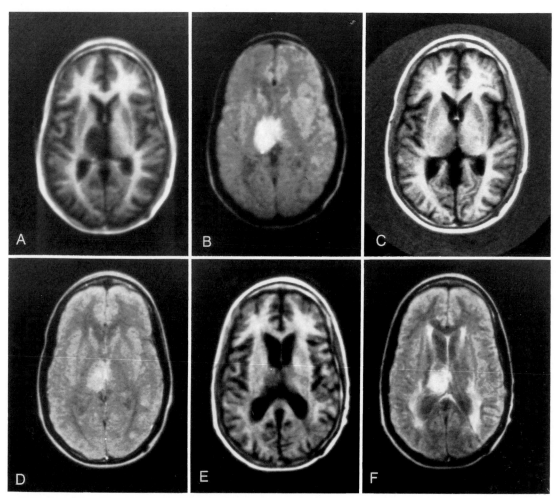

Figure 11–27. Astrocytoma, Grade III: IR 1500/500/44, (*A*) and SE 1500/80, (*B*) scans before radiotherapy, after initial response (*C–D*), and after recurrence (*E–F*). The tumor is smaller and shows a decrease in *T1* and *T2* in *C* and *D* but has increased in size and shows periventricular changes in *E* and *F*.

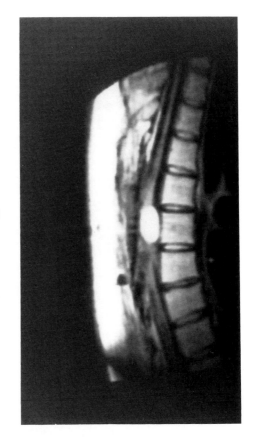

Figure 11–28. Epidermoid tumor in the upper thoracic region: SE 544/44, scan. The tumor is highlighted.

The choice of sequence is important not only to demonstrate the spinal cord but also to display the discs and vertebrae of the spinal column. Fat-suppression sequences are useful to develop contrast between tumors and red marrow. Short *TE* SE sequences may be helpful in demonstrating lipid-containing tumors.

In the spinal cord, Gd-DTPA is used in a way comparable to its use in the brain.[44] All extramedullary tumors examined to date have demonstrated contrast enhancement (Fig. 11–29). This has been of value in defining the extent of the lesion as well as in distinguishing solid tumors from cystic lesions, such as arachnoid cysts. Fifteen intramedullary tumors have been examined with Gd-DTPA to date, and all have shown at least some degree of contrast enhancement (Fig. 11–30).

The general features of spinal cord tumors are similar to those of brain, with an increased *T1* and *T2*. Cystic conditions also occur, and it may be difficult to distinguish a tumor from complicated hydromyelia. The presence of increased *T2* components in the brain seems a valuable indicator of tumor as does the presence of contrast enhancement.

Differential Diagnosis

The differential diagnosis of CNS tumors covers a large and important area of conventional neuroradiology. Much of this can be transposed directly to MRI. For example, mass effects are characteristic of tumors, but they may also be seen with other pathologic processes. Besides hemorrhage and abscess these include some multiple sclerosis lesions and cases of infarction. Conversely, tumors may occur without mass effects. This is seen with some infiltrating tumors, including primary lymphomas.

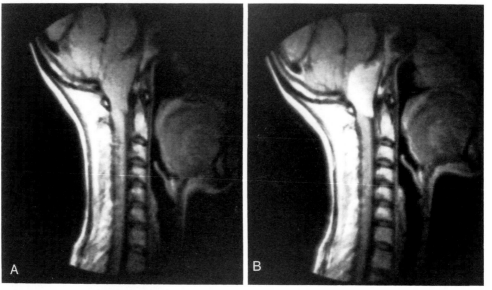

Figure 11–29. Meningioma: SE 544/44, scans before (A) and after (B) intravenous Gd-DTPA. The tumor shows a high level of enhancement.

An increase in *T1* and *T2* is frequently seen with tumors, but in 12 percent of 278 tumors significant short *T1* or short *T2* components were seen. These include examples of acoustic neuromas, meningiomas, malignant melanoma metastases, hemorrhage into tumors, tumors treated with radiotherapy, and pediatric tumors.

There are major difficulties in assessing tumor recurrence, particularly following radiotherapy and chemotherapy.

We have also had difficulty in distinguishing cases of diffuse viral infection within

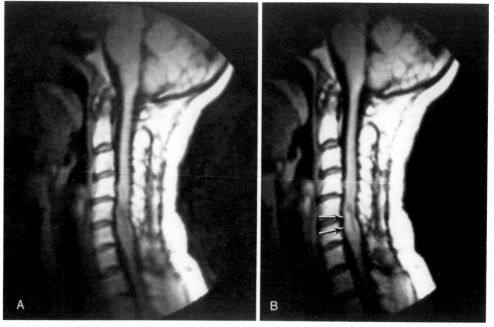

Figure 11–30. Ependymoma: SE 544/44 scans before (A) and after (B) Gd-DTPA. The intramedullary tumor shows enhancement (arrows), differentiating it from surrounding edema.

the brainstem from tumor. A case of sarcoidosis was thought to represent tumor but resolved following steroid therapy. Two cases of primary lymphoma initially were thought to represent diffuse demyelinating disease. Before we began using Gd-DTPA to enhance cord tumors we were left in doubt about whether cases of complicated syringomyelia were, in fact, cystic tumors.

When we began MRI imaging we thought that CT was so effective in tumor diagnosis that if MRI turned out to be merely another tumor-localizing technique, it would have little future. Over the last five years the problems with CT have become increasingly apparent, and there no longer seems to be any doubt that MRI will have a significant role in routine tumor diagnosis within the CNS in the foreseeable future. Some problems are likely to remain, however. One is the insensitivity of MRI to the presence of calcification. Another is the fact that the specificity of the technique is much less impressive than its sensitivity.

References

1. Bydder GM, Butson PR, Harman RR, Gilderdale DJ, Young IR: Use of spherical receiver coils in magnetic resonance imaging of the brain. J Comput Assist Tomogr 2:413, 1985.
2. Bydder GM, Curati WL, Gadian DG, Hall AS, Harman RR, Butsen RR, Gilderdale DJ, Young IR: Use of closely coupled receiver coils in MRI: Practical aspects. J Comput Assist Tomogr 5:987, 1985.
3. Axel L: Surface coil magnetic resonance imaging. J Comput Assist Tomogr 8:361, 1984.
4. Bydder GM, Young IR: Clinical use of the partial saturation and saturation recovery sequences in MR imaging. J Comput Assist Tomogr 9:1020, 1985.
5. Dixon WT: Simple proton spectroscopic imaging. Radiology 153:189, 1984.
6. Bydder GM, Young IR: MRI: Clinical use of the inversion recovery sequence. J Comput Assist Tomogr 9(4):659, 1985.
7. Sepponen RE, Pohjonen JA, Sipponen JT, Tanttu JI: A method for $T1\rho$, imaging. J Comput Assist Tomogr 9(6):1007, 1985.
8. Weinmann H-J, Brasch RC, Press WR, Wesbey GE: Characteristics of gadolinium-DTPA complex: a potential NMR contrast agent. AJR 143:619, 1984.
9. Felix R, Schorner W, Laniado M, Niendorf HP, Claussen C, Fiegler W, Speck U: Brain tumours: MR imaging with gadolinium-DTPA. Radiology 156:681, 1985.
10. Carr DH, Brown J, Bydder GM, Weinmann H-J, Speck U, Thomas DJ, Young IR: Intravenous chelated gadolinium as a contrast agent in NMR imaging of cerebral tumours. Lancet 1:484, 1984.
11. Claussen C, Laniado M, Schorner W, et al: Gadolinium DTPA in MR imaging of glioblastomas and intracranial metastases. AJNR 6:669, 1985.
12. Gadian DG, Payne JA, Bryant DR, Young IR, Carr DH, Bydder GM: Gd^{3+}-DTPA as a contrast agent in MR imaging—theoretical projections and practical observations. J Comput Assist Tomogr 9(2):242, 1985.
13. Thomas DGT, Davis CH, Ingram S, Olney JS, Bydder GM, Young IR: Stereotactic biopsy of the brain under magnetic resonance imaging control. AJNR 7:161, 1986.
14. Hawkes RC, Holland GN, Moore WS, Worthington BS: Nuclear magnetic resonance tomography of the brain: a preliminary clinical assessment with demonstration of pathology. J Comput Assist Tomogr 4:577, 1980.
15. Bydder GM, Steiner RE, Young IR, Hall AS, Thomas DJ, Marshall J, Pallis CA, Legg NJ: Clinical NMR imaging of the brain: 140 cases. AJR 139:215, 1982.
16. Brant-Zawadski M, Davis PL, Crooks LE, Mills CM, Norman D, Newton TH, Sheldon P, Kaufman L: NMR demonstration of cerebral abnormalities: comparison with CT. AJR 140(5):847, 1983.
17. Zimmerman RA, Bilaniuk LT, Goldberg HI, Grossman RI, Levine RS, Lynch R, Edelsteing W, Bottomley P, Redington R: Cerebral NMR imaging: early results with a 0.12T resistive system. AJR 141:1187, 1983.
18. Bradley WG, Waluch V, Yadley RA, Wycoff RR: Comparison of CT and MR in 400 patients with suspected disease of the brain and cervical spinal cord. Radiology 152:695, 1984.
19. Worthington BS: NMR imaging of intracranial and orbital tumours. Br Med Bull 40:179, 1984.
20. Lee BCP, Kneeland JB, Cahill PT, Deck MDF: MR recognition of supratentorial tumors. AJNR 6:871, 1985.
21. Huelft MG, Han JS, Kaufmann B, Benson JE: MR imaging of brain stem gliomas. J Comput Assist Tomogr 9:262, 1985.
22. Brant-Zawadski M, Bodami JP, Mills CM, et al: Primary intracranial tumor imaging; a comparison of magnetic resonance and CT. Radiology 150:435, 1984.
23. Damadian R, Zaner K, Hor D, Di Maio T: Human tumors detected by nuclear magnetic resonance. Proc Natl Acad Sci 171:1471, 1974.

24. Young IR, Bydder GM, Hall AS, Steiner RE, Worthington BS, Hawkes RC, Holland GN, Moore WS: The role of NMR imaging in the diagnosis and management of acoustic neuroma. AJNR 4(3):223, 1983.
25. Daniels DL, Herfkens R, Fochler PR, et al: Magnetic resonance imaging of the internal auditory canal. Radiology 151:105, 1984.
26. Kingsley DPE, Brooks GB, Leung AW-L, Johnson MA: Acoustic neuromas: evaluation by MRI. AJNR 6(1):1, 1985.
27. New PFJ, Boekow TB, Wisner GL, Rosen BR, Brady JT: MR imaging of the acoustic nerves and small acoustic neuromas at 0.6T: prospective study. AJNR 6:165, 1985.
28. Curati WL, Graif M, Kingsley DPE, Sholtz CL, King T, Steiner RE: Acoustic neuromas: a review of 35 cases. Neuroradiology 28:208, 1986.
29. Zimmerman RD, Fleming CA, Saint-Louis LA, Lee BCP, Manning JJ, Deck MDF: Magnetic resonance imaging of meningiomas. AJNR 6:149, 1985.
30. Kean DM, Smith MA, Douglas KHB, Matyn CH, Best JJK: Two examples of CNS lipomas demonstrated by computed tomography and low field (0.08T) MR imaging. J Comput Assist Tomogr 9:494, 1985.
31. Davidson HD, Ouchi T, Steiner RE: NMR imaging of congenital intracranial germinal layer neoplasms. Neuroradiology 27:301, 1985.
32. Price AC, Runge VM, Allen JH, Partain CL, James AE: Magnetic resonance imaging of the pituitary at 0.5T update after one year. Scientific Program, Society of Magnetic Resonance in Medicine, Third Annual Meeting. New York, August 1984, p 603.
33. Bilaniuk LT, Simmerman RA, Wehrli FW, et al: Magnetic resonance imaging of pituitary lesions using 1.0 to 1.5T field strength. Radiology 153:415, 1985.
34. Oot R, New PFJ, Buonanno FS: MR imaging of pituitary adenoma using a prototype resistive magnet; preliminary assessment. AJNR 5:131, 1984.
35. MacKay IM, Bydder GM, Young IR: MR imaging of central nervous system tumours that do not display increase in T1 or T2. J Comput Assist Tomogr 9(6):1055, 1985.
36. Graif M, Bydder GM, Steiner RE, Niendorf HP, Thomas DGT, Young IR: Contrast enhanced MRI of malignant brain tumors. AJNR 6:855, 1985.
37. McGinnis BD, Brady TJ, New PFJ, Buonanno FS, Pykett IL, DeLaPaz RL, Kistler JP, Tavernas JM: Nuclear magnetic resonance (NMR) imaging of tumors in the posterior fossa. J Comput Assist Tomogr 7:575, 1983.
38. Randall CP, Collins AG, Young IR, Hayward R, Thomas DJ, McDonnell MJ, Orr JS, Bydder GM, Steiner RE: Nuclear magnetic resonance imaging of posterior fossa tumours. AJR 141:489, 1983.
39. Aaron J, New PFJ, Stand R, Veaulieu P, Elwarden K, Brady TJ: NMR imaging in temporal lobe epilepsy due to gliosis. J Comput Assist Tomogr 8:608, 1984.
40. Peterman SB, Bydder GM, Steiner RE: NMR imaging of brain tumors in children and adolescents. AJNR 5(6):703, 1984.
41. Kucharcyk W, Brant-Zawadski M, Sobel D, et al: Central nervous system tumors in children: detection by magnetic resonance imaging. Radiology 155:131, 1985.
42. Han JS, Benson JE, Kaufman B, et al: MR imaging of pediatric cerebral abnormalities. J Comput Assist Tomogr 9:103, 1985.
43. Di Chiro G, Doppman JL, Dwyer AJ, Patronas HJ, Knop RH, Bairamian D, Vermess M, Oldfield EH: Tumors and arteriovenous malformation of the spinal cord: assessment using MR. Radiology 156:689, 1985.
44. Bydder GM, Brown J, Niendorf HP, Young IR: Enhancement of cervical intraspinal tumors in MR imaging with intravenous gadolinium-DTPA. J Comput Assist Tomogr 9:847, 1985.

12

Tumor Imaging with Gd-DTPA

ANN C. PRICE
VAL M. RUNGE
JOSEPH H. ALLEN

Magnetic resonance imaging (MRI) rapidly has achieved a premier position as an imaging modality in the evaluation of normal and pathologic states of the central nervous system (CNS).[1] Superior resolution of soft tissue planes, absence of bone artifact, direct multiplanar imaging capability, and the availability of multiple imaging parameters have resulted in a sensitive, versatile imaging technique. These factors have led to earlier and more accurate diagnosis of demyelinating diseases, tumors, and various disorders of the posterior fossa and brainstem.[2-4]

Despite the wide variety of pulse sequences, the consistent visualization of meningiomas and the differentiation of tumor nidus from the associated edema have not been possible.[5] The development and use of intravascular MR contrast agents promises to overcome these major drawbacks, leading to the selection of MR as the primary imaging modality in tumor evaluation and diagnosis.

The principal agents of interest in MR have been the paramagnetic ions of manganese, iron, chromium, and gadolinium chelated to ethylenediamine tetraacetic acid (EDTA), glucoheptonic acid, or desferrioxamine.[6] Gadolinium diethylenetriamine pentaacetic acid (Gd-DTPA) is the paramagnetic pharmaceutical agent that has received the most attention and use, both clinical and laboratory, as an MR contrast agent. The details of chemistry, toxicology, and pharmacology are more thoroughly addressed in Chapters 46 to 52.

The strong paramagnetic properties of gadolinium, an element from the lanthanide rare earth series, results from the seven unpaired electrons. The lower orbital position of these electrons protects the paramagnetic properties by preventing combination with other substances.[7] In its ionic form, gadolinium is highly toxic. Chelation neutralizes this toxicity by forming stable in vivo complexes. DTPA is the preferred chelating complex, since it appears to be less toxic than the alternatives, e.g., EDTA. Chelation reduces the paramagnetism. As compared with other chelating agents, DTPA results in less reduction of this very important property.[7,8]

Gd-DTPA is distributed throughout the vascular system and is excreted by the kidneys by glomerular filtration. Renal excretion is rapid, with 90 percent recovered after 24 hours in laboratory animals.[8] This suggests an additional imaging application in MR investigation of the genitourinary tract.

The in vivo stability and rapid renal excretion contribute to the low observed clinical toxicity. None of the 30 patients studied at Vanderbilt University as a part of the Phase II USA Clinical Trials experienced any toxic (headache, nausea, or vomiting) or allergic (hives or urticaria) reaction. This was also true of the other centers involved in this clinical trial.[9] This is not surprising, since Gd-DTPA is a poor activator of the body's complement system. It is the activation of this system by iodinated contrast that results in anaphylactoid reactions.[8,10]

One patient in this series with a planum meningioma had experienced a severe anaphylactic reaction with iodinated CT contrast but had no difficulty with Gd-DTPA. The postcontrast MR study added significantly to his operative management (Fig. 12–1).

Comprehensive laboratory and clinical examinations were obtained before and after injection of Gd-DTPA (0.1 mm/kg). Of these extensive hematologic, serologic, ECG, EEG, and physical examinations, only the serum iron showed any significant change after intravenous Gd-DTPA administration. Serum iron increased in 25 patients, seven of whom showed values 15 μg/dl above the upper limits of normal laboratory values. These returned to normal within 24 to 48 hours. No explanation for this change has been offered.

The mechanism of tumor enhancement with iodinated contrast agents is the result of alteration both in vascularity and in the blood-brain barrier.[11,12] Histologic studies confirm the breakdown in the blood-brain barrier. There is a structural alteration in the capillary walls of tumors that allows extravascular or interstitial accumulation of contrast.[13] The more aggressive the tumor, the greater the enhancement.[13]

The enhancement by paramagnetic compounds is on a similar basis. This was documented by Runge and coworkers[14] by intravenous infusion of hyperosmolar mannitol into the internal carotid artery of dogs. A reversible disruption of the blood-brain barrier (BBB), limited to the area of perfusion, occurred. Following intravenous Gd-DTPA administration, localized enhancement corresponded to the tissue perfused with mannitol. This was documented pathologically by injection of Evans blue dye prior to animal sacrifice. Post-mortem studies showed correspondence of the dye-stained brain to the area of contrast enhancement.[14]

Blood-brain barrier disruption in intracranial disease processes has been further documented with animal studies of experimentally induced brain abscesses. A localized disruption of the BBB could be documented in the early cerebritis stage of abscess formation as a focal area of Gd-DTPA enhancement.[7,15]

The degree of vascularity plays an important role in those tumors that do not arise within the brain parenchyma (autochthonous). These include meningiomas, neurinomas, pituitary origin tumors, and some parasellar tumors, such as chordomas.[16] Eight of 11 extraparenchymal tumors in this series exhibiting expansile growth, including two craniopharyngiomas, three chromophobe adenomas, one clivus chordoma (Fig. 12–2), and a large convexity meningioma were adequately delineated on *T1* and/or *T2*

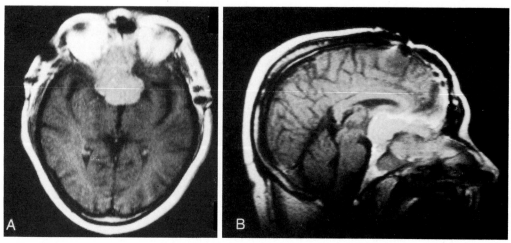

Figure 12–1. Planum meningioma. Axial (*A*) and direct sagittal (*B*) postcontrast sections demonstrate the suprasellar and anterior extent of the meningioma. Note the associated osseous irregularity (SE 500/32).

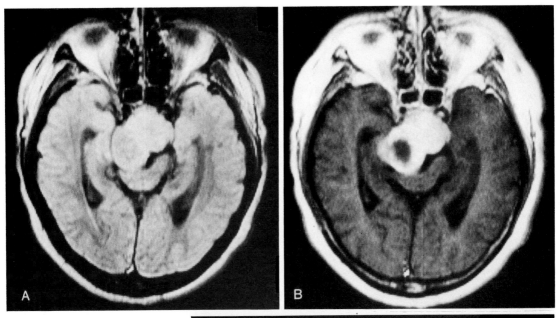

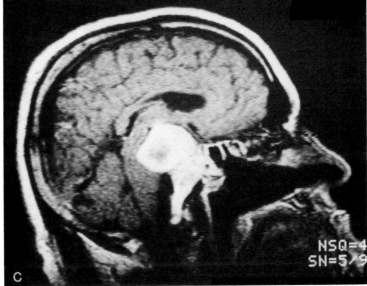

Figure 12–2. Clivus chordoma. *A*, Slight *T2* weighting before contrast adequately delineates the tumor and secondary brainstem changes (SE 2000/32). *B*, Following Gd-DTPA contrasting, there is dense enhancement, better than that which occurred with iodinated CT contrast (SE 250/32). *C*, The sagittal postcontrast section shows to better advantage the brainstem mass effect, particularly involving the midbrain (SE 500/38).

sequences without contrast. The three tumors not adequately evaluated without contrast included two meningiomas (Fig. 12–3) and one recurrent acoustic neurinoma.

Prior to MR contrast agents, meningiomas were not consistently visualized unless of sufficient size to produce a mass effect due to the tumor, parenchymal edema, or signal intensity change as a result of the edema.[17] The enhancement of meningiomas with Gd-DTPA overcomes one of the major drawbacks of MR as the primary imaging modality in intracranial tumor evaluation (Fig. 12–3).

Separation of tumor nidus from the associated edema is also necessary for adequate tumor evaluation, particularly for presurgical localization. It has been suggested that for higher grade tumors the nidus can be localized as a relative area of decreased signal intensity within an area of high signal intensity on heavily *T2* weighted sequences (Fig. 12–4).[1,3] Despite this and the variety of pulse-sequence selections, consistent separation

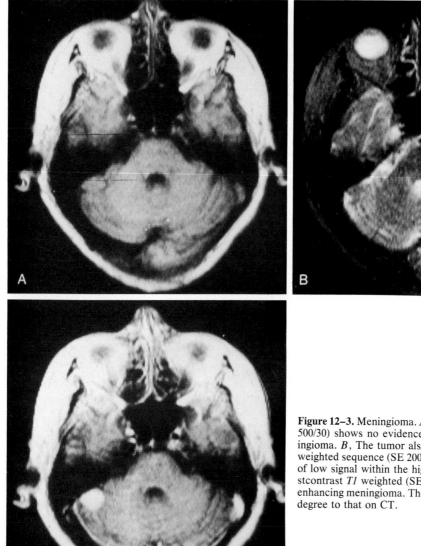

Figure 12–3. Meningioma. *A*, The *T1* weighted study (SE 500/30) shows no evidence of the right CP angle meningioma. *B*, The tumor also is not visualized on the *T2* weighted sequence (SE 2000/180) except as a vague area of low signal within the higher signal CSF. *C*, The postcontrast *T1* weighted (SE 300/32) sequence shows the enhancing meningioma. The enhancement was similar in degree to that on CT.

of tumor nidus from the associated edema has not been possible.[1,3,6] Gd-DTPA results in precise localization of the tumor nidus (Fig. 12–5).

In this series of 14 patients with infiltrative tumors, Gd-DTPA was necessary to separate tumor nidus from edema in four patients with gliomas and in three patients with six metastatic lesions. The remaining patients had lower grade tumors or focally enhancing lesions with little associated edema.

Optimum sequence selection has been discussed in greater detail in Chapters 6 to 9. Contrast enhancement curves, calculations of contrast to noise, calculation of *T1* and *T2* relaxation parameters, and clinical images indicate that *T1* weighted images (i.e., $TE = 30$ ms, $TR = 55$ ms) show the greatest contrast enhancement (Figs. 12–4B and 12–5B–C).[18]

Although contrast enhancement can be seen on *T2* weighted images, this generally occurs in those patients with little or no signal intensity change on *T2* weighted se-

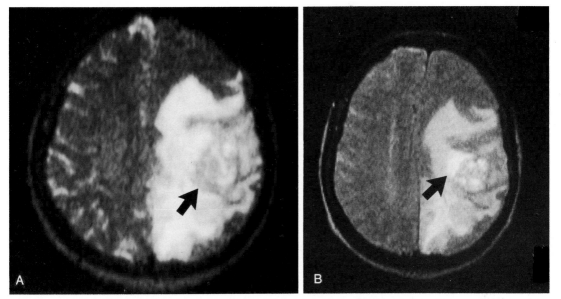

Figure 12–4. Glioblastoma multiforme. *A*, *T2* weighted image, SE 1500/180, without contrast. Although the tumor nidus is suggested by an area of low signal (arrow), it is not clearly separated from the edema. *B*, *T2* weighted image, SE 1500/90, 50 minutes after contrast enhancement. The contrast-enhanced image demonstrates superior contrast resolution between tumor border and edema (arrow).

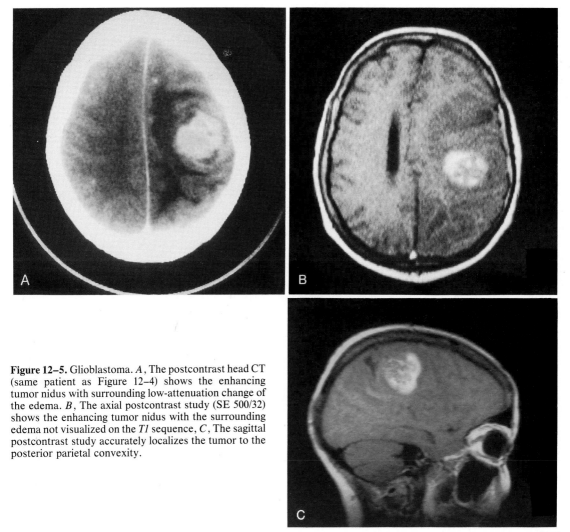

Figure 12–5. Glioblastoma. *A*, The postcontrast head CT (same patient as Figure 12–4) shows the enhancing tumor nidus with surrounding low-attenuation change of the edema. *B*, The axial postcontrast study (SE 500/32) shows the enhancing tumor nidus with the surrounding edema not visualized on the *T1* sequence, *C*, The sagittal postcontrast study accurately localizes the tumor to the posterior parietal convexity.

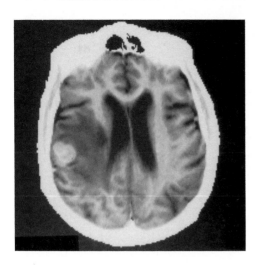

Figure 12–6. Metastic tumor. Heavily *T1* weighted IR image shows the enhancing metastatic nidus within the low signal intensity edema.

quences without contrast (i.e., meningiomas and pituitary origin tumors).[18] Heavily *T1* weighted images, such as inversion recovery (IR), show excellent contrast enhancement if the region is surrounded by edema or adjacent to cisterns (Fig. 12–6). If the lesion is parenchymal with little surrounding edema, the enhancement may blend with the high signal intensity of the adjacent white matter (Fig. 12–7). IR is the one sequence that depicts both tumor nidus and edema in a single sequence acquisition (Fig. 12–6).[18] Shorter *TE* and *TR* sequences (at 0.5 tesla) tend to suffer from lack of anatomic detail despite the adequacy of tumor enhancement (Fig. 12–7).[19]

The time course of Gd-DTPA enhancement differs from that of iodinated contrast. An earlier peak and relatively rapid decline over a one-hour period occurs with iodinated CT contrast agents[20] as compared with Gd-DTPA, which shows a rapid rise to maximum at 4 minutes and nearly flat enhancement curve to 60 minutes with only a slight decline from maximum. This suggests greater leeway in scanning time as compared with CT.

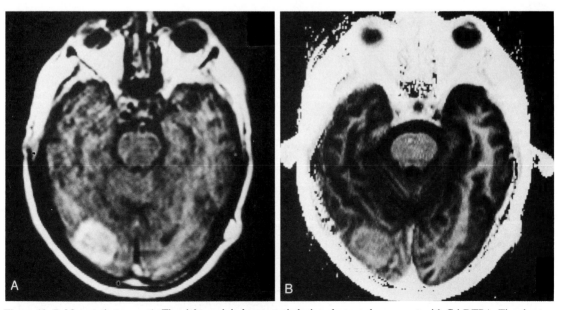

Figure 12–7. Metastatic tumor. *A*, The right occipital metastatic lesion shows enhancement with Gd-DTPA. The shorter SE volume sequence (250/40) shows slight loss of anatomic resolution. *B*, The IR sequence only vaguely demonstrates the lesion, which blends with the high signal of the white matter since there is little surrounding edema.

Normal brain shows little, if any, enhancement in SE sequences, veins, or sinuses. The choroid plexus and nasal mucosa enhance, with marked enhancement of the nasal mucosa (see Fig. 12–12C). Arterial enhancement can be seen on SE and IR but is less prominent as compared with venous enhancement.[7]

The enhancement of the cavernous sinus shows promise in evaluation of parasellar pathology, i.e., meningiomas and hemangiomas.

GLIOMAS

Eight of the 30 intracranial tumors were gliomas of varying grade, with four of these being higher grade tumor pathologies (Grades II to IV). All of these showed dense enhancement with Gd-DTPA and only one true ring enhancement. As compared with CT, three showed greater enhancement (Fig. 12–8) and the remainder were equivalent. As previously indicated, tumor nidus could be separated from the surrounding edema with Gd-DTPA in these higher grade tumors (Fig. 12–5).

The remaining four gliomas were lower grade tumors, with the enhancement the same or only slightly greater than with iodinated contrast. In each of these tumors, additional information was available with the MR study. Invasive properties were more evident in a recurrent frontal glioma and a corpus callosum tumor. Although improved localization is generally greater with MR as a result of direct multiplanar potential, the superior resolution of soft tissue planes in comparable axial MR projections was helpful in the assessment and localization of lower grade tumors in the temporal lobe and corpus callosum.

One patient was re-evaluated two months following surgery. A part of her clinical symptoms could be attributed to the presence of hemorrhage not demonstrated on CT (Fig. 12–9).

METASTASES

Six patients with intracranial metastatic disease were studied. In one patient the metastatic lesions were more densely enhanced with MR (Fig. 12–10). The metastatic disease was sufficiently aggressive in three patients with six lesions that tumor nidus could be separated from edema. One tumor with a hemorrhagic metastasis showed little

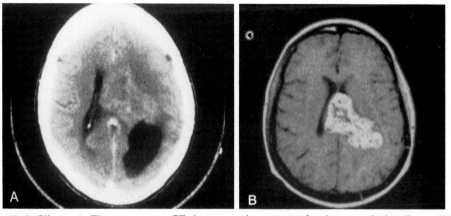

Figure 12–8. Glioma. *A*, The postcontrast CT shows no enhancement of an intraventricular glioma. *B*, The postcontrast MR study shows dense enhancement of the tumor. The section is at a slightly higher level and different angle so that the trapped occipital horn is not seen in the MR section.

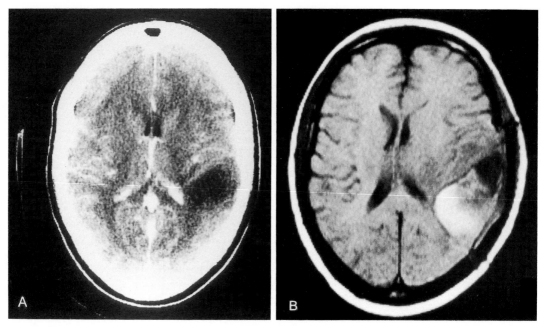

Figure 12–9. Recurrent glioma. A, There is a left temporal area of low attenuation in the postoperative Grade II–III glioma (contrast-enhanced CT). B, The MR study without contrast shows a rather extensive area of hemorrhage in the left temporal lobe.

enhancement with either imaging modality. The remaining metastatic lesions enhanced equally by CT and MR.

In this series of patients, no additional lesions were demonstrated with Gd-DTPA than with *T2* sequences without contrast. One group in the multicenter study, however, found additional metastasis with MR enhancement.[20] This suggests an important application in the exclusion of multiple lesions when solitary metastases have been demonstrated by CT or MR without contrast. For those patients with multiple lesions, Gd-DTPA offers little further clinical information unless precise localization is necessary for anticipated stereotactic or open biopsy.

MENINGIOMA

Five patients with meningioma were examined with Gd-DTPA. One patient with a planum origin tumor had no corresponding CT owing to a previous anaphylactic reaction to iodinated contrast (see Fig. 12–1). The Gd-DTPA enhancement was excellent, and the anterior extent along the frontal bone with the associated osseous irregularity was well demonstrated, particularly with the direct sagittal section.

Contrast enhancement was similar but not dense with either CT or MR in an intrasellar meningioma. The intrasellar and parasellar extent were better shown with MR, principally because of the superior soft tissue resolution.

The remaining three tumors densely enhanced with Gd-DTPA. One of these could not be seen on MR without contrast except in longer *TR* sequences, in which it appeared as a vague negative signal in the CSF of the cerebellar pontine angle cistern (see Fig. 12–3). A large convexity meningioma was better demonstrated by MR owing, in part, to the poor quality of the CT scan.

A planum origin tumor was better localized by MR. The CT study showed a large enhancing suprasellar mass. With the sagittal post–Gd-DTPA contrast examination,

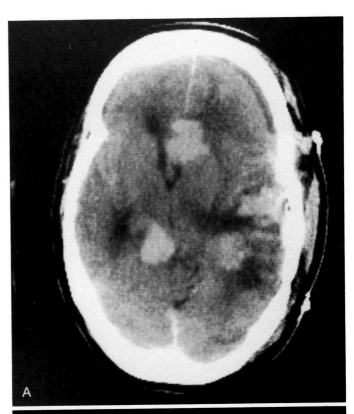

Figure 12–10. Metastases. *A*, The contrast-enhanced CT shows multiple metastatic lesions. *B*, The MR study shows precontrast sections on the left and postcontrast views on the right. Gd-DTPA enhancement is much denser.

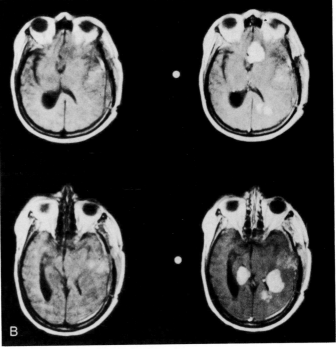

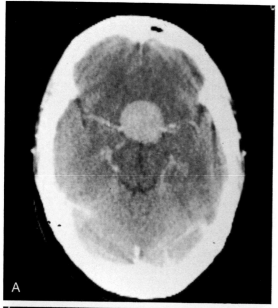

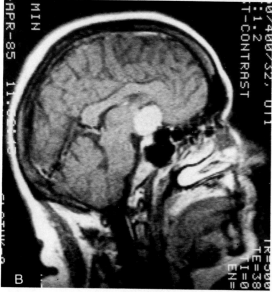

Figure 12–11. Planum meningioma. *A*, A large enhancing suprasellar lesion was thought to be of pituitary origin on this axial postcontrast CT section. *B*, The sagittal enhanced MR view shows a densely enhancing pituitary with a thin division between the enhancing pituitary and the planum meningioma. The absence of sellar enlargement also favors a nonpituitary origin.

the densely enhancing pituitary could be separated from the densely enhancing tumor, resulting in a more precise localization and thereby a more accurate diagnosis (Fig. 12–11).

The meningioma in the small series represented larger or osseous-based tumors that could be diagnosed on MR without contrast. For the smaller convexity or base of skull meningioma, MR contrast agents represent a major advance in diagnosis (see Fig. 12–3), since these are the tumors not consistently visualized on MR without contrast.

PITUITARY AND PARASELLAR REGION TUMORS

This subject is discussed in Chapter 16. A few of the assets of Gd-DTPA enhancement in this region are reviewed here. The intrinsic enhancement of the pituitary and most pituitary origin tumors assists in assessing intrinsic pathology and distinguishing those abnormalities arising adjacent to the sella (Fig. 12–11). This intrinsic enhancement, in combination with the multiplanar potential and the more recent thin-section capability, is of paramount importance in the diagnostic evaluation of pituitary and parasellar region pathology.

The evaluation of secondary mass effect on adjacent structures, such as the brainstem and optic chiasm, is also of considerable importance in parasellar tumor evaluation (see Fig. 12–2).

POSTOPERATIVE TUMORS

The CT evaluation of tumors that recur following surgery may be difficult owing to the lack of enhancement, the subtle mass effect, and the need to distinguish postoperative encephalomalacia from tumor edema. MR without contrast (*T1* sequences) has an advantage over CT in the resolution of soft tissue planes, often showing irregular soft tissue change and mass effect that would indicate tumor recurrence.[3] Signal intensity changes on the *T2* weighted sequences are not helpful in distinguishing postoperative change from tumor edema, since both show signal intensity increase.

Gd-DTPA enhancement may offer additional assistance in evaluation of tumor recurrences, since enhancement was better than with CT in 50 percent of patients (three of six patients) (Fig. 12–12). The delineation of tumor margins was superior with MR as was the demonstration of tumor nidus (Fig. 12–13).

MR offered additional information in one recurrent meningioma with a contrast allergy (see Fig. 12–1) and one recurrent glioma with underlying hemorrhage (see Fig. 12–9).

No tumor enhanced by CT that did not enhance by MR. Several tumor pathologies did not enhance with either CT or MR contrast agents. These included a hypothalamic hamartoma, a hemorrhagic metastasis, and an epidermoid of the posterior fossa. The hypothalamic tumor was most clearly seen with *T2* weighted sequences without contrast (Fig. 12–14).

In conclusion, Gd-DTPA shows promise as a MR contrast agent. It overcomes two major drawbacks of MR. These are the enhancement of meningiomas and the separation of tumor nidus from surrounding edema. Gd-DTPA enhancement was superior to iodinated contrast in 30 percent of the patients in this study.

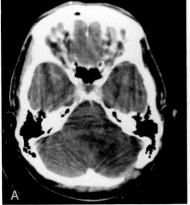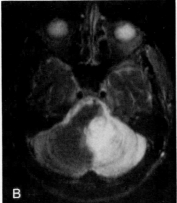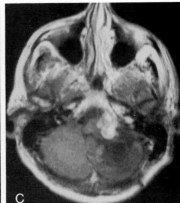

Figure 12–12. Recurrent neurinoma. *A*, The recurrent acoustic tumor only faintly enhances on the postcontrast CT. *B*, The *T2* weighted sequence does not separate tumor from postoperative encephalomalacia or edema. *C*, There is excellent visualization of the tumor following MR contrast enhancement. Note nasal mucosa.

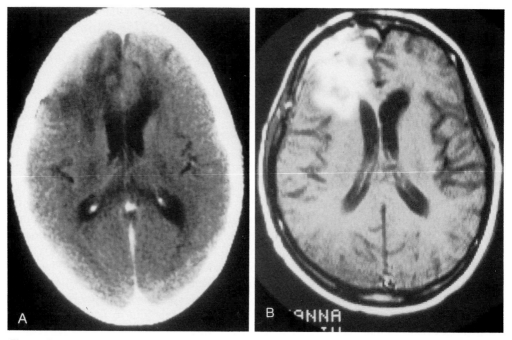

Figure 12–13. Recurrent glioma. *A*, There is only low-attenuation change and vague mass effect on the postcontrast CT. *B*, Excellent tumor enhancement occurs with Gd-DTPA with sharp margin definition.

The contrast enhancement was equivalent with both modalities. MR offered additional clinical information, such as tumor localization, associated hemorrhage, and infiltrative properties. For those patients with iodinated contrast allergies, Gd-DTPA offers a safer alternative in tumor evaluation.

Little benefit may be realized in evaluation of intracranial metastatic disease with Gd-DTPA over *T2* weighted studies without contrast. There may be applications for Gd-DTPA enhancement in therapy planning by excluding multiplicity of lesion and in precise nidus localization.

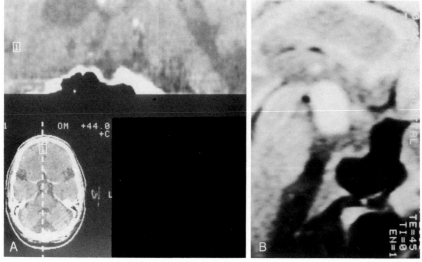

Figure 12–14. Hypothalamic hamartoma. *A*, The sagittal reformatted postcontrast CT study shows the nonenhancing tumor. *B*, The *T2* weighted sequence (no contrast) clearly demonstrates the tumor and was the optimum sequence since there was little, if any, MR enhancement.

One of the greatest benefits seems to be in the evaluation of postoperative tumor recurrences. Enhancement is generally better than with CT, the margins are more clearly defined, and secondary mass effect is more clearly shown.

With the advent of Gd-DTPA in combination with the other technological advances of MR, this modality may soon replace CT in the evaluation of intracranial neoplastic disease.

References

1. Brant-Zawadzki M, Badami JP, Mills CM: Primary intracranial tumor imaging: A comparison of magnetic resonance and CT. Radiology *150*:435, 1984.
2. Runge VM, Price AC, Kirshner HS, Allen JH, Partain CL, James AE Jr: The evaluation of multiple sclerosis by magnetic resonance imaging. AJR *143*:1015, 1984.
3. Price AC, Runge VM, Allen JH, James AE Jr: Primary glioma: Diagnosis with magnetic resonance imaging. Comput Tomogr. In press.
4. Randall CP, Collins AG, Young IR, et al: Nuclear magnetic resonance imaging of posterior fossa tumors. AJR *141*:4809, 1983.
5. Felix R, Schorner W, Laniado M, et al: Brain tumors: MR imaging with gadolinium DTPA. Radiology *156*:681, 1985.
6. Carr DN, Brown J, Bydder GM, et al: Gadolinium-DTPA as a contrast agent in MRI: Initial clinical experience in 20 patients. AJR *143*:215, 1984.
7. Brasch RC, Weinmann HJ, Wesby G: Contrast-enhanced NMR imaging: Animal studies using gadolinium-DTPA complex. AJR *142*:625, 1984.
8. Weinmann HJ, Brasch RC, Press WR, Wesby GE: Characteristics of gadolinium-DTPA complex: A potential NMR contrast agent. AJR *142*:619, 1984.
9. Bradley WG, Brant-Zawadzki M, Brasch RC, Knop R, Maravilla KR, Price AC, Runge VM, Yang W: Initial clinical experience with Gd DTPA in North America: MR contrast enhancement of brain tumors. Radiology *157*(P):125, 1985.
10. Lang JH, Saser EC, Kolb WP: Activation of the complement system by x-ray contrast media. Invest Radiol *11*:303, 1976.
11. Ambrose J: Computerized transverse axial scanning (tomography) II: Clinical application. Br J Radiol *46*:1023, 1973.
12. Butler AR, Passalaqua AM, Berenstein A, Kricheff II: Contrast enhanced CT scan and radionuclide brain scan in supratentorial gliomas. AJR *1132*:606, 1979.
13. Front D, Israel O, Kohn S, Nir I: The blood-tissue barrier of human brain tumors: Correlation of scintigraphy and ultrastructure findings: concise communication. J Nucl Med *25*:461, 1984.
14. Runge VM, Price AC, Wehr CJ, Atkinson JB, Tweedle MF: Contrast enhanced MRI: Evaluation of a canine model of osmotic blood-brain barrier disruption. Invest Radiol *20*:830, 1985.
15. Runge VM, Clanton JA, Price AC, Herzer WA, Allen JH, Partain CL, James AE Jr: Evaluation of contrast enhanced MR imaging in a brain abscess model. AJNR *6*:139, 1985.
16. Zulck KJ: Principles of the new world health (NHO) classification of brain tumors. Neuroradiology *19*:59, 1980.
17. Bydder GM, Steiner RE, Young IR, et al: Clinical NMR imaging of the brain, 140 cases. AJR *139*:215, 1982.
18. Price AC, Runge VM: Optimization of pulse sequence in Gd DTPA tumor enhanced MRI. *In* Runge VM, Claussen C, Felix R, James AE (eds): Contrast Agents in Magnetic Resonance Imaging. New York, Excerpta Medica, 1986, pp 99–102.

13

Inflammatory Disease of the Brain

WILLIAM G. BRADLEY, JR.
KEITH E. KORTMAN

Inflammation is the "reaction of living tissues to all forms of injury."[1] In the brain, acute inflammation produces breakdown of the blood-brain barrier with secondary formation of vasogenic edema. As healing occurs, the blood-brain barrier defect is repaired, vasogenic edema is resorbed, and the injured brain becomes encephalomalacic and occasionally calcified.

Inflammation is classified[2] as "primary" (when brought about by penetration of the central nervous system [CNS] by an infective agent or a toxic substance) or "symptomatic or resorptive" (when due to tumors, infarcts, mechanical and thermal insults, or foreign bodies). Inflammation can involve vascular changes as well as humoral factors and cellular elements. Arterial narrowing with secondary stasis of blood flow (and occasionally thrombosis) can lead to infarction and selective neuronal necrosis in the region of vascular supply. Erythrodiapedesis and leukodiapedesis are frequently noted in acute inflammation. Early in the inflammatory process, lymphocytes collect around venules and capillaries. If the pathologic process is severe enough to rupture the perivascular glial limiting membrane, lymphocytes can enter the CNS. These cells are the most common manifestation of inflammation. Later in the inflammatory process, histiocytes in the vascular sheath may be transformed into macrophages. Macrophages can also originate from monocytes in the blood stream, from pericytes, and from Hortega microgliocytes.

The details of the inflammatory response depend to a significant degree on the specific offending organism. Bacterial infections result in a purulent reaction. Some fungi and protozoans (e.g., *Plasmodium falciparum*) evoke an immune response. Other fungi (e.g., *Histoplasma capsulatum*) produce a granulomatous response. Viruses tend to produce a nonpurulent CNS response.

The detection of acute inflammation by magnetic resonance (MR) is based on the high sensitivity to the presence of increased water content (i.e., edema). *T2* weighted (long *TR*, long *TE*) images (Fig. 13–1) are the most sensitive of all MR pulsing sequences for the detection of the edema associated with inflammation.[3,4] Such sequences have rendered MRI more sensitive than CT, particularly in the middle and posterior cranial fossae, where CT is relatively degraded by beam hardening artifact.[5] Chronic inflammation (including granulomatous reactions) results in local encephalomalacia, which is also better evaluated by MRI than by CT. On the microscopic level, this appears as small cystic spaces in the parenchyma, i.e., "microcystic encephalomalacia."[6] The water molecules in this environment are attracted to the hydrophilic side groups of the proteins on the membrane surfaces in hydration layers. In contrast to its natural "bulk phase" state like CSF, water in this environment has a relatively short *T1* relaxation time while maintaining a long *T2* relaxation time.[7] This increases the intensity of mi-

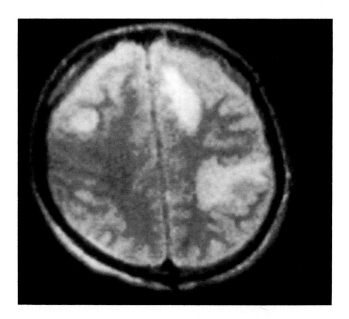

Figure 13–1. Toxoplasmosis. *T2* weighted MR image (*TR* = 2.0 sec, *TE* = 56 ms) causes vasogenic edema associated with inflammatory lesions to have high contrast.

crocystic encephalomalacia on the most clinically useful, moderately *T2* weighted sequences (e.g., *TR* 1.5 to 2.0 sec, and *TE* 30 to 60 ms).[8]

While MRI may be more sensitive than CT in the detection of microcystic encephalomalacia, CT is more sensitive in the detection of calcification.[8] CT may also demonstrate enhancement following administration of iodinated contrast. Enhancement due to blood-brain barrier breakdown can also be seen following administration of paramagnetic compounds in MR (e.g., gadolinium-DTPA); however, such intravenous contrast agents are not yet generally available for MR.[9]

Although MR is generally considered to be the most sensitive imaging modality for the detection of inflammation in the brain, it may be nonspecific. A large number of disease processes result in vasogenic edema; primary and metastatic tumors, trauma, hemorrhage, and infarction.[10] Encephalomalacia may occur after surgery (or other trauma) and in chronic infarction.[6] Differentiation of inflammatory vasogenic edema from other processes may be possible on the basis of clinical presentation and laboratory findings, although, in some cases, biopsy undoubtedly will still be necessary.

Inflammation in the brain generally accompanies infectious processes, but noninfectious and autoimmune diseases can also produce an inflammatory response, e.g., sarcoid (Fig. 13–2) and eosinophilic granuloma. Autoimmune diseases, such as systemic lupus erythematosus, are covered elsewhere. Autoimmune processes related to prior infection, e.g., postinfectious or postvaccinal leukoencephalopathy, are discussed below.

As long as the blood-brain barrier is intact, the brain is generally resistant to infection.[11] Following breakdown of the blood-brain barrier, however, the brain has greater susceptibility to infection than other tissues. Infection can gain access to the brain through four routes: (1) through hematogenous dissemination (e.g., from pneumonia or endocarditis); (2) through contiguous spread from sinusitis, otitis media, mastoiditis, or osteomyelitis of the calvarium; (3) following penetrating trauma or as a complication of surgery; or (4) via the meninges and CSF. After intracranial infection is established in one compartment, it can spread easily to a second. For example, parenchymal abscesses can rupture into the ventricles or other CSF spaces. Cerebritis can complicate a subdural empyema.

A variety of organisms can affect the brain and meninges.[2] The most fulminant

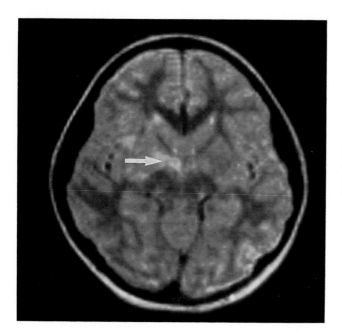

Figure 13–2. Sarcoidosis. Patient with positive angiotensin-converting enzyme and inflammatory lesions in diencephalon and hypothalamus (arrow). Strongly suspicious for sarcoidosis.

infections tend to be bacterial. Viral infections can be acute (e.g., herpes simplex), "slow" (e.g., Jakob-Creutzfeldt, or subacute sclerosing panencephalitis, and possibly multiple sclerosis); or postinfectious-autoimmune. Tuberculosis tends to cause a granulomatous meningitis with secondary tuberculoma formation. Sarcoid, certain fungal diseases (e.g., cryptococcosis), and certain helminthic infections (e.g., cysticercosis) can cause a granulomatous meningitis that may be difficult to distinguish from tuberculosis by MRI. Other fungal infections (e.g., actinomycosis, aspergillosis, candidiasis, and mucormycosis) are generally associated with immunosuppression. While this category generally has been limited to patients with chronic debilitating disease, lymphoproliferative disorders, and severe diabetes, patients with acquired immune deficiency states (AIDS) are now acquiring certain infections that were previously considered to be quite rare. In addition, protozoan infections (e.g., toxoplasmosis) are becoming increasingly common with the increasing prevalence of AIDS.[12,13]

Infection in the brain can involve the meninges or the brain parenchyma, or both. Viruses tend to cause diffuse nonpurulent meningoencephalitis while pyogenic bacterial infections tend to be more focal.[2] Bacterial infections may initially produce diffuse cerebritis, but eventually a capsule is formed with central suppuration, i.e., an abscess is formed. Intracranial infections can be loculated in the epidural or subdural spaces as empyemas. Alternatively, subdural effusions can complicate meningitis, particularly in children infected with *Haemophilus influenzae*.[11]

MENINGITIS

The organism involved in pyogenic meningitis generally depends on the patient's age.[11] Newborns are most often infected with pneumococcus or gram-negative bacilli, whereas older children acquire *Haemophilus influenzae*. The meningococcus is the most common organism affecting young adults, and the pneumococcus again is the most common cause of meningitis in the elderly (generally secondary to pneumococcal pneumonia). Meningitis is usually diagnosed from a combination of clinical findings (fever, headache, and nuchal rigidity) and CSF analysis. CT or MRI is indicated if a mass lesion is to be excluded prior to lumbar puncture. Most patients with uncomplicated acute bacterial meningitis will have a normal MRI and normal CT (with or without intravenous contrast). We have occasionally noted diffusely increased signal from the meninges in patients recovering from bacterial meningitis (Fig. 13–3).

MRI or CT may demonstrate a benign subdural effusion, which is a normal inflammatory response to certain causes of meningitis, i.e., *Haemophilus influenzae* meningitis in young children.[13] Unless these are associated with mass effect, they do not require treatment. Occasionally, however, they may be symptomatic, necessitating a subdural tap. Aseptic meningitis is generally diagnosed from a combination of clinical findings and analysis of CSF. MRI and CT in such patients is generally normal.

Chronic granulomatous forms of meningitis have a predilection for the basilar meninges. Such basal arachnoiditis is generally associated with ventricular enlargement secondary to obstruction of fourth ventricular outlet foramina. Cerebral infarction may result from compromise of the perforating arteries originating at the base of the brain (Fig. 13–4). Meningeal enhancement is more often seen by CT following administration of intravenous contrast in chronic granulomatous meningitis than in acute bacterial forms of meningitis. Such patients may have cranial nerve dysfunction as well owing to involvement of the interpeduncular, pontine, and medullary cisterns. Such diffuse meningeal enhancement on CT or increased intensity on MRI can be seen with the chronic granulomatous meningitides (e.g., tubercular and fungal). This appearance can also be seen when there is subarachnoid seeding of primary CNS (medulloblastoma, ependymoma) and metastatic (breast) tumors and in chemical meningitis secondary to subarachnoid hemorrhage. Tuberculous meningitis generally follows a primary pulmonary infection with hematogenous spread to the leptomeninges.[11] Small granulomas form in the leptomeninges or brain parenchyma. Should these rupture into the adjacent CSF spaces, tuberculous meningitis results.

Tuberculomas within the brain may demonstrate ring enhancement following administration of contrast on CT and eventually may calcify. Both findings are currently

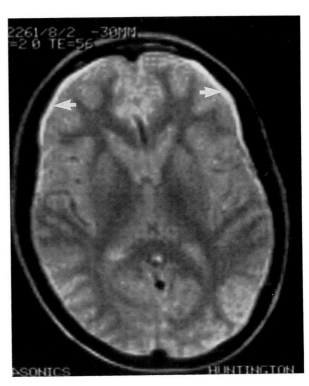

Figure 13–3. Meningitis. The meninges have increased intensity (arrowheads) in this patient several weeks after treatment for bacterial meningitis.

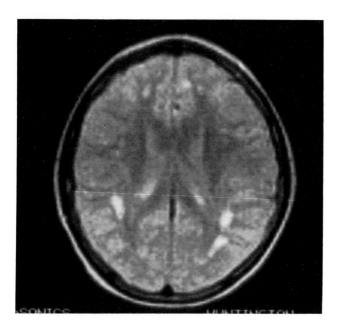

Figure 13–4. Deep white matter infarction following childhood meningitis. High-intensity lesions in periventricular region represent old infarcts due to compromise of the lenticulostriate arteries originating in the basal cisterns.

more easily made by CT than by MRI. While gadolinium-DTPA should be capable of demonstrating ring enhancement in the future,[14] CT will probably always remain more sensitive in the detection of subtle calcification. Sarcoid granulomas may be distinguished from tuberculomas on CT by the pattern of enhancement. Since sarcoid granulomas do not caseate, enhancement tends to be homogeneous and nodular rather than ringlike, as seen in the centrally caseating tuberculomas.[11] Again, this distinction requires the administration of intravenous contrast, which is currently more available for CT than for MRI.

Cryptococcus is the most common fungus that produces a basilar granulomatous meningitis. While half of the cases of cryptococcal meningitis are found in patients with AIDS or other forms of immunosuppression, the other half are found in ostensibly healthy individuals. Occasional findings by CT include meningeal enhancement with

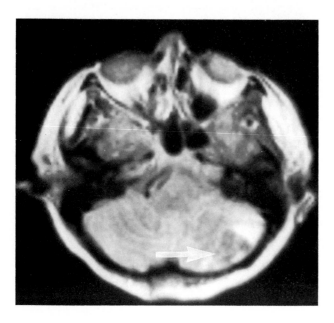

Figure 13–5. Cryptococcal granuloma in AIDS patient.

contrast. MRI findings may be normal or may demonstrate thickened meninges with increased intensity. Intracranial cryptococcal granulomas or "torulomas" (Fig. 13–5) have an appearance similar to tuberculomas or sarcoid granulomas.

ENCEPHALITIS

Encephalitis is generally due to viral infection. The most common causative organism is herpes simplex, which has a predilection for young children.[15] Medial temporal lobe involvement is most common, with bilateral involvement noted in approximately two thirds of the cases. The insular or orbitofrontal regions may also be involved. High intensity with mass effect is noted on MR, reflecting generalized increase in brain water content as a result of vasogenic edema. When hemorrhagic, herpes encephalitis may have a short $T1$ component in the subacute phase, which would have high intensity on $T1$ weighted images. Contrast enhancement has been noted in 50 percent of the herpes encephalitis patients studied by CT; similar findings would be expected using Gd-DTPA and MR. Diagnosis must be established by brain biopsy prior to administration of specific antiviral agents, such as adenine arabinoside. Biopsy prior to treatment with this agent is important, since other viral encephalitides will not respond to this agent. The most common cause of viral encephalitis (after the herpes simplex virus) is the arbovirus group, which causes the eastern, western, and Vene-

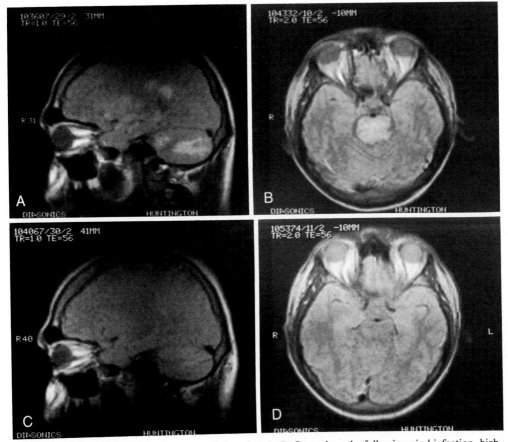

Figure 13–6. Postinfectious viral leukoencephalopathy. A–B, Several weeks following viral infection, high-intensity areas with mass effect are noted in the brainstem, cerebellum, and diencephalon. C–D, Following steroid therapy, inflammatory lesions have largely resolved.

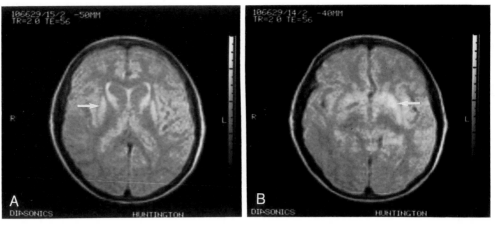

Figure 13–7. A–B Jakob-Creutzfeldt disease. Bilateral high-intensity lesions noted in basal ganglia and subcaudate regions in patient with strong clinical suspicion of Jakob-Creutzfeldt disease.

zuelan equine encephalitides.[11] Coxsackie virus may also cause encephalitis. Diagnosis is generally based on CSF titers or biopsy.

In some cases, encephalitis may follow a viral infection, particularly the exanthems such as measles, varicella, and rubella. This is thought to be an allergic or autoimmune reaction rather than a primary viral infection and is thus known as acute toxic dysimmune postinfectious leukoencephalopathy.[16] Such inflammatory states can also follow smallpox vaccination. Focal areas of high intensity in the periventricular white matter (Fig. 13–6), in the diencephalon, or in the brainstem may be noted on MRI, corresponding to foci of demyelination noted at post-mortem examination.

Slow virus infections, though much less common, tend to be uniformly lethal. These include Jakob-Creutzfeldt (Fig. 13–7) and other spongiform encephalopathies.[17] MRI may be more sensitive than CT in detecting the early basal ganglial involvement

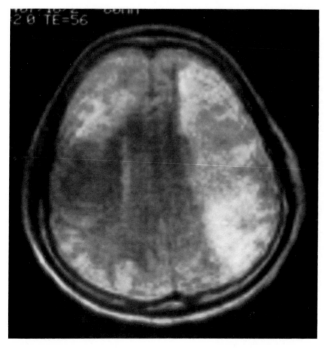

Figure 13–8. Progressive multifocal leukoencephalopathy. Diffuse high intensity is noted within the white matter, most pronounced on the left side in this AIDS patient.

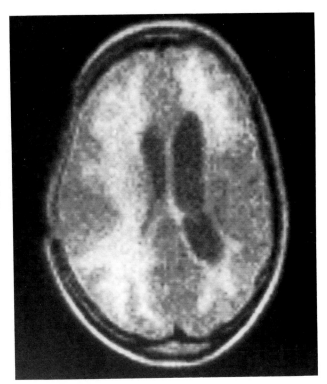

Figure 13–9. Methotrexate leukoencephalopathy. Diffuse white matter edema is noted following intrathecal administration of methotrexate for astrocytoma.

in Jakob-Creutzfeldt disease (Fig. 13–7). Subacute sclerosing panencephalitis (SSPE) is believed to represent a slow viral manifestation of measles infection. Measles antigen has been demonstrated in the brain tissues, and high titers of antimeasles antibodies have been noted in the serum of patients with SSPE. Progressive multifocal leukoencephalopathy (PML) is most often seen in chronically debilitated patients, particularly those with lymphoproliferative disorders or those receiving chemotherapy.[18] PML is being recognized with increasing frequency in patients with AIDS (Fig. 13–8). MR studies in such patients demonstrate extensive periventricular abnormalities, primarily in the white matter. Similar inflammatory findings can be seen following intrathecal administration of methotrexate (Fig. 13–9).

CEREBRITIS AND ABSCESS

Cerebritis and abscess tend to be more focal infections of brain parenchyma than encephalitis. When such infections are bacterial, they may result from hematogenous spread (generally from sepsis, subacute bacterial endocarditis, bronchiectasis, or pneumonia) or from contiguous extension (from sinusitis, mastoiditis, otitis media, or osteomyelitis). MRI findings in such patients demonstrate nonspecific high intensity with mass effect (Fig. 13–10). When contiguous and resulting from spread of infection, the lesion can generally be related to the offending structure. When distributed throughout the brain at the gray–white matter junction, infection may be confused with hematogenously spread metastatic disease.

Over a period of several weeks, a capsule forms at the periphery of the cerebritis, surrounding the necrotic central portion of what is now considered an abscess (Fig. 13–11). While cerebritis and abscess may not be distinguishable by MRI, contrast enhancement of the capsule may be demonstrable by CT. Abscesses larger than 3 cm

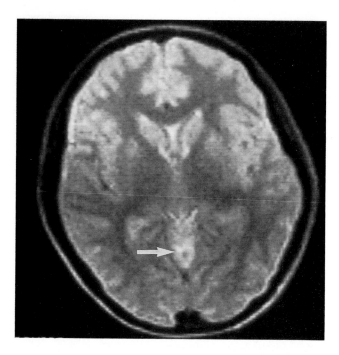

Figure 13–10. Vermian abscess. High intensity and mass effect noted in patient with vermian signs following episode of sepsis.

in diameter are generally not amenable to treatment by systemic antibiotics and require surgical drainage.[11] Since the capsule tends to be thicker on the superficial cortical side than on the deep ventricular side, rupture into the ventricular system is not uncommon. Secondary ventriculitis or ependymitis results. While ependymal enhancement may be noted following administration of contrast on CT, generalized increased intensity and ventricular enlargement may be apparent by MRI. When gadolinium-DTPA is generally available, ependymal enhancement should also be apparent by MRI.

Cerebritis and abscess formation may also be noted in nonbacterial infections.

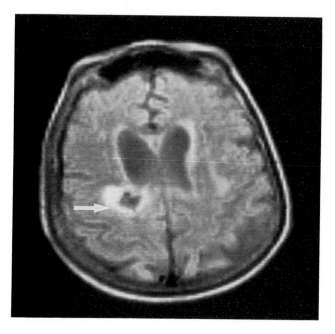

Figure 13–11. Bacterial brain abscess. Pneumococcal abscess in patient with pneumococcal pneumonia.

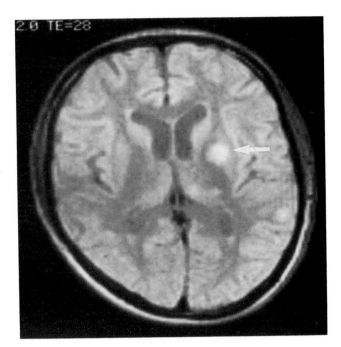

Figure 13–12. Toxoplasmosis. AIDS patient with diffuse toxoplasmosis.

Toxoplasmosis (protozoan) is a known cause of intrauterine infection (one of the TORCH organisms) and is an opportunistic infection in immunosuppressed individuals. Recently, toxoplasmosis has been found to be the most common CNS complication of AIDS.[12] The disease generally begins as a subacute meningoencephalitis with secondary formation of multiple scattered necrotic granulomas throughout the cerebral hemispheres. Ring enhancement is generally noted on CT, and a central area of low intensity[12] may be noted by MRI (Fig. 13–12). Biopsy is generally required for diagnosis. In AIDS patients, toxoplasmosis may not be distinguishable from other opportunistic infections, such as cryptococcosis, or from other diseases, such as lymphoma. Coexistence of toxoplasmosis with lymphoma (Fig. 13–13) and toxoplasmosis with PML (Fig. 13–14) has also been noted in AIDS patients, further complicating therapeutic intervention.[12]

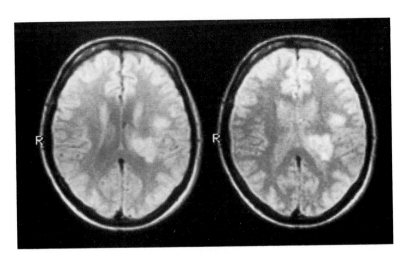

Figure 13–13. AIDS patient with biopsy-proven toxoplasmosis (superficial lesion) and lymphoma (deeper lesion).

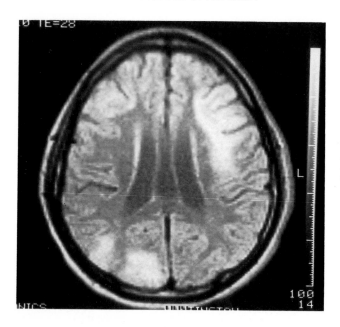

Figure 13–14. AIDS patient with toxoplasmosis and progressive multifocal leukoencephalopathy (PML) (biopsy-proven).

CYSTICERCOSIS

Cysticercosis results from intermediate host infection by the pork tapeworm *Taenia solium*.[11] Cysticercosis can exist in three locations in the brain: intraventricular, parenchymal, and arachnoidal. When the ventricles, aqueduct, or basilar meninges are involved with large cysts, hydrocephalus may result (Fig. 13–15). Aqueductal scarring and obliteration may result from the inflammatory response to a cyst and may remain after the disease has been treated (Fig. 13–16). Parenchymal involvement (Fig. 13–17) results in mental deterioration and seizures. Diagnosis is based on the history of travel within an endemic area and is documented by the presence of serologic or CSF titers. Calcification, which is quite obvious on CT, may be subtle or inapparent by MRI. The fluid within the cysts tends to have a lower protein content than other pathologic cystic processes (e.g., cystic astrocytomas) and potentially may be confused with arachnoid cysts.

EPIDURAL AND SUBDURAL EMPYEMAS

Epidural empyemas have a characteristic lenticular shape on both CT and MR.[11] On MRI, the dura is recognized as a low-intensity structure between the high-intensity epidural collection and the subjacent brain parenchyma (Fig. 13–18). Epidural empyemas may result from contiguous frontal sinusitis or osteomyelitis of the calvarium. They may also follow penetrating trauma or result as a complication of a craniotomy. Epidural empyema may be indistinguishable from epidural hematoma by MRI alone.

Subdural empyemas may result from secondary infection of a subdural hematoma or sudural effusion.[11] They may also result from extension of infection through the dura from an epidural empyema or contiguous sinusitis or osteomyelitis. Subdural empyema may also result from septic thrombophlebitis involving the emissary veins into the dural space. CT or MRI is generally performed in such cases prior to lumbar puncture to exclude mass effect. As above, it may not be possible to distinguish an infected from a noninfected subdural hematoma by MRI alone.

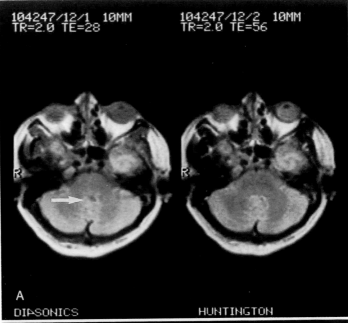

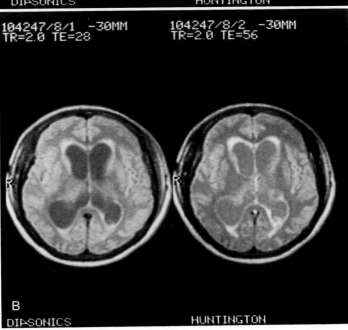

Figure 13–15. Cysticercosis. *A*, Cysticercotic cyst in fourth ventricle (arrow). *B*, Secondary hydrocephalus.

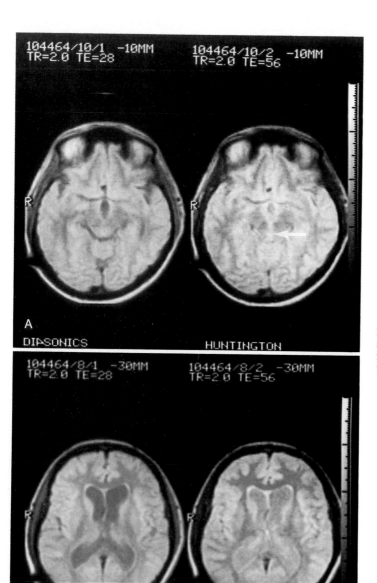

Figure 13–16. Cysticercosis. *A*, Obliteration of aqueduct due to inflammation from earlier cyst. *B*, Secondary obstructive hydrocephalus.

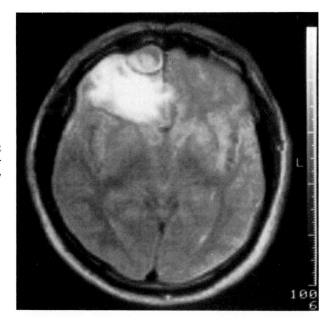

Figure 13–17. Parenchymal cysticercosis. Right frontal cyst (with surrounding edema) is in a somewhat unusual location for parenchymal disease, which tends to be more periventricular.

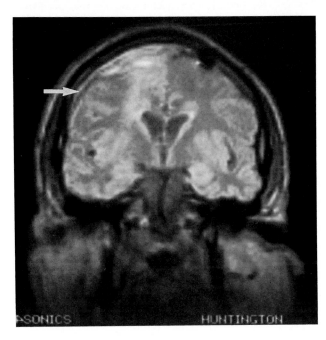

Figure 13–18. Epidural empyema. Postoperative/post-trauma infection in epidural space (arrow). Note also subdural fluid collection and subjacent vasogenic edema.

References

1. Robbins SL, Angell M: Inflammation and repair. *In* Robbins SL, Angell M (eds): Basic Pathology, 2nd ed. Philadelphia, WB Saunders, 1976, pp. 31–53.
2. Lindenberg R: Inflammation. *In* Haymaker W, Adams RD (eds): Histology and Histopathology of the Nervous System, Vol 1. Springfield, IL, Charles C Thomas, 1982, pp. 1150–1170.
3. Brant-Zawadzki M, Norman D, Newton TH, Kelly WM, Kjos B, et al: Magnetic resonance of the brain: The optimal screening technique. Radiology *152*:71, 1984.
4. Davidson HD, Steiner RE: Magnetic resonance imaging in infections of thhe central nervous system. AJNR 6:499, 1985.
5. Bradley WG, Waluch V, Yadley RA, Wycoff RR: Comparison of CT and MR in 400 patients with suspected disease of the brain and cervical spinal cord. Radiology *152*:695, 1984.

6. Bradley WG: Pathophysiologic correlates of signal alterations. *In* Brant-Zawadzki M, Norman D (eds): MRI of the CNS. New York, Raven Press, 1986, pp 23–42.
7. Fullerton GD, Cameron IL, Ord VA: Frequency dependence of magnetic resonance spin-lattice relaxation of protons in biological materials. Radiology *151*:135, 1984.
8. Bradley WG: Fundamentals of MR image interpretation. *In* Bradley WG, Adey WR, Hasso AN (eds): Magnetic Resonance Imaging of the Brain, Head and Neck: A Text Atlas. Rockville, MD, Aspen, 1985.
9. Carr DH, Brown J, Bydder GM, et al: Intravenous chelated gadolinium as a contrast agent in NMR imaging of cerebral tumors. Lancet *1*:484, 1984
10. Bradley WG: Magnetic resonance imaging of the central nervous system. Neurol Res 6:91, 1984
11. Weisberg L, Nice C, Katz M: Infectious inflammatory conditions. *In* Weisberg L, Nice C, Katz M (eds): Cerebral Computed Tomography, 2nd ed. Philadelphia, WB Saunders, 1984, pp. 229–248.
12. Levy RM, Bredesen DE, Moore S, Mills C: Cranial magnetic resonance imaging in the acquired immunodeficiency syndrome (AIDS): Superiority to CT. Presented at the Fourth Annual Meeting, Society of Magnetic Resonance in Medicine, London, England, August 19–23, 1985.
13. Floris R, De La Paz, RL, Brant-Zawadzki M, Norman D, Newton TH: MRI findings in acquired immune deficiency syndrome (AIDS). Presented at the Fourth Annual Meeting of the Society of Magnetic Resonance in Medicine, London, England, August 19–23, 1985.
14. Runge VM, Clanton JA, Price AC, et al: Evaluation of contrast-enhanced MR imaging in a brain-abscess model. AJNR 6:139, 1985.
15. Benator RM, Magill HL, Gerald B, Igarashi M, Fitch SJ: Herpes simplex encephalitis: CT findings in the neonate and young infant. AJNR 6:539, 1985.
16. Dunn V, Bale JF, Bell WE, Ehrhardt JC: MRI in children with post-infectious disseminated encephalomyelitis. Presented at the Fourth Annual Meeting of the Society of Magnetic Resonance in Medicine, London, England, August 19–23, 1985.
17. Kovanen J, Erkinjuntti T, Iivanainen M, Ketonen L, Haltia M, Sulkava R, Sipponen JT: Cerebral MR and CT imaging in Creutzfeldt-Jakob disease. J Comput Assist Tomogr 9(1):125, 1985.
18. Fernandez RE, Kishore PRS: White matter disease of the brain. *In* Lee SH and Rao KCVG (eds): Cranial Computed Tomography. New York, McGraw-Hill 1983, pp. 662–663.

14

Ischemic Cerebrovascular Disease

ROBERT M. KESSLER
MARK P. FREEMAN

Cerebrovascular disease is a widespread health problem in many societies. In the United States an estimated 2 million strokes occurred in 1985.[1] Before discussing the evaluation of stroke with nuclear magnetic resonance imaging, it is important to review the progression of metabolic and structural changes that occur in stroke. Oxygen and glucose[2] are the substrates normally utilized for brain energy metabolism. The loss of these substrates can be caused by a loss of blood flow to the brain, ischemia, or deficient delivery of energy substrates with normal blood flow, hypoxia, or hypoglycemia. Although there is rapid failure of energy metabolism with total ischemia or hypoxia,[3–5] tissue death may not occur until many minutes later[6,7]; in regional ischemia there appears to be an evolution of metabolic changes that can last an hour or more.[8] The sensitivity of the brain to either ischemic or hypoxic insult varies greatly from region to region.[6,9] This differential sensitivity may be due to a number of factors, which include vascular anatomy[10] and the density of specific neurotransmitter innervation.[11] The development of edema following a cerebrovascular insult has important consequences for the appearances of stroke on nuclear magnetic resonance studies.[12] These three aspects of cerebrovascular disease—metabolic changes, regional sensitivity, and edema—will be discussed in some detail. Magnetic resonance imaging (MRI) in cerebrovascular disease will then be discussed in reference to these mechanisms and to clinical imaging results.

METABOLIC CHANGES IN STROKE

Both behavioral and metabolic studies have demonstrated that the brain possesses limited energy reserves in the face of a loss of blood flow or oxygen delivery. The studies of Lowry et al.[3] have demonstrated that total ischemia in mice (due to decapitation) leads to a loss of 18 μmol of high-energy phosphates per gram brain tissue in the first ten minutes following total hypoxia. Over three fourths of this loss occurs in the first minute, and just under 90 percent occurs within two minutes; phosphocreatine and ATP fall by 85 and 50 percent, respectively, within 30 seconds. Thus, in total ischemia, few energy reserves remain within two minutes. In studies of both total cerebral ischemia[13] and total anoxia,[9] unconsciousness occurs within six seconds, suggesting rapid depletion of energy and oxygen reserves. Despite the rapid failure of energy metabolism in total ischemia, recovery of neurologic function has been seen in man as long as 15 to 18 minutes following circulatory arrest[7]; animal studies have demonstrated neuronal viability after one hour of total ischemia.[14,15] It would appear that neuronal viability persists for many minutes following failure of energy metabolism.

Regional ischemia is more frequently encountered in man than total ischemia or anoxia. With the exception of long perforating end-arteries, such as the lenticulostriate arteries, significant collateral circulation exists in the brain through pial anastomoses. As a result, most vascular occlusions lead to incomplete ischemia. Siesjo[2] reviewed experimental findings in incomplete ischemia and concluded that cerebral metabolism is maintained with blood flow decreases of 50 percent. Below this level, failure of cerebral energy metabolism starts to occur. In man, Powers et al.[16] reported a threshold for viability of 15 ml/100 gm/min using positron emission tomography (PET). Interestingly, Finnerty et al.[17] demonstrated that in man the threshold of arterial blood pressure for behavioral symptoms varies with the subject's blood pressure history. This threshold generally occurred at blood pressure levels that corresponded to cerebral blood flows 60 to 70 percent of normal flow; for normotensive individuals this was at a mean arterial blood pressure of 29 to 35 mm Hg. For those with essential hypertension, the threshold for behavioral changes was 47 mm, and for those with malignant hypertension, 89 mm. This indicates a significant change in autoregulation of cerebral blood flow in hypertension.

Animal studies of middle cerebral artery occlusion have shown a range of blood flow decrements varying from no significant changes from normal levels in some studies to over 80 percent reductions in other studies, with near-total cessation of flow in the center of the lesion.[8] Middle cerebral artery obstruction in the squirrel monkey led to blood flow decrements of 20 to 50 percent compared with normal control values.[18] Cerebral ATP concentrations fell from 2 μmol per gm to about 0.4 μmol per gm over a three-hour period. Lactate levels doubled over the same period. Studies in cats have shown 60 to 80 percent decrements in blood flow in the middle cerebral distribution, with flow reductions of up to 40 percent in the border zone.[8] Metabolic changes similar to those described in the squirrel monkey were found in the cat model; falls in phosphocreatine levels (60 percent reduction), ATP levels (50 percent reduction), and rises in lactate occurred over a one- to three-hour period. A decrease in flow in the border zone developed over a period of one hour; after an hour, further decreases did not occur. Simultaneous measurements of regional NADH, ATP, and glucose concentrations using fluorescence and bioluminescence techniques reveal a characteristic pattern of regional changes following middle cerebral occlusion in cats.[19] Centrally, abnormal concentrations of all three metabolites—NADH, ATP, and glucose—were seen, with an increase in NADH concentration and a decrease in glucose and ATP concentrations. Surrounding this central region was a larger zone characterized by decreased ATP and glucose concentrations but normal NADH levels. A third and larger surrounding zone with decreased glucose levels but more normal ATP and NADH levels was noted. These findings are consistent with deoxyglucose studies demonstrating increased glycolytic activity at the periphery of infarcts and decreased glucose metabolism centrally.[20,21] At four hours this appears to be due to increased glycolysis in neurons in the border zone. The metabolic findings in the middle cerebral artery model of regional ischemia indicate that with incomplete ischemia there is a gradient of increasing levels of flow and decreasing metabolic impairments from the center of the ischemic region outward.

SELECTIVE VULNERABILITY

Certain regions of brain appear much more sensitive to the effects of ischemia.[6,9] These include boundary regions falling between major vascular territories and certain vulnerable regions—hippocampus; basal ganglia; Purkinje cells of the cerebellum; layers 3, 5, and 6 of cortex; and, in some cases, white matter. Boundary zones, e.g., between middle and posterior cerebral arteries corresponding to lateral parieto-occipital cortex, and between anterior and middle cerebral arteries corresponding to lateral frontal cortex, often are affected by infarction following periods of hypotension or following total ischemia due to circulatory arrest. Experimental models of cerebral hypoperfusion have failed to show selective flow or metabolic deficits in boundary zones.[10] Paschen et al.,[22] using a cat brain model of total ischemia followed by recirculation, demonstrated impaired recovery of energy metabolism in boundary zones, implying that selective hypoperfusion may occur in boundary zones during recirculation.

Welsh et al.,[10] in attempting to create a model of cerebral hypoperfusion to study border-zone infarctions, demonstrated that the greatest derangements in energy metabolism occurred in white matter with hypoperfusion. With cerebral oligemia, there were no signficant changes in ATP levels in boundary zones of frontal cortex or caudate in the cat, but there was a 30 percent fall in ATP levels in white matter. Phosphocreatine levels fell from 15 to 28 percent in cortex and caudate but declined 87 percent in white matter. Similarly, lactate levels rose greater than nine fold in white matter. In cortex, the changes ranged from two to three fold. Interestingly, the caudate, where the arterial supply consists of long perforating branches similar to those in the deep white matter, had a sixfold increase in lactate levels. During arterial hypotension, the white matter suffers disproportionately decreased cerebral blood flow.[23] It is of interest that in carbon monoxide poisoning, white matter lesions are common and can be disproportionate to damage seen in gray matter.[9] White matter appears to be vulnerable to reductions in flow or, in the case of carbon monoxide poisoning, to a hypoxic insult.

It has been known for some time that specific gray matter regions and cell types appear to be far more sensitive to ischemia than other regions of the brain. These regions include the hippocampus, particularly the CA1 subfield; cerebellar Purkinje cells, small and medium-sized striatal neurons; and layers 3, 5, and 6 of the cerebral cortex.[6,9] These regions undergo delayed necrosis after as little as five minutes of ischemia. With restitution of flow after an appropriate ischemic period, delayed cell death in these regions may not occur for a period of days. The mechanism of this delayed necrosis is not completely understood. Recent evidence strongly points to excitatory amino acid neurotransmitters as a factor in this regional sensitivity.[11] Transection of the perforant pathway, the principal pathway for excitatory amino acid input into hippocampus greatly reduced ischemic damage in the hippocampus after hypoxia.[24] Similarly, destruction of the anterior neocortex, the source of excitatory neurotransmitter input to the caudate, greatly decreased the effects of 30 minutes of hypoglycemia.[25] Selective excitatory amino acid receptor antagonists have been shown to be protective against the effects of 30 minutes of ischemia.[11] While there may be additional factors responsible for the vulnerability of these regions, excitatory amino acid neurotransmitters appear to be a major factor. Hossman[6] has recently reviewed a number of other factors implicated in delayed necrosis, including the role of calcium, postischemic hypoperfusion, protein synthesis, energy metabolism, acidosis, and water and ion homeostasis. Although these factors may have a role in this phenomenon, the importance of each is not clear at present.

EDEMA ASSOCIATED WITH STROKE

In stroke, there are rapid changes in water and ion homeostasis. An increase in brain volume can be detected as early as one minute following a middle cerebral artery occlusion.[26] This rapid change in brain volume is thought to be due to vasodilation, with a resulting increase in cerebral blood volume. Beneath a cerebral blood flow of 10 to 15 ml/100 gm/min, there is a rapid onset of cytotoxic edema followed three to four hours later by vasogenic edema.[27,28] With milder degrees of ischemia, edema may occur at a slower rate and progress with time.

The initial cytotoxic edema is due to failure of energy metabolism and the sodium-potassium membrane pump.[26] There is resultant increase in intracellular sodium content, a decrease in tissue potassium content, and a marked rise in the sodium:potassium ratio in tissue. Intracellular ions may be released from binding sites. With incomplete ischemia, lactate will accumulate. These events lead to an increase in tissue osmolality. Following middle cerebral artery occlusion, these changes increase in magnitude for at least a four-hour period. Associated with these changes is an actual decrease in the size of the extracellular fluid space.[8] The total water content within the central area of the stroke is, however, increased at one hour: This change reaches statistical significance by two hours.[12] Similarly, tissue pressure in the center of the stroke rises from 7 mm Hg to 12 mm Hg by two hours and continues to rise. In the initial few hours there is no significant breakdown of the blood-brain barrier. The major change in the first few hours is intracellular accumulation of fluid with an increase in intracellular sodium and a loss of potassium. This cellular swelling affects the glial cells adjacent to the microvasculature, and the swelling of these cells may compress the microvasculature, thus increasing the degree of ischemia.[28]

Depending on the duration and severity of ischemia, breakdown of the blood-brain barrier will start at from 3 to 24 hours.[27] In the cytotoxic phase of cerebral edema, the gray matter tends to be affected more than the white matter. With the onset of vasogenic edema, there is leakage of larger molecules, e.g., proteins, and water across the blood-brain barrier. Studies in cats and rhesus monkeys indicate that maximum vasogenic edema occurs at two days and four days, respectively.[29] Vasogenic edema spreads into the white matter; water content may rise to 80 percent in the white matter,[30] and local tissue pressure may rise to 80 mm Hg.[31] In cats and monkeys, maximal opening of the blood-brain barrier does not occur until about four days in cats and seven to ten days in monkeys.[29] The barrier remains open when water content returns to normal levels. Although the onset of vasogenic edema appears to be related to opening of the blood-brain barrier, barrier opening and vasogenic edema are not tightly coupled during the resolution of edema.

NMR IMAGING STUDIES OF CEREBRAL ISCHEMIA—EXPERIMENTAL STUDIES

Multiple studies have now shown that proton nuclear magnetic resonance imaging studies can detect stroke within hours after its onset (Fig. 14–1). Experimental stroke studies in primates, cats, and rats have shown that in some cases strokes may be visible as early as 30 minutes to two hours after the event.[32–35] Spetzler et al.[32] reported changes on saturation recovery images as early as 90 minutes after middle cerebral artery occlusion in the baboon. Brant-Zawadzki and colleagues,[33] using an acute middle cerebral artery occlusion model in cats, demonstrated changes on NMR imaging studies by 30 minutes in two of five animals. The other three animals showed equivocal or no changes over a three-hour period of study. Eight other cats were imaged at four or more hours, and all showed definite changes. These changes always involved the caudate and usually the globus pallidus and temporoparietal cortex. Lesions were best seen as areas of increased signal intensity on a *T2* weighted (SE 2000/56) pulse sequence. The lesions were not apparent in seven of ten cats studied with a *T1* weighted sequence (SE 500/28) but showed decreased signal intensity in three of ten animals. Mass effect was most pronounced at about the time of maximum vasogenic edema at three days. The lesion did not change in configuration over this period. Calculated *T1* values were

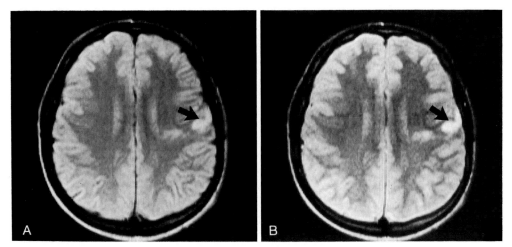

Figure 14–1. Acute nonhemorrhagic stroke. *A*, Transverse SE 3000/32 MR image; increased intensity in the cortex of the left hemisphere (arrow). *B*, Transverse SE 3000/64 MR image. Notice further increase in intensity in region of acute nonhemorrhagic stroke (arrow.)

lengthened by 12 to 42 percent in ischemic gray matter, while calculated $T2$ values were increased by 6 to 24 percent. Using a feline model of middle cerebral artery occlusion, McNamra et al.[36] recently published a study of enhancement in stroke following gadolinium-DTPA administration. Enhancement was seen in six cats at 16 hours following occlusion (best seen on a SE 500/28 pulse sequence). Imaging studies were performed for various time periods up to one week. At 16 to 24 hours, shortening of $T1$ occurred more rapidly than at three or seven days. Encephalomalacia from chronic ischemia is exquisitely demonstrated by MRI (Fig. 14–2).

Studies have been performed using various models of ischemia in rodents. Buonanno and colleagues[34] performed both proton spectroscopic and imaging studies in gerbils and rats. Gerbils were subjected to carotid ligation. In rats the carotid artery was catheterized, ligated, and injected with 0.1 ml of autologous clot. Spectroscopic measurement of $T1$ and $T2$ of the affected hemisphere within three hours following carotid ligation revealed a mean prolongation of 16 percent for $T1$ and 25 percent for

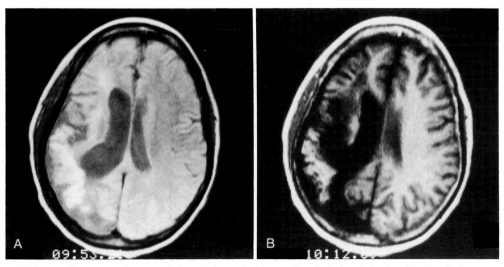

Figure 14–2. Chronic stroke, encephalomalacia secondary to chronic ischemia in the right hemisphere. *A*, Transverse SE 3000/32 MR image. *B*, Transverse inversion recovery 1800/400/32 MR image.

T2. At three hours after carotid ligation, 11 of 28 gerbils showed recognizable alterations in imaging studies; by 24 hours, 10 of 11 gerbils had abnormal imaging studies. Studies in rats showed imaging abnormalities in some animals by two hours but more frequently by 24 hours. The area of abnormal signal was largest and mass effect greatest at 44 hours in the rat; signal abnormalities persisted up to 3.5 months. Bryan and colleagues[35] have also studied ischemia in the rat induced by cauterization of the middle cerebral artery. Prolongation of *T2* in the affected area was seen at six hours but not at one hour. These changes persisted for the length of the study (30 days). Calculated *T2* values were prolonged by more than two fold.

Levy and colleagues[37] used proton NMR imaging to study the effect of naloxone (2 mg/kg) and morphine sulfate (10 mg/kg) on the evolution of acute stroke in the gerbil. Following occlusion of the right carotid artery, gerbils were imaged at about 3 hours, 12 hours, and 24 hours. *T1* values and *T2* values in the ischemic hemisphere were significantly prolonged by three hours and continued to increase up to 24 hours, reaching values of 130 percent of controls for *T2* and 147 percent of controls for *T1* by 24 hours. Neither drug had a significant effect on *T1* or *T2* at any time point.

The relationship of proton NMR imaging changes in ischemia to changes in water content and electrolytes in brain has been examined by Kato et al.[38] Two models of ischemia were utilized. In the rat, four-vessel ischemia for one hour was followed by a one-hour period of restored blood flow. In vitro spectroscopic measurements of *T1* and *T2*, water content, sodium concentration, and potassium concentration were performed. *T1* was prolonged by 7.1 to 9.2 percent and *T2* by 8.8 to 13.0 percent, water content increased 2.4 to 3.4 percent in ischemic regions. Sodium levels rose and potassium levels fell in all ischemic regions. In both normal and ischemic regions, *T1* was highly correlated with water content (r=0.987); *T2* was also significantly correlated with water content, but the correlation coefficient was only 0.734. Factors other than total water content appear to influence *T2*. Imaging studies were performed with gerbils following cauterization of the right common carotid artery. Increased signal intensity was seen on the SE 1600/106 images at 30 minutes in the region of the thalamus. The difference in signal intensities between the ischemic and control sides increased from a ratio of 1.07 at 30 minutes to 1.13 at four hours. Calculated *T1* and *T2* values were lengthened in both cortex and thalamus by four hours. For the thalamus, the *T1* and *T2* showed a monoexponential decay. The major conclusion in this study was that the visibility of cerebral ischemia on NMR studies appears to be due largely to increased water content. *T1* appears linearly dependent on water content; *T2* is largely but not totally dependent on water content. The contribution of ionic shifts to protein NMR imaging in stroke was thought to be minor. The rapid visibility of stroke on proton NMR appears to be due to the sensitivity of proton NMR to edema. As increased water content appears to be a major reason for the visibility of early stroke, areas of ischemia may not be readily distinguishable from the edema associated with stroke on unenhanced proton NMR studies.

CLINICAL IMAGING

In ischemic stroke in man, the findings are consistent with experimental studies of pathophysiology and imaging.[39–42] These findings are decreased signal on *T1* weighted sequences, indicating a prolonged *T1*, and increased signal on *T2* weighted sequences, indicating a prolonged *T2*. These findings appear within hours of the onset of stroke at a time when CT findings are negative (see Fig. 14–1). These findings have been reported as early as six hours[40] and are believed to be due to the rapid onset of cytotoxic edema. With the onset of vasogenic edema within several hours, the area of increased *T1* and *T2* tends to increase in size and spread into the white matter. This edema and mass effect tend to peak within the first week, when vasogenic edema is maximal. As the edema subsides the area of abnormality and mass effect decreases. In subacute and chronic stroke a residual area of prolonged *T1* and *T2* remains, with no mass effect or atrophy. It has not proved possible to differentiate areas of edema from infarction.

This sequence of changes can be modified by the presence of hemorrhage (Fig. 14–3).[43] Hemorrhagic infarction occurs in 10 to 20 percent of cases of stroke. The cortex is the usual site of hemorrhage. It is believed to occur when recently infarcted

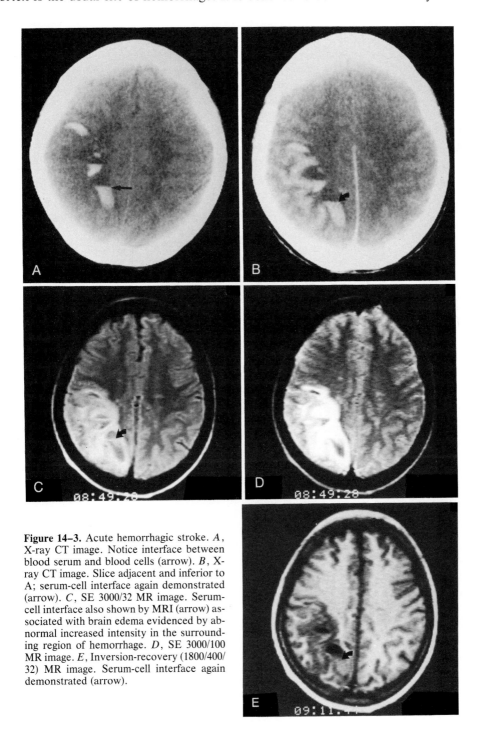

Figure 14–3. Acute hemorrhagic stroke. *A*, X-ray CT image. Notice interface between blood serum and blood cells (arrow). *B*, X-ray CT image. Slice adjacent and inferior to A; serum-cell interface again demonstrated (arrow). *C*, SE 3000/32 MR image. Serum-cell interface also shown by MRI (arrow) associated with brain edema evidenced by abnormal increased intensity in the surrounding region of hemorrhage. *D*, SE 3000/100 MR image. *E*, Inversion-recovery (1800/400/32) MR image. Serum-cell interface again demonstrated (arrow).

brain is exposed to normal levels of arterial blood pressure, e.g., following rapid lysis of an embolus, following a hypotensive episode, or with watershed infarctions with good collateral blood supply. Hecht-Leavitt et al.,[43] using a 1.5 tesla scanner, reported nine patients with hemorrhagic infarction. In all but one case reported, the infarction was in a watershed zone. The patients were studied no later than five days after the clinical event. The appearance of the stroke was modified by the presence and evolution of the hemorrhagic zone. In the acute phase (5 to 18 days following stroke), there was "mildly low intensity" on *T2* weighted pulse sequences (SE 8/2500/80) and isointensity with brain on *T1* weighted sequences (SE 600/25). This appearance was believed to be due to the presence of deoxyhemoglobin. In the subacute phase (5 to 24 days) there was an apparent shortening of *T1* and a normal, followed by a prolonged, *T2* value. In a single chronic case (five years), the area of infarction was isointense on *T1* but showed a shortened *T2*, presumably owing to *T2* relaxation induced by residual hemosiderin. The findings in hemorrhagic infarction appear to be similar to those described for intracerebral hematomas.[44]

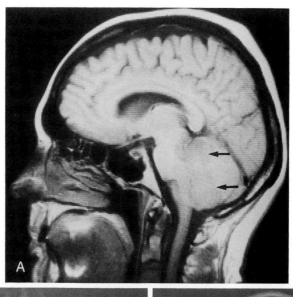

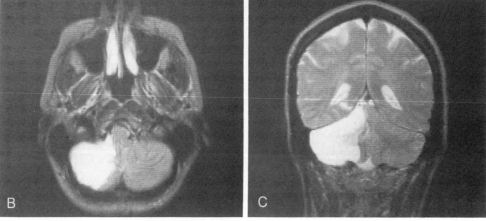

Figure 14–4. Posterior fossa stroke. *A*, Midline sagittal SE 500/32 MR image; area of infarction in cerebellum indicated by region of abnormal intensity (arrows). *B*, Transverse SE 3000/100 MR image; right cerebellar stroke evidenced by abnormal increased intensity. *C*, Coronal SE 3000/100 MR image; right cerebellar infarct again demonstrated by abnormal increased intensity.

The ability of magnetic resonance imaging to visualize infarction within hours of the clinical event is one advantage in comparison with x-ray computed tomography. In the posterior fossa, the absence of bone artifacts and the high inherent contrast in magnetic resonance studies have made MRI the modality of choice for cerebral infarction in the posterior fossa and brainstem (Figs. 14–4 and 14–5). Kistler et al.[45] presented 16 cases of vertebral-basilar territory infarctions; MRI identified the infarcted zones in 15 of 16 cases. Of the 16 cases, 14 had posterior fossa infarctions and all 14 were identified. Biller et al.[46] presented ten cases of pontine infarction studied with a 0.5 tesla imager. In all ten cases the zone of infarction was well seen on both *T1* weighted and *T2* weighted pulse sequences. In one case, a large infarction in the right "basis pontis" was not seen at 12 hours and subsequently was seen at six days. In 40 percent of Biller's cases, MRI showed more extensive abnormalities than would be clinically predicted. The inability of MRI to distinguish edema from infarction was believed to be responsible for this dichotomy. Fox et al.,[47] using a 1.5 tesla scanner, reported five patients with small lateral medullary infarctions. Three of the five showed areas of infarction just a few millimeters in size. These were identified more easily on *T1* than on *T2* weighted pulse sequences; the noise encountered on *T2* weighted sequences made identification of small infarcts difficult. A high-signal area ipsilateral to the medulla was noted in two cases, suggesting a vertebral occlusion that was confirmed angiographically in one case. Combining the studies of Biller and Fox, MRI detected 13 of 15 pontine and medullary infarctions, whereas CT detected only one. It should be noted that in Biller's series, CT was performed within hours of the patient's hospitalization.

Thrombosis of the dural sinuses (Fig. 14–6) or a cortical vein may produce infarction in the brain.[9] On NMR imaging the infarction itself appears to be similar to that described earlier for stroke due to arterial disease, i.e., prolongation of *T1* and *T2* in the area of infarction.[48,49] Hemorrhage within the venous infarction produces changes in signal intensity that appear to be similar to those described for hemorrhagic infarction. MRI allows direct visualization of the thrombus.[48–50] There seem to be some differences in the appearance of acute venous thrombosis observed at intermediate field strength (0.35 tesla) and high field strength (1.5 tesla). Both McMurdo[48] and Erdman[50] have observed an increase in signal intensity of venous thrombi on both *T1* and *T2* weighted images with use of a 0.35 tesla scanner. Macchi,[49] using a 1.5 tesla scanner, has reported an evolution of signal abnormalities in a thrombus similar to that

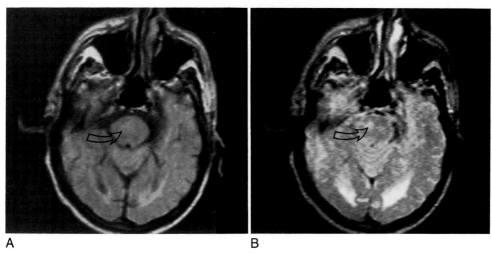

A   B

Figure 14–5. Brainstem stroke. *A*, Transverse SE 3000/32 MR image; poorly defined area of slightly increased intensity demonstrated on the right side of the brainstem (open arrow). *B*, Transverse SE 3000/100 MR image; right brainstem stroke better visualized as area of increased intensity (open arrow).

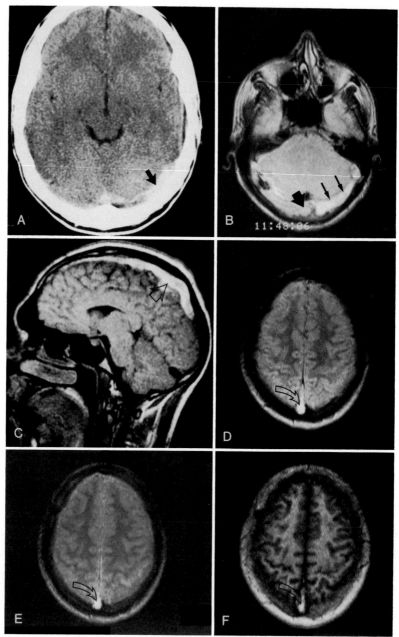

Figure 14–6. Superior sagittal sinus thrombosis. *A*, Transverse x-ray CT image; left posterior region of increased density (arrow) initially thought to represent artifact. *B*, Transverse SE 3000/64 MR image; increased intensity in left transverse sinus (arrows) and torcular Herophili (large arrow) represent dural sinus thrombosis *C*, Midline sagittal SE 777/30 MR image; increased intensity in superior sagittal sinus (open arrow) representing thrombosis. *D*, Transverse SE 3000/32 (odd-echo) MR image; increased intensity in superior sagittal sinus (open arrow) representing thrombosis. *Caution*: Increased intensity in veins also may be due to odd-echo dephasing, and the suspicion of thrombosis must be confirmed, for example, by evaluating the image intensity during the even echo or with correlative imaging modality. *E*, Transverse SE 3000/64 (even-echo) MR image; abnormal intensity in superior sagittal sinus persists, failing to demonstrate odd-echo rephasing and hence supporting the diagnosis of superior sagittal sinus thrombosis. *F*, Transverse inversion-recovery 1800/400/32 MR image; abnormal intensity again seen, representing superior sagittal sinus thrombosis (open arrow).

described for intracerebral hemorrhage. Acute thrombosis produced a signal isointense with brain on *T1* weighted sequences and hypointense on *T2* weighted sequences. In the subacute phase (starting at four to five days after the event), there was increased signal on both *T1* and *T2* weighted sequences. Macchi[49] reported only three patients, and McMurdo[48] six, while Erdman[50] reported 13 patients with extracerebral thrombosis.

MRI has also proved to be a sensitive tool in the evaluation of ischemia caused by vasculitis and vasculopathies (Fig. 14–7). Aisen et al.[51] reported three different types of lesions in eight cases of cerebral lupus erythematosus. The first is a large area of elongated *T1* and *T2* corresponding to areas of infarction seen on CT. The second is small areas of increased signal intensity seen best on *T2* weighted sequences in the white matter. These were usually not well seen on CT. The third pattern was gyral areas of increased signal intensity in the gray matter. The third pattern resolved over time in two of three patients. Vermess et al.[52] reported cerebral findings with MRI and CT in nine patients with systemic lupus erythematosus. All lesions seen on CT were seen on MRI; two patients had negative CT studies and positive MRI studies. In three of the remaining six patients with positive CT and MRI studies, the MRI studies demonstrated additional lesions. Both small white matter lesions and large areas with the CT appearance of infarction were seen. Holland et al.[53] also reported one case of meningovascular syphilis studied by CT and MRI. The MRI showed additional lesions both in the white matter and in the basal ganglia not seen on CT. It appears that MRI is an indicator of ischemia in cerebral vasculitis and vasculopathy, particularly in the white matter. The finding of reversible cortical lesions again points out the apparent inability of proton MRI to separate a reversible ischemia with edema from infarction.

To date, little clinical literature has been published regarding the use of gadolinium-DTPA in stroke. Virapongse et al.[54] reported 11 patients with stroke imaged from 4 to 30 days after the clinical event. Maximal enhancement was seen from 4 days to 18 days after stroke, with lesser enhancement at 28 to 30 days. MRI failed to show enhancement in one patient at 5 days. One patient who did not show CT enhancement at 8 days, did show MRI enhancement at 11 days. Maximal increases in signal due to contrast enhancement on SE 500/30 pulse sequences ranged from 10 percent for early infarctions

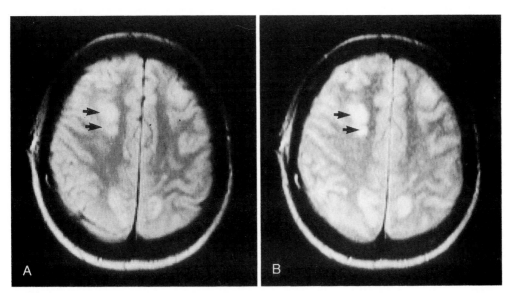

Figure 14–7. Ischemic infarcts in patient with vasculitis. *A*, Transverse SE 3000/32 MR image; infarct demonstrated in right hemisphere as area of increased intensity (arrows). *B*, Transverse SE 3000/64 MR image; further increased intensity noted in area of infarction (arrows).

to 37 percent for infarctions studied in the second week. Averaging all lesions studied, maximal enhancement occurred at 30 minutes. Overall, *T2* weighted nonenhanced studies were believed to be superior to CT. Gadolinium did not greatly improve the sensitivity of NMR imaging to the presence of stroke. Of 20 infarctions, only one thalamic lacune not seen on *T2* weighted pulse sequences was detected with gadolinium-enhanced *T1* imaging. Gadolinium studies may offer information regarding the state of neuronal viability in stroke, as breakdown of the blood-brain barrier has been associated with irreversible infarction.

White Matter Disease in the Elderly

The sensitivity of nuclear magnetic resonance imaging to pathologic changes in the white matter has enabled the frequent diagnosis of "deep white matter disease" in the elderly (Fig. 14–8).[55] The usual findings are areas of increased signal intensity on *T2* weighted sequences in the periventricular region and in the deep white matter of the cerebral hemispheres. These changes frequently are found in elderly subjects without other conditions that might produce changes in the white matter, e.g., cerebral neoplasms, trauma, radiation therapy, methotrexate therapy, obstructive hydrocephalus, multiple sclerosis, or leukodystrophies, and can occur in elderly subjects who are clinically normal. The etiology and significance of these white matter changes is the subject of the following discussion.

It is desirable to define first the range of normal for white matter signal characteristics on MRI. Zimmerman et al.[56] noted some periventricular hyperintensity in 93.5 percent of 365 consecutive cerebral NMR imaging studies. Small foci of increased signal intensity at the angles of the frontal horns and around occipital horns were considered a normal finding. A pencil-thin line of increased intensity around the lateral ventricles

Table 14–1. INCIDENCE OF DEEP WHITE MATTER DISEASE

Study	Modality	Incidence of Deep White Matter Disease (%)	Number of Subjects	Age Range (Years)
Lotz et al.[66]	CT and autopsy	22	82	56–93*
Kinkel et al.[57]	CT	1.7	1633	Consecutive CT studies "Adult patients"
George et al.[64]	CT	6.7	45	Normal: age 55–69
		24.4	45	Normal: age 70–85
		18.4	49	Alzheimer's disease: age 55–69
		35.3	102	Alzheimer's disease: age 70–85
Zeumer et al.[68]	CT	2.7	473	Consecutive CT examinations of patients 60–85 without other pathology
Goto et al.[61]	CT	0	529	0–49
		3.1	225	50–59
		12.0	250	60–69
		28.6	175	70–79
		38.1	21	80–89
Bradley et al.[55]	NMR	30	20	Over 60
Brant-Zawadzki[58]	NMR	0†	5	Normal: age 59–66
		44	9	Normal: age 74–81
Brun and Englund[67]	Autopsy	60	48	Alzheimer's disease: aged 52–92

* Age of subjects with deep white matter disease; ages of total number of subjects not given.
† Brant-Zawadzki's Class 1, punctate foci at the angles of the frontal horns, is considered not pathologic.

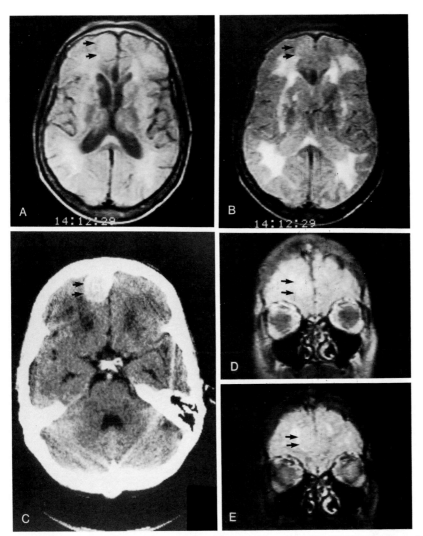

Figure 14–8. Ischemic deep white matter disease of the elderly. *A*, Transverse SE 3000/32 MR image. Bilateral deep white matter disease as illustrated by area of abnormal increased intensity. Incidentally, a right frontal meningioma is illustrated (arrows), but the soft tissue contrast delineation is poor. *B*, Transverse SE 3000/80 MR image. Deep white matter disease is more apparent. Again, the meningioma in the right frontal lobe is poorly delineated on the basis of soft tissue contrast (arrows). If meningioma is suspected, more heavily *T1* weighted pulse sequences (inversion recovery, for example) are required for improved soft tissue contrast discrimination. *C*, Transverse x-ray CT image. White matter disease is poorly demonstrated by comparison with MRI. However, right frontal meningioma is better demonstrated on this contrast-enhanced CT image. *D*, Coronal SE 3000/32 MR image. Incidentally, a meningioma poorly demonstrated (arrows). *E*, Coronal 3000/80 MR image. Meningioma again poorly demonstrated (arrows). *T1* weighted imaging is required to visualize meningioma on the basis of soft tissue contrast.

is nonspecific and may be seen commonly in normal older persons. The presence of a thick periventricular rind of increased intensity or small foci removed from the periventricular region is abnormal and may be seen in a variety of disorders, including trauma, hydrocephalus, tumors, and diseases of the white matter.

The incidence of deep white matter disease without an obvious cause has varied considerably depending on the population studied and the methods used. The incidence has varied (Table 14–1) from as low as 1.7 percent in Kinkel's[57] studies of consecutive CT examinations in adult subjects to as high as 44 percent in Brant-Zawadzki's[58] NMR study of nine normal subjects aged 74 to 81 years. Interestingly, careful autopsy studies have given still higher incidences.[66,67] The etiology of these changes appears to be subcortical arteriosclerotic encephalopathy in most pathologically examined cases.

Subcortical arteriosclerotic encephalopathy, also known as Binswanger's disease, has been considered a rare clinical entity.[9] Pathologically, it has been characterized by a loss of white matter with demyelination, a loss of axons, gliosis, and an associated hyaline thickening of the walls of the small penetrating arteries and arterioles in the deep white matter.[59-61] The pathologic changes in white matter often have been ascribed to "incomplete infarction," although Feigin and Popoff[62] have suggested that these changes can result from chronic edema. The subcortical U fibers are generally spared, as is the overlying cortex. These changes in the white matter frequently but not always from associated with lacunar infarction in the basal ganglia and white matter as well as atherosclerotic narrowing of the larger cerebral vessels (Fig. 14–9). The clinical features of this disorder vary depending on the report. Caplan and Schoene[59] presented 11 patients, including five autopsied cases. They emphasized the presence of dementia, hypertension, systemic vascular disease, acute strokes, the subacute evolution of focal neurologic deficits over weeks, plateau periods, a long clinical course averaging more

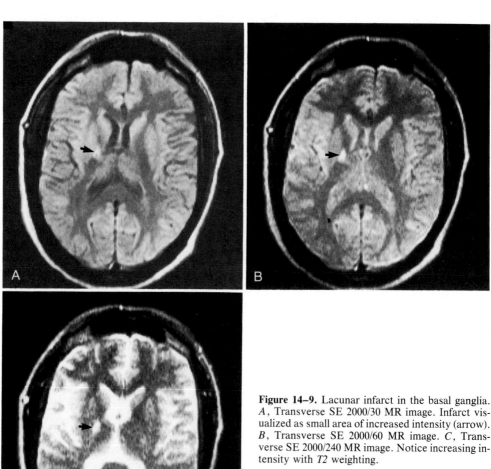

Figure 14–9. Lacunar infarct in the basal ganglia. *A*, Transverse SE 2000/30 MR image. Infarct visualized as small area of increased intensity (arrow). *B*, Transverse SE 2000/60 MR image. *C*, Transverse SE 2000/240 MR image. Notice increasing intensity with *T2* weighting.

than six years, psychologic changes, motor signs including pseudobulbar palsy, and hydrocephalus. The five cases that were pathologically examined revealed extensive white matter lesions with arterial and arteriolar sclerosis, demyelination, loss of axons, and gliosis as well as lacunar infarctions in the white matter, basal ganglia, and thalamus. These changes were not seen in the cortex. Atherosclerosis of the larger vessels and cortical strokes were seen as well, although the cortex was much less affected than were white matter and the diencephalon.

Loizou et al.[63] reported 15 patients with subacute arteriosclerotic encephalopathy. They reported clinical features similar to those described by Caplan and Schoene.[59] The principal clinical features were stated to be as follows: onset from 50 to 70 years of age, hypertension and/or atherosclerotic vascular disease; and focal neurologic deficits. The last can develop acutely or subacutely, particularly gait abnormalities and motor abnormalities, including pseudobulbar palsy, dementia with memory loss, psychologic changes, and stepwise deterioration. As with Caplan's[59] patients, the motor abnormalities were as clinically prominent or more marked than the dementia. Loizou emphasized the presence on CT of symmetric areas of low attenuation in the periventricular white matter, particularly in the frontal and parietal regions.[63] Mild to moderate hydrocephalus was seen in 12 of the 15 patients, mild to moderate cortical atrophy in six, cortical infarcts in three, and subcortical lacunar infarcts in three. Loizou[60] separately reported a normotensive case of subcortical arteriosclerotic encephalopathy for which autopsy correlation was available. The findings consisted of a hyaline arteriosclerosis of the small arteries and arterioles throughout the deep white matter, demyelination, cyst formation in the white matter, and discrete areas of cortical infarctions. The U fibers were preserved, as was the cortex overlying areas of affected white matter.

Goto et al.,[61] using first- and second-generation CT scanners, reported ten patients with deep white matter disease who had a CT examination and were subsequently autopsied. The age at onset of disease ranged from 44 to 80 with a mean of 67.6 years. The length of illness was shorter than that in Caplan's or Loizou's series, being 2.8 years. Prominent clinical features included dementia (10 of 10), motor abnormalities (8 of 10), pseudobulbar palsy (5 of 10), urinary incontinence (7 of 10), hypertension (8 of 10), and acute strokes (8 of 10). Pathologically, all patients had atherosclerotic changes in the larger arteries, hyaline thickening of the walls of the deep medullary arteries, ventricular enlargement, and extensive lesions in the deep white matter. These lesions were characterized by demyelination, loss of axons, and gliosis. Multiple cystic infarctions were seen in the white matter in eight cases. The subcortical U fibers and the overlying cortex were largely spared. These pathologic features are similar to those reported by Caplan and Schoene,[59] Loizou et al.,[63], Kinkel et al.,[57] and George et al.[64] Goto also reported two series of 1200 CT studies from Fukuska and 3542 CT studies from Akita. In the Fukuska series, no patients with white matter disease were seen under 50 years of age. The incidence rose steadily with age being 3.1 percent (7 of 225) in the sixth decade, 12.0 percent (30 of 250) in the seventh decade, 28.6 percent (50 of 175) in the eighth decade, and 38.1 percent (8 of 21) in the ninth decade. The age range was 54 to 89 years in these 95 subjects. Dementia was seen in 21 subjects. Motor abnormalities including pseudobulbar palsy, urinary incontinence, and emotional lability were seen in 47. In the Akita series, 152 cases of white matter disease were seen in 3542 studies from a hospital specializing in cerebrovascular disease. No age breakdown was given. The mean age of subjects with white matter disease was 67.1 years with a range of 42 to 86 years. Of 152 patients, 141 were hypertensive. Strokes (70 of 152), motor abnormalities (77 of 152), mental deterioration (44 of 152), and urinary incontinence (38 of 152) were the most common neurologic abnormalities.

Kinkel et al.[57] studied 23 of 28 patients (54–86 years of age) identified by CT (from

1633 consecutive adult studies) as having white matter disease of unexplained etiology. These investigators noted the presence of hypertension in 18 subjects. Three of eight neurologically normal subjects were not hypertensive. Of the fifteen individuals with neurologic abnormalities, fourteen had motor deficits and seven had strokes with acute motor deficits. Thirteen patients presented with slowly progressive dementia not characterized by language impairment; 5 of these 13 patients had gait disturbances and urinary incontinence. Of the 13 patients with dementia, seven had ventricular enlargement and four of these had reversal of normal CSF flow patterns. Of the four patients with abnormal CSF flow patterns, two were incontinent. One patient with severe dementia, normal ventricular size, and a severe degree of white matter disease was autopsied three months following CT and MRI. "Numerous cystic infarcts" measuring 1 to 6 mm in diameter and small areas of early infarction were seen throughout the centrum semiovale, thalamus, and basal ganglia. Demyelination was noted in the centrum semiovale. Only minimal atherosclerotic changes were seen in the circle of Willis, but an obliterative arteriosclerosis was noted in the white matter, basal ganglia, and thalamus.

In a CT study of white matter disease, George et al.[64] reported decreased white matter attenuation in 6.7 percent of normal subjects aged 55 to 69 and 24.4 percent (11 of 45) of normal subjects from 70 to 85 years. Interestingly, white matter lesions were more common in Alzheimer's subjects, being seen in 18.4 percent (9 of 49) of patients aged 55 to 69 years and 35.3 percent (36 of 102) of subjects aged 70 to 85 years. Overall, 16 percent of normal subjects over 55 and 30 percent of Alzheimer's patients over 55 had CT evidence of white matter disease. Autopsy examinations were performed in five subjects with Alzheimer's disease; changes of demyelination, hyaline thickening of white matter arteries, and "cystic lucencies" were described. In four of the five patients there was a lack of correspondence between the changes due to Alzheimer-related pathologic changes and the severity of clinical dementia, suggesting that the white matter disease may have contributed to the severity of the dementia. Correlation with clinical data showed that in normal subjects, white matter disease was significantly correlated with hypertension. Hypertension was found in 57 percent of normal patients with white matter disease and in 25 percent of normal patients without white matter disease. In the Alzheimer's subjects there was no significant correlation with hypertension; 22 percent of subjects without, and 24 percent of subjects with, white matter disease were hypertensive. Gait abnormalities were correlated with white matter disease in Alzheimer's subjects. George et al.[65] reported a limited number of MRI examinations in normal subjects and those with Alzheimer's disease (nine normal and eight Alzheimer's subjects). All nine of the normal group over the age of 60 had some degree of white matter change. Ignoring minimal changes, 25 percent (2 of 8) of normal subjects and 75 percent (6 of 8) of Alzheimer's subjects had mild or moderate white matter changes.

Lotz et al.[66] has reported autopsy correlation in a group of 20 patients aged 56 to 93 years with CT evidence of reduced x-ray attenuation in the deep white matter. These 20 were from a group of 82 autopsied patients with ante-mortem CT studies. Eighteen of the 20 had evidence of subcortical arteriosclerotic encephalopathy and demonstrated demyelination, loss of axons, and thickening of the walls of small arteries in the white matter walls. The findings on CT were totally periventricular in 15 cases, limited to areas separated from the ependyma by uninvolved white matter in two cases, and a combination of findings in one case. The periventricular disease tended to be located at the angles of the frontal horns and to spare the region medial to the trigone and occipital horns. Seventeen of the 18 patients were hypertensive, and 16 had evidence of focal infarction at autopsy. Seven subjects were demented. There was an apparent correlation of cerebral arteriosclerosis and nephrosclerosis. Interestingly, autopsy study of ten subjects aged 54 to 89 years with normal CT studies showed microscopic evidence of pathologic changes in the white matter in seven instances. These changes were less severe than in CT positive cases.

MRI studies have shown a high incidence of deep white matter disease in elderly and demented subjects. In addition to the study reported by George et al.,[65] Bradley et al.[55] found a 30 percent incidence in 20 consecutive subjects over the age of 60. Brant-Zawadzki et al.[58] reported MR findings in patients aged 65 to 79 with a "non-Alzheimer's" dementia and two control groups. The first control group included five active professionals age 59 to 66 years in excellent health, while the second group included nine retired professionals aged 74 to 81 in good health. Of the dementia patients, four had diffuse white matter changes and the fifth had subependymal disease. Two of the five were hypertensive, and a third had cardiovascular disease. None of the younger control group had significant white matter disease, whereas four of the nine in the older control group had evidence of white matter disease. Of note is the absence of any history of hypertension or vascular disease in three of four subjects with white matter disease in the older control group and in two of five demented subjects.

In addition to the clinical and imaging studies discussed above, Brun and Englund[67] recently published a post-mortem study of white matter disease in subjects with an Alzheimer's type dementia. Of 20 patients with Alzheimer's disease and 28 with senile dementia of the Alzheimer's type, 60 percent had evidence of white matter disease with loss of axons, myelin sheaths, oligodendroglial cells, and fibrohyaline thickening of the walls of small arterioles and capillaries. No infarctions or cavitations were noted. These findings were periventricular in location and were more severe frontally. Hypertensive changes with spiraling of vessels, microaneurysms, and lacunes were not seen in this group. There was no evidence of nephrosclerosis in the patients studied. One demented patient, without hypertension or Alzheimer's disease, had severe white matter changes identical to those seen in Alzheimer's subjects. Presumably his dementia was due to these changes. The changes in the white matter are believed by Brun to be ischemic in nature, perhaps arising from hypotension and hypoperfusion.

The pathologic, clinical CT, and early NMR imaging studies of subcortical arteriosclerotic encephalopathy have been remarkably consistent over the past decade in studies done on three continents. The clinical and radiographic manifestations of this disease appear in the sixth decade, and the incidence increases with age, rising from 3 to 5 percent in the sixth decade to about 40 percent in the eighth decade. It is associated clinically with dementia, motor abnormalities, urinary incontinence, hypertension, vascular disease, stroke, and psychological disturbances. While hypertension and vascular disease frequently are seen, this is not invariably the case. Differential diagnosis must include other causes of increased signal in the white matter, as discussed earlier: multi-infarct dementia, the lacunar state, and normal pressure hydrocephalus. The pathophysiology of this disorder generally is believed to be related to ischemia caused by arteriosclerosis. The susceptibility of white matter to reduced flow or anoxia is supported by both animal and clinical studies of white matter changes in anoxia and carbon monoxide poisoning. A similar disorder or a portion of the spectrum of this disorder appears to occur more frequently in subjects with Alzheimer's disease than in non-Alzheimer's subjects.

In conclusion, NMR imaging has proved to be a sensitive indicator of stroke and has heightened our awareness of ischemic white matter disease. It is hoped that future developments in phosphorus,[69–71] sodium,[72,73] and lactate imaging[74] will enable a more precise delineation of the metabolic status of ischemic tissue and may allow therapeutic interventions to minimize extension of infarction into the surrounding ischemic border zone. In subcortical arteriosclerotic encephalopathy, additional research remains to elucidate the etiology and progression of this disorder.

References

1. Cardiovascular Fact Sheet, American Heart Association, 1985.
2. Siesjo BK: Brain Energy Metabolism. New York, John Wiley & Sons, 1978.
3. Lowry OH, Passonneau JV, Hasselberger FX, Schulz DW: Effect of ischemia on known substrates and cofactors of the glycolytic pathway in brain. J Biol Chem *239*:18, 1964.
4. Goldberg ND, Passonneau JV, Lowry OH: Effects of changes in brain metabolism on the levels of citric acid cycle intermediates. J Biol Chem *241*:3997, 1966.
5. Welsh FA: Regional evaluation of ischemic metabolic alterations. J Cereb Blood Flow Metab *6*:1, 1986.
6. Hossman KA: Post-ischemic resuscitation of the brain: selective vulnerability versus global resistance. Prog Brain Res *63*:3, 1985.
7. Gilston A: Complete cerebral recovery after prolonged circulatory arrest. A report of two cases. Intensive Care Med *5*:193, 1979.
8. Hossman KA: Experimental aspects of stroke. *In* Russell RWR (ed): Vascular Disease of the Central Nervous System. New York, Churchill Livingstone, 1983, pp. 73–100.
9. Brierly JB, Graham DI: Hypoxia and vascular disorders of the central nervous system. Adams JH, Corsellis J, Duncan LW (eds): Greenfield's Neuropathology, 4th ed. New York, John Wiley & Sons, 1984.
10. Welsh FA, O'Connor MJ, Marcy VR: Effect of oligemia on regional metabolite levels in cat brain. J Neurochem 31:311, 1978.
11. Wilock T: Neurochemical correlates to selective neuronal vulnerability. *Prog Brain Res 63*:69, 1985.
12. Hatashita S, Hoff JT: Cortical tissue pressure gradients in early ischemic brain edema. J Cereb Blood Flow Metab *6*:1, 1986.
13. Rossen R, Kabat H, Anderson JP: Acute arrest of cerebral circulation in man. Arch Neurol Psychiatr *50*:510, 1943.
14. Hossman KA, Ophoff BG: Recovery of monkey brain after prolonged ischemia. I. Electrophysiology and brain electrolytes. J Cereb Blood Flow Metab *6*:15, 1986.
15. Bodsch W, Barbier A, Oehmichen M, Ophoff BG, Hossman KA: Recovery of monkey brain after prolonged ischemia. II. Protein synthesis and morphological alterations. J Cereb Blood Flow Metab *6*:23, 1986.
16. Powers WJ, Grubb RL Jr, Darriet D, Raichle ME: Cerebral blood flow and cerebral metabolic rate of oxygen requirements for cerebral function and viability in humans. J Cereb Blood Flow Metab *5*:600, 1985.
17. Finnerty FA, Wilkins L, Fazekas JF: Cerebral hemodynamics during cerebral ischemia induced by acute hypotension. J Clin Invest *33*:1227, 1954.
18. Michenfelder JD, Sundt TM Jr: Cerebral ATP and lactate levels in the squirrel monkey following occlusion of the middle cerebral artery. Stroke *2*:319, 1971.
19. Paschen W, Matsuoka Y, Niebuhr I, Hossman KA: Regional biochemistry of the energy producing metabolism of the cat brain following middle cerebral artery occlusion. *In* Cervos-Navarro J, Fritschka E (eds): Cerebral Microcirculation and Metabolism. New York, Raven Press, 1981, pp 337–342.
20. Diedrich WD, Ginsberg MD, Bush R, Waten BD: Photochemically induced cortical ischemia in the rat. 2. Acute and subacute alteration in local glucose utilization. J Cereb Blood Flow Metab *6*:195, 1986.
21. Kuhl DE, Phelps ME, Kowell AP, et al: Effects of stroke on local cerebral metabolism and perfusion: mapping by emission computed tomography of 18FDG and 13 WHz. Ann Neurol *8*:47, 1982.
22. Faschen W, Hossman KA, van Kerkhoff W: Regional assessment of energy-producing metabolism following prolonged ischemia of cat brain. J Cereb Blood Flow Metab *3*:321, 1983.
23. Mueller SM, Heistad DD, Marcus ML: Total and regional cerebral blood flow during hypotension, hypertension and hypocapnia. Circ Res *41*:350, 1977.
24. Wieloch T, Lindvall O, Blomquist P, Gage F: Evidence for amelioration of ischemic neuronal damage in the hippocampal formation by lesions of the perforant path. Neurol Res *7*:24, 1985.
25. Simon RP, Swan JIH, Grifith T, Meldrun BS: Blockade of *N*-methyl-D-aspartate receptors may protect against ischemic damage in the brain. Science *226*:850, 1984.
26. Hossman KA, Schurier FJ: Experimental brain infarcts in cats. I. Pathophysiological observations. Stroke *11*:583, 1980.
27. Olsson Y, Crowell RM, Klatzo I: The blood-brain barrier to protein tracers in focal ischemia and infarction caused by occlusion of the middle cerebral artery. Acta Neuropathol *18*:82, 1971.
28. Little JR: Microvascular alterations and edema in focal cerebral ischemia. *In* Pappius HM, Feindel W (eds): Dynamics of Brain Edema. New York, Springer-Verlag, 1976, pp 243–256.
29. O'Brien MD: Ischemic cerebral edema. *In* Russell RWR (ed): Vascular Disease of the Central Nervous System. New York, Churchill Livingstone, 1983, pp 128–138.
30. O'Brien MD, Waltz AG, Jordon MM: Ischemic cerebral edema. Distribution of water in brains of cats after occlusion of the middle cerebral artery. Arch Neurol *30*:456, 1974.

31. O'Brien MD, Waltz AG: Intracranial pressure gradients caused by experimental cerebral ischemia and edema. Stroke *4*:694, 1973.
32. Spetzler RF, Zabrawski J, Kaufman B, Young HN: Acute NMR changes during MCA occlusion: a preliminary study of primates. Stroke *14*:185, 1983.
33. Brant-Zawadzki M, Pereria B, Weinstein P, et al: MR imaging of acute experimental ischemia in cats. AJNR *7*:7, 1986.
34. Buonanno FS, Pykett IL, Brady TJ, et al: Proton NMR imaging in experimental ischemic infarction. Stroke *14*:178, 1983.
35. Bryan RN, Willcott MR, Schneiders NJ, Rose JE: NMR evaluation of stroke in the rat. AJNR *4*:242, 1983.
36. McNamara MT, Brant-Zawadzki M, Berry I, et al: Acute experimental cerebral ischemia: MR enhancement using Gd DTPA. Radiology *158*:701, 1986.
37. Levy RM, Stryker M, Hosobuchi Y: Studies of nuclear magnetic resonance imaging and regional glucose metabolism in acute cerebral ischemia: possible mechanism of opiate antagonist therapeutic activity. Life Sci *33*(Suppl I):763, 1983.
38. Kato H, Kogure K, Ohtomo H, et al: Characterization of experimental ischemic brain edema using proton nuclear magnetic resonance imaging. J Cereb Blood Flow Metab *6*:212, 1986.
39. Sipponen JT: Visualization of brain infarction with nuclear magnetic resonance imaging. Neuroradiology *26*:387, 1984.
40. Sipponen JT, Kaste M, Ketoneu L, et al: Serial nuclear magnetic resonance (NMR) imaging in patients with cerebral infarction. J Comput Assist Tomogr *7*:585, 1983.
41. Bryan RN, Willcott MR, Schneiders NJ, et al: Nuclear magnetic resonance evaluation of stroke. Radiology *149*:198, 1983.
42. DeWitt LD, Buonanno FS, Kistler JP, et al: Nuclear magnetic resonance imaging in evaluation of clinical stroke syndromes. Ann Neurol *16*:535, 1984.
43. Hecht-Leavitt C, Gomori JM, Grossman RI, et al: High-field MRI of hemorrhagic cortical infarction. AJNR *7*:581, 1986.
44. Gomori JM, Grossman RI, Goldberg HI, et al: High field magnetic resonance imaging of intracranial hematomas. Radiology *157*:87, 1985.
45. Kistler JP, Buonanno FS, Dewitt LD, et al: Vertebral-basilar posterior cerebral territory stroke—delineation by proton nuclear magnetic resonance imaging. Stroke *15*:417, 1984.
46. Biller J, Adams HP, Dunn V, et al: Dichotomy between clinical findings and MR abnormalities in pontine infarction. J Comput Assist Tomogr *10*:379, 1986.
47. Fox AJ, Bogousslavsky J, Carey LS, et al: Magnetic resonance imaging of small medullary infarctions. AJNR *7*:229, 1986.
48. McMurdo SK, Brant-Zawadzki M, Bradley WG, et al: Dural sinus thrombosis: study using intermediate field strength MR imaging. Radiology *161*:83, 1986.
49. Macchi PJ, Grossman RI, Gomori JM, et al: High field MR imaging of cerebral venous thrombosis. J Cereb Blood Flow Metab *10*:10, 1986.
50. Erdman WA, Weinreb JC, Cohen JM, et al: Venous thrombosis: clinical and experimental MR imaging. Radiology *161*:233, 1986.
51. Aisen AM, Gabrielson TO, McCune WJ: MR imaging of systemic lupus erythematosus involving the brain. AJNR *6*:197, 1985.
52. Vermess M, Bernstein RM, Bydder GM, et al: Nuclear magnetic resonance (NMR) imaging of the brain in systemic lupus erythematosus. J Comput Assist Tomogr *7*:461, 1983.
53. Holland BA, Perrett LV, Mills CM: Meningovascular syphilis: CT and MR findings. Radiology *158*:439, 1986.
54. Virapongse C, Mancuso A, Quisling R: Human brain infarcts: Gd-DTPA–enhanced Mr imaging. Radiology *161*:785, 1986.
55. Bradley WG, Waluch V, Brant-Zawadzki M, et al: Patchy periventricular white matter lesions in the elderly: common observation during NMR imaging. Noninvas Med Imag *1*:35, 1984.
56. Zimmerman RD, Fleming CA, Lee BEP, et al: Periventricular hyperintensity as seen by magnetic resonance: prevalence and significance. AJNR *7*:13, 1986.
57. Kinkel WR, Jacobs L, Ploachini H, et al: Subcortical arteriosclerotic encephalopathy (Binswanger's disease), computed tomographic nuclear magnetic resonance, and clinical correlations. Arch Neurol *42*:951, 1985.
58. Brant-Zawadzki M, Fein G, Van Dyke C, et al: MR imaging of the aging brain: patchy white matter lesions and dementia. AJNR *6*:675, 1985.
59. Caplan LR, Schoene WC: Clinical features of subcortical arteriosclerotic encephalopathy (Binswanger's disease). Neurology *28*:1206, 1978.
60. Loizou LA, Jefferson JM, Smith WT: Subcortical arteriosclerotic encephalopathy (Binswanger's disease) and cortical infarcts in a young normotensive patient. J Neurol Neurosurg Psychiatr *45*:409, 1982.
61. Goto K, Ishii N, Fukasawa H: Diffuse white-matter disease in the geriatric population. Radiology *141*:687, 1981.
62. Feigin I, Popoff N: Neuropathological changes late in cerebral edema: the trauma, hypertensive disease and Binswanger's encephalopathy. J Neuropathol Exp Neurol *22*:500, 1963.
63. Loizou LA, Kendall BE, Marshall J: Subcortical arteriosclerotic encephalopathy: a clinical and radiological investigation. J Neurol Neurosurg Psychiatr *44*:294, 1981.

64. George AE, deLeon MJ, Gentes CL, et al: Leukoencephalopathy in normal and pathologic aging: 1. CT of brain lucencies. AJNR 7:561, 1986.
65. George AE, deLeon MJ, Kalnin, A et al: Leukoencephalopathy in normal and pathologic aging: 2. MRI of brain lucencies. AJNR 7:567, 1986.
66. Lotz PR, Ballinger WE, Quisling RG: Subcortical arteriosclerotic encephalopathy: CT spectrum and pathologic correlation. AJNR 7:817, 1986.
67. Brun A, Englund E: A white matter disorder in dementia of the Alzheimer type: a pathoanatomical study. Ann Neurol 19:253, 1986.
68. Zeumer H, Schonsky B, Sturm KW: Predominant white matter involvement in subcortical arteriosclerotic encephalopathy (Binswanger's disease). J Comput Assist Tomogr 4:14, 1980.
69. Bottomley PA, Drayer BP, Smith LS: Chronic adult cerebral infarction studied by phosphorus NMR spectroscopy. Radiology 160:763, 1986.
70. Youkin DP, Delivoria-Papadopoulos M, Leonard JC, et al: Unique aspects of human newborn cerebral metabolism evaluated with phosphorus nuclear magnetic resonance spectroscopy. Ann Neurol 16:581, 1984.
71. Hope PL, Costello AM de L, Cady EB, et al: Cerebral energy metabolism studied with phosphorus NMR spectroscopy in normal and birth-asphyxiated infants. Lancet 2:366, 1984.
72. Hilal SK, Maudsley AA, Ra JB, et al: In vivo NMR imaging of sodium-23 in the human head. J Comput Assist Tomgr 9:1, 1985.
73. Turski PA, Perman WH, Hald JK, et al: Clinical and experimental vasogenic edema: in vivo sodium MR imaging. Radiology 160:821, 1986.
74. Roseu BR, Weeden VJ, Brady TJ: Selective saturation NMR imaging. J Comput Assist Tomogr 8:813, 1984.

15

Intracranial Hemorrhage

WILLIAM G. BRADLEY, JR.

The earliest reports of intracranial hemorrhage[1,2] suggested a relatively intense magnetic resonance (MR) appearance of the hemorrhage relative to surrounding brain. This was attributed to the short *T1* of presumably paramagnetic, iron-containing hemoglobin. Figure 15–1 demonstrates this appearance in a patient imaged one week after rupture of an anterior communicating artery aneurysm with resultant intraparenchymal hematoma and subarachnoid hemorrhage. The short *T1* character of the lesion is enhanced relative to surrounding brain on a *T1* weighted spin-echo image.

As experience was gained, subsequent reports[3,4] indicated that *acute* intracranial hemorrhage could be much more difficult to detect on MR images. This was attributed by Sipponen et al.[3] to a lack of *T1* shortening during the acute phase; however, no explanation of this phenomenon was attempted. Acute subarachnoid hemorrhage in particular was said to be difficult to detect, particularly in comparison with CT.[4] Although DeLaPaz et al.[4] agree with Sipponen et al.[3] that acute intracranial hemorrhage is difficult to detect on MR images, they disagree as to the mechanism of the later MR intense appearance. While the data of Sipponen et al.,[3] Bailes et al.,[1] Bydder et al.,[2] and Bradley and Schmidt[5] suggest a *T1* shortening process, the data of DeLaPaz et al.[4] suggest no change in *T1* but rather a prolongation of *T2*, both of which would increase the intensity on spin-echo images. Recently Gomori et al.[6] and Brooks et al.[7] described the short *T2* appearance of an acute intracranial hematoma at 1.5 and 0.5 tesla, respectively. They note that the subsequent intensity increase in the hematoma reflects *both* a shortening of *T1* and a prolongation of *T2*. Recently Sipponen et al.[8] reported a short *T1* appearance of an acute ("8 hours") intraparenchymal hematoma, which was evident only at 0.02 tesla, the effect decreasing at 0.17 tesla (and presumably higher fields). Despite the apparent disagreement, it should be noted that the authors often are describing different types of intracranial hemorrhage, often at quite different field strengths.

While it now seems that there is agreement on the *appearance* of intracranial hemorrhage, the biochemical mechanisms for this appearance continue to be a matter of some debate. Not only does the MR appearance of intracranial hemorrhage change over time, but also it depends on the field strength of the particular MR imaging system being used. A working understanding of this complex topic requires a basic knowledge of MR relaxation mechanisms. The purpose of this chapter is to review these mechanisms in an attempt to explain the changing MR appearance of the various forms of intracranial hemorrhage.

MECHANISMS OF PROTON RELAXATION ENHANCEMENT

The mechanisms of proton relaxation enhancement (PRE) have been described in detail previously.[6-10] In biologic substances, the dipole-dipole interaction between nu-

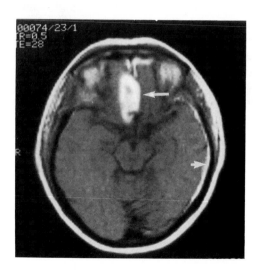

Figure 15–1. Subacute subarachnoid hemorrhage. Intraparenchymal hematoma (arrow) and subarachnoid hemorrhage (arrowhead) noted one week following rupture of anterior communicating artery aneurysm. The contrast between the lesions and the surrounding brain is enhanced on this *T1* weighted spin-echo image (*TR* = 0.5 sec, *TE* = 28 ms). (From Bradley WG, Schmidt, PC: Radiology *156*:99, 1985. Used by permission.)

clear magnetic moments is the principal mechanism for *T1* and *T2* relaxation. The magnitude of these nuclear magnetic moments is small and depends upon having an odd number of neutrons or protons (or both) in the nucleus.[11] This is referred to as nuclear paramagnetism. The hydrogen nucleus has a magnetic moment because it consists of a single, unpaired proton. This property is the basis of all clinical proton magnetic resonance imaging. The interaction between hydrogen nuclei is quite dependent upon their proximity and falls off as the sixth power of the distance between them. The electron has a magnetic moment 700 times greater than that of the proton, primarily on the basis of its smaller size. Only the unpaired electrons result in a magnetic moment. This is referred to as electronic paramagnetism, although the modifier "electronic" is usually dropped in our MR imaging literature. The greater the number of unpaired electrons, the greater the magnetic moment of the particular atom. Unpaired electrons in the outer shell of an atom are constantly flipping "up" and "down" (in a quantum mechanical sense) relative to the main magnetic field. This results in temporal change in the electronic magnetic moment, which is called the electron spin relaxation time. This can be considered the *T1* of an electron. How rapidly the unpaired electrons flip back and forth is a major determinant of the magnetic influence of the paramagnetic substance on the water protons in the environment.[5] Since the interaction between the dipole of the electron and that of a local hydrogen nucleus still falls off as the sixth power of the distance between them, hydrogen nuclei must be able to approach the paramagnetic center within a distance of several angstroms,[6] or there will be no enhancement of relaxation. The paramagnetic center produces local magnetic "turbulence," enhancing the return to equilibrium magnetization (i.e., shortening of the *T1* and *T2*) of all accessible water protons.

When discussing the properties of paramagnetic substances, it is useful to consider the reciprocal of the *T1* or *T2* relaxation times, called the R1 and R2 *relaxation rates*, respectively.[10] Adding a paramagnetic substance to an aqueous solution affects the R1 and R2 relaxation rates to the same degree, i.e.,

$$R_{net} = R_{substance} + R_{paramagnetic\ agent}$$

where R = R1 or R2. The effect on the *T1* or *T2* relaxation times differs markedly, however. For example, if a substance has a *T1* of 600 ms and a *T2* of 50 ms, then, R1 = 1/*T1* = 1.66 sec^{-1} and R2 = 1/*T2* = 20 sec^{-1}. If the paramagnetic agent increases both relaxation rates by 1 sec^{-1}, then, R1$_{net}$ = 2.66 sec^{-1} and R2$_{net}$ = 21 sec^{-1}. The resultant $T1 = 1/2.66 = 376$ ms, and the resultant $T2 = 1/21$ sec$^{-1} = 48$ ms. Thus $T1$ has decreased by 37.4 percent, while $T2$ has decreased by only 4 percent, despite the "equal" effect on the *relaxation rates*.

This relation applies to proton-electron–dipole-dipole interactions when the water protons in an aqueous solution have access to the paramagnetic center. Since the $T1$ of most biologic tissues is significantly longer than the $T2$, the effect of adding a paramagnetic agent is initially one of $T1$ shortening and, as the concentration increases, $T2$ shortening.[12] The effect of $T1$ shortening, of course, is to increase the intensity, particularly on $T1$ weighted spin-echo images. At higher concentrations, however, the effect of $T2$ shortening is to decrease the intensity, as a result of increased dephasing and loss of coherence.[12]

When considering paramagnetic substances in aqueous solutions, $T1$ shortening always occurs prior to $T2$ shortening. There are other mechanisms of relaxation, however, in which $T2$ can be selectively shortened without affecting $T1$.[6] The $T2$ relaxation time of the substance reflects the randomly fluctuating internal magnetic fields, which lead to irreversible loss of phase coherence.[11] The fixed nonuniformities in the main static magnetic field cause even greater loss of coherence in the free induction decay (FID) at a rate $T2^*$.[11] The loss of coherence due to these fixed nonuniformities, however, can be reconstituted by the 180 degree rf pulse of a spin-echo sequence. Several additional examples of dephasing (and subsequent spin-echo signal loss) have appeared in the MR imaging literature. Autodiffusion through a magnetic field gradient causes dephasing, decreasing the intensity of the spin echo.[13] Thus $T2$ values of fluids (with high autodiffusion coefficients) calculated from MR images (obtained with slice-selecting, phase-encoding, and read-out gradients) will be lower than $T2$ values calculated from spectrometers that do not use gradients.[13] When blood in a vessel flows slowly through a gradient, signal is lost as a result of dephasing.[14] If flow through the gradient continues slowly (i.e., is laminar) for a multiecho sequence, then the even echoes will demonstrate rephasing, and thus increased intensity.[14] The dephasing in these cases is proportional to the square of the local magnetic field gradient.[15]

An additional cause of dephasing is caused by slowly tumbling molecules or cells with high magnetic susceptibility.[6] Iron-containing, paramagnetic substances, such as hemosiderin, become strongly magnetized when placed in a magnetic field, the magnetic susceptibility reflecting the relationship between the *applied* and *induced* magnetic fields. If free in solution, such substances will cause both $T1$ and $T2$ shortening if there is free access to the paramagnetic center. If water protons are unable to approach the paramagnetic center within a distance of several angstroms, there will be no enhanced proton relaxation. When paramagnetic deoxyhemoglobin is free in solution, for example, it does not enhance proton relaxation, i.e., there is neither $T1$ nor $T2$ shortening.[16] When such substances are contained within a slowly tumbling red blood cell, however, the strong induced magnetic field varies quite slowly, creating regions of local magnetic nonuniformity.[6] Diffusion of water molecules through these regions causes dephasing that is proportional to the square of the local magnetic field gradient.[15] Since the local magnetic nonuniformity was induced in the magnetically susceptible substance by the main magnetic field, the dephasing that results increases with the square of the applied static magnetic field. The dephasing, of course, results only in $T2$ shortening, $T1$ remaining unchanged. This $T2$ shortening effect is most noticeable at higher field strength (e.g., 1.5 tesla), although it has certainly been noted at intermediate field strengths as well.[7] The $T2$ shortening effect has also been reported for paramagnetic hemosiderin in macrophages[6,12] and for ferritin that is deposited in various structures in the brain, namely the globus pallidus, the red nucleus, the reticular substantia nigra, the putamen, and the dentate nucleus of the cerebellum.[17]

OXIDATION OF HEMOGLOBIN

In order to attempt an understanding of the variable MR appearance of intracranial hemorrhage, the structure of hemoglobin and its various breakdown products must be considered in some detail. In its circulating form, hemoglobin alternates between the oxy and deoxy forms as oxygen is exchanged during transit through the high-oxygen environment of the lungs and the low-oxygen environment of the capillary circulation. In order to bind oxygen reversibly, the iron in the hemoglobin (the "heme iron") must be maintained in the reduced ferrous (Fe^{++}) state.[18] To do this, the red cell maintains several metabolic pathways to prevent various oxidizing agents from converting its heme iron to the nonfunctional ferric (Fe^{+++}) state. When removed from the circulation, these metabolic pathways fail and the hemoglobin begins to undergo oxidative denaturation.

The heme iron is normally suspended in a nonpolar crevice in the center of the hemoglobin molecule. It is held in this position by a covalent bond with a histidine at the so-called F8 position of the globin chain and by four planar hydrophopic Van der Waals bonds with various nonpolar groups on the globin molecule. The sixth coordination site of the heme iron is occupied by molecular oxygen in the oxyhemoglobin and is vacant in deoxyhemoglobin (Fig. 15–2). As oxidative denaturation of hemoglobin proceeds, the ferrous heme iron is oxidized to the ferric state and methemoglobin is formed.[5] Although the five bonds to the globin molecule are unchanged, the sixth coordination site is now occupied by either a water molecule or a hydroxyl ion, depending on whether the methemoglobin is in the acid or base form, respectively. At physiologic pH, the acid form predominates. With continued oxidative denaturation, methemoglobin is converted to derivatives known as hemichromes.[18] While the iron is these compounds remains in the ferric state, alteration of the tertiary structure of the globin molecule occurs such that the sixth coordination site of the heme iron is

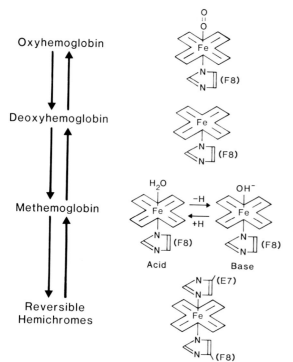

Figure 15–2. Oxidative denaturation of hemoglobin. In the circulating oxy- and deoxyhemoglobin forms the heme iron is in the reduced ferrous state, which can reversibly bind molecular oxygen. Following oxidation to the paramagnetic ferric form as methemoglobin, the heme iron can no longer bind oxygen and is thus nonfunctional. Continued oxidative denaturation produces hemichromes, which are ferric compounds with the sixth coordination site occupied by a ligand from the now-denatured globin chain. (From Bradley WG, Schmidt PC: Radiology *156*:99, 1985. Used by permission.)

occupied by a ligand from within the globin molecule (most likely the distal histidine at E7).

The magnetic properties of blood were first evaluated by Faraday 140 years ago.[19] He considered blood only in the dried, solid state; not until 90 years later did Pauling and Coryell[20] consider the magnetic properties of blood in the fluid state. By using a capillary tube filled with either oxy- or deoxyhemoglobin suspended between the poles of an electromagnet, they were able to determine that deoxyhemoglobin was paramagnetic, i.e., attracted to the stronger part of the magnetic field, whereas oxyhemoglobin was diamagnetic, i.e., repelled from the stronger part of the magnetic field. These observations led them to describe the various electron spin states of oxy- and deoxyhemoglobin. In deoxyhemoglobin, the heme iron is in the "high-spin" ferrous state characterized by six electrons in the outer shell, four of which are unpaired. When oxygen is added, one of the electrons is partially transferred to the oxygen molecule, resulting in a low-spin form with a single unpaired electron in the outer shell.[18]

Although the static susceptibility test performed by Pauling and Coryell demonstrates that deoxyhemoglobin is paramagnetic, this does not ensure a proton paramagnetic enhancement effect in aqueous solution. Such an effect, originally described by Bloembergen et al.,[9] requires not only that a paramagnetic center be present but also that it be accessible to surrounding water protons. As noted earlier, the quantitation of this effect requires consideration of the magnitude of the magnetic moment of the paramagnetic dipole (i.e., the number of unpaired electrons); the electron spin relaxation rate (in effect, the $T1$ of the electron); the concentration of paramagnetic dipoles; the average distance from surrounding water protons; and the relative motion of the proton and paramagnetic centers.[5,9,10] Such theories of proton relaxation by paramagnetic solute ions are based on translational diffusion and the distance of closest approach of the proton and paramagnetic ions, which determines an "outer sphere" of influence.[21] It has also been shown that there can be a contribution to the relaxation from exchange between solvent and water ligands in the first coordination sphere of the paramagnetic ion, i.e., "inner sphere effects."[21] Thus, while deoxyhemoglobin is considered "paramagnetic" from static susceptibility experiments,[20] the $T1$ relaxation times of aqueous solutions of oxy- and deoxyhemoglobin do not demonstrate a difference in the proton paramagnetic relaxation effects.[16] Methemoglobin, on the other hand, causes significant $T1$ shortening in aqueous solution owing to a combination of both "inner sphere" and "outer sphere" effects.[21] Thus $T1$ relaxation by methemoglobin is due to a combination of ligand exchange effects (from the water molecule at the sixth coordination site) and from outer sphere diffusional effects, perhaps by virtue of increased access of solvent protons to the heme iron through the nonpolar crevice.[21]

SUBARACHNOID HEMORRHAGE

Figure 15–3*A* illustrates the rather subtle increased intensity present in acute subarachnoid hemorrhage 17 hours post ictus. One week following the acute subarachnoid hemorrhage, the appearance is significantly more intense (Fig. 15–3*B*).

When considering subarachnoid hemorrhage, one must evaluate the interaction between water protons in the CSF and the iron-containing hemoglobin within the red cell. A trivial explanation for the observed $T1$ shortening that occurs over a matter of days following subarachnoid hemorrhage might be red cell lysis, which can certainly result from exposure to phospholipases in the CSF. Unfortunately, such a mechanism for enhanced proton relaxation can be readily excluded, since water molecules are already allowed access to the hemoglobin by virtue of rapid transit across the red cell

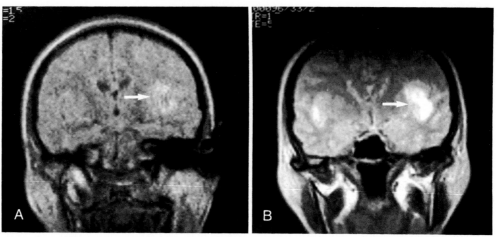

Figure 15–3. Subarachnoid hemorrhage. *A*, Seventeen hours post ictus. Coronal section demonstrates minimally increased intensity in the left sylvian cistern (arrow) on this *TR* = 1.5 sec, *TE* = 28 ms image. *B*, One week post ictus, intensity of the CSF in the left sylvian cistern has increased significantly. (From Bradley WG, Schmidt PC: Radiology *156*:99, 1985. Used by permission.)

membrane.[9,22] Thus, changing proton relaxation enhancement effects can be directly attributed to the changes in the interactions between CSF water protons and the heme iron that occur during the course of oxidative denaturation of hemoglobin.

Quantitation of subarachnoid hemorrhage is generally performed using light spectroscopy.[23] Such spectrophotometric analysis provides the ''xanthochromic'' index that is used to quantitate the degree of hemorrhage. The xanthochromic index is the sum of the absorption values at 415 nm (oxyhemoglobin) and 460 nm (bilirubin). All samples are prepared for spectrophotometric analysis by centrifugation with examination only of the supernatant. By such analysis, little methemoglobin has been found either acutely or within several weeks of subarachnoid hemorrhage.[23,24]

Bradley and Schmidt[5] modeled subarachnoid hemorrhage in vitro by addition of fresh venous human blood to artificial CSF, producing a 10 percent (by volume) solution. *T1* and *T2* relaxation times were evaluated using an IBM Minispec desktop spectrometer operating at 20 MHz. The effect of red cell concentration on *T1* and *T2* was evaluated by measuring the relaxation times at concentrations varying from 0 percent (i.e., pure CSF) to 10 percent by volume. The effect of red cell lysis was evaluated by mechanically lysing the red cells by repeated passage of fresh venous blood through a 25-gauge needle prior to mixing with CSF. The effect of concentration of blood in CSF is demonstrated in Figure 15–4, which shows a small (10 percent) decrease in *T1* and *T2* as the concentration is increased from 0 percent (pure CSF) to 10 percent. Such *T1* shortening is clearly not the primary mechanism for the increased intensity observed in subarachnoid hemorrhage clinically. Figure 15–4 also demonstrates that the effect of red cell lysis is negligible.

The magnetic relaxation times of oxy- and deoxyhemoglobin were compared by bubbling either oxygen or nitrogen through fresh solutions of bloody CSF. Methemoglobin was produced by treatment with $NaNO_2$. Prior to measurement, all samples were agitated to suspend the red cells. All measurements were performed at 38 degrees C. Figure 15–5 demonstrates that the *T1* measurements of oxy- and deoxyhemoglobin are quite similar, confirming what had been reported previously.[16] Methemoglobin in a 10 percent solution of lysed red cells in CSF is seen to have a significantly lower *T1* than oxy- or deoxyhemoglobin. No significant *T2* difference was found among oxy-, deoxy-, and methemoglobin at 20 MHz (0.47 tesla). Figure 15–5 also shows the sequential decrease in *T1* for the 10 percent ''unknown'' solution of lysed red cells in

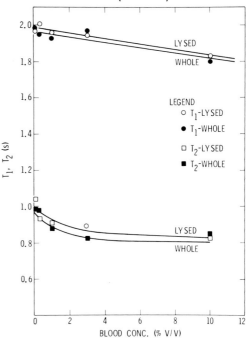

BLOOD IN CSF CONCENTRATION DEPENDENCE OF RELAXATION TIMES (20 MHz)

Figure 15–4. Change in magnetic relaxation times as a function of red cell concentration in CSF and red cell lysis. A 10 percent decrease in the $T1$ (above) and $T2$ (below) times is noted as a function of increasing concentration of red cells in the CSF from pure CSF to 10 percent. There is no significant effect of red cell lysis on $T1$ or $T2$. (From Bradley WG, Schmidt PC: Radiology 156:99, 1985. Used by permission.)

CSF over 84 hours of measurement. Figure 15–6 demonstrates $T1$ shortening of a 20 percent solution of whole red cells in CSF stored hypoxically for 160 hours. The $T1$ value continues to shorten for 90 hours before reaching a plateau.

The solutions of oxy- and deoxyhemoglobin and methemoglobin were then analyzed using a Perkin-Elmer UV-visible spectrophotometer. To assess the change in magnetic relaxation times for bloody CSF stored hypoxically, a 10 percent solution was measured over several days. $T1$ shortening was demonstrated. In a second experiment, a 20 percent solution of whole red cells in CSF was again stored hypoxically

RELAXATION TIMES FOR BLOOD IN CSF (20 MHz)

Figure 15–5. Relaxation times for blood in CSF at 20 MHz. The $T1$ times for oxy- and deoxyhemoglobin are similar: The $T1$ time for methemoglobin (produced by treatment with $NaNO_2$) is significantly less than that of oxy- and deoxyhemoglobin. The $T1$ time of the 10 percent solution of lysed blood and CSF is followed over a period of 84 hours during hypoxic storage and is seen to decrease. (From Bradley WG, Schmidt PC: Radiology 156:99, 1985. Used by permission.)

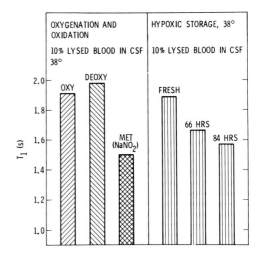

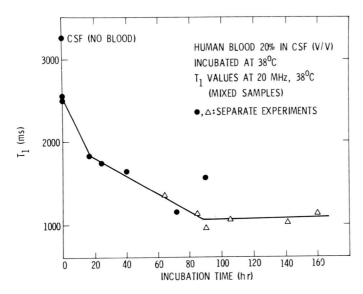

Figure 15–6. Change in *T1* relaxation time during subarachnoid hemorrhage. Changing *T1* relaxation time for solution of 20 percent whole blood in CSF is followed for 160 hours and is seen to decrease to a plateau value at approximately 90 hours. (From Bradley WG, Schmidt PC: Radiology *156*:99, 1985. Used by permission.)

for several days with sequential measurement of *T1* and *T2* relaxation times. Spectrophotometric analysis was performed on the "unknown" (bloody CSF) and compared with the known standards previously produced. Spectrophotometry of known solutions of oxy-, and deoxy-, and methemoglobin and of both unknown solutions of bloody CSF demonstrated strong absorption at 360 nm, called the Soret band (Fig. 15–7). Strong absorption is present for all forms of hemoglobin in this region; thus it is not specific. The portion of the spectrum that is more specific for methemoglobin is the 630 nm region (Fig. 15–8). Here temporal increase in a broad peak is observed in the "un-

UV - VIS ABSORPTION SPECTRA

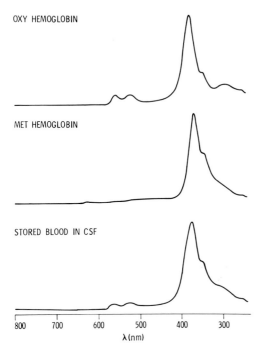

Figure 15–7. Spectrophotometry of oxy- and methemoglobin and hypoxically stored blood in CSF. Strong absorption is noted near 400 nm (Soret band), which is nonspecific. The specific absorption for methemoglobin is perceptible at 630 nm in both the methemoglobin and the unknown bloody CSF solution. (From Bradley WG, Schmidt PC: Radiology *156*:99, 1985. Used by permission.)

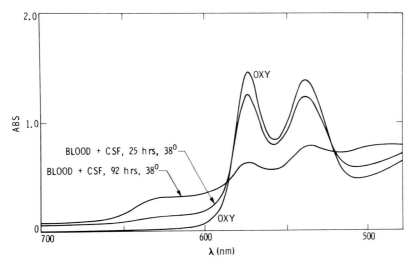

Figure 15–8. Spectrophotometry at 630 nm. Oxyhemoglobin is seen to have no absorption at 630 nm. During hypoxic storage of a solution of blood and CSF, *a broad-based peak develops at 630 nm. By comparison with known standards, the peak at 92 hours was shown to correspond to 90 percent methemoglobin. Differences in peak height reflect differences in extinction coefficients. (From Bradley WG, Schmidt PC: Radiology 156:99, 1985. Used by permission.)*

known'' 20 percent bloody CSF solution, which corresponds to increasing methemoglobin concentration. Although there is significant difference in the height of the 630 nm and 360 nm peaks, this reflects differences in the extinction coefficients rather than differences in concentration. Thus, by comparison with known standards, the peak observed at 92 hours at 631 nm is shown to correspond approximately to 90 percent methemoglobin.

Sequential spectrophotometric analysis of the solution thus demonstrated a corresponding increase in the concentration of methemoglobin during the period of *T1* shortening. Since oxy- and deoxyhemoglobin were known to have an insignificant proton relaxation enhancement effect in aqueous solutions,[9] it was presumed that methemoglobin was responsible for the *T1* shortening observed during the in vitro experiments as well as that observed clinically.[5] In vivo methemoglobin has now been demonstrated spectroscopically in a subacute subdural hematoma in this laboratory. Thus methemoglobin formation is felt to be the principal determinant of *T1* shortening during evolution of subarachnoid hemorrhage.

INTRAPARENCHYMAL HEMATOMA

The MR appearance of intraparenchymal hematomas (IPH) has been described by several authors[1–4,8] and more recently by Gomori et al.,[6] who have noted additional findings at higher fields. When describing IPH, it is useful to consider four separate factors: the age of the hematoma, separate zones within and surrounding the hematoma, the MR technique (i.e., *T1* or *T2* weighted), and the strength of the imaging field (Table 15–1). Three stages in the aging of the hematoma are described: acute (0 to 2 days), subacute (2 to 14 days), and chronic (greater than two weeks). Four zones are described: inner core, outer core, rim, and reactive brain. Acutely (0 to 2 days) the hematoma consists of deoxyhemoglobin within intact red cells (Fig. 15–9). This has been demonstrated by Gomori et al.[6] in material aspirated from a recent IPH. Over the subacute period from 2 to 14 days, the deoxyhemoglobin undergoes oxidative denaturation, form-

Table 15–1. MR APPEARANCE OF INTRAPARENCHYMAL HEMATOMAS

	T1 Weighted Images		
	Acute	*Subacute*	*Chronic*
Inner core	0	0	+
Outer core	0	+ +	+ +
Rim	NP	NP	NP
Reactive brain	−	−	0

	T2 Weighted Images (0.35/1.5 Tesla)		
	Acute	*Subacute*	*Chronic*
Inner core	−/− −	−/− −	+/+
Outer core	−/− −	+ +/+ +	+ +/+ +
Rim	NP/NP	NP/−	−/− −
Reactive brain	+ +/+ +	+ +/+ +	0/0

Scale + +: much more intense than brain
      +: more intense than brain
      0: isointense with brain
      −: less intense than brain
   − −: much less intense than brain
  NP: not present

ing methemoglobin, first at the periphery (outer core) and then in the center (inner core).[6] During this phase, red cell lysis occurs as well (Fig. 15–10). At the end of the first two weeks, modified macrophages (gitter cells) have begun to remove the iron from the hemoglobin within the hematoma.[25] This marks the beginning of the "chronic" phase. The heme iron is deposited at the periphery as a rim of hemosiderin within the

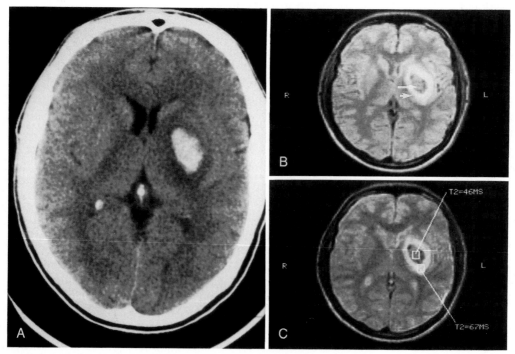

Figure 15–9. Acute intraparenchymal hematoma (two days post ictus). *A*, Noncontrast CT. *B*, MR image demonstrates lower intensity centrally (arrow) with surrounding rim of higher intensity vasogenic edema (arrowhead) (*TR* = 2.0 sec, *TE* = 28 ms). *C*, As *T2* weighting increases (*TR* = 2.0 sec, *TE* = 56 ms), the intensity of the central short-*T2* hematoma decreases relative to the surrounding brain and vasogenic edema. The *T2* relaxation times are indicated for the central hematoma and surrounding vasogenic edema.

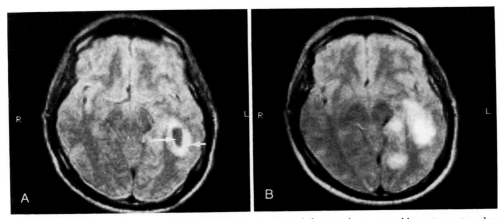

Figure 15–10. Resolving intraparenchymal hematoma. *A*, Acute left posterior temporal hematoma, two days post ictus. The central deoxyhemoglobin is decreased in intensity (arrow) with surrounding high-intensity rim of vasogenic edema (arrowhead) (*TR* = 2.0 sec, *TE* = 56 ms). *B*, Two months post ictus, the center of the hematoma has "filled in" as the red cells have lysed and the deoxyhemoglobin has undergone oxidative denaturation, forming methemoglobin, with shortening of the *T1* relaxation time.

macrophages surrounding the hematoma (Fig. 15–11).[6,25] The center of the hematoma[25] is left with a non–iron-containing, nonparamagnetic, heme pigment (e.g., hematoidin). During the acute phase the hematoma is surrounded by vasogenic edema, which gradually resorbs during the subacute phase and is essentially absent during the chronic phase.

On *T1* weighted images, the hematoma is acutely isointense with brain, whereas the reactive vasogenic edema is somewhat less intense than brain owing to its longer

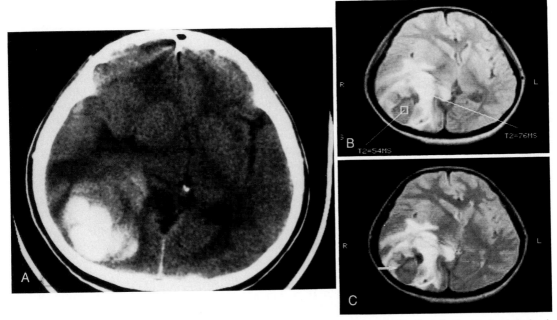

Figure 15–11. Recurrent intraparenchymal hemorrhage. *A*, Nonenchanced CT study. *B*, Complex hemorrhagic lesion in right temporal-occipital lobe, with regions of acute, subacute, and chronic hemorrhage and surrounding vasogenic edema (*TR* = 2.0 sec, *TE* = 28 ms). *C*, As *T2* weighting increases the acute hemorrhage becomes less intense owing to the short *T2* relaxation time, and a rim of low intensity is noted secondary to chronic hemosiderin deposition (arrow) (*TR* = 2.0 sec, *TE* = 56 ms).

T1 value. As the deoxyhemoglobin is oxidized to methemoglobin during the subacute phase, the *T1* is markedly shortened, resulting in increased intensity on *T1* weighted images (see Fig. 15–1).[5] During the chronic stage the deoxyhemoglobin in the inner core is oxidized to methemoglobin, and the vasogenic edema is resorbed.[6]

On *T2* weighted images, the changing appearance of a hematoma depends on the field strength of the MR imaging system.[6–8] Acutely, there is decreased intensity centrally, particularly at higher fields (Figs. 15–9 to 15–11). This reflects *T2* shortening due to the presence of the highly magnetically susceptible deoxyhemoglobin within intact red cells.[6] The dephasing (*T2* decay) that occurs as a result of the local magnetic nonuniformities increases as the square of the local field gradients. Since the induced magnetic moment in magnetically susceptible, paramagnetic substances depends on the strength of the applied magnetic field, *T2* shortening also increases as the square of the applied magnetic field. Thus, the low-intensity appearance in the center of an acute hematoma is much more obvious at 1.5 tesla than at 0.35 tesla.[6] Vasogenic edema surrounding the hematoma in the acute and subacute stages results in a high-intensity appearance on *T2* weighted images (Figs. 15–9 to 15–11).

In the early subacute phase, deoxyhemoglobin has been oxidized to methemoglobin, but the red cells are still intact. Since methemoglobin is magnetically susceptible, this produces *T2* shortening. In the late subacute stage, the red cells in the outer core have lysed and methemoglobin has formed. This results in shortening of *T1* and lengthening of *T2*, both of which will increase the intensity on *T2* weighted images (Fig. 15–10). While deoxyhemoglobin or methemoglobin is present in intact red cells in the inner core, a low-intensity appearance will persist.

In the chronic stage, hemosiderin is found within macrophages (gitter cells) in the rim surrounding the hematoma.[25] Like deoxyhemoglobin, the intracellular, magnetically susceptible, paramagnetic hemosiderin causes preferential *T2* shortening (Fig. 15–10).[6] Since this is also a magnetic susceptibility effect, the low-intensity rim is much more noticeable at higher fields. The persistent low-intensity center in chronic hemorrhage may reflect the removal of paramagnetic iron by the macrophages.[25]

SUBDURAL AND EPIDURAL HEMATOMAS

Subdural hematomas (SDH) have three distinct stages of evolution and three distinct appearances on MR. Acute subdural hematomas contain deoxyhemoglobin within intact red cells. As noted previously, this results in *T2* shortening. Thus, acute SDHs will have low intensity on *T2* weighted images, particularly at higher fields.[6] They will be isointense with brain on *T1* weighted images.

During the subacute stage (CT isointense), the red cells lyse and deoxyhemoglobin becomes oxidized to methemoglobin. These effects tend to shorten the *T1* and lengthen the *T2*, both of which will increase the intensity on either *T1* weighted or *T2* weighted images (Fig. 15–12).

The definition of a chronic SDH depends on whether the determination is being made clinically or by CT hypointensity (both of which suggest onset at three weeks), or by MR. Continued oxidative denaturation of methemoglobin forms hemichromes, which are low-spin, nonparamagnetic ferric compounds.[18] The *T1* of such compounds is increased relative to that of paramagnetic methemoglobin; thus the intensity of chronic subdural hematomas (Fig. 15–12) is decreased relative to that of subacute subdural hematomas, particularly on *T1* weighted images.[26] As the chronic SDH continues to age over many years, the fluid contents may be partially resorbed and the protein content of the fluid may decrease, approaching that of CSF.

Epidural hematomas age in a similar manner to SDHs. They are distinguished from

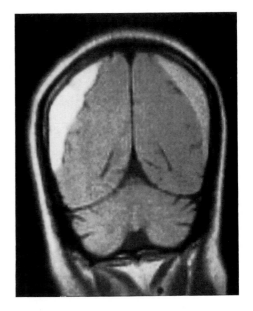

Figure 15–12. Bilateral subdural hematomas. Right-sided subacute subdural hematoma has increased intensity relative to the more chronic left-sided subdural hematoma. The subacute hematoma contains short-$T1$ methemoglobin, while the chronic subdural hematoma contains hemichromes that are nonparamagnetic and have longer $T1$ values (TR = 1.0, TE = 28 ms).

SDHs by the low-intensity appearance of the fibrous dura between the hematoma and the brain. Like an acute subdural hematoma, an acute epidural hematoma will have deoxyhemoglobin within intact red blood cells, resulting in $T2$ shortening and low intensity on $T2$ weighted images, particularly at high fields. On the basis of intensity characteristics alone, it may be difficult to separate the low-intensity dura from the low-intensity hematoma in this situation and to accurately distinguish a subdural from an epidural collection (Fig. 15–13). In the subacute phase of an epidural hematoma, methemoglobin is formed and the diagnosis is obvious on both $T1$ and $T2$ weighted sequences, regardless of field strength.

In conclusion, understanding the MR appearance of intracranial hemorrhage requires a basic knowledge of the pathophysiology and the paramagnetic MR phenomena that are occurring. Subacute hemorrhage in any compartment leads to methemoglobin formation, which has high intensity on any sequence and is therefore easily detectable. In the acute phase, however, the MR appearance of the hemorrhage changes rapidly and depends on the location (e.g., intraparenchymal, subarachnoid, subdural, or epidural), on the sequence parameter times (e.g., $T1$ or $T2$ weighted), and on the field strength. Although acute intraparenchymal hematomas can be recognized on the basis of a particularly low-intensity appearance on $T2$ weighted images at high field, these

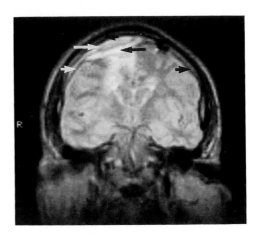

Figure 15–13. Epidural hematoma. Following surgery, three extra-axial structures are noted: epidural hematoma (white arrow), dura mater (white arrowhead), and subdural hematoma (black arrow). Note also calvarial marrow (black arrowheads), which potentially can be confused for extra-axial fluid collection (TR = 2.0 sec, TE = 56 ms).

observations do not apply to less well defined regions of hemorrhage, i.e., hemorrhagic infarcts or contusions, in which the blood is much more dispersed. For these reasons, we and others still recommend CT as the most sensitive imaging modality for the detection of intracranial hemorrhage within 48 hours of onset.

ACKNOWLEDGMENT

I thank Jay Mericle, Terry Andrews, Leslie Watson, and Ken Bishop for technical assistance, Kaye Finley and Louise Evans for manuscript preparation, and Keith Kortman, M.D., and Paul Schmidt, Ph.D., for review of the manuscript.

References

1. Bailes DR, Young IR, Thomas DJ, Straughan K, Bydder GM, Steinere RE: NMR imaging of the brain using spin-echo sequences. Clin Radiol *33*:395, 1982.
2. Bydder GM, Steiner RE, Young IR, et al: Clinical NMR imaging of the brain: 140 cases. AJR *139*:215, 1982.
3. Sipponen JT, Sepponen RE, Sivula A: Nuclear magnetic resonance (NMR) imaging of intracerebral hemorrhage in the acute and resolving phases. J Comput Assist Tomogr *7*(6):954, 1983.
4. DeLaPaz RL, New PFJ, Buonanno FS, Kistler JP, et al: NMR imaging of intracranial hemorrhage. J Comput Assist Tomogr *8*(4):599, 1983.
5. Bradley WG, Schmidt PC: Effect of methemoglobin formation on the MR appearance of subarachnoid hemorrhage. Radiology *156*:99, 1985.
6. Gomori JM, Grossman RI, Goldberg HI, Zimmerman RA, Bilaniuk LT: Intracranial hematomas: Imaging by high field MR. Radiology *157*:87, 1985.
7. Brooks RA, Di Chiro G, Girton M, Caporale D, et al: The changing appearance of blood: An in vivo and in vitro study. Presented at the Fourth Annual Meeting, SMRM, London, 1985.
8. Sipponen JT, Sepponen RE, Tanttu JI, Sivula A: Intracranial hematomas studied by MR imaging at 0.17 and 0.02 T. J Comput Assist Tomogr *9*(4):698, 1985.
9. Bloembergen N, Purcell E, Pound RV: Relaxation effects in nuclear magnetic resonance absorption. Phys Rev *73*:679, 1948.
10. Wolf GL, Burnett KR, Goldstein EJ, Joseph PM: Contrast agents for magnetic resonance imaging. *In* Kressel HY (ed): Magnetic Resonance Annual 1985. New York, Raven Press, 1985, pp 231–266.
11. Bradley WG, Crooks LE, Newton TH: Physical principles of NMR. *In* Newton TH, Potts DG (eds): Modern Neuroradiology: Advanced Imaging Techniques. Vol II. San Francisco, Clavadel Press, 1983.
12. Bradley WG: Fundamentals of MR image interpretation. *In* Bradley WG, Adey WR, Hasso AN (eds): Magnetic Resonance Imaging of the Brain, Head, and Neck: A Text Atlas. Rockville, MD, Aspen, 1985.
13. Wesbey GE, Moseley ME, Ehman RL: Translational molecular self-diffusion in magnetic resonance imaging: Effects and applications. *In* James TL, Margulis AR (eds): Biomedical Magnetic Resonance. San Francisco, University of California Press, 1984, pp 63–78.
14. Waluch V, Bradley WG: NMR even echo rephasing in slow laminar flow. J Comput Assist Tomogr *8*:594, 1984.
15. Packer KJ: The effects of diffusion through locally inhomogeneous magnetic fields on transverse nuclear spin relaxation in heterogeneous systems: Proton transverse relaxation in striated muscle tissue. J Magn Reson *9*:438, 1973.
16. Singer JR, Crooks LE: Some magnetic studies of normal and leukemic blood. J Clin Eng *3*:237, 1978.
17. Drayer BP, Burger P, Riederer S, et al: High-resolution magnetic resonance for mapping brain iron deposition. Presented at the 23rd Annual Meeting of the American Society of Neuroradiology, New Orleans, February 18–23, 1985.
18. Wintrobe MM, Lee GR, Boggs DR, Bithell TC, Foerster J, Athens JW, Lukens JN: Clinical Hematology. Philadelphia, Lea & Febiger, 1981, pp 88–102.
19. Pauling L, Coryell C: The magnetic properties and structure of hemoglobin, oxyhemoglobin and carbonmonoxyhemoglobin. Proc Natl Acad Sci *22*:210, 1936.
20. Pauling L, Coryell C: The magnetic properties and structure of the hemochromogens and related substances. Proc Natl Acad Sci *22*:159, 1936.
21. Koenig SH, Brown RD, Lindstrom TR: Interactions of solvent with the heme region of methemoglobin and fluoro-methemoglobin. Biophys J *34*:397, 1981.
22. Brooks RA, Battocletti JH, Sances A, Larson SJ, Bowman RL, Kudravcev V: Nuclear magnetic relaxation in blood. IEEE Trans Biomed Eng *1*:12, 1975.
23. Vermeulen M, van Gijn J, Blijenberg BG: Spectrophotometric analysis of CSF after subarachnoid hemorrhage: Limitations in the diagnosis of rebleeding. Neurology *33*:112, 1983.
24. Van der Meulen JP: Cerebrospinal fluid xanthochromia: An objective index. Neurology *16*:170, 1966.
25. Whisnant JP, Sayer GP, Millikan CH: Experimental intracerebral hematoma. Arch Neurol *9*:586, 1963.
26. Bradley WG: Magnetic resonance imaging of the central nervous system. Neurol Res *6*:91, 1984.

16

Pituitary and Parasellar Region

ANN C. PRICE
VAL M. RUNGE
JOSEPH H. ALLEN

Magnetic resonance imaging (MRI) of the pituitary and parasellar disorders has rapidly progressed from an adjunctive examination to one of primary diagnostic significance. This has occurred primarily as the result of the acquisition of thin-section imaging capability (see Chapter 97), which allows the visualization of smaller structures and more precise characterization of the intrinsic features of various lesions. This important development augments the inherent advantages of MRI, which include direct multiplanar imaging capability, absence of bone or dental artifact, absence of ionizing radiation, superior resolution of soft tissue planes, and multiple sequence potential.[1–5]

Multiplanar MR imaging allows sections in the axial, coronal, and sagittal planes without alteration of patient position and thereby a greater degree of patient comfort. Direct coronal CT examinations often can be difficult, particularly when imaging an obese individual with a short neck. When a true coronal position cannot be assumed, CT images are usually further degraded by dental artifact. Sagittal and coronal images reformatted from thinner (1.5 mm) axial sections suffer from lack of resolution and motion artifact due to longer scan times. Additional time is required by the technician both in performing the study and in obtaining the reformatted images.

The absence of ionizing radiation is an important consideration. Serial examinations of younger patients are often warranted or mandated in many types of pituitary pathology, such as in chromophobe adenomas or other tumors without secondary visual or chemical changes, in prolactinomas undergoing medical therapy, and in postoperative pituitaries to exclude recurrences.

Perhaps the most important feature of MRI in pituitary and parasellar evaluation is the superior resolution of soft tissue planes (Fig. 16–1). Precise anatomic delineation of pituitary lesions is of utmost importance because of the proximity of the optic chiasm and other parasellar structures, such as the cavernous sinus and sphenoid sinus.[6,7]

The full implication of multiple-sequence potential has yet to be realized and awaits further experience and investigation. To date, *T2* weighted sequences have been most useful in characterization of craniopharyngioma and necrosis associated with larger tumors.[8] Most other pituitary tumor pathology is adequately characterized and localized with *T1* sequences.

The material in this chapter represents an accumulation of experience with MR pituitary imaging over the past two and one-half years. The images were obtained with a 0.5 tesla system (Technicare).

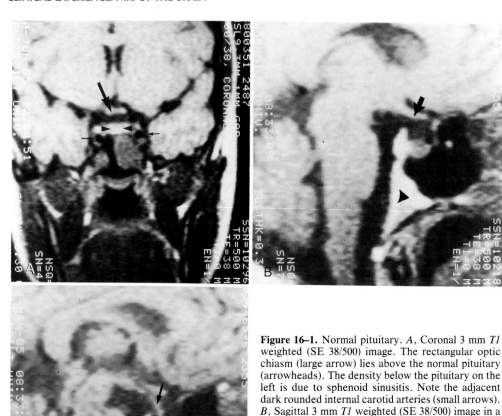

Figure 16–1. Normal pituitary. *A*, Coronal 3 mm *T1* weighted (SE 38/500) image. The rectangular optic chiasm (large arrow) lies above the normal pituitary (arrowheads). The density below the pituitary on the left is due to sphenoid sinusitis. Note the adjacent dark rounded internal carotid arteries (small arrows). *B*, Sagittal 3 mm *T1* weighted (SE 38/500) image in a different patient. Note the obliquely oriented optic chiasm (arrow). The pituitary is normal and rounded in appearance. The clivus has a high signal (arrowhead); the sphenoid sinus is clear and has a low signal. *C*, Three mm adjacent slice in the same patient (SE 38/500) shows nearby vertically oriented pituitary stalk (arrow). LV = Lateral ventricle; TV = third ventricle; T = thalamus; SF = sylvian fissure; P = pons.

THE NORMAL PITUITARY

MRI assessment of the size and appearance of the pituitary gland compares favorably with CT[8] but offers the advantage of excellent visualization without the use of intravenous or intrathecal contrast agents (Fig. 16–1). A wide variation in size, configuration, and regularity of enhancement has been demonstrated with both CT[9,10] and MRI.[8]

The optic chiasm and pituitary stalk are well visualized, particularly with thin-section imaging and, owing to the superior resolution of soft tissue planes, are usually better demonstrated with MRI than with CT. These structures are of similar signal intensity to white matter in the brain, so they contrast well with the low signal intensity of CSF in the suprasellar cistern. In coronal sections the optic chiasm is seen above the pituitary and is flat and rectangular, whereas, in the sagittal view it is linear and directed downward from the brainstem. The pituitary stalk is a fine and nearly vertical structure that can be visualized in both planes using thin sections (Fig. 16–1).

Adjacent to the sella laterally are the cavernous sinuses. The smooth, rounded, low-signal structures are the internal carotid arteries. Below the pituitary lies the sphenoid sinus with its varying degree of pneumatization. The clivus is usually a bright signal intensity structure, reflecting its fatty bone marrow content.

The sellar floor is not usually well seen owing to the lack of signal intensity from cortical bone. In those cases in which the sphenoid sinus is incompletely pneumatized, the lamina dura is seen as a thin line of decreased signal, especially at high field strengths (1.5 tesla).[11] In pituitary evaluation, the relative importance of bony change has diminished greatly with the ability to visualize the gland directly.[10] The inconsistent visualization of sphenoid sinus septa may be viewed as a relative drawback by the neurosurgeon who utilizes the trans-sphenoidal approach.

T1 weighted sequences ($TR = 500$ ms, $TE = 30$ ms) are superior for anatomic definition in both the normal and the abnormal pituitary. The signal is similar to that of the brain white matter regardless of the sequence utilized.[8] The normal pituitary densely enhances with intravenous gadolinium-DTPA.[12] This contrast material has many diagnostic implications in pituitary and parasellar evaluation, as discussed later in this chapter.

EMPTY SELLA

The empty sella, which is attributed to intrasellar herniation of the suprasellar cistern, is a benign condition. An enlarged sella often is discovered on plain films usually obtained for unrelated cranial complaints, such as trauma or headaches.[13] Prior to CT, evaluation was extensive and costly, requiring hospitalization and pneumoencephalography. With high-resolution CT, direct coronal postcontrast studies show the infundibulum or pituitary stalk extending to the sellar floor or to a thin rim of residual pituitary tissue. The finding is termed the positive infundibular sign and excludes an intrasellar cystic abnormality.[14] Occasionally, the infundibulum is not midline or artifacts are present, necessitating the intrathecal injection of water-soluble contrast followed by CT to confirm the abnormality by observing contrast within the sella.

During the early utilization of MRI, alternation of sequences was necessary for diagnosis (Fig. 16–2). At present, using thin-section imaging (*T1* weighted sequence),

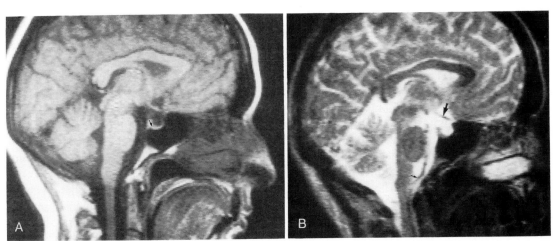

Figure 16–2. Empty sella. *A*, Sagittal *T1* weighted section (10 mm) showing a thin rim of pituitary tissue (arrow) with low-signal CSF above. *B*, With heavy *T2* weighting (SE 180/2000), the CSF is reversed from *A* and is increased in signal intensity, particularly within the sella. Note the low signal of the optic chiasm (large arrow) and vertebral artery (small arrow).

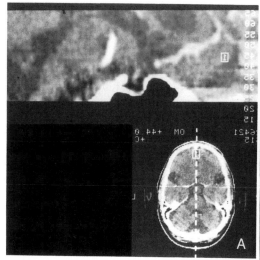
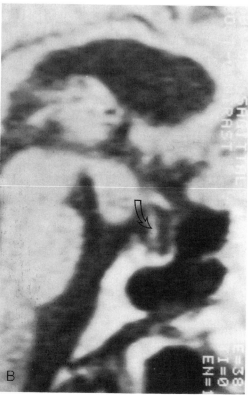

Figure 16–3. Partially empty sella. *A*, Contrast-enhanced sagittal reformatted CT shows questionable empty sella. The pituitary stalk cannot be identified to the sella floor, nor is there identifiable pituitary tissue. *B*, The pituitary stalk (open arrow) is identified to the rim of pituitary tissue. Also, note the better demonstration of the hypothalamic hamartoma (arrow) with the 3 mm direct sagittal (SE 38/500) MRI section.

the thin rim of residual pituitary tissue within the empty sella can be demonstrated (Fig. 16–3).

PROLACTINOMA

Thin-section imaging is of paramount importance in the visualization of these small (up to 10 mm) intrasellar tumors. With thicker sections (0.75 to 1.0 cm), only 50 percent of these tumors can be diagnosed, owing principally to volume averaging (Fig. 16–4).[8] More recent technology providing thin-slice imaging at 0.2 to 0.3 cm has increased sensitivity.

These nonenhancing or low-attenuation abnormalities at CT examination are generally low-signal intensity changes on *T1* weighted MRI (Fig. 16–4).[8,15] The coronal examination may demonstrate the prolactinoma more effectively than the sagittal, since in some patients the anteroposterior dimension of the sella is greater than the width. As a result, in a small gland the 3 mm section may result in sufficient volume averaging to obscure the abnormality.

For those small tumors not clearly defined, Gd-DTPA may offer some assistance in diagnosis. Since the normal pituitary gland densely enhances with gadolinium, the prolactinoma should be readily seen as an area without enhancement, assuming that enhancement patterns follow those of CT in this abnormality. This should be the case, since enhancement, although better in most cases, generally follows that of CT for abnormalities in this region.[12]

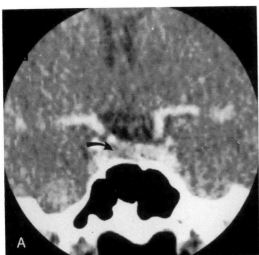

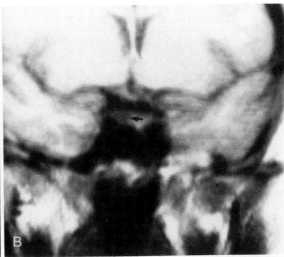

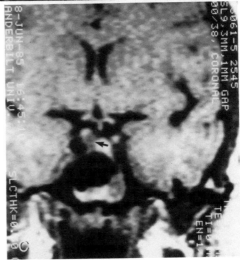

Figure 16–4. Prolactinoma. *A,* Direct coronal contrast-enhanced CT shows nonenhancing microadenoma on right (arrow). *B,* Coronal 10 mm *T1* weighted (SE 38/500) sequence shows low-signal microadenoma corresponding to the CT study (arrow). *C,* Coronal 3 mm *T1* weighted (SE 38/500) sequence showing the low-signal abnormality on the right (arrow). The apparent increase in signal to the normal gland on the left is photographic, for optimal visualization of the low signal-intensity prolactinoma. A short upper segment of the pituitary stalk is seen.

CHROMOPHOBE ADENOMAS

Larger adenomas are well demonstrated by MRI (Fig. 16–5). Thin-section imaging more closely compares with thin-section CT than does thicker section (0.75 to 1.0 cm) MRI, in which volume averaging often obscures the small associated areas of necrosis (Fig. 16–6). With better resolution of soft tissue planes, MRI is superior to CT in demonstration of the parasellar relationships of these tumors, particularly for the suprasellar extent toward the optic chiasm.

Those tumors without associated liquefaction, necrosis, or previous radiation therapy display little, if any, signal intensity change on *T2* weighted sequences, so that the primary sequence for anatomic evaluation is the *T1* weighted sequence. If there is sufficient necrosis, increase in *T2* signal intensity occurs and may diffusely involve the gland so that it can be confused with a craniopharyngioma (Fig. 16–6). Larger bulk, irregular tumor margins, and secondary enlargement of the sella are distinguishing characteristics of the chromophobe adenoma.

CT contrast enhancement of chromophobe adenomas is generally good to excellent with iodinated contrast agents (see Fig. 16–5). Three patients were studied at Vanderbilt

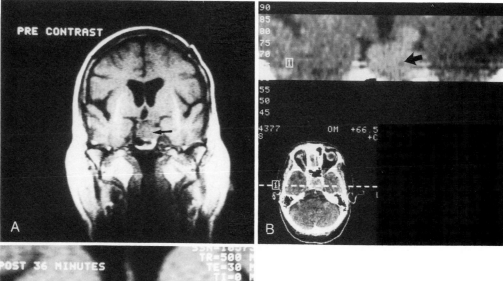

Figure 16–5. Chromophobe adenoma. *A*, Direct coronal *T1* weighted sequence (SE 38/500). This large bulky tumor (arrow) is well demonstrated, as is the suprasellar and sphenoid sinus extent to the left. *B*, Postcontrast coronal CT reformation shows similar findings. With contrast, the suprasellar extent (arrow) is somewhat better demonstrated, while the inferior extent is better shown by MRI. *C*, The gadolinium enhancement is superior to the CT enhancement as is the parasellar extent, particularly into the left suprasellar region (arrow).

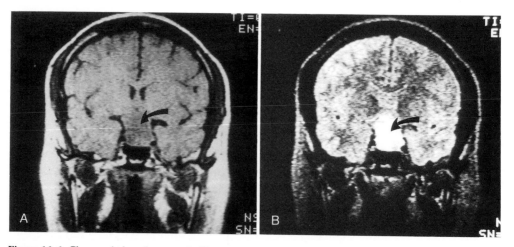

Figure 16–6. Chromophobe adenoma. *A*, Three mm coronal (SE 38/500) sequence showing a large chromophobe adenoma. The central portion of the tumor is lower in signal (arrow). *B*, With *T2* weighting (SE 90/2000) there is diffuse increase in signal, presumably due to associated tumor necroses. Bulky contour, irregularity, and secondary increase in size of the sella are features that distinguish this tumor from a craniopharyngioma (arrow).

University with Gd-DTPA. In two patients the gadolinium contrast enhancement was similar to CT; in the remaining patient, enhancement was much denser than on CT. In each case, MRI showed a greater clarity of parasellar relationships.

CRANIOPHARYNGIOMA

Of all the pituitary region tumors, craniopharyngioma produces the most profound and easily recognizable changes (Figs. 16–7 and 16–8). It is the only tumor that has such a bright and diffuse signal intensity change on *T2* weighted sequences. The margins are smooth, rounded, and well defined. There may be adjacent smaller areas of similar configuration and signal intensity change so that the abnormal region appears as small adjacent or superimposed rounded structures separated by linear areas of low signal intensity. These are consistent with multiple areas of lobulation or loculation demonstrated by CT in the larger tumors of this type.[16]

Since the majority of these tumors are suprasellar in origin, there is usually little secondary alteration in size or appearance of the sella turcica (Figs. 16–7 and 16–8). Although presumed intrasellar origin craniopharyngiomas can occur rarely, these usually become clinically apparent relatively early, before they can enlarge the sella, because of mild prolactin elevation with associated symptoms of amenorrhea and galactorrhea.

With *T1* weighted sequences a low signal intensity abnormality is usually seen. Smaller tumors may have sufficient tissue density in the margins to display suprasellar extent. In larger lobulated tumors, it may be more difficult to differentiate tumor from adjacent low-signal CSF in the suprasellar cistern. Here, a *T2* weighted sequence is helpful. The mechanism of the *T2* signal intensity increase in craniopharyngioma is unknown but may be related to the protein content of the cyst fluid.[16]

Enhancement with Gd-DTPA is similar to CT contrast enhancement. A low signal intensity center corresponds to the low attenuation CT change, with a surrounding rim of contrast enhancement. The advantage of postcontrast MRI in these tumors is the increased intensity of the normal pituitary below the cystic suprasellar tumor, which is more easily appreciated than with CT. Otherwise, little diagnostic information is added by the postcontrast MRI study of craniopharyngiomas.

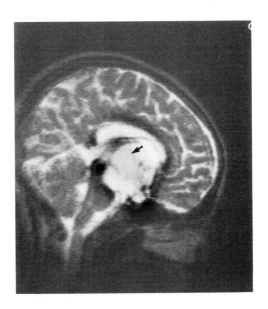

Figure 16–7. Craniopharyngioma. *T2* weighted sequence shows multiloculated craniopharyngioma with small adjacent rounded areas of increase in signal intensity separated by linear area of low signal intensity (arrow).

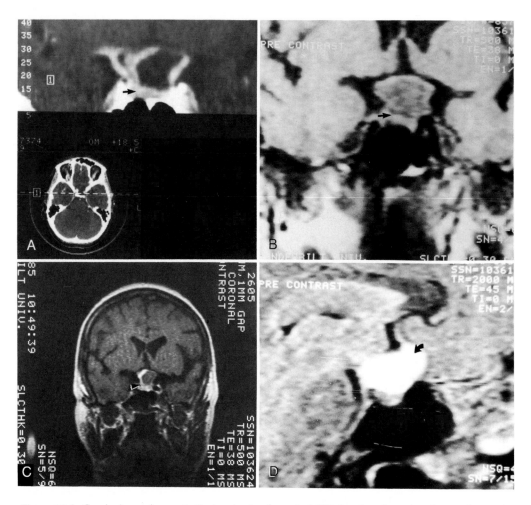

Figure 16–8. Craniopharyngioma. *A*, Postcontrast reformatted CT showing rim enhancing cystic cranio-pharyngioma (arrow). The enhancing pituitary appears slightly compressed on left. *B*, *T1* weighted (SE 500/38) coronal 3 mm section shows findings similar to CT study. The rim is not quite as dense as with contrasted CT (arrow). The suprasellar origin and extent are better shown than with CT. *C*, Postcontrast, *T1* weighted (SE 500/38) MRI, coronal view. Note enhancement of the pituitary and rim enhancement of the cystic su-prasellar tumor (arrow). *D*, Direct sagittal *T2* weighted (SE 90/2000) sequence (3 mm) shows characteristic diffuse signal intensity increase (arrow). Note smooth, rounded, well-marginated contour.

The occurrence of the characteristic increase in *T2* signal intensity change in this tumor is helpful in differential diagnosis, although *T2* signal increase can be seen in other tumors with necrosis or liquefaction, empty sella, or postradiation changes as well as in epidermoids (Figs. 16–7 and 16–8).

GROWTH HORMONE TUMOR

A single growth hormone tumor was examined by MRI prior to the availability of thin-section imaging (Fig. 16–9). This tumor showed low signal intensity changes suggesting necrosis on the *T1* weighted sequences, corresponding to the lower attenuation abnormality on CT. Little significant signal intensity change occurred with *T2* weighting.

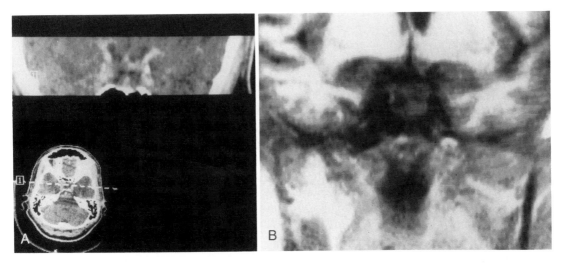

Figure 16–9. Growth hormone tumor. *A*, Coronal reformatted contrast-enhanced CT shows an H-shaped area of low attenuation in this slightly enlarged growth hormone tumor. *B*, Direct coronal heavily *T1* weighted IR shows low signal intensity abnormality that is quite similar to the CT study even in this thicker 10 mm section.

CUSHING'S ADENOMA

A wide range of CT presentation is exhibited by the Cushing pituitary tumor,[18] varying from larger enhancing tumors to the smaller ones that cannot be distinguished from normal pituitary owing to isoenhancement. This variable presentation is also seen with thicker section (10 mm) MRI imaging. Larger tumors could be demonstrated with good correspondence in size of the tumor by both modalities. Low signal intensity change on *T1* sequences were similar but did not closely correspond to CT. No signal intensity change was noted on the *T2* weighted sequences (Fig. 16–10).

Imaging of these tumors would be expected to improve with thin-section MR imaging, especially for the small intrasellar abnormalities that are difficult, if not impos-

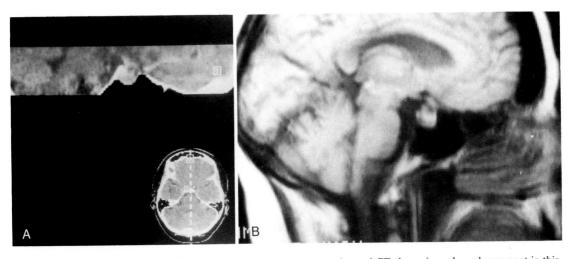

Figure 16–10. Cushing's tumor. *A*, The sagittal reformatted contrast-enhanced CT shows irregular enhancement in this Cushing's tumor. *B*, The *T1* weighted (SE 30/500) direct sagittal view is similar in appearance to CT in this 10 mm section. A low-signal area in the upper portion of the tumor is similar to the CT.

sible, to visualize by CT. *T1* or *T2* characteristics may become apparent with thinner sections. Gd-DTPA, with its greater tumor enhancement, may also improve diagnosis in these tumors.

POSTOPERATIVE PITUITARY

Postoperative changes in and about the pituitary often result in a confusing image owing to scarring, transsphenoidal fascia lata grafts with their associated fat, osseous defects, and irregular or cystic tumor recurrences. The postoperative pituitaries were examined prior to the availability of thin-section capability. Even with thicker section images, however, MRI was helpful in confirming the presence of soft tissue planes, separation of postsurgical changes from intrinsic abnormalities would be expected and augmented by thin-section MR images (Fig. 16–11).

CONTRAST ENHANCEMENT

Gd-DTPA should further improve the diagnostic sensitivity of MRI in evaluation of pituitary and parasellar disorders. Eleven patients with pituitary and parasellar region abnormalities were evaluated at Vanderbilt University. Tumor enhancement and better definition of surrounding soft tissue structures added helpful information in each case (Fig. 16–12).[12]

Separating intrinsic pituitary abnormalities from those of parasellar origin, (e.g., meningioma) is facilitated by demonstrating intrinsic lesions with greater clarity (Fig. 16–12). The excellent enhancement of the cavernous sinus aids in distinguishing intrinsic (aneurysms) and adjacent (neuroma, meningioma) lesions. This is an area that has been notoriously "silent" for smaller abnormalities examined by CT (Fig. 16–13).

In conclusion, since few pituitary abnormalities result in *T2* signal intensity change, the *T1* weighted sequence is usually more important in pituitary and parasellar assessment. Despite this, both sequence parameters (*T1* and *T2*) should be obtained for

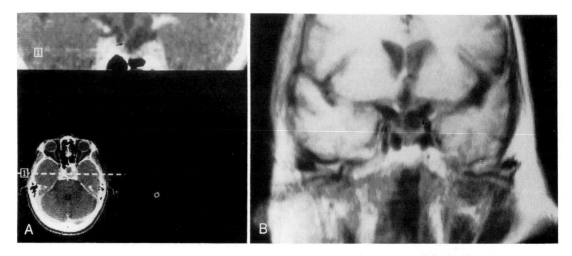

Figure 16–11. Postoperative pituitary tumor. *A*, Coronal reformatted contrast-enhanced CT in a postoperative pituitary tumor. There is no tumor recurrence in this partially empty sella with the pituitary stalk extending toward the right (arrow). *B*, The direct coronal *T1* weighted sequence is essentially identical in appearance to the CT study and confirms the absence of tumor recurrence.

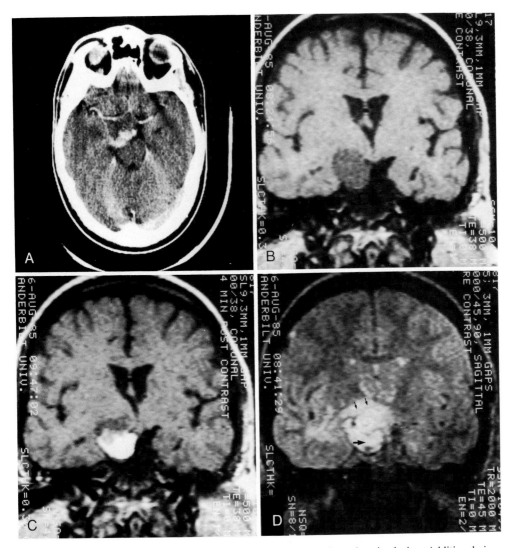

Figure 16–12. Suprasellar mass. *A*, Axial CT section shows a suprasellar enhancing lesion. Additional views were not obtained at the referring hospital, so the precise tumor origin was not ascertained. *B*, The 3 mm direct MRI (SE 500/38) control section accurately localizes this hypothalamic glioma with associated mass effect. *C*, The gadolinium-enhanced MRI shows the enhancing pituitary in a normal-sized sella, with the enhancing tumor just above this abnormality. *D*, The *T2* weighted sequence (SE 90/2000) shows that gadolinium does separate tumor (arrow) from the edema (arrows) it produces.

greater accuracy. The effect of higher field strength and even narrower slice widths (1.5 mm) may result in an increasing role for *T2* weighted sequence in smaller lesions.

Balanced images (*TR* = 1000 and *TE* = 30 where *T1* and *T2* effects cancel) have sufficient *T2* weighting so that cystic or low-signal abnormalities may be obscured; therefore, true *T1* images (SE 315/30 or SE 500/30) are recommended. Inversion recovery, a heavily *T1* weighted sequence, may result in confusing images, since many low-signal pituitary abnormalities will blend with the low signal of the CSF, resulting in a formless area of low signal intensity change. In addition, the IR sequence is one of the least efficient in terms of time.

Acquisition of thin-section imaging has accelerated the role of MR as a primary imaging modality in the parasellar region. Relative lack of experience with this modality is currently the major limiting factor. This drawback is rapidly being remedied by the

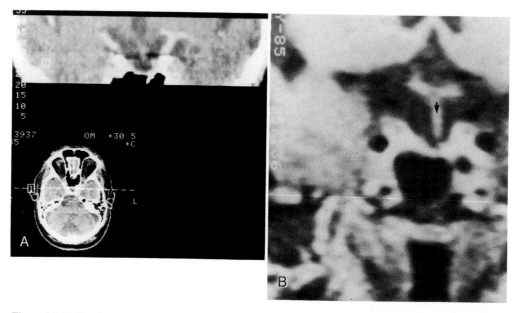

Figure 16–13. Cystic tumor. *A*, The postcontrast CT in coronal reformation raises the question of a cystic tumor. The contents of the cavernous sinus are not well seen. *B*, The gadolinium contrast study confirms the empty sella with the density enhancing pituitary stalk extending to a thin rim of pituitary tissue (arrow). Note the enhancement of the adjacent cavernous sinus with clear resolution of the soft tissue planes.

increased utilization of the modality both nationwide and worldwide. The effect of high field strength examination is not completely elucidated, but the greater signal has the potential for decreasing slice thickness to those obtainable with CT (1.5 mm or less).

Contrast agents show promise in further expanding the diagnostic potential of an already highly sensitive imaging modality so that MRI may eventually replace CT in the examination of this small but very important anatomic region.

References

1. Hawkes RC, Holland GN, Moore WS, Corston R, Kean DM, Worthington BS: The application of NMR imaging to the evaluation of pituitary and juxtasellar tumors. AJNR 4:221, 1983.
2. Danoff BF, Prepsteine S, Croce N, Kramer S, Lees KF: The value of computerized tomography in delineating suprasellar extension of pituitary adenoma for radiotherapeutic management. Cancer 42:1066, 1978.
3. Bydder GM, Steiner RE, Young IR, Hall AS, Thomas DJ, Marshall J, Pallis CA, Legg NJ: Clinical NMR imaging of the brain: 140 cases. AJR 139:215, 1982.
4. Worthington BS: Clinical prospects for nuclear magnetic resonance. Clin Radiol 34:3, 1983.
5. Pykett IL, Newhouse JH, Buonanno FS, Brady TJ, Goldman MR, Kistler JP, Pohost GM: Principles of nuclear magnetic resonance imaging. Radiology 143:157, 1982.
6. Oot R, New PJF, Buonanno FS, et al: MR imaging of pituitary adenomas using a prototype resisting magnet, preliminary assessment. AJNR 5:131, 1984.
7. Bilaniuk LT, Zimmerman RA, Wehrli FW, et al: Magnetic resonance imaging of pituitary lesions using 1.0 to 1.5T field strength. Radiology 153:415, 1984.
8. Price AC, Runge VM: Pituitary and thyroid diseases evaluated by magnetic resonance imaging. In Mettler F, Muroff L, Kulkarni M (eds): Magnetic Resonance Imaging and Spectroscopy. New York, Churchill Livingstone, 1986.
9. Wolpert SM, Molitch ME, Goldman JA, Wood JB: Size, shape and appearance of the normal female pituitary gland. AJR 143:377, 1984.
10. Taylor S: High resolution computed tomography of the sella. Radiol Clin North Am 20(1):207, 1982.
11. Mark L, Pech P, Daniels D, et al: The pituitary fossa: A correlative anatomic and MR study. Radiology 153:453, 1984.
12. Price AC, Runge VM, Allen G, James AE: MR imaging contrast enhancement with Gd DTPA: Imaging experience with 30 intracranial neoplasms at 0.5 T. Radiology 157(P):37, 1985.

13. Roppolo HNM: Intrasellar and parasellar abnormalities. *In* Latchaw RE (ed): Computed Tomography of the Head, Neck and Spine. Chicago, Year Book Medical Publishers, 1985.

14. Haughton VM, Rosenbaum AE, Williams AL, Drayer B: Recognizing the empty sella by CT: The infundibulum sign. AJR *136*:293, 1981.

15. Syvertsen A, Haughton VM, Williams AL, Cusick JF: The computed tomographic appearance of the normal pituitary gland and pituitary microadenomas. Radiology *133*:385, 1979.

16. Fitz CR, Wortzman G, Harwood-Nash DC, Holgate RC, Barry JF, Boldt DW: Computed tomography in craniopharyngiomas. Radiology *127*:687, 1978.

17. Nakasu Y, Nakasu S, Handa J, Takeuchi J: Amenorrhea—galactorrhea syndrome with craniopharyngioma. Surg Neurol *13*:154, 1980.

18. Houston LW, Thomas C, Normal D, Tyrell JB, Newton TH: High resolution CT findings in the diagnosis of pituitary dependent Cushing's syndrome. Presented at the American Society of Neuroradiology, 21st Annual Meeting, San Francisco, 1983.

IV

CLINICAL EXPERIENCE: MRI OF THE SPINE, FACE, AND NECK

17

Spinal Cord

MADAN V. KULKARNI

Magnetic resonance (MR) imaging has demonstrated its ability in the diagnosis of diseases of the central nervous system.[1-4] Since MR affords excellent inherent contrast between the spinal cord and surrounding structures, it currently is being utilized as an imaging modality in the evaluation of diseases of the spine. In addition to the transverse imaging, similar to that performed using computed tomography (CT), MR can acquire images in the sagittal or coronal plane, allowing evaluation of the spine and spinal cord along their long axis. Hence, MR provides unique imaging advantages in the evaluation of the spinal cord. Unlike CT and myelography, in which the cord is demonstrated as a negative shadow after intrathecal injection of contrast material, MR provides direct noninvasive visualization of the spinal cord.

NORMAL ANATOMY

The spinal cord is approximately 43 to 45 cm long in an adult. The cord begins at the craniovertebral junction as a continuation of the medulla. Until the third month of intrauterine life the cord occupies the entire length of the spinal canal.[5] However, the spinal canal grows faster than the cord and the lower end of the cord terminates at various levels around the first lumbar vertebra. In adults the cord usually terminates either at the lower end of the first lumbar or at the upper end of the second lumbar vertebra. The normal cord has two areas of expansion: one at the lower end of the cervical spine (Fig. 17–1) to accommodate the brachial plexus and the other at the thoracolumbar region to accommodate the lumbosacral plexus. Since the spinal cord is shorter than the vertebral column, the spinal segments below the lower cervical cord are at a higher level compared with corresponding vertebral bodies.

The appearance of the spinal cord on MR images depends on the pulse sequence utilized. On spin-echo (SE) sequences with short *TE* and short *TR* parameters, the cord (Fig. 17–2) has relative increased signal intensity compared with that of cerebrospinal fluid (CSF). As the *TE* and *TR* values increase the relative signal from the cord starts decreasing while the signal intensity from the CSF starts increasing (Fig. 17–3). On SE images with long *TE* and *TR* values (i.e., SE 120/2000) the cord has relative decreased signal intensity compared with that of CSF. On sagittal SE images with short *TE/TR* parameters there is an area of decreased signal intensity in the center of the cord along its longitudinal axis. This is more frequently seen with high-resolution images (Fig. 17–4) using surface coils. This most likely represents decreased signal from the central gray matter.

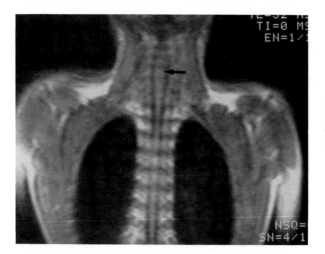

Figure 17–1. Angled coronal image of cervicothoracic spine demonstrates normal expansion of the spinal cord (arrow) at the lower portion of the cervical spine.

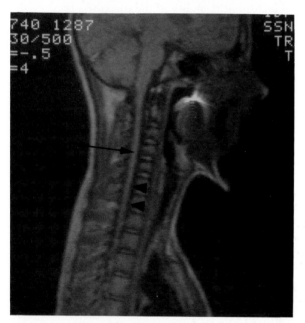

Figure 17–2. Sagittal image of the cervical spinal cord using SE sequence with short *TE* and *TR* parameters (SE 30/500). Spinal cord (arrow) has relative increased signal intensity compared with CSF (arrowheads). On this image it is difficult to detect the posterior margin of foramen magnum, since cortical bone and CSF both have decreased signal intensity. Body coil has relatively poor resolution, and details of normal anatomy of the cord are not adequately displayed.

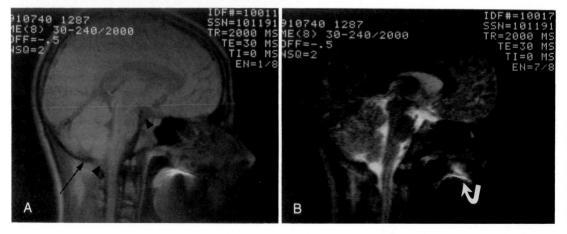

Figure 17–3. Head-coil sagittal image of the cervical spine and the foramen magnum with SE 45/2000. *A*, CSF (arrowheads) has increased signal intensity compared with that of the cortical bone of the foramen magnum (arrow). *B*, Increasing *TE* to 210 ms provides more *T2* weighting, and CSF has brighter signal intensity compared with the signal intensity of the spinal cord. Field-distortion artifact (curved arrow) is caused by metallic dental fillings.

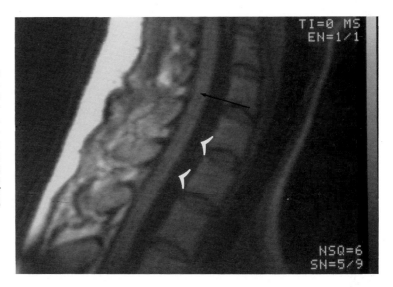

Figure 17–4. High-resolution surface coil image of the spinal cord. The central area of decreased signal (arrow) intensity most likely represents gray matter. On SE 38/500 the CSF (arrowheads) has decreased signal intensity because of its long *T1* relaxation times. The slice thickness is 4 mm and the pixel size is 0.7><1.5 mm, using surface coil. Body coil cord image (see Fig. 17–2) has slice thickness of 10 mm and pixel size of 1.8><3.6 mm.

IMAGING TECHNIQUES

Since the long axis of the cord is along the sagittal plane, we prefer this plane of imaging as a routine screening technique. At least two, but preferably three, pulse sequences are required not only to detect the abnormality but also to characterize it. Once the abnormality is detected, it can be further evaluated by using other pulse sequences or different imaging planes. The selection of the radio frequency (rf) coil for imaging of the cord depends on the length of the cord to be examined. The use of surface coils in examination of the cord has demonstrated improved lesion detectability. Since signal-to-noise received using surface coil is improved significantly when compared with those ratios associated with conventional head and body coils, the slice thickness and field of view can be decreased. This results in diminished partial volume averaging and improvement in the spatial resolution, respectively.

Using surface coils, the slice thickness can be reduced to 3 to 4 mm. The long segment of the spine can be evaluated with conventional head or body coils, but once the abnormality is located, the use of the surface coil for further evaluation is advantageous. As surface coil technology improves, we will see additional types of coils, necessitating the selection of the proper coil and technique for individual clinical situations.[6]

CONGENITAL ANOMALIES

MRI has been extremely useful in evaluating congenital anomalies of the spine. Arnold-Chiari malformations are examined in the sagittal plane. Spin-echo images with short *TE* and *TR* parameters demonstrate herniation of cerebellar tonsils into the spinal canal (Fig. 17–5). These pulse sequences are also useful in evaluating the fourth ventricle. Associated changes of hydrocephalus or syringomyelia are also seen on these sequences. These SE sequences are relatively *T1* weighted, and, because of its long *T1* relaxation times, CSF demonstrates decreased signal intensity compared with that of the cord. Since cortical bone has diminished signal intensity on all pulse sequences, it is sometimes difficult to detect the posterior border of the foramen magnum. In these situations, SE sequences with long *TE* and *TR* values will provide bright signal from CSF owing to its prolonged *T2* relaxation times, while cortical bone has decreased

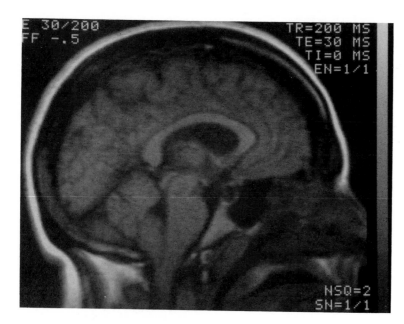

Figure 17–5. Type I Arnold-Chiari malformation on SE 30/2000 image. Herniation of cerebellar tonsils and inferior displacement of the fourth ventricle are seen.

signal intensity. This creates contrast between CSF and the posterior margin of the foramen magnum (see Fig. 17–3).

MRI can demonstrate tethered cord and associated anomalies on the sagittal plane (Fig. 17–6). *T1* weighted images are useful in differentiating varying tissue components of lipomeningocele (Fig. 17–6). Associated changes of hydromyelia (Fig. 17–7) can be diagnosed using MR, and follow-up evaluation after surgery also can be performed. In patients with extensive scoliosis the cord cannot be evaluated in a single tomographic plane, but using multislice acquisition, the entire cord can be examined in a piecemeal fashion. Imaging in the sagittal plane is usually sufficient for most diseases of the cord, but occasionally coronal or transverse images (Fig. 17–8) are required to make the diagnosis.

In pediatric patients, MRI is extremely useful, since it does not require either ionizing radiation or intrathecal contrast material. Because of the prolonged imaging times, sedation is essential when MRI is undertaken in infants and children. We have

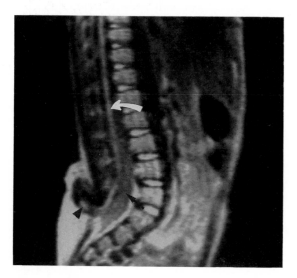

Figure 17–6. Sagittal SE 30/2000 image in a patient with tethered cord and lipomeningocele. Fat in the lipomeningocele (arrowhead) has higher signal intensity than CSF (arrow), while cord has intermediate signal (curved arrow).

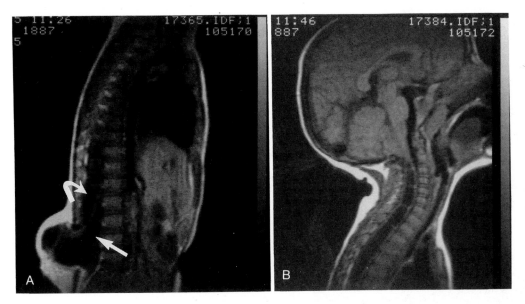

Figure 17–7. Myelomeningocele with tethered cord and hydromyelia (*A*). CSF (arrow) and the cystic portion of the hydromyelia (curved arrow) have similar signal intensity. *B*, The junction of the normal brainstem and the beginning of the hydromyelia are demonstrated.

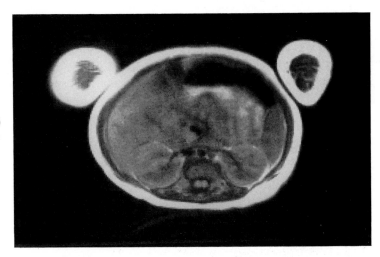

Figure 17–8. Transverse SE 30/500 image in a child with diastematomyelia.

had success with the oral administration of chloral hydrate (50 mg per kg) in infants and young children and with intramuscular Demerol (2 mg per kg) and Seconal (2 mg per kg) in older children.

INTRAMEDULLARY LESIONS

With the advent of MRI the diagnosis of syringomyelia and hydromyelia is more easily made. MRI demonstrates not only the cord enlargement but also the cystic cavity within the cord. On a *T1* weighted pulse sequence the cystic cavity has decreased signal intensity compared with the cord (Fig. 17–9). The margin of the syrinx cavity usually is sharply defined. When imaging is performed using relatively thick tomographic sections, the walls of the syrinx may appear irregular owing to partial volume averaging. Use of thinner sections diminishes the partial volume averaging, and the margins of

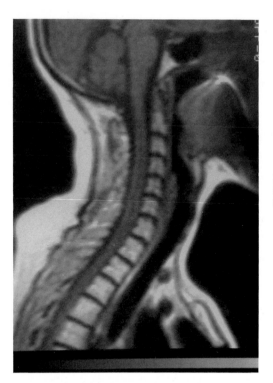

Figure 17–9. Minimal cord enlargement in a patient with syringomyelia. Syrinx cavity is poorly resolved in this body coil image.

the syrinx cavity can be better defined (Fig. 17–10). *T2* weighted images (i.e., long *TE* and *TR*) demonstrate change in signal intensity within the syrinx cavity, often similar to that observed in the CSF in the subarachnoid space. Syringomyelia more frequently involves the cervicothoracic cord and sometimes has multiple cavities.[7] Traumatic syringomyelia may have different signal intensity (Fig. 17–11) compared with CSF. Use

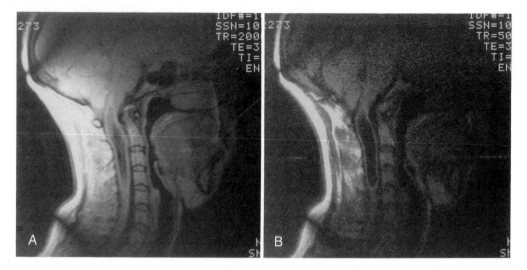

Figure 17–10. Large cavity of a syringomyelia is demonstrated in this SE 32/2000 sagittal image. The walls of the cavity appear slightly irregular on a 10 mm thick slice (*A*), whereas the same syrinx cavity has smooth walls in a 4 mm slice (*B*) owing to decrease in partial volume averaging.

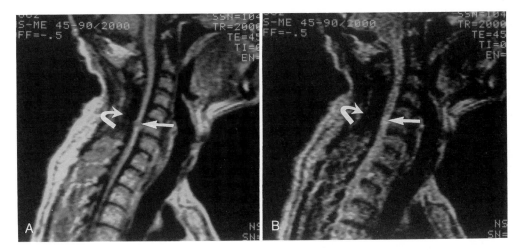

Figure 17–11. Traumatic cavitation in the cervical cord in a 47-year-old patient. *A*, The cavity (arrow) has increased signal intensity on SE 45/2000 (*A*) as well as on SE 90/2000 (*B*) sequence. Also noted are the changes of laminectomy (curved arrows).

of a body coil can decrease imaging time, since large segments of the cord can be examined with a single acquisition. However, surface coils have better spatial resolution and they can demonstrate craniocaudal extension of the syrinx cavity more clearly. In one study MR provided additional diagnostic information in patients with syringomyelia when compared with CT and myelography.[8]

As with the diagnosis of syrinx abnormalities, MRI has demonstrated superior ability in the diagnosis of cord neoplasms. It is also extremely useful in detecting cord enlargement (Fig. 17–12) and differentiating it from the normal anatomic expansions. Because of its multiple pulse sequences, MR frequently can differentiate between tumor and normal cord on the basis of the signal intensity, particularly on *T2* weighted images.

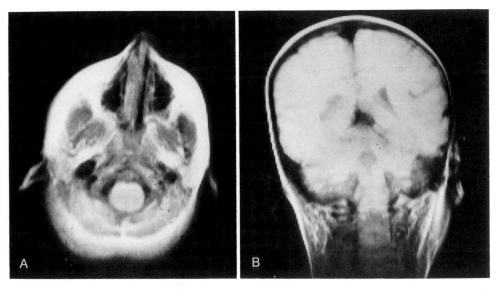

Figure 17–12. Enlargement of the cervical cord (*A*) in a patient with glioma of the cord. Extention of the tumor in the brainstem is seen on coronal imaging plane (*B*).

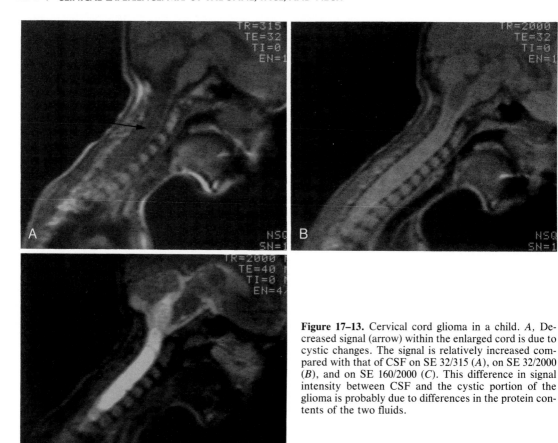

Figure 17–13. Cervical cord glioma in a child. *A,* Decreased signal (arrow) within the enlarged cord is due to cystic changes. The signal is relatively increased compared with that of CSF on SE 32/315 (*A*), on SE 32/2000 (*B*), and on SE 160/2000 (*C*). This difference in signal intensity between CSF and the cystic portion of the glioma is probably due to differences in the protein contents of the two fluids.

Many astrocytomas and other infiltrative tumors show uniform signal intensity on *T1* as well as *T2* weighted sequences, but cystic changes in some gliomas (Fig. 17–13) and hemangioblastomas often are seen and sometimes are due to necrotic or hemorrhagic foci. When cystic lesions are detected in a focal area of cord enlargement, it is often necessary to distinguish between benign syringomyelia and cystic neoplasm. Because of relatively poor spatial resolution with use of the body coil, this differentiation is often difficult (Fig. 17–14). The resolution can be significantly improved with the use of surface coils (Fig. 17–14). Early experience suggests that the cystic portion of the cord neoplasm has a different signal intensity compared with CSF on *T1* and *T2* weighted pulse sequences (Fig. 17–14), and the margins of the cyst and solid portion of the tumor are ill defined. Similar observations have been made by a group of independent investigators.[9] Further experience with a larger patient series is needed to confirm these findings, but similar findings have been noted in the cystic lesions in the brain.

MRI is useful in the follow-up of patients with cord tumors after therapy (Fig. 17–15). Metastatic disease of the spinal cord is difficult to diagnose with conventional radiographic procedures. With MRI the diagnosis of intramedullary metastasis can be made by detecting focal signal abnormality in the absence of significant cord enlargement (Fig. 17–16). Similarly, diagnosis of multiple sclerosis plaques is made with MRI by diagnosing increased signal intensity on *T2* weighted sequences (Fig. 17–17). These findings are similar to those seen in intracranial multiple sclerosis.[2]

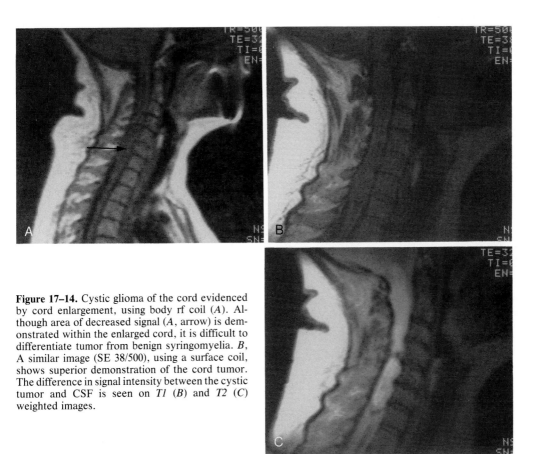

Figure 17–14. Cystic glioma of the cord evidenced by cord enlargement, using body rf coil (*A*). Although area of decreased signal (*A*, arrow) is demonstrated within the enlarged cord, it is difficult to differentiate tumor from benign syringomyelia. *B*, A similar image (SE 38/500), using a surface coil, shows superior demonstration of the cord tumor. The difference in signal intensity between the cystic tumor and CSF is seen on *T1* (*B*) and *T2* (*C*) weighted images.

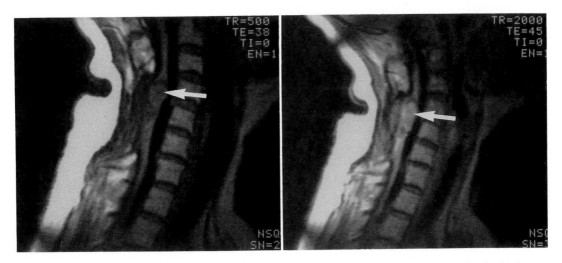

Figure 17–15. Postoperative changes in a cord glioma (arrow). The tumor and the cord are tethered at the laminectomy site (*A*). The tumor shows persistent increased signal intensity after surgery and radiation treatment on *T2* weighted sequence (*B*).

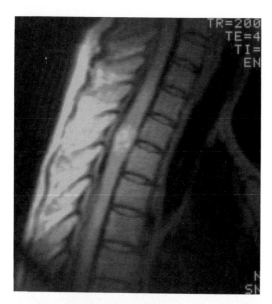

Figure 17–16. Metastatic disease of the spinal cord in a patient with primary breast carcinoma. The myelogram and CT scan were normal.

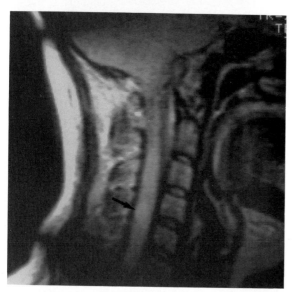

Figure 17–17. Multiple sclerosis plaque in the cervical cord (arrow) in a patient with extensive intracranial MS.

INTRADURAL EXTRAMEDULLARY LESIONS

Currently, spatial resolution of the MR systems does not allow visualization of the normal dura apart from the surrounding structures. The diagnosis of the intradural extramedullary lesion can be made because of its location and its relationship to the spinal cord, which is well identified with MR (Fig. 17–18). The most commonly seen lesions in this category are Arnold-Chiari malformations. Sagittal images are useful in diagnosis of this abnormality (see Fig. 17–5). Modic et al.[8] reported that, in a small group of patients with Arnold-Chiari malformation, MRI was superior to CT and myelography in the diagnosis.[8] The associated abnormalities with Arnold-Chiari malformation have been reported.[10]

The vascular anomalies of the spinal canal and the spinal cord are also included in this classification. The large arteriovenous malformation (AVM) can be identified (Fig. 17–19) with the use of a body coil, but smaller AVMs need to be evaluated using

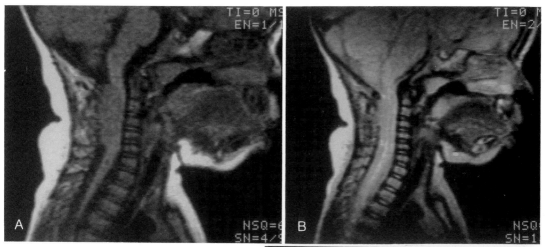

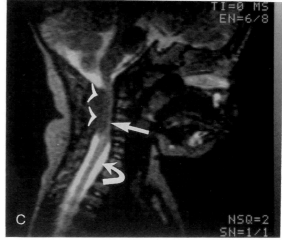

Figure 17–18. Extramedullary intradural mass (histiocytosis X) of the cervical spine in a child. *A*, The mass and its extrinsic mass effect are demonstrated on SE 38/500 sequence. *B*, Increasing echo line (*TE*) makes the lesion isointense with the cord and CSF on SE 32/2000 pulse sequence. *C*, However, on SE 190/2000 the tumor (arrowheads), spinal cord (arrow), and CSF (curved arrow) have different signal intensities.

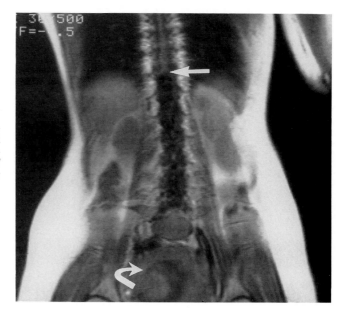

Figure 17–19. Large arteriovenous malformation of the thoracolumbar spine in a pregnant patient. The AVM and the junction of the normal cord are demonstrated (arrow) on SE 30/500 coronal image. Intrauterine pregnancy (curved arrow).

surface coils. MRI is helpful in determining the junction of normal cord and the AVM.[11] Magnetic resonance has successfully demonstrated the intramedullary nidus of AVM and post-treatment thrombosis.[9]

Other commonly seen intradural extramedullary lesions such as meningioma, lipoma, meningocele, and lipomeningocele have been reported in the literature. Further developments in surface coil technology will enhance the ability of MRI in the diagnosis of these lesions.

EXTRADURAL LESIONS

Multiplanar imaging with MR and surface coils has been used in the diagnosis of disc herniation.[12] Surface coils can be effectively utilized in imaging extradural manifestations on the spinal cord. Early clinical experience using conventional head and body coils in imaging extradural lesions has shown encouraging results.[8,13,14] Owing to continuing improvement in MR technology the spatial resolution has improved markedly,[15–17] and increased sensitivity of MR in detecting small extradural lesions is expected.

In addition to tomographic anatomy, MRI has an advantage of inherent soft tissue contrast, which demonstrates a different signal from that of the cord and CSF, and use of intrathecal contrast is not necessary. The use of proper pulse sequences is essential in determining encroachment of the spinal subarachnoid space. Sometimes disc herniation or ligamentous hypertrophy can be seen on *TI* weighted images (Fig. 17–20), but sequences with long *TE* and *TR* parameters demonstrate contrast between bright signal from CSF and decreased signal from the fibrous anuli or hypertrophied ligaments (Fig. 17–20). The contrast between cord and CSF is lost on these pulse sequences, and *TI* weighted images are useful in demonstrating cord morphology (Fig. 17–20).

Inflammatory changes due to rheumatoid arthritis and the mass effect due to pannus can be identified (Fig. 17–21). The changes in subluxation at the C1–C2 junction can be identified on MRI, similar to conventional radiography. MRI has been shown to be more specific in demonstrating soft tissue mass in the region of the joint synovium and transverse ligament posterior to the dens.[13] Vertebral osteomyelitis and the mass effect from the abscess on the cord as well as its extension in the retropharyngeal space can be depicted with MR (Fig. 17–22).

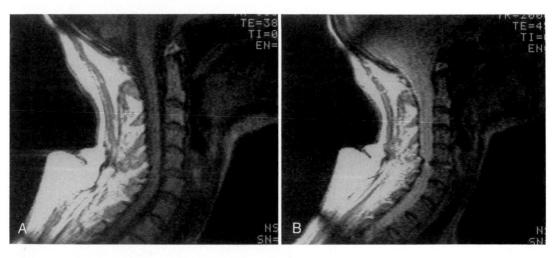

Figure 17–20. Extradural defect on the spinal cord and the spinal subarachnoid space is shown in a patient with cervical spine trauma (*A*). The extent of the encroachment is better documented on SE 90/2000 sequence (*B*).

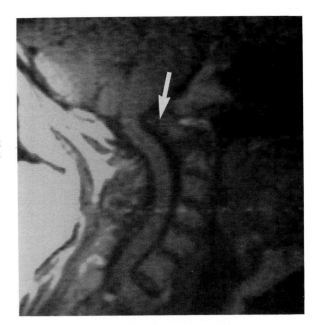

Figure 17–21. Rheumatoid arthritis pannus causing mass effect (arrow) on the junction of the brainstem and the cord.

MRI has great potential in imaging patients with kyphoscoliosis. Owing to the tomographic nature of the imaging modality, large portions of the spine and the cord cannot be seen on a single tomographic section. But pressure effects of the gibbus on the cord (Fig. 17–23) or other associated changes are well demonstrated on MRI. By calculating Euler angles and thus changing the angular orientation of the next data collection, large sections of the cord and spinal canal may be examined with MR.

Disc herniation is relatively uncommon in the cervical and thoracic spine as compared with the lumbar spine (details of MR imaging of the spine are described in Chapter 18). Magnetic resonance also allows evaluation of anatomy in the parasagittal plane.

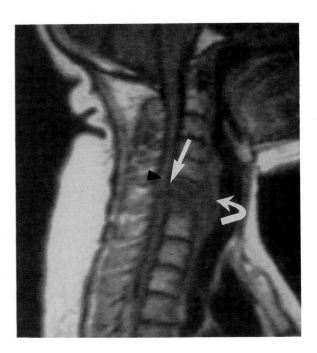

Figure 17–22. Vertebral osteomyelitis and abscess formation (TB) in the cervical spine. Extradural extension of the inflammatory process (arrow) is demonstrated anterior to the cord (arrowhead), and extension into retropharyngeal space (curved arrow) also is noted.

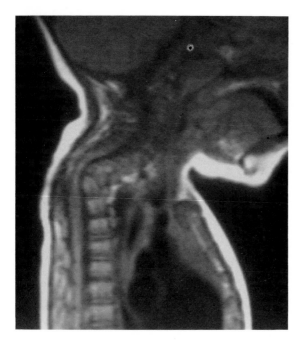

Figure 17–23. Impingement of the thoracic cord due to extensive kyphosis in a child.

Disc herniation is demonstrated on *T2* weighted images (Fig. 17–24), since contrast between CSF and fibrous anuli is best demonstrated with these sequences.

Metastatic tumor in the extradural space is a frequent cause of cord compression in the oncology patient population. Early experience suggests that MRI is excellent in detecting cord compression due to benign or malignant tumor (Fig. 17–25). *T1* weighted images using surface coils have an excellent combination of spatial resolution and proper contrast between CSF and tumor. This contrast is usually diminished with pulse

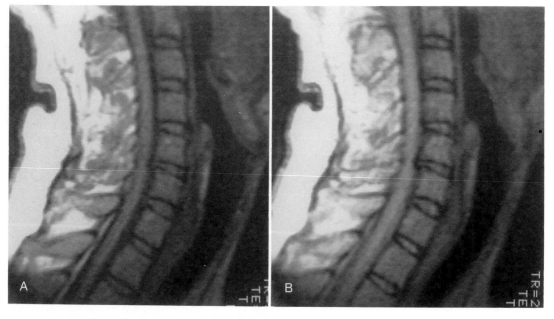

Figure 17–24. Disc herniation is shown (*A*) as an anterior extradural defect in the cervical spine. *B*, The encroachment of the subarachnoid space is demonstrated superiorly on *T2* weighted image.

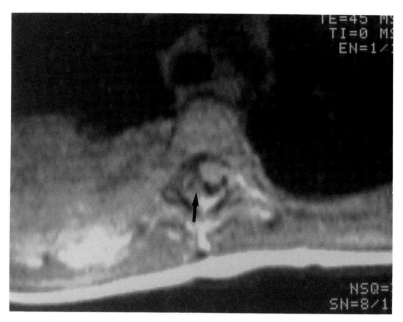

Figure 17–25. Intraspinal extension (arrow) from radiation-induced mediastinal chondrosarcoma. CSF, tumor, and cord have different signal intensity on SE 45/2000 transverse image.

sequences having relatively long *TE* and *TR* parameters. These *T2* weighted images also diminish contrast between CSF and normal cord.[9] Since signal-to-noise (S/N) ratio is somewhat poor on *T2* weighted images, the depiction of the anatomy is also poor. Although most of the benign and malignant tumors have increased signal intensity on *T2* weighted sequences, the *T1* weighted images, in our early experience, are more useful in determining intraspinal extension.

Postoperative changes, small dural AVMs, and spinal canal stenosis diagnosed by MRI previously have been reported in the literature.[8,9] Other disease processes such as epidural hematoma and abscesses currently are being studied to determine the clinical utility of MR in these disorders.

In summary, magnetic resonance imaging has demonstrated its superior ability in the diagnosis of diseases of the spinal cord. Large clinical trials are necessary to determine the role of MR in comparison with current imaging modalities such as CT and myelography. Since MR technology continues to improve, it is essential to evaluate its diagnostic limits with regard to soft tissue contrast and spatial resolution. Development in surface coil technology in particular has enhanced imaging of the spinal cord. The marked improvement in S/N ratio that is obtained using surface coils can be exploited to decrease the slice thickness and to diminish partial volume averaging and use of smaller field of view, resulting in improvement in spatial resolution.[6]

In comparison with CT, the soft tissue contrast and multiple-plane imaging are superior with MRI. With surface coil techniques the spatial resolution of MR images should approach that of CT. For imaging of spinal cord lesions, our experience has demonstrated MR to be the modality of choice. The real test of MRI is its comparison with myelography. Because of its inherent contrast, MRI does not require insertion of intrathecal contrast material. Although its spatial resolution will probably never match that of myelography, MRI still could be used as a screening modality, since it is a noninvasive procedure and has practically no morbidity. Early experience suggests that MRI is definitely the preferred modality compared with myelography, and it has replaced myelograms in many situations, particularly with pediatric patients.

In addition to its imaging advantages, MR has potential in tissue characterization. Development in spectroscopic imaging as well as in vivo chemical shift analysis using multiple nuclei could improve tissue characterization. Use of paramagnetic contrast agents may improve sensitivity and specificity of diagnosis. Thus MRI has demonstrated its potential in the diagnosis of diseases of the spinal cord, and its accuracy in clinical diagnosis continues to improve.

ACKNOWLEDGMENTS

The author gratefully acknowledges the editorial help of Ms. Margaret Moore and the technical assistance of Mr. Oscar Wolfe.

References

1. Bydder GM, Steiner RE, Young IR, et al: Clinical NMR imaging of the brain: 140 cases. AJNR *3*:459, 1982.
2. Runge VM, Price AC, Kirshner HS, Allen JH, Partain CL, James AE: Magnetic resonance imaging of multiple sclerosis: A study of pulse technique efficiency. AJR *143*:1015, 1984.
3. Han JS, Kaufman B, Alphidi RJ, et al: Head trauma evaluated by magnetic resonance and computed tomography: A comparison. Radiology *150*:71, 1984.
4. Lee BC, Kneeland JB, Deck MD, Cahill PT: Posterior fossa lesions: Magnetic resonance imaging. Radiology *153*:137, 1984.
5. Meschan I: The Vertebral Column and the Spinal Cord. An Atlas of Anatomy Basic to Radiology. Philadelphia, WB Saunders, 1975.
6. Kulkarni MV, Patton JA, Price RR: Surface coils: Optimization of technique and clinical applications. AJR *147*:373, 1986.
7. Escourolle R, Poirier J: Syringomyelia. *In* Manual of Basic Neuropathology. Philadelphia, WB Saunders, 1978.
8. Modic MT, Weinstein MA, Pavlicek W, Starnes DL, Duchesneau PM, Boumphrey F, Hardy RJ: Nuclear magnetic resonance imaging of the spine. Radiology *148*:757, 1983.
9. Di Chiro G, Doppman JL, Dwayer AJ, et al: Tumors and arteriovenous malformation of the spinal cord: Assessment using MR. Radiology *156*:689, 1985.
10. DeLaPaz RL, Brady TJ, Buonanno FS, et al: Nuclear magnetic resonance (NMR) imaging of Arnold Chiari type I malformation with hydromyelia. J Comput Assist Tomogr *7*(1):126, 1983.
11. Kulkarni MV, Burks DD, Price AC, Cobb C, Allen JH: Diagnosis of spinal arteriovenous malformation in a pregnant patient by MR imaging. J Comput Assist Tomogr *9*:171, 1985.
12. Edelman RR, Shoukimas GM, Stark DD, et al: High resolution surface coil imaging of lumbar disc disease. AJR *144*:1123, 1985.
13. Modic MT, Weinstein MA, Pavlicek W, Boumphrey F, Starnes D, Duchesneau PM: Magnetic resonance of the cervical spine: Technical and clinical observations. AJR *141*:1129, 1983.
14. Hyman RA, Edwards JH, Vacirca SJ, Stein HL: 0.6 t MR imaging of the cervical spine: Multislice and multiecho techniques. AJNR *6*:229, 1985.
15. Bilaniuk T, Shenck JF, Zimmerman RA, et al: Ocular and orbital lesions. Surface coil MR imaging. Radiology *156*:669, 1985.
16. Daniels DL, Schenck JF, Foster T, et al: Surface coil magnetic resonance imaging of the internal auditory canal. AJR *145*:469, 1985.
17. Shenck JF, Hart HR, Foster TH, et al: Improved MR imaging of the orbit at 1.5 t with surface coils. AJR *144*:1033, 1985.

18

The Spine

BRADFORD J. RICHMOND
HARRY K. GENANT

Early in the development of total-body magnetic resonance (MR) imaging the spine was extensively investigated.[3,13,21,23] Initially, spin-echo technique with body coils was used to image the spine; at present, surface coils are used almost exclusively. MR imaging of the spine has contributed much to current MR technology.

ADVANTAGES AND DISADVANTAGES

MR has several advantages over CT[19,38]; the most obvious is the absence of ionizing radiation. MR can acquire coronal, sagittal, axial, and oblique images directly without requiring additional postscan reformatting. *TE* and *TR* changes can vary contrast between soft tissues to enhance evaluation of the tissue of interest without the use of contrast agents, giving soft tissue contrast that is superior to that of CT. Beam hardening or streak artifacts do not occur; with the exception of ferromagnetic aneurysm clips, most surgical metallic devices cause only a light local distortion of the MR image that does not affect interpretation.[18,34]

There are several disadvantages to MR.[19] Imaging time is significantly longer than with CT. *T1* imaging techniques may take 3 to 8 minutes, intermediate acquisitions take 12 to 18 minutes, and *T2* weighted technique requires 17 to 30 minutes depending on the software and magnet strength.[20,21] The evaluation of bone, specifically cortex, is still better performed with CT. Four and 5 mm contiguous section thicknesses are available with MR,[23] and 1.2 to 5 mm thick sections can be obtained experimentally (Fig. 18–1). This is an improvement over thick sections with intervening gaps but cannot compete with the 1.5 mm thick contiguous images available with CT. Within the section, resolution is better with CT (0.5 to 0.6 mm) than with MR (0.9 to 1.0 mm) at present. Patients with cardiac pacemakers cannot undergo MR imaging. Although possible, imaging patients from the intensive care unit who require life support mechanisms is very difficult with MR. Cost and maintenance of most MR systems has been reported to exceed that of CT on an annual basis, partly owing to low patient throughput, maintenance downtime, and cryogen costs. MR is more expensive and has a higher patient charge and less clinical demand than CT had after equivalent development time.[9]

Advances have been rapid with MR. Further advances in surface coil design as well as other coil design, 3D volume imaging,[10] 512 × 512 (high-resolution) matrix imaging, and software should overcome the few advantages that CT has over MR.

TECHNIQUES

MR, using spin-echo technique, started at a disadvantage because of low resolution, in part due to section thickness (7 to 15 mm).[12] Furthermore, body coils were

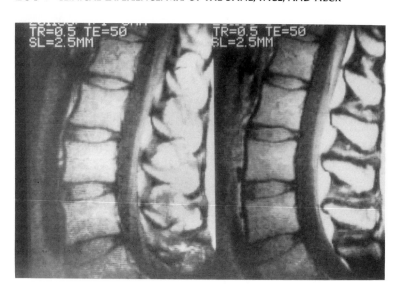

Figure 18–1. Sagittal images of the lumbar spine. Experimental 2.5 mm thick sections, with *T1* weighting, provide both anatomic high resolution and high contrast, allowing evaluation of cortical bone as well as ligamentous structures.

originally the only useful coils; therefore, the signal-to-noise ratio was not optimal and images were degraded. Originally, only single-section/single-echo acquisition was available with no localization capabilities. Finally, when multi-imaging first became available, there were gaps of up to 3 mm between sections so that subtle and sometimes not so subtle disc herniations could often not be diagnosed.[3] Recent advances, including better coil design and widespread availability of high signal-to-noise surface coils, allow for thinner image sections (2.5 to 5 mm) and interleaving so that no gap is present.[27] Improvements in technique parameters, both in defining *TE* and *TR* selection and in multiselection/multiecho capability,[34] have significantly improved utility of MR in the evaluation of both disc herniation and the postoperative back. Direct multiplanar imaging also enhances the utility of MR.

Imaging techniques are variable,[3,11,21,23,24] and determining the best technique depends on the problem being evaluated, time constraints, and image capabilities. *T1* weighted techniques are relatively universal and generally use *TE* of around 30 ms and a *TR* range of 300 to 600 ms for heavy *T1* weighting. *TR* times of 1.0 to 1.5 sec can be used for *T1* weighting. Intermediate weighting has selective usefulness (described below) and is achieved using a *TE* of 30 to 60 ms with a *TR* of 1.5 to 2.0 sec. This signal technique gives an additional echo when multiecho technique with *TE* 30 to 60 ms is used. Multiecho technique, as a form of acquiring *T2* weighted images, allows added information from the first echo. Multiecho sequences have ranged from *TE* 30 to 60 ms to 60 to 120 ms with *TR* 2.0 to 3.0 sec. Asymmetric multiecho techniques have been employed to assure good signal-to-noise ratio using a longer *TR*, 2 sec, and a *TE* of 30 to 75 ms, giving an anatomic image and a more heavily weighted *T2* image. *T2* weighted imaging of the spine has been performed with *TE* 60 to 120 ms and *TR* 2.0 to 3.0 sec.

Body coils are useful for localization of vertebral bodies in order to position surface coils. Short sequences, *TE* 30 ms with *TR* 250 to 300 ms, have been used for localization on MR. These techniques vary between manufacturers and can result in a second image or a compressed uniplanar image. Acquiring this localizing move takes approximately 1 to 2.5 minutes. Body coils are also useful for searching the entire spine for diffuse bony processes and metastases. Head coils are not adequate for cervical spine evaluation at this stage of technology, since the shoulders usually preclude the visualization of the lower cervical spine.

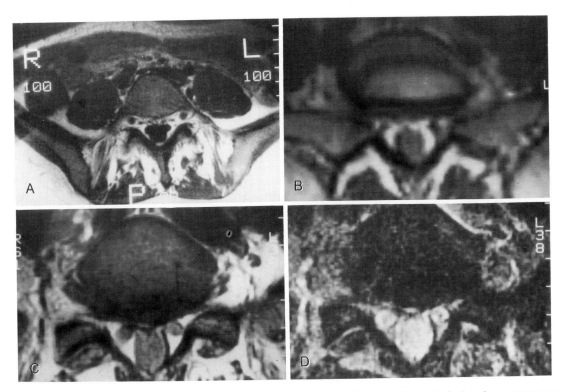

Figure 18–2. Normal axial images of the lumbar spine show low to intermediate signal intensity in thecal sac, nerve root sheaths, and anterior spinal vessels. *A,* High signal intensity in epidural fat on *T1* images provides contrast in the canal and neuroforamina. *B–C,* The vertebral body and paraspinal structures are also visualized. Intermediate or slightly weighted *T2* images have signal intensities similar to *T1* weighting. (*D*) *T2* weighting results in high signal intensity from CSF in the thecal sac, which is a higher signal than the intermediate-high epidural fat signal. Nerve roots may be seen in the nerve root sheath as a low signal intensity on *T2* images. Chemical-shift artifact (*B–D*) is a low signal intensity line along the thecal sac and nerve root sheath dependent on the direction of sampling in the y-axis. (*C* Courtesy of Dr. Meredith Weinstein, The Cleveland Clinic Foundation.)

Axial images have improved markedly over the past year and images now can be acquired using surface coils (Fig. 18–2).

NORMAL SPINE

The superior contrast of MR has been very useful for evaluating the spine with *T1* and *T2* acquisition technique. Signal intensity characteristics of various tissues are listed in Table 18–1. Fat content in the cancellous portion of the vertebral body has high signal intensity on *T1* weighted images.[34] Anterior and posterior ligamentous structures and cortical bone have low signal intensity, blending together.[14] Anulus fibrosus blends imperceptibly with nucleus pulposus at an intermediate signal intensity.[35] The outermost fibers of the anulus fibrosus have low signal. CSF in the canal is low signal intensity in contrast to the spinal cord, which is well visualized at an intermediate signal intensity; this allows for evaluation of impingement on the cord by extradural lesions and paraspinal fat, which have high signal intensity. Fat is seen in the spinal canal, most prominently in the dorsal thoracic canal and ventral lumbar canal on sagittal images. Increased signal from fat is also seen in the neural foramina on parasagittal images. This allows detection of the low signal intensity nerve root sheath. Soft tissues around the spine are generally of intermediate signal intensity (Fig. 18–3).

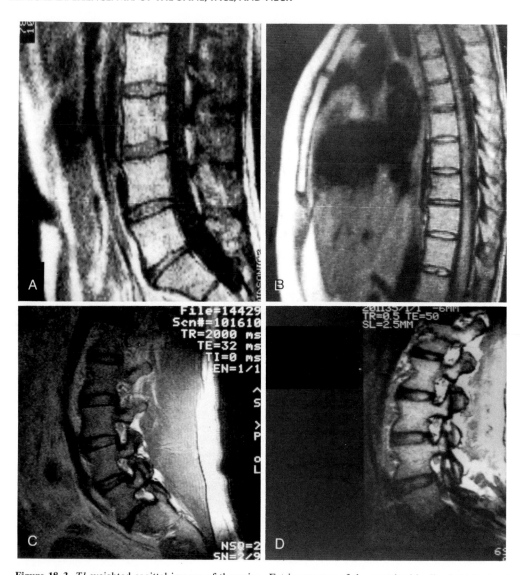

Figure 18–3. *T1* weighted sagittal images of the spine. Fat in marrow of the vertebral bodies is high signal intensity. Cortical bone, ligaments, and CSF are low signal intensity. Spinal cord, intervertebral discs, and paraspinal soft tissues are intermediate signal intensity. Epidural fat has high signal intensity. *A,* Normal *T1* sagittal image of the lumbar spine. *B,* Normal *T1* sagittal image of the thoracic spine and spinal cord is seen. Parasagittal images demonstrate nerve root sheath surrounded by epidural fat with 5 mm thick section (*C*) and 2.5 mm section (*D*).

T2 weighting[34] results in an intermediate signal intensity of the cancellous vertebral body, whereas cortical bone and ligaments remain low. Anulus fibrosus, low in signal intensity, can be easily differentiated from nucleus pulposus in the nondegenerated disc.[35] The anulus is asymmetric, with the anterior portion of the ring thicker than the posterior portion. The normal nucleus pulposus is of high signal intensity, with a thin horizontal linear area of low signal intensity through the centrum of the nucleus. This is the intranuclear cleft,[1] a fibrous band seen after the age of 30 years. The spinal cord is not seen with heavy *T2* weighting because the increased CSF signal intensity blends with the cord signal. With intermediate *T2* weighting (*TE* 28 to 60 ms and *TR* 2.0 sec),

Table 18–1. TISSUE SIGNAL CHARACTERISTICS

Signal Intensity	T1 Weighting	T2 Weighting
Low signal	CSF Cortical bone Ligaments Lytic metastases Degenerated disc Osteophytes Spinal vessels Osteomyelitis Blastic metastases	Cortical bone Ligaments Degenerated disc Osteophytes Spinal vessels Blastic metastases Nerve root
Intermediate signal	Spinal cord Paraspinal soft tissue Intervertebral disc Nerve root sheath Spinal vessels Osteophytes	Paraspinal soft tissue Spinal vessels Osteophytes

High signal	Epidural, marrow, and
	  paraspinal fat
	End-plates around a
	  degenerated disc
	Acute fracture
		Osteomyelitis
		Intervertebral disc
		Lytic metastases
		CSF
		Acute fracture

spinal cord, nerve roots, and CSF may be visualized. Increased CSF signal on *T2* weighting results in a "contrast myelographic"[4] effect (Fig. 18–4), allowing for evaluation of impingement by bulging anulus or disc on the thecal sac. In general, fat and soft tissues are intermediate in signal intensity. Nerve root sheaths are high in signal intensity and the nerve roots within them are of intermediate signal intensity (Fig. 18–

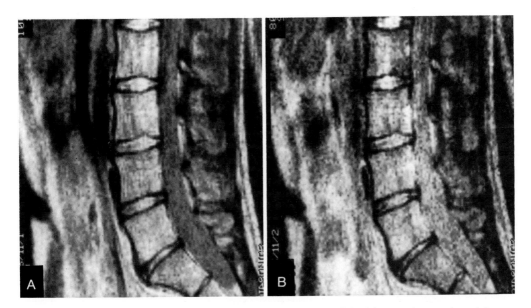

Figure 18–4. Intervertebral discs have high signal intensity on *T2* weighted images; intranuclear clefts are seen after age 30 years. High-spinal nucleus pulposus is readily separated from low signal intensity anulus fibrosis. CSF has high signal intensity (*A*), which increases with increasing *T2* weighting (*B*)—the "contrast myelographic" effect.

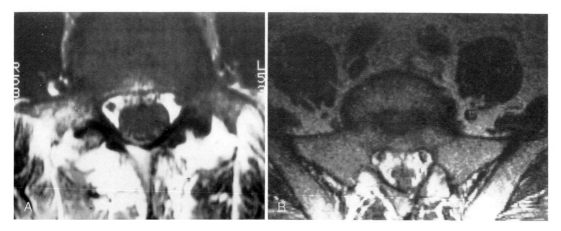

Figure 18–5. Normal axial images of the lumbar spine with intermediate or slightly *T2* weighted technique (*A–B*). Thecal sac, nerve root sheath, and anterior spinal vessels are low to intermediate signal intensity; epidural fat is high signal intensity.

5). The nerve root sheath is surrounded by intermediate signal fat, which makes the sheath plainly visible.

Intermediate or slightly *T2* weighted images (*TE* 30 to 60 ms, *TR* 2.0 sec) are used for axial acquisitions (Fig. 18–6). Whether this pulse sequence is intermediate or slightly *T2* weighted depends on the magnet field strength. With high field strength, *T1* relaxation time is longer. Low field strength magnets will therefore have more *T2* weighting at this pulse sequence, and signal intensities will reflect this. The cancellous bone in the vertebral body is of high to intermediate signal intensity. The bone and ligaments are of low signal intensity. Thecal sac and spinal cord are of intermediate signal intensity. Individual nerve root sheaths may be seen as low to intermediate signal intensity.[8]

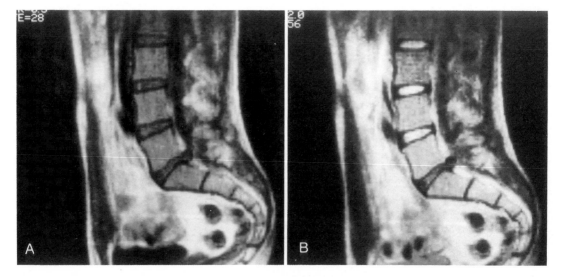

Figure 18–6. Disc herniation at L5–S1 level, surrounded by high-signal epidural fat (*A*). *T2* weighted images, with CSF high-signal ''contrast myelographic'' effect, demonstrate impingement on the thecal sac by the herniated disc. High-signal areas within the nonherniated and herniated portions of the disc indicate that the disc has not totally degenerated.

DISC HERNIATION/DEGENERATION

CT has proved to be a very accurate tool and one difficult to supplant in the diagnosis of disc herniation.[38,42] MR has recently made large strides, not only equaling the diagnostic capabilities of CT in disc herniation,[38] but also, in some instances, possibly surpassing it, e.g., in postoperative backs.

Imaging for disc evaluation generally is performed in the sagittal plane using *T1* and *T2* techniques (Fig. 18–6). Axial images are obtained using intermediate and *T2* technique.

Sagittal images readily demonstrate midline herniation of the nucleus pulposus and/or bulge of anulus fibrosus. Intermediate signal intensity is seen in both the nucleus pulposus and the inner fibers of the anulus fibrosus on *T1* weighted images. The outermost fibers of the anulus fibrosus are of low signal intensity. The relationship between the annular bulge or nucleus herniation and the cervical spinal cord is easily appreciated on midline *T1* images using surface coils. Thoracic disc herniations or annular bulges are not very frequent and are more difficult to localize using surface coils (Fig. 18–7). Lumbar midline herniations or bulges are readily appreciated with respect to ventral epidural canal fat on *T1* weighted images (Fig. 18–8). *T2* weighted images allow for further differentiation since herniation of the nucleus pulposus shows high signal intensity and anulus fibrosus has low signal intensity. Acute disc herniations are readily recognized with *T2* weighting (Fig. 18–8); herniation of degenerated disc is more difficult to diagnose since both the nucleus and the anulus have low signal intensities in this condition. Free fragments may have variable signal intensity depending on the length

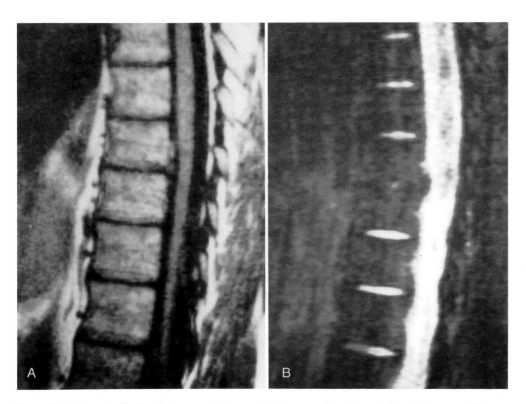

Figure 18–7. Thoracic disc herniation on a *T1* image (*A*) does not affect the spinal cord, but on a *T2* image (*B*), impression on the thecal sac by the disc is appreciated.

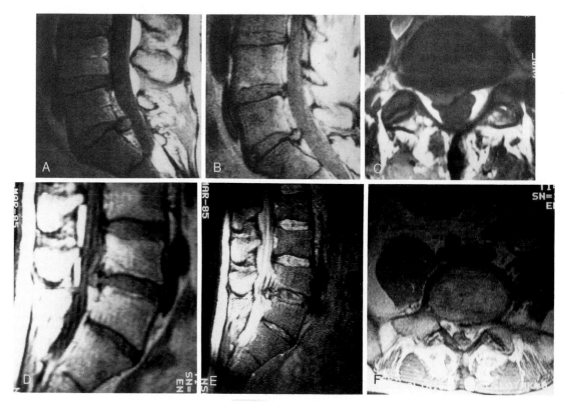

Figure 18–8. Herniated L5–S1 disc, of the same signal intensity as nonherniated disc, (*A*) is seen in high-signal ventral epidural fat. Intermediate signal intensity ventral spinal vessels are also seen on this sagittal image. A small disc herniation and anulus bulge is present at the L4–L5 level. *T2* weighted image with acute herniated disc at L5–S1 demonstrating the same high signal intensity as the nonherniated disc (*B*). Acute disc herniation on axial image (*C*); right side of thecal sac impinged upon. *T1* weighted image (*D*) and *T2* weighted image (*E*) demonstrate acute disc herniation. Acute disc herniation on axial image (*F*) affects left side of thecal sac and left nerve root. (*D–F* Courtesy of Dr. Meredith Weinstein, The Cleveland Clinic Foundation.)

of time they have been present and their state of hydration (Fig. 18–9). Lateral disc herniations, away from the neuroforamina, may be difficult to distinguish from large osteophytes (Fig. 18–10). CT at present appears to be more specific in making this differentiation, but as surface coil technology advances, MR imaging may approach its specificity.

Lateral recesses are not easily assessed on sagittal images.[4] The lateral recesses[6] and neural foramen are frequently seen on parasagittal images. Obliteration of the fat signal in the neural foramen indicates impingement (Fig. 18–11).[8] This finding is sensitive but not specific. Intraspinal Pantopaque (iophendylate) has been shown to have increased signal on *T1* and decreased signal on *T2*.[2] The decreased *T2* signal may prove confusing when one is looking for other pathologic conditions, e.g., disc fragment, and plain radiographic correlation is required.

Edelman et al.,[8] using a surface coil, demonstrated 29 disc bulges or herniations in 17 patients. Surgery, CT, or myelography was used to diagnose 19 focal disc herniations and 10 diffuse bulges. MR results agreed with those of CT and myelography for normal discs, but one free disc fragment was missed on MR. Sagittal images were useful in multilevel disc bulges. Calcified disc herniations were demonstrated in two patients; however, the extent of calcification demonstrated on MR was less than on CT. Continuity of a herniation in the neural foramen with disc could be seen on MR, whereas on CT it could not be distinguished from an osteophyte.

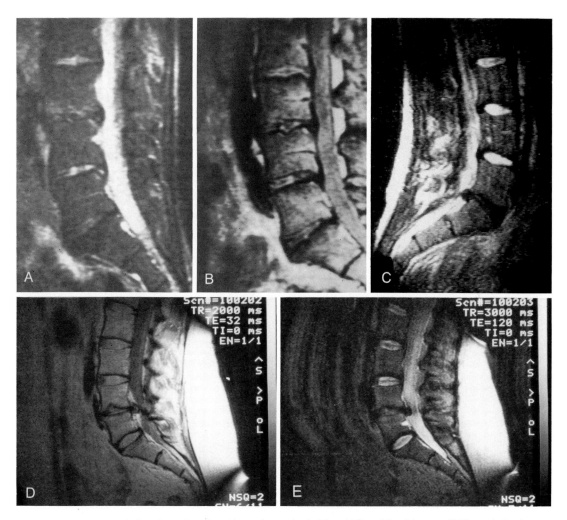

Figure 18–9. Degenerated discs have low signal intensity on both *T1* and *T2* weighted images. Differentiation between degenerated disc herniation and bulge of the anulus fibrosus may be difficult. *A*, L3–L4 and L5–S1 degenerated disc with partially degenerated disc at L4–L5 on a *T2* weighted image. Sagittal *T2* weighted image with multilevel bulging of the anulus fibrosus impinging on the thecal sac in the lumbar spine (*B*) and with normal discs. *C*, Degenerated disc herniation at L5–S1 (sagittal plane with *T2* weighting). *D*, Disc fragment with herniated degenerated disk (intermediate weighting). *E*, Same patient as in *D* with parasagittal orientation and *T2* weighting does not demonstrate the free fragment. (*C–E* Courtesy of Dr. Meredith Weinstein, The Cleveland Clinic Foundation.)

Early studies by Maravilla et al.[20] of 60 intervertebral discs indicated that CT gave better information than MR at 17 percent of the disc levels evaluated. This study was performed with a body coil using 7 mm thick sections with 3 mm gaps. In a recent abstract,[42] the same group reported the second study using surface coil with 5 mm thick sections. Thirteen cases of disc bulges and an additional 14 abnormalities of intervertebral discs were demonstrated on MR but not on CT. Their reappraisal was that MR gives more information than CT in evaluating lumbar disc disease.

Modic et al.[21] evaluated ten patients with disc herniation by MR with myelographic, CT, or surgical correlation. Herniated discs were demonstrated to have a variably decreased signal intensity, and extruded portions were indistinguishable from CSF. In an additional study[21] with 17 patients, herniated discs were demonstrated to have decreased signal intensity. Multiple levels of disc herniation were demonstrated on sagittal images. Five patients had encroachment demonstrated on axial images that was not

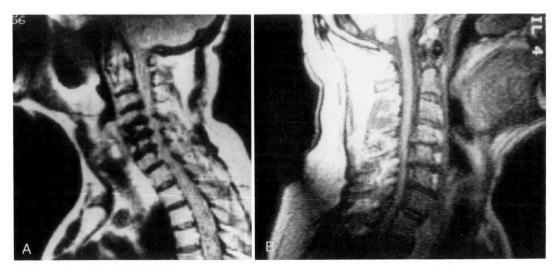

Figure 18–10. Large osteophytes at the end-plates of several levels of the cervical spine impinge on the thecal sac (*A*) on these *T2* weighted images. Smaller osteophytes may mimic degenerated disc herniations. *T1* weighted image (*B*) shows osteophyte plainly, with impression on the spinal cord. (*B* Courtesy of Dr. Meredith Weinstein, The Cleveland Clinic Foundation.)

seen on sagittal images. An error in one patient's diagnosis was attributed to inadequate axial images at L5. MR was concluded to be as accurate as CT or myelography in the evaluation of disc herniation. Subtle changes in disc herniations were best evaluated on axial images. A third study[29] utilizing a surface coil with 4 mm thick contiguous sections to evaluate cervical and lumbar spine for disc disease, canal stenosis, and neural foraminal disease confirmed that MR is now as accurate as CT or myelography when axial images are used. In this study, however, only 85 percent of the examinations were useful because of the high motion sensitivity of the surface coil and its inability to evaluate large patients adequately.

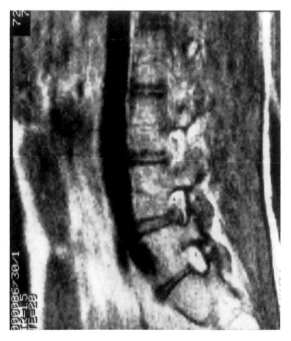

Figure 18–11. Parasagittal *T1* weighted image demonstrates lateral disc herniation into a neural foramen with partial obliteration of epidural fat signal but no displacement of the nerve root sheath.

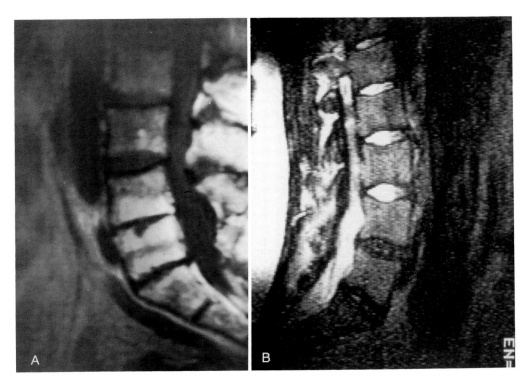

Figure 18–12. Degenerated discs have low signal intensity on *T1* and *T2* weighted images. L4–L5 and L5–S1 degenerated discs on *T1* (*A*) and *T2* (*B*) weighted images. On *T1* weighted images (*A*), high signal intensity in the end-plates adjacent to a degenerated disc is often present. This may represent fatty replacement in the end-plates as a response to altered stress secondary to the degenerated disc. (*B* Courtesy of Dr. Meredith Weinstein, The Cleveland Clinic Foundation.)

Advances in surface coils have allowed MR evaluation in the axial plane to be comparable to or better than CT. The inherent contrast on MR of epidural fat, thecal sac, and nerve roots with sheath on 2.5 to 5.0 mm thick images allows evaluation of the lateral recesses and neuroforamina. MR is superior in sensitivity to any other imaging modality in the evaluation of disc degeneration.[12,24,33] Normal discs on *T1* and *T2* images are described above. Degenerated discs have low signal intensity on *T1* and *T2* (Fig. 18–12). They may be associated with disc bulge or herniation. Disc degeneration is a natural phenomenon; in youth there is high water content (85 to 90 percent) of the nucleus pulposus and low water content (78 percent) of the anulus fibrosus. With aging, the water content of the nucleus approaches that of the anulus, probably as a result of proteoglycan and collagen breakdown in the nucleus.[17,24] The result is overall low signal intensity in aged discs of an asymptomatic patient. Some patients do have low back pain with degenerated discs but without herniation of a disc.

SPINAL STENOSIS

Small spurs or osteophytes were not easily appreciated on early MR images, but with the relatively rapid development of surface coils, resolution has improved (Fig. 18–13).[7] Cortical bone blends imperceptibly with posterior longitudinal ligament, which makes differentiation between these two structures difficult when stenosis is recognized. Anterior epidural fat in the lumbar spine has high signal intensity on *T1* images,

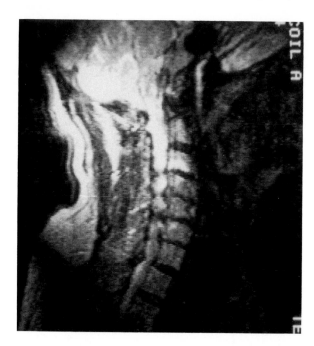

Figure 18–13. *T2* weighted image of the cervical spine demonstrates multiple levels of osteophytes and posterior element hypertrophy causing canal stenosis (see also Fig. 18–19*A*). (Courtesy of Dr. Meredith Weinstein, The Cleveland Clinic Foundation.)

which acts as a contrast to low or intermediate signal intensity structures impinging on the spinal canal.

Spinal stenosis can be diagnosed in two ways on MR. On *T1* weighted images, the spinal cord is visualized in its entire length with sagittal images.[16] Impingement on the cord is easily recognized on midsagittal images but less readily appreciated on parasagittal images, in part because of partial averaging. Incursion on the thecal sac, both anteriorly and posteriorly, is determined with the use of *T2* weighted images, which provide a "contrast myelographic" effect (Fig. 18–13).[16] Evaluating disease metastatic to the spine and involving subarachnoid and spinal cord compression, MR is helpful in assessing canal stenosis and can preclude the use of myelography.[37] Complete block can be defined at both its highest and lowest extents.[33]

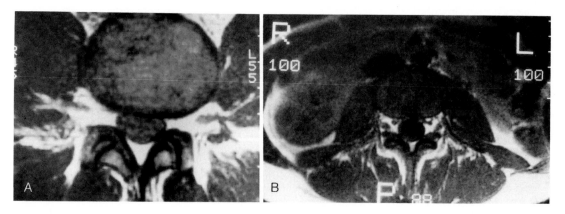

Figure 18–14. *A–B*, Axial images of the lumbar spine show facet joints in detail. Cortical bone is low signal intensity, and fat in marrow of cancellous bone is intermediate signal intensity.

Posterior elements and facet joints are better visualized on MR with surface coils, although CT provides better imaging at this time (Fig. 18–14).

POSTOPERATIVE BACK

Postoperative back assessment has been a problem for both CT and MR. The use of bolus contrast enhancement to distinguish between fibrosis and disc or disc fragment frequently has been unrewarding. Both fibrosis and edge of disc may enhance, making distinction between them difficult, or neither may enhance. MR can demonstrate fibrosis as an intermediate signal intensity with *T1* weighted imaging and intermediate signal intensity weighting. With *T2* weighting, scar tissue has both increased and intermediate signal intensity (Fig. 18–15). Partially desiccated disc fragment or herniated disc may have the same signal intensity as fibrosis. Our experience has been that MR is superior to unenhanced CT in evaluating the postoperative back and is comparable to intravenous or intrathecal contrast-enhanced CT. Further assessment of this complex problem is needed for both CT and MR.

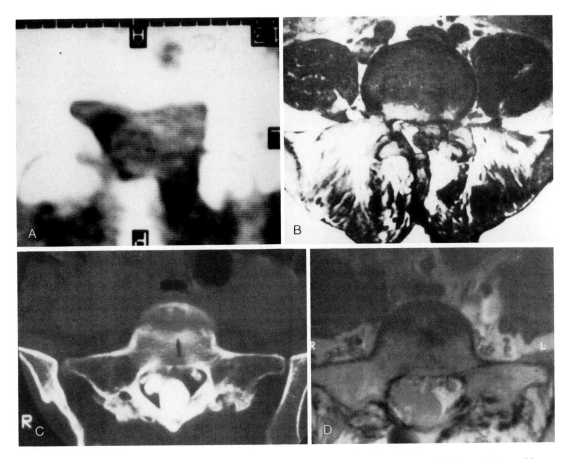

Figure 18–15. On both CT and MR the thecal sac impingement and laminectomy defect with fat pad interposition are seen. *A,* CT with intravenous contrast demonstrates enhancement around the periphery of, and including the mass impinging on, the thecal sac. *B,* MR with *T1* weighting shows the area of fibrosis impinging on the thecal sac, having intermediate to high signal intensity. *C,* Intravenous and intrathecal enhanced CT demonstrates a postsurgical dilatation of the right nerve root sheath and a small area of enhancement in the right lateral recess. *D,* MR, slightly *T2* weighted, demonstrates the same findings but in addition shows nerve root entrapment in the right lateral recess by low-intermediate signal intensity fibrosis.

CERVICAL SPINE

Surface coils have significantly changed in utility of MR in the evaluation of the cervical spine.[7,16,28] High-resolution thin axial images have allowed consistent visualization of the dorsal and ventral root ganglia. Impingement on the spinal cord can be appreciated on *T1* weighted images. Disc herniations and extradural masses are readily identified (Fig. 18–16). Disc degeneration demonstrates decreased signal intensity on *T1* and *T2* weighted images.[15] Bony encroachment (Fig. 18–17) may not be directly visualized, but its effect can be demonstrated on *T2* weighted images as a result of the "contrast myelographic" effect on the high signal intensity CSF.[15]

Normal cervical spine anatomy is similar to that of the rest of the spine, as described earlier, with the following exceptions (Fig. 18–18)[14,22]: The dens is of low signal intensity on *T1* images in contrast to high signal of the other vertebral bodies. There is a normal small soft tissue mass at the C1–C2 synovium seen along with the transverse ligament. *T1* weighted images of the intervertebral discs are of intermediate signal intensity with no differentiation between the anulus and nucleus. On *T2* weighted images, the nucleus is increased in signal intensity, differentiating it from anulus, but the intranuclear cleft seen in the lumbar disc after the age of 30 is not seen in the cervical discs. *T2* images are useful in evaluating subtle disc abnormalities, since the low-signal anulus fibrosus and high-signal nucleus pulposus are readily distinguished from each other.[43] Inability to image the entire cervical spine because of constrictions for the head coil is no longer a problem with surface coils. Small calcifications are not easily imaged with MR. This also may be the case for small disc fragments.

In patients with rheumatoid arthritis, stability of C1–C2 as well as other levels can be assessed with MR using flexion and extension sagittal images.[14,22,23] The soft tissue mass at the synovium can be visualized (Fig. 18–19) along with the transverse ligament, and their potential for cord compression can be assessed with C1–C2 subluxation, if present, on the sagittal image.

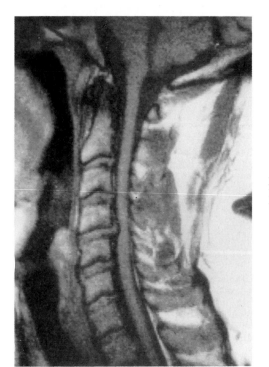

Figure 18–16. *T1* weighted sagittal image of cervical spine with herniation of the C4–C5 intervertebral disc and impingement on the spinal cord.

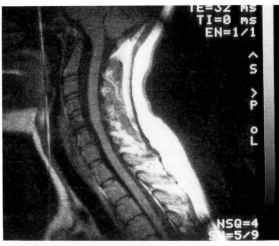

Figure 18–17. Moderate-sized osteophyte at the inferior end-plate of C6 causing minimal impingement on the spinal cord (see also Figs. 18–9 and 18–13). (Courtesy of Dr. Meredith Weinstein, The Cleveland Clinic Foundation.)

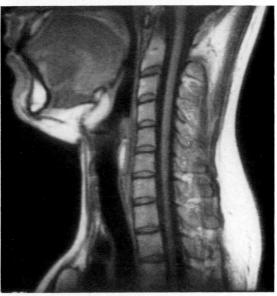

Figure 18–18. Normal cervical spine. The dens has low signal intensity, unlike the high-signal fat in the marrow of the vertebral bodies. Cortical bone, ligaments, and CSF are low signal intensity on *T1* weighted images. Intervertebral discs and spinal cord are intermediate signal intensity.

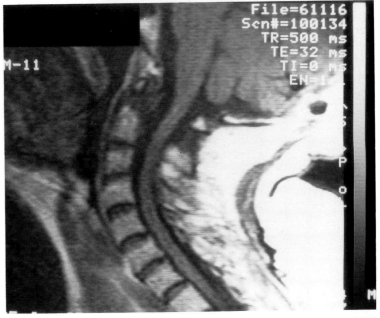

Figure 18–19. *T1* weighted sagittal image of the cervical spine demonstrates an intermediate signal intensity mass at the dens, a synovial mass seen in rheumatoid arthritis. The mass presses on the CSF space but not the spinal cord. (Courtesy of Dr. Meredith Weinstein, The Cleveland Clinic Foundation.)

INFECTION AND INFLAMMATION

Vertebral osteomyelitis with intervertebral disc space infection has a characteristic appearance on MR images.[25] Changes of vertebral osteomyelitis are best evaluated on sagittal acquisitions. *T1* weighted images demonstrate a low signal from the affected disc and low signal from the end-plates of the adjacent vertebral bodies. Intervertebral disc edge is no longer distinguishable from vertebral end-plate. *T2* weighting demonstrates higher signal intensity than normal in disc. Configuration of the disc is abnormal; the internuclear cleft is not seen in the disc space infection, whereas it is seen in normal lumbar discs after the age of 30 years. Adjacent vertebral body end-plates also have increased signal intensity on *T2* weighting (Fig. 18–20). With resolution of the infection, decreased signal is seen in the center high signal intensity of the disc. This finding is thought to represent healing with disc degeneration. In 6 weeks to 3 months, with complete resolution of the infection, disc signal intensity is either returned to normal or becomes decreased on *T2* images secondary to degeneration. Once there is a stable

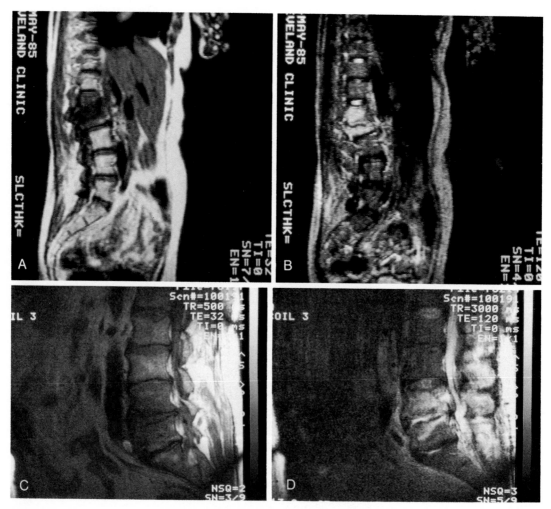

Figure 18–20. Intervertebral disc space and adjacent end-plates have decreased signal intensity on *T1* weighted images (*A* and *C*) with disc space infection–osteomyelitis. On *T2* weighted images (*B* and *D*) the disc space is higher than normal signal intensity with loss of the intranuclear cleft. Adjacent end-plates are also high signal intensity. (Courtesy of Dr. Meredith Weinstein, The Cleveland Clinic Foundation.)

pattern of signal intensity, recurrence of infection can be diagnosed by the reappearance of abnormal high signal intensity in the affected disc on *T2* weighted images.

MR is more anatomically accurate than radionuclides, i.e., technetium and gallium, in imaging vertebral osteomyelitis–intervertebral disc space infection. A greater appreciation of vertebral body, disc, and paravertebral soft tissue involvement is achieved with MR than with radionuclides or single-photon emission computed tomography (SPECT). Antibiotic therapy may alter the MR signal intensity of vertebral osteomyelitis but does not obscure the diagnosis, as gallium may. Using *T2* weighted imaging defines the high signal intensity of CSF in the thecal sac, allowing evaluation of the effect of vertebral osteomyelitis on this structure. Parasagittal *T1* weighted images demonstrate any effect on the neural foramen.

Extravertebral soft tissue or osseous involvement is better appreciated using radionuclides. Unless additional sagittal images are acquired, the usual 9 to 15 images obtained (*TR* dependent) may not allow visualization of the sacroiliac joints, thereby potentially missing infection.

MR is more sensitive and specific than plain radiographs or CT in disc space infection with vertebral osteomyelitis. Accuracy and sensitivity of MR equals that of the combined radionuclides of technetium and gallium. Gallium, however, may allow detection of changes from osteomyelitis before MR does.

Differential diagnostic[25,26] considerations for vertebral osteomyelitis include severe degenerative disease, metastatic disease, and acute reaction to chymopapain therapy. Patients who have undergone chymopapain therapy have increased end-plate signal intensity with *T2* weighting. With time, the end-plate signals return to normal. The disc signal may be normal or may have decreased signal intensity, with small areas of increased signal intensity remaining.

The foregoing findings are based on work performed on adults. Children have a separate blood supply to the intervertebral disc. This may result in different findings related to intervertebral disc space infection with or without osteomyelitis in this patient population. Further work in young patients with these infections is required.

MARROW REPLACEMENT/NEOPLASM

High soft contrast makes MR a more sensitive imaging modality than CT. CT is generally better for evaluation of bone; however, replacement of bone marrow is readily appreciated on MR to a much greater extent than on CT.

Leukemic infiltration of vertebral bodies changes the normally high signal intensity of marrow fat on *T1* images to an intermediate signal intensity (Fig. 18–21).[32] Whether this is a result of marrow fat replacement or due to the inherent prolonged *T1* value of the infiltrating leukemic cells is uncertain at this time. Perhaps both the leukemic cells and the fat replacement combine to produce the intermediate signal intensity on *T1* images seen in new cases of acute lymphocytic leukemia and in relapse. Children in remission have normal *T1* values and signal intensity. On *T2* weighted images, there is no statistical difference in *T2* or in signal intensity appearance between leukemic infiltrated marrow and normal marrow. Chemical shift imaging may prove to be of further value in assessing marrow infiltration of both fat and other cells.[34,39] Other marrow replacement diseases that have a decreased signal intensity on *T1* and *T2* weighted images are β-thalassemia[31] and Gaucher's disease.[41]

Fatty replacement of vertebral body red marrow has been demonstrated in marrow aplasia[5] and implicated in postradiation changes of vertebral bodies (Fig. 18–22). Radiation doses were greater than 4000 rads (40 Gy).[36] Fat replacement of the vertebral

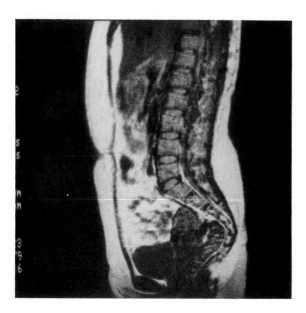

Figure 18–21. *T1* weighted image demonstrates diffuse decrease in marrow fat signal intensity of vertebral bodies as a result of leukemic infiltration of the marrow.

body red marrow is recognized as an easily detectable increase in marrow signal intensity on *T1* weighted images.

Neoplastic processes, either primary or metastatic,[11,33] have been demonstrated to have a long *T1* time with either intermediate or low signal intensity, as in the case of lytic and blastic lesions (Fig. 18–23).[5,15,30] On *T2* weighted images, blastic lesions remain of low signal intensity. Lytic lesions have high signal intensity and a prolonged *T2* time. Chordoma of the sacrum[40] and C1 have been evaluated by MR. Use of MR in this tumor has demonstrated the ability of the superb soft tissue contrast in this

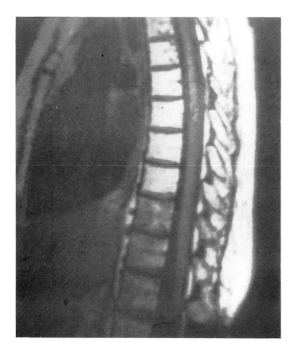

Figure 18–22. Postradiation changes resulting in increased high signal intensity of vertebral body marrow, on a *T1* weighted image, probably as a result of fat replacement of red marrow. Vertebral bodies with low signal intensity are involved with metastatic disease.

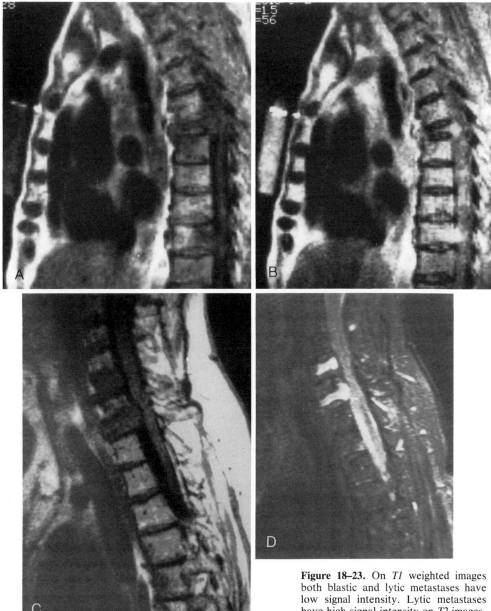

Figure 18–23. On *T1* weighted images both blastic and lytic metastases have low signal intensity. Lytic metastases have high signal intensity on *T2* images, whereas blastic metastases remain low signal intensity. Lytic metastases in midthoracic spine with intracanalicular mass impinging on the spinal cord; *T1* (*A*) and *T2* (*B*) weighted images. Sagittal *T1* (*C*) and *T2* (*D*) images of the cervical spine show metastases at two levels, with one metastatic mass displacing the spinal cord posteriorly.

modality to define the entire extent of the chordoma, both about the vertebral body and in the soft tissue (Fig. 18–24). Direct coronal and sagittal images also enhance the ability of MR to delineate the extent of a tumor in a way that is not attainable by CT. In addition, MR is much more sensitive to recurrence of tumor in soft tissues. Recurrence is seen as a high *T2* signal intensity. Postsurgical changes (edema early and scar later) may make the diagnosis of recurrence more difficult on MR.

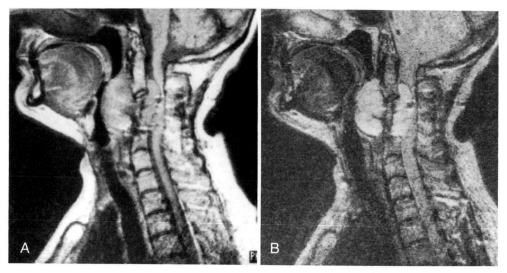

Figure 18–24. A large chordoma of the cervical spine on *T1* weighted image (*A*) has an intermediate signal intensity, destroyed cortical bone of C2 and C3, a large posterior pharyngeal mass, and a large posterior intracanalicular mass pushing the cervical spinal cord posteriorly. On *T2* weighted image (*B*) the chordoma has a high-intermediate signal intensity. (Courtesy of Dr. Klaus Bhondorf, West Germany.)

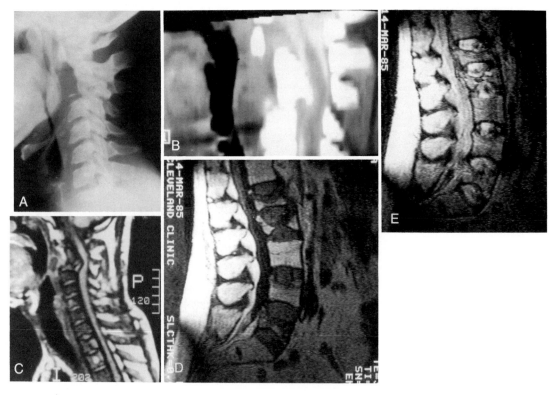

Figure 18–25. Plain radiograph (*A*) demonstrates fracture and posterior displacement of C2–C3 vertebral bodies, with narrowing of the spinal canal. CT sagittal reformation (*B*) confirms the information on the plain radiograph and more accurately reflects the decreased space in the spinal canal. Sagittal *T1* MR image (*C*) clearly demonstrates the fractures and displacement of the vertebral bodies but in addition provides direct evaluation of the result of the changes on the spinal cord. Compression deformities of the lumbar spine (*D*) are present, on a *T1* weighted image, with normal disc and vertebral body signal intensities but with evident anatomic alterations in the vertebral bodies. *T2* weighting demonstrates normal disc and vertebral body signal intensity (*E*), but the discs have an altered shape to conform to the compression deformity of the vertebral body. The dorsal L2 compression fracture fragment impinges on the thecal sac owing to slight posterior displacement. (*D* and *E* Courtesy of Dr. Meredith Weinstein, The Cleveland Clinic Foundation.)

OTHER CONDITIONS

Trauma to vertebral bodies that causes compression or fracture results in decreased signal intensity on *T1* and increased signal intensity on *T2* images (Fig. 18–25). Post-traumatic spinal cord impingement can be demonstrated on *T1* images and thecal sac involvement on *T2* images.[21] Minimal compression fracture has been reported to produce no change on vertebral body signal intensity on *T1* images; the signal intensity remains high.

Spinal dysraphism can be diagnosed on MR by imaging the tethered spinal cord using *T1* weighting. An associated, isolated, or post-traumatic[21] meningocele can be demonstrated with *T2* weighting, which causes the CSF to have a "contrast myelographic" effect. We have demonstrated an intrasacral meningocele by using sagittal images with *T1* and *T2* weighting to prove contiguity of the meningocele with the thecal sac (Fig. 18–26). Significant benign erosion of the bony sacrum was demonstrated on both MR and CT in this case.

Neurofibromas and schwannomas have been demonstrated to have a decreased signal intensity on *T1* images, although we have seen neurofibromas with intermediate signal intensity.[44] Signal intensity is increased on *T2* images. Widening of the neural foramen is readily demonstrated as well as paraspinal and intracanal extension (Fig. 18–27).

Chemical shift spectroscopy may be useful in the quantitation of the fat:water ratio of the vertebral body. This form of analysis could add a dimension in evaluation of osteoporosis. Work in this area has begun recently.

In conclusion, since the first edition of this text, MR has improved greatly in evaluation of the spine. Surface coil technology with high contrast, high resolution, and sagittal and axial images has made MR equal to CT in evaluation of disc disease. MR is superior to CT in the diagnosis of osteomyelitis–intervertebral disc infection, spinal cord impingement, and marrow infiltration. CT shows cortical bony changes in the spine and lateral disc herniation (out of the neuroforamina) better than MR does.

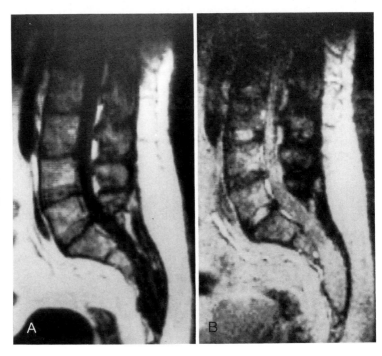

Figure 18–26. Intrasacral meningocele is demonstrated to be contiguous with the CSF space on sagittal *T1* (*A*) and *T2* (*B*) images. Erosion of the sacrum is readily apparent as a loss of high-intensity marrow fat signal on the *T1* image.

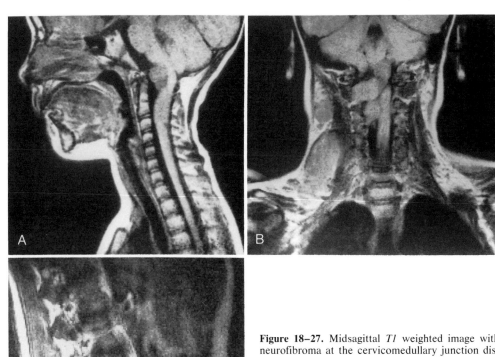

Figure 18–27. Midsagittal *T1* weighted image with neurofibroma at the cervicomedullary junction displacing the spinal cord posteriorly (*A*). Coronal *T1* weighted image demonstrates lateral displacement of the spinal cord; the neurofibroma exists in a high cervical neural foramen with part of its mass in the soft tissue of the neck (*B*). In a different patient the epidural fat signal and nerve root sheath of the L3 neural foramen are totally obliterated by the intermediate signal intensity neurofibroma (*C*). (*C* Courtesy of Dr. Meredith Weinstein, The Cleveland Clinic Foundation.)

MR is superior to CT in evaluation of the postoperative back unless intrathecal or intravenous contrast material is used; with contrast enhancement they are equal.

Further advances in surface coil and other coil technology as well as software should produce greater image resolution, making MR equal to or better than CT in evaluation of the spine.

ACKNOWLEDGMENT

The authors wish to thank Miss Cathy Stine, Ms. Denice Nakano, and Julie Ann George for their help in the preparation of this manuscript.

References

1. Aquila LA, Piraino DW, Modic MT, et al: The intranuclear cleft of the intervertebral disk. Magnetic resonance imaging. Radiology *155*:155, 1985.
2. Braun IF, Hoffman JC, Malko JA, et al: MR imaging of intraspinal Pantopaque (Abstr 55). Radiology *157*(P):39, 1985.

3. Chafetz NI, Genant HK, Moon KL, et al: Recognition of lumbar disk herniation with NMR. AJR *141*:1153, 1983.
4. Chafetz NI: Evaluation of lumbar spine: MR vs CT. *In* Clinical Magnetic Resonance Imaging Syllabus; Review Course. San Francisco, UCSF School of Medicine, October 21–25, 1985.
5. Cohen MD, Klatte EC, Baehner R, et al: Magnetic resonance imaging of bone marrow disease in children. Radiology *151*:715, 1984.
6. Cranshaw C, Kean DM, Mulholland RC, et al: The use of nuclear magnetic resonance in the diagnosis of lateral canal entrapment. J Bone Joint Surg 66-B:711, 1984.
7. Davis PC, Hoffman JC, Brown IF, Spencer T: MR imaging of cervical disk disease and spondylosis: potentials and limitations (Abstr 689). Radiology *157*(P):248, 1985.
8. Edelman RR, Shoukimas GM, Stark DD, et al: High resolution surface coil imaging of lumbar disk disease. AJNR 6:479, 1985.
9. Evens RG, Jost RG, Evens RG Jr: Economic and utilization analysis of magnetic resonance imaging units in the United States in 1985. AJR *145*:393, 1985.
10. Feinberg DA, Honninger JC, Crooks LE, et al: Inner volume MR imaging: technical concepts and their application. Radiology *156*:743, 1985.
11. Genant HK, Moon KL, Helms CA: Nuclear magnetic resonance: musculoskeletal applications. Spine Update, 1984. San Francisco, Radiology Research and Education Foundation, 1984.
12. Gillespy T, Genant HK, Chafetz NI: Magnetic resonance imaging of the spine. *In* Katz, W (ed): The Diagnosis and Management of Rheumatic Disease. Philadelphia, JB Lippincott. In press.
13. Han JS, Kaufman B, El Yousef SJ, et al: NMR imaging of the spine. AJR *141*:1137, 1983.
14. Han JS, Benson JE, Yoon YS: Magnetic resonance imaging in the spinal column and craniovertebral junction. Radiol Clin North Am *22*(4):805, 1984.
15. Hyman RA, Edwards HJ, Vacirca SJ, Stein HL: 0.6T MR imaging of the cervical spine: multislices and multiecho techniques. AJNR 6:229, 1985.
16. Hyman RA, Carras R, Epstein J, et al: The role of MR in initial evaluation and postoperative management of cervical spinal stenosis (Abstr 690). Radiology *157*(P):249, 1985.
17. Jenkins JPR, Hickey DS, Zhu XP, et al: MR imaging of the intervertebral disc: a quantitative study. Br J Radiol 58:705, 1985.
18. Laakman RW, Kaufman B, Han JS, et al: MR imaging in patients with metallic implants. Radiology *157*:711, 1985.
19. Margulis AR: Current status and the future of MRI. *In* Clinical Magnetic Resonance Imaging Syllabus; Review Course. San Francisco, UCSF School of Medicine, October 21–25, 1985.
20. Maravilla KR, Lesh P, Weinreb JC, et al: Magnetic resonance imaging of the lumbar spine with CT correlation. AJNR 6:237, 1985.
21. Modic MT, Weinstein MA, Pavlicek W, et al: Nuclear magnetic resonance imaging of the spine. Radiology *148*:757, 1983.
22. Modic MT, Weinstein MA, Pavlicek W, et al: Magnetic resonance imaging of the cervical spine: technical and clinical observations. AJR *141*:1129, 1983.
23. Modic MT, Weinstein MA: Nuclear magnetic resonance of the spine. Br Med Bull *40*(2):183, 1984.
24. Modic MT, Pavlicek W, Weinstein MA, et al: Magnetic resonance of intervertebral disc disease. Radiology *152*:103, 1984.
25. Modic MT, Feiglin DH, Piraino DW, et al: Vertebral osteomyelitis: assessment using MR. Radiology *157*:157, 1985.
26. Modic MT: Magnetic resonance of brainstem, spinal cord, and vertebral column. *In* Clinical Magnetic Resonance Imaging Syllabus; Review Course. San Francisco, UCSF School of Medicine, October 21–25, 1985.
27. Modic MT: Surface coil imaging. *In* Clinical Magnetic Resonance Imaging Syllabus; Review Course. San Francisco, UCSF School of Medicine, October 21–25, 1985.
28. Modic MT, Masaryk TJ, Mulopulos G, et al: MR surface coil imaging in cervical radiculopathy: a prospective study (Abstr 688). Radiology *157*(P):248, 1985.
29. Modic MT, Masaryk TJ, Weinstein MA, et al: Magnetic resonance surface coil imaging of the spine. Paper #3, Program of the 85th Annual Meeting of the American Roentgen Ray Society, Boston, April 21–26, 1985.
30. Moon KL, Genant HK, Helms CA, et al: Musculoskeletal applications of nuclear magnetic resonance. Radiology *147*:161, 1983.
31. Moon KL, Genant HK, Davis PL, et al: Nuclear magnetic resonance imaging in orthopaedics: principles and applications. J Orthop Res *1*:101, 1983.
32. Moore SG, Gooding C, Brasch RC, et al: Bone marrow in children with acute lymphocytic leukemia: MR relaxation times. Radiology *160*:237, 1986.
33. Paushter DM, Modic MT, Borkowski GP, et al: Magnetic resonance: principles and applications. Med Clin North Am *68*(6):1393, 1984.
34. Paushter DM, Modic MT, Masaryk TJ: Magnetic resonance imaging of the spine: applications and limitations. Radiol Clin North Am *23*(3):551, 1985.
35. Peck P, Haughton VM: Lumbar intervertebral disc: correlative MR and anatomic study. Radiology *156*:699, 1985.
36. Ramsey RG, Zacharias CE: MR imaging of the spine after radiation therapy: easily recognized effects. AJNR 6:247, 1985.

37. Ramsey RG, Geremia GK, Foust R, et al: MR imaging in disease metastatic to the spine (ex 311). Radiology *157*(P):370, 1985.
38. Richardson ML, Genant HK, Helms CA, et al: Magnetic resonance imaging of the musculoskeletal system. Orthop Clin North Am *16*(3):569, 1985.
39. Rosen BR, Wismer GL, Buxton R, Brady TJ: Chemical shift imaging of bone marrow (Abstr 547). Radiology *157*(P):202, 1985.
40. Rosenthal DI, Scott JA, Mankin HJ, et al: Sacrococcygeal chordoma: magnetic resonance imaging and computed tomography. AJR *145*:143, 1985.
41. Scott JA, Rosenthal DI, Dopplet SH, et al: MR imaging evaluation of marrow involvement in Gaucher disease (Abstr 545). Radiology *157*(P):202, 1985.
42. Sory C, Maravilla KR, Lesh P, et al: Updated comparison of MR imaging with CT of the lumbar spine (Abstr 694). Radiology *157*(P):250, 1985.
43. Steinbach LS, Gillespy T, Richardson ML, et al: Magnetic resonance imaging of the cervical spine. Paper #4, Program of the 85th Annual Meeting of the American Roentgen Ray Society, Boston, April 21–26, 1985.
44. Zee C, Segall HD, Boswell WD, et al: MR imaging in the diagnosis of spinal schwannomas and neurofibromas (Abstr 401). Radiology *157*(P):149, 1985.

19

Face, Orbit, and Temporomandibular Joint

STEVEN E. HARMS

In the early years of magnetic resonance imaging (MRI), it was recognized that the high contrast inherent in this technique was advantageous in the diagnosis of disease in the brain.[1-8] MRI had difficulty resolving many facial lesions despite high contrast because of the limited spatial resolution available on early systems. Most structures in facial imaging practice require higher resolution and thinner slices than are needed for routine brain imaging. Owing to the reduced signal-to-noise (S/N) ratio, images suffered from "data starvation" when high-resolution, thin-slice imaging was attempted.[9-18]

The biggest single factor changing the application of MRI for the diagnosis of facial disease was the advent of surface coil imaging.[19-23] Surface coils dramatically improved the S/N so that adequate signal was available for the high-resolution, thin-slice images needed to resolve many facial structures. Most facial anatomy is easily penetrated by relatively small coils near the skin surface. Surface coils limit the signal to a small volume so that direct gradient magnification can be used for high spatial resolution images.

Despite the anatomic proximity of facial structures, the clinical problems are quite varied. In this chapter, the region will be divided into MRI applications in the TMJ, orbit, and face.

PRINCIPLES

Technique selection for imaging facial structures requires some special considerations. The general principles of MR imaging are treated in more depth elsewhere.[24-31] Technique strategies for the imaging of specific facial diagnostic problems are outlined in the following discussion.

Coil Selection

The physics of surface coils are covered in Chapter 73. As a general rule, the optimal coil is one that will cover only the area of interest, since the use of a larger coil will reduce the S/N. Additionally, one of the best ways to improve resolution without increasing the scan time is to decrease the field of view with gradient magnification. If a larger coil is used, the gradient magnification will have to be reduced to avoid image aliasing. Some of the surface coils that have been used at Baylor University Medical Center are shown in Figure 19–1.

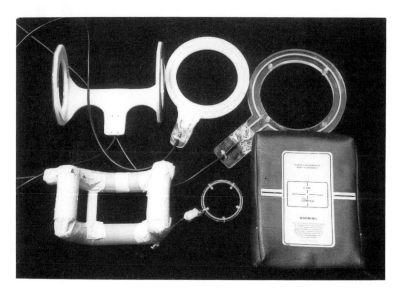

Figure 19–1. Surface coils.

Acquisition Selection

Acquisition techniques are rapidly improving and will change greatly in the future. Currently the most widely used method commercially is 2DFT multislice.[33] This method takes advantage of the fact that the time needed for recovery of a tissue is much greater than the time needed to obtain a spin-echo signal owing to the generally long $T1$ of most tissues. This recovery time is used to excite additional slices while the initial slice recovers.

Since a selective excitation is used for each slice, the thinness of each slice is limited by the strength of the slice selection gradient and the narrowness of the bandwidth of the rf pulse. The signal distribution is also affected by this approach. The signal contribution within a slice will tend to decrease toward the edge of the slice compared with the center. The slice thickness is usually defined by the full width half maximum (FWHM) value of the excitation. By definition, a portion of the excitation and signal will lie outside the described slice thickness. If contiguous slices are attempted, the "tails" of the excitation outside the FWHM slice thickness will overlap and saturate the signal. This problem is reduced by the use of a "square" rf pulse, but since no rf pulse is perfectly square, it is not entirely eliminated. Some manufacturers interleaf slices so that the odd slices are excited and the gaps then filled with the even slices at $\frac{1}{2}$ TR. This technique reduces the signal saturation by adjacent slices, but the uneven signal contribution of the slice is not eliminated because the effective TR of the overlap is one half that of the non-overlapped region.

The selective 3DFT acquisition method is emerging as a means of solving some of the problems encountered with a 2DFT multislice acquisition when imaging small anatomic parts.[34–36] In 3DFT, slices are defined by phase-encoding gradients instead of the selective excitation used in 2D methods. The thinness of the slice is not limited by the gradient or excitation pulse bandwidth. Very thin slices are easily achieved by most commercial hardware. This method eliminates the slice gap and the signal fall-off toward the slice edge that are experienced in 2D methods. The S/N in the central slices is improved by more even tip angles across the slice. The overall S/N of the acquisition improves with the square root of the number of slices.

Pulse Sequence Selection

The optimal pulse sequence (see Chapters 7, 8, 74 and 100) will depend upon the clinical setting, the normal *T1* and *T2* relaxation times of the desired anatomy, and the acquisition method.

Much of the normal anatomy of the face, orbit, and temporomandibular joint will have short *T2*'s and moderate to short *T1*'s with the exception of the vitreous humor and aqueous humor of the eye.[37] The visualization of normal anatomy, therefore, will be best with a very short *TE* and shorter *TR*. Since most disease has a longer *T1* and *T2*, additional *N(H)* or *T2* weighted images may be necessary. A great deal of signal will be lost from normal tissue with short *T2* values (10 to 100 ms) if a short *TE* is not used. Many commercial instruments require a lengthening of the *TE* when very thin slices are requested with a 2D multislice acquisition. It is not necessary to lengthen the *TE* in thin-slice 3D acquisitions. Thin slices can be obtained by a 3D acquisition with a shortened *TE*.

Because of the generally shorter *T1* values of normal tissues in this area, *T1* weighted images require a shorter *TR* compared with a usual *T1* weighted brain scan. *TR* values in the range of 200 to 300 ms will enhance the *T1* contrast between fat, muscle, and fibrous tissue. Longer *TR* values will result in a substantial loss in contrast. When evaluating image contrast at a variety of *TR* settings, it is important to normalize the scan times. For example, a *TR* 200 scan employing five times the number of excitations as a *TR* 1000 scan would have the same scan time but may have much better contrast to noise value. If the same number of excitations are used, then the shorter scan time of the short *TR* examination will reduce the signal-to-noise ratio, which may result in poorer contrast-to-noise.

Short *TR* scans reduce the number of slices available per scan in 2D multislice techniques. For example, a *TR* 500, *TE* 30 examination with a duty cycle of 100 ms would provide a maximum of five slices. If the *TR* is decreased to 200, then only two slices could be obtained. If the duty cycle could be reduced to half, then twice the number of slices could be obtained. The number of slices available in a 3D acquisition is not limited by the *TR* or duty cycle of the gradients.

The manipulation of timing parameters for *T2* weighted images of this region requires some different considerations compared with other body parts. *T2* weighted images are often useful for enhancing tumors, abscesses, edema, or fluid collections with long *T2* values. The high signal often contributed by fat in the image can mask the *T2* weighted signals from the abnormal tissue. The high signal of fat is primarily due to its short *T1*. The *T1* weighting of the scan is reduced by a longer *TR*, resulting in a relatively lower signal from fat. The signal of the long *T2* structures can be increased relative to normal structures by increasing the *TE*. A *TE* 120, *TR* 2000 image will have moderate-signal fat compared with high-signal fluid or tumor. If a shorter *TR* (more *T1* weighting) is used, then a longer *TE* (more *T2* weighting) must be used to achieve similar contrast. Long *TR* sequences are efficiently produced by 2D multislice acquisitions. The scan times in 3D acquisitions are considerably longer with long *TR* sequences. A shorter *TR* and longer *TE* would be a more efficient sequence for *T2* weighted 3D acquisitions.

TEMPOROMANDIBULAR JOINT IMAGING

Pain and dysfunction of the temporomandibular joint (TMJ) is a common problem in the adult population. Up to an estimated 28 percent of the population of the United

States have some form of TMJ disease.[38,39] Internal derangements of the TMJ are a major cause of symptoms in this area.[40–42]

Because of the inherently high soft tissue contrast of MRI, superb anatomic definition of the TMJ is possible.[22,34,43–46] Early attempts to image the TMJ by MR were limited by a poor S/N ratio, resulting in low resolution and thick slices.[17] Recently, surface coils have been employed to improve the S/N for marked improvement in the definition of small parts, such as the TMJ. The slice thickness and resolution available from surface coil images allow reproducible visualization of TMJ anatomy in a clinical setting.[22,34] MRI is considered a very safe examination, since it uses no ionizing radiation and has no known biologic hazards.[47,48] In contrast, plain films and tomography cannot directly image the disc.[41,42,49,50] Arthrography provides indirect visualization of the disc, but there is associated morbidity with the procedure.[51–55] Pain is often experienced by patients undergoing arthrography. Symptoms can last for weeks, even when the study is performed by experienced radiologists.[55] The technical difficulty of TMJ arthrography can produce unsatisfactory results, especially when it is performed by inexperienced workers. CT can directly visualize the disc, but the definition of TMJ anatomy is frequently suboptimal compared with MR.[56–59] All x-ray–based methods have well-known biologic hazards.[60] These factors have contributed to the impact of MRI in the diagnosis of TMJ disorders. MRI is currently the method of choice for the evaluation of the TMJ at Baylor University Medical Center.

Physiology

The temporomandibular joint is a complex structure, having both rotation and translation movements. In the closed-mouth position the condyle and disc lie in the articular fossa with the posterior band of the disc lying at 12 o'clock relative to the mandibular condyle. With opening, the disc and condyle translate anteriorly, and the disc, attached to the condyle by the capsule, rotates on the condyle (Fig. 19–2).

An internal derangement of the TMJ usually implies abnormal disc position or morphology. Since the anterior band of the disc is attached to the superior belly of the lateral pterygoid muscle and opposed not by another muscle but by the elastic fibers of the bilaminar zone, discs are usually anteriorly or anteromedially displaced. In more minor internal derangements, the disc can be reduced with opening. The reduction of the disc often results in a click that can be observed on physical examination (Fig. 19–

**Normal TMJ
Articulating Relationship
During Opening Movement**

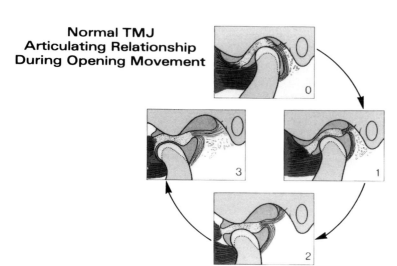

Figure 19–2. Normal TMJ articulating relationships. On the closed-mouth image (0), the posterior band of the disc lies at 12 o'clock relative to the mandibular condyle. The disc and condyle translate anteriorly on partial opening (1), the condyle translates anteriorly with further opening (2), and the disc rotates on the condyle to a position of maximum opening (3). (From Harms SE, Wilk RM: RadioGraphics 7: 521, 1987. Used by permission.)

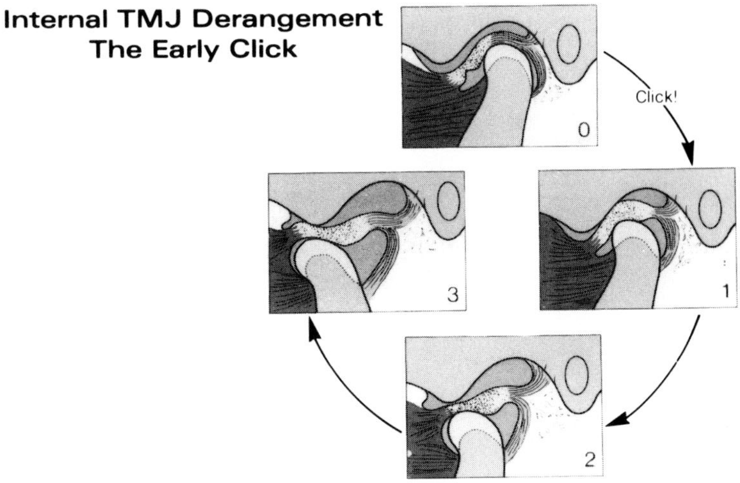

Internal TMJ Derangement
The Early Click

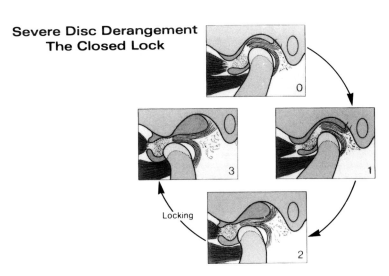

Figure 19–3. Mild internal derangement. The disc is anteriorly displaced on the closed-mouth view (0). On physical examination a click is noted with opening, in which the condyle translates under the anteriorly displaced disc and the disc is reduced (1, 2). At maximum opening, the condyle and disc have a normal position (3). (From Harms SE, Wilk RM: RadioGraphics. 7: 521, 1987. Used by permission.)

3). When the disc remains displaced even with opening, the internal derangement is considered more severe (Fig. 19–4). Perforations that are diagnosed by arthroscopy when contrast crosses into both upper and lower joint compartments are usually not disruptions of the disc itself but of the thin elastic tissue of the bilaminar zone. Perforations of the disc itself can rarely occur.

Anatomy

The mandibular condyle and articular eminence are recognized as high-intensity marrow surrounded by low-intensity cortical bone on *T1* or *N(H)* weighted images (Fig. 19–5). As described under the pulse sequence selection, *T2* weighted images are designed for enough *T2* weighting that fat has a moderate signal relative to high-signal fluid or edema. Normally there is no high-signal fluid around the TMJ on *T2* weighted images. The fibrocartilage of the articular disc has very low signal on current *T1*, *T2*, and *N(H)* weighted images owing to a very short *T2*. If *TE* values significantly shorter than *T2* were possible, disc signal could be observed, but currently this is not possible on most commercial imagers. The disc is divided into an anterior band, a posterior

Severe Disc Derangement
The Closed Lock

Figure 19–4. Severe internal derangement. For an example of a severe internal derangement, the disc is anteriorly displaced in the closed-mouth position (0) and remains displaced even with opening (1–3). The range of opening is limited because of the anteriorly displaced disc that is not reducing. On physical examination, this situation presents as a closed-locked joint. (From Harms SE, Wilk RM: RadioGraphics. 7: 521, 1987. Used by permission.)

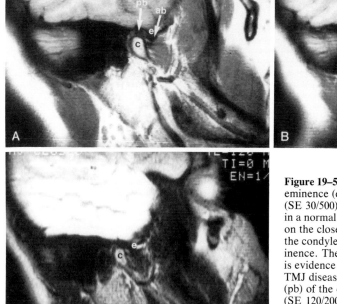

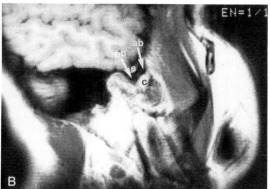

Figure 19–5. Normal disc. Fat within the condyle (c) and eminence (e) has high signal on the *T1* weighted images (SE 30/500). *A,* The posterior band (pb) of the disc lies in a normal position at 12 o'clock relative to the condyle on the closed-mouth view. *B,* On the open-mouth view, the condyle and disc translate anteriorly beyond the eminence. The marked anterior translation of the condyle is evidence of a hypermobile joint, which predisposes to TMJ disease. The anterior band (ab) and posterior band (pb) of the disc are labeled. *C,* The *T2* weighted images (SE 120/2000) show no evidence of high-signal fluid in the TMJ.

band, and a thin or intermediate zone lying between the two bands and representing the weight-bearing region of the disc. The anterior band of the disc is attached to the superior belly of the lateral pterygoid muscle. The posterior band of the disc is attached to the temporal bone by elastic fibers of the bilaminar zone or retrodiscal tissues. The inferior head of the lateral pterygoid muscle inserts on the condyle.

Pathology

Displaced discs of increasing severity are shown in Figures 19–6 to 19–8. A morphologically normal-appearing disc with mild displacement and reduction on opening

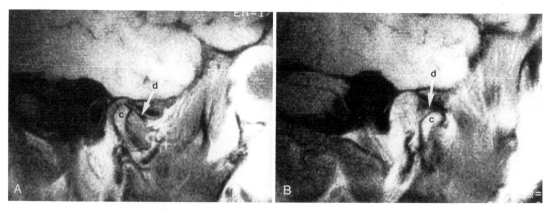

Figure 19–6. Anterior displacement with reduction. The disc (d) is anteriorly displaced on the closed-mouth view (*A*) and reduces with opening (*B*). The condyle (c) is labeled. (SE 30/500.)

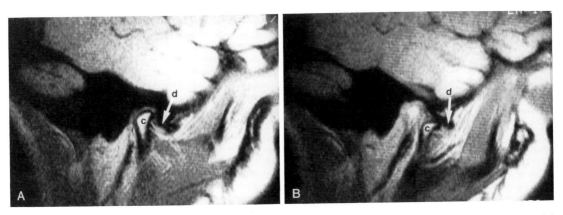

Figure 19–7. Anterior displacement without reduction. The disc (d) is anteriorly displaced on the closed-mouth view (A) and remains displaced on the open-mouth view (B). The condyle (c) is labeled. (SE 30/500.)

is usually treated conservatively. If symptoms do not fit with the imaging findings, further work-up may be necessary. Myositis, mastoiditis, intracerebral tumors, and bony metastases have been found in patients with TMJ-related symptoms. In these patients, the MR examination aided in reaching the correct diagnosis and spared the patient inappropriate management.

Discs that are more severely displaced or patients who have failed conservative management may require surgery. If the disc is not thickened or distorted, a plication procedure can be performed to salvage the disc and bring it into a more normal anatomic position. Follow-up MR scans are useful after plication, especially if new symptoms

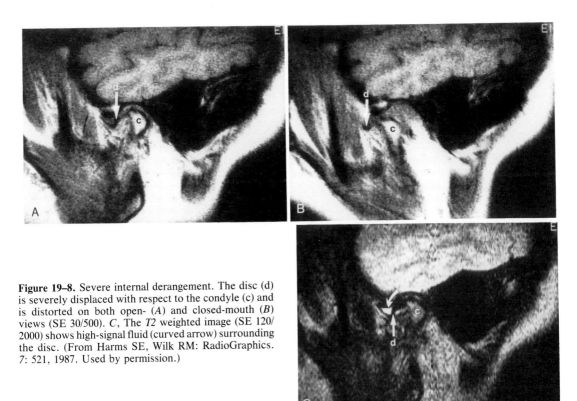

Figure 19–8. Severe internal derangement. The disc (d) is severely displaced with respect to the condyle (c) and is distorted on both open- (A) and closed-mouth (B) views (SE 30/500). C, The T2 weighted image (SE 120/2000) shows high-signal fluid (curved arrow) surrounding the disc. (From Harms SE, Wilk RM: RadioGraphics. 7: 521, 1987. Used by permission.)

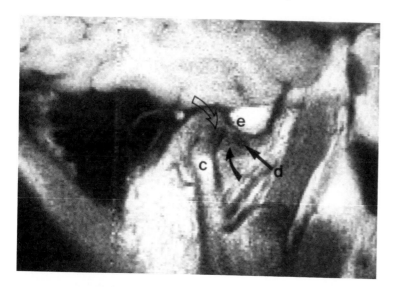

Figure 19–9. Adhesion. An adhesion (straight arrow) is visualized between the disc (d) and condyle (c). The eminence (e) and joint space soft tissue (curved arrow) are labeled. The condyle is sclerotic (open arrow). The disc moved with the condyle on open- and closed-mouth views. (From Harms SE, Wilk, RM, Wolford LM, et al: Radiology *157*: 133, 1985. Used by permission.)

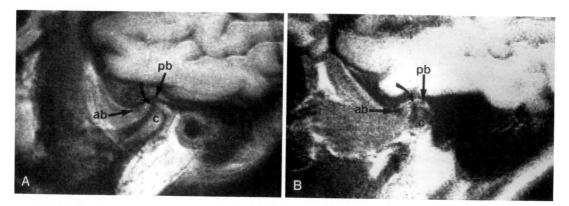

Figure 19–10. Disc perforation. An osteophyte (curved arrow) from the condyle (c) projects through a tear in the disc. The separated anterior band (ab) and posterior band (pb) of the disc are labeled on the medial (*A*) and lateral (*B*) images of the TMJ. (From Harms SE, Wilk RM, Wolford LM, et al: Radiology *157*: 133, 1985. Used by permission.)

develop, since adhesions are a common complication of this procedure. Adhesions are diagnosed by the direct visualization of low-signal fibrous bands or the absence of disc movement with respect to either the condyle or the eminence (Fig. 19–9).

Thickened or distorted discs have correlated with stiff or fragmented discs at surgery. Plication procedures usually are not used in these patients. Removal of the disc with insertion of a prosthetic implant is a common surgical approach. Before the advent of MRI of the TMJ, the preoperative evaluation of disc morphology for surgical planning purposes was difficult.

Severely displaced discs, degenerated discs, or perforated discs (Fig. 19–10) frequently require surgery for relief of symptoms. The physical examination findings may be confusing in these patients. MRI can provide the anatomic definition of the problem that is needed for proper clinical management.

ORBITAL IMAGING

MR has certain inherent advantages over CT in orbital imaging. MR avoids the use of ionizing radiation and the well-known hazards of radiation exposure to the lens.[60]

Multiplanar imaging of the orbit is almost a necessity for anatomic definition of orbital lesions. The direct acquisition of planes other than axial by MRI improves the diagnostic effectiveness of the examination. Beam-hardening artifacts often cause problems in orbital CT studies, particularly in the coronal plane where metal dental fillings are present.

The advent of surface coils has made MRI of orbit competitive with CT in terms of resolution.[19,20] Selective 3D acquisitions produce high-resolution, thin-slice images without gaps between the slices. These factors make MRI a superb method for defining orbital anatomy.[61] Recent reports indicate that MRI provides improved specificity for certain orbital lesions.[19,61–63]

Anatomy

T1 and *T2* weighted images are shown in Figure 19–11. With *T1* weighting, the orbital fat has high signal because of the short *T1* of fat. The vitreous humor and aqueous humor have low signal because of the long *T1* of fluid. Extraocular muscles have moderate signal. The retina and choroid have higher signal than sclera. Cortical bone has low signal on *T1*, *T2*, and *N(H)* weighted images because of a short *T2* and low *N(H)*.

For *T2* weighting, we prefer an image with enough *T2* weighting and reduced *T1* weighting to lower the relative signal of fat compared with fluid so that tumors in the orbital fat will not be lost in the high-signal fat. At 0.6 tesla, timing parameters of *TE* 120 and *TR* 2000 will result in sufficient *T2* weighting that fat signal is moderated. Tumors are then enhanced compared with surrounding orbital fat because of a generally longer *T2*. A shorter *TR* or *TE* would increase the signal from fat, and some tumors could be masked. If a shorter *TR* is desired, a longer *TE* can be used. The vitreous and aqueous humors have very high signal on a *TE* 120, *TR* 2000 scan. Muscle has very low signal because of a short *T2*.

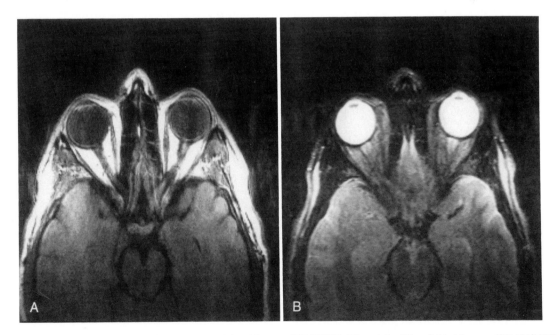

Figure 19–11. Normal orbital MRI. The *T1* weighted images (SE 30/500) (*A*) and the *T2* weighted images (SE 120/2000) (*B*) demonstrate the relative increase in fluid signal and relative decrease in fat signal (*T2* weighting compared with *T1* weighting).

Less contrast is seen on N(H) weighted images. The muscle has a moderate signal because the TE is short, resulting in less signal loss due to T2. Vitreous humor has higher signal compared with T1 weighted images because the longer TR results in less signal loss due to T1 weighting. Fat has the highest signal, but the contrast is not as great as on the T1 weighted images.

Pathology

Orbital pathology can usually be divided according to the site of origin of the lesion. The three anatomic regions are ocular, extraconal, and intraconal. Extraconal and intraconal refer to lesions outside or inside the extraocular muscles, respectively. The differential diagnosis is principally determined by most imaging methods on anatomic grounds. MRI signal intensities can provide additional help in differentiating certain lesions.

EXTRACONAL LESIONS

Extraconal lesions originate from tissues outside the extraocular muscles, such as the lacrimal gland, skin, bone, and paranasal sinuses. Lacrimal gland tumors comprise dermoid, epidermoid, carcinoma, adenocarcinoma, adenocystic carcinoma, and pleomorphic adenoma. Lesions involving the sinuses include mucocele, bacterial abscess, mucormycosis, and carcinoma. Bone tumors can involve the orbit, particularly osteomas in patients with Gardner's syndrome.

Magnetic resonance can aid in the differential diagnosis of extraconal lesions. Table 19–1 lists a variety of extraconal lesions and their relative signal intensities on T1, T2, and N(H) weighted images.

Dermoid cysts have a characteristic appearance on MRI. These lesions frequently have fluid-fluid levels that can be seen on MRI but not on CT. Because of the high fat content of these lesions, high signal is seen on the T1 weighted images from the higher level fluid that has moderate signal on T2 weighted images. The lower level fluid has lower signal than fat on the T1 weighted images but high signal on the T2 weighted images because of a higher fluid content.[19]

Because of their high protein content, mucoceles have homogeneous high signal on T1, T2, and N(H) weighted examinations (Fig. 19–12). Subacute hemorrhage also can have high signal on all images but is typically less homogeneous.[19,61]

Epidermoids can be distinguished from most other tumors because of the tendency to nearly follow fluid signal intensity. These tumors, like most other tumors, have low

Table 19–1. EXTRACONAL LESIONS

Lesion	T1*	T2*	N(H)*
Carcinoma	L	H	H
Lymphoma	L	H	H
Hemangioma	L	H	H
Epidermoid	L	H	M
Encephalocele	L	H	M–L
Lipoma	H	M	H
Dermoid†	H/M	M/H	H/M
Tolosa-Hunt syndrome	L	L	L
Hemorrhage (subacute)	H	H	H
Mucocele	H	H	H

* Low (L), moderate (M), or high (H) signal relative to surroundings.
† Nondependent/dependent levels.

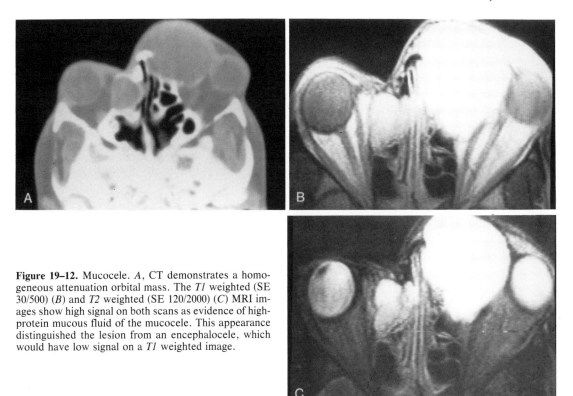

Figure 19–12. Mucocele. *A*, CT demonstrates a homogeneous attenuation orbital mass. The *T1* weighted (SE 30/500) (*B*) and *T2* weighted (SE 120/2000) (*C*) MRI images show high signal on both scans as evidence of high-protein mucous fluid of the mucocele. This appearance distinguished the lesion from an encephalocele, which would have low signal on a *T1* weighted image.

signal on *T1* weighted images and high signal on *T2* weighted images. On *N(H)* weighted images and crossover images in which fluid and brain are isointense (*TE* 60, *TR* 2000 at 0.6 tesla), most tumors have higher signal than fluid, but epidermoids are almost isointense. The easiest way to examine these patients is to use a multiecho sequence in which the first echo is *N(H)* weighted and each additional echo provides additional *T2* weighting. The middle echoes through the crossover between fluid and brain will be most helpful, since most other tumors will have considerably higher signal than fluid or brain on these images.[61]

Encephaloceles have homogeneous signal exactly matching CSF fluid signal in almost all cases.

Lipomas have homogeneous fat signal. Fat has high signal on *T1* and *N(H)* weighted images and moderate signal on *T2* weighted images. Low-grade liposarcomas have been difficult to differentiate from lipomas. Higher grade liposarcomas, however, are usually not difficult to separate from lipomas in terms of signal intensity.

Tolosa-Hunt syndrome is a rare granulomatous disease, pathologically similar to orbital pseudotumor, that involves the superior orbital fissure and cavernous sinus. The disease produces painful ophthalmoplegia, a symptom that should alert the clinician to the possibility of its presence. This lesion has low signal on *T1*, *T2*, and *N(H)* weighted images.

Most other tumors have low signal on *T1* weighted images and high signal on *T2* and *N(H)* weighted images. Hemangiomas are usually well-defined, localized, homogeneous masses without evidence of local invasion. Carcinomas of this region typically arise from the skin (like basal cell carcinoma) or lacrimal gland (carcinoma, adenocarcinoma, or adenocystic carcinoma). Carcinomas usually are poorly circumscribed and, if large enough, have mixed signal intensities. Evidence of invasion of surrounding tissues and edema may be helpful signs in distinguishing these lesions from the more well-defined hemangiomas.[19,61,62]

INTRACONAL LESIONS

The signal intensities of a variety of intraconal lesions are outlined in Table 19–2.

The most common intraconal lesion not involving the optic nerve is a hemangioma (Fig. 19–13). Hemangiomas have homogeneous low signal on *T1* weighted images and high signal on *T2* weighted images. Hemangiomas are well-circumscribed lesions that produce a mass effect but do not invade adjacent structures. Lymphoma has a similar homogeneous low signal on *T1* weighted images, with high signal on *T2* weighted images. Lymphomas (Fig. 19–14) are usually poorly circumscribed and invade adjacent structures. Carcinomas and sarcomas (rhabdomyosarcoma) can be similar to lymphomas but are usually less homogeneous.

Optic gliomas occur with a peak incidence at age four to six years. They typically have homogeneous low signal on *T1* weighted images and high signal on *T2* weighted images. The high-contrast lesion can be separated from the normal optic nerve by MRI. The exact definition of the mass is more difficult on CT because of reduced contrast. The tumor involves the optic nerve and sometimes extends into the chiasm and brain parenchyma. The ability of MR to define the abnormal signal is very useful in staging this lesion. Optic neuritis secondary to a demyelinating disease, such as multiple sclerosis, or secondary to radiation has similar signal intensities on both *T1* and *T2* weighted images, but a focal mass lesion is not usually associated with these entities.[19,61,62]

A number of intraconal lesions have low-signal *T2* weighted images. Meningiomas have signal intensities that nearly follow brain on all images or have lower signal than brain on all images. Meningiomas can arise from the optic nerve sheath, but some have no dural attachment or extend from adjacent intracranial meningiomas. Meningiomas can be differentiated from optic gliomas, which have high signal on *T2* weighted images. Meningiomas also usually occur in an older age group than do optic gliomas.

Orbital pseudotumors (Fig. 19–15) can be distinguished from most orbital tumors, since the chronic inflammatory changes of orbital pseudotumor result in low signal on *T1* and *T2* weighted images.[19,61]

Endocrine ophthalmopathy (Grave's disease) also has low signal on both *T1* and *T2* weighted images (Fig. 19–16). It is important to distinguish these entities from a malignancy such as lymphoma or rhabdomyosarcoma, which has high signal on *T2* weighted images.

Table 19–2. INTRACONAL LESIONS

Lesion	T1*	T2*
AVM	L	L
Meningioma	L–M	L
Pseudotumor	L	L
Endocrine	L	L
Hemangioma	L	H
Lymphoma	L	H
Metastases	L	H
Neuroma	L	H
Optic neuritis	L	H
Hemorrhage (subacute)	H	H
Lipoma	H	M

* Low (L), moderate (M), or high (H) signal relative to surroundings.

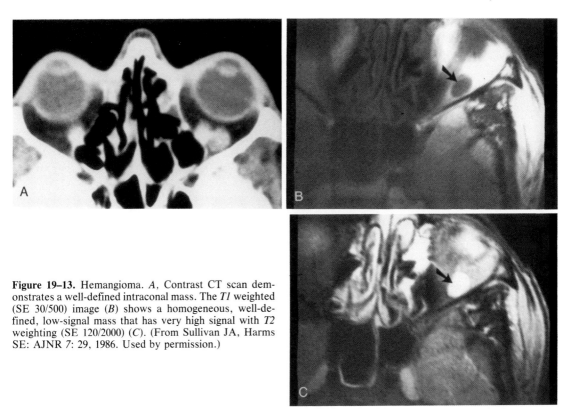

Figure 19–13. Hemangioma. *A,* Contrast CT scan demonstrates a well-defined intraconal mass. The *T1* weighted (SE 30/500) image (*B*) shows a homogeneous, well-defined, low-signal mass that has very high signal with *T2* weighting (SE 120/2000) (*C*). (From Sullivan JA, Harms SE: AJNR 7: 29, 1986. Used by permission.)

Arteriovenous malformations (AVMs) have low signal on both *T1* and *T2* weighted images owing to the signal void of the rapidly flowing blood. The ropelike appearance of the vascular malformation distinguishes it from other low-signal lesions such as pseudotumor and Grave's disease.[19,61]

Hemorrhage usually secondary to trauma can occur in the intraconal region. Subacute hemorrhage has high signal on both *T1* and *T2* weighted images.

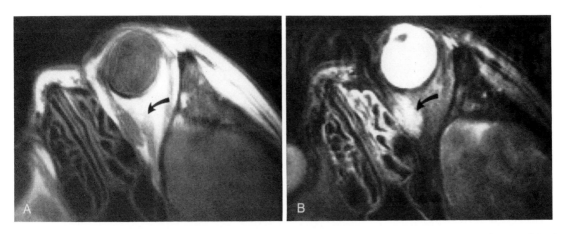

Figure 19–14. Lymphocytic lymphoma. The medial rectus muscle is enlarged by low-signal lymphoma on the *T1* weighted image (SE 30/500) (*A*). Lymphoma enhances on the *T2* weighted images (SE 120/2000) (*B*). (From Sullivan JA, Harms SE: AJNR 7: 29, 1986. Used by permission.)

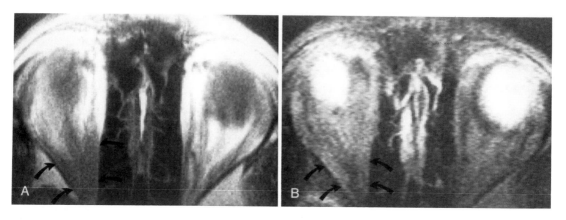

Figure 19–15. Orbital pseudotumor. Orbital pseudotumors (arrows) have low signal on both *T1* weighted (SE 30/500) (*A*) and *T2* weighted (SE 30/500) (*B*) images.

OCULAR LESIONS

MRI can provide very useful diagnostic information about a variety of ocular lesions (Table 19–3).

In the adult population, the most common primary ocular tumor by far is melanoma. Melanoma has high signal on *T1* weighted images and low signal on *T2* weighted images (Fig. 19–17). The signal appearance is dramatically different from that of most other tumors. The short *T1* and *T2* is presumably due to the paramagnetic relaxation enhancement effect of the stable free radicals with melanin. Melanomas are usually associated with a high-signal subretinal effusion on *T1* and *T2* weighted images. This subretinal effusion may obscure the lesion from ophthalmoscopic examination. Early reports indicating high signal from melanoma on *T2* weighted images may reflect the inability to separate the tumor mass from the subretinal effusion on the thick slices. It is important to have the ability to achieve thin slices in order to resolve the small melanoma lesions within the larger subretinal effusion. The cure rate is substantially lower for melanomas that extend beyond the globe.[65] Clinically the major differential diagnosis for primary melanoma is choroidal metastases. Most metastatic carcinomas have low signal on *T1* weighted images and high signal on *T2* weighted images. These lesions can also have a retinal detachment and a large subretinal effusion, which in our experience has a similar appearance to the subretinal effusions of melanoma. Resolution

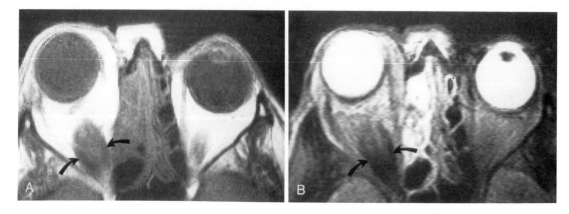

Figure 19–16. Endocrine ophthalmopathy. This patient with Graves' disease shows enlargement of the inferior rectus muscle by a low-signal process on both *T1* weighted (SE 30/500) (*A*) and *T2* weighted (SE 120/2000) (*B*) images.

Table 19–3. OCULAR LESIONS

Lesion	T1*	T2*
Retinoblastoma	H	L
Melanoma	H	L
Coats' disease	H	H
PHPV	H	H
Hemorrhage (subacute)	H	H
Metastases	L	H
Phthisis bulbi	L	L
Posterior scleritis	L	L

* Low (L), moderate (M), or high (H) signal relative to surroundings.

of the mass itself has to be done before a diagnosis based on signal intensities can be made. With melanomas, the lesion is seen as a dark spot surrounded by high-signal subretinal effusion on the *T2* weighted images. On the *T1* weighted images the melanoma is isointense with the high-signal subretinal effusion. Carcinomas, on the other hand, present as low-signal masses surrounded by high-signal effusion on the *T1* weighted images and are nearly isointense with the high-signal subretinal effusion on the *T2* weighted images.[61,63] These lesions are important to distinguish because melanomas confined to the globe should be treated by enucleation, whereas patients with carcinomas would not benefit from enucleation.

In childhood the ocular lesion of primary concern is retinoblastoma. Staging of

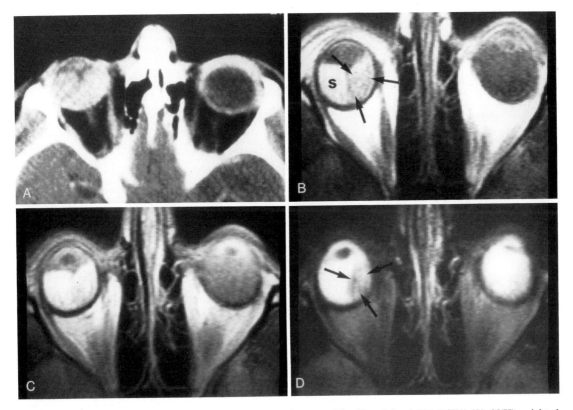

Figure 19–17. Melanoma. *A,* CT scan shows a large intraocular mass. The *T1* weighted (SE 30/500) (*B*), N(H) weighted (SE 30/1000) (*C*), and *T2* weighted (SE 120/2000) (*D*) images show the melanoma (arrows) best as a low-signal mass on the *T2* weighted images. The mass can be difficult to separate from the high-signal subretinal effusion on the *T1* and N(H) weighted images. (From Sullivan JA, Harms SE: AJNR 7: 29, 1986. Used by permission.)

this lesion is important, since tumors confined to the globe have a cure rate approaching 90 percent. Once the lesion extends beyond the globe, the cure rate drops to below 20 percent.[66,67] In addition, bilateral tumors are relatively common. MRI provides excellent contrast between the tumor and the adjacent normal structures for accurate staging. Like melanoma, retinoblastomas have high signal on *T1* weighted images and low signal on *T2* weighted images (Fig. 19–18). These lesions are often associated with retinal detachments and proteinaceous subretinal effusions that have homogeneous high signal on *T1* and *T2* weighted images. Retinoblastomas are treated quickly and aggressively with enucleation and/or radiation therapy.

Several rare lesions can mimic retinoblastoma. These lesions include Coats' disease, toxocariasis, and persistent hyperplastic primary vitreous. Because the diagnosis of retinoblastoma often mandates a rapid enucleation, accurate distinction between retinoblastoma and potential look-alike lesions is important. Thin sections without slice gaps are often necessary in correctly evaluating the child with an ocular mass. Currently, we prefer a 1.6 mm slice 3D acquisition.

Coats' disease is a primary retinal anomaly characterized by telangiectasia of the retina with a lipoproteinaceous exudate in the retina and subretinal space.[68] Coats' disease has homogeneous high signal on both *T1* and *T2* weighted images. It presents in similar-aged patients as retinoblastoma and can look like a necrotic retinoblastoma by ophthalmic sonography. Coats' disease can be treated by laser therapy, with preservation of vision.

Persistent hyperplastic primary vitreous (PHPV) is a congenital, frequently uni-

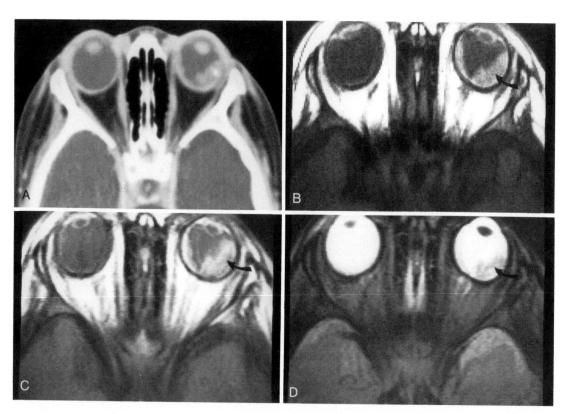

Figure 19–18. Retinoblastoma. *A,* The retinoblastoma and associated calcifications are seen on the CT scan. The lesion itself (curved arrow) is difficult to separate from the high-signal subretinal effusion on the *T1* weighted (SE 30/500) (*B*) and N(H) weighted (SE 30/1000) (*C*) images but is easily defined as a low-signal mass surrounded by high-signal subretinal effusion on the *T2* weighted (SE 120/2000) (*D*) images. (From Sullivan JA, Harms SE: AJNR 7: 29, 1986. Used by permission.)

lateral disorder related to a persistence and hyperplasia of the embryonic hyaloid vascular system.[69] PHPV is usually noticed at birth or during infancy, whereas retinoblastoma is usually diagnosed later. In PHPV the globe is smaller than the opposite normal globe and is filled with high-signal hemorrhage on both *T1* and *T2* weighted images. Fluid levels may sometimes be present.

Chronic inflammatory processes such as phthisis bulbi and posterior scleritis have low signal on both *T1* and *T2* weighted images.

Subacute hemorrhage has high signal on both *T1* and *T2* weighted images. Unlike Coats' disease, hemorrhage is usually not homogeneous.[19,61]

FACIAL IMAGING

Initially, the use of MRI in the evaluation of diseases involving the face did not appear promising for several reasons. Cortical bone produces little signal and small bony defects or erosions could not be visualized. Early machines did not provide thin sections or high-resolution imaging capability. The motion of facial structures posed a significant problem, especially with the longer scan times of early instruments.

The advent of surface coils and high-resolution imaging with reasonable scan times makes facial imaging much more attractive. The muscles and surrounding fat provide excellent soft tissue anatomy. The salivary glands and their ducts are well visualized as different signal from adjacent soft tissues. Even small vessels can be defined because of the high contrast resulting from the flow void of moving blood.[70]

Pathology

Unfortunately, most squamous cell carcinomas of the head and neck region do not produce the dramatic contrast typically seen on MRI scans of brain tumors. Squamous cell carcinoma typically has moderate signal on *T2* weighted images and is best defined on an anatomic basis rather than by signal differences alone.

Arteriovenous malformations have a characteristic appearance of a tangle of low-intensity vessels on *T1*, *T2*, and *N(H)* weighted images. AVMs can be differentiated from other tumors that have more signal on *N(H)* and *T2* weighted images.

MRI may provide useful information on mandibular tumors. The medullary extent of many mandibular tumors is difficult to assess on conventional imaging studies. The high-signal marrow fat provides excellent contrast on *T1* weighted images with a typically lower signal tumor. Accurate staging is essential for correct surgical planning. In Figure 19–19, a mandibular fibromyxoma staged with MRI defines an unaffected mandibular condyle that can be used to form a functional mandibular prosthesis. If the condyle were removed at surgery, preservation of normal function would have been difficult.

The diagnosis of salivary gland disorders should become a useful area for MRI application. Excellent soft tissue contrast and multiplanar imaging capability are advantageous. There is potential for distinguishing a variety of lesions involving the salivary glands on the basis of anatomy and signal intensity changes. Sarcoid typically does not have high signal on *T2* weighted images. Lymphoma and most metastatic lesions (not including squamous cell carcinoma) have high signal on *T2* weighted images. There is potential for differentiating acute inflammation from chronic inflammatory and autoimmune diseases.

The paranasal sinuses and their mucoperiosteal lining are well seen by MRI. Since the sinuses are also well seen on radiographs, the routine use of MRI for sinus disease

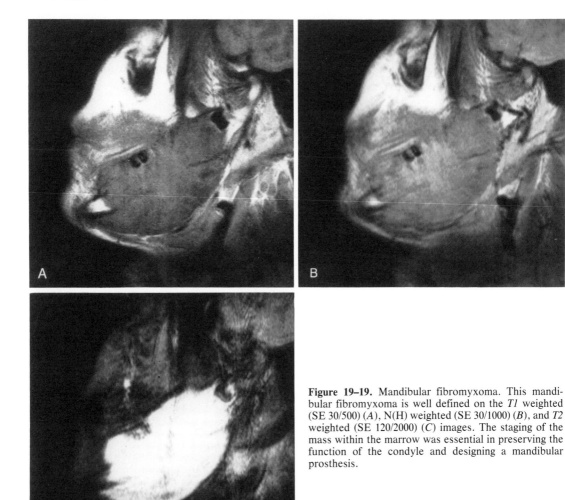

Figure 19–19. Mandibular fibromyxoma. This mandibular fibromyxoma is well defined on the *T1* weighted (SE 30/500) (*A*), N(H) weighted (SE 30/1000) (*B*), and *T2* weighted (SE 120/2000) (*C*) images. The staging of the mass within the marrow was essential in preserving the function of the condyle and designing a mandibular prosthesis.

is not expected. MRI can provide useful information, however, in certain clinical circumstances. Mucus retention cysts and mucoceles (see Fig. 19–12) often have very proteinaceous fluid that has high signal on both *T1* and *T2* weighted images. Other cysts and polyps do not have high signal on *T1* weighted images. Cholesteatomas usually nearly follow CSF in signal intensity and can be distinguished from most other tumors on the *N(H)* weighted or crossover images. Fibrous dysplasia, osteomas, ossifying fibroma, osteoblastoma, and Paget's disease have low signal on both *T1* and *T2* weighted images. Chronic granulomatous diseases, such as sarcoid, typically do not enhance on *T2* weighted images. Most squamous cell carcinomas, unfortunately, do not enhance on *T2* weighted images. Metastatic disease and lymphoma usually have high signal on *T2* weighted images. Meningiomas tend to follow brain signal on all images. Traumatic injuries are usually best examined by radiographs or CT, in which better bone definition is provided.

The soft tissue contrast has been used to produce excellent anatomic detail of the tongue and oral cavity.[71] Intrinsic disease of the tongue could potentially be defined more accurately by MRI.

Conclusion

MRI has made tremendous progress toward imaging facial disorders in the last few years, with the availability of commercial surface coils. Acquisition methods such as selective 3D imaging and square-pulse 2D imaging are further improving image quality. Scan times are being reduced by higher S/N systems. The hybrid echo planar[72] and 3D multislab[73] acquisition methods should considerably reduce the scan time and the associated motion artifacts. New pulse sequences such as FLASH[74] and STEAM[75] can be implemented to shorten the acquisition time still further. These advances are expected to broaden MRI applications in the facial region because of the critical link between scan time and motion-related artifacts. When the examination times are shortened, the improved patient throughput should result in lower costs per scan. MRI has the potential for replacing other imaging modalities in the routine evaluation of the facial region for most clinical diagnostic applications.

References

1. Randell CP, Collins AG, Young IR, Haywood R, Thomas DJ, McDonnell MJ, Orr JS, Bydder GM, Steiner RE: Nuclear magnetic resonance imaging of posterior fossa tumors. AJR *141*:489, 1983.
2. Crooks LE, Mills CM, Davis PL, Brant-Zawadzki M, Hoenninger J, Arakawa M, Watts J, Kaufman L: Visualization of cerebral and vascular abnormalities by NMR imaging: The effects of imaging parameters on contrast. Radiology *144*:843, 1982.
3. Bydder GM, Steiner RE, Young IR, Hall AS, Thomas DJ, Marshall J, Pallis CA, Legg NA: Clinical NMR imaging of the brain: 140 cases. AJR *139*:215, 1982.
4. Bydder GM, Pennock JM, Steiner RE, Orr JS, Bailes DR, Young IR: The NMR diagnosis of cerebral tumors. Magn Reson Med *1*:15, 1984.
5. Brant-Zawadzki M, Davis PL, Crooks LE, Mills CM, Norman D, Newton TH, Sheldon P, Kaufman L: NMR demonstration of cerebral abnormalities: Comparison with CT. AJR *140*:847, 1983.
6. Weinstein MA, Modic MT, Pavlicek W, Keyser CK: Nuclear magnetic resonance for the examination of brain tumors. Semin Roentgenol *19*:139, 1984.
7. Harms SE, Siemers PT, Hildenbrand P, Plum G: Multiple spin echo magnetic resonance imaging of the brain. RadioGraphics *1*:117, 1986.
8. Feinberg DA, Mills CM, Posin JP, Ortendahl DA, Hylton NM, Crooks LE, Watts JC, Kaufman L, Arakawa M, Hoenninger JC, Brant-Zawadzki M: Multiple spin echo magnetic resonance. Radiology *155*:437, 1985.
9. Li KC, Poon PY, Hinton P, Willinsky R, Pavlin CJ, Hurwitz JJ, Buncic JR, Henkelman RM: MR imaging of orbital tumors with CT and ultrasound correlations. J Comput Assist Tomogr *8*(6):1039, 1984.
10. Hawkes RC, Holland GN, Moore WS, Rizk S, Worthington BS, Kean DM: NMR imaging in the evaluation of orbital tumors. AJNR *4*:254, 1983.
11. Han JS, Benson JE, Bonstelle CT, Alfidi RJ, Kaufman B, Levine M: Magnetic resonance imaging of the orbit: A preliminary experience. Radiology *150*:755, 1984.
12. Sobel DF, Kelly W, Kjos BO, Char D, Brant-Zawadzki M, Normal D: MR imaging of orbital and ocular disease. AJNR *6*:259, 1985.
13. Edward JH, Hyman RA, Vacirca SJ, Boxer MA, Packer S, Kaufman IH, Stein HL: 0.6T magnetic resonance imaging of the orbit. AJNR *6*:253, 1985.
14. Sobel DF, Mills C, Char D, Norman D, Brant-Zawadzki M, Kaufman L, Crooks L: NMR of the normal and pathologic eye and orbit. AJNR *5*:345, 1984.
15. Moseley I, Brant-Zawadzki M, Mills C: Nuclear magnetic resonance imaging of the orbit. Br J Ophthalmol *67*:333, 1983.
16. Dillon WP, Mills CM, Kjos B, DeGroot J, Brant-Zawadzki M: Magnetic resonance imaging of the nasopharynx. Radiology *152*:731, 1984.
17. Harms SE, Kramer DM: Fundamentals of magnetic resonance imaging. CRC Crit Rev Diagn Imag *25*:1:79, 1985.
18. Lufkin RB, Larsson SG, Hanafee WN: Work in progress: NMR anatomy of the larynx and tongue base. Radiology *148*:173, 1983.
19. Sullivan JA, Harms SE: Surface coil MR imaging of orbital neoplasms. AJNR *7*:29, 1986.
20. Schenck JF, Hart HR, Foster TH, et al: Improved MR imaging of the orbit at 1.5T with surface coils. AJNR *6*:193, 1985.
21. Schenck JF, Foster TH, Henkes JL, et al: High-field surface-coil MR imaging of localized anatomy. AJNR *6*:181, 1985.
22. Harms SE, Wilk RM, Wolford LM, Chiles DG, Milam SB: The temporomandibular joint: Magnetic resonance imaging using surface coils. Radiology *157*:133, 1985.

23. Lufkin RB, Hanatee WN: Application of surface coils to MR anatomy of the larynx. AJR *145*:483, 1985.
24. Harms SE, Kramer DM: Fundamentals of magnetic resonance imaging. CRC Crit Rev Diagn Imag *25*:79, 1985.
25. Fullerton GD: Basic concepts for nuclear magnetic resonance imaging. Magn Reson Imag *1*:39, 1982.
26. Hoult DI: An Overview of NMR in Medicine. Washington DC, National Center for Health Care Technology, DHEW, 1981.
27. Rosen BR, Brady TJ: Principles of nuclear magnetic resonance for medical application. Semin Nucl Med *13*:308, 1984.
28. Pykett IL: NMR imaging in medicine. Sci Am *246*:78, 1982.
29. Pykett IL, Newhouse JH, Buonanno FS, et al: Principles of nuclear magnetic resonance imaging. Radiology *143*:157, 1982.
30. Kramer DM: Basic principles of magnetic resonance imaging. Radiol Clin North Am *22*:765, 1984.
31. Peterson SB, Muller RN, Rinck PA: An Introduction to Biomedical Nuclear Magnetic Resonance. New York, Thieme-Stratton, 1985.
32. Harms SE, Morgan TJ, Yamanashi WS, Harle TS, Dodd GD: Principles of nuclear magnetic resonance imaging. RadioGraphics *4*:26, 1984.
33. Crooks LE, Ortendahl PA, Kaufman L, et al: Clinical efficiency of nuclear magnetic resonance imaging. Radiology *146*:123, 1983.
34. Harms SE, Wilk RM: Magnetic resonance imaging of the temporomandibular joint. RadioGraphics. In press.
35. Harms SE, Wilk RM: Magnetic resonance of the temporomandibular joint. NMR update series. In press.
36. Harms SE, Kramer DM: Selective three-dimensional imaging of neurological disorders using a surface coil. Book of Abstracts, Society of Magnetic Resonance in Medicine, 1985, pp 359–360.
37. Beall PT, Amtey SR, Kasturi SR: NMR Data Handbook for Biomedical Applications. New York, Pergamon Press, 1984.
38. Guralnick W, Kaban LB, Merril RG: Temporomandibular joint afflictions. N Engl J Med *229*:123, 1978.
39. Solberg WK, Woo MW, Houston JB: Prevalence of mandibular dysfunction in young adults. J Am Dent Assoc *98*:25, 1979.
40. Bell WE: Clinical Management of Temporomandibular Joint Disorders. Chicago, Year Book Medical Publishers, 1982.
41. Helms CA, Katzberg RW, Dolwick MR (eds): Internal Derangements of the Temporomandibular Joint. San Francisco, Radiology Research and Education Foundation, 1983.
42. Katzberg RW, Keith DA, Guralnick WC, Manzione JV, Ten Eick WR: Internal derangements and arthritis of the temporomandibular joint. Radiology *146*:107, 1983.
43. Roberts D, Schenck J, Joseph P, Hart H, Pettigrew J, Kundel H, Edelstein WA, Foster T: Magnetic resonance imaging of temporomandibular joint tissues. Radiology *154*:829, 1985.
44. Katzberg RW, Schenck J, Roberts D, et al: Magnetic resonance imaging of the temporomandibular joint meniscus. Oral Surg Oral Med Oral Pathol *59*:4:332, 1985.
45. Katzberg RW, Bessette RW, Tallents RH, Plewes DB, Manzione JV, Schenck JF, Foster TH, Hart HR: Normal and abnormal temporomandibular joint: MR imaging with surface coil. Radiology *158*:183, 1986.
46. Harms SE, Wilk RM: Magnetic resonance imaging of the temporomandibular joint. RadioGraphics *7*:521, 1987.
47. Budinger TF, Cullander C: Health effects of in vivo nuclear magnetic resonance. *In* James TL, Margulis AR (eds): Biomedical Magnetic Resonance. San Francisco, Radiology Research and Education Foundation, 1984, pp 421–441.
48. Saunders RD, Smith H: Safety aspects of NMR clinical imaging. Br Med Bull *40*:148, 1984.
49. Campbell W: Clinical radiographic investigations of the temporomandibular joint. Br J Radiol *38*:401, 1964.
50. Stanson AW, Baker HL: Routine tomography of the temporomandibular joint. Radiol Clin North Am *14*:105, 1976.
51. Katzberg RW, Dolwick MF, Helms CA, Bales DJ, Coggs GC: Arthrotomography of the temporomandibular joint. AJR *134*:995, 1980.
52. Dolwick MF, Katzberg RW, Helms CA, Bales DJ: Arthrotomographic evaluation of the temporomandibular joint. J Oral Surg *37*:793, 1979.
53. Westesson PL: Double contrast arthrotomography of the temporomandibular joint. J Oral Maxillofac Surg *41*:163, 1983.
54. Blaschke DD, Solberg WK, Sanders B: Arthrography of the temporomandibular joint: review of current status. J Am Dent Assoc *100*:388, 1980.
55. Lydiatt D, Kaplan P, Tu H, Sleder P: Morbidity associated with temporomandibular joint arthrography in clinically normal joints. J Oral Maxillofac Surg *44*:8, 1986.
56. Helms CA, Morrish R, Kircos L, Katzberg RW, Dolwick MF: Computed tomography of the meniscus of the temporomandibular joint: preliminary observations. Radiology *145*:719, 1982.
57. Helms CA, Katzberg RW, Morrish R, Dolwick MF: Computed tomography of the temporomandibular joint meniscus. J Oral Maxillofac Surg *41*:512, 1983.
58. Manzione JV, Seltzer SE, Katzberg RW, Hammerschlag SB, Chiango BF: Direct sagittal computed tomography of the temporomandibular joint. AJR *140*:165, 1983.
59. Manzione JV, Katzberg RW, Brodsky GL, Seltzer SE, Mellins HZ: Internal derangements of the temporomandibular joint: diagnosis by direct sagittal computed tomography. Radiology *150*:111, 1984.
60. Hall EJ: Radiobiology for the Radiologist. New York, Harper & Row, 1978.

61. Sullivan JA, Harms SE: Characterization of orbital lesions by surface coil MR imaging. RadioGraphics. In press.
62. Bilaniuk LT, Schenck JF, Zimmerman RA, Hart HR, Foster TH, Edelstein WA, Goldberg HI, Grossman RI: Ocular and orbital lesions: surface coil MR imaging. Radiology *156*:669, 1985.
63. Peyster RG, Augsburger JJ, Shields JA, Satchell TV, Markoe AM, Clarke K, Haskin ME: Choroidal melanoma: comparison of CT, fundoscopy, and US. Radiology *156*:675, 1985
64. Glaser JS: Neuro-ophthalmology. New York, Harper & Row, 1978.
65. Hogan MJ: Clinical aspects, management, and prognosis of melanomas of the uvea and optic nerve. *In* Boniuk M (ed): Ocular and Adnexal Tumors: New and Controversial Aspects. St Louis, CV Mosby, 1964.
66. Brown DH: The clinicopathology of retinoblastoma. Am J Ophthalmol *61*:508, 1966.
67. Reese AB, Ellsworth RM: The evaluation and current concept of retinoblastoma therapy. Trans Am Acad Ophthalmol Otolaryngol *67*:164, 1963.
68. Sherman JL, McLean IW, Brallier DR: Coats' disease, CT-pathologic correlation in two cases. Radiology *146*:77, 1983.
69. Mafee MF, Goldberg MF, Valvassori GE, Capek V: Computed tomography in the evaluation of patients with persistent hyperplastic primary vitreous (PHPV). Radiology *145*:713, 1982.
70. Harms SE: Magnetic resonance imaging of neoplasms involving the head. Semin Surg Oncol *1*:188, 1985.
71. Unger JM: The oral cavity and tongue: magnetic resonance imaging. Radiology *155*:151, 1985.
72. Haacke EM, Bearden FH, Clayton JR, Linga NR: Reduction of MR imaging time by the hybrid fast-scan technique. Radiology *158*:521, 1986.
73. Kramer DM, Compton RA, Yeung HN: A volume (3D) analogue of 2D multislice or "multislab" MR imaging. Book of Abstracts, Society of Magnetic Resonance in Medicine, 1985, pp 162–163.
74. Frahm J, Hasse A, Matthari W: Rapid three-dimensional MR imaging using the FLASH technique. J Comput Assist Tomogr *10*:363, 1986.
75. Hasse A, Frahm J, Matthari W, Hanicke KD: Rapid images and NMR movies. Program of Society of Magnetic Resonance in Medicine, 1985, pp 980–981.

20

Malignant Lesions of the Paranasal Sinuses

B. G. ZIEDSES DES PLANTES
R. G. M. DE SLEGTE
G. J. GERRITSEN
M. SPERBER
J. VALK
M. C. KAISER
F. C. CREZEE

Among head and neck cancers, approximately 3 percent are tumors of the paranasal sinuses.[1,2] The diagnostic work-up of these tumors demands an assessment of the exact location of the tumor, the extension to adjacent areas, and the involvement of bony structures, such as the skull base, the walls of the sinuses, and the borders of the orbit. Conventional radiology, especially multidirectional tomography, was the method of choice in the pre–CT scan era. Conventional tomography has been helpful in establishing the presence of bone destruction and in showing the air-tissue contours of the lesion. However, tumors extending beyond the bony limits of the sinuses into the brain, the orbit, and neighboring soft tissues are often difficult to visualize by this method.[3] The application in recent years of high-resolution CT scanning led to a significant improvement in the depiction of anatomic details of the initial lesion, its extent, and the degree of bony and soft tissue involvement.[4,5] Areas previously insufficiently visualized, such as the infratemporal fossa and the parapharyngeal space, can be accurately shown by CT. However, there is often not enough soft tissue contrast in these areas to allow the demonstration of the borders between tumor and normal tissues.[6–8]

With the development of MRI a greater soft tissue contrast resolution has been achieved[9] combined with multiplanar imaging. Without the use of contrast material, vascular structures are easily identified and the solid component of a tumoral mass can be differentiated from mucosal swelling. In this chapter we will discuss the use of MRI in malignant lesions of the paranasal sinuses, with special attention to the choice of pulse sequences for optimal imaging. A description of various tumor extensions as visualized by MRI is also presented.

MRI TECHNIQUES

This chapter summarizes our experience in the study of the paranasal sinuses by MRI based on examination performed with a 0.6 tesla superconductive system.

Between April and November 1985, 17 patients with tumors of the paranasal sinuses were examined at our institution. In all patients the diagnosis was confirmed by biopsy and/or surgery. The histologic diagnosis is listed in Table 20–1. In all cases, high-resolution CT examinations performed in transverse and coronal planes were available for comparison.

Slice Direction

In the MRI examinations, transverse, coronal, and sagittal slices were used routinely. Transverse and coronal slices provided all the information needed in most cases. For the investigation of tumor extent to the anterior fossa, however, sagittal slices were obtained.

Pulse Sequence

The patients were studied with a series of pulse sequences, as follows:
Inversion recovery/spin echo (IR):
   TI 400, TR 1400, TE 30 ms (multiple slice)
Saturation recovery/spin echo (SE):
   TR 500, TE 30 and 60 ms (two echoes, multiple slice)
   TR 1500, TE 30 and 60 ms (two echoes, multiple slice)
   TR 2000, TE 30 to 240 ms (eight echoes, single slice)
This series runs in gradual steps from TI dependency (for IR: TI 400, TR 1400, TE 30 ms) to extreme $T2$ dependency (for SE: TR 2000, TE 240 ms). Some patients were also scanned with an SE sequence: TR 3000, TE 30 and 60 ms (multiple slice).

The TI dependent pulse sequences (such as IR: TI 400, TR 1400, TE 30) outlined the tumors in this region as dark areas. The signal strength was not sufficient for proper imaging of the anatomic details of the paranasal region. For this reason, we felt that IR was not the pulse sequence of choice in the examination of tumors of the paranasal area. Moderate TI dependent pulse sequences (such as SE: TR 500, TE 30 ms; and SE: TR 1500, TE 30 ms) usually outlined the investigated area. This group of pulse sequences permitted adequate differentiation between tumor, facial fat, and surrounding muscles in a short period of time (2 to 6 minutes). However, differentiation between tumor and mucosal swelling was not possible.

Changing to moderate $T2$ weighted pulse sequences (such as SE: TR 1500, TE 60 ms; and SE: TR 2000, TE 60 ms) resulted in relatively increased signal intensity compared with neighboring muscular structures. Consequently, the contrast between tumor and muscles improved. However, delineation of the tumor from the neighboring mucosal swelling requires heavily $T2$ dependent pulse sequences (Fig. 20–1). We obtained

Table 20–1. TUMORS OF THE PARANASAL SINUSES

Clinical Diagnosis	Number of Patients
Squamous cell carcinoma	4
Adenocarcinoma	3
Adenocystic carcinoma	3
Melanoma	2
Fibrosarcoma	1
Chondrosarcoma	1
Rhabdomyosarcoma	1
Malignant fibrous histiocytoma	1
Ameloblastoma	1

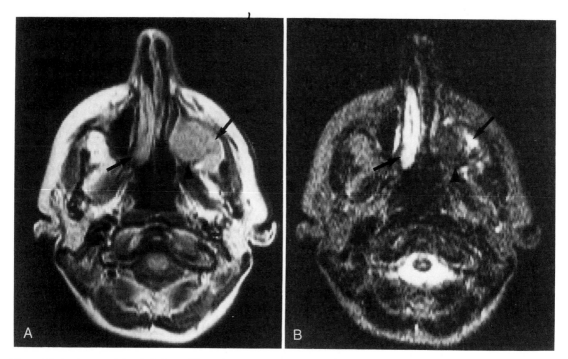

Figure 20–1. Tumor arising in left maxillary sinus. *A,* Spin-echo image: *TR* 2000, *TE* 30 ms. The tumor has the same signal intensity as the mucosal swelling. *B,* Spin-echo image: *TR* 2000, *TE* 240 ms. In this heavily weighted *T2* image, good contrast is obtained between mucosal swelling and tumor. The mucosal swelling is bright (arrows). The tumor is dark (arrowhead).

good results with SE: *TR* 2000, *TE* 180–240 ms. Delineation of tumor from arteries was, in our experience, hardly influenced by the choice of pulse sequence.

Other Parameters

The choice of other parameters, such as slice thickness, matrix size, number of signal averages, and rf coil, is directly related to the signal strength or to the signal-to-noise (S/N) ratio. There are two major factors to be taken into consideration when selecting the slice thickness. These are the partial volume averaging and the signal intensity of the image. The partial volume effect is less prominent when thin slices are used. The signal intensity is diminished with decreased slice thickness. Therefore, slice thickness seems to be the factor that determines both the presence or absence of partial volume effect and the signal intensity. In our series, the slice thickness varied between 0.4 and 1 cm.

Other parameters such as matrix size, number of signal averages, and rf coil selection depend on the spatial resolution desired, the maximum examination time, and the signal strength or the S/N ratio to be obtained. All these parameters are interdependent. We commonly used an acquisition matrix of 128 × 256, interpolated to a display matrix of 256 × 256. The signal was averaged two to four times. All these parameters are expected to change with future technical development.

Paramagnetic Contrast Media

The role of paramagnetic contrast media in the study of paranasal sinus lesions has not yet been established. One of the problems we have encountered is the massive enhancement of the mucosa together with enhancement of the tumor (in *T1* weighted images). For that reason, it was impossible to separate tumor from mucosal swelling. In our experience, heavily weighted *T2* images are superior in separating the mucosal swelling from tumor.

CARCINOMAS OF THE NOSE AND PARANASAL SINUSES

Squamous cell carcinomas account for 50 to 80 percent of all malignant neoplasms in the sinonasal tract.[2,11] The lesions originate from the respiratory mucosa. Endoscopic procedures are usually limited in their ability to determine the exact anatomic site of the tumor and its extension to adjacent areas. In the experience of our institution, 90 percent or more of these lesions have invaded adjacent bony structures before the diagnosis is made. Early diagnosis often is made difficult by the initial lesion's being masked by inflammatory disease or by location inaccessible to visual evaluation. Therefore, surgical procedures sometimes are required for diagnostic evaluation and biopsy.[2] Squamous cell carcinoma of the paranasal sinus is primarily a disease of men in the mid-50s and older. Metastases are reported in less than 25 percent of cases. The overall prognosis is nevertheless poor, owing to local aggressive behavior of the tumor with involvement of adjacent vital areas. A review of the literature supports a five-year survival rate of 10 to 30 percent for all varieties of squamous cell carcinoma.[11,12]

Adenocarcinomas represent the second most frequent malignant lesion of the sinonasal tract. They are characterized by a glandular or adenomatous architecture. The upper nasal cavity and the ethmoidal sinuses are the most common primary sites. Also, these lesions are usually first recognized as a result of destructive manifestations, and clinical evaluation may be problematic. To date the survival rate has not been adequately assessed. However, patients with poorly differentiated adenocarcinomas seem to have only a 20 percent five-year survival rate.[11]

Treatment of Carcinomatous Lesions

Squamous cell carcinomas and adenocarcinomas of the nose and paranasal sinuses are treated by radical surgery at the time of the initial diagnosis, if the lesion is found to be resectable. A less aggressive approach often leads to recurrence and eventually to additional mutilating surgery. Radiation therapy usually follows surgery. However, in most series, patients who are poor surgical risks or who have lesions too extensive for block resection are treated with radiation therapy alone.

The surgical treatment of choice for carcinomas confined to the antrum is total maxillectomy. Inferiorly located carcinomas of the maxillary sinus have the best chance for definitive cure. Lesions confined to the ethmoidal region are treated by local removal via lateral rhinotomy. Preoperative determination of tumor extent in both locations is of major importance in the selection of the surgical approach.

MISCELLANEOUS TUMORS

Other lesions, such as melanomas, malignant bone tumors, malignant lymphoepithelial tumors, and sarcomas are relatively rare.[2,10–12] Since a number of these rare tumors are present in our series, and the MRI findings have not been described, it seems appropriate to discuss some aspects of the MRI findings of these rare tumors.

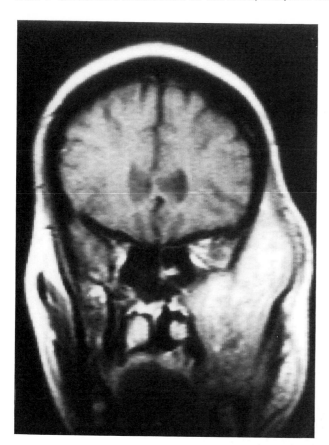

Figure 20–2. Fibrosarcoma originating from the infratemporal fossa. The tumor could be adequately delineated by MRI.

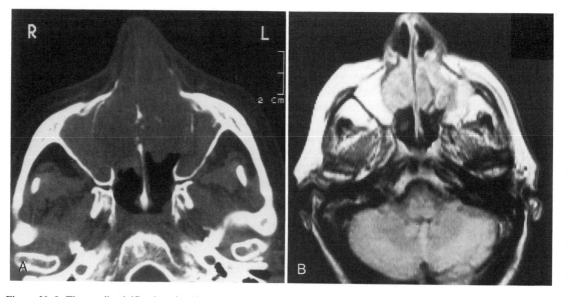

Figure 20–3. The small calcifications in this chondrosarcoma of the nose as demonstrated by CT (*A*) are not discernible on the MR image (*B*). Spin echo: *TR* 1500, *TE* 30 ms.

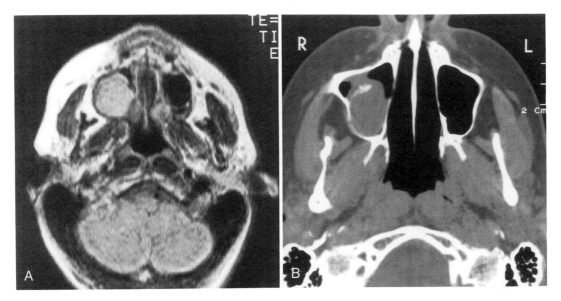

Figure 20–4. Involvement of the maxilla by an adenocystic carcinoma. *A,* MRI displays the relationship to the lateral pterygoid muscle. Spin-echo image: *TR* 1500, *TE* 60 ms. *C,* The bony destruction is well depicted by CT.

Case I is an 20-year-old female presenting with headache. Other than a slight soft tissue swelling at the right cheek, clinical examination revealed no abnormalities. The CT scan demonstrated a soft tissue swelling in the infratemporal fossa but, although the swelling was obvious, could not delineate a tumoral mass. However, the tumor, a fibrosarcoma, could be adequately outlined by MRI, owing to good contrast with surrounding soft tissues (Fig. 20–2). This case illustrates that tumors in the infratemporal fossa, such as this fibrosarcoma, can be present without clinical signs.

The presence of calcified material can be helpful in the differential diagnosis of a tumoral process, such as is demonstrated in Cases II and III.

Case II is a 68-year-old male in whom a chondrosarcoma of the nasal septum was diagnosed. The characteristic small amorphous parenchymal calcifications were demonstrated by CT. These calcifications were not reproducible with MRI. However, MRI provided better distinction between tumor and mucosal swelling (Fig. 20–3).

Case III is a 42-year-old female with an ameloblastoma. The rests of a dental element in the tumor could be visualized by CT, but MRI failed to demonstrate it (Fig. 20–4). CT is known to be superior for the purpose of demonstrating hyperdense material, such as calcifications or dental elements.

In general, for all these lesions, demonstration of the extension of the tumor is important for treatment planning, as in the previously described conditions. In the majority of cases, MRI could not provide clues for the histologic diagnosis.

MRI FINDINGS CONCERNING TUMOR EXTENSION

The majority of patients presenting in our hospital with tumors of the paranasal sinuses are beyond TNM Stages T1 and T2.[13] The resectability of the tumors in Stages T3 and T4 is dependent on the direction of the extension. For instance, extension into the pterygoid muscle is a contraindication to surgery, whereas extension into the cribriform plate or orbit still allows surgical resection. Therefore, extension according to the different levels, which will be described below, seems to be a more appropriate method for evaluation of tumor extent in Stages T3 and T4 tumors.

Level of the Maxillary Sinus

Caudal Extension. In case of tumor extension into the maxilla or the hard palate, a total maxillectomy has to be performed. Although invasion of the upper jaw or palatum is well demonstrated by MRI, the presence of ferromagnetic material is a source of disturbing artifacts (Fig. 20–5). Compared with CT, however, the MR image is not deteriorated by streak artifacts caused by nonferromagnetic dental elements and filling material (Fig. 20–6).

Anterior and Lateral Extension. If the lesion has broken through the anterior wall of the maxillary sinus, all soft tissues under the cutaneous cheek must be removed; occasionally the skin of the cheek must be included in the resected specimen. Therefore, extension into the soft tissues of the cheek results in surgical defects of the overlying facial skin and demands reconstructive surgical procedures. The lateral and anterior extensions can be well demonstrated by coronal and transverse MR images (Fig. 20–7).

Medial Extension. Tumor extension in a medial direction results in invasion of the nasal cavity and nasal septum. Although this type of tumor extension can be easily visualized by rhinoscopy, it is well demonstrated by MRI (Fig. 20–8).

Posterior Extension. Destruction of the posterior wall and extension beyond the pterygoid process and hamulus makes radical surgical treatment impossible. Although the anatomic landmark of the hamulus pterygoideus is not visualized on MRI, the soft tissue extension is clearly shown. Since erosion of the pterygoid process and hamulus is an indirect sign, and extension into the soft tissues as imaged by MRI is a direct sign, of tumor involvement, MRI seems to be a better method for assessment of extension into the pterygopalatine fossa and the infratemporal fossa (Fig. 20–9).

Tumors that extend posteriorly through the skull base have a poor prognosis.

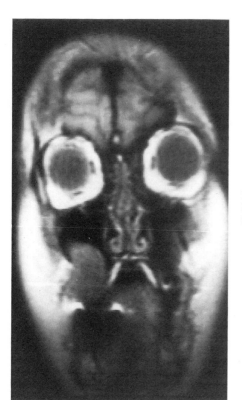

Figure 20–5. The MR image of the inferior part of the tumor is altered by artifacts caused by neighboring ferromagnetic material. Spin-echo image: *TR* 1500, *TE* 30 ms.

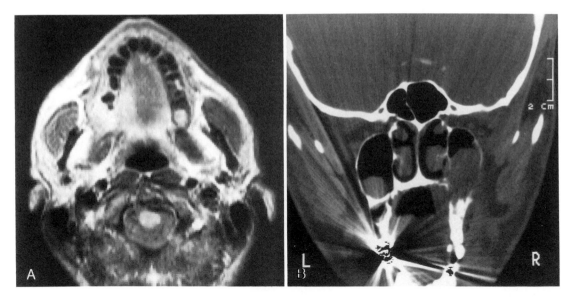

Figure 20–6. MR image at the level of dental elements. There are no disturbing artifacts at this level. *A,* Spin-echo image: *TR* 1500, *TE* 30 ms. *B,* Direct coronal CT section of the same patient. The high-density material in the teeth causes streak artifacts.

Surgery in these cases is not the treatment of choice. Cancellous bone is imaged by MRI as a low signal intensity area and, as a result, is hard to visualize. However, by direct visualization of tumor extent, invasion into the skull base can be determined. In cases of involvement of structures containing bone marrow, such as the clivus, the high signal intensity of bone marrow will permit accurate imaging (Fig. 20–10). However, in the early stages of tumor protrusion through the skull base, it appears that CT is the investigative method of choice, since even small defects in the skull base can be identified (Fig. 20–11). At times, direct extension through the skull base into the middle cranial fossa can raise a false suspicion of the presence of a primary brain tumor or

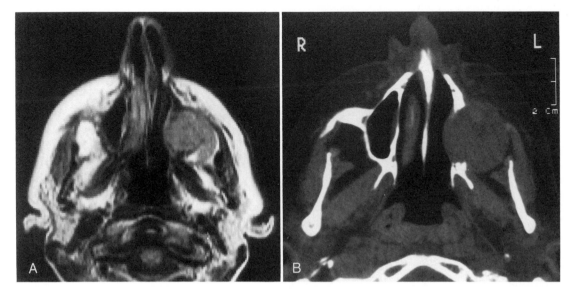

Figure 20–7. The lateral extension of this malignant fibrous histiosarcoma to the subcutaneous soft tissue is well depicted by (*A*) MRI (spin-echo image: *TR* 1500, *TE* 30 ms) and (*B*) CT.

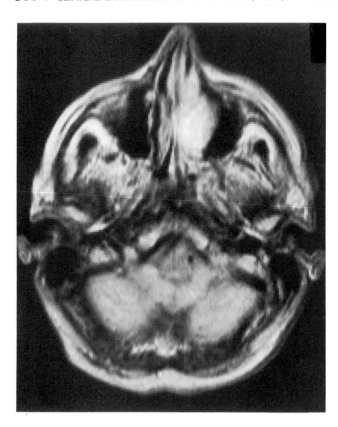

Figure 20–8. Extension of the tumor (malignant melanoma) to the nasal cavity. Spin-echo image: *TR* 3000, *TE* 30 ms.

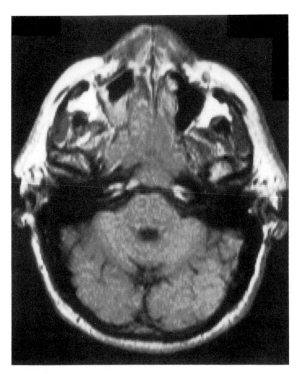

Figure 20–9. Extension of tumor (adenocystic carcinoma) to the pterygopalatine fossa and the clivus. Spin-echo image: *TR* 1500, *TE* 30 ms.

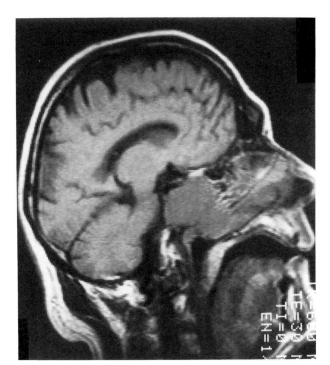

Figure 20–10. Direct visualization of tumor extension (adenocystic carcinoma) into the clivus. Spin-echo image: *TR* 600, *TE* 30 ms.

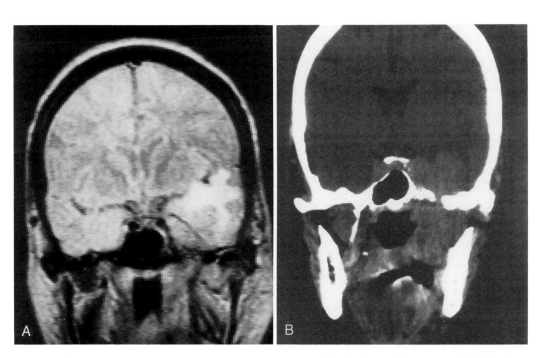

Figure 20–11. Tumor (squamous cell carcinoma) ingrowth into the middle fossa. In contrast to CT, MRI failed to demonstrate the small bony defect in the skull base. *A*, Spin-echo image: *TR* 1500, *TE* 60 ms. *B*, CT image.

metastasis on MRI (Fig. 20–12). In such cases, CT will be able to demonstrate the small bony defect in the skull base.

Level of the Ethmoid Region

Lamina Papyracea. Invasion or destruction of the lamina papyracea stresses the need for orbital enucleation. Coronal and sagittal images are required to demonstrate this extension properly. Extension from the orbital apex to the cavernous sinus usually represents a contraindication to surgical extirpation (Fig. 20–13).

Lamina Cribrosa. Destruction of the lamina cribrosa makes adequate radical surgery extremely difficult and requires a combined neurosurgical–ENT approach.

Level of the Frontal Sinus

Destruction of the bony contours of the frontal sinus sometimes indicates the need for a combined neurosurgical–ENT approach and even makes radical surgery impossible, particularly when the posterior wall of the frontal sinus is destroyed, with tumor invasion into the dura. Extension through the ethmoid and frontal sinuses into the skull base is well visualized by MRI (Fig. 20–14). However, for the demonstration of parasellar extension into the middle cranial fossa, especially when the defect is small, CT is at present the method of choice.

Metastases

Finally, it is of importance to know whether or not cerebral metastases are present. If they are, the surgical approach is eliminated. An additional advantage of MRI is the

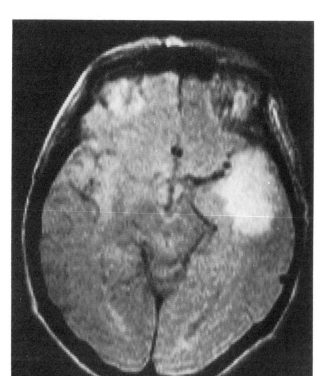

Figure 20–12. Tumor extension (squamous cell carcinoma) into the temporal lobe, mimicking a brain tumor. Spin-echo image: *TR* 1500, *TE* 60 ms.

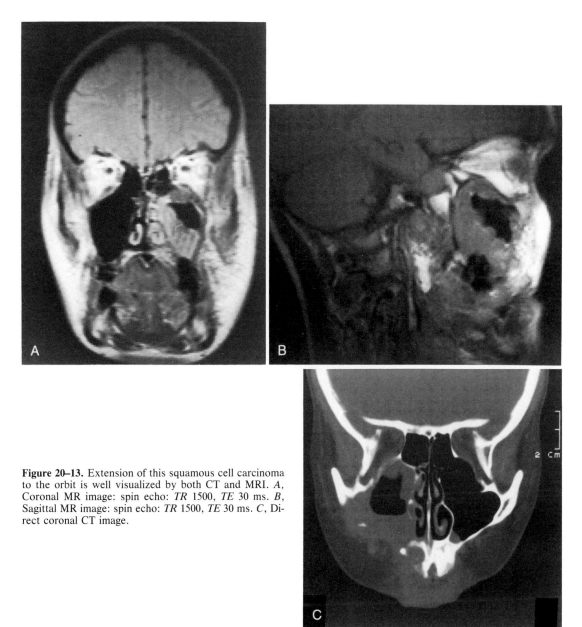

Figure 20–13. Extension of this squamous cell carcinoma to the orbit is well visualized by both CT and MRI. *A*, Coronal MR image: spin echo: *TR* 1500, *TE* 30 ms. *B*, Sagittal MR image: spin echo: *TR* 1500, *TE* 30 ms. *C*, Direct coronal CT image.

possibility of visualizing the brain in routine studies of the paranasal sinuses.[14] Lymph node metastases can usually be diagnosed by palpation of the neck, making imaging techniques unnecessary.

Conclusion

In summary, preoperative visualization of the tumor by CT or MRI is important in treatment planning. We feel that MRI has the capacity to select those patients who are suitable for surgery. It particularly selects those cases in which extension of the lesion into the soft tissues is still within the margins of operability. In most cases examined in our institution, MRI and CT were complementary or basically demon-

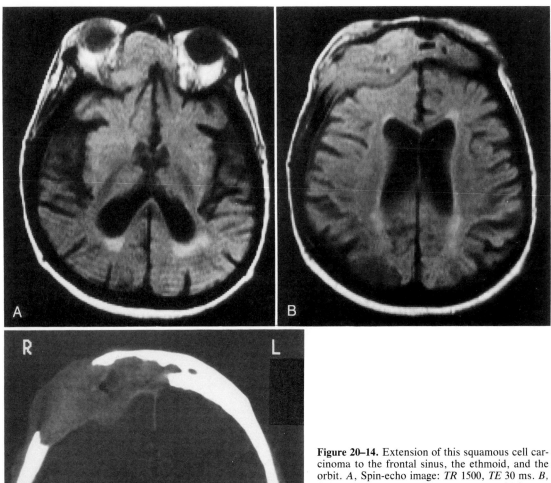

Figure 20–14. Extension of this squamous cell carcinoma to the frontal sinus, the ethmoid, and the orbit. *A*, Spin-echo image: *TR* 1500, *TE* 30 ms. *B*, Spin-echo image: *TR* 1500, *TE* 60 ms. *C*, CT image.

strated the same degree of accuracy. Extension to the skull base was more accurately depicted by CT, with the possible exception of tumor invasion into the clivus. For the visualization of posterior extension into the infratemporal fossa and the pterygopalatine region, MR images were of greater diagnostic value. Tumor extension is well depicted by moderately *T2* weighted pulse sequences (e.g., SE: *TR* 1500, *TE* 60 ms). Heavily *T2* weighted pulse sequences (such as SE: *TR* 2000, *TE* 180–240 ms) produce the best contrast between tumor and mucosal swelling.

References

1. Weber AL, Tadmor R, Davis R, et al: Malignant tumors of the sinuses. Neuroradiology *16*:443, 1978.
2. Jackson RF, Fitz-Hugh GS, et al: Malignant tumors of the nasal cavities and the paranasal sinuses. Laryngoscope *87*:726, 1977.

3. Potter GD: Radiology of the paranasal sinuses and facial bones. *In* Valvassori GE, Potter GD, Hanafee WN, et al (eds): Radiology of the Ear, Nose and Throat. Stuttgart, Thieme Verlag, 1982.
4. Valk J, Olislagers de Slegte R: High resolution CT scanning in nontraumatic maxillo-facial-oral pathology. Medicamundi *29*(2):45, 1984.
5. Hasso AN: CT of tumors and tumor-like conditions of the paranasal sinuses. Radiol Clin North Am *22*(1):119, 1984.
6. Getenby RA, Mulhern CB, Strawitz J: Comparison of clinical and computed tomographic staging of head and neck tumors. AJNR *6*:399, 1985.
7. Kondo M, Masatoshi H, Stiga H, et al: Computed tomography of malignant tumors of the nasal cavities and paranasal sinuses. Cancer *50*:226, 1981.
8. Silver AJ, Maward ME, Hilal SK: Computed tomography of the nasopharynx and related spaces. Radiology *147*:733, 1983.
9. Han JS, Huss RG, Benson JE, et al: MR imaging of the skull base. J Comput Assist Tomogr *8*(5):944, 1984.
10. Hyans VJ: Pathology of the nose and paranasal sinuses. *In* English G (ed): Otolaryngology. New York, Harper & Row, 1981.
11. Batsakis JG: Tumors of the Head and Neck. Baltimore, Williams & Wilkins, 1974.
12. Batsakis JG: Mucous gland tumors of the nose and paranasal sinuses. Ann Otol Rhinol Laryngol *79*:557, 1970.
13. American Joint Committee for Cancer Staging and End-Result Reporting: Manual for Staging of Cancer. Chicago, AJC, 1978.
14. Mancuso AA, Hanfee WH: Computed Tomography and Magnetic Resonance Imaging of the Head and Neck, 2nd ed. Chapter 1. Baltimore, Williams & Wilkins, 1985.

21

Neck

CHARLES B. HIGGINS
MADELEINE R. FISHER

Magnetic resonance imaging (MRI) has several characteristics that suggest clinical utility for imaging the neck. The hydrogen (spin) density and $T1$ and $T2$ relaxation times are sufficiently different among the various tissues of the neck to permit discrimination of muscles, fat, lymph nodes, blood vessels, salivary glands, and thyroid. Moreover, tumors and lymphadenopathy can be clearly delineated from adjacent structures, since they have distinctly different imaging characteristics compared with fat, muscle, and blood vessels. Early clinical experience with MRI of the neck has been reported.[1,2] This latter experience provides some insight into the utility of MRI for the evaluation of diseases of the neck.

The outstanding contrast among soft tissues afforded by MRI is probably the most important feature for visualizing the neck. Additional advantages are the natural contrast for the blood pool,[3] obviating the need for contrast media, and the ability to obtain direct images in the coronal and sagittal planes. Imaging in the coronal plane seems to be particularly useful for evaluating the cervicothoracic junction and the extent of neck mass spreading into the mediastinum.

However, at the current stage of development of MRI there are limitations, including spatial resolution, slice thickness, and the need for immobility during the several-minute imaging procedure. High spatial resolution images (0.8 mm) and thinner slices (2.5 and 5.0 mm) are possible and useful in studying diseases of the neck. Others have also achieved excellent signal-to-noise ratio (S/N) with thin slices and high-resolution images by employing collar-shaped surface coils for the neck.[4]

This chapter describes the technique of MRI of the neck as well as normal anatomy of the neck depicted by MRI and summarizes early experience in imaging of neck pathologies. It should be noted at the outset that current experience with MRI of the neck is still limited; consequently, conclusions are tentative at this time.

TECHNIQUE

The standard plane for MRI of the neck is the transverse. The coronal plane was used in some instances, especially when the cervicothoracic junction was examined. Both $T1$ weighted (TR 0.5 sec, TE 30 ms) and $T2$ weighted (TR 2.0 sec, TE 60 to 80 ms) images are employed. All studies are done using the multislice technique, whereby 5 to 20 anatomic levels are obtained during an imaging run. Most studies have been done using an elliptical neck coil. Surface coils either were of the transmit-receiver type or served only as the signal receiver; the latter configuration is now considered to be superior.[5] The surface coils provide an increase in S/N compared with the neck and body coils. The 10 cm diameter surface coil provided 4.6 to 1 increase in S/N compared with the body coil.[5] Collar-shaped surface coils have been particularly useful for imaging of the neck.[4]

NORMAL ANATOMY

The high contrast resolution with MR produces excellent discrimination among various tissues and sharply displays the multiple tissue planes in the neck. No contrast medium is required to differentiate blood vessels from lymph nodes. Under most imaging conditions the lumens of blood vessels are black owing to the signal void produced by flowing blood. However, the blood entering sections at the ends of an imaging volume may generate bright signal (intensity equal to or greater than fat). The internal jugular and other veins may contain intraluminal signal at the cranial end of the imaging volume, while the carotid and other arteries may contain signal on the section at the caudal end. Since patients are supine during MRI, blood flow in the internal jugular vein is apparently slowed to the extent that intraluminal signal is frequently observed in these vessels.

Contrast between tissues can be enhanced with variations in imaging parameters. An example of this is the situation for lymph nodes, in which they are best contrasted from surrounding fat on *T1* weighted images (inversion recovery or spin echo with short *TR*, SE 500/28). On the other hand, lymph nodes can be clearly distinguished from adjacent muscle using *T2* weighted images (spin echo with long *TR* and *TE*, SE 2000/56). Contrast between thyroid gland and fat is best on *T1* weighted images, whereas the contrast relative to the strap muscles is optimal on *T2* weighted images.

Anatomic boundaries of the neck are, cranially, the plane extending from the lower margin of the mandible to the superior line of the occipital bone and, caudally, the plane extending from the suprasternal notch to the first thoracic vertebral body.

The major anatomic components demonstrated on MR images in the neck are:
1. Muscle groups
2. Carotid sheath
3. Larynx-trachea-esophagus
4. Thyroid-parathyroid glands
5. Lymph node groups
   a. jugular chain
   b. spinal accessory chain
   c. submandibular
   d. submental
   e. retropharyngeal

TRANSVERSE IMAGES

For the interpretation of transverse images, the neck has been divided into three anatomic compartments: visceral, posterior, and lateral. The anteriorly located visceral compartment contains the larynx, trachea, esophagus, and thyroid and parathyroid glands. These structures are surrounded anteriorly and laterally by the strap muscles (superficially the sternohyoid and omohyoid and, deeper, the sternothyroid and thyrohyoid muscles) and the sternocleidomastoid muscle (SCM). Skeletal muscle has intermediate intensity on *T2* weighted images because of its short *T2* relaxation time.

The lateral compartment contains the neurovascular bundles (carotid sheaths) consisting of the carotid arteries, jugular veins, vagus nerve, and sympathetic chain. The vascular structures are easily distinguished as circular black structures, whereas the

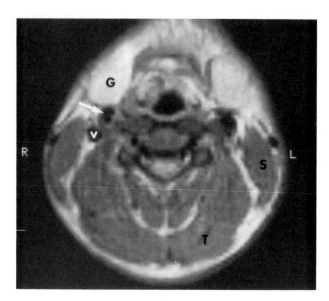

Figure 21–1. Transverse MRI image at the base of the tongue. Submandibular gland (G). Sternocleidomastoid muscle (S). Trapezius muscle (T). Jugular vein (V). Internal and external carotid arteries (arrow).

neural structures are not visualized on standard-resolution MR images. Small lymph nodes in the jugular and spinal accessory chain are visible in many normal subjects.

The posterior compartment includes the cervical vertebrae and the flexor muscles (scalenes and longus colli) on the anterior aspect and the extensor muscles on the posterior aspect of the vertebrae. Cortical bone of the vertebrae produces very low MR signal, while the marrow space has a high intensity, slightly less than fat.

Hyoid bone (Fig. 21–1). Slightly cranial to the hyoid, located anteriorly, are the myelohyoid and the geniohyoid muscles. The lateral muscles are the sternocleidomastoid, and the posterior muscles are the longus colli (capitus) and the trapezius. The muscle groups and associated ligaments (nuchal ligament) are especially well delineated on MR images. Fat between muscles, around blood vessels, and between muscles shows high signal. The submandibular gland has lower intensity than fat and, like lymph nodes, is best distinguished from fat on short *TR* images. The gland has higher intensity than muscle, and the contrast between them is accentuated with longer *TE* (*TE* = 56 ms). This is frequently the level of bifurcation of the carotid artery.

The air in the valleculae and hypopharynx has no signal intensity and identifies these structures. The valleculae are separated by the median glossoepiglottic fold and are frequently asymmetric in size and configuration. Even slight tilting or rotation of the neck accentuates this asymmetry. The epiglottis cut transversely at this level divides the vallecula from the pharyngeal space. Likewise, the internal carotid artery, branches of the external carotid artery, and jugular vein are recognized as low-intensity rounded structures situated laterally, as are the vertebral arteries lying in the transverse vertebral processes. The hyoid bone may be recognized owing to the high intensity produced by marrow.

Pyriform Sinuses (Fig. 21–2). The infrahyoid strap muscles (sternohyoid and thyrohyoid) separate the high-intensity fat of the pre-epiglottic space (PES) from the subcutaneous fat. The air in the pyriform sinuses is separated from the medial vestibule by the aryepiglottic folds. Laterally, the sinuses abut the laminae of the thyroid cartilage. Because of fat within the aryepiglottic folds they have high intensity and blend anteriorly into the fatty PES. The carotid sheath lies just beneath the SCM muscle. This sheath is separated from the laryngeal vestibule medially and SCM muscle laterally by fat planes. Because of the long time required to obtain MR images, variation in the size of the pyriform sinus and vestibule with respiration and phonation is not seen.

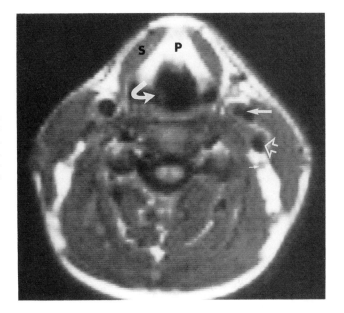

Figure 21–2. Transverse image at the level of the pyriform sinus. Pre-epiglottic space (P). Entrance from vestibule to pyriform sinuses (curved arrow). Carotid artery (long arrow). Jugular vein (open arrow). Infrahyoid strap muscles (S). Normal-sized lymph nodes (small arrow) are visible in the internal jugular and spinal accessory chains.

Vocal Cords (Fig. 21–3). The thyroid laminae may be identified owing to the central medullary fat. The margins of the thyroid and other laryngeal cartilages produce very low intensity because of cartilaginous or calcified tissues. The false cords have higher signal intensity than the true cords. The true cords have a lower intensity than the false cords because of partial replacement of fatty paralaryngeal fat by the vocalis muscle. Because of the slice thickness currently being used, the true and false cords are not always imaged separately. Within the posterior end of the true and false cords lie portions of the low-intensity cortex and high-intensity medullary cavity of the arytenoid cartilages and posterior lamina of the cricoid cartilage. Visualization of the intrinsic muscle of the larynx as well as separate visualization of the true and false cords has been demonstrated using thin slices and collar-shaped surface coils[4] or head coils with specially designed extensions that also encompass the neck (Fig. 21–4).

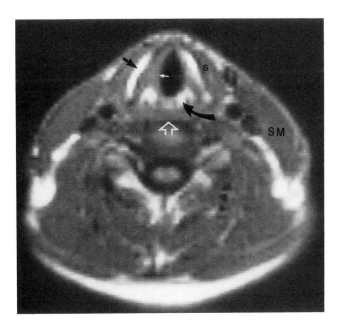

Figure 21–3. Transverse image at the level of the true cords. Central medullary fat in laminae of thyroid cartilage (black arrow). Arytenoid cartilages (curved arrow). True cords (small white arrow). Muscle complex consisting of pharyngeal constrictors, cricopharyngeus, and cricoarytenoid muscles (open arrow). Strap muscles (S). Sternocleidomastoid muscle (SM).

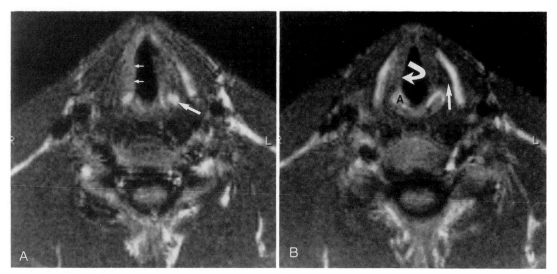

Figure 21–4. Thin section (5 mm thickness) images through the level of the false (*A*) and true (*B*) cords. Foot process of arytenoids (long arrow). False cords (small arrow). True cords (curved arrow). Thyroarytenoid muscle (long arrow). Arytenoid cartilage (A).

Approximately 1 cm further caudad, the medullary cavity of the cricoid cartilage produces a high-intensity ring surrounding the now-circular airway (Fig. 21–5). Posterolateral to the laryngeal and cricoid cartilages, and deep to the SCM muscle, the jugular vein and internal carotid artery can be easily identified.

Thyroid Glands (Fig. 21–6). Beneath the subcutaneous fat and immediately abutting the thyroid gland, the relatively low-intensity sternothyroid and sternohyoid muscles can be discerned. There the strap muscles can best be distinguished from the thyroid on *T2* weighted images (SE 2000/60). The two lobes of the thyroid surround the anterior and lateral circumference of the trachea and extend over three or four transverse images. The esophagus may be identified behind the trachea; usually the mucosa can be

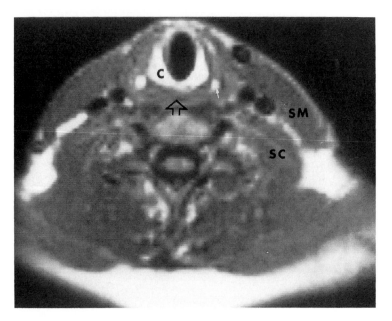

Figure 21–5. Transverse image at the end of the cricoid cartilage. Inferior cornu of thyroid cartilage (white arrow). Posterior lumina of cricoid cartilage (C). Complex of muscles composed of cricopharynges and inferior pharyngeal constrictors (open arrow). Scalene muscles (SC). Sternocleidomastoid muscle (SM).

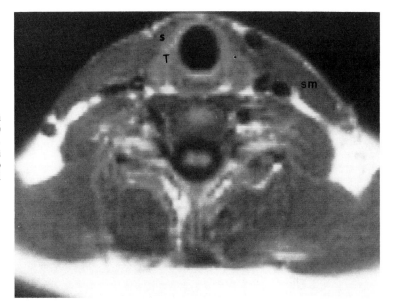

Figure 21–6. Transverse image (spin echo with *TR* = 0.5 sec, *TE* = 30 ms) at the level of the thyroid gland (T). The thyroid has lower intensity than does fat and higher intensity than do surrounding strap muscles (S) and sternocleidomastoid muscles (sm).

distinguished as being of higher intensity than the muscular walls on SE 2000/60 images. Superficially between the two lobes, a prominent venous structure (distal portion of the inferior thyroid vein) is frequently identified.

The inferior parathyroid glands are usually located at the lower poles of the thyroid gland. High-quality images at this site display the vascular components of the minor neurovascular bundle (inferior thyroid artery and vein) lying within high-intensity fat (Fig. 21–7). In nearly all individuals there is a substantial layer of fat between the lower pole of the thyroid lobes and the longus colli muscle. This is the site at which the inferior parathyroid glands are located. The recurrent laryngeal nerve is not visible on standard images. The small vessels may be seen in the fat located between the posterior aspect of the thyroidal poles and the longus colli muscles. The normal-sized parathyroid glands are located here but are usually too small to identify.

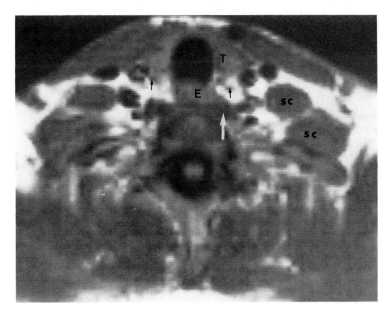

Figure 21–7. Transverse image at lower pole of thyroid gland. Components of the minor neurovascular bundle (black arrows) are seen at this level. The inferior parathyroid glands and adenomas are frequently found at this location. Thyroid (T). Esophagus (E). Anterior and middle scalene muscles (sc). Longus colli muscle (white arrow).

CORONAL IMAGES

The anatomy of coronal images at four important levels is described.

Thyroid Gland (Fig. 21–8A–D). The most anterior of the useful coronal tomograms display the lobes of the thyroid gland medially. At this level the strap muscles and SCM muscles lie laterally. However, the SCM muscles are located posterior to this plane at more cranial levels. Superior to the thyroid gland, the anterior portions of the thyroid and cricoid cartilage produce midline high-intensity regions (medullary cavities) above the thyroid gland. The low-intensity valleculae are usually also visualized at this plane.

Larynx (Fig. 21–9). Farther posterior, coronal images display the internal components of the larynx in the midline. These include the false vocal cords, true vocal

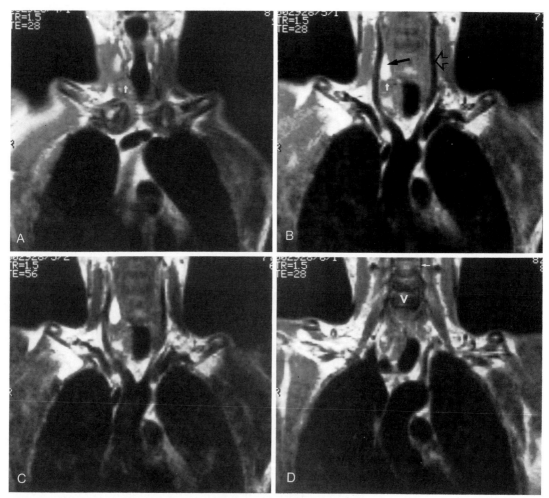

Figure 21–8. Coronal image of the neck and thorax, *A*, The most ventral image shows the thyroid (t), trachea, and a portion of the sternocleidomastoid muscles. *B*, A section 1 cm farther dorsal shows the enlarged right lobe of this thyroid goiter, which contains a region of high-signal intensity (black arrow) representing a site of colloid degeneration. The carotid arteries (open arrow) in the neurovascular bundle are seen lateral to the thyroid lobe. *C*, The second-echo image at the same level shows an even greater contrast between the colloid degeneration and the remainder of the thyroid. *D*, A section 1 cm farther dorsal shows the vertebral bodies (V), vertebral artery (arrow), and insertion of the anterior scalene muscles into the first rib.

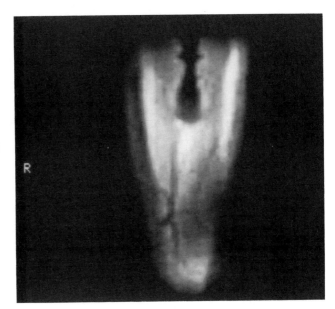

Figure 21–9. Coronal image of the larynx obtained with a surface coil.

cords, and ventricle between the false and true cords and the vestibule of the larynx. Lateral to these midline structures is a region of high intensity resulting from the fat in the paralaryngeal spaces and in the medullary cavity of the thyroid laminae and cricoid cartilage.

Carotid Sheath (Fig. 21–8C). The neurovascular bundle lies in the groove between the airway and the esophagus. The jugular vein is positioned anterior and lateral to the carotid artery. The vagus nerve is usually not resolved on MRI. This bundle has a slightly ventral-to-dorsal course—proceeding from caudal to cranial levels in the neck. Consequently, these vessels as a rule are not included over the entire length of any coronal image. Fat usually surrounds these vessels. The SCM muscles lie lateral to the vessels. Medium-intensity muscle is generally identified medial to these vessels. At cranial levels these muscles are the pharyngeal constrictors, cricopharyngeus muscle, and/or longus capitis muscles; at inferior levels they are the wall of the collapsed esophagus and longus colli muscles. The posterior portion of the thyroid lobe may be identified between the carotid sheath and the esophagus. The intensity of the thyroid is greater than the esophagus; this contrast is accentuated on *T2* weighted images (SE 2000/60).

Cervicothoracic Junction. The cervicothoracic junction, delineated by the sternoclavicular junction and the sternal notch, is the region at which the three longitudinal compartments of the thorax narrow markedly as they more or less continue into the neck. These three longitudinal compartments are the prevascular (anterior), the vascular (middle), and the postvascular or aeroesophageal space (posterior). While these spaces are truly anterior, middle, and posterior in the mediastinum, the vascular space wraps around the aeroesophageal compartment at the cervicothoracic junction and the neck. The prevascular space at the cervicothoracic junction is very narrow and contains areolar tissue, small veins, lymph nodes, and a portion of the thymus glands. The vascular component includes the brachiocephalic vein and its branches as well as the major arch vessels. These lie lateral and anterior to the trachea and esophagus. Tomographic sections through this region demonstrate the origin of several muscles from the upper ribs, sternum, and clavicles (SCM, sternothyroid, sternohyoid, and scalenes).

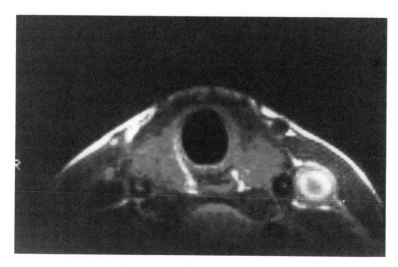

Figure 21–10. Transverse image of the thyroid obtained with a surface coil.

SURFACE COILS IN THE NECK

Surface coils can be extremely useful in the neck since the structures are close to the surface. Surface coils increase S/N compared with standard body and neck coils. With our unit a flat 10 cm (diameter) coil achieves a 4.6-fold S/N compared with the standard body coil.[5] A shaped (collar or solenoid) coil for the neck has been used by Lufkin and Hanafee[4] for neck imaging. This type of coil has produced uniform signal intensity through the regions of interest of the neck. The MR images of the larynx produced by this group demonstrated the intrinsic muscle and smaller cartilage of the larynx. Using these collar-shaped surface coils, they found MRI superior to thin-section CT for the staging of laryngeal tumors. The improvement in S/N gained by these coils has permitted the use of thin sections (4 mm) and high spatial resolution (0.5 mm).

Surface coils have produced sharp delineation of the carotid artery, larynx (Fig. 21–9) and thyroid (Fig. 21–10). The normal surface nodularity of the thyroid gland has been recognized on surface coil images (Fig. 21–10) but not on images using standard neck coils.

NECK PATHOLOGY

Lymphadenopathy. Lymph nodes in the neck are usually embedded in fat and frequently are situated adjacent to blood vessels or skeletal muscle. Because of the flow void in blood vessels, lymph nodes are readily discerned from adjacent vessels. Since lymph nodes have a distinctly longer $T1$ relaxation time compared with fat, the best contrast of nodes to fat is achieved on $T1$ weighted images (SE 500/28) on which the nodes have low signal intensity (Fig. 21–11).[6] Compared with muscle, the $T1$ relaxation time is not very different, whereas the $T2$ relaxation time is considerably longer for nodes compared with muscle.[6] Consequently, the best contrast between nodes and muscle is achieved on $T2$ weighted images (SE 2000/56), in which nodes have a higher intensity than the adjacent muscle (Fig. 21–11). The percent contrast for nodes versus fat and nodes versus muscle is shown for various TR and TE parameters in Figure 21–12. Thus there is high contrast between lymph nodes and adjacent tissues, and this contrast can be accentuated by manipulating the imaging parameters TR and TE. This is an advantage over CT, in which the lymph nodes have an attenuation equivalent to muscle and different from blood vessels only after adequate contrast enhancement of the vessels.

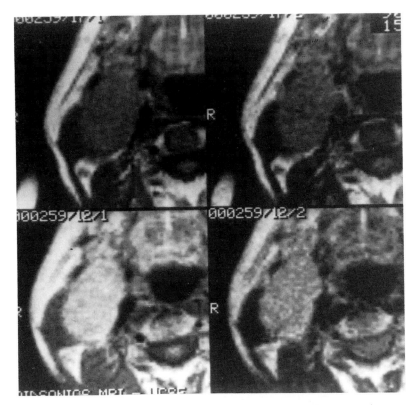

Figure 21–11. Transverse images of the same anatomic level using four different imaging parameters. SE 500/28, left upper panel. SE 500/56, right upper panel. SE 2000/28, left lower panel. SE 2000/56, right lower panel. Contrast between the enlarged lymph node and fat is maximal on SE 500/28, while contrast between node and muscle is maximal on SE 2000/56. (From Dooms GC et al: Radiology *153*:719, 1984. Used by permission.)

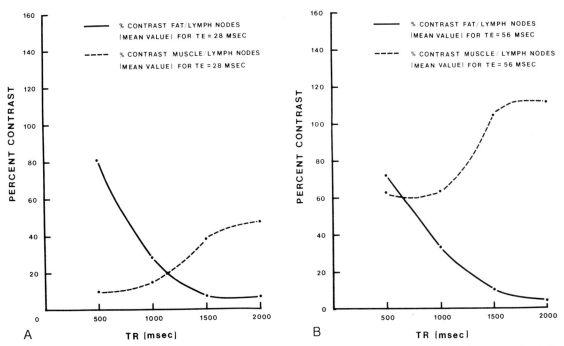

Figure 21–12. Percent contrast as a function of *TR* is plotted for lymph node vs. fat and lymph node vs. muscle. *A–B*, This is shown for the first (*TE* = 28 ms) and second (*TE* = 56 ms) spin-echo images. (From Dooms GG et al: Radiology *153*:719, 1954. Used by permission.)

There is widespread distribution of lymph nodes in the neck. A detailed description of the anatomy of cervical nodes is available.[7] Figure 21–13 shows the sites and particular names of these nodes. Normal lymph nodes are less than 10 mm in diameter and are not visible at most sites even by CT. CT depiction of normal nodes in the internal jugular and spinal accessory chain is possible in most individuals. Nodes measuring 1 cm in diameter are to be expected in the internal jugular chain in 20 percent of normal patients. The largest normal node in this chain is usually the jugulodigastric node. With the current spatial resolution and slice thickness of MRI, normal lymph nodes are occasionally visualized in the jugular and spinal accessory chain (see Fig. 21–2).

Pathologic lymph nodes ranging in size from 13 to 50 mm are clearly demonstrated on MRI (Figs. 21–11 and 21–14). MRI has depicted cervical lymphadenopathy caused by acute inflammation, lymphoma, and metastasis. Figure 21–14 shows nodes in the internal jugular and spinal accessory chain in a patient with autoimmune deficiency syndrome (AIDS). The variations in signal intensity of nodes and contrast relative to adjacent tissues for varying *TR* and *TE* values are shown in Figure 21–11. MRI has also demonstrated nonhomogeneous intensity of signal in metastatic lymph nodes due to regions of necrosis of portions of the nodes.

The comparative advantages of MRI and CT for identifying lymph nodes must remain tentative at this early stage in development of MRI. CT has the advantage in the neck of slightly better spatial resolution and slice thickness. MRI has considerably better contrast resolution. Lymph nodes show signal contrast relative to muscle, fat, and blood vessels without the need for contrast medium. Since comparative prospective studies with large numbers of patients are not yet available, the role of MRI compared with CT cannot be stated with any certitude.

Laryngeal Disease. Magnetic resonance imaging, like computed tomography, is an effective method for evaluating the cartilage and soft tissue composing and surrounding the larynx (Figs. 21–3 to 21–5). The spatial resolution and slice thickness routinely employed with MRI are not optimal for evaluation of small intraluminal lesions of the larynx. Diagnosis of such mucosal lesions is clearly within the province of laryngoscopy, which MRI and CT are intended to supplement. Excellent images of the larynx have been achieved with collar-shaped surface coils[2] and with a cranial coil extending to the shoulders (see Fig. 2–4). While section thickness can now be as thin as 2.5 mm and "in-plane" spatial resolution can be 0.9 mm, such images still have poor S/N unless such specialized coils are used. With the use of these coils the intrinsic muscle of the

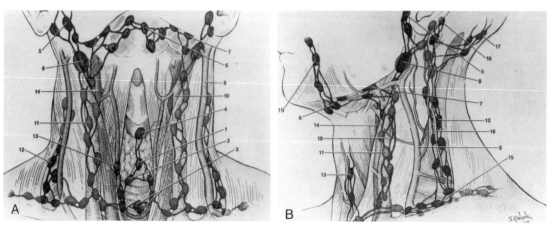

Figure 21–13. *A* and *B*, Diagram shows the location of the lymph node chains in the neck. (From Reede DL, et al: RadioGraphics *3*(2):339, 1983. Used by permission.)

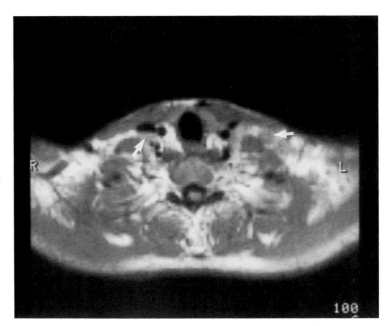

Figure 21–14. Transverse SE 500/28 image shows multiple enlarged lymph nodes (arrows) in the jugular chain and supraclavicular region.

larynx can be identified. Although the cortex of the cartilage is invisible on MRI, the laryngeal cartilage is visible owing to the high-intensity medullary cavity.

As has been found with CT of the larynx, precision in the technique of the MRI study is critical in order to avoid misdiagnosis. Maintenance of the neck in extension, the chin in midline, and the body aligned exactly along the Z axis is even more difficult to attain with MRI than with CT because of the longer acquisition time of MRI. Slight tilting or rotation of the neck complicates interpretation of intrinsic anatomy by introducing asymmetry.

Benign Conditions. Benign endolaryngeal lesions consist mostly of inflammatory granulomas, papillomas, and polyps. Granulomas are usually small and appear on the posterior third of the true cords or, less frequently, on the aryepiglottic folds. The spatial thickness and slice thickness, as well as the laryngeal motion that occurs during the relatively long image acquisition time, render MRI impractical for evaluating such lesions.

Polyps are the most commonly occurring endolaryngeal lesions; they arise from unusual vocal stress in singers and self-appreciating politicians. For the same reasons stated earlier, MRI has no role here. On the other hand, MRI may be very useful for defining the extent of large infiltrative tumors of the neck, such as hemangioma and lymphangioma. The wide field of view available with coronal and sagittal images affords this information (Fig. 21–15).

Congenital cysts of the larynx arise most frequently from the aryepiglottic folds and lie in the paralaryngeal tissue. The larger ones, measuring several centimeters in diameter, are distended with mucus; mucus usually produces high signal intensity on MRI. Because of their relatively large size and mucous content, they should be readily identified by MRI. The extensions of such lesions into the paralaryngeal tissues should be well defined by MRI. The cysts bulge the aryepiglottic fold and project into the vestibule; when very large, they extend into the ipsilateral vallecula or project through the thyrohyoid membrane lateral to the larynx.

Laryngeal Trauma. Trauma to the larynx, especially external trauma, has been evaluated by CT with increasing frequency in recent years.[8] Evaluation of fractures and dislocations of laryngeal cartilage is an essential part of the CT evaluation; similar

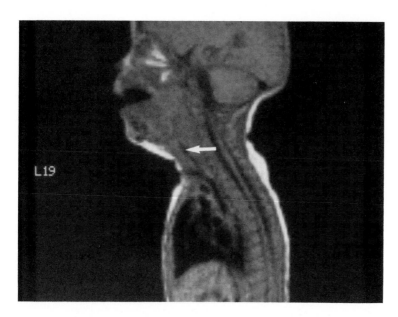

Figure 21–15. Sagittal image of a child with an invasive lymphangioma of the neck (arrow). The pharynx and airway are nearly obliterated by the mass.

information should be attainable with MRI. Since MRI can specifically identify hematoma and optimally defines blood vessels without contrast medium, it may be the ideal technique for defining vascular injuries of the neck, such as the site and extensiveness of deep hemorrhages, possible vascular occlusion, compression, or disruption.

MRI is usually not indicated in the acutely traumatized patient with pain or respiratory distress, since such patients cannot be expected to remain sufficiently immobile to permit good images. Finally, because of the motion caused by respiratory and cardiac motion during the image acquisition period, the diameter of the airway is underestimated by MRI. This may be an important consideration in patients with laryngeal edema and hemorrhage.

Table 21–1. CLASSIFICATION OF PRIMARY TUMOR (T)

Primary Tumor	TX	Tumor that cannot be assessed
	T0	No evidence of primary tumor
Supraglottis	TIS	Carcinoma in situ
	TI	Tumor confined to site of origin with normal mobility
	T2	Tumor involves adjacent supraglottic site(s) or glottis without fixation
	T3	Tumor limited to/or extension to involve postcricoid area, medial wall of piriform sinus, or pre-epiglottic space
	T4	Massive tumor extending beyond the larynx to involve oropharynx, soft tissues of neck, or thyroid cartilage
Glottis	TIS	Carcinoma in situ
	TI	Tumor confined to vocal cord(s) with normal mobility (includes involvement of anterior or posterior commissures)
	T2	Supraglottic and/or subglottic extension of tumor with normal or impaired cord mobility
	T3	Tumor confined to the larynx with cord fixation
	T4	Massive tumor with thyroid cartilage destruction and/or extension beyond the confines of the larynx
Subglottis	TIS	Carcinoma in situ
	T1	Tumor confined to the subglottic region
	T2	Tumor extension to vocal cords with normal or impaired cord mobility
	T3	Tumor confined to larynx with cord fixation
	T4	Massive tumor with cartilage destruction or extension beyond the confines of the larynx, or both

Table 21–2. CLASSIFICATION OF REGIONAL NODES (N)

NX	Nodes cannot be assessed
N0	No clinically positive node
N1	Single, clinically positive, homolateral node 3 cm or less in diameter
N2	Single, clinically positive, homolateral node more than 3 cm but not more than 6 cm in diameter; or multiple, clinically positive, homolateral nodes, none more than 6 cm in diameter
N2a	Single, clinically positive, homolateral node more than 3 cm but not more than 6 cm in diameter
N2b	Multiple, clinically positive, homolateral nodes, none more than 6 cm in diameter
N3	Massive homolateral node(s), bilateral nodes, or contralateral node(s)
N3a	Clinically positive, homolateral node(s), one more than 6 cm in diameter
N3b	Bilateral, clinically positive nodes (in this situation, each side of the neck should be staged separately, e.g., N3b, N2a, left N)
N3c	Contralateral, clinically positive node only

Carcinoma. Carcinoma of the larynx (95 percent of which is squamous cell) has been evaluated extensively by CT. Although the results of CT should be transferable to MRI, only early experience with MRI in laryngeal carcinoma has been reported to date.[9] However, this experience has been extremely encouraging and suggests some advantages for MRI compared with CT.

Carcinoma of the larynx has been classified into four groups, based upon site of origin: supraglottic (25 percent), glottic (55 percent), subglottic (5 percent), and piriform sinus (15 percent). Nodal metastasis is frequently seen with carcinoma of the piriform sinus, occurring in more than 50 percent of patients at the time of presentation. It is also frequent with supraglottic carcinoma. Therapeutic decisions are based upon initial staging. The TNM staging classification is based on assessment of extent of the primary tumor (T); status of regional lymph nodes (N); and presence of distant metastases (M). The criteria for each stage are provided in Tables 21–1 and 21–2.

The evaluation of endolaryngeal tumor and mobility of laryngeal structures is done by laryngoscopy. At the current time, MRI is considered to have limited capability in this regard. Because of the partial volume effect imposed by 5 to 10 mm thick sections, the true and false cords are not resolved separately in many subjects and the ventricle is usually not visualized. These structures are reasonably well depicted on coronal images using surface coils.

The role of MRI in the evaluation of laryngeal carcinoma can be predicted based upon the experience of CT. Both modalities assist in the staging of laryngeal carcinoma, especially by defining invasion of laryngeal cartilages and paralaryngeal soft tissues. The potential of MRI is indicated by its success in defining the hyoid bone and thyroid, arytenoid, and cricoid cartilages in normal subjects aged 30 to 35 years studied in our laboratory (see Figs. 21–3 to 21–5). MRI demonstrated the high-intensity medullary and low-intensity cortical rim of each cartilage (see Figs. 21–3 to 21–5). Lymphadenopathy in the neck is also well depicted by MRI.

THYROID PATHOLOGY

The thyroid gland, usually situated between the oblique line of the thyroid cartilage and the sixth ring of the trachea, is surrounded by a fibrous capsule and enclosed in a fascial compartment formed by the sheath of pretracheal fascia. The thyroid varies in size with age, sex, and general nutrition, being larger in youth, in women, and in the well nourished.[10] Average dimensions for the thyroid are 5 cm in height, 6 cm in width, and 1 to 2 cm in thickness for each lobe. Usually the thyroid lobes are homogeneous in signal intensity and conical, united by the isthmus portion anteriorly. Occasionally, in elderly females and men, the lobe is horseshoe-shaped, while in young women it is more rounded. A pyramidal lobe is reported to be present in 40 percent of people[10]; this is a process of the thyroid that extends upward from the upper border of the isthmus, anterior to the cricoid and thyroid cartilages. This process usually is found more on the left than on the right.

The gland is optimally delineated with the spin-echo technique on the *T2* weighted image, in which it has higher signal intensity than the overlying sternothyroid and sternohyoid muscles anteriorly and the SCM muscles laterally. The best contrast between fat and thyroid is attained with *T1* weighted images, whereas the best contrast relative to muscle is observed on *T2* weighted images (Fig. 21–16). Each lobe approaches posteriorly the prevertebral fascia covering the longus colli muscle, and laterally the carotid sheath. At the lower pole, fat separates the gland from the longus colli muscles; vessels of the minor neurovascular bundle are visible on MRI in this fat (see Fig. 21–7).

Benign Diseases

Thyroiditis may be secondary to infectious agents, trauma, radiation, autoimmune disease, and unknown etiologies, such as granulomatous thyroiditis. In each, the gland anatomically enlarges acutely. Limited experience with the MR appearance of thyroiditis exists. To date, this entity is demonstrated by a diffusely enlarged gland that has increased signal intensity both on the short (i.e., 0.5 sec) and on the long (i.e., 2.0 sec) repetition time (*TR*) images relative to the normal gland.

Goiterous enlargement includes the diffuse primary enlargement and the multiple, nodular goiter. The simple goiter initially is composed of hypertrophy and hyperplasia of the gland, which later may undergo involution with colloid accumulation.[11] Hemorrhage and calcification may be present. Nodular enlargement of the thyroid is the end result of hyperplasia, asymmetric focal involution, hemorrhages, and scarring.[12] On MRI, multinodular goiters have similar or slightly increased signal intensity relative to normal thyroid on the short *TR* images (*T1* weighted) and substantially increased

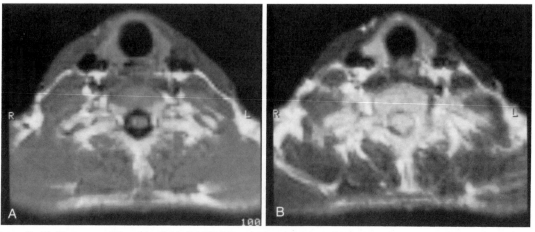

Figure 21–16. Transverse *T1* weighted (*A*, SE 500/28) and *T2* weighted (*B*, SE 2000/56) images through the thyroid gland of a normal subject. Contrast is maximal between thyroid and fat on *T1* weighted image, whereas contrast relative to muscle is best on the *T2* weighted image.

intensity on the long *TR* images (*T2* weighted). All goiters encountered to date have been nonhomogeneous on *T2* weighted images and include foci of high signal intensity (Fig. 21–17). Goiters produce low signal intensity on *T1* weighted images but occasionally contain areas of high signal intensity. The high-intensity foci in goiters probably represent colloid cysts or hemorrhage into cysts. Sites of cystic degeneration have lower intensity than the remainder of the gland on *T1* weighted images and increase in intensity relative to the remainder of the gland on *T2* weighted images. Regions of calcification are seen as low intensity on both the short and the long *TR* images. MRI is especially useful for the evaluation of substernal goiters, to define their full extent into the cervicothoracic junction (Fig. 21–17).

The most common benign tumor of the thyroid is the adenoma. The pathologic criteria of an adenoma are complete fibrous encapsulation, a clear distinction between the architecture of the adenoma inside and outside the capsule, a uniform histologic architecture within the capsule, and compression of the surrounding thyroid substance.[12] Adenomas are either follicular or papillary.

Follicular adenomas usually are solitary, spherical masses, less than 3 to 4 cm in diameter. There is marked variability in the composition of follicular adenomas. At one end of the spectrum they are composed of solid cords of small cuboidal cells separated by fibrous stroma, while at the other end of the spectrum they are composed of large, cystically dilated glands containing abundant colloid separated by little stroma. Between these extremes, all gradations may be found.[12] Colloid, a proteinaceous material, most likely causes shortening of *T1*, which likely accounts for the slightly higher signal intensity of some adenomas compared with normal thyroid on the short *TR* images. Those follicular adenomas composed of solid cords of tissue account for the MRI appearance of adenomas seen with an intensity similar to that of the normal thyroid on the short *TR* image and higher intensity than the normal thyroid on the long *TR* image (Fig. 21–18). This appearance is consistent with the adenoma's having a *T1* longer than or similar to the normal thyroid tissue and a prolonged *T2*. A distinct pattern for the papillary or atypical adenoma had not been seen with MR. Coronal images are useful for demonstrating the overall size of the adenoma (Fig. 21–19).

The contrast between thyroid cyst, adenoma, and carcinoma compared with normal thyroid tissue is greatest on the *T2* weighted images. No specific MRI appearance has been recognized that would specify the histologic diagnosis of a thyroidal mass.

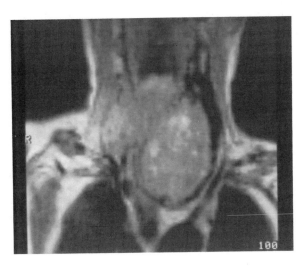

Figure 21–17. Multinodular goiter. The extent of the huge goiter extending below the sternal notch into the mediastinum is shown on the coronal image. On this *T2* weighted image, foci of high signal intensity are seen within the goiter.

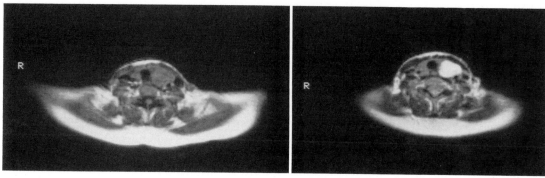

Figure 21–18. Transverse images of a patient with a follicular adenoma of the left lobe of the thyroid. *A,* The *T1* weighted images show enlargement of the left lobe but similar intensity to normal thyroid. *B,* The *T2* weighted image displays markedly greater intensity of the adenoma compared with normal thyroid.

Malignant Diseases

Several histologic forms of thyroid carcinoma occur: papillary, follicular, anaplastic, and medullary. The most common type is papillary. Papillary carcinoma usually is composed of papillary and follicular components. Papillary carcinoma spreads by the lymphatics to regional lymph nodes within the neck and, uncommonly, spreads hematogeneously. The MRI evaluation should encompass not only the thyroid bed with short and long *TR* sequences but also lymph node regions in the neck.

Limited experience with the various types of carcinoma on MRI allows only tentative description of their MR image. Carcinoma has had the same or slightly lower signal intensity than the normal thyroid on the short *TR* images and increased signal intensity relative to the normal thyroid tissue on a long *TR* image (Fig. 21–20). Anaplastic thyroid carcinoma is highly malignant and invasive, extending beyond the thy-

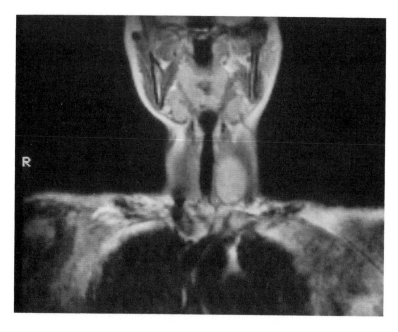

Figure 21–19. Coronal image of the neck in same patient shown in Figure 21–17. The extent of the nodule with higher intensity than normal thyroid is depicted in this plane.

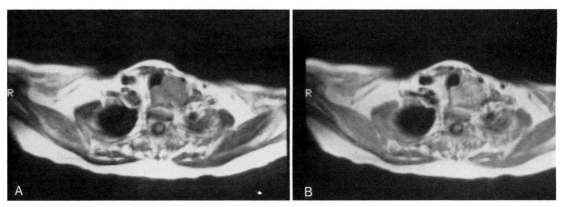

Figure 21–20. Transverse images with *TR* 0.5 sec (*A*) and *TR* 2.0 sec (*B*) show the recurrent carcinoma of the left thyroid bed with invasion of the trachea. The carcinoma increases in signal intensity with the longer *TR*.

roid bed and producing large bulky masses. The anaplastic carcinomas encountered to date have shown low intensity on *T1* weighted images and high intensity on *T2* weighted images compared with normal thyroid tissue (Figs. 21–21 and 21–22).

MRI has advantages over any other technique for evaluating bulky and invasive tumors of the neck; it provides excellent contrast between the mass and surrounding tissue, thereby delineating involvement of muscles, esophagus, larynx, and other structures in the neck (Figs. 21–21 to 21–23). Distinction between the mass and surrounding fat is best seen on the *T1* weighted images (Fig. 21–21). Distinction between mass and muscle is excellent on *T2* weighted images; invasion of muscle can be recognized as regions of abnormally increased signal intensity within the SCM or strap muscles. Differentiation of the large mass from the remainder of the thyroid is best attained on *T2* weighted images (Fig. 21–21). For defining the extent of large bulky tumors of the neck and assessing invasion of the mediastinum, the coronal images are especially useful (Figs. 21–22 and 21–24). These coronal images provide a wide field of view and demonstration of the cervicothoracic junction and superior mediastinum (Figs. 21–22 and 21–24).

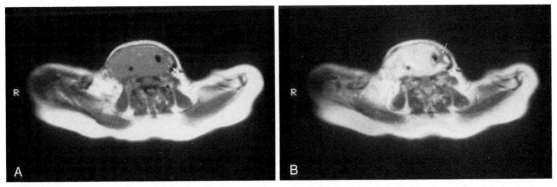

Figure 21–21. Transverse *T1* (*A*) and *T2* (*B*) weighted images in a patient with anaplastic carcinoma. The carcinoma increases markedly in signal intensity on the *T2* weighted image. The left neurovascular bundle (*A*, arrowhead) is displaced posteriolaterally by the tumor. The right jugular vein is occluded and the right carotid artery surrounded by tumor. Delineation of tumor from fat is possible in the *T1* weighted image but not on the *T2* weighted image. The small portion of normal thyroid (*B*, arrow) can be distinguished from tumor only on the *T2* weighted image.

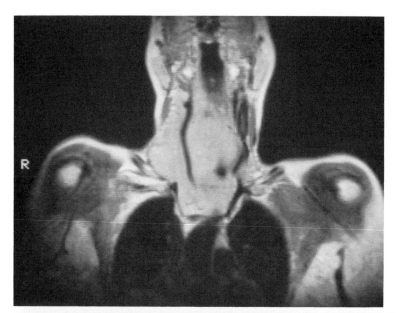

Figure 21–22. Coronal image in same patient as shown in Figure 21–21. The extent of this large bulky tumor and its extension into the mediastinum is displayed on the coronal image.

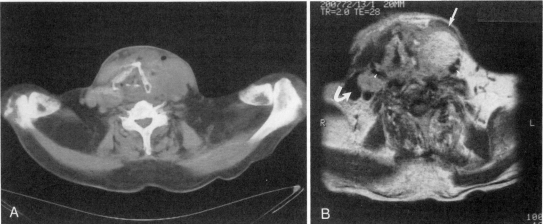

Figure 21–23. The contrast-enhanced CT scan (*A*) and transverse MR image (*B*) in a patient with a large invasive anaplastic carcinoma of the thyroid. *B*, The differentiation of the mass from muscle (arrow) and blood vessels (arrowheads) is more definitively shown by MR. Note the markedly dilated right jugular vein (curved arrow). The neurovascular bundles are displaced both laterally and posteriorly by the tumor.

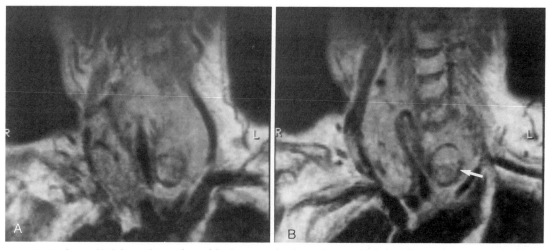

Figure 21–24. Coronal MR image in a patient with a huge anaplastic carcinoma widely invading the neck and mediastinum. Image on *A* is 1 cm ventral to the one on *B*. Note the low signal rim surrounding a nodule of tumor (*B*, arrow); this was shown to be calcium on the CT scan. MR scan shows the displacement of the neurovascular bundles and extension of the mass into the superior mediastinum.

340

PARATHYROID PATHOLOGY

The parathyroid glands are two pairs of small glands, superior and inferior, closely applied to the posterior surface of each thyroid lobe. They are lentiform, with average dimensions of 3 to 5 mm length, 2 to 4 mm width, and from 0.5 to 2 mm thickness.[10] The usual location of the superior parathyroid glands is about the midportion of the posterior aspect of the thyroid lobe, and the inferior parathyroid glands are situated at the posteroinferior aspect of each thyroid lobe. It should be remembered that the parathyroids can have variable locations, and knowledge of these sites is important in the evaluation of the patient with a suspected adenoma. The superior parathyroid may be located behind the pharynx or esophagus; in the fibrous tissue at the side of the larynx, above the level of the thyroid gland; behind any part of the corresponding lobe of the thyroid; or within the thyroid itself.[10] The inferior parathyroid may be located near the bifurcation of the common carotid artery; behind any part of the corresponding lobe of the thyroid; on the side of the trachea at the cervicothoracic junction; or in the thorax near the thymus.[10]

Current techniques for demonstration of parathyroid tissue employ an extended head coil or surface coils in order to augment S/N so that thin sections and larger image voxels can be used. For imaging of small structures, such as the parathyroid adenomas, it is very helpful to have in-plane spatial resolution of less than 1 mm and section thickness of 5 mm or less. Our current technique is to obtain thin-section (5 mm) high-resolution (0.8 mm) transverse images; both *T1* and *T2* weighted images are acquired. For patients who have had unsuccessful neck surgery for hyperparathyroidism, gated transverse images are also obtained, encompassing the cervicothoracic junction and superior mediastinum.

An important anatomic landmark for localizing parathyroid glands with MRI is the retrothyroidal fat between the thyroid and longus colli muscles (see Figs. 21–6 and 21–7). This fat plane is observed behind the middle and lower portions of the thyroid lobes; it has been seen in all normal volunteers, even in very slim individuals. This region is the most common site for the superior and inferior parathyroid glands, respectively, to lie. The normal structures situated in this fat plane are inferior thyroidal vessels and recurrent laryngeal nerves; these structures compose the minor neurovascular bundle lying between the dorsal aspect of the thyroid gland and the longus colli muscles. The esophagus separates the right and left sides of the fat plane, which are bounded laterally by the carotid artery and jugular vein.

Benign Diseases

Hypoparathyroidism is characterized and diagnosed by metabolic and clinical findings and not by morphologic changes. Primary hyperparathyroidism is characterized not only by metabolic and clinical findings but also by morphologic changes within the parathyroid glands. A single adenoma is the most common cause (76 percent) of primary hyperparathyroidism. Hyperplasia of the glands (chief cell type) accounts for 12 percent, and double adenoma, hyperplasia (clear cell type), and carcinoma account for 4 percent each.[12]

Most parathyroid adenomas arise in the lower glands. Usually, the adenoma arising in the inferior gland is located posterior to the inferior aspect of the thyroid. Occasionally, ectopic adenomas occur in the mediastinum. There is marked variation in the cell composition of adenomas and in the degree of vascularity, which may influence the MRI appearance.

Radiologic identification of parathyroid adenomas has been fraught with error, and consequently a number of modalities have been used to investigate this difficult clinical problem. In recent years, high-resolution (10 MHz), real-time sonography has achieved 90 percent accuracy in preoperative detection of parathyroid adenomas in patients with primary hyperparathyroidism at some centers[13,14]; others have reported a sensitivity of 69 percent and specificity of 94 percent.[15] In the latter series,[15] only 35 percent of abnormal glands weighing less than 200 mg were identified by sonography. Parathyroid adenomas located in areas of acoustic shadowing behind the trachea or beneath the clavicles were generally not detectable by sonography.[15]

Although the localization of adenomas by CT has usually shown a lower accuracy than has ultrasonography, the use of thin-slice, higher-resolution CT in recent years has attained a sensitivity of 70 to 80 percent.[16–18] Indeed, two comparative studies showed slightly better sensitivity for CT compared with ultrasonography.[17,18] Localization in previously explored necks was decidedly superior for CT.[18] While little experience currently exists with MRI for localization of parathyroid adenoma in hyperparathyroidism, initial results do show considerable promise.

A potential benefit of MRI compared with CT for the detection of parathyroid adenomas is the absence of streak artifacts from bone and surgical clips and the ease of identification of the surrounding vasculature. The distinctive tissue intensity of the longus colli muscle may aid in unequivocally distinguishing adenomas from this muscle, which is frequently nearby. Additionally, the superior soft tissue contrast with MR allows differentiation of the muscles, fat, blood vessels, and thyroid gland from parathyroid tissue. The delineation of parathyroid adenomas or other parathyroid pathology generally entails the acquisition of *T1* weighted images for contrast with fat and *T2* weighted images for better contrast with adjacent muscles.

Parathyroid adenomas have a variable appearance on MRI. They are usually lower in signal intensity relative to the normal thyroid on a *T1* weighted image (Fig. 21–25) and are the same or slightly higher in signal intensity on the *T2* weighted images. One adenoma was higher in intensity relative to thyroid even on the *TR* 0.5 image. Since the parathyroid adenoma commonly arises in the inferior glands or, occasionally, in the mediastinum, the short *TR* image is optimal for delineating the adenoma located within either the retrothyroid or the mediastinal fat, respectively (Figs. 21–25 and 21–26). On the long *TR* images the adenoma increases in signal intensity and may blend with fat. The excellent demonstration of vessels in the neck has been useful for distinguishing adenoma from the carotid artery lying in an unusual location and with an

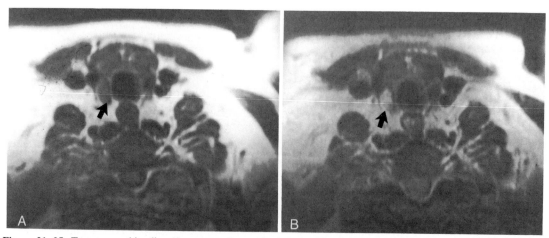

Figure 21–25. Transverse thin slice (5 mm) section at the lower pole of the thyroid gland in a patient with primary hyperparathyroidism. The adenoma (arrow) is situated behind the right lobe of the thyroid. The signal intensity of the parathyroid adenoma is low on the *T1* weighted image (*A*) and high on the *T2* weighed image (*B*).

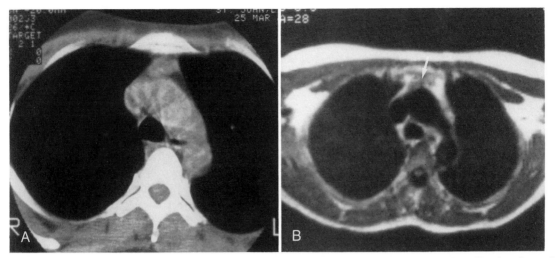

Figure 21–26. CT (*A*) and MR (*B*) images in a patient with recurrent hyperparathyroidism. On both studies there is good contrast between the adenoma and surrounding fat (*B*, arrow).

atypical shape caused by extreme tortuosity (Fig. 21–25). It is also important to obtain a long *TR* sequence to differentiate those adenomas embedded in or immediately adjacent to the thyroid. Enlargement of at least two glands should be sought to establish the diagnosis of hyperplasia; this observation has been made in a number of patients with chronic renal failure and secondary hyperparathyroidism.

In patients with recurrent hyperparathyroidism, MR images must extend into the superior mediastinum. Figure 21–26 shows the CT scan and MR image in a patient with ectopic parathyroid adenoma.

POSTOPERATIVE NECK

CT and MRI are utilized to detect recurrence after surgery for tumors of the neck. Experience with MRI for this purpose is very limited at present. Familiarity with the distorted anatomy of the postoperative neck is necessary to properly interpret such studies. In contrast to CT, surgical clips do not result in degradation of MR images.

After thyroidectomy, tissue with MR characteristics of fibrosis is observed in the paratracheal region. Consistent with fibrosis, this tissue has relatively low intensity and decreases in signal intensity on the second, compared with the first, echo image. On the other hand, recurrent tumor and lymphadenopathy show an increase in signal from first to second echo images. The signal intensity of fibrous tissue is usually less than muscle, while recurrent tumor and lymphadenopathy are greater than muscle. The extent of the recurrent tumor and the effect on the trachea and esophagus can be defined by MRI (see Fig. 21–20). Small recurrent deposits of tumor in lymph nodes are frequent in patients treated for medullary carcinoma. The level of suspicion for such recurrences is raised by elevated serum thyrocalcitonin levels; this increases sensitivity in interpretation of even small tissue collections in the tracheoesophageal groove or the presence of prominent lymph nodes.

Recurrence of chemical abnormalities after surgery for hyperparathyroidism raises the suspicion of parathyroid adenoma left behind in the initial exploration. In such instances MRI has revealed adenomas within the neck and superior mediastinum. Experience to calculate the accuracy of MRI for this purpose is insufficient. One study has stated a sensitivity of 76 percent for CT employing 5 mm thick sections and contrast-enhanced dynamic scanning with improved patient immobilization.[18] MRI is also now done using 5 mm contiguous sections for the evaluation of persistent parathyroid pathology after operation. It is not yet clear if the greater contrast resolution of MRI will compensate for the lesser spatial resolution compared with CT in the evaluation of persistent parathyroid disease.

After neck dissection the absence of the SCM muscle, jugular vein, and submandibular gland is demonstrated on MRI. After total laryngectomy, fat surrounds and separates the surgically reconstructed pharynx (neopharynx) and carotid sheath.[19] A fat plane beneath the SCM muscle can be expected to be intact. Tumor recurrence is usually located in (or obliterates) the fat plane of the carotid sheath within the internal lymph node chain. Tumor recurrence has also been shown by CT to occasionally produce enlargement of the SCM muscle. Since the signal intensity of muscle increases when it is infiltrated by neoplastic or inflammatory processes, MRI should prove very effective in demonstrating this type of recurrence. Other areas to be evaluated for recurrence are the upper mediastinum, tracheostomy site and tracheal lumen, and esophagus.

COMPARISON WITH OTHER IMAGING MODALITIES

It is too early in the experience with MRI to state or even predict its role in evaluation of neck pathology. Our early experience indicates three potential advantages: All tissues in the neck can be unequivocally distinguished without using contrast medium; coronal images facilitate evaluation of the cervicothoracic junction; and wide field of view and multiple imaging planes contribute importantly to defining the limits of extensive and bulky tumors.

Experience with MRI of the neck is still very limited. Its advantages compared with ultrasonography are undetermined owing to small numbers of patients studied by both techniques. It seems to have distinct promise for imaging of the cervicothoracic junction and for defining the anatomic extent and infiltration of muscles by large tumors of the neck.

References

1. Higgins CB, McNamara MT, Fisher MR, Clark OH: MR imaging of the thyroid. AJR *147*:1255, 1985.
2. Peck WW, Higgins CB, Fisher MR, Ling M, Okerlund MD, Clark OH: Hyperthyroidism: Comparison of MR imaging with radionuclide scanning. Radiology *163*:415, 1987.
3. McNamara MT, Higgins CB: Cardiovascular application of magnetic resonance imaging. Magn Reson Imag *2*:167, 1984.
4. Lufkin RB, Hanafee WN: Application of surface coils to MR anatomy of the larynx. AJR *145*:483, 1985.
5. Fisher MR, Barker B, Amparo EG, Brandt G, Brant-Zawadzki M, Hricak H, Higgins CB: MR imaging using specialized coils. *Radiology 157*:443, 1985.
6. Dooms GC, Hricak H, Crooks LE, Higgins CB: Magnetic resonance imaging of the lymph nodes: comparison with CT. Radiology *153*:719, 1984.
7. Mancuso AA, Harnsberger HR, Muraki AS, Stevens MH: Computed tomography of cervical and retropharyngeal lymph nodes. Normal anatomy. Radiology *148*:709, 1983.
8. Sagel SS, Aufderheide JF, Aronberg DJ, Stanley RJ, Archer CR: High resolution computed tomography in the staging of carcinoma of the larynx. Laryngoscope *91*:292, 1981.
9. Lufkin RB, Hanatee WN, Wortham D, Hoover L: Larynx and hypopharynx: MR imaging with surface coils. Radiology *158*:747, 1986.
10. Harrison RG: The ductless glands. *In* Romanes GT (ed): Cunningham's Textbook of Anatomy. London, Oxford University Press, 1972, pp 565–568.
11. Ingbar SH, Woeber KA: Disease of the thyroid. *In* Petersdorf RG, Adams RD, Brunswald E, et al (eds): Harrison's Principles of Internal Medicine. New York, McGraw-Hill, 1983, pp 620–621.
12. Robbins SL: Pathologic Basis of Disease. Philadelphia, WB Saunders, 1974, pp 1320–1354.
13. Schieble W, Deutsch AL, Leopold GR: Parathyroid adenoma: accuracy of preoperative localization by resolution real-time sonography. J Clin Ultrasound *9*:325, 1981.

14. Simeone JF, Mueller PR, Ferrucci JT, von Sonsnberg E, Wang C, Hall D, Wittenberg J: High resolution real-time sonography of the parathyroids. Radiology *14*:745, 1981.
15. Reading CC, Charboneau JW, James RM, Karsell PR, Purnell DC, Grant CS, van Herden JA: High resolution parathyroid sonography. Radiology *139*:539, 1982.
16. Ovenfors CO, Stark DD, Moss AA, Goldberg HI, Clark OK, Galante M: Localization of parathyroid adenoma by computed tomography. J Comput Assist Tomogr *6*:1094, 1982.
17. Sommer B, Welter HF, Spelsberg F, Scherer U, Lissner J: Computed tomography for localizing enlarged parathyroid glands in primary hyperparathyroidism. J Comput Assist Tomogr *6*:521, 1982.
18. Stark DD, Gooding GAW, Moss AA, Clark O, Ovenfors CO: Parathyroid imaging: comparison of high resolution CT and high resolution sonography. AJR *141*:633, 1983.
19. DiSantis DJ, Balfe DM, Hayden RE, Sagel SS, Sessions D, Lee JKT: The neck after total laryngectomy: CT study. Radiology *153*:713, 1984.

22

Thyroid and Parathyroid Glands

MARTIN P. SANDLER
JAMES A. PATTON
GLYNIS A. SACKS

Thyroid and parathyroid disorders affect a wide spectrum of our population from the fetus and neonate through the adolescent and young adult to the middle-aged adult and the elderly. Numerous imaging modalities, including nuclear medicine, ultrasonography, x-ray fluorescence, computerized tomography, and, more recently, magnetic resonance imaging (MRI), have been used in an attempt to provide a pathophysiologically related diagnosis in patients with diseases of the thyroid and parathyroid glands.

THYROID

Embryology

The thyroid gland can be recognized in the human by the end of the first month after conception, when the embryo is 3.5 to 4 mm in length. The gland evolves from a medial primordium arising from two lateral primordia derived from the fourth and fifth branchial pouch complex. Toward the end of the fourth week of development the thyroid gland is bilobed, joined by the thyroglossal duct, which is attached to the ventral floor of the pharynx. The duct becomes a solid stalk and begins to atrophy by the sixth week, maintaining its pharyngeal connection in the form of a permanent pit (foramen caecum) situated at the apex of the V-shaped sulcus terminalis on the dorsum of the tongue. Toward the end of the seventh week the gland assumes a new position at the level of the developing trachea, while the pharynx grows forward. The thyroid gland at this stage consists of two lobes situated on either side of the trachea joined by a narrow isthmus of developing thyroid tissue. Cells of the lower portion of the duct differentiate into thyroid tissue forming the pyramidal lobe.

At the completion of the normal thyroid's migration, it is still attached to the floor of the pharynx by the thyroglossal duct. A total arrest of thyroid migration results in a lingual thyroid, and a partial migration results in a nonlingual, yet ectopic, thyroid. Whereas the majority of the thyroid tissue may assume a typical bilobed configuration at the usual level of final development, significant remnant tissue may separate from the main migrating body and result in aberrant rest tissues: accessory thyroid and thyroglossal duct cyst (Fig. 22–1).

Part of the lateral lobe of the thyroid is derived from the ventral portion of the last branchial pouch, which remains as a separate gland known as the ultimobranchial body.[1] This tissue is the origin of the parafollicular cells, or C-cells, that secrete calcitonin.[2] The hormone calcitonin inhibits osteoclastic activity in bone and tends to decrease bone turnover and to lower serum calcium.[3] Thyroid follicles begin developing

346

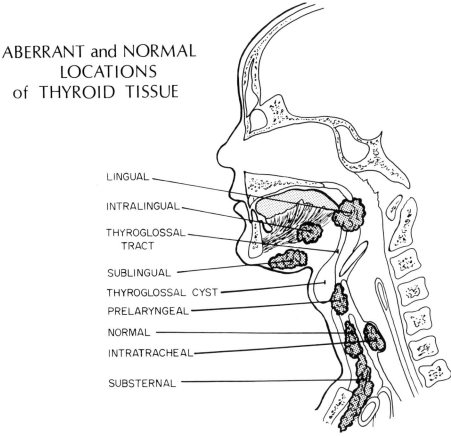

ABERRANT and NORMAL
LOCATIONS
of THYROID TISSUE

LINGUAL

INTRALINGUAL

THYROGLOSSAL
TRACT

SUBLINGUAL

THYROGLOSSAL CYST

PRELARYNGEAL

NORMAL

INTRATRACHEAL

SUBSTERNAL

Figure 22–1. Normal and aberrant locations of thyroid tissues. (Modified from Netter FH: *In* the Ciba Collection of Medical Illustrations. Endocrine System and Selected Metabolic Diseases, Vol. 4. Summit, N.J., Ciba Pharmaceutical Company, 1981. Used by permission.)

by the eighth week and acquire colloid material by the third month.[4] The human fetal thyroid gland exhibits the full spectrum of organically bound iodinated products, including thyroxine (T4), by approximately ten and a half weeks.[5] A variety of congenital abnormalities of the thyroid gland may occur in relation to its embryologic development, including numerous hereditary deficiencies affecting enzymes involved in the biosynthesis of thyroxine.[6]

Anatomy

The thyroid gland is normally situated in the lower neck and consists of two lobes joined by an isthmus that crosses the anterior tract of the second and third tracheal rings.[7,8] The thyroid is one of the largest endocrine organs, weighing approximately 20 gm, and rests in the pretracheal fascia. The isthmus is approximately 0.5 cm thick, 2 cm wide, and 2 cm high. The individual lobes have an ellipsoid configuration, with a pointed superior pole and poorly defined inferior pole merging medially toward the isthmus. Each lobe is approximately 2.0 to 2.5 cm in both thickness and width at its largest diameter and is approximately 4.0 cm in length. A pyramidal lobe is frequently present and in most instances is attached to the left lobe.

The thyroid gland is closely fixed to the anterior and lateral aspects of the trachea by loose connective tissue. A fibrous capsule, which invests the gland, is connected to the pretracheal fascia, causing the thyroid to move upward with deglutition. In most cases the upper margin of the isthmus lies just below the cricoid cartilage, which provides an excellent landmark for locating the thyroid gland. Lying lateral to the gland are the carotid arteries and sternocleidomastoid muscles.

Blood supply to the gland is largely from the superior thyroidal artery derived from the external carotid artery (enters superior pole). The right lobe of the thyroid is frequently more vascular than the left and is often the slightly larger of the two. It tends to enlarge more in disorders associated with a diffuse increase in gland size. A wide capillary network surrounds each follicle, and veins are derived from a perifollicular plexus. The thyroid is richly supplied with lymphatics.

Physiology

The function of the thyroid gland includes the concentration of iodine, the synthesis of thyroid hormones, the storage of the various hormones, and their release into the circulation as required. Dietary sources of iodine include sea fish, milk, eggs, and iodized products (e.g., salt). The average iodide intake is between 100 and 150 μg per day. Sites of iodide absorption include the stomach and the upper small bowel. Approximately two thirds of the iodide in the blood is excreted in the urine, and one third is trapped by the thyroid. About 95 percent of the body's iodine stores are situated in the thyroid, with the remainder circulating as thyroid hormones in the blood and tissues. The ability to trap iodide is not unique to the thyroid gland because trapping also occurs in the salivary glands and gastric mucosa and in the milk of lactating women, but none of these tissues is able to use the trapped iodide to form thyroid hormones. The gland is composed of clusters of follicles or acinar units, which are lined by a single layer of spherical follicular cells with their apices directed toward the lumen of the follicle and their base toward a basement membrane. The center of each follicle contains colloid made up largely of protein, especially the iodinated glycoprotein thyroglobulin.

Thyroid Imaging

Nuclear Medicine

Thyroid scintigraphy is an important diagnostic modality in the evaluation of patients with thyroid disorders and can be used for in vivo evaluation of thyroid size, position, architecture, and function. Thyroid scintigraphy, however, only provides a guideline for the diagnosis and management of thyroid disease, and correlation of scan results with clinical history, physical examination, and laboratory data is essential for correct patient management.

Radionuclides. Numerous radionuclides have been used for thyroid imaging, including technetium-99m pertechnetate (Tc-99m), iodine-123 (I-123), and I-131. X-ray fluorescence, which can be used to assess intrathyroidal iodine content, is not used routinely.

^{99m}Tc is the most popular radionuclide employed for thyroid imaging. The pertechnetate ion (TcO_4^-) is trapped by the thyroid in the same manner as iodine through an active transport mechanism but is not organified by the thyroid gland.[9-13] Radiation dose to the thyroid is low—even lower than that obtained with I-123; however, whole-body radiation dose is greater than that obtained with studies using I-13. ^{99m}Tc is a pure gamma emitter with a principal photon energy of 140 keV.

I-123 is the ideal thyroid imaging agent because it is both trapped and organified by the thyroid gland, allowing assessment of overall thyroid function. I-123 decays by

Table 22–1. CLASSIFICATION OF HYPERTHYROIDISM

Thyroid Gland (95)%
Diffuse toxic goiter (Graves' disease)
Toxic nodular goiter
      Multinodular (Plummer's disease)
      Solitary nodule
Thyroiditis (subacute)
Exogenous Thyroid Hormone/Iodine (4%)
Iatrogenic
Factitious
Iodine-induced (jodbasedow)
Rarely Encountered Causes (1%)
Hypothalamic-pituitary neoplasms
Struma ovarii
Excessive HCG production by trophoblastic tissue
Metastatic thyroid carcinoma

electron capture, emitting gamma rays with the principal photon energy of 159 keV, an ideal energy for imaging with the gamma camera.

In the assessment of physiologic organification, imaging should not be performed less than eight hours following oral administration because early images represent only trapping of the radionuclide by the thyroid gland. Total radiation dose to the thyroid is greater than that of pertechnetate; overall total radiation dose to the body is less.

I-131, although frequently used in the past, now plays a minor role in the routine investigation of the thyroid, with the exception of metastatic thyroid disease, owing to its unacceptably high thyroid and total-body radiation dose.

The choice of radiopharmaceutical for imaging thyroid disorders, especially thyroid nodules, lies between ^{99m}Tc and I-123. A disadvantage of imaging with pertechnetate is that it is only trapped and not organified by the thyroid gland. In addition, early imaging following intravenous administration is associated with high background activity. Imaging with ^{99m}Tc, however, provides a large amount of information and serves as an acceptable alternative to I-123. In those instances in which it is thought essential to assess both organification and trapping, I-123 scanning can be performed subsequently.

Hyperthyroidism. Hyperthyroidism, a clinical syndrome that results from supraphysiologic levels of thyroid hormones, may occur as a consequence of numerous diseases (Table 22–1). Clinical history and physical examination combined with thyroid scintigraphy, thyroid uptake, and antibodies usually allow identification and differentiation of the various disease processes (Table 22–2). Magnetic resonance imaging has limited value in the assessment of patients with Graves' disease (see p. 158).

Nonfunctioning Solitary Thyroid Nodules. The management of patients with a solitary thyroid nodule remains controversial and relates to the high incidence of nodules, the relative infrequency of cancer (Table 22–3), and the low morbidity and mortality

Table 22–2. I-131 THYROID UPTAKE IN THYROTOXICOSIS

Increased	Normal	Decreased
Graves' disease (diffuse goiter)	Trophoblastic disease	Thyroiditis (subacute, chronic)
Plummer's disease (multinodular goiter)		Iatrogenic/factitious
Trophoblastic disease (HCG)		Jodbasedow (iodine-induced)
		Functioning thyroid metastases

Table 22–3. INCIDENCE OF THYROID NODULES AND THYROID CANCER

	Nodules	Cancer
Autopsy	50% of population	4% of nodules
Clinical	4%	4%
"High-risk" radiation (800 r)	20%	25%

From A Review of Endocrinology: Diagnosis and Treatment. Bethesda, MD, The Foundation for Advanced Education in the Sciences Inc, National Institutes of Health. October 12–16, 1981, p 191. Used by permission.

associated with thyroid malignancy. Thyroid nodules may contain normal thyroid tissue; benign inactive tissue that may be solid, cystic, or mixed solid and cystic; autonomously functioning benign tissue; or malignant tissue.

Investigation of the Solitary Thyroid Nodule. The investigation of a solitary thyroid nodule should be directed toward differentiating benign lesions of many etiologies from the malignant nodule, preventing indiscriminate surgical intervention (Table 22–4).

COLD OR COOL NODULES. Cold or cool nodules, as identified by thyroid scintigraphy, are regions that have impaired function and cannot concentrate radioisotopes relative to the rest of the thyroid gland (Fig. 22–2). Although thyroid malignancies do not effectively concentrate radioisotopes, only 20 percent or less of cold nodules are caused by cancerous lesions.[14-16] The remaining 80 percent of cold nodules arise from thyroid adenomas, colloid nodules, degenerative nodules, nodular hemorrhage, cysts, inflammatory nodules (including Hashimoto's thyroiditis or de Quervain's thyroiditis), infiltrative disorders (including amyloid or hemochromatosis), or nonthyroid neoplasms. A functioning TSH-dependent adenoma may appear as a cold nodule in patients with Graves' disease. This entity is known as the Marine-Lenhart syndrome, and impaired radionuclide uptake by the nodule is secondary to low TSH levels. Confirmation of the diagnosis can be made by TSH stimulation.[17] The presence of a cold nodule on scintigraphy is totally nonspecific, and its value is primarily to differentiate "hot" from "cold" nodules. The detection of extrathyroidal activity on a routine thyroid scan in a patient with palpable lymph nodes and a solitary thyroid nodule most likely indicates metastatic thyroid disease.

HOT OR WARM NODULES

EUTHYROID. A nodule that concentrates the administered radioisotope to a greater degree than the surrounding tissue appears either "hot" or "warm" relative to the thyroid gland. A hot thyroid nodule, in most cases, is benign because, as previously

Table 22–4. ETIOLOGY OF THE SOLITARY PALPABLE NODULE

Benign	Malignant	
	Primary	*Secondary*
Adenoma	Carcinoma	Kidney
Adenomatous hyperplasia	Papillary adenocarcinoma	Pancreas
in a goiter	Follicular carcinoma	Esophagus
Adenomatous nodule	Clear cell carcinoma	Rectum
Cyst	Oxyphil carcinoma	Melanoma
Colloid nodules	Medullary carcinoma	Lung
Chronic thyroiditis	Undifferentiated carcinoma	Lymphoma
Subacute thyroiditis	Small cell carcinoma	
	Giant cell carcinoma	
Miscellaneous	Epidermoid carcinoma	
Amyloid	Other malignant tumors	
Hemochromatosis	Lymphoma	
	Sarcoma	
	Malignant teratoma	

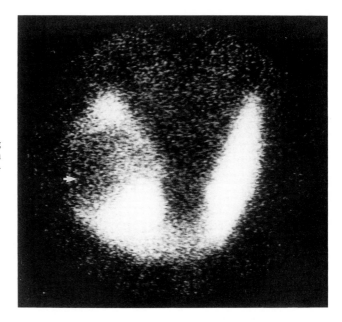

Figure 22–2. Solitary nonfunctioning cold nodule situated in the midportion of the right lobe (arrow). Image by Tc-99m radionuclide scan.

mentioned, malignant tissue rarely demonstrates scintigraphic activity (Fig. 22–3).[18-20] The incidence of hot nodules in patients with discrete thyroid nodules varies from 6.6 to 25 percent.[18-20]

Hot functioning nodules (i.e., nodules that exhibit both trapping and organification) in the euthyroid patient can be classified as either an autonomous adenoma or a hypertrophic (reactive) nodule. Both these nodules are benign.

HYPERTHYROID. The truly toxic solitary nodule accounts for 4 percent of solitary nodules and 4 percent of all cases of thyrotoxicosis.[21] Patients with a solitary toxic nodule are easily recognized by scintigraphic imaging, because only the nodule concentrates the radioisotope without evidence of trapping in the remainder of the gland, which becomes suppressed owing to the excessive thyroid hormone production by the toxic nodule. These patients are suitable candidates for treatment with radioactive

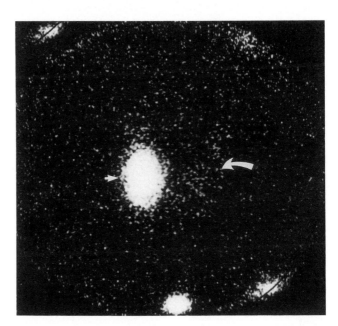

Figure 22–3. Solitary right-sided functioning autonomous nodule post Cytomel suppression (straight arrow). Imaged by Tc-99m radionuclide scan. Minimal activity is noted in the left lobe of the thyroid (curved arrow).

iodine, which results in the ablation of the toxic nodule and allows the previously suppressed thyroid gland to recover function and resume normal thyroid hormone synthesis.

Disparate Thyroid Imaging. Disparate thyroid imaging is a dissociation between trapping and organification, measured respectively with ^{99m}Tc and I-123. It occurs in 2 to 3 percent of individuals with thyroid disorders and is not specific for malignant disease, having been described in patients with adenomatous goiter and follicular adenoma.[22-24] A common subcellular defect has been postulated to account for the nonspecificity of this finding.

In view of the low incidence of disparity between trapping and organification, initial thyroid imaging in patients with solitary thyroid nodule using I-123 should be reserved for those who have an increased risk of thyroid malignancy, i.e., individuals with a previous history of head and neck irradiation during childhood, prepubertal patients, adult males, and patients with a positive family history of thyroid malignancy. Similarly, if a hot or warm nodule is demonstrated by ^{99m}Tc imaging, it should be reimaged with I-123 to ascertain the true functioning status of the nodule.[16]

ULTRASOUND

The traditional use of ultrasound in thyroid imaging has been an attempt to differentiate benign from malignant thyroid nodules. Two signs have been proposed by the ultrasonographer as markers of benignancy: pure cystic lesions and the halo sign (Fig. 22–4).[25,26] Hypoechogenicity of the nodule compared with the surrounding tissue has been presented as a sign indicative of malignancy.[27] Simple cysts less than 4 cm in diameter are virtually diagnostic of benign lesions, with an accuracy of 98 percent, whereas the probability of malignancy in a mixed nodule approaches 25 percent.[27,28] High-resolution real-time ultrasound has demonstrated that pure cysts of the thyroid may be rare; most cystic lesions are probably complex, containing both solid tissue

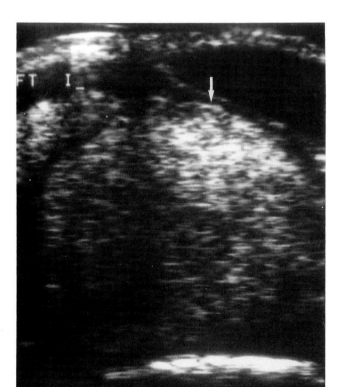

Figure 22–4. Solitary echogenic solid nodule with surrounding sonolucent "halo" (arrow).

and fluid.[27] The halo sign and hypoechogenicity of solid nodules have failed to demonstrate specificity for either benign or malignant lesions.

The introduction of high-resolution real-time sonography has allowed the identification of adenomas of 2 to 3 mm in size, increasing the detection of multinodular goiter when only solitary thyroid nodules were suspected clinically.[27] The significance of this capability relates to the lower incidence of malignancy in patients with multinodular goiter (1 to 6 percent) compared with those having single nodules (15 to 25 percent).[29]

Serial sonograms have also been used to follow changes in the size of solid nodules, facilitating precise evaluation in the growth patterns of these nodules. This has proved to be particularly useful when a conservative approach has been adopted in the management of patients with solitary thyroid nodules, i.e., long-term administration of thyroid hormone.[30]

X-RAY FLUORESCENT SCANNING

Quantitative x-ray fluorescent scanning is an established technique for the investigation of thyroid disorders and has proved to be especially useful in the evaluation of solitary cold thyroid nodules.[31–33] With this technique, the in vivo iodine content of a solitary thyroid nodule and that of a corresponding region of normal thyroid tissue in the contralateral lobe are measured. The iodine content ratio (ICR) of the nodule versus the normal tissue is calculated and used as a predictor of benignancy. This technique is valid only when investigating single nodules (Fig. 22–5).

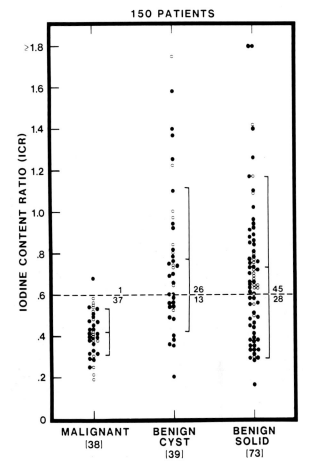

Figure 22–5. Iodine content ratios determined by x-ray fluorescent tomography before surgery from 150 patients with solitary "cold" thyroid nodules. Groupings are based on histologic study of surgical specimens. Open circles correspond to 42 patients in original retrospective study. (From Patton JA, Sandler MP: J Nucl Med 26(5):461, 1985. Used by permission.)

Fluorescent thyroid scanning has proved to be both a sensitive and a noninvasive method for determining the incidence of benignancy of solitary cold thyroid nodules. This technique does not require the administration of a radioisotope and thus becomes the method of choice in the evaluation of thyroid nodules in both pediatric and pregnant patients.

MAGNETIC RESONANCE IMAGING (MRI)

The basic physics and imaging principles of MRI have been described in detail in Chapters 3, 6, and 7 and will not be discussed here.

Clinical Application. Magnetic resonance imaging is suitable for demonstrating neck pathology, since it offers excellent soft tissue contrast without the need for intravenous contrast material. It is resistant to motion-related artifacts and can be used to examine the entire neck and thoracic inlet. MRI can achieve resolution of structures comparable to that of ultrasound and CT. Yet, the method is based upon the observation of hydrogen nuclei and their interaction within their chemical environment. This provides a physiologic basis for MRI, enabling tissue discrimination not possible with ultrasound or standard x-ray–based techniques. In this way, MRI shares a basis with the functional type of examination provided by the field of nuclear medicine.

In vitro studies on thyroid biopsy specimens performed by de Certaines and co-workers revealed abnormal *T1* and *T2* values in both benign and malignant lesions.[34] Nodules demonstrating increased radionuclide uptake showed a marked degree of variability in *T1* values, but all (N = 10), with a single exception, had significantly increased *T2* values compared with normal extranodular tissue. Solitary benign cold nodules (N = 9) all showed increased *T1* and *T2* values. *T1* and *T2* values showed considerable variation in four patients with thyroid carcinoma. An increase in *T1* was observed in two patients, and a decrease was noted in one. *T1* was not measured in the fourth patient. *T2* values increased in two cases and declined in two. There was no significant difference in the relaxation times between nodular and extranodular tissue in patients with multinodular goiter.

The normal thyroid gland and mass lesions, including both benign adenomas and neoplasms, can be identified with MRI (Figs. 22–6 to 22–11). Benign and malignant tissue may, in part, be distinguished by the degree of disruption of normal thyroid structure, invasion of normal thyroid tissue, and the surrounding anatomy.[35] Figure 22–10 illustrates the MRI of a metastatic melanoma compressing the trachea in a patient with a history of a left hemilobectomy for benign multinodular goiter.

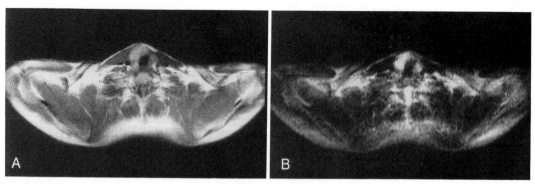

Figure 22–6. Transverse section through a benign Hürthle cell adenoma using (*A*) a spin echo 500/30 (proton density with slight *T1* weighting where *TR* = 500 ms and *TE* = 30 ms) sequence, and (*B*) a spin echo 2000/120 (*T2* weighting). The abnormality is seen as an area of high signal intensity on the *T2* weighted image in the right lobe of the thyroid (From Sandler MP et al: Thyroid and Parathyroid Imaging. East Norwalk, CT, Appleton-Century-Crofts, 1986. Used by permission.)

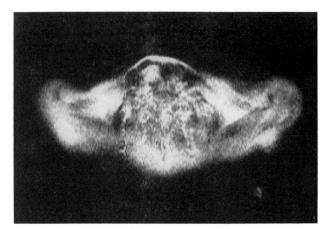

Figure 22–7. Benign functioning hypertrophic nodule is seen by MRI as an area of increased signal intensity in the right lobe of the thyroid using a spin-echo 1000/120 pulse sequence.

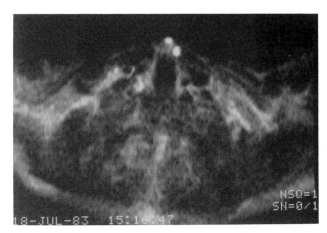

Figure 22–8. A thyroglossal ductal cyst on MRI transverse section using a spin echo 1000/120 (*T2* weighting). At surgery, this patient was noted to have a papillary carcinoma. The lesion is seen as two discrete areas of high signal intensity in the midline and in the left lobe of the thyroid. (From Sandler MP et al: Thyroid and Parathyroid Imaging. East Norwalk, CT, Appleton-Century-Crofts, 1986. Used by permission.)

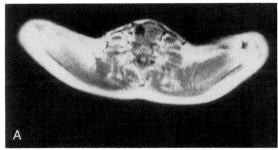

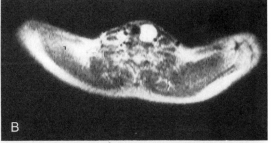

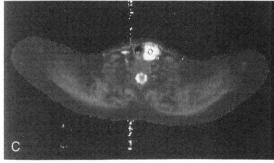

Figure 22–9. Transverse MRI sections through a benign follicular adenoma. *A*, A spin-echo 500/30 pulse sequence (proton density with slight *T1* weighting. *B*, A spin-echo technique 2000/120 (*T2* weighting). *C*, Calculated OT1 value = 1647 ms ± 300.4 ms in 23 picture elements with an area of 0.59 cm^2.

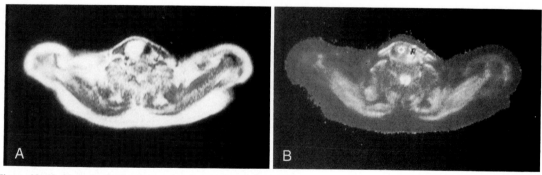

Figure 22–10. Note tracheal compression in a patient with melanoma metastatic to the right lobe of the thyroid. There was a history of left hemilobectomy for benign multinodular goiter. *A*, MRI spin-echo 2000/120 pulse sequence (*T2* weighting). *B*, calculated OT1 value = 428 ms ± 61.8 in 29 picture elements with an area of 0.74 cm^2.

Colloid cysts exhibit greatly prolonged *T1* values characteristic of simple fluids. Hemorrhage into a cyst should lower the *T1* value. Adenomas exhibit a wide range of *T1* values, although generally prolonged, encompassing those of thyroid carcinomas.

The in vivo differentiation between malignant and benign lesions appears to be unlikely on the basis of *T1* and *T2* measurements alone (Figs. 22–6 to 22–10). The ability of in vivo spectroscopy to differentiate benign from malignant thyroid nodules is not yet known.

Multinodular goiters are identifiable by MRI on the basis of their anatomic appearance. Figures 22–11 and 22–12 illustrate a normal thyroid gland and multiple cystic areas in a benign multinodular goiter, respectively.

Graves' disease can be distinguished on the basis of *T1* measurements from normal thyroid tissue (Fig. 22–13).[36] Table 22–5 reveals the prolonged *T1* values present in Graves' disease, the physiologic basis of which remains unexplained. MRI of patients with Graves' disease, however, is of limited value when compared with the numerous modalities currently available to diagnose this disorder.

RETROSTERNAL GOITER

Although substernal aberrant thyroid accounts for only 10 percent of all mediastinal masses, it remains one of the major diagnostic considerations in the assessment of mediastinal abnormalities.[37]

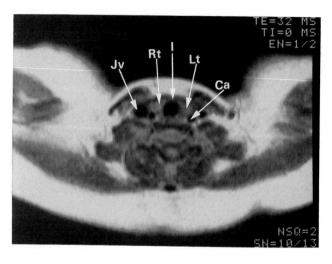

Figure 22–11. Transverse MRI section through a normal thyroid gland using a spin echo 3000/32 (*T2* weighting). Thyroid isthmus (I), right lobe (Rt), left lobe (Lt), carotid artery (Ca), and jugular vein (Jv). (From Sandler MP et al.: Thyroid and Parathyroid Imaging. East Norwalk, CT, Appleton-Century-Crofts, 1986. Used by permission.)

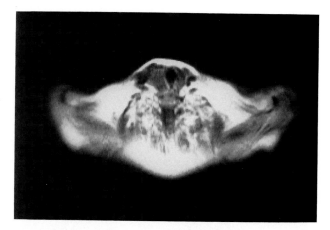

Figure 22–12. Transverse MRI section through a multinodular goiter with a spin-echo technique 500/30 (primary proton density with *T1* weighting). The thyroid is seen to be enlarged and lobular.

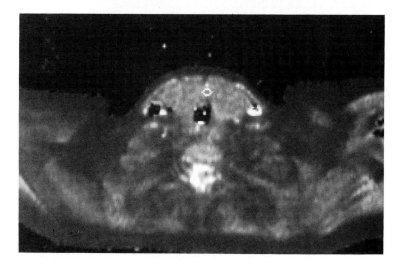

Figure 22–13. Transverse MRI section through a symmetrically enlarged thyroid gland in a patient with Graves' disease. Calculated OT1 value = 477 ms.

Goiters in the superior mediastinum generally arise from one or both lower poles of the thyroid gland or from the isthmus.[38] Although clear continuity between the cervical and intrathoracic components should be present in cases of mediastinal goiter extension,[39] the connection may be only a narrow fibrous band or vascular pedicle.[40] In such cases as well as in the presence of a primary intrathoracic goiter, lack of continuity between the cervical gland and the thoracic mass does not exclude the diagnosis of mediastinal goiter. The clinical presentation of symptoms of mediastinal compression associated with a palpable goiter and mediastinal mass on chest radiograph are suggestive of, but not specific for, the diagnosis of a thyroidal mediastinal mass.[41–43] The preoperative diagnosis of a thyroidal mediastinal mass frequently requires the

Table 22–5. T1 OF NORMAL AND ABNORMAL THYROID TISSUE AT 1.7 MHz

	T1 (ms)
Normal	150–195
Graves' disease	195–265
Thyroid cyst	260–700
Adenoma	190–350

From Sandler MP, Patton JA, Partain CL: Thyroid and parathyroid imaging. ACC, 1986, p 354. Used by permission.

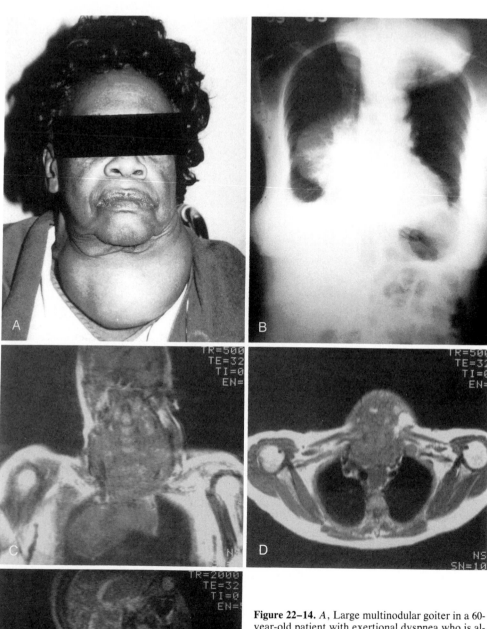

Figure 22–14. *A*, Large multinodular goiter in a 60-year-old patient with exertional dyspnea who is allergic to contrast media. *B*, X-ray reveals a large right-sided chest mass. *C*, A sagittal spin-echo 500/32 MRI reveals a large multinodular goiter extending into the mediastinum. *D*, Transverse spin-echo 500/32 MRI identifies involvement of both anterior and posterior mediastinum. *E*, MRI with spin echo 1000/160 pulse sequence (*T2* weighting) shows diffuse increase in signal intensity in most areas of the multinodular goiter that is most likely related to colloid and hemorrhage.

use of more sophisticated imaging techniques, including, either alone or in combination, radionuclide thyroid scintigraphy, computed tomography (CT), and MRI.[43-45]

Radionuclide scanning has been the standard method for evaluating whether or not a mediastinal mass represents functioning thyroid tissue.

The choice of radionuclide for imaging retrosternal thyroid masses lies between I-131 and I-123. For I-131, the principal gamma photon is 364 keV, representing an energy suitable for retrosternal imaging. The use of I-131, however, has fallen into disfavor because of the high radiation dose to the thyroid (50 rads) associated with its beta decay.[46] The principal photon energy of I-123, 159 keV, is suitable for imaging mediastinal thyroid masses even though they may be situated outside the anterior mediastinum.

False negative thyroid scans in mediastinal goiter may occur when there is too little uptake of radioactive iodine by the goiter either because of low iodine concentrating capacity of the tissue or because of recent exposure of the patient to exogenous iodines. Although false positive thyroid scans theoretically may occur in rare mediastinal teratoma similar to ovarian struma, only one false positive scan has been reported; this was in a patient with poorly documented papillary adenocarcinoma of the lung.[47]

Computed tomographic studies of intrathoracic goiter have noted the continuity with the cervical gland, focal calcifications, high noncontrast attenuation values of the goiter, and post–intravenous contrast enhancement.[48,49] These features, although suggestive of intrathoracic goiter, are not specific for the diagnosis of a thyroid mediastinal mass. The early enhancement of intrathoracic masses following intravenous contrast more than likely represents the vascularity of the mass rather than significant trapping and organification of iodine by the thyroid gland.[50] This is supported by cases reported in the literature demonstrating marked contrast enhancement in mediastinal masses other than thyroid tissue. Contrast-enhanced CT as the initial diagnostic procedure may occasionally prove counterproductive in the noninvasive work-up of the mediastinal mass because expansion of the body pool of iodine by contrast infusion interferes with normal thyroid uptake of the scanning dose of radioiodine. This reduces the sensitivity of detection of mediastinal thyroid uptake beyond the blood pool phase, a scintigraphic finding specific for mediastinal thyroid.

The ability to produce high-resolution tomographic or three-dimensional images without the use of ionizing radiation (Fig. 22–14) makes MRI an excellent modality to study the mediastinum. The success of MRI in the mediastinum is further enhanced by its superior ability to differentiate vascular structures from solid hilar or mediastinal masses without the use of contrast agents.[51] Volume calculations of thyroid mediastinal masses are also possible, with MRI permitting quantitative assessment of the response of mass to TSH suppression with levothyroxine (Synthroid).

PARATHYROID

Embryology

The parathyroid glands originate from the third and fourth pharyngeal pouches and are usually designated parathyroid glands III and IV. The inferior parathyroid glands (III) arise from the third branchial pouch and migrate caudally with the thymus gland. The superior parathyroid glands (IV) arise from the dorsal portion of the fourth branchial pouch and migrate a lesser distance together with the thyroid (Fig. 22–15). The position of the superior parathyroid glands is fairly constant, with 99 percent located either behind the upper pole of the thyroid lobes or adjacent to the cricoid cartilage. Aberrant superior glands may be found between the thyroid and esophagus,

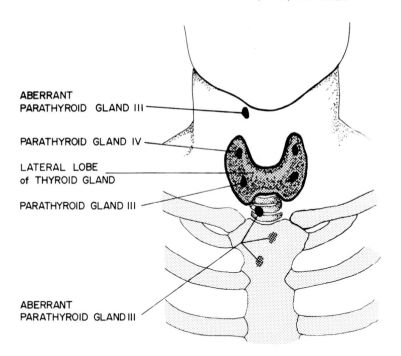

ABERRANT
PARATHYROID GLAND III

PARATHYROID GLAND IV

LATERAL LOBE
of THYROID GLAND

PARATHYROID GLAND III

ABERRANT
PARATHYROID GLAND III

Figure 22–15. Normal and abnormal distribution of parathyroid glands.

within the carotid sheath, behind the innominate vein, or occasionally in the posterior mediastinum. The position of the inferior parathyroid glands is less constant than that of the superior glands, with 95 percent of them located in the immediate vicinity of the lower pole of the thyroid. Ectopic sites of the inferior parathyroid glands include the superior pole of the thymus (39 percent) and the mediastinum (2 percent); an additional 2 percent occupy miscellaneous positions.

Anatomy and Histology

The parathyroid glands normally measure about 6 mm in length, 3 to 4 mm in breadth, and 0.2 to 2 mm in thickness. They have a variable location, and each gland weighs approximately 35 mg. There are usually four parathyroid glands: two upper and two lower. Extra parathyroid glands either may be involved in diffuse glandular hyperplasia or may be the site of a primary adenoma. The superior pair of parathyroid glands are often significantly larger and therefore easier to find. The parathyroid glands receive their blood supply from the inferior thyroidal vessels or from the anastomoses between the superior and inferior thyroidal arteries. Identification of the inferior thyroid artery serves as a landmark to help localize the parathyroid glands at surgery.

Histology

Histologically, the gland is made up of chief cells, oxyphil cells, and water clear cells.

CHIEF CELLS

The parathyroid gland in the infant and child is composed of sheets of closely packed chief cells with little intervening stroma. In the adult there are two forms of chief cells: light and dark. The light chief cells are rich in glycogen; they have a small Golgi apparatus, scanty endoplasmic reticulum, a few secretory granules, dark nuclei, and a definite chromatin network. The function of these cells is the secretion of parathyroid hormone. Dark chief cells, on the other hand, are poor in glycogen; these cells have a prominent Golgi apparatus, a dense endoplasmic reticulum, and numerous secretory granules. The dark chief cells are the primary source of parathyroid hormone.

OXYPHIL CELLS

The oxyphil cells first make their appearance after puberty. Typically, these cells are devoid of glycogen and have granular cytoplasm and small dense nuclei. They vary in size but are generally larger than the chief cells. The function of the oxyphil cells is the secretion of parathyroid hormone.

WATER CLEAR CELLS

The water clear cells appear after puberty and are large polygonal cells with inconspicuous vacuolated cytoplasm. The primary function of these cells is uncertain, but they have the potential to secrete parathyroid hormone.

Physiology

Parathyroid hormone is an 84 amino acid straight-chain polypeptide. The molecular weight of the hormone is 9500, and it has no disulfide bridges. The main function of parathyroid hormone is the regulation and maintenance of a normal serum calcium level (9 to 11 mg/al) by its actions on bone, small intestine, and kidney.

There are four principal actions of the parathyroid hormone (Fig. 22–16): (1) increased calcium absorption from the gastrointestinal tract; (2) osteoclastic stimulation with resultant resorption of calcium and phosphate from bone; (3) inhibition of phosphate reabsorption by the proximal renal tubule and the resultant phosphaturia; and

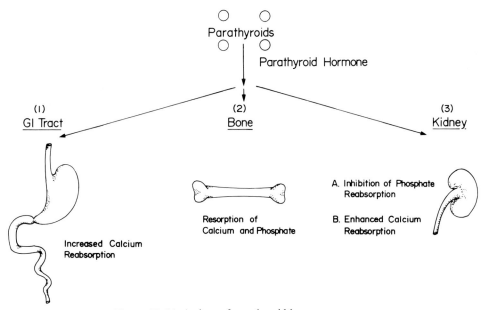

Figure 22–16. Actions of parathyroid hormone.

(4) enhancement of renal tubular calcium reabsorption (exact site unknown). The biochemical changes that result from excess parathyroid hormone secretion include hypercalcemia, hypophosphatemia, hyperphosphaturia, hypocalciuria, and increased urinary hydroxyproline secretion.

Classifications of Hyperparathyroidism

Hyperparathyroidism may be classified as primary, secondary, or tertiary. Primary hyperparathyroidism may be characterized as a primary dysfunction of the parathyroid glands. Secondary hyperparathyroidism includes reactive hyperplasia of the glands secondary to chronic renal failure, osteomalacia, or rickets. Tertiary hyperparathyroidism is considered secondary hyperparathyroidism with resultant autonomy of the parathyroid glands.

PRIMARY HYPERPARATHYROIDISM

Etiology. The syndrome of primary hyperparathyroidism may result from a single adenoma, diffuse hyperplasia, or carcinoma (Table 22–6).

Incidence. There has been a generalized increase in the number of patients reported with primary hyperparathyroidism during the past decade.[54-57] This increase has been attributed to the routine determination of serum calcium by new automated methods and the development of sensitive radioimmunoassay techniques for the detection of parathyroid hormone (Table 22–7). The routine screening of serum calcium has had a significant influence on the clinical presentation of patients with primary hyperthyroidism. The incidence of urolithiasis has fallen to less than 10 percent of its former rate, and three times as many patients now have no obvious symptoms or adverse effects of the disease.

Therapy. Treatment of patients with primary hyperparathyroidism is usually surgical and includes the following: (1) subtotal parathyroidectomy (3.5 glands); (2) adenomectomy plus three-gland biopsy; (3) total parathyroidectomy plus autotransplantation[59]; and, more recently, (4) ethanol injection into parathyroid adenomas in patients with chronic renal failure.[57] In experienced hands, surgery leads to a 90 to 95 percent cure rate without any preoperative localizing procedure. However, even the best techniques result in a 5 to 10 percent recurrence rate, usually related to aberrant or ectopically located glands or recurrent hyperplasia.[60-64] Re-exploration is technically more difficult, with a higher morbidity and poorer success rate than for the initial operative procedure. Diseased parathyroid glands are frequently aberrantly located, and the availability of an accurate, noninvasive test for the preoperative localization of these glands would be of great assistance to the surgeon.

Table 22–6. PATHOLOGIC CLASSIFICATION OF PARATHYROID LESIONS IN PATIENTS WITH PRIMARY HYPERPARATHYROIDISM (PERCENT)

Adenomas	
Single	80
Hyperplasia	
Chief Cell	15
Clear Cell	1
Carcinoma	4

Table 22–7. INCIDENCE OF PRIMARY HYPERPARATHYROIDISM

Relevant Factors	No. of Cases per 100,000	Study Period
Pre–routine Ca^{++} screening	7.8 ± 1.2	1965–1974
Post–routine Ca^{++} screening	51 ± 9.6	1975–1980
Age and sex: ≤39	<10	
≥40 female	188	
≤40 male	92	

Modified from Heath H, et al: Primary hyperparathyroidism: N Engl J Med *302*(4):955, 1980. Used by permission.

Parathyroid Imaging

Nuclear Medicine

Selenomethionine-75. Potchen and colleagues introduced the use of selenomethionine-75 (Se-75) labeled amino acid analogue of methionine, selenomethionine, in which there is an amorphous substitution of selenium for the naturally occurring sulfur as a scintigraphic agent for parathyroid scanning.[65] Although imaging with Se-75 is a noninvasive technique, the suboptimal imaging characteristics associated with its low sensitivity and specificity (Table 22–8) have made it a poor diagnostic test for detecting parathyroid adenomas. Modifications to improve the diagnostic yield of this test, including both Cytomel suppression and ^{99m}Tc subtraction, have proved unsuccessful, and the test has now been abandoned.[66]

Technetium-Thallium Subtraction. Ferlin and colleagues[67] and Young and colleagues[68] have described the successful utilization of combined technetium-thallium subtraction (^{99m}Tc/T1-201) imaging for the localization of parathyroid adenomas in patients with primary hyperparathyroidism. Modifications of this technique have been described by Basarab and associates.[69]

The ^{99m}Tc/T1-201 subtraction technique is based on the fact that the thyroid traps ^{99m}Tc and T1-201. It has been shown that parathyroid adenomas also take up T1-201. The accumulation of T1-201 in a parathyroid adenoma is nonspecific and is most likely related to the cellularity or vascularity of the lesion. Thus, T1-201 is administered to identify the thyroid and any parathyroid adenomas that may be present. ^{99m}Tc is administered to identify only the thyroid. The thyroid can then be subtracted out of the

Table 22–8. COMPARATIVE SENSITIVITY/SPECIFICITY OF TECHNIQUES USED FOR PARATHYROID IMAGING

Technique	Sensitivity(%)	Specificity(%)
Nuclear medicine		
Se-75/^{99m}Tc	40	51
T1-201/^{99m}Tc	95	94
I-131 RTB/^{99m}Tc	93	80
Real-time sonography		
Computerized tomography		
Conventional	63	95
High-resolution	70	96
Angiography		
SPA	69	*
NSADA	44	*
VDA	31	*
MRI*	*	*

SPA = Selective parathyroid angiography; NSADA = nonselective arterial digital anteriography; VDA = venous digital anteriography.
* Includes visualization of hyperplastic glands.

combined image by subtracting the ^{99m}Tc image from the T1-201 image. Any remaining areas of T1-201 concentration are probably markers for identification of parathyroid adenomas (Fig. 22–17).

There are several advantages to ^{99m}Tc/T1-201 subtraction for the detection of a parathyroid adenoma. It is a noninvasive technique and has a high sensitivity and specificity (Table 22–8) for the detection of parathyroid adenomas. In addition, it has the potential to identify both aberrant and ectopic glands. The disadvantages of this technique are its inability to determine adenoma depth, its inability to determine the relationship of the adenoma to adjacent structures, and its inability to detect four-gland hyperplasia with any degree of accuracy.[68] False positive results have been reported in patients with thyroid nodules, including hypertrophic[68–70] and malignant nodules,[71] multinodular goiter,[72] and sarcoid lymph nodes.[68]

Modifications to improve the sensitivity include taking oblique views,[73] administration of oral phosphates (1 gm per day in divided doses for three weeks),[74] and iodine-123/thallium-201 (I-123/T1-201) subtraction.[69] A disadvantage of I-123/T1-201 subtraction is that salivary glands will routinely appear positive, since iodine does not accumulate significantly in the salivary gland, whereas T1-201 does.

Iodine-131 Toluidine Blue/Tc-99m Imaging. Iodinated toluidine blue (RTB) is an organic, histologic radiopharmaceutical that is concentrated selectively in the parathyroid glands as opposed to the thyroid. Zwas et al.[74a] have documented a high sensitivity for detecting small hyperplastic parathyroid glands (30 mg) as well as parathyroid adenomas with superimposed I-131 TB/Tc-99m imaging (Table 22–8). False positive results with RTB have been reported secondary to lymph node uptake and focal thyroidal abnormalities.[74a] Labeling TB with radionuclides such as I-123 or Tc-99m will help optimize and enhance the use of RTB as a diagnostic parathyroid radiopharmaceutical.

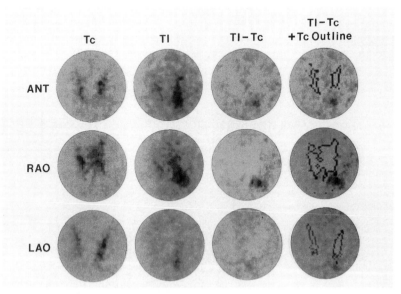

Figure 22–17. Tc-99m, Ti-201, and Tc-99m/Ti-201 subtraction images in the anterior, left anterior oblique (LAO), and right anterior oblique (RAO) projections using the pinhole collimator from a patient with a parathyroid adenoma situated at the base of the left lobe of the thyroid. Subtraction images with an overlay of the thyroid obtained from the Tc-99m image are also shown for localization purposes. (From Sandler MP et al: Thyroid and Parathyroid Imaging. East Norwalk, CT, Appleton-Century-Crofts, 1986. Used by permission.)

SONOGRAPHY

Sonographic imaging of the parathyroid gland has assumed increased clinical importance with the greater availability of high-resolution real-time sonography. Although normal parathyroids can only occasionally be imaged, abnormally enlarged parathyroids can be reliably detected with currently available scanners. Failure to delineate the gland is most likely due to the variable location of the small (2 to 3 mm) glands as well as their similar echogenicity to normal thyroid and surrounding tissue.

Enlarged parathyroid glands (75 mm), resulting from hypertrophy, adenoma, or neoplasia, can be identified with high-resolution real-time imaging.[76] Adenomatous, hyperplastic, and neoplastic glands demonstrate a texture that is less echogenic than surrounding thyroid tissue (Fig. 22–18).[76–79] Enlarged parathyroids tend to be fusiform. This is related to their dissection through longitudinally oriented tissue planes as they enlarge. Adenomas frequently measure approximately 1 cm in length in patients with clinical signs of hyperparathyroidism. Thus, parathyroid adenomas in normotopic glands are not difficult to detect. Problems occur when the abnormal gland is located in an ectopic position or in a sonographically inaccessible area, such as in a retroesophageal, substernal, or mediastinal position.

Hyperplasia of the parathyroids usually can be differentiated from an adenoma in that hyperplasia typically involves all four glands, whereas adenomas tend to involve one or two glands. Demonstration of the origin of these masses depends on careful localization of the masses to the regions of the parathyroids. Occasionally, thyroid nodules that are found in the expected location of parathyroid glands can mimic the appearance of parathyroid masses. Similarly, degenerated parathyroid adenomas may mimic partially cystic thyroid masses.

Sonographic identification of abnormally enlarged parathyroid glands may be helpful to the neck surgeon, since the abnormal gland can be localized preoperatively, thus decreasing the operating time and the need for intraoperative exploration of each of the glands. Sonography has been shown to be of particular help in evaluation of patients with persistent or recurrent hyperparathyroidism, since the abnormal gland(s) in the neck can be identified. However, false negative studies may occur when the abnormal gland is retroesophageal, substernal, or mediastinal in position.

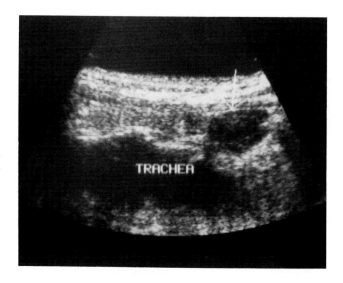

Figure 22–18. Longitudinal sonogram showing parathyroid adenoma, 1 cm in diameter, inferior to the left thyroid lobe. (From Sandler MP et al: Thyroid and Parathyroid Imaging. East Norwalk, CT, Appleton-Century-Crofts, 1986. Used by permission.)

COMPUTED TOMOGRAPHY

The accuracy of computerized tomography (CT) in the detection of parathyroid adenomas is largely dependent on tumor size.[80-85] The use of specially designed positioning maneuvers, bolus contrast administration, and dynamic CT scanning has improved the ability of this modality to detect parathyroid lesions. The use of intravenous contrast material is necessary to distinguish vessels from adjacent soft tissue structures and parathyroid masses. Stark and colleagues[88] have demonstrated contrast enhancement in 25 percent of parathyroid tumors and noted that large adenomas were more likely to enhance than small adenomas and that large hyperplastic glands were more likely to enhance than small hyperplastic glands (Fig. 22–19). Disadvantages of high-resolution CT scanning include the use of ionizing radiation, requirement for contrast enhancement, and anatomic distortion from scarring and metal clips in those patients who have a history of previous thyroid or parathyroid surgery. The major advantage of CT is its ability to locate parathyroid tumors that may be situated in either the retrosternal or the retroclavicular position.

ANGIOGRAPHY

Angiographic techniques used to locate parathyroid adenomas include selective parathyroid arteriography and venous sampling,[86] nonselective arterial digital arteriography,[87] and venous digital arteriography. Selective arteriography is not an ideal technique for assessing the parathyroid glands because of its low sensitivity (see Table 22–8) and its requirement for considerable expertise to perform the procedure. In addition, the possibility of stroke or spinal cord infarction has limited the examination to only a few centers. Other problems include prolonged catheterization time, significant radiation exposure, and large contrast loads in some patients with a history of compromised renal function. Although both digital and arterial venous angiography offer several advantages over conventional arteriography, they remain significantly less sensitive than noninvasive imaging modalities currently available for the detection of parathyroid lesions.

MAGNETIC RESONANCE IMAGING (MRI)

Although the spatial resolution of MRI is currently a limiting factor, the use of specialized surface coils provides imaging with sharp detail in a superficial structure such as the parathyroid glands (Fig. 22–20). A variety of parathyroid lesions have been

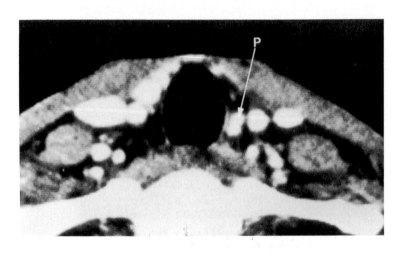

Figure 22–19. Contrast-enhancing parathyroid adenoma. Axial CT section with tumor at left lower pole of thyroid gland (arrow). At operation, adenoma measured 20 × 9 × 5 mm. (From Stark DD et al: AJR *141*:633, 1983. Used by permission.)

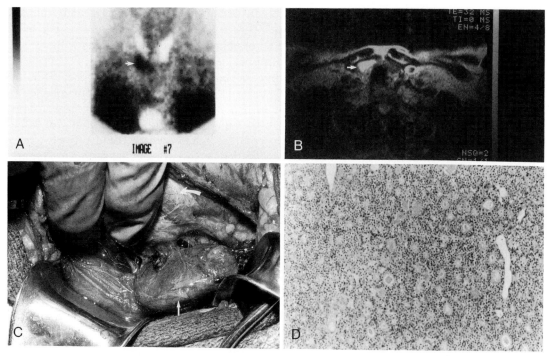

Figure 22-20. *A*, Tc-99m/Ti-201 subtraction image in the anterior projection, using a converging collimator, from a patient with a parathyroid adenoma situated at the base of the right lobe of the thyroid (arrow). *B*, Transverse view of the neck, MRI surface-coil image, 2000/128, 1 cm slice thickness. Parathyroid adenoma (arrow) situated at the inferior pole of the right lobe of the thyroid. *C*, Intraoperative view of parathyroid adenoma identified in *A* and *B*. Parathyroid adenoma (straight arrow), inferior pole of the right lobe of thyroid (curved arrow). *D*, Microscopy of adenoma reveals a typically highly cellular lesion made up of uniformly eosinophilic finely granular cells. In some areas, characteristic small acini are present. (*C*, Courtesy of W. Scott, M.D. *D*, Courtesy of J. Baxter, M.D.)

identified using MRI, some of which were 0.5 cm in size.[88] Although the lesions could be separated from adjacent structures, it was not possible to distinguish reliably between the various types of parathyroid tumors. Spritzer et al.,[89] in a limited study of 23 hyperparathyroid patients, calculated the overall sensitivity and specificity of high-resolution MRI in the detection of parathyroid abnormalities to be 77.8 percent and 95.4 percent, respectively. However, the inability of *T1* and *T2* weighted images to differentiate parathyroid disorders from a wide range of thyroid pathology,[90] as well as lymph nodes in the neck, may result in a significant decrease in the specificity of MRI to detect parathyroid lesions.[88] Routine preoperative evaluation of patients with suspected hyperparathyroidism remains to be established.

In conclusion, technetium-99m/thallium-201 subtraction imaging has proved to be an accurate, noninvasive procedure for the detection of parathyroid adenomas. The sensitivity and specificity of dual subtraction parathyroid scintigraphy is equal to or better than that of other noninvasive imaging modalities. Tc-99m/Ti-201 subtraction should be the investigative modality of choice in both pre- and postoperative localization of parathyroid tissue. Ultrasound and CT, within limits, should be used as complementary procedures to help identify those adenomas missed by radionuclide subtraction imaging, enabling increased diagnostic accuracy. Angiography, because of its invasiveness, should be reserved for finding recurrence of ectopic adenomas not detected by the previously mentioned modalities following failed initial surgery.

The role of MRI in parathyroid lesions remains to be defined. Care must be exercised in the use of *T1* measurements in patients with thyroid nodules because calibration of an MR imager must be continually performed to assure precise determination of *T1*. In addition, the absolute value of *T1* is dependent upon the strength of the magnetic field utilized. Thus, comparison of values between instruments with different magnetic field strengths and resonant frequencies is complex.

Rapid improvements in image quality are being achieved in MRI. These, in addition to improvements in the precision of *T1* determinations, will undoubtedly enhance the use of MRI in all fields. Determination of tissue *T2* values, and in vivo spectroscopy, in addition to *T1* measurements, may further improve the diagnostic ability of MRI.

The development of paramagnetic contrast agents, which could provide greater tissue discrimination on the basis of vascularity, is still in its initial stages.[52] Paramagnetic metal ion chelates may potentially be linked to more site-specific ligands, providing the chemical basis for tissue-specific contrast agents. Development of this class of compounds could have impact, especially upon imaging of the thyroid and parathyroid glands by MR and differentiation between benign and malignant disease. Optimization of pulse sequence techniques to provide the greatest contrast between tissue structures (as discussed in Chapter 8) and development of surface coil technology could significantly improve MRI of the thyroid and parathyroid. Future comparative studies will define the role of MRI in the diagnosis of thyroid and parathyroid disease. Cost-effectiveness may limit its application, despite the ability of MR to display both anatomic and functional information with high resolution and excellent quality. Other chapters review the evolving role of MRI in endocrinologic studies of the pituitary (Chapter 16), the adrenal (Chapter 32), the ovaries (Chapter 34), and the testicles (Chaper 33).

ACKNOWLEDGMENT

The authors extend their grateful appreciation to Ms. Sharon Phillips for her patience and perseverance during the preparation of the manuscript.

References

1. Shepard TH: The thyroid. *In* Dehann AC, Ursprung H (eds): Organogenesis. New York, Holt, Rinehart & Winston, 1965.
2. Pearse AGE, Carvalheira AF: Cytochemical evidence for an ultimobranchial origin of rodent thyroid C cells. Nature *214*:929, 1967.
3. Raisz LG: Bone metabolism and calcium regulation. *In* Avioli LV, Krane SM (eds): Metabolic Bone Disease. Vol 1. New York, Academic Press, 1977.
4. Toran-Allerand CD: Normal development of the hypothalamic-pituitary-thyroid axis: Ontogeny of the neuroendocrine unit. *In* Werner SC, Ingbar SH (eds): The Thyroid. New York, Harper & Row, 1978, p 403.
5. Villee DB: Development of endocrine function in the human placenta and fetus (second of two parts). N Engl J Med *281*:533, 1969.
6. Villee DB: Human Endocrinology. A Developmental Approach. Philadelphia, WB Saunders, 1975.
7. Feind CR: Surgical anatomy. *In* Werner SC, Ingbar SH (eds): The Thyroid. New York, Harper & Row, 1978, p 426.
8. Sloan LW: Surgical anatomy of the thyroid. *In* Werner SC, Ingbar SH (eds): The Thyroid, 3rd ed. New York, Harper & Row, 1971, p 323.
9. Andros G, Harper PV, Lathrop KA, et al: Pertechnetate 99m localization in man with applications to thyroid scanning and the study of thyroid physiology. J Clin Endocrinol Metab *25*:1067, 1965.
10. Sodee DB: The study of thyroid physiology utilizing intravenous sodium pertechnetate. J Nucl Med *7*:564, 1966.
11. Atkins HL, Richard P: Assessment of thyroid function and anatomy with technetium 99m pertechnetate. J Nucl Med *9*:7, 1968.
12. Burke GA, Halko A, Silverstein GE, et al: Comparative thyroid uptake studies with I-131 and 99m-Tc04. J Clin Endocrinol Metab *34*:630, 1972.
13. dos Remedios LV, Weber PM, Jasko IA: Thyroid scintiphotography in 1,000 patients: Rational use of 99m-Tc and I-131 compounds. J Nucl Med *12*:673, 1971.
14. Wang CA, Vickery AL, Maloof F: The role of needle biopsy in evaluating solitary cold thyroid nodules. *In* Robbins J, Braverman LE (eds): Thyroid Research. Amsterdam, Excerpta Medica, 1976, p 568.

15. Psarra A, Papadopoulos SN, Livada D, et al: The single thyroid nodule. Br J Surg *59*:545, 1974.
16. Mazzaferri EL, Young RL, Oertel JE, et al: Papillary thyroid carcinomas: The impact of therapy in 576 patients. Medicine *56*:171, 1977.
17. Park HM, Zieverink S, Ransburg RC, et al: Marine-Lenhart syndrome: Graves' disease with poorly functioning nodules. Proceedings of VIII International Thyroid Congress. Canberra, Australian Academy of Science, 1980, p 641.
18. Jackson IMD, Thomson JA: The relationship of carcinoma to the single thyroid nodule. Br J Surg *54*:1007, 1967.
19. Sisson JC, Bartold SP, Bartold SL: The dilemma of the solitary thyroid nodule: Resolution through decision analysis. Semin Nucl Med *8*:59, 1978.
20. Goldsmith SJ: Thyroid in vivo tests of function and imaging. *In* Rothfeld B (ed): Nuclear Medicine Endocrinology. Philadelphia, JB Lippincott, 1978, p 19.
21. Roualle HLM: The solitary thyroid nodule and thyrotoxicosis. Br J Surg *36*:312, 1949.
22. Strauss HW, Hurley PJ, Wagner HN Jr: Advantages of 99m Tc pertechnetate for thyroid scanning in patients with decreased radioiodine uptake. Radiology *97*:307, 1970.
23. Atkins HL, Klopper JF, Laubrerit RM, et al: A comparison of technetium 99m and iodine for thyroid imaging. Am J Roentgenol Radium Ther Nucl Med *117*:195, 1973.
24. Shambaugh GE III, Quinn JL, Oyasu R, et al: Disparate thyroid imaging: Combined studies with sodium pertechnetate Tc-99m and radioactive iodine. JAMA *228*:886, 1974.
25. Sykes D: The solitary thyroid nodule. Br J Surg *68*:510, 1981.
26. Propper RA, Skolnick ML, Weinstein BJ, et al: The nonspecificity of the thyroid halo sign. J Clin Ultrasound *8*:129, 1980.
27. Simeone JR, Daniels GH, Mueller RP, et al: High-resolution real-time sonography of the thyroid. Radiology *145*:431, 1982.
28. Gobien RP: Aspiration biopsy of the solitary thyroid nodule. Radiol Clin North Am *17*:543, 1979.
29. Brown CL: Pathology of the cold nodule. J Clin Endocrinol Metab *10*:235, 1981.
30. Miller JM: Carcinoma and thyroid nodules: The problem in an endemic goiter area. N Engl J Med *252*:247, 1955.
31. Patton JA, Hollifield JW, Brill AB, et al: Differentiation between malignant and benign solitary thyroid nodules by fluorescent scanning. J Nucl Med *17*(1):17, 1976.
32. Patton JA, Sandler MP, Sacks GA, et al: Prediction of benignancy of solitary "cold" thyroid nodules using x-ray fluorescent scanning. Endocr Soc *64*:281, 1982.
33. Patton JA, Sandler MP, Partain CL: Prediction of benignancy of the solitary "cold" thyroid nodule by fluorescent scanning. J Nucl Med *26*:461, 1985.
34. de Certaines J, Herry JY, Lancien G, et al: Evaluation of human thyroid tumors by proton nuclear magnetic resonance. J Nucl Med *23*:48, 1982.
35. Smith FW, Runge VM, Sandler MP, et al: Magnetic resonance imaging in thyroid disease. *In* Sandler MP, Patton JA, Partain CL: Thyroid and Parathyroid Imaging. ACC, 1986, p 339.
36. Runge VM, Smith FW: NMR imaging of the thyroid. J Nucl Med *24*(5):P46, 1983.
37. Daniel RA Jr, Diveley WL, Edwards WH, et al: Mediastinal tumors. Ann Surg *151*:783, 1960.
38. Sweet RH: Intrathoracic goiter located in the posterior mediastinum. Surg Gynecol Obstet *89*:57, 1949.
39. Glazer GM, Axel L, Moss AA: CT diagnosis of mediastinal thyroid. AJR *138*:495, 1982.
40. McCort JJ: Intrathoracic goiter: Its incidence, symptomatology and roentgen diagnosis. Radiology *53*:227, 1949.
41. Ellis FH Jr, Good CA: Intrathoracic goiter. Ann Surg *135*:79, 1952.
42. Leigh TF: Mass lesions of the mediastinum. Radiol Clin North Am *1*:377, 1983.
43. Burkell CC, Cross JM, Kent HP, et al: Mass lesions of the mediastinum. Curr Probl Surg *2*:57, 1969.
44. Bashist B, Ellis K, Gold RP: Computed tomography of intrathoracic goiters. AJR *140*:455, 1983.
45. Cohen AM, Crevistom S, LiPuma JP, et al: NMR evaluation of hilar and mediastinal lymphadenopathy. Radiology *148*:739, 1983.
46. Pizzarello D, Witrofski R: Medical Radiation Biology. Philadelphia, Lea & Febiger, 1972, p 83.
47. Fernandez-Ulloa M, Maxon HR, Mehta S, et al: Iodine 131 uptake by primary lung adenocarcinoma: Misinterpretation of I-131 scan. JAMA *236*:857, 1976.
48. Benjamin SP, McCormack LJ, Effler DB, et al: Primary tumors of the mediastinum. Chest *62*:297, 1972.
49. Brasch RC, Boyd DP, Gooding CA: Computer tomographic scanning in children: Comparison of radiation dose and resolving powers of commercial CT scanners. AJR *131*:95, 1978.
50. Sekiya T, Tada S, Kawakami K, et al: Clinical application of computed tomography to thyroid disease. Comput Tomogr *3*:185, 1979.
51. Sandler MP, Patton JA, Sacks GA, et al: Evaluation of intrathoracic goiter with I-123 scintigraphy and nuclear magnetic resonance imaging. J Nucl Med *25*:874, 1984.
52. Runge VM, Clanton JA, Lukehart CM, et al: Paramagnetic agents for contrast enhanced NMR imaging: A review. AJR *141*:1209, 1983.
53. Runge VM, Clanton JA, Herzer WA, et al: Intravascular contrast agents suitable for magnetic resonance imaging. Radiology *153*:171, 1984.
54. Boonstra CE, Jackson CE: Serum calcium: Survey for hyperparathyroidism: Results in 50,000 clinic patients. Am J Clin Pathol *55*:523, 1971.
55. Preisman RA, Mehnert JH: A plethora of primary hyperparathyroidism. Arch Surg *103*:12, 1971.
56. Johansson H, Thoren L, Werner I: Hyperparathyroidism: Clinical experiences from 208 cases. Ups J Med Sci *77*:41, 1972.

57. Heath H, Hodgson SF, Kennedy MA: Primary hyperparathyroidism: Incidence, morbidity, and potential economic impact in a community. N Engl J Med *302*(4):955, 1980.
58. Solbiati L, Montali G, Crace F, et al: Parathyroid tumors detected by fine-needle aspiration biopsy under ultrasonic guidance. Radiology *148*:793, 1983.
59. Coffey RJ, Lee TC, Canary JJ: The surgical treatment of primary hyperparathyroidism: A 20 year experience. Ann Surg *185*:518, 1981.
60. Clark OH, Way LW, Hunt TK: Recurrent hyperparathyroidism. Ann Surg *184*:391, 1976.
61. Brennan MR, Marx SJ, Doppman J, et al: Results of reoperation for persistent and recurrent hyperparathyroidism. Ann Surg *194*:671, 1981.
62. Martin JK, van Heerden JA, Edis AJ, et al: Persistent postoperative hyperparathyroidism. Surg Gynecol Obstet *151*:164, 1980.
63. Wang CA: Parathyroid re-exploration: A clinical and pathological study of 112 cases. Ann Surg *186*:140, 1977.
64. Livesay JJ, Mulder DG: Recurrent hyperparathyroidism. Arch Surg *111*:688, 1976.
65. Potchen EJ, Adelstein SJ, Dealy JB: Radiographic localization of the overactive human parathyroid. AJR *93*(4):955, 1965.
66. Waldorf JC, van Heerden JA, Gorman CA, et al: [^{75}Se] Selenomethionine scanning for parathyroid localization should be abandoned. Mayo Clinic Proc *59*:534, 1984.
67. Ferlin G, Borsato N, Camerani M, et al: New perspectives in localizing enlarged parathyroids by technetium-thallium subtraction scan. J Nucl Med *24*:438, 1983.
68. Young AE, Gaunt JI, Croft DN, et al: Location of parathyroid adenoma by thallium-201 and technetium-99m subtraction scanning. Br Med J *286*:1384, 1983.
69. Basarab RM, Manni A, Harrison TS: Dual isotope subtraction parathyroid scintigraphy in the preoperative evaluation of suspected hyperparathyroidism. Clin Nucl Med *10*(4):100, 1985.
70. McKusick KA, Palmer EL, Hergenrother J, et al: Is there a role for dual tracer imaging in detection of parathyroid disease? J Nucl Med *25*:P19, 1984.
71. Punt CJA, DeHooge P, Hoekstra JBL: False-positive subtraction scintigram of the parathyroid glands due to metastatic tumor. J Nucl Med *26*:155, 1985.
72. Fukuchi M, Hyodo K, Tachibana K, et al: Marked thyroid uptake of thallium-201 in patients with goiter: Case report. J Nucl Med *18*:1199, 1977.
73. Urgancioglu I, Hatemi H, Seyahi V, et al: Letter to the editor. J Nucl Med *26*(1):99, 1985.
74. Gupta SM, Belsky JL: Letter to the editor. J Nucl Med *26*(1):99, 1985.
74a. Zwas ST, Czerniak A, Boruchowsky S, et al: Preoperative parathyroid localization by superimposed iodine-131 toluidine blue and technetium-99m pertechnetate imaging. J Nucl Med *29*:298, 1987.
75. Simeone J, Mueller P, Ferrucci J, et al: High-resolution real-time sonography of the parathyroid. Radiology *141*:745, 1981.
76. Sample W, Mitchell S, Bledsoe R: Parathyroid ultrasonography. Radiology *127*:485, 1978.
77. Duffy P, Picker R, Duffield S, et al: Parathyroid sonography: A useful aid to preoperative localization. J Clin Ultrasound *8*:113, 1980.
78. Reading C, Charboneau JW, James EM: High resolution parathyroid sonography. AJR *139*:539, 1982.
79. Scheible W, Deutsch A, Leopold G: Parathyroid adenoma: Accuracy of preoperative localization by high-resolution real-time sonography. J Clin Ultrasound *9*:325, 1981.
80. Stark DD, Gooding GAW, Moss AA, et al: Parathyroid imaging: Comparison of high-resolution CT and high-resolution sonography. AJR *141*:633, 1983.
81. Ovenfors CO, Stark D, Moss AA, et al: Localization of parathyroid adenoma by computed tomography. J Comput Assist Tomogr *6*:1094, 1982.
82. Friedman M, Mafee MF, Shelton VK, et al: Parathyroid localization by computed tomographic scanning. Arch Otolaryngol *109*:95, 1983.
83. Takagi H, Tominaga Y, Uchida K, et al: Preoperative diagnosis of secondary hyper-parathyroidism using computed tomography. J Comput Assist Tomogr *6*:527, 1982.
84. Sommer B, Welter HF, Spelsberg F, et al: Computed tomography for localizing enlarged parathyroid glands in primary hyperparathyroidism. J Comput Assist Tomogr *6*:521, 1982.
85. Stark DD, Moss AA, Gooding GAW, et al: Parathyroid scanning by computed tomography. Radiology *148*:297, 1983.
86. Krudy AG, Doppman JL, Brennan MF, et al: The detection of mediastinal parathyroid glands by computed tomography, selective arteriography and venous sampling. Radiology *140*:739, 1981.
87. Brennan MF, Doppman JL, Krudy AG, et al: Assessment of techniques for preoperative parathyroid gland localization in patients undergoing reoperation for hyperparathyroidism. Surgery *91*:6, 1982.
88. Stark DD, Moss AA, Gamsu G, Clark OH, Gooding GAW, Webb WR: Magnetic resonance imaging of the neck, part 2: Pathologic findings. Radiology *150*:455, 1984.
89. Spritzer CE, Gefter WB, Hamilton R, et al: Abnormal parathyroid glands: High-resolution MR imaging. Radiology *162*:487, 1987.
90. Sandler MP, Patton JA: Multimodality imaging of the thyroid and parathyroid glands. J Nucl Med *28*(1):122, 1987.

V

CLINICAL EXPERIENCE: MRI OF THE HEART AND THORAX

23

Ischemic Heart Disease

ROBERT C. CANBY
RUSSELL C. REEVES
WILLIAM T. EVANOCHKO
GERALD M. POHOST

A major problem facing medicine today is ischemic heart disease (IHD). Approximately 1 million deaths annually in the United States are due to cardiovascular disease; one half of these deaths result from myocardial infarction. At the present time, non-invasive methods that are helpful in the assessment of patients with possible IHD include electrocardiographic stress testing, radionuclide techniques, and echocardiography. Although all are useful, each has certain serious limitations. In exercise electrocardiography, the patient's inability to exercise maximally is a frequent cause for an indeterminant result. The incidence of false negative and false positive tests is relatively high. Radionuclide procedures provide a means for evaluating relative regional myocardial perfusion as well as global and regional ventricular function at rest and with exercise. A major limitation of the radionuclide methods is their low resolution. The incidence of false negative and false positive tests is moderate. Echocardiography can generate relatively high-resolution images of the heart and can be used to assess regional ventricular wall motion, but bone and lung obstruct transmission of ultrasound and frequently obscure a view of the entire heart. Since IHD is usually regional in its distribution, an obstructed view can be a serious impediment to diagnostic evaluation.

In the early 1970s, methods for generating images using the principles of MR were described[1]; and in 1978 the first MR image of the heart was published.[2] Today, electrocardiographically gated proton MR imaging can generate images with excellent morphologic detail and contrast. Nevertheless, since radionuclide and ultrasound methods usually provide adequate morphologic information, it is most likely that other aspects of MR imaging will ultimately determine its relative importance as a cardiovascular diagnostic tool.

Many different cardiologically relevant nuclei are MR-sensitive. For a given nucleus, the intensity of the MR signal is related to its concentration, motion, and the relaxation properties of the imaged tissue. Accordingly, MR methods provide several avenues for diagnosis and assessment of IHD. Thus, clinical MR applications have been largely in proton imaging for assessment of cardiac and large vessel morphology. This chapter will focus on the important diagnostic problems in IHD that MR methods have the potential to address. These applications can be divided into five categories: (1) noninvasive angiography, (2) assessment of the extent and severity of coronary artery disease on regional myocardial perfusion, (3) detection of myocardial infarction, (4) evaluation of the complications of myocardial infarction, and (5) assessment of the effects of pharmacotherapy on IHD.

NONINVASIVE ANGIOGRAPHY

Owing to its prevalence and the considerable morbidity and mortality associated with it, atherosclerotic involvement of the coronary arteries is one of the most important diseases facing modern cardiology. Currently, no adequate noninvasive methods exist for direct detection of coronary artery disease. MRI, however, exhibits potential for providing useful definition of the coronary vessels. The contrast generated within proton MR images by motion, hence to blood flow, suggests that it will be a powerful tool for delineating the internal structure of the vasculature and cardiac chambers without the need for contrast medium. The reduction of MR signal intensity related to more rapid proton motion accounts for the contrast between arterial lumen and surrounding wall. In general, faster flow results in a greater reduction in signal. Accordingly, contrast between arterial vessels and surrounding tissue can be maximized by synchronizing, or gating, acquisition to the portion of the cardiac cycle with highest flow. In addition to images of the abdominal aorta and iliac vessels,[3] glimpses of the proximal portions of the coronary arteries have been visualized using gated MR techniques (Fig. 23–1).[4] Furthermore, MR techniques may provide a means to take quantitative measurements of flow velocity and assess the impact of obstructions on flow velocity.[5–7] Van Dijk[8] has developed a method to generate velocity-encoded images by measuring the phase shifts induced by the motion of the spins.

Proton MR imaging has the potential to detect atherosclerotic disease involving the arterial vasculature by depicting (1) the physical distortion of the arterial lumen, (2) anomalies in the intra-arterial signal resulting from turbulence or variations in intra-arterial velocity profile, and (3) gross MR characterization of plaque. The protons of aliphatic lipids are characterized by relaxation properties that differ substantially from those of the protons of normal cell water. Such fats have short *T1* and long *T2* values. Accordingly, signal intensity is increased in *T2* sensitive spin-echo images. Such lipid-sensitive increased signal intensity may allow visualization of early atherosclerotic plaque. Indeed, atherosclerosis in iliac and femoral arterial vessels has been demonstrated in vivo.[9]

Proton MR imaging has the inherent resolution required for visualization of the lumen of the proximal coronary arteries; however, several factors make such imaging technically difficult. Electrocardiographic gating provides images with sufficient res-

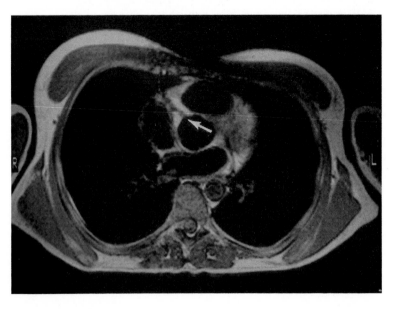

Figure 23–1. Gated transverse spin-echo image visualizing the descending aorta and cardiac outflow vessels (aorta centrally and pulmonary outflow anteriorly). Loss of signal intensity caused by blood flow in the right coronary artery can be observed (arrow). (Courtesy of Philips Medical Systems, Best, The Netherlands.)

olution to depict the cardiac chambers and great vessels, with glimpses of proximal coronary arterial lumen. However, variations in coronary artery position, due to respiratory motion and changes in the size of the heart from fluctuation in ventricular filling caused mainly by changes in cardiac cycle length, reduce the resolving potential of this imaging method. Respiratory gating may improve resolution but will substantially increase imaging time and will not overcome the image degradation related to heart rate–dependent changes in heart size. High-speed image acquisition techniques, such as the echo planar method of Mansfield, may be helpful by reducing the acquisition period to the 30 ms range.[10] However, at present such methods have limited resolution.

A second problem with the coronary artery imaging techniques is their tortuous nature. Consequently, tomographic sections are inadequate for diagnostic study. The three-dimensional imaging possibilities of MR could overcome the sampling problems of other methods, including coronary angiography but would also increase the complexity and duration of the procedure. In conclusion, imaging and characterization of the coronary arteries will be technically difficult. Nevertheless, because of the clinical importance of detecting coronary artery atherosclerosis, especially that involving the left main and proximal vessels, successful MR coronary angiography would be unique and would justify cost.

ASSESSMENT OF CORONARY ARTERY DISEASE

Assessment of relative regional myocardial blood flow during exercise or with administration of the vasodilator dipyridamole has been of considerable clinical value for physiologic determination of the severity of coronary artery disease. Radionuclide methods, including thallium-201 gamma camera imaging and rubidium-82 positron-emission computed tomographic imaging, are used currently to provide a clinical assessment of relative regional myocardial blood flow and to determine the pathophysiologic consequences of coronary atherosclerosis. However, resolution is limited, and with thallium-201, gamma photon energy is low, resulting in frequent artifacts from attenuation by overlying soft tissue and bone. Despite these technical problems, thallium imaging is of clinical importance in the detection and prognosis of coronary artery disease.[11–14] MR imaging has substantially better resolution than radionuclide methods, and image intensity is not attenuated by overlying tissue. However, it will be necessary to develop an MR contrast agent comparable to thallium-201, which localizes in myocardium.

Paramagnetic relaxation reagents are being examined for their clinical utility for assessing IHD. Paramagnetic agents have unpaired electrons that accelerate relaxation of MR-sensitive nuclei and thereby shorten $T1$ and $T2$. Accordingly, these substances can be used as contrast agents for MR imaging studies. For example, manganous (Mn^{++}) ion is strongly paramagnetic, and its radionuclide Mn-54 has been shown to distribute in the myocardium in proportion to blood flow.[15] Lauterbur et al.[16] demonstrated that the relaxation times of normal myocardium were significantly reduced after intravenous administration of manganous chloride ($MnCl_2$) in dogs. To assess the potential utility of paramagnetic contrast enhancement in the evaluation of IHD, Goldman et al.[17] studied dogs that were infused with intravenous $MnCl_2$ after 24 hours of left circumflex coronary artery ligation. Excised hearts were imaged using the steady-state–free-precession (SSFP) technique in a 7 inch 1.44 tesla prototype imaging system. Hearts from animals that did not receive the Mn^{++} infusion revealed no differences in the intensities between normal and ischemic zones, whereas those with Mn^{++} showed a clearly defined zone of reduced signal intensity. Deficits in Mn^{++} distribution were compared with deficits in the uptake of the supravital dye, triphenyltetrazolium chloride (TTC), which indicates infarct size. Infarct size, as measured by TTC, correlated well with that defined by proton MR Mn^{++} distribution. Although Mn^{++} appears to be a reasonable myocardial perfusion imaging agent, the toxicity of the manganese ion in doses needed to alter image appearance seems to preclude clinical use.

To reduce the toxicity of ions of such paramagnetic metals as manganese and of gadolinium (Gd), the paramagnetic element with the greatest effect on the relaxation times of hydrogen nuclei,[18] these agents are complexed with ligands such as diethylenetriaminepentaacetic acid (DTPA). Wesbey et al.[19] administered Gd-DTPA to dogs after 24 hours of coronary artery ligation. Nonischemic zones from hearts in animals injected with Gd-DTPA had significantly shorter myocardial relaxation times than did infarcted zones excised 90 seconds after injection. In contrast, at five minutes after injection, infarcted myocardium had shortened relaxation times and noninfarcted myocardium returned toward control, suggesting early accumulation in and clearance from normal myocardium and delayed accumulation in and clearance from infarcted myocardium. In another study,[20] spin-echo images of dogs infused with Gd-DTPA one minute following coronary ligation demonstrated regions of increased signal intensity in the anterior wall of the left ventricle, reflecting the longer *T2* values in the ischemic zones versus the adjacent normal myocardium. No differences in signal intensities between ischemic and normal myocardium were observed in spin-echo images following one minute of left anterior descending (LAD) coronary artery ligation in dogs without Gd-DTPA infusion.

These studies suggest that Gd-DTPA may be useful to outline regional myocardial blood distribution in experimental coronary occlusion; however, the short time course of the relaxation rate enhancement precludes clinical usefulness. Furthermore, Gd-DTPA is an extracellular and nonspecific marker of myocardial perfusion. To be clinically useful, it would be desirable to develop an agent that could be extracted by viable or nonischemic myocardial cells. Like thallium-201, such an agent could be administered during exercise or other stress and provide a means for detecting coronary artery disease without the low resolution and attenuation problems of thallium.[21]

Other approaches to produce contrast agents are under investigation and may have relevance in myocardial imaging. Elgavish et al.[22] have developed a strongly paramagnetic complex of bis-dihydroxyphosphonylmethyl phosphinate and gadolinium (Gd-BDP) and are now investigating to determine its suitability as a myocardial imaging agent. Brasch[23] is evaluating stable free radicals as MR contrast agents. Unlike paramagnetic inorganic ions, the unpaired electron in the free radical is contained in an outermost molecular orbital path. Because of their potential for chemical bonding, nitroxide stable free radicals (NSFR) are well suited for labeling target specific biomolecules. These agents have been covalently attached to several drugs, such as propranolol and steroids.[24,25] By complexing NSFR compounds to substances of known specificity, tissue and receptor selectivity may be possible.

In conclusion, there are no paramagnetic agents suitable for myocardial perfusion imaging at the present time. A paramagnetic metal such as gadolinium will need to be complexed with a chelating agent to reduce toxicity to clinically applicable levels. Such an agent will have to have specificity for myocardial cells to depict the perfusion pattern. That is, it must remain within the myocardium long enough to allow administration during exercise and imaging over a 30 to 60 minute period.

MYOCARDIAL INFARCT DETECTION

In recent years, efforts to limit the extent of myocardial necrosis associated with acute myocardial infarction (MI) have intensified with the appreciation that prognosis is dependent on the amount of myocardial destruction. Reperfusion of ischemic myocardium early in the course of infarction by administration of intracoronary or intravenous streptokinase or tissue plasminogen activator, or by transluminal coronary angioplasty or immediate surgical revascularization, has been shown to be feasible. Pharmacologic intervention with beta blockers, calcium channel blockers, and nitrates has been used early in the course of MI in an attempt to limit the size of the infarction. To demonstrate the benefit of such procedures, it is necessary to identify at a very early stage the ischemically insulted myocardium and to accurately and reproducibly quantify the size of the infarct. Proton MR is emerging as a high-resolution, noninvasive technique that is potentially useful for infarct sizing.

MR spectroscopic and imaging methods can be used to evaluate the proton relaxation times, $T1$ and $T2$, in tissues. These MR parameters are affected by the concentration and compartmentalization of water, the concentration and type of lipid, macromolecular environment, temperature, and other factors affecting the chemical milieu.[26–29] In virtually all models of myocardial disease, $T1$ and/or $T2$ become abnormal. Measurement of bulk tissue relaxation rates of biopsy material from animal models of disease can help evaluate the utility of proton MR imaging techniques to depict these relaxation times in vivo. Among the first such studies were those of Buonanno et al.[30] of ischemic stroke in gerbils. They demonstrated substantial increases in $T1$ and $T2$ in the cerebral hemispheres with ischemic strokes within two hours after carotid ligation. Studies of the changes in proton relaxation parameters in myocardial ischemic insult are currently being explored. The earliest study, by Williams et al.,[31] reported $T1$ prolongation in the myocardium of dogs within 30 minutes of LAD ligation. $T1$ increased as the duration of ischemia increased to 120 minutes. These $T1$ increases were not directly related to tissue levels of high-energy phosphates, lactate, or hydrogen ions but appeared to reflect the increased water content in the regionally ischemic myocardium.

During ischemia, certain physical and biochemical changes occur that may alter the magnetic relaxation times. These include changes in (1) tissue concentrations of oxygen, high-energy compounds, and electrolytes; (2) content and distribution of tissue water; and (3) pH. Water content appears to play an important role in the rise of $T1$ and $T2$ after coronary occlusion. Jennings et al.[32] have demonstrated that myocardial ischemia following acute coronary artery ligation results in a time-dependent increase in tissue water and sodium content. In very early ischemia, only intracellular water content, not total water content, rises.[33] If the ischemia persists, total myocardial water content increases,[34,35] but it remains primarily intracellular owing to disrupted cell membrane function; however, some interstitial edema occurs.

Reperfusion affects myocardial water content and electrolytes as a function of the severity of ischemic damage. Following irreversible myocardial cell injury, massive swelling and ion concentration changes occur with reperfusion.[36] In reversibly injured tissue, ion and water changes observed with reflow are much smaller in magnitude and are sometimes in a different direction.[37] Thus, viable but damaged reperfused myocardium has a characteristic electrolyte and water distribution that differs greatly from that of reperfused irreversibly damaged myocardium.

Later in the course of an infarct, additional pathologic changes are observed. For example, lipid accumulation and fibrosis are seen. Post-mortem human studies show that acute inflammatory changes predominate in the first week after MI, chronic inflammatory mechanisms predominate during the second week, and fibrosis predominates during the third week. By five weeks after MI, scar tissue has largely replaced the damaged myocardium.

To determine the relationship between proton relaxation times and acute myocardial damage, Ratner et al.[38,39] measured $T1$ and $T2$ in myocardial tissue subjected to 30 or 60 minutes of coronary occlusion with and without 15 minutes of reflow. Their data suggest that the degree of elevation of $T1$ and $T2$ is related to the severity of the ischemic insult during occlusion and to the extent of reperfusion with reflow. Following 30 minutes of coronary artery occlusion, endocardial samples demonstrated significant inverse correlations between both $T1$ and $T2$, and radiolabeled microsphere determined myocardial blood flow during occlusion. If 15 minutes of reflow followed the ischemic period, $T1$ and $T2$ were directly related to the blood flow during reperfusion. Johnston et al.[40] examined $T1$ and $T2$ parameter changes in dog myocardium following three hours of occlusion of the LAD with and without reperfusion. In the models with and without reflow, modest inverse correlations existed between $T1$ and $T2$ and regional myocardial blood flow in regions where ischemia was sufficient to cause increased relaxation times. Although a slight further increase in $T1$ and $T2$ occurred after reperfusion, marked changes were not observed. These studies demonstrate the association between $T1$ and $T2$ and the severity of myocardial ischemia.

To assess the effects of acute and chronic ischemic injury on myocardial $T1$ values in dogs, Brown et al.[41] evaluated infarcts for water content and $T1$ values at 3 hours and 4, 21, and 56 days following MI created by LAD ligation. Tissue water content in early infarcts was increased, and $T1$ was prolonged. Old infarcts, where fibrosis had replaced the damaged tissue and where water concentrations subsequently were lower, had shortened $T1$ values. At 21 days, water content and $T1$ were variably affected. Thus, the study suggests that proton MR techniques that depict relaxation parameters would distinguish between acute MI, myocardial scar, and normal myocardium and the extent and progression of fibrosis.

In vitro $T1$ and $T2$ studies indicate that proton relaxation properties are affected by myocardial ischemic damage and suggest that images weighted for proton relaxation times will reflect the extent and severity of myocardial ischemic insult. In vitro studies also suggest that $T1$ is an earlier indicator of myocardial damage than $T2$. Accordingly, an imaging approach that is weighted for $T1$ contrast, i.e., an inversion recovery (IR) pulse sequence, would be more likely to define the region of early myocardial damage. Although cardiac-gated IR imaging is not currently technically possible, studies comparing IR and spin-echo (SE) imaging with a short echo delay time (16 ms) on excised canine hearts have been done.[40] Following one hour of LAD coronary artery occlusion and one hour of reperfusion, SE imaging depicted no contrast between normal and damaged myocardium. However, IR imaging defined the damaged myocardium. Additional $T2$ contrast by increasing the echo delay time may provide the means to depict the infarct using $T2$ changes. Several groups have observed contrast clinically in areas of acute MI using gated SE imaging approaches. Such $T2$ changes occur later during the course of MI (after 30 to 60 minutes).[42,43]

In vitro studies indicate that imaging parameters change as a function of the time following an ischemic insult. To assess the ability of MR imaging methods to detect ischemic myocardial damage at 24 hours after initial insult, Higgins et al.[44] ligated the LAD coronary artery in canine models and obtained cross-sectional images of the excised hearts using an SE pulse sequence. The MR signal intensity of the region of myocardial infarction was perceptibly increased on images of all dogs, reflecting prolongation of $T2$. The contrast between the normal and damaged myocardium varied as a function of the echo delay time and the repetition time. This study suggests that in the 24 hour infarct model, $T2$ changes occur that can be depicted by a gated SE proton MR imaging approach.

To demonstrate the potential utility of gated proton MR imaging methods for assessing the sequelae of coronary artery occlusion, the effects of 30 minutes of LAD coronary artery occlusion followed by 15 minutes of reperfusion were studied in dogs. Gated serial tomographs taken at a level that depicted right and left ventricles and interventricular septum were obtained using an arterial pulse synchronized spin-echo pulse sequence. During coronary artery occlusion, myocardial thinning and left ventricular dilatation were well defined. A region of increased signal intensity was frequently evident subjacent to the ischemic myocardial zone and within the left ventricular cavity. This observation suggests that anomalous blood motion associated with regional ventricular asynergy occurred. With reflow, myocardial thickness, ventricular size, and interventricular blood pool signal reverted toward normal.[45] Using this gated SE pulse sequence (echo delay time of 16 ms), where signal intensity is primarily a function of proton density and $T2$, no consistent change in the myocardial signal of the ischemic zone relative to the normal zones was observed.

To determine the usefulness of gated MR imaging methods to characterize myocardial infarction at two to seven days after LAD coronary artery ligation, Wesbey et al.[46] imaged canine hearts in vivo using an ECG-gated SE pulse sequence. The gated MR images of all hearts with post-mortem evidence of myocardial infarction demonstrated areas of distinctly increased signal intensity in the anterior segment of the left ventricle. Subendocardial regions in the anterior segments were noted to have greater signal intensity. Such increases in signal are related to an increase in $T2$. Calculated $T2$ estimations derived from these images also demonstrated the $T2$ prolongation in the infarct region as compared with normal myocardium.

Using SE imaging with ECG gating, McNamara et al.[47] detected acute MI in humans as regions of high signal intensity compared with that of adjacent normal myocardium. All patients had suffered an acute MI within 5 to 12 days before the MR imaging studies were performed. Discrimination between the normal and infarcted myocardium on the images was sufficient to estimate the location of the infarct (Fig. 23–2).

The mechanisms for $T1$ and $T2$ elevation associated with acute ischemic damage remain uncertain. The $T1$ and $T2$ prolongations are believed to be due primarily to increases in tissue water content. While $T1$ is a function of absolute tissue water content, it is also dependent on other parameters. Water proton relaxation is affected by the macromolecular (largely protein) and ionic milieu. Furthermore, changes in cation concentrations can alter relaxation times. It has been suggested that the $T1$ and $T2$ relaxation times are sensitive to the relative amounts of water in the compartments. Canby et al.[48] examined the relationship between relaxation rates and myocardial water content in a four-hour severe ischemic insult in dogs. The relationship between bulk proton $T1$ relaxation and water content was observed to vary depending upon the severity of the insult. As stated earlier, the perturbation of the ionic milieu is a function of the

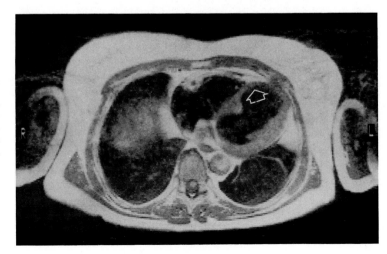

Figure 23–2. Anteroapical and septal wall thinning on a gated transverse spin-echo image in a patient with a previous anterior myocardial infarction (arrowhead). (Courtesy of Professor Kutzim, Institut für Klinische und experimentelle Nuklearmedizin der Universität Köln.)

severity of the ischemic insult. Thus, a contribution to relaxation by mechanisms additional to the simple diluting effects of edema is suggested by these data.

Water content cannot be assumed to be the only factor contributing to relaxation parameter changes observed in ischemic damage in vivo. Other factors being considered include change in lipid form and content and reduction in wall motion (similarly shown in blood flow stasis). Ratner et al.[49] have demonstrated that triglyceride accumulation correlates well with *T2* relaxation time elevation in hepatic steatosis. Increased triglyceride is present and can be demonstrated by NMR spectroscopy at 24 hours after coronary ligation in dogs. Preliminary data suggested that such triglyceride increases have no effect on *T2*,[50] while more recent data suggest that such triglyceride accumulation may be responsible, in part, for alterations in transverse relaxation times.[51]

Detection of Infarction With Paramagnetic Agents

Previous clinical studies have demonstrated that patient prognosis depends on the size of the myocardial infarct.[52–54] Accurate measurement of infarct size is essential for determining the efficacy of interventions designed to limit the extent of infarction. Clinically used methods to quantify infarct size include radioisotopic labeling of necrotic myocardium (technetium-99m stannous pyrophosphate), myocardial perfusion (thallium-201), assessment of ventricular wall motion using ultrasound and radionuclide methods, and release of intracellular enzymes into the blood stream (CK-MB). MR imaging can provide contrast for defining areas of MI using relaxation parameter alterations.

Another MR approach to provide or enhance contrast between infarcted and normal myocardium involves the use of paramagnetic agents (Fig. 23–3). A paramagnetic agent coupled to an agent such as pyrophosphate may provide a proton MR "hot spot" approach for depicting zones of MI.[55] Specific demarcation of infarcted myocardium has been achieved in dogs by intracoronary administration of a specific manganese-

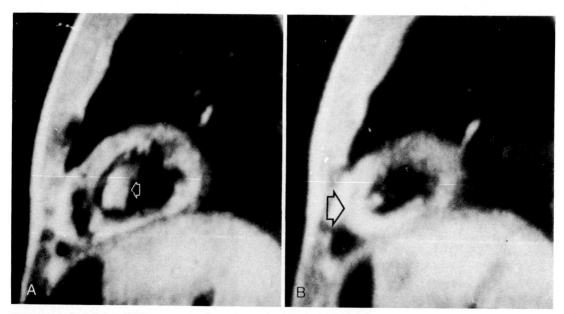

Figure 23–3. Gadolinium-DTPA contrast-enhanced, gated spin-echo oblique images of a patient with a previous anterior myocardial infarct. *A*, Mural thrombus formation gives rise to an intracavitary signal (arrowhead). *B*, increased signal intensity in the anteroseptal, septal, and diaphragmatic regions of the heart (arrowhead). (Courtesy of Richard Bauer, Technische Universität München.)

labeled antibody to cardiac myosin.[56] It appears that this complex binds to the exposed myosin of the necrotic myocytes, causing a selective decrease in the *T1* of infarcted tissue. Although of great academic interest, the clinical relevance of this approach remains undefined.

In summary, MRI may be useful for demonstrating the size and possibly the severity of myocardial ischemic and/or infarct zones. Noninvasive, high-resolution tomographic or three-dimensional imaging without ionizing radiation and without contrast agents makes proton MR techniques potentially advantageous over other imaging modalities for assessing the extent and severity of myocardial ischemic damage.

ASSESSING THE SEQUELAE OF MYOCARDIAL INFARCTION

The complications of MI can include thromboembolism, ventricular aneurysm, ventricular pseudoaneurysm, mitral regurgitation, pericardial effusion, and septal perforation. Early detection and evaluation of the complications is frequently important for determining proper medical and surgical intervention. Higgins et al.[57] have studied patients with chronic IHD with ECG-gated SE images. Regions of myocardial scar

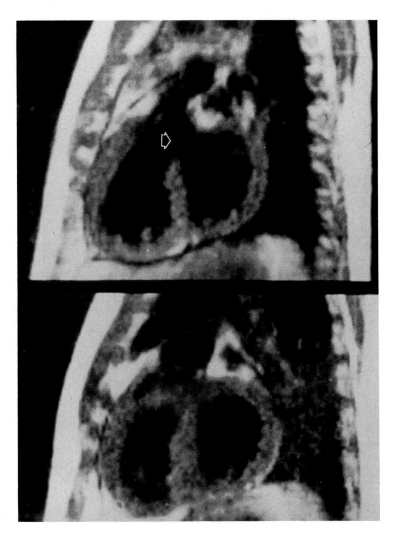

Figure 23–4. Gated oblique spin-echo images of a patient with a congenital high ventricular septal defect. The upper image visualizes the communication between the ventricles (arrowhead). The lower image demonstrates right ventricular enlargement and hypertrophy. (Courtesy of Richard Bauer, Technische Universität München.)

demonstrated ventricular wall thinning, with the transition between normal wall thickness and wall thinning being well defined. Signal intensity in zones of myocardial scar was similar to that of normal myocardium. Ventricular aneurysms and anomalous blood motion within the aneurysm were clearly depicted. Mural thrombi were noted as structures of medium signal intensity projecting into the signal void of the left ventricular chamber.

Although pericardial effusion and ventricular septal defect (Fig. 23–4) have not been specifically reported in patients with IHD, these abnormalities have been reported in patients with other pathology with the use of MR imaging.[58,59] Evidence of mitral insufficiency may be detected by aberrations in heart chamber sizes as shown on MR images.

MYOCARDIAL METABOLISM AND RESPONSE TO INTERVENTION

NMR spectroscopy provides a unique means for direct monitoring of myocardial metabolic function. There is an increasing body of data describing the effect of ischemic or ischemia-like insults on myocardial high-energy phosphate metabolism. Most of these studies have been performed in vitro with spectroscopy of the isolated perfused rat or rabbit heart model. The myocardial phosphorus-31 (P-31) spectrum allows quantification of the metabolically important phosphates: phosphocreatine, adenosine triphosphate, sugar phosphates, and inorganic phosphate. Additionally, it is possible to determine intracellular pH because the resonance position of the inorganic phosphate peak is affected by the local pH. By observing pH-dependent splitting of the inorganic phosphate peak, Hollis et al.[60] demonstrated that P-31 NMR could be used to characterize regional myocardial ischemia. High-energy phosphate concentrations and intracellular pH have been quantified during hypoxia, anoxia, and ischemia with and without pharmacologic intervention.[61,62] For example, Pieper et al.[62] demonstrated that the intracellular acidosis that develops during ischemic arrest could be substantially reduced by adding the beta-adrenergic blocking agent propranolol.

Surface coils have been applied by several groups to study high-energy phosphate metabolism in skeletal muscle and myocardium. Nunnally and Bottomley[63] have applied the surface coil method to the myocardium. Using such coils placed on the epicardial surface of excised rabbit hearts, the protective effects of pretreatment with verapamil hydrochloride and chlorpromazine hydrochloride on sustaining myocardial high-energy phosphate levels after coronary ligation were demonstrated. Kantor et al.[64] have developed a technique to acquire P-31 spectra from a localized area of myocardium in dogs using a catheter with a small radio frequency coil at its tip. This approach permits phosphorus spectra of myocardium to be obtained in close proximity to the coil. However, such an approach might not be easily applied clinically to coronary artery disease, in which ischemic myocardium tends to be focal. Because surface coil spectroscopy provides a means to evaluate tissue immediately subjacent to the coil, left ventricular myocardium will not be easily accessible using surface coils. On the other hand, it would be most valuable to be able to evaluate the regional distribution of high-energy phosphate and/or inorganic phosphate.

Maudsley et al.[65] have produced two-dimensional images of separate P-31–containing compounds and the P-31 density distribution in the cat head and human leg. Although the acquisition time was long (four hours at 2.7 tesla), this study demonstrated the feasibility of P-31 imaging. Although P-31 NMR has great potential and possible advantages over other nuclei, considerable progress will be needed to develop clinically relevant methods for monitoring myocardial high-energy phosphate metabolism.

High-resolution proton spectroscopy applied to the myocardium may also assist in the staging of myocardial ischemic insults. Chemical shift imaging studies have demonstrated the ability to separate the aqueous and aliphatic peaks within the proton spectrum. The ability to distinguish between water and fat signal may be clinically useful in staging myocardial infarction, since lipid accumulation is demonstrable within several hours after coronary occlusion. Lactic acid is a metabolically important moiety that can be detected using high-resolution spectroscopy. Its presence in elevated concentrations suggests metabolic insult. Images of myocardial lactate distribution would be of great value for demonstrating the regional distribution of metabolically important ischemia. However, owing to the low concentration of lactate and its relatively close resonance position to the fat (—CH$_2$—) resonance, clinically relevant lactate imaging will be technically difficult.

THE FUTURE OF MR IMAGING IN ISCHEMIC HEART DISEASE

Three-Dimensional Imaging

Today, most gated proton imaging methods acquire one or more tomographic cuts such that the heart is divided into several parallel slices about 10 mm in thickness. The coronary arteries cannot be properly imaged with such thick-slice sampling. Unlike other modalities, MR imaging is inherently three-dimensional, and acquisition of three-dimensional data sets is feasible. Such acquisitions using present techniques will require substantial increases in image acquisition time. Furthermore, technical problems with three-dimensional display of the images need to be addressed.

High-Speed MR Imaging

Gated tomographic imaging of the heart, as currently applied, requires several minutes for the acquisition of enough cardiac cycles to generate high-quality images. If image acquisition is rapid relative to cardiac periodicity (e.g., less than 100 ms), gating would be unnecessary. Innovative approaches are being developed. The pioneering work of Mansfield's group at the University of Nottingham has led to the echo planar method, which acquires a single tomographic image within a 30 ms interval. Thus, its clinical application does not require cardiac gating. Although images produced thus far demonstrate limited spatial resolution, the approach could provide the basis for rapid proton MR imaging in the future.

Imaging of Other Nuclei

In vitro and in vivo spectroscopic studies have demonstrated that clinically useful information can be obtained using nuclei other than protons and P-31. Sodium-23 (Na-23) is abundant in the extracellular fluid and is also relatively MR-sensitive. DeLayre et al.[66] generated gated blood pool images of an isolated beating rat heart using the resonance of blood sodium. While this study demonstrated the feasibility of gated Na-23 imaging of the heart, it is unlikely that sodium blood pool studies will have any clinical relevance, since gated proton images of the cardiac blood pool are technically good. Nevertheless, Na-23 imaging of the myocardium has some potential for being clinically relevant. Under normal conditions, sodium remains in the extracellular space;

with infarction, however, sodium will distribute into the intracellular space. Taking advantage of pathophysiology, Hilal et al.[67] obtained images of regions of cerebral infarction associated with ischemic stroke. Imaging time is approximately one hour at 1.5 tesla. With the gating required for cardiac imaging, Na-23 myocardial imaging will necessitate very lengthy acquisition periods. Regions of myocardial infarction in excised canine hearts have been depicted by Na-23 MR imaging.[68]

Carbon-13–enriched glucose or fatty acids may provide a means for in vivo assessment of myocardial substrate metabolism. However, low sensitivity and low concentration continue to present technical difficulties that must be overcome before carbon-13 MR will be useful for clinical assessment of the myocardium.

In conclusion, magnetic resonance techniques applied to the detection of IHD have the potential to provide important diagnostic information. High-resolution proton MR tomography can generate detailed cardiovascular images. Nevertheless, more important than its potential to generate high-resolution images of the heart are its other potentials, which include (1) noninvasive angiography, (2) regional perfusion measurements, (3) direct tissue characterization, and (4) determination of regional cardiac metabolism.

At the present time, detection of coronary artery atherosclerosis is restricted to catheterization techniques. MR angiography has some potential to depict the proximal coronary arteries noninvasively. Evaluation of myocardial perfusion is limited to radionuclide approaches, using either thallium-201 with gamma camera imaging or positron-emission tomography (PET). Gamma camera methods, although performed at a moderate cost, require administration of radiopharmaceuticals and have relatively poor resolution. PET imaging also has relatively poor intrinsic resolution and requires a cyclotron for production of most of the radionuclides used. Rubidium-82, a positron-emitting radionuclide potassium analogue with a half-life of 75 seconds, is available by eluting a generator, obviating the need for a cyclotron for studies restricted to that tracer. For assessing the sequelae of MI, echocardiography and high-speed x-ray computed tomography can provide similar anatomic information to MR, and two-dimensional echocardiography can provide this information at a considerably lower cost than MR and high-speed CT. Of course, MR techniques and high-speed CT are not susceptible to the considerable bone and lung attenuation that interferes with the technical quality of ultrasound. Finally, direct noninvasive evaluation of myocardial metabolism is possible only with MR techniques at the present time.

The success of the unique potential applications of MR methods in ischemic heart disease will ultimately decide its clinical utility and cost-effectiveness. Despite the fact that the clinical applications of MR techniques to the cardiovascular system are in their infancy, and more basic and clinical research and development are needed, it is apparent that this modality may have an enormous impact on the diagnosis of cardiovascular diseases and the assessment of the response to intervention. A noninvasive modality that has the potential to combine imaging with high spatial resolution and direct assessment of tissue metabolism and function is unparalleled in imaging technology; these factors make clinical MR one of the most exciting advances in medical science.

References

1. Lauterbur PC: Image formation by induced local interactions: examples employing nuclear magnetic resonance. Nature 242:190, 1973.
2. Lauterbur PC: NMR imaging technique provides high resolution. Phys Today May 1978, p 18.
3. Herfkens RJ, Higgins CB, Hricak H, et al: Nuclear magnetic resonance imaging of the cardiovascular system: Normal and pathologic findings. Radiology 147:749, 1983.
4. Higgins CB, Lanzer P, Herfkens RJ, et al: Cardiovascular systems. In Margulis AR, Higgins CB, Kaufman A, et al (eds): Clinical Magnetic Resonance Imaging. San Francisco, Radiology Research and Education Foundation, 1983, pp 159–184.

5. Kaufman L, Crooks LE, Sheldon PE, et al: Evaluation of NMR imaging for detection and quantification of obstructions in vessels. Invest Radiol *17*:554, 1982.
6. Crooks LE, Mills CM, Davis PL, et al: Visualization of cerebral and vascular abnormalities by NMR imaging: the effects of imaging parameters on contrast. Radiology *144*:843, 1982.
7. Bradley WG Jr, Waluch V, Lai K, et al: The appearance of rapidly flowing blood on magnetic resonance images. AJR *143*:1167, 1984.
8. Van Dijk P: Direct cardiac NMR imaging of heart wall and blood flow velocity. J Comput Assist Tomogr *8*(3):429, 1984.
9. Herfkens RJ, Higgins CB, Hricak H, et al: Nuclear magnetic resonance imaging of atherosclerotic disease. Radiology *148*:161, 1983.
10. Rzedzian R, Doyle M, Mansfield P, et al: Echo planar imaging in paediatrics: real-time nuclear magnetic resonance. Ann Radiol *27*:182, 1984.
11. Massie BM, Botvinick EH, Brundage BH: Correlation of thallium-201 scintigrams with coronary anatomy: factors affecting region by region sensitivity. Am J Cardiol 44:616, 1979.
12. Verani MS, et al: Sensitivity and specificity of Tl-201 perfusion scintigrams under exercise in the diagnosis of coronary artery disease. J Nucl Med *19*:773, 1978.
13. Pohost GM, Alpert NM, Ingwall JS, et al: Thallium redistribution: mechanisms and clinical utility. Semin Nucl Med *10*:79, 1980.
14. Dunn R, et al: Noninvasive prediction of multivessel disease after myocardial infarction. Circulation *62*:726, 1980.
15. Chauncey DM Jr, Schelbert HR, Halpern SE, et al: Tissue distribution studies with radioactive manganese: A potential agent for myocardial imaging. J Nucl Med *18*:933, 1977.
16. Lauterbur PC, Dias MHM, Rudin AM: Augmentation of tissue water proton spin-lattice relaxation rates by in vivo addition of paramagnetic ions. *In* Dutton LP, Leigh JS, Scarpa A (eds): Frontiers of Biological Energetics. New York, Academic Press, 1979, p 752.
17. Goldman MR, Brady TJ, Pykett IL, et al: Quantification of experimental myocardial infarction using nuclear magnetic resonance imaging and paramagnetic ion contrast enhancement in excised canine hearts. Circulation 66:1012, 1982.
18. Pople JA, Schneider WG, Bernstein HJ: High-Resolution Nuclear Magnetic Resonance. New York, McGraw-Hill, 1959, p 209.
19. Wesbey GE, Higgins CB, McNamara MT, et al: Effect of gadolinium-DTPA on the magnetic relaxation times of normal and infarcted myocardium. Radiology *153*:165, 1984.
20. McNamara MT, Higgins CB, Ehman RL, et al: Acute myocardial ischemia: Magnetic resonance contrast enhancement with gadolinium-DTPA. Radiology *153*:157, 1984.
21. Pohost GM, Ratner AV: Nuclear magnetic resonance: Potential applications in clinical cardiology. JAMA *251*:1308, 1984.
22. Elgavish GA, Pohost GM: Evaluation of Gd(BDP)$_2$, a non-hydrolizable aqueous NMR relaxation reagent, as a contrast agent for NMR imaging. Scientific Program of Society of Magnetic Resonance in Medicine, 1984, p 215.
23. Brasch RC: Work in progress: methods of contrast enhancement for NMR imaging and potential applications. Radiology *147*:781, 1983.
24. Benson WR, Maienthal M: Synthesis of spin-labeled nitroxyl ester of steroids. J Med Chem *20*:1308, 1977.
25. Burkett DJ, Dwek RA, Radda GK, et al: Probes for the conformational transitions of phosphorylase b. Eur J Biochem *20*:494, 1981.
26. Ling GN, Tucker M: Nuclear magnetic resonance relaxation and water contents in normal mouse and rat tissues and in cancer cells. J Natl Cancer Inst *64*:1199, 1980.
27. Block RE, Maxwell GP, Prudhomme DL, et al: High resolution proton magnetic resonance spectral characteristics of water, lipid and protein signals from three mouse cell populations. J Natl Cancer Inst *58*:151, 1977.
28. Inch WR, McCredie JA, Knispel RR, et al: Water content and proton spin relaxation time for neoplastic and non-neoplastic tissues from mice and humans. J Natl Cancer Inst *52*:353, 1974.
29. Beall PT, Asch BB, Chung DC, et al: Distinction of normal, preneoplastic, and neoplastic mouse mammary primary cell cultures by water nuclear magnetic relaxation times. J Natl Cancer Inst *64*:335, 1980.
30. Buonanno FS, Pykett IL, Brady TJ, et al: Proton NMR imaging in experimental ischemic infarction. Stroke *14*:178, 1983.
31. Williams ES, Kaplan JI, Thatcher F, et al: Prolongation of proton spin lattice relaxation times in regionally ischemic tissue from dog hearts. J Nucl Med *21*:449, 1980.
32. Jennings RB, Ganote CE, Reimer KA, et al: Ischemic tissue injury. Am J Pathol *81*:179, 1975.
33. Kloner RA, Reimer KA, Jennings RB: Distribution of collateral flow in acute myocardial ischemic injury: effect of propranolol therapy. Cardiovasc Res *10*:81, 1976.
34. Willerson JT, Scales F, Mukherjee A, et al: Abnormal myocardial fluid retention as an early manifestation of ischemic injury. Am J Pathol *87*:159, 1977.
35. Buja LM, Willerson JT: Abnormalities of volume regulation and membrane integrity in myocardial tissue slices after early ischemic injury in the dog: Effects of mannitol, polyethylene glycol, and propranolol. Am J Pathol *103*:79, 1981.
36. Whalen DA, Hamilton DG, Ganote CE, et al: Effect of a transient period on myocardial cells. I. Effects on cell volume regulation. Am J Pathol *74*:381, 1974.
37. Jennings RB, Schaper J, Hill ML, et al: Effect of reperfusion late in the phase of reversible ischemic injury. Circ Res *56*:262, 1985.

38. Ratner AV, Goldman MR, Pohost GM: Visualization of myocardial ischemic damage using nuclear magnetic resonance imaging. Clin Res (abstr) *31*(2):213A, 1983.
39. Ratner AV, Okada R, Newell J, et al: The relationship between proton NMR relaxation parameters and myocardial perfusion with acute coronary artery occlusion and reperfusion. Circulation *71*(4):823, 1985.
40. Johnston DL, Brady TJ, Ratner AV, et al: Assessment of myocardial ischemia with proton magnetic resonance: effects of a three hour coronary occlusion with and without reperfusion. Circulation *71*:595, 1985.
41. Brown JJ, Peck WW, Gerber KH, et al: NMR analysis of acute and chronic myocardial infarction in dogs: Alterations in spin-lattice relaxation times. Am Heart J *108*:1292, 1984.
42. Ratner AV, Okada RD, Goldman MR, et al: Early detection of myocardial ischemic damage using proton NMR techniques. Circulation (abstr) *68*:III-387, 1983.
43. Plugfelder PW, Wisenberg G, Prato FS, et al: Early detection of canine myocardial infarction by magnetic resonance imaging. Circulation *71*:587, 1985.
44. Higgins CB, Herfkens R, Lipton MJ, et al: Nuclear magnetic resonance imaging of acute myocardial infarction in dogs: Alterations in magnetic relaxation times. Am J Cardiol *52*:184, 1983.
45. Pohost GM, Goldman MR, Pykett IL, et al: Gated NMR imaging in myocardial infarction. Circulation (abstr) *66*:II-39, 1982.
46. Wesbey G, Higgins CB, Lanzer P, et al: Imaging and characterization of acute myocardial infarction in vivo by gated nuclear magnetic resonance. Circulation *69*:125, 1984.
47. McNamara MT, Higgins CB, Schechtmann N, et al: Detection and characterization of acute myocardial infarction in man with use of gated magnetic resonance. Circulation *71*:717, 1985.
48. Canby RC, Reeves RC, Evanochko WT, et al: Proton nuclear magnetic resonance relaxation times in severe myocardial ischemia. J Am Coll Cardiol *10*:412, 1987.
49. Ratner AV, Carter EA, Pohost GM: Noninvasive quantification of hepatic steatosis by proton NMR (abstr). American Federation of Clinical Research, 1984.
50. Reeves RC, Evanochko WT, Pohost GM: NMR studies of 24 hour canine myocardial infarction. Clin Res (abstr) *33*:220A, 1985.
51. Reeves RC, Evanochko WT, Pohost GM: Myocardial triglycerides (TG) with infarction: NMR detection and effects on proton relaxation. Circulation (abstr) *72*:391, 1985.
52. Sobel BE, Bresnahan GF, Shell WE, et al: Estimation of infarct size in man and its relation to prognosis. Circulation *46*:610, 1972.
53. Geltman EM, Ehsani AA, Campbell MK, et al: The influence of location and extent of myocardial infarction on long-term ventricular dysrhythmia and mortality. Circulation *60*:805, 1979.
54. Hillis LD, Braunwald E: Myocardial ischemia. N Engl J Med *296*:1034, 1977.
55. Elgavish GA, Sakai TT, Reeves RC, et al: *T1* differentiation between infarcted and noninfarcted myocardium by the contrast agent Gd(BDP)$_2$. Proceedings of Society of Magnetic Resonance in Medicine, 4th Annual Meeting (abstr), 852, 1985.
56. Lauffer R: The design of NMR contrast agents. Scientific Program of Society of Magnetic Resonance in Medicine, 1984, p 446.
57. Higgins CB, Lanzer P, Stark D, et al: Imaging by nuclear magnetic resonance in patients with chronic ischemic heart disease. Circulation *69*:523, 1984.
58. Higgins CB, Lanzer P, Stark D, et al: Assessment of cardiac anatomy using nuclear magnetic resonance imaging. J Am Coll Cardiol *5*:77S, 1985.
59. Fletcher BD, Jacobstein MD, Nelson AD, et al: Gated magnetic resonance imaging of congenital cardiac malformations. Radiology *150*:137, 1984.
60. Hollis DP, Nunnally RL, Jacobus WE, et al: Detection of regional ischemia in perfused beating hearts by phosphorus nuclear magnetic resonance. Biochem Biophys Res Commun *75*:1086, 1977.
61. Flaherty JT, Weisfeldt ML, Bulkley BH, et al: Mechanisms of ischemic myocardial cell damage assessed by phosphorus-31 nuclear magnetic resonance. Circulation *65*:561, 1982.
62. Pieper GM, Todd GL, Wu ST, et al: Attenuation of myocardial acidosis by propanolol during ischemic arrest and reperfusion: Evidence with P-31 nuclear magnetic resonance. Cardiovasc Res *14*:646, 1980.
63. Nunnally RL, Bottomley PA: Assessment of pharmacological treatment of myocardial infarction by phosphorus-31 NMR with surface coils. Science *220*:1170, 1983.
64. Kantor HL, Briggs RW, Balaban RS: In vivo ^{31}P nuclear magnetic resonance measurements in canine heart using a catheter-coil. Circ. Res *55*:261, 1984.
65. Maudsley AA, Hilal SK, Simon HE, et al: In vivo MR spectroscopic imaging with P-31: Work in progress. Radiology *153*:745, 1984.
66. DeLayre JE, Ingwall JS, Malloy C, et al: Gated sodium-23 nuclear magnetic images of an isolated perfused working rat heart. Science *212*:935, 1981.
67. Hilal SK, Maudsley AA, Bonn J, et al: NMR imaging of tissue sodium in vivo and in resected organs. Scientific Program of the Society of Magnetic Resonance in Medicine (abstr) 1983, p 155.
68. Cannon PJ, Maudsley AA, Hilal SK, et al: NMR imaging of Na-23 in myocardium following coronary artery occlusion and reperfusion. Circulation (abstr) *68*:III-177, 1983.

Gated MRI in Congenital Cardiac Malformations

MURRAY J. MAZER
MARTIN P. SANDLER
MADAN V. KULKARNI
THOMAS P. GRAHAM, JR.
JACK TISHLER

Imaging with magnetic resonance (MRI) provides natural inherent contrast between flowing blood and the myocardium, since nuclei of blood flowing at normal velocities generally produce minimal signal relative to the surrounding cardiac tissues[1-5] during standard pulse sequences. Considerable contrast also occurs between the epicardial surface and pericardial fat, since fat produces a much stronger magnetic resonance imaging signal than the myocardium.[6]

Gating of magnetic resonance images of the beating heart reduces, if not eliminates, motion artifacts.[4,5] Technology also now exists to obtain multiple, thinner sections simultaneously to provide more precise anatomic detail in a shorter time. Investigators have been successful in obtaining high-quality gated MR images, demonstrating normal cardiac anatomy and cardiovascular pathology, including a variety of congenital abnormalities.[7-17] It is important to evaluate MR gated images in patients with congenital cardiac disorders and, in particular, to assess the advantages and disadvantages of MRI compared with echocardiography as a noninvasive imaging modality in this group of patients.

MATERIAL AND METHODS

Patient Population. Fifty-three patients (33 males and 20 females) with a variety of 81 congenital cardiac malformations (Table 24–1) were imaged with gated magnetic resonance. Ages varied from 3 months to 38 years (mean, 11.6 years). The accuracy of this evolving new imaging technique was compared with the known results of cineangiography, available on all patients, as well as with the results of echocardiography, available on 48 patients.

Magnetic resonance imaging was performed with a 0.5 tesla superconducting magnet (Teslacon, Technicare, Solon, Ohio). Infants and small children were studied using a radio frequency (rf) coil with a diameter of 28 cm. The images were reconstructed on a 256 × 256 display matrix with spatial resolution of 2.2 mm. The slice thickness varied from 5.0 mm to 15 mm. Older children who could not be accommodated in a 28 cm diameter rf coil were examined in a 55 cm diameter rf coil and the images displayed on a 256 × 256 matrix with a spatial resolution of 3.6 mm. Gated cardiac

Table 24–1. CONGENITAL CARDIAC MALFORMATIONS IMAGED BY MR

Diagnosis	Number
Tricuspid atresia	3
Tetralogy of Fallot	8
Transposition of great vessels	20 (4 L-type; 16 D-type)
Single ventricle	6
Double outlet right ventricle	2
Ebstein's malformation	1
Total anomalous pulmonary venous return	1 (S/P repair)
Coarctation	10 (including 1 aneurysm, 1 restenosis complication, and S/P surgery)
ASD	6
VSD	11
Pulmonary stenosis: supravalvar, valvar, and subvalvar	10
Aortic and subaortic stenoses	3

Total: 81 defects in 53 patients

images were acquired by telemetric detection of the "R" wave of an electrocardiogram using a telemeter (Model 78100 A, Hewlett-Packard, Waltham, Massachusetts). The transmitter was placed just outside the magnetic bore connected to the three nonferromagnetic leads attached to the patient's arms and right lower leg, and the signal was transmitted outside the room into the gating module receiver (Technicare, Solon, Ohio) located near the computer console. The interval between the occurrence of the QRS complex and the time the echo is read varies for each pulse sequence. The delay between the QRS complex and the 90 degree pulse is determined by the patient's heart rate. In small infants, the forearms with their ECG lead wires were placed anterior and lateral to the body wall to eliminate field artifacts from the metallic wires in the parasagittal and coronal planes. Also, by keeping the leads on the most distal aspect of the forearms, the wires were beyond the planes of the transverse tomograms, which again eliminated metallic artifacts.

The spin-echo images were acquired using an echo interval (TE) of 20 ms. The effective pulse repetition time (TR) in cardiac gated MRI is the R-R interval when the set TR is shorter than the R-R interval. In our first few cases, the TR was 500 ms. In the later studies, the TR was increased or decreased depending on the R-R interval.

Cardiac gated images were obtained using a multislice format. The number of slices acquired in the multislice protocol depends on the TR interval. The image initiated with the "R" wave pulse is in the end-diastolic phase of the cardiac cycle. After the detection of the "R" wave, the first slice from multislice data collection is initiated. The subsequent slices are at a different level and also in a different phase of the cardiac cycle. By presetting the level of slice to begin after detection of the "R" wave signal, the chamber anatomy can be evaluated near the end-diastolic phase, i.e., the ventricles are imaged in the end-diastolic phase for evaluating the ventricular septum and myocardium, while atria are examined in ventricular systole. In patients with rapid heart rates we were able to diminish cardiac motion artifacts by decreasing the number of slices in a multislice acquisition.

The multislice cardiac-gated acquisitions required from 5.5 to 8.5 minutes, depending upon the R-R interval. Total imaging time varied from 20 minutes to 1 hour, depending on the number of projections desired. Infants less than six months of age were sedated with oral chloral hydrate, 50 to 75 mg per kg. The remainder of the infants and young children were sedated with intramuscular meperidine (Demerol) 2 mg per kg, and secobarbital (Seconal) 2 mg per kg.

Images were performed routinely in the transverse, coronal, or parasagittal plane. In some cases, oblique images were studied by placing patients in the left posterior oblique or right posterior oblique position in the magnetic gantry and then performing parasagittal or coronal sections. Later, electronic axis angulation was used to accomplish the same angled views while leaving the patients undisturbed in a supine position.

RESULTS

Normal Anatomy

Transverse images from the aortic arch downward to the superior aspect of the liver provided the best initial analysis of cardiac anatomy; subsequent decisions were made to obtain coronal and/or parasagittal views or angled views if these were considered necessary. Preferred projections for visualizing intracardiac and extracardiac anatomy are listed in Table 24–2.

Abnormal Cardiovascular Anatomy

Aorta and Pulmonary Artery

Aortic and pulmonary artery relationships were clearly identified in transverse imaging planes, with the mid–ascending aorta being anterior and to the right of the mid–main pulmonary artery in uncorrected D-transposition of the great vessels (D-TGVs), and anterior and to the left of the pulmonary artery in uncorrected L-transposition of the great vessels (L-TGVs); the two are side by side in double outlet right ventricle (DORV) (Fig. 24–1).

The actual size of the main pulmonary artery and its right and left pulmonary artery branches can be analyzed with exceptional clarity in the transverse plane, revealing poststenotic dilation in pulmonary valvar stenosis, the varying degrees of underdevelopment in severe right heart obstructive disease, and patency and degree of ongoing growth after temporary surgical shunting or definitive reconstruction (Fig. 24–2).

Right-sided versus left-sided aortic arches and descending thoracic aortas are very clearly documented with transverse imaging. However, more complex presurgical analysis of aortic abnormalities (coarctation and postrepair aneurysm and restenosis complication) requires additional assessment of great vessel relationships that is better provided by coronal or parasagittal imaging or angled nonorthogonal views (Fig. 24–3). Systemic (bronchial, intercostal, and subclavian) arterial collaterals from the aorta

Table 24–2. PREFERRED PROJECTIONS FOR VISUALIZATION OF INTRACARDIAC AND GREAT VESSEL ANATOMY

Transverse Projection
   Right atrium, coronary sinus, right ventricle, main pulmonary artery and main branches, pulmonary veins, left atrium, left ventricle, atrial septum, ventricular septum, A-V valves, aortic arch.
Coronal Projection
   Superior and inferior vena cava, azygous vein. (Also helpful for right atrium, left atrium, and aortic arch.)
Parasagittal Projections
   Ascending and descending aorta, aortic and pulmonary valves. (Also helpful for venae cavae, right ventricle, left ventricle, and ventricular septum.)

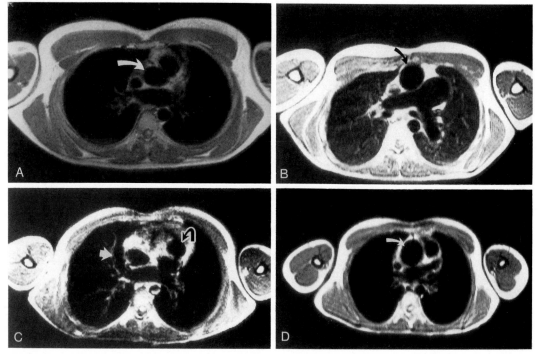

Figure 24–1. *A,* Normal relationship of aorta (curved arrow) to the right and posterior to the pulmonary artery at the base of the heart. *B,* Aorta (curved arrow) anterior and to the right of the pulmonary artery in D-transposition of the great vessels. *C,* Aorta (curved arrow) anterior and to the left of the pulmonary artery in the L-transposition of the great vessels; also note the right subclavian to right pulmonary artery (Blalock-Taussig) shunt (horizontal white arrow). *D,* Aorta (curved arrow) and right pulmonary artery side by side at base of heart in double-outlet right ventricle.

to each lung were adequately imaged with coronal and transverse sectioning in the mediastinum but could not be imaged beyond the mediastinum in the low-signal intra-pulmonary tissue.

ATRIA

Atrial septal defects (ASD) were best assessed in the transverse plane. The septum is thin and often mobile in the region of the fossa ovalis. As with echocardiography, the potential for false positive results in ASD remains a problem. With thin sectioning we noted a sudden focal dropout in signal intensity in the region of the ASD with prominent signals in the adjacent cranial and caudal intact septum (compared with gradually decreasing signal intensity about the region of the fossa ovalis in patients with an otherwise intact septum). Repeat imaging with a second series of offset inter-leaved adjacent slices reduces the error of partial volume averaging and increases the accuracy of analysis. Further commercial development of thinner multislicing tech-niques (as thin as 1 mm) for more accurate immediate evaluation of this area may be on the horizon.

Absent cranial atrial septum followed by intact midseptum indicated sinus venosus ASD. Absent midseptum and intact uppermost and lowermost septum indicated se-cundum ASD (Fig. 24–4). Absent lowermost septum and right atrial–left ventricular septal barrier indicated ostium primum ASD.

Overall dilation of the right atrium and large obligatory ASDs were well appreciated in tricuspid atresias. Right atrial dilation and ASD plus atrialization of the proximal inflow portion of the right ventricle was well appreciated in Ebstein's malformation.

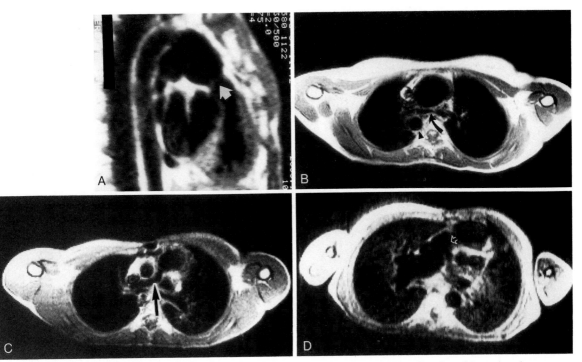

Figure 24–2. Parasagittal projection of pulmonary valve stenosis (arrow) and poststenotic dilatation of the main pulmonary artery. *B*, Severe tetralogy of Fallot with pulmonary atresia; hypoplastic entire right pulmonary artery (curved arrow) behind dilated ascending aorta; right-sided descending aorta (arrowhead). *C*, Patent Rastelli conduit, distal anastomosis to native pulmonary artery; right pulmonary artery (arrow) still somewhat underdeveloped. *D*, Waterston conduit from anteriorly transposed ascending aorta to dilated right pulmonary artery (open arrow).

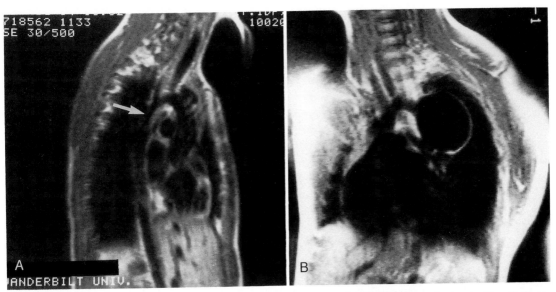

Figure 24–3. *A*, Tubular coarctation (arrow) beyond left subclavian artery takeoff; LPO parasagittal projecttion. *B*, Status postoperative coarctation repair with patch graft aneurysm sequela; normal proximal anastomosis; no intraluminal thrombus; RPO coronal projection.

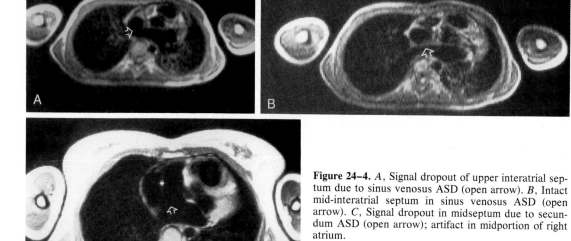

Figure 24–4. *A*, Signal dropout of upper interatrial septum due to sinus venosus ASD (open arrow). *B*, Intact mid-interatrial septum in sinus venosus ASD (open arrow). *C*, Signal dropout in midseptum due to secundum ASD (open arrow); artifact in midportion of right atrium.

Displacement of the septal leaflet into the right ventricular chamber may be identified on transverse views.

A dilated coronary sinus entering the posterior aspect of the lower portion of the right atrium was frequent in patients with right heart obstructive disease and some patients with large left-to-right ASD shunts. The most dilated coronary sinus was noted with persistent left SVC draining through the sinus to the right atrium. All were best assessed with transverse imaging (Fig. 24–5).

Whenever coronal imaging was performed, the situs of the atria and viscera was well defined. Morphology and disposition of the tracheobronchial tree, i.e., situs of

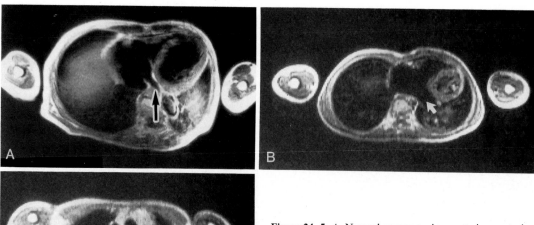

Figure 24–5. *A*, Normal coronary sinus entering posterior aspect of caudal portion of right atrium (arrow). *B*, Dilated coronary sinus receiving venous inflow from the persistent left SVC (arrow). *C*, Persistent left SVC draining to coronary sinus (curved arrow); right SVC (arrowhead).

the longer and more horizontal left (hypoarterial) than the right (epiarterial) bronchus, could also be defined and, in so doing, predict atrial situs (Fig. 24–6).

VENTRICLES AND VENTRICULOARTERIAL CONNECTIONS

Membranous ventricular septal defect (VSD) was well assessed with transverse imaging. Multiple membranous and muscular VSDs were imaged successfully in one patient. Differentiation between complete absence of the ventricular septum and some residual septal remnant was readily apparent on transverse MRI (Fig. 24–7).

Overall chamber size and wall thickness response to the strains of shunt and obstruction abnormalities were well assessed by transverse imaging and long-axis oblique angled views. Outflow tract subvalvar thickening was not always fully appreciated in earlier cases, when electronically angled nonorthogonal views were not available; parasagittal imaging for the right ventricular outflow tract (RVOT) and coronal imaging for the left ventricular outflow tract (LVOT) were most useful for these earlier evaluations. Transverse imaging outside the heart clearly identified TGVs, as previously mentioned, but their precise communication with each ventricle was better identified with coronal or sagittal imaging (Fig. 24–8). Atretic right ventricle due to tricuspid atresia was well assessed via transverse imaging. A second case of tricuspid atresia with atretic right ventricular inflow tract and a better developed outflow tract, maintained via a VSD, was well identified via transverse and parasagittal imaging (Fig. 24–9).

SYSTEMIC AND PULMONARY VEINS

Central pulmonary veins entering the mediastinum and then the left atrium were well assessed in patients with normal venous return and one patient with patent reanastomosed, previously anomalous pulmonary veins. Diverted pulmonary veins, superior vena cava (SVC) and inferior vena cava (IVC) in Mustard and Senning repair

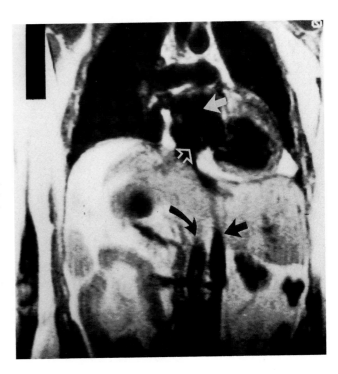

Figure 24–6. Discordant visceroatrial relationship; visceral situs inversus (left-sided liver, right-sided stomach, mirror-image abdominal aorta [curved arrow] and IVC [straight black arrow]); atrial situs solitus (open arrow = lower portion of right atrium; closed white arrow = left atrium).

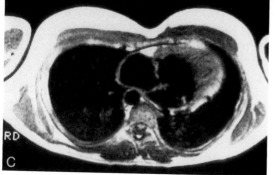

Figure 24–7. *A*, Membranous VSD (open arrow). *B*, Muscular VSD (open arrow). *C*, Two atria; two AV valves; single ventricle.

of D-TGVs were well assessed with transverse and coronal MRI, respectively (Fig. 24–10). However, partial anomalous right upper lobe pulmonary vein drainage to the SVC (and associated with sinus venosus ASD) could not be identified with coronal and transverse MRI. Midpulmonary veins in each hemithorax could not be separated from the low signals of each aerated lung.

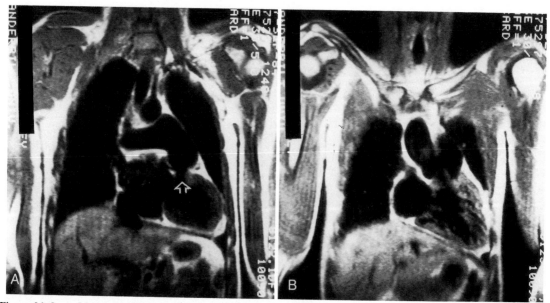

Figure 24–8. *A*, Morphologic left ventricle with mild LVOT narrowing (open arrow) below a continuing transposed pulmonary artery. *B*, Morphologic, trabeculated right ventricle with outlet into a transposed aorta.

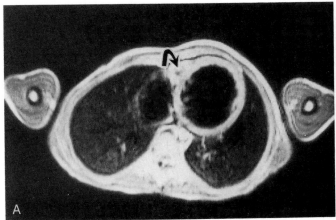

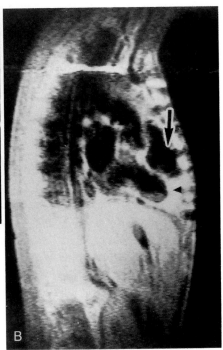

Figure 24–9. *A*, Atretic right ventricular inflow tract (curved arrow). *B*, Right ventricular inflow tract atresia (arrowhead); still developed right ventricular outflow tract (straight arrow), maintained via obligatory right-to-left ASD, and then left-to-right VSD (not shown).

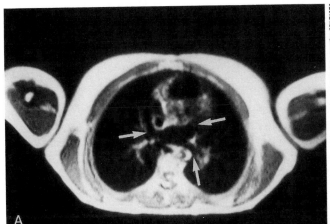

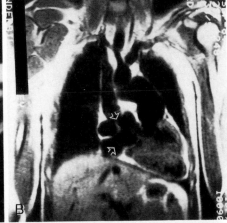

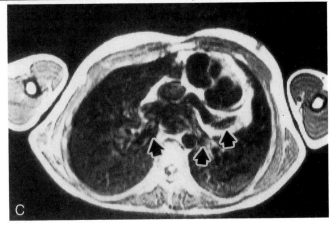

Figure 24–10. Normal pulmonary veins entering left atrium (arrows)—transverse projection. *B*, Status post Mustard repair of D-TGVs with patent SVC and IVC diversion toward the venous (morphologic left) atrium (open arrows)—coronal projection. *C*, Mustard repair of D-TGVs with diversion of pulmonary veins to systemic (morphologic right) atrium (arrows)—transverse projection.

VALVES

A four-chamber transverse image in the midheart defines the atrioventricular (A-V) valves leading from one or two atrial chambers to one or two ventricles (see Fig. 24–7). However, with the exception of one adult with pulmonary valvar stenosis and one patient with Ebstein's malformation and a displaced septal leaflet, MRI generally could not provide clear detail of most normal, and some abnormal, pulmonary and aortic valves. Real-time echocardiography was superior in these instances.

Comparison of MRI and Echocardiography Findings

In assessment of the 48 cases with both echocardiography and gated MRI comparisons (in which there were a total of 66 congenital defects), the instances in which MRI provided more anatomic information were as follows:
1. Right heart obstructive disease (tetralogy of Fallot [8]; tricuspid atresia [3]).
2. Sinus venosus ASD (1).
3. Differentiation between large VSD and single ventricle (6).
4. Aortic anomalies (coarctation [10]).
5. Pulmonary artery anomalies (dilatation [3], banding [3], postoperative growth [6]).
6. Pulmonary artery shunts (temporary and permanent [6]).
7. Central pulmonary veins (postanomalous return repair [1]; transposition repair [16]).
8. Persistent left SVC [1].
9. Visceroatrial situs [2].

DISCUSSION

Gated magnetic resonance cardiac imaging can delineate congenital cardiovascular abnormalities in a noninvasive manner without requiring contrast medium or ionizing radiation.[7-17] High-resolution two-dimensional echocardiography, however, has already established itself for such a purpose.[18-25] Precatheterization echocardiography provides highly accurate evaluation of congenital cardiac malformations to better plan the subsequent cineangiographic projections, thus minimizing catheter manipulation, avoiding excess radiation, and reducing contrast volume. In selected lesions, such as atrial septal defect, hypoplastic left heart syndrome, and critical aortic stenosis in infancy, detailed echocardiography coupled with an understanding of the natural history and surgical alternatives can eliminate the need for preoperative catheterization. More detailed comparison of 2D-echocardiography and MRI of congenital cardiac malformations than has previously been reported is therefore necessary to better assess the relative advantages of each imaging discipline in the context of specific lesions and management alternatives.

There are several general advantages of MRI over echocardiography. First, there is a greater ability to transport a signal through air or bone than with echocardiography. There is therefore no limitation of view through the sternum and no hindrance to imaging in the presence of pneumomediastinum, pneumothorax, or emphysema. Adult congenital heart disease, in particular, is not always easy to evaluate with echocardiography, since the presence of an ossified sternum and a greater degree of substernal air produce limitations on traditional echocardiographic projections. Furthermore, without significant attenuation of signals by increasing distance from the energy source, resolution of remote structures deep within the body is unimpaired with MRI, unlike ultrasonography.

An additional advantage of MRI over echocardiography is the wider field of view in the older child and teenager, with comparable spatial resolution. Thus, the right ventricle and pulmonary artery branches can be identified more completely; this is unlike the echocardiographic evaluation of older patients, in whom these structures frequently cannot be assessed satisfactorily owing to "piecemeal" imaging. In addition, MRI provides improved great vessel and distal pulmonary vein visualization as well as gross assessment of coronary arteries. Finally, visceroatrial situs and atrioventricular and ventriculoarterial connections may be delineated in complex congenital heart disease in a more definitive manner with MRI in situations in which echocardiographic analysis is inconclusive.

Conversely, there are several general disadvantages of MRI as compared with echocardiography. First, the installation and maintenance are very expensive and contribute to the high patient cost. Second, imaging time to produce satisfactory signal-to-noise ratios is considerably longer for MRI. However, continuing improvement in early, prototype MRI equipment may ameliorate this temporary disadvantage, as faster imaging techniques appear to be emerging on the horizon. Certainly, there is a greater potential for image degradation from body motion and rapid and deep respiration with MRI than with echocardiography. Therefore, more patient cooperation and possibly sedation may be necessary. Unlike echocardiography, at the time of writing, real-time imaging is not possible with MRI, and evaluation of valvular function is limited to static imaging. However, once again, this statement may be obsolete if faster imaging progresses to a capability for dynamic MRI. Combined echocardiographic-Doppler studies provide an estimated pressure gradient in valvular lesions, whereas comparable information is not possible as yet with MRI (although there may be a potential for quantitation of blood flow by MRI).[26-29] In the critically ill infant and child the presence of support equipment, such as monitoring devices, pacing apparatus, and oxygen supply, produces a ferromagnetic interference that prohibits the MRI study entirely. Improved shielding by some manufacturers suggests that this drawback will be overcome in the future. Nevertheless, portable studies at the bedside will not be possible with MRI; the presence of arrhythmias negates the advantages of ECG gating; and, finally, there is a 2 to 5 percent incidence of claustrophobia encountered in the early clinical experience with MRI.

The relative simplicity of echocardiographic equipment compared with that for MRI and the numerous above-mentioned advantages make echocardiography the obvious noninvasive imaging procedure of choice for most congenital cardiac malformations. It is therefore not as important to assess the accuracy rate for MRI of lesions that echocardiography already images very well. To better determine the role for MRI of congenital cardiac malformations it is more important to assess what it images better than, rather than equal to, echocardiography. A more detailed evaluation of the 48 cases in our series with echocardiographic and MRI comparisons provides the following analysis of the main potential for MRI in this field.

Global assessment of the right ventricular outflow tract, right ventricular wall thickness, and, especially, pulmonary artery development were consistently better with MRI than with echocardiography in patients with right heart obstructive disease (eight cases of tetralogy of Fallot, three cases of tricuspid atresia). After the initial echocardiographic and/or angiographic diagnosis of tetralogy of Fallot, pulmonary atresia, or tricuspid atresia, follow-up MRI prior to definitive surgery may negate the need in some patients for additional preoperative cardiac catheterizations.

Sinus venosus ASD (one case), which is frequently difficult to assess by echocardiography, was noted only by MRI. However, the partial anomalous right upper lobe pulmonary vein draining to the SVC could be identified neither by MRI nor by echocardiography. This drawback warrants further evaluation with oblique views (not performed in this case) that should be able to image the anomalous pulmonary vein.

Differentiation between a very large VSD, in which a small septal remnant may still provide the foundation for surgical repair, and a single ventricle (six cases), in which a surgical attempt to separate it into two ventricles is less likely, was felt to be more definitive with MRI.

Aortic arch anomalies (coarctation, pre- and postoperative evaluation [ten cases]) and adjacent great vessel takeoffs were more clearly assessed with MRI in older children and adults, in whom echocardiographic windows frequently are suboptimal. There is a real potential for MRI assessment of coarctation (along with complementary echocardiography of intracardiac anatomy) to negate preoperative intravenous digital subtraction angiography or selective intra-arterial angiography in this lesion. The critical coarctation of infancy may, however, still require catheterization for definitive assessment while maintaining critical monitoring and support devices during the imaging procedure.

A persistent left SVC (one case) draining to the coronary sinus was visualized only by MRI (although the dilated coronary sinus on echocardiography did indirectly point to its presence). While this lesion is potentially visualized with echocardiography, the important presurgical information of relative size of the right and left SVC and the presence or absence of an intercommunicating left innominate vein are more easily obtainable (short of catheterization) by MRI.

Blalock-Taussig (three of three cases) and Waterston shunt (one case) evaluation was superior by MRI. Follow-up evaluation of shunt patency with MRI could obviate catheterization follow-up in some cases.[12]

Patency of Rastelli (one case) and Fontan (one case) conduits after repair of severe right ventricular outflow tract narrowings and tricuspid atresia was better appreciated by MRI, which could obviate some follow-up catheterizations. Incorporation of a right ventricular conduit into the sternotomy defect was noted only by MRI and could be a significant anatomic finding should reoperation be necessary.

Patency of repaired anomalous pulmonary venous return that has been reanastomosed into the left atrium (one case) and diversion of systemic and venous channels in Mustard and Senning correction of D-TGVs (12 cases) were better assessed by MRI, which could obviate some follow-up catheterizations.

Finally, a complex case of visceroatrial situs abnormality was better assessed by MRI.

On the other hand, pulmonary (seven of eight cases) and aortic and subaortic valvar (two of two cases) stenosis were generally not adequately identified by MRI as compared with echocardiography (with the exception of one adult pulmonary valvar stenosis). Distal hilar left pulmonary artery occlusive changes were also missed by MRI (two cases). These abnormalities should be visualized with MRI and warrant further study with axial and/or obliquely angulated views.

In conclusion, the role of MRI in the clinical evaluation of patients with congenital cardiac malformations is not well established. Our study was limited mainly to older patients, and most of those examined by MRI had a known anatomic diagnosis established by angiocardiography and/or echocardiography. A prospective study with no knowledge of the diagnosis would better assess the true efficacy of MRI. On the other hand, it is quite likely that most lesions to be examined by MRI will have prior echocardiography and, hence, an established clinical diagnosis.

It is unlikely that MRI will replace echocardiography as the simplest and most definitive method of establishing a noninvasive diagnosis in patients with congenital cardiac malformations. MRI is more likely to become a complementary additive noninvasive imaging procedure to answer some questions left in doubt by echocardiography (mainly extracardiac artery and vein assessments) and as a preferred follow-up imaging method in certain clinical circumstances. Angiocardiography will remain necessary to provide vital physiologic data, i.e., chamber pressures, shunt volumes, oxygen saturations, and pulmonary vascular resistance. However, MRI could negate some follow-up catheterization in appropriate clinical circumstances. The potential for MR evaluation of tissue characterization,[30-32] noninvasive blood flow measurements,[26-29] and even myocardial metabolism assessment[33,34] is intriguing and awaits clinical evaluation. In addition, dynamic cine MRI of the heart, dynamic contrast-enhanced functional imaging, and metabolic correlative imaging with cardiac positron-emission tomography (PET) are at the threshold of meaningful clinical utility.

ACKNOWLEDGMENTS

The secretarial, photographic, and editorial assistance of Vivian Fletcher, John Bobbitt, and Holly Pelton, respectively, is gratefully acknowledged.

References

1. Hawkes RC, Holland GH, Moore WB, et al: Nuclear magnetic resonance (NMR) tomography of the normal heart. J Comput Assist Tomogr 5:605, 1981.
2. Kaufman L, Crooks L, Sheldon P, et al: The potential impact of nuclear magnetic resonance imaging on cardiovascular diagnosis. Circulation 67:251, 1983.
3. Ratner AV, Okada RD, Brady TJ: Nuclear magnetic resonance imaging of the heart. Semin Nucl Med 13:339, 1983.
4. Go RT, MacIntyre WJ, Yeunz HN, et al: Volume and planar gated cardiac magnetic resonance imaging: a correlative study of normal anatomy with thallium-201, SPECT and cadaver sections. Radiology 150:129, 1984.
5. Lanzer P, Botvinick EH, Schiller NB, et al: Cardiac imaging using gated magnetic resonance. Radiology 150:121, 1984.
6. Stark DD, Higgins CB, Lanzer P, et al: Magnetic resonance imaging of the pericardium: Normal and pathological findings. Radiology 150:469, 1984.
7. Herfkens RJ, Higgins CB, Hricak H, et al: Nuclear magnetic resonance imaging of the cardiovascular system: normal and pathologic findings. Radiology 147:749, 1983.
8. Higgins CB, Stark D, McNamara M, et al: Multiplane magnetic resonance imaging of the heart and major vessels: studies in normal volunteers. AJR 142:661, 1984.
9. Lieberman JM, Alfidi RJ, Nelson AD, et al: Gated magnetic resonance imaging of the normal and diseased heart. Radiology 152:465, 1984.
10. Fletcher BD, Jacobstein MD, Nelson AD, et al: Gated magnetic resonance imaging of congenital cardiac malformations. Radiology 150:137, 1984.
11. Jacobstein MD, Fletcher BD, Nelson AD, et al: ECG-gated nuclear magnetic resonance imaging: appearance of the congenitally malformed heart. Am Heart J 107:1014, 1984.
12. Jacobstein MD, Fletcher BD, Nelson AD, et al: Magnetic resonance imaging: evaluation of palliative systemic-pulmonary artery shunts. Circulation 70:650, 1984.
13. Didier D, Higgins DB, Fisher MR, et al: Congenital heart disease: Gated MR imaging in 72 patients. Radiology 158:227, 1986.
14. Higgins CB, Byrd BF, Farmer DW, et al: Magnetic resonance imaging in patients with congenital heart disease. Circulation 70:851, 1984.
15. Schulthess RL, Higashino SM, Higgins SS, et al: Coarctation of the aorta: MR imaging. Radiology 158:469, 1986.
16. Soulen RL, Donner RM: Advances in noninvasive evaluation of congenital anomalies of the thoracic aorta. Radiol Clin North Am 23(4):727, 1985.
17. Soulen RL, Donner RM: Magnetic resonance imaging of rerouted pulmonary blood flow. Radiol Clin North Am 23(4):737, 1985.
18. Tajik AJ, Seward JB, Hagler DT, et al: Two dimensional realtime ultrasonic imaging of the heart and great vessels: technique, image orientation, structure identification and validation. Mayo Clin Proc 53:271, 1978.
19. Henry WL, Maron BJ, Griffith JM: Cross-sectional echocardiography in the diagnosis of congenital heart disease: identification of the relation of the ventricles and great arteries. Circulation 56:267, 1977.
20. Allen HD, Goldberg SJ, Ovitt TW, Goldberg BB: Suprasternal notch echocardiography: assessment of the clinical utility in pediatric cardiology. Circulation 55:605, 1977.
21. Silverman NH, Snider AR: Two-Dimensional Echocardiography in Congenital Heart Disease. Norwalk, Connecticut, Appleton-Century-Crofts, 1982.

22. Goldberg SJ, Allen HD, Sahn DJ: Pediatric and Adolescent Echocardiography—A Handbook, 2nd ed. Chicago, Year Book Medical Publishers, 1980.
23. Weyman AE: Cross-Sectional Echocardiography. Philadelphia, Lea & Febiger, 1982.
24. Bierman FZ: Two-dimensional echocardiography and its influence on cardiac catheterization. Cardiovasc Intervent Radiol 7:140, 1984.
25. Sahn DJ: Two-dimensional echocardiography as an aid to planning cardiac catheterization. Cardiovasc Intervent Radiol 7:154, 1984.
26. Morse O, Singer JR: Blood velocity measurements in intact subjects. Science 170:440, 1970.
27. Kaufman L, Crooks LE, Sheldon P, Rowan W: Evaluation of NMR imaging for detection and quantitation of obstructions in vessels. Invest Radiol 17:554, 1982.
28. Crooks LE, Sheldon P, Kaufman L, Rowan W: Quantification of obstruction in vessels by nuclear magnetic resonance (NMR). IEEE Trans Nucl Sci 29:1181, 1982.
29. Mills CM, Brant-Zawadzki M, Crooks LE, et al: Nuclear magnetic resonance: Principles of blood flow imaging. AJR 142:165, 1984.
30. Higgins CB, Herfkens R, Lipton MJ, Sheldon P, Kaufman L, Crooks LE: Nuclear magnetic resonance imaging of acute myocardial infarctions in dogs: alterations in magnetic relaxation times. Am J Cardiol 52:184, 1983.
31. Herfkens RJ, Sievers R, Kaufman L, et al: Nuclear magnetic resonance imaging of the infarcted muscle: A rat model. Radiology 147:761, 1983.
32. Wesbey G, Higgins CB, Lanzer P, Botvinick E, Lipton MJ: Imaging and characterization of acute myocardial infarction in vivo using gated nuclear magnetic resonance. Circulation 69:125, 1984.
33. Jacobus WF, Taylor GI, Hollis DP, et al: Phosphorus NMR of perfused working hearts. Nature 26:756, 1977.
34. Nunnally RL, Bottomley PA: 31P NMR studies of myocardial ischemia and its response to drugs. J Comput Assist Tomogr 5:296, 1981.

25

Magnetic Resonance Imaging of the Heart

GARY R. CAPUTO
CHARLES B. HIGGINS

Magnetic resonance imaging (MRI) is a new technique that permits noninvasive imaging of the heart.[1-3] It does not require the use of ionizing radiation or contrast media. MRI of the heart offers the advantages of the natural contrast between the blood pool and cardiac structures, because flowing blood produces minimal MR signal[2,4]; high soft tissue contrast, enabling sharp delineation of the myocardium, pericardium, and pericardial fat[1,3,5]; and the ease of synchronization of pulse sequences to a fixed segment of the cardiac cycle.[6]

TECHNICAL CONSIDERATIONS

Physiologic Gating of MRI

Cyclic cardiac motion causes myocardial protons (such as the flowing nuclei in blood) to experience a "distorted" pulse sequence; consequently, under standard imaging conditions, myocardial signals are weak. Typical MRI acquisition times range from 4 to 18 minutes, and specific structures occupy different positions at different times during the acquisition period. The motion results in a blurred, averaged image of the cardiac cycle that represents neither end-diastole nor end-systole. Therefore, cardiac MRI requires that signals be acquired in a fixed relationship to the cardiac cycle.

An ECG sensing device compatible with a 0.35 tesla MR imager was developed to synchronize the imaging sequences with a specific phase of the cardiac cycle. The system was designed to sense the ECG signal and to generate an MR-sequence triggering pulse. To protect the patient from power-line leakage currents, the electrical ECG signal is converted into an optical signal by an isolated acquisition module and is transmitted by a fiberoptic cable. The isolated acquisition module is powered by an internal 6-volt battery.[6]

With the imaging technique used in our laboratory (spin-echo), each pulse sequence can be completed in 28 ms or 56 ms. These periods are called echo delay times, denoted *TE*. When using ECG gating the MR repetition rate (*TR*) is defined by the R-R interval of the ECG. With a heart rate of 60/min, the *TR* is 1.0 sec. If the acquisition sequence utilizes every second R wave at the same heart rate, then the *TR* is 2.0 sec.

Cardiac Imaging Techniques

With multisection imaging, after the first section is acquired a second section is done, and so on, for a fixed amount of time that must not exceed the R-R interval. If two spin echoes with a *TE* of 28 ms and 56 ms are obtained, five sections are easily fitted within a cardiac cycle. Advancing from section to section, however, the time interval between the R wave and the initiation of pulse sequences changes. The first section is initiated with the R wave of the ECG, the second is initiated 100 ms later, and so on, to the fifth section, which is delayed 400 ms after the R wave.

Thus, five sections are sampled per heartbeat, each at a different but fixed point in the cardiac cycle (Fig. 25–1). The point in the cardiac cycle when the first section will begin to be acquired is hardware-selectable by varying the ms delay after the R wave. If the second echo is sacrificed, sections can be advanced every 50 ms and ten sections can be acquired within one R-R interval.

Multisection imaging can be implemented so as to allow the imaging of each section at multiple times in the cardiac cycle. The technique, called a rotating gated sequence, obtains each anatomic section at five phases of the cardiac cycle.[7] Each of five sections is imaged at end-diastole and then at four 100 ms intervals extending into the cardiac cycle. The total imaging time required to achieve this multiphase-multisectional imaging is approximately 35 to 40 minutes (Figs. 25–2 and 25–3).

ECG-gated volume imaging of the heart is also possible. With this three-dimensional mode of image acquisition, tomographic images of the heart in any plane may be reconstructed by the computer.[8] All images from a given acquisition will be at the same phase of the cardiac cycle, solving the current multiplanar imaging problem of sequential tomograms, each 100 ms out of phase with the next. Evaluation of ventricular mechanics through end-diastolic measurements of mass, volume, and wall stress will be easily accomplished with volume imaging. Quantitative analysis of myocardial hypertrophy and regional wall thinning will be improved when each section of the heart

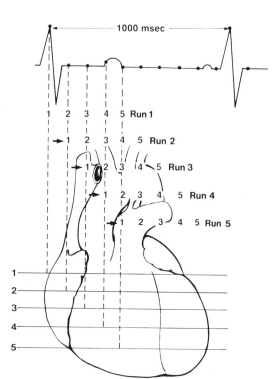

Figure 25–1. Diagram of multisection imaging of the heart shows runs 1 through 5 synchronized with the ECG, each with a different time delay. Each run encompasses five sequences corresponding to anatomic levels 1 through 5. The first sequence of run 1 is triggered from the ECG R wave and corresponds to imaging anatomic level 1 at end-diastole and anatomic level 5 at end-systole, with each level being offset by 100 ms and 7 mm. Run 5, with a delay of 400 ms, images anatomic level 5 late in the diastolic phase. (From Lanzer P, et al: Radiology *155*:681, 1985. Used by permission of the Radiological Society of North America.)

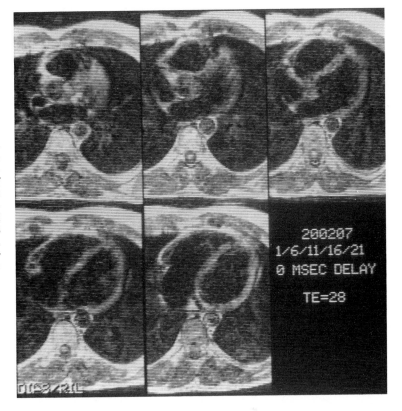

Figure 25–2. Diagram of five adjacent isophasic sections at end-diastole, selected from five cycled multisection acquisitions consisting of five sections imaged at five different times in the cardiac cycle. The signal in the aorta indicates slow blood flow at end-diastole. (From Crooks LE, et al: Radiology *153*:459, 1984. Used by permission of the Radiological Society of North America.)

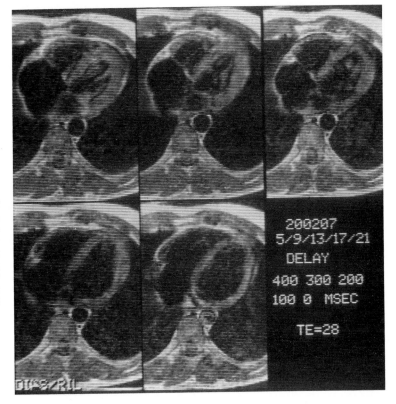

Figure 25–3. Transverse images through the left ventricle obtained in a rotated, gated, five-section, dual-echo mode. The left upper image is obtained at 400 ms after the R wave of the ECG, with subsequent images (left to right) delayed 300, 200, 100, and 0 ms after the R wave (end-diastole). The image delayed 300 ms after the R wave is near end-systole, and comparison of this image with the end-diastolic image shows considerable and uniform thickening of the left ventricular and, to a lesser extent, the right ventricular myocardium. (From Crooks LE, et al: Radiology *153*:459, 1984. Used by permission of the Radiological Society of North America.)

is assessed at the same phase in the cardiac cycle. It will also be possible to reorient tomographic images for analysis along the long or short axis of the heart.

A real-time MR imaging modality that allows the acquisition of a tomographic image in approximately 30 to 50 ms has been developed.[9] Called echo-planar imaging, it is accomplished by rapidly switching magnetic field gradients, and it allows rapid imaging of the heart. Although this technique has potential for evaluating cardiac function, it is limited by its low spatial resolution and, owing to technical limitations, is currently adapted only for imaging the thorax of infants or small children.

NORMAL CARDIAC MORPHOLOGY

Magnetic resonance imaging of the heart is most often performed with the patient supine. The Z-axis imaging plane is aligned with the patient in a head-to-toe orientation, which uses the patient as a frame of reference for imaging (i.e., coronal, sagittal, and transaxial image orientations). The transaxial images obtained are most easily compared with the subcostal long-axis view obtained using two-dimensional echocardiography, since both ventricular septum and posterolateral wall are imaged on transaxial magnetic resonance images (Fig. 25–4).

The natural contrast between blood and myocardium as imaged using magnetic resonance is evident in Figure 25–5. The sharp contrast between moving blood and the walls of the cardiac chambers results in clear discrimination of the ventricular and atrial septa. With the degree of spatial resolution demonstrated, wall thickness and chamber dimensions may be measured easily. MRI does not have the difficulties with gain-related artifacts or coarse lateral resolution that occur with two-dimensional echocardiography. The moderator band of the right ventricle and papillary muscles are regularly seen in MR images (Fig. 25–6). However, the atrioventricular valves are so thin and mobile that they are visualized only intermittently. The pericardium is com-

MAGNETIC RESONANCE IMAGING PLANES

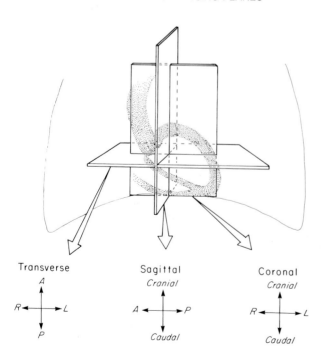

Transverse

Sagittal

Coronal

Figure 25–4. Schematic representation of the tomographic imaging planes in relation to cardiac anatomy when the patient is used as a frame of reference for imaging. The terms transverse and transaxial are used interchangeably. (From Higgins CB, et al: *55*:1121, 1985. Used by permission.)

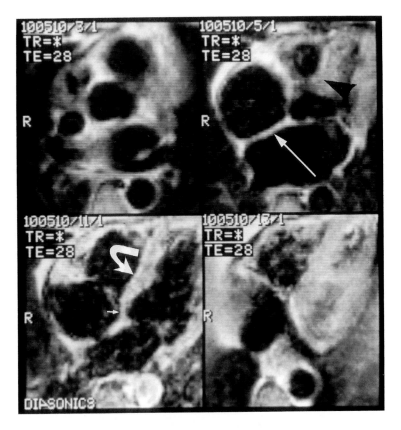

Figure 25–5. Multiple transverse MR images, extending from the level of the great vessels to the middle portion of the ventricles, demonstrate the normal relationship of the great vessels, atrial septum, and outflow (anterior) and inflow (posterior) portions of the ventricular septum. Atrial septum (long arrow), outflow septum (arrowhead), inflow septum (curved arrow), atrioventricular portion of the septum (small arrow). (From Higgins CB, et al: Radiology *155*:671, 1985. Used by permission of the Radiological Society of North America.)

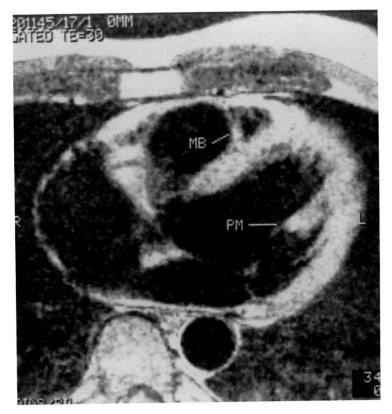

Figure 25–6. Transverse MR image at the midventricular level of a normal volunteer shows all four cardiac chambers. Internal topography of the ventricles is demonstrated, including the moderator band (MB) of the right ventricle and a papillary muscle of the left ventricle (PM).

posed of fibrous tissue with little proton signal because of its low water content. The normal pericardium frequently is visualized anterior to the right ventricle and cardiac apex only as a thin dark line between myocardium, epicardial fat, and pericardial fat (Fig. 25–7). Proximal portions of the coronary arteries may be seen using MRI without using contrast medium because of the high contrast between moving intraluminal blood and the surrounding epicardial fat.

Complete evaluation of the left ventricle by MRI is achieved by also obtaining images in the sagittal and coronal planes. The sagittal plane demonstrates the thickness of the anteroseptal and posterior walls of the left ventricle (Fig. 25–8). The coronal plane will depict another region of the septum as well as the diaphragmatic and lateral walls of the left ventricle (Fig. 25–9).

MR techniques allowing the use of the heart as a frame of reference (i.e., long-axis and short-axis image orientations) facilitate definition of cardiac structural detail and functional status (Fig. 25–10). The transverse, sagittal, and coronal sections using the patient as a frame of reference rarely coincide with the long or short axis of the heart unless this occurs fortuitously, with the septum lying in a standard orthogonal projection and the left ventricle in a truly transverse plane.

Recently, these oblique axis reorientations were accomplished by selection of electronic angulation of the magnetic fields for each subject rather than by attempting to approximate the cardiac axes by altering the position of the patient.[10] The standard transverse section provides information on angulation of the septum from the horizontal plane so that new reoriented sagittal or coronal images can be obtained (Fig. 25–11). These reoriented images should improve accuracy and reproducibility of cardiac measurements such as wall thickness, chamber volume, and mass.

In general, signal in the left ventricle of normal individuals occurs in diastole, and the intraluminal second echo signal resulting from slow flow is stronger than the first echo signal. End-diastolic slow flow occurs because left ventricular filling at heart rates of 50 to 60 beats per minute is virtually complete approximately 200 to 300 ms before the onset of the next systole. In the latter part of diastasis there is little inflow to the left ventricle, resulting in relatively static blood. During the ejection phase, blood at the left ventricular apex undergoes acceleration late, resulting sometimes in intraventricular signal near the apex in late systole. In normal persons, intraluminal signal on MR images appear to be merely a reflection of normal physiologic events. At higher

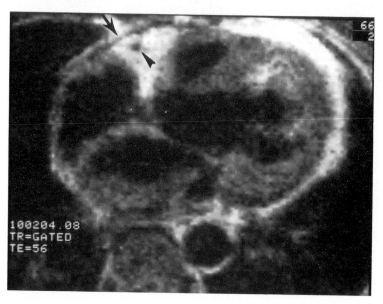

Figure 25–7. Gated transverse image in patient with a normal pericardium. The pericardium is represented by a rim of low signal intensity (arrow) separating the subepicardial fat tissue (high signal intensity) from the pericardial fat tissue. The image also shows the right coronary artery (arrowhead) and thinning of the posterior myocardial wall in this patient with a prior myocardial infarction. (From Higgins CB, et al. *In* Pohost GM (ed): New Concepts in Cardiac Imaging. Boston, GK Hall Medical Publishers, 1985. Used by permission.)

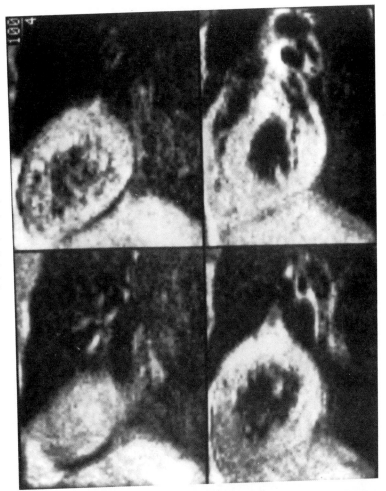

Figure 25–8. Sagittal MR images of the left ventricle in a normal volunteer show similar thickness of the anteroseptal, diaphragmatic, and posterior walls. (From Higgins CB, et al: *In* Pohost GM (ed): New Concepts in Cardiac Imaging. Boston, GK Hall Medical Publishers, 1985. Used by permission.)

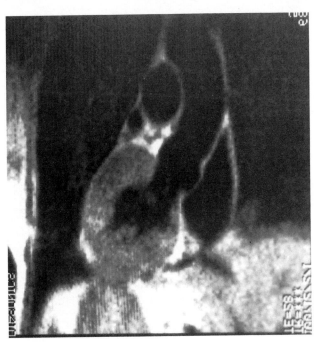

Figure 25–9. Coronal MR image of the left ventricle in a normal volunteer shows similar thickness of the diaphragmatic and lateral walls.

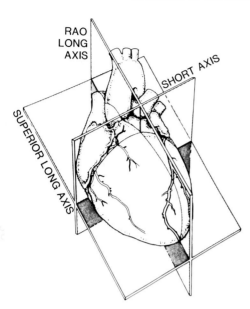

Figure 25–10. Schematic representation of the tomographic imaging planes in relation to cardiac anatomy when the heart is used as a frame of reference. These planes, similar to those used in two dimensional echocardiography, are either parallel or perpendicular to the long axis of the left ventricle. RAO = right anterior oblique. (From Caldwell JH, et al: *In* Pohost GM (ed): New Concepts in Cardiac Imaging. Boston, GK Hall Medical Publishers, 1985. Used by permission.)

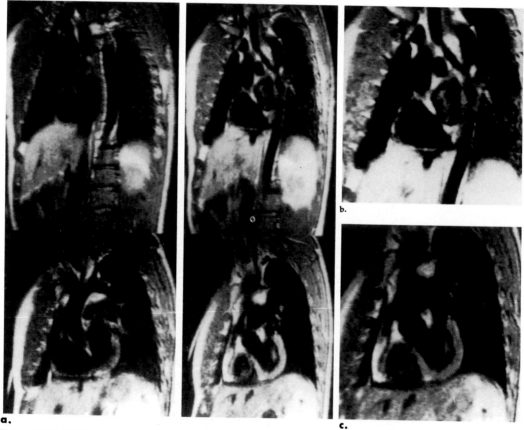

Figure 25–11. MR images corresponding to the short axis imaging plane defined in Figure 25–10. *a*, The short-axis images at 12 mm intervals demonstrate: (top panels) right atrium, vena cava, descending thoracic aorta, right and left atria, and atrial septum; (bottom left panel) both ventricles, aortic arch, and left pulmonary artery; (bottom right panel) a more anterior view of both ventricles. *b*, Magnified top right panel from *a*. *c*, Magnified bottom right panel from *a*. (From Feiglin DH, et al: Radiology *154:*129, 1985. Used by permission of the Radiological Society of North America.)

heart rates diastasis shortens; inflow and outflow of blood in the left ventricle alternate more rapidly, causing intraventricular blood to remain in constant motion; and left ventricular intraluminal signal is decreased to absent.

Left atrial signal is prominent during systole in normal subjects, when blood flow into the atrium is slow. The right-sided heart chambers show little signal throughout the cardiac cycle compared with the left-sided chambers. This probably is the result of the different prevailing pressures of the systemic and pulmonary circulations, the right ventricle showing lower peak but higher minimum velocities, earlier onset of ejection, and a different chamber configuration.[11]

CARDIAC ABNORMALITIES

Acute Myocardial Infarction

Magnetic relaxation times in canine models of myocardial infarction have been extensively investigated. In general, these studies have shown that *T1* and *T2* relaxation times are prolonged by ischemic myocardial damage. Such studies suggest that acute infarcts should be readily depicted by MRI in vivo. Because patient prognosis is greatly dependent on the amount of myocardium that is destroyed in the setting of an acute myocardial infarction, great attention has been directed toward methods for direct visualization of the extent of myocardial necrosis. A noninvasive means for detecting ischemia early in the course of myocardial infarction would be desirable.

In another canine model, *T1* and *T2* values were determined from spin-echo MRI studies of excised hearts imaged within one hour after sacrifice of animals with 24-hour-old anterior infarctions.[12] In each heart, the area of infarction exhibited increased signal intensity compared with normal myocardium (Fig. 25–12). When the animals with experimental myocardial infarction were considered as a group, the mean value for *T1* relaxation times of infarcted myocardium (728 $\pm$ 95 ms [standard deviation])

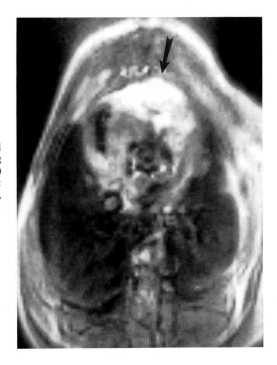

Figure 25–12. Transaxial MR image at a left ventricular level in a dog at 24 hours after ligation of the left anterior descending coronary artery. The infarct has high signal intensity (arrow) compared with normal myocardium. (From Higgins CB, et al: *In* Pohost GM (ed): New Concepts in Cardiac Imaging. Boston, GK Hall Medical Publishers, 1985. Used by permission.)

was higher than the value for normal myocardium (650 ± 87 ms). There was overlap of *T1* values between infarcted and normal myocardium. On the other hand, the *T1* value of the infarcted myocardium was higher than that of the normal myocardium for each individual animal. The mean value for *T2* relaxation time of infarcted myocardium (48.4 ± 2 ms) was significantly greater (p < .01) than of normal myocardium (42.1 ± 1 ms). There was a narrow range of *T2* values for normal myocardium (40 to 43 ms) and no overlap of individual values between infarcted and normal groups.

Gated spin-echo MRI performed in vivo on dogs with one- to seven-day-old myocardial infarctions has also shown that the infarcted myocardium could be distinguished from normal myocardium without the use of contrast medium.[13] The infarcted myocardium exhibited high signal intensity compared with normal myocardium in these images, and the *T2* relaxation time of infarcted myocardium was significantly longer than in normal myocardium.

Seven patients were studied by MR at four to ten days after documented acute myocardial infarctions.[14] Infarctions were documented by ECG changes and a diagnostic rise in the creatinine phosphokinase level. An inadequate MR study was obtained on one of these patients. The MR images in the other six patients demonstrated distinct regions of high signal intensity of the myocardium in the area corresponding to the site of infarction as predicted by the ECG changes (Fig. 25–13). The regions of high intensity demonstrated a further increase in intensity relative to adjacent myocardium on the second spin-echo image. This pattern of response of the infarcted region is similar to observations made in canine models of acute infarctions and is consistent with a longer *T2* relaxation time of infarcted compared with normal myocardium.

The question arose as to how soon after coronary occlusion MRI can detect the region of myocardial ischemic injury. Therefore, in vivo gated magnetic resonance imaging was performed in nine dogs with acute myocardial infarctions immediately after coronary artery occlusion and serially up to five hours.[15] MR images and measurements indicated that the signal intensity of the infarcted myocardium was significantly greater than that of normal myocardium at three (29.1 ± 8.4 percent), at four (77.5 ± 24.6 percent), and at five hours (91.8 ± 41.7 percent) post occlusion. A sig-

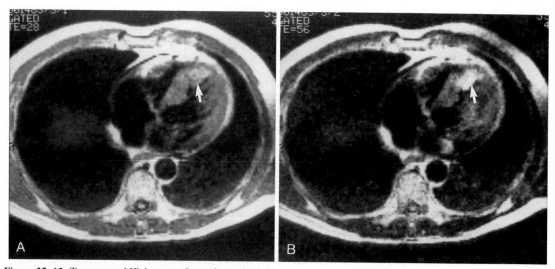

Figure 25–13. Transverse MR images of a patient who had an acute myocardial infarction show high regional intensity (arrow) in the anterior wall of the left ventricular myocardium. There is a relative increase in signal intensity on the second spin-echo image (*B, TE* = 56 ms) compared with that of the first spin-echo image (*A, TE* = 28 ms). (From Higgins CB, et al: *In* Pohost GM (ed): New Concepts in Cardiac Imaging. Boston, GK Hall Medical Publishers, 1985. Used by permission.)

nificant prolongation of the *T2* relaxation time was found in the region of myocardial infarct at three (49.2 ± 9.9 ms), at four (57.1 ± 11.6 ms), and at five hours (58.8 ± 13.6 ms) post occlusion compared with normal myocardium (36.8 ± 4.2 ms). In vivo gated MRI displayed acute myocardial infarction as a region of high signal intensity with additional myocardial wall thinning and increased intracavitary flow signal after three hours of coronary occlusion.

In another study, 15 dogs were studied with MRI before and serially for up to six hours after coronary occlusion.[16] By four hours after coronary artery occlusion, the signal in the infarct zone increased to 36 ± 20 percent greater than that in adjacent normal myocardium on first-echo images and to 116 ± 100 percent for second-echo images, clearly delineating ischemic myocardium. Changes observed on MRI correlated well with the location of ischemic changes noted on pathologic examination of the excised hearts.

Chronic Myocardial Infarction

In addition to abnormalities in *T1* and *T2* parameters, old myocardial infarctions are demonstrated as regions of wall thinning in magnetic resonance images.[17] Figure 25–14 demonstrates both anteroseptal and posterior wall infarctions with thinning in that region on the transaxial image. Measurement of the spatial distribution of such thinned regions allows estimation of the extent of infarction. These estimates correlate with angiographic and echocardiographic findings.[17] Marked wall thinning and dilation of thinned areas on MRI were found in patients with left ventricular aneurysms.

Regions of unusually high signal intensity may appear on MRI of infarcted hearts within the left ventricular aneurysm, suggesting blood flow stasis as a consequence of regional akinesis or dyskinesis. The signal from stagnant blood adjacent to a dysfunctional region of the left ventricle has been most pronounced on second-echo images (*TE* = 56 ms) (Fig. 25–15).

Left ventricular thrombus was demonstrated on magnetic resonance images in

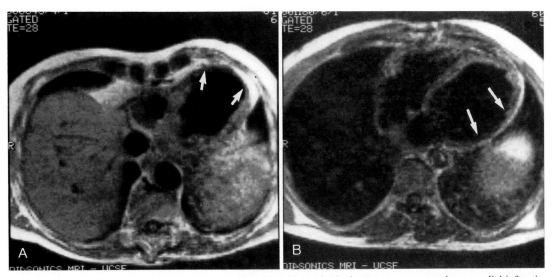

Figure 25–14. *A*, Transverse MR image (*TE* = 28 ms) of a patient who had remote anteroseptal myocardial infarction showing regional thinning of the anterior wall of the left ventricle (arrows). *B*, Transverse MR image (*TE* = 28 ms) of a patient who had multiple previous infarctions, including a posterior myocardial infarction, demonstrating thinning of the posterolateral wall of the left ventricle (arrows). (From Higgins CB, et al: Radiology *155*:671, 1985. Used by permission of the Radiological Society of North America.)

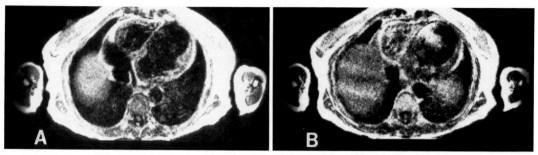

Figure 25–15. Transverse images near the apex of the left ventricle in a patient with a remote transmural infarction. First spin-echo image (*TE* = 28 ms) (*A*), and second spin-echo image (*TE* = 56 ms) (*B*). There is prominent signal intensity in the chamber, presumably due to blood flow stasis in a region of dyskinesis. (From Higgins CB, et al: Circulation 69:523, 1984. Used by permission of the American Heart Association.)

several patients confirmed to have this abnormality on either two-dimensional echocardiography or CT scans.[17] Mural thrombus was noted on MRI as a structure of medium signal intensity projecting into the left ventricular chamber. The signal intensity of the thrombus increased on the images formed with the second spin echo (*TE* = 56 ms) compared with those from the first spin echo (*TE* = 28 ms). The presence of signal within the left ventricular cavity on both spin-echo images helps to differentiate thrombus from stagnant blood, in which intraluminal signal is usually observed on only the second (*TE* = 56 ms) spin-echo image. The increase in intensity of the thrombus on the second spin-echo image tends to accentuate the interface between the thrombus and the myocardial wall (Fig. 25–16).

Magnetic resonance images in patients with ischemic cardiomyopathy have shown left and often right ventricular enlargement with regional wall thinning (Fig. 25–17). The nonischemic cardiomyopathies have shown more uniform wall thickness than the ischemic cases. Measurement of wall thickness and chamber dimensions by MRI may in the future allow assessment of ventricular wall stress in the cardiomyopathies.

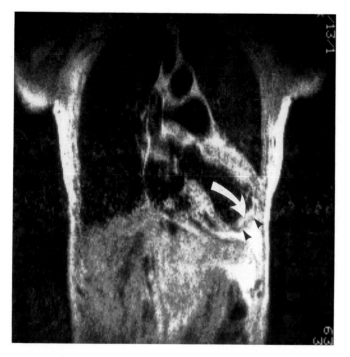

Figure 25–16. Coronal MR image (*TE* = 28 ms) of a patient who had an anteroseptal myocardial infarction shows severe thinning of the apical wall (arrowheads) and mural thrombus (curved arrow). (From Higgins CB, et al: Radiology *155*:671, 1985. Used by permission of the Radiological Society of North America.)

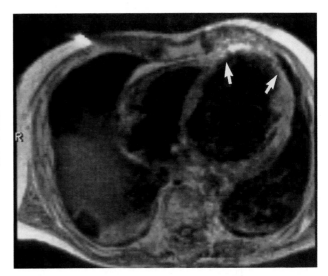

Figure 25–17. Transverse MR image in a patient with ischemic cardiomyopathy and an anteroapical aneurysm (arrows). (From Higgins CB, et al: *In* Pohost GM (ed): New Concepts in Cardiac Imaging. Boston, GK Hall Medical Publishers, 1985. Used by permission.)

Cardiomyopathies

Magnetic resonance imaging provides accurate definition of the extent, location, and severity of left ventricular hypertrophy in patients with hypertrophic cardiomyopathy.[18] The variable presentation and course of hypertrophic cardiomyopathy may be better understood in light of the great variability in ventricular morphology found in these patients. In some patients, hypertrophy exists only in the outflow septum (Fig. 25–18). In others, the entire septum is hypertrophied, and in still others hypertrophy may extend from the septum into the free wall or apex (Fig. 25–19). Observations on the patterns of hypertrophic cardiomyopathy in images made with magnetic resonance correspond well with those made with two-dimensional echocardiography (Fig. 25–20).[18] Often the resolution of MRI is superior to echocardiography, although ultrasonic Doppler analysis does add information about outflow tract gradients and mitral regurgitation in hypertrophic cardiomyopathy.

In addition to morphologic analysis, tissue characterization of hypertrophic cardiomyopathy with spin-echo MRI has been investigated in our laboratory. No significant difference in $T2$ relaxation time has been noted in hypertrophic cardiomyopathy compared with the myocardium of normal volunteers.

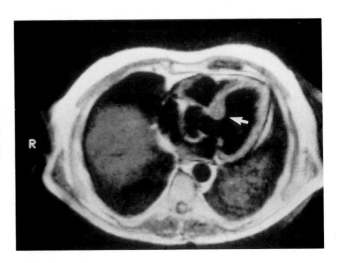

Figure 25–18. Transverse MR image obtained at a level just beneath the aortic valve in a patient with hypertrophic cardiomyopathy shows focal hypertrophy of the upper portion of the septum (arrow). (From Higgins CB, et al: Am J Cardiol *55*:1121, 1985. Used by permission.)

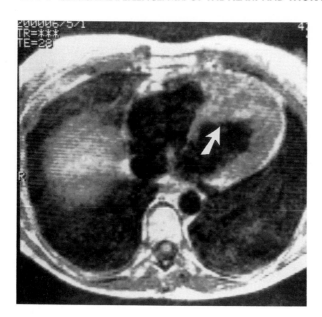

Figure 25–19. Transverse image in a patient with hypertrophic cardiomyopathy demonstrating hypertrophy involving the anteroseptal (arrow) and anterolateral segments of the left ventricle. (From Higgins CB, et al: Am J Cardiol 55:1121, 1985. Used by permission.)

In congestive cardiomyopathy, MR has demonstrated dilation of the left ventricle and, in some instances, left atrial and right ventricular enlargement. MR has shown normal or mildly reduced wall thickness as well as disproportionate thinning of the ventricular septum in patients with idiopathic congestive cardiomyopathy (Fig. 25–21). As was the case in hypertrophic cardiomyopathy, no alterations in *T2* relaxation time were noted in congestive cardiomyopathy when compared with the myocardium of normal volunteers.

Pericardial Disease

Since it is composed of fibrous tissue, the normal pericardium appears on magnetic resonance images only as a curvilinear line of low signal intensity situated between the epicardial fat or myocardium and pericardial fat (see Fig. 25–7). The small amount of fluid normally present in the pericardial space may also contribute to the thickness of this low-intensity curvilinear line. In chronic constrictive pericarditis, MRI shows increased thickness of the dark rim of fibrotic pericardium between myocardium and epicardial fat (Fig. 25–22). The right atrium and inferior vena cava are dilated in relationship to the small to normal-sized right ventricle. Pericardial cysts have also been demonstrated with magnetic resonance imaging.[5] In patients with pericardial effusion,

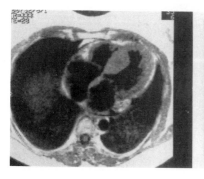 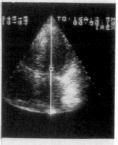

Figure 25–20. MR (*TE* = 28 ms) and two-dimensional echocardiographic images at comparable levels. The marked hypertrophy of the ventricular septum is more sharply defined on the MR image because of better definition of the endocardial borders of the septum on MR. (From Higgins CB, et al: Radiology 155:671, 1985. Used by permission of the Radiological Society of North America.)

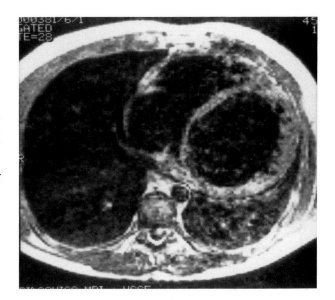

Figure 25–21. Transverse MR image (TE = 28 ms) of a patient who had idiopathic congestive cardiomyopathy shows disproportionate thinning of the septal segment of the left ventricular myocardium. (From Higgins CB, et al: Radiology *155*:671, 1985. Used by permission of the Radiological Society of North America.)

this technique shows the size of the effusion and the atrial and ventricular chambers within that effusion. Two-dimensional echocardiography, when technically adequate, is preferable in the unstable patient with pericardial effusion, because it allows a real-time search for the right-sided chamber compression suggestive of the hemodynamic compromise of tamponade.[19] In the stable patient, however, magnetic resonance imaging provides anatomic information about the diseased pericardium which is at least comparable to that obtained with computed tomography[20] or echocardiography. MRI may also give some indication of the composition of the pericardial effusion. In this regard, it has clearly defined the presence of intrapericardial blood, which produced a much higher regional intensity than other pericardial effusions (Fig. 25–23).

A potential advantage of MRI in pericardial disease is that signal intensity may provide unique insights into the pathologic process involved. In patients with uremic pericarditis, magnetic resonance imaging has demonstrated a moderate pericardial effusion and abundant inflammatory exudate of the pericardium (Fig. 25–24). Unlike normal pericardium, the inflamed or uremic pericardium produced strong magnetic

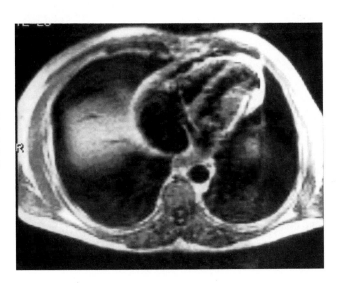

Figure 25–22. Transverse MR image in a patient with constrictive pericarditis. The thickened pericardium is represented by a thick rim of low signal intensity surrounding the right side of the heart. Note also the enlarged right atrium and small ventricular chambers.

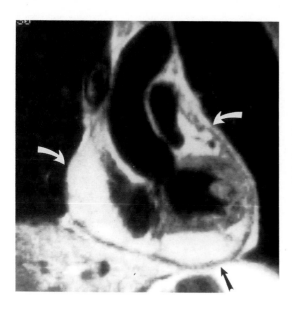

Figure 25–23. Coronal MR image in a patient with a pericardial hematoma. Note the very high signal intensity (white arrows) created by blood in the pericardial sac. The pericardium is demonstrated by a thin line of decreased signal intensity (black arrow).

resonance signal intensity, as did adhesions between the visceral and parietal pericardium. Also, the signal intensity of uremic pericardium is greater, with a longer echo delay time ($TE = 56$ ms), which is consistent with the long $T2$ relaxation time previously observed in other edematous tissues.[16,21] Initial clinical experience with imaging of the pericardium suggests that MRI may provide both anatomic and tissue-characterizing information about pericardial disease.

Intracardiac and Paracardiac Masses

MRI has been useful for demonstrating intracardiac and paracardiac masses affecting the heart (Fig. 25–25). Comparison of MR studies with two-dimensional echocardiography showed that MR more clearly demonstrated the presence, location, and

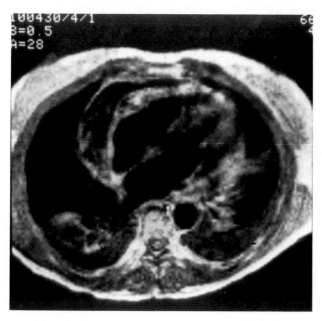

Figure 25–24. Transverse MR image of the heart in a patient with uremic pericarditis. Image shows shaggy thickened pericardium with high signal intensity. The thickened edematous visceral and parietal pericardial layers are separated by effusion. (From Higgins CB, et al: *In* Pohost GM (ed): New Concepts in Cardiac Imaging. Boston, GK Hall Medical Publishers, 1985. Used by permission.)

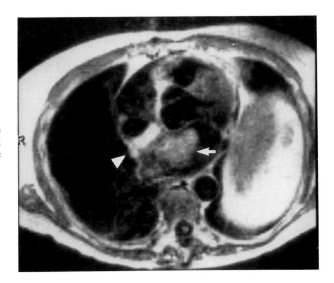

Figure 25–25. Transverse MR image (TE = 28 ms) shows a large globular mass in the cavity of the left atrium (arrow). The myxoma is attached to the atrial septum (arrowhead).

extent of the mass. The large field of view, the capability to image noncardiac mediastinal structures, and the definition of the limits of cardiac walls were decided advantages of MR. MR provides at least as definitive an evaluation of paracardiac masses as angiography and contrast-enhanced CT but does so in a completely noninvasive manner.[22]

Congenital Heart Disease

Magnetic resonance imaging has been used to define congenital cardiovascular anomalies.[23] Atrial and ventricular septal defects have been demonstrated by gated MR imaging (Fig. 25–26). Visceroatrial situs and the type of bulboventricular loop can

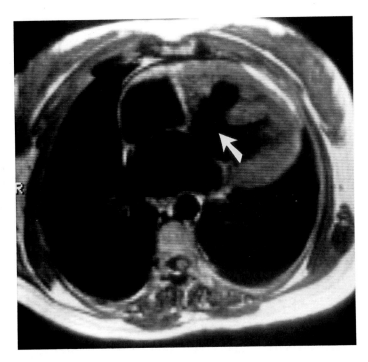

Figure 25–26. Transverse MR image (TE = 30 ms) showing a ventricular septal defect (arrow). (From Higgins CB, et al: Radiology *155*:671, 1985. Used by permission of the Radiological Society of North America.)

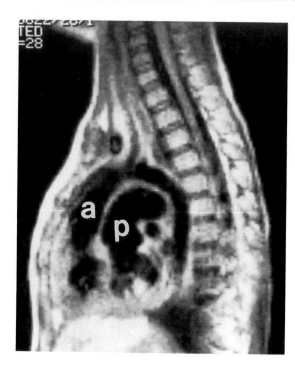

Figure 25–27. Sagittal MR image (*TE* = 28 ms) shows the origins of the aorta (a) from the right ventricle and the pulmonary (p) artery from the left ventricle. (From Higgins CB, et al: Radiology *155*:671, 1985. Used by permission of the Radiological Society of North America.)

be clearly defined by transverse MR images. Likewise, the relationship of the great vessels is demonstrated; the sagittal images show the anterior position of the aorta in transposition (Fig. 25–27). Coarctation of the aorta can be demonstrated on both non-gated and gated sagittal images of the thorax (Fig. 25–28).

Abnormalities of the bulboventricular loop can also be seen on coronal MR images. Evaluation of the relationships of the great vessels and cardiac chambers can be important in a patient's preoperative assessment. Single ventricle and levo-transposition of the great vessels is demonstrated in Figure 25–29.

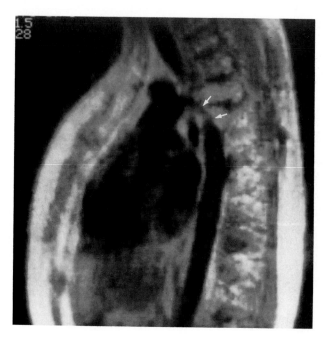

Figure 25–28. Sagittal MR image (*TE* = 28 ms) of the aorta shows a long segment coarctation (arrows). (From Higgins CB, et al: Radiology *155*:671, 1985. Used by permission of the Radiological Society of North America.)

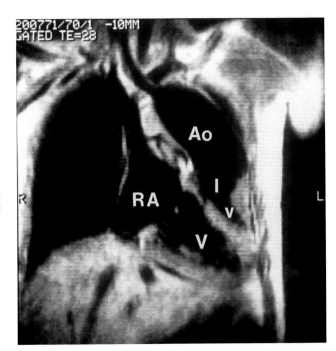

Figure 25–29. Coronal MR image of a patient with levotransposition of the great vessels and single ventricle. The aorta (Ao) arises from the infundibulum (I) communicating with a small subaortic ventricular chamber (v). The single ventricle (V) is seen communicating with the right atrium (RA).

Magnetic resonance imaging is perhaps the most accurate modality for defining right ventricular wall thickness. In patients with Eisenmenger's syndrome, the right ventricular myocardium has been shown to be equivalent to or to exceed the thickness of the left ventricle (Fig. 25–30). Likewise, MRI has shown substantial wall thickening in patients with obstruction of the right ventricular outflow tract.

Pulmonary Hypertension

MRI characterizes pulmonary hypertension by enlargement of the main pulmonary artery and by right ventricular hypertrophy (Fig. 25–31). In the presence of severe

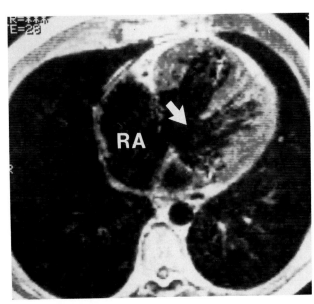

Figure 25–30. Transverse image through the middle of the ventricles of a patient with ventricular septal defect complicated by Eisenmenger's syndrome. The defect in the ventricular septum (arrow) is evident. Note that the right atrium (RA) is enlarged and that the wall thickness of the right ventricle is equal to that of the left ventricle.

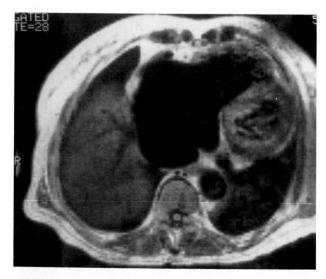

Figure 25–31. Transverse MR image (TE = 28 ms) of a patient who had pulmonary hypertension complicated by substantial tricuspid regurgitation. There is substantial right ventricular and atrial enlargement and an enormous degree of dilation of the inferior vena cava. (From Higgins CB, et al: Radiology *155*:671, 1985. Used by permission of the Radiological Society of North America.)

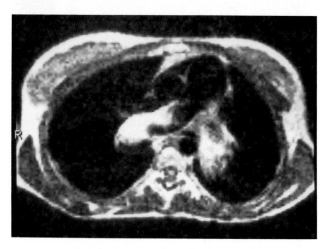

Figure 25–32. Transverse MR image of a patient who had pulmonary arterial hypertension, showing enlargement of the pulmonary artery and substantial intraluminal signal in the pulmonary arteries during systole. (From Higgins CB, et al: Radiology *155*:671, 1985. Used by permission of the Radiological Society of North America.)

pulmonary hypertension complicated by tricuspid regurgitation, there was massive enlargement of the right atrium and inferior vena cava (Fig. 25–32). In patients with severe pulmonary hypertension (pulmonary arterial systolic pressure greater than 90 mm Hg), MR studies showed considerable signal within the pulmonary artery on images obtained during systole as well as the intraluminal signal expected on the end-diastolic image (Fig. 25–31). This finding suggested the presence of slow flow in the pulmonary circulation.[22]

MRI COMPARED WITH OTHER CARDIAC IMAGING MODALITIES

The major advantages and disadvantages of MRI relative to other tomographic cardiac imaging techniques may be briefly summarized. Unlike two-dimensional echocardiography, magnetic resonance imaging is not dependent on operator technique or the patient's body habitus. MRI also has a larger field of view than does echocardiography. However, echocardiography also has distinct advantages: It is portable, obtains images in unlimited and easily adjustable planes, and can estimate pressure gradients using Doppler techniques.

Unlike cardiac CT, magnetic resonance imaging does not employ ionizing radiation and does not require injection of contrast medium to distinguish blood vessels and myocardium from the blood pool. Thrombus and mass within the cardiac chamber are better visualized by MRI, since they are not partially obscured by contrast medium. The direct demonstration of cardiac anatomy with MRI is superior to both conventional contrast angiography and radionuclide scans, which visualize only the intracardiac blood pool. Disadvantages of magnetic resonance imaging at its present stage of development include (1) the requirement that the patient lie quietly during gated acquisition over a five- to ten-minute period; (2) the high cost; and (3) the difficulty in studying critically ill patients and patients on cardiorespiratory assist devices.

FUTURE PERSPECTIVES

Intraluminal magnetic resonance signal intensity is related to the velocity of blood flow at a given cross-sectional area, suggesting the capacity of MRI to measure blood

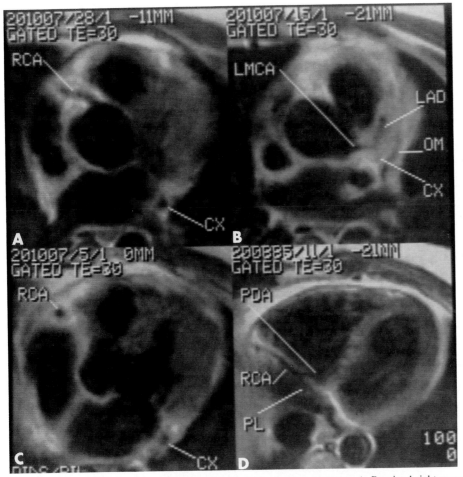

Figure 25–33. Transverse MR images demonstrating normal coronary anatomy. *A*, Proximal right coronary artery (RCA) and circumflex (CX). *B*, Left main coronary artery (LMCA), giving rise to the left anterior descending coronary artery (LAD), running in the anterior interventricular groove, and the circumflex (CX) seen with an obtuse marginal branch (OM). *C*, Anatomic level including the mid-right and circumflex coronary arteries. *D*, Anatomic level passing through the inferior wall of the left ventricle, including the distal right coronary artery (RCA), posterior descending artery (PDA), and posterolateral branches (PL).

flow. This capability has been only partially explored and incompletely exploited.[2,24] Clinical applications in this area are few but include distinction by imaging at $TE =$ 56 ms of the true and false lumina in aortic dissection.[1] Attempts to use MRI to measure aortic or even coronary blood flow are beyond current capabilities, yet the former possibility should soon be achieved.

Metabolic magnetic resonance imaging using nuclei other than hydrogen holds promise for future clinical application. Most of the experimental work to date has utilized phosphorus-31 magnetic resonance to study the metabolism of high-energy phosphate in isolated, working hearts.[25] In vivo phosphorus-31 spectroscopy has demonstrated high-energy phosphate shifts between diastole and systole,[26] depletion of high-energy phosphate stores during myocardial ischemia,[27–29] and a preservation of high-energy phosphate compounds after therapeutic interventions to alleviate ischemia.[28] Recently, utilizing phosphorus-31 nuclear magnetic resonance spectroscopy, a metabolic disorder was demonstrated in vivo in both myocardium and skeletal muscle of an infant with congenital cardiomyopathy.[30] A phosphocreatine:inorganic phosphate ratio of half of that for a normal control infant was found, demonstrating the feasibility of using phosphorus-31 nuclear magnetic resonance spectroscopy to evaluate the biochemistry of the human myocardium in vivo. While the use of surface coil magnetic resonance to study cardiac metabolism will have very limited clinical application, a combination of the large, superconducting magnet necessary for cross-sectional imaging and phosphorus-31 magnetic resonance spectroscopy has a great deal of potential.

Our initial efforts to image coronary atherosclerosis noninvasively using MRI have been encouraging. Normal proximal and distal right and proximal left coronary arteries have been successfully visualized (Fig. 25–33). Left main coronary artery stenoses characterized by angiography as being greater than 50 percent have been detected by

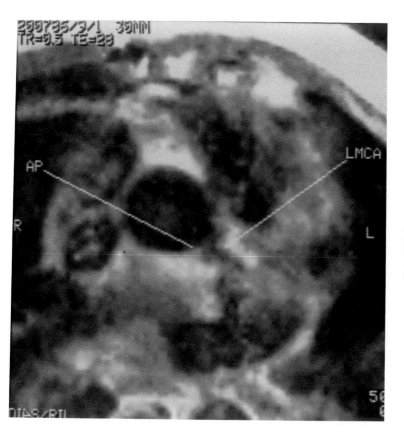

Figure 25–34. Transverse MR image through the left main coronary artery of a patient who was demonstrated by angiography to have an atheromatous plaque (AP) causing a proximal 60 percent narrowing of this vessel.

MRI (Fig. 25–34), and noninvasive characterization of coronary atherosclerosis preceding and following angioplasty is currently under investigation.

Magnetic resonance imaging is a completely noninvasive technique for the visualization of the cardiovascular system. The excellent resolution of cardiac and vascular structures provided without ionizing radiation or contrast medium makes MRI an attractive addition to other noninvasive imaging methods such as echocardiography and cardiac scintigraphy. Magnetic resonance imaging can clearly define the anatomy of pericardial disease and myocardial abnormalities such as infarction and hypertrophy. MRI provides enormous potential for cardiovascular diagnosis and research, since it has the potential for direct tissue characterization and blood flow measurements. Recent developments in dynamic cardiac imaging allow cardiac imaging in a cine mode and provide a new noninvasive imaging technique for the evaluation of the heart and great vessels.[31,32] The accurate measurement of intracardiac blood flow by metabolic phosphorus-31 imaging of the human heart awaits significant technical advances. However, as further development ensues, it is expected to provide a nonperturbing method for in vivo assessment of myocardial metabolism.

References

1. Herfkens RJ, Higgins CB, Hricak H, Lipton MJ, Crooks LE, Lanzer P, Botvinick EH, Brundage B, Sheldon PE, Kaufman L: Nuclear magnetic resonance imaging of the cardiovascular system: normal and pathological findings. Radiology *147*:749, 1983.
2. Kaufman L, Crooks L, Sheldon P, Hricak H, Herfkens R, Bank W: The potential impact of nuclear magnetic resonance imaging on cardiovascular diagnosis. Circulation *67*:251, 1983.
3. Hawkes RC, Holland GN, Moore WS, Roebuck EJ, Worthington BS: Nuclear magnetic resonance (NMR) tomography of the normal heart. J Comput Assist Tomogr *5*:605, 1981.
4. Crooks LE, Sheldon P, Kaufman L, Rowan W: Quantitation of obstructions in vessels by nuclear magnetic resonance. IEEE Trans Nucl Sci *29*:1181, 1982.
5. Stark DD, Higgins CB, Lanzer P, et al: Magnetic resonance imaging of the pericardium: normal and pathologic findings. Radiology *150*:469, 1984.
6. Lanzer P, Barta C, Botvinick EH, Wiesendanger HU, Modin G, Higgins CB: ECG-synchronized cardiac MR imaging: method and evaluation. Radiology *155*:681, 1985.
7. Crooks LE, Barker B, Chang H, Feinberg D, Hoenninger J, Watts J, Arakawa M, Kaufman L, Sheldon PE, Botvinick E, Higgins CB: Magnetic resonance imaging strategies for heart studies. Radiology *153*:459, 1984.
8. Alfidi RJ, Haaga JR, Yousef SJ, Bryan PJ, Fletcher BD, LiPuma JP, Morrison SC, Kaufman B, Richey JB, Hinshaw WS, Kramer DM, Yeung HN, Cohen AM, Butler HE, Ament AE, Lieberman JM: Preliminary experimental results in humans and animals with superconducting, whole body, nuclear magnetic resonance scanner. Radiology *143*:175, 1982.
9. Ordidge RJ, Mansfield P, Coupland RD: Rapid biomedical imaging by NMR. Br J Radiol *54*:850, 1981.
10. Feiglin DH, George CR, MacIntyre WJ, O'Donnell JK, Go RT, Pavlicek W, Meaney TF: Gated cardiac magnetic resonance structural imaging: optimization by electronic axial rotation. Radiology *154*:129, 1985.
11. vonSchulthess GK, Fisher M, Crooks LE, Higgins CB: The nature of intracardiac signal on gated NMR images in normals and patients with abnormal left ventricular function. Radiology *156*:125, 1985.
12. Higgins CB, Herfkens R, Lipton MJ, Sievers R, Sheldon P, Kaufman L, Crooks L: Nuclear magnetic resonance imaging of acute myocardial infarction in dogs: alterations in magnetic relaxation times. Am J Cardiol *52*:184, 1983.
13. Wesbey G, Higgins CB, Lanzer P, Botvinick EH, Lipton MJ: Imaging and characterization of acute myocardial infarction in vivo using gated nuclear magnetic resonance. Circulation *69*:125, 1984.
14. McNamara MT, Higgins CB, Schechtmann N, Botvinick EH, Lipton MJ, Chatterjee K, Amparo EG: Detection and characterization of acute myocardial infarction in man with use of gated magnetic resonance. Circulation *71*:717, 1985.
15. Tscholakoff D, Higgins CB, McNamara MT, Derugin N: Early-phase myocardial infarction: Evaluation by MR imaging. Radiology *159*:667, 1986.
16. Pflugfelder PW, Wisenberg G, Prato FS, Carroll SE, Turner KL: Early detection of canine myocardial infarction by magnetic resonance imaging in vivo. Circulation *71*:587, 1985.
17. Higgins CB, Lanzer P, Stark D, Botvinick EH, Schiller NB, Crooks L, Kaufman L, Lipton MJ: Imaging by nuclear magnetic resonance in patients with chronic ischemic heart disease. Circulation *69*:523, 1984.
18. Higgins CB, Byrd BF III, McNamara MT, Lipton MJ, Lanzer PA, Schiller NB, Botvinick EH, Chatterjee K: Magnetic resonance imaging of hypertrophic cardiomyopathy. Circulation *70*:II–248, 1984.
19. Schiller NB, Botvinick EH: Right ventricular compression as a sign of cardiac tamponade. Circulation *56*:774, 1977.

20. Moncada R, Baker M, Salinas M, Demos TC, Churchill R, Love L, Reynes C, Hale D, Cardoso M, Pifarre R, Gunnar RM: Diagnostic role of computed tomography in pericardial heart disease. Congenital defects, thickening, neoplasms, and effusions. Am Heart J *103*:263, 1982.
21. Herfkens R, Davis P, Crooks L, Kaufman L, Price D, Miller T, Margulis AR, Watts J, Hoenninger J, Arakawa M, McRee R: NMR imaging of the abnormal live rat and correlations with tissue characteristics. Radiology *141*:211, 1981.
22. Higgins CB, Byrd BF III, McNamara MT, Lanzer P, Lipton MJ, Botvinick E, Schiller NB, Crooks LE, Kaufman L: Magnetic resonance imaging of the heart: a review of the experience in 172 subjects. Radiology *155*:671, 1985.
23. Fletcher RD, Jacobstein MD, Nelson AD, Riemenschneider TA, Alfidi RJ: Gated magnetic resonance imaging of congenital cardiac malformations. Radiology *150*:137, 1984.
24. Singer JR: Blood flow measurements by NMR. *In* Kaufman L, Crooks LE, Margulis AR (eds): Nuclear Magnetic Resonance in Medicine. New York, Igaku-Shoin, 1981, p 11.
25. Jacobus WE, Taylor GJ, IV, Hollis DP, Nunnally RL: Phosphorus nuclear magnetic resonance of perfused working rat hearts. Nature *265*:756, 1977.
26. Fossel ET, Morgan HE, Ingwall JS: Measurement of changes in high-energy phosphate in the cardiac cycle by using gated P-31 nuclear magnetic resonance. Proc Natl Acad Sci USA *77*:3654, 1980.
27. Hollis DP, Nunnally RL, Jacobus W, Taylor GJ: Detection of regional ischemia in perfused beating hearts by phosphorus nuclear magnetic resonance. Biochem Biophys Res Comm *75*:1086, 1977.
28. Nunnally RL, Bottomley PA: P-NMR studies of myocardial ischemia and its response to drug therapies. J Comput Assist Tomogr *5*:296, 1981.
29. Pernot AC, Ingwall JS, Menasche P, Grousset C, Bercot M, Piwnica A, Fossel ET: Evaluation of high energy phosphate metabolism during cardioplegic arrest and reperfusion: A phosphorus-31 nuclear magnetic resonance study. Circulation *67*:1296, 1983.
30. Whitman GJ, Chance B, Bode H, Maris J, Haselgrove J, Kelley R, Clark BJ, Harken AH: Diagnosis and therapeutic evaluation of a pediatric case of cardiomyopathy using phosphorus-31 nuclear magnetic resonance spectroscopy. J Am Coll Cardiol *5*:745, 1985.
31. Utz JA, Herfkens RJ, et al: Cine MRI determination of left ventricular ejection fraction. AJR *148*:839, 1987.
32. Utz JA, Herfkens RJ: Dynamic and physiologic cardiac MR. *In* Stark DD, Bradley WG Jr (eds): Magnetic Resonance Imaging. St. Louis, CV Mosby, 1988, pp 921–933.

26

Lungs

FRANK E. CARROLL, JR.

Magnetic resonance imaging has opened a new window into the chest, through which we are just beginning to glimpse anatomic, physiologic, and biochemical information that previously has been unavailable to us—and to do it in a totally noninvasive way. At this time, we have barely touched the surface of MR's potential in this region. This chapter will review some of the difficulties encountered in attempting to use MR on the lung, and offer tested and potential solutions to overcome such problems. It will look at clinically useful techniques, list conditions wherein MR may be useful in the chest, correlate MR with other imaging modalities, and explore some of the future pathways that this exciting technology opens to us.

SURMOUNTABLE DIFFICULTIES IN LUNG IMAGING

The lung tends to have the dubious distinction of being the most difficult organ to image, always offering the toughest test to any imaging modality. Of course, this is partially due to its unique structure and the incessant vascular and ventilatory dynamics occurring therein.

Lung Parenchyma

The lung is subdivided by physiologists into four zones of capillary perfusion.[1] Zone I, located in the least dependent portion of the lung, has most of its capillaries closed or not perfusing owing to the fact that the air pressure in the alveoli is higher than the pressure in the feeding pulmonary arteriole. An intermediate zone (Zone II), in midlung, has about half of the capillaries open and perfusing and half of them closed. In the third zone, which includes the most dependent one third of the lung, most of the capillaries are open. A rather small Zone IV is postulated as that thin area slightly compressed by the weight of the lung above. In any patient assuming the supine or prone position, a redistribution of blood in the lung takes place almost immediately into a similar pattern of zones from the least dependent to the most dependent areas. In addition, it has been shown[2] that the pulmonary blood not only shifts to the dependent area but also slowly decreases in volume over a 30-minute period following assumption of a recumbent position. All of this leads to a reproducible gravity-dependent gradient of signal intensity in the lung in MR images.[3]

Since the most frequently used MR process depends upon the presence of protons, the fact that the lung consists only of solid tissue equivalent to 20 percent of that of other solid organs starts us off at a great disadvantage when attempting to study pulmonary parenchyma by this method. Variations in the degree of inflation of the lung will cause marked alteration in signal intensity. During expiration less air and more blood, interstitial fluid, and lung parenchyma are compressed into the same volume of interest, increasing mobile proton density.

Water in the lung not only is compartmentalized but also exhibits a markedly different composition in each of its intravascular, interstitial, and cellular parenchymal subdivisions. The *T1* and *T2* relaxation behavior of each of these fluids is somewhat different.

Normally the interstitium of the lung contains interstitial fluid, which is a variable filtrate of the capillary blood. In animals and in man its protein content has been shown to average approximately 60 percent that of plasma. It has few formed elements within it.[4] Although formed peripherally, it is collected by lymphatics slightly more centrally, as there are no lymphatics in the alveolar wall itself.

With elevation of hydrostatic pressure in the pulmonary circuit, there is an increase in lymph production, with a slight reduction in protein content lowering the lymph/plasma protein ratio.[4] In vitro experiments on such lymph from sheep show an inverse linear relationship between lymph/plasma protein ratio and *T1* with no concomitant alteration in *T2*. The interstitial fluid in hydrostatic pulmonary edema, therefore, has a longer *T1* than that of normal lung lymph, and signal intensity will rise with the accumulation of interstitial fluid.

If, on the other hand, the pulmonary capillary membrane undergoes an alteration in the permeability ("capillary leak") secondary to a diffuse insult (such as exposure to endotoxin), there will be subsequent leakage of greater quantities of protein and fluid as well as leakage of proteins of larger size. This lymph demonstrates an increase in the lymph/plasma protein ratio and a shorter *T1* than that seen in the baseline state.

These observations hold promise for the noninvasive identification of these disease states. They offer a potential research tool that will help us to better understand the mechanisms of lung injury, to follow the progression of the disease, and to establish animal models that may be used to seek therapeutic modalities to pre-empt formation of full-blown disease or offer more effective therapy once the abnormality is present.

Just as alterations in lymph composition will change the observed *T1* values from lung, changes in the capillary bed may vary the observed *T1*'s obtainable from lung in several ways. An increase in pressure in the pulmonary circuit causes recruitment of nonperfused capillaries in Zones I and II. In addition, capillaries already perfused in Zones III and IV may undergo distention, along with arterioles and venules. The net result of such engorgement with blood will be movement of the observed *T1* value of lung more toward that of blood; the previous balance between blood, lymph, lung parenchyma, and air (each having a different *T1*) no longer exists. Needless to say, signal intensity will also rise owing to the increase in mobile proton density. Eventually, alveolar flooding will occur, causing a progressive increase in signal intensity and further alteration of *T1*.

In the periphery of the lung there is another mechanism in play that alters the signal returned from the lung with MR. Streaming of blood in the capillaries results in a change in the effective hematocrit (Hct) far peripheral in the capillary bed, such that it is lower than the central venous packed cell volume. Since this may amount to a 5 to 7 percent difference, assumptions as to the *T1* and *T2* of the blood present in these different body locations should not be made. Pulsed NMR analysis of blood reconstituted to various hematocrits from 5 to 72 percent shows an inverse relationship between *T1* and Hct.

These and other factors, such as variations in peripheral blood flow, alterations in blood plasma proteins and fat after meals, and translational molecular self-diffusion, act synergistically to complicate the usefulness of signals received from the lung. Multispectral whole-image analysis,[5] calculations with information received at various inversion times with dual pulse sequences,[6] and other novel postprocessing of obtained data hold promise in unraveling this complex information. These methods will yield three-dimensional separation of tissue parameters and quantitation of protons in the various compartments for better comprehension of these disease states.

Motion

The effect of motion on two-dimensional Fourier transformation magnetic resonance images is nicely documented by Schultz and others.[7] Respiratory and cardiac motion, patient motion, blood flow, and molecular diffusion may all contribute to image degradation.

PATIENT MOTION

The easiest motion to control during most examinations is patient motion. A thorough, reassuring explanation of the imaging process stressing the importance of immobility usually suffices for all but the least cooperative patients. In those exhibiting claustrophobic tendencies, assumption of the prone position may be of help.

RESPIRATORY MOTION

Respiratory movement is most troublesome when one is imaging near the diaphragm or in the upper abdomen (Fig. 26–1). As the diaphragm descends, the chest wall moves anteriorly and laterally. Sixty percent of an individual's vital capacity is secondary to diaphragmatic movement. Men have a tendency to be "belly breathers" and have been shown to utilize a greater degree of diaphragmatic descent by midinspiration and less chest wall movement than females. Respiratory artifacts, therefore, are less of a problem in men, particularly higher in the chest where little chest wall motion occurs.

Respiratory "ghosting" consists of multiple, shifted, superimposed, and foldedover images of the anatomic parts in motion, but also a similar displacement and multiplication of stationary body parts or even reference phantoms outside the patient (Fig. 26–2).

Hedlund et al.[8] have shown that the magnitude of the MR respiratory artifact is partially rate-dependent. The closer the respiratory rate to the heart rate and pulse repetition rate (particularly if the study is cardiac gated) the less visible is the respiratory "ghosting."

Depth of respiratory excursion, however, is also a factor to be considered,[7] since greater movement tends to displace ghost images farther from the center of the image plane in the direction of the phase-encoding gradient.

Respiratory Gating. To overcome the respiratory "ghosting" artifact, several types of respiratory gates have been developed.[9] Warmed air in expiration may be sensed by a thermistor within a small plastic mask or nasal cannula; however, these devices are uncomfortable to wear and sensitive to small displacements in position. An abdominal belt with a fiberoptic passive light-modulation device has also been used with success. One that we have found most useful is a bellows-type sensor strapped to the upper abdomen, transmitting a pneumatic signal via tubing to a nearby transducer. This transducer allows conversion of ventilatory movement into a gating-enabling voltage.[10] The MR gate is "opened" in end-expiration and remains open throughout the expiratory "pause." Imaging is therefore performed essentially at functional residual capacity (FRC) (Fig. 26–3). The use of such a gate approximately doubles data acquisition time,

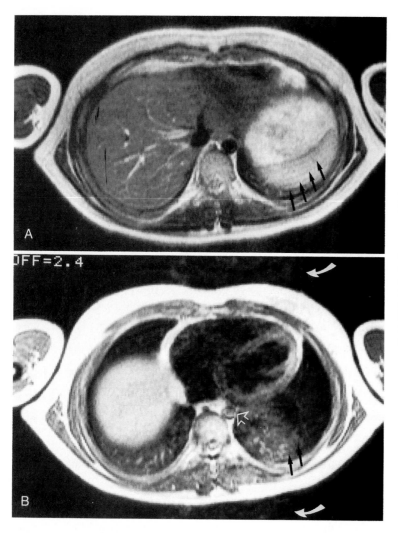

Figure 26–1. *A*, Respiratory artifacts (arrows) caused by diaphragmatic movement and chest wall motion in upper abdomen. *B*, "Ghosting" artifacts superimposed upon dependent areas of lungs (solid arrows). Artifact from cardiac action seen best outside of patient image (curved arrows). This artifact extends through entire image as a broad band of "noise." Flow artifact (open arrow) in descending thoracic aorta.

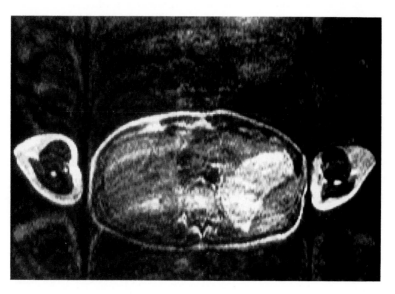

Figure 26–2. Severe ghosting artifacts secondary to respiratory motion. These are multiple, displaced, and folded-over images of the patient.

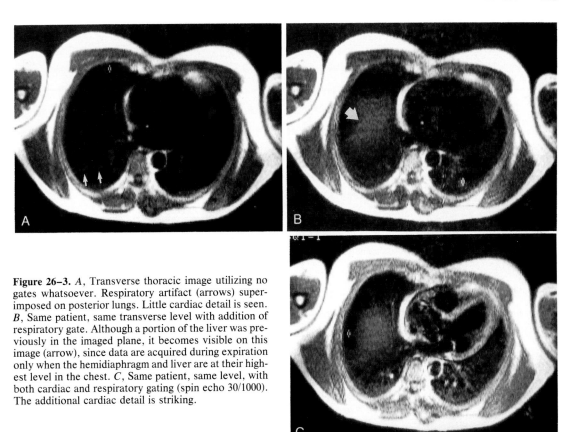

Figure 26–3. *A*, Transverse thoracic image utilizing no gates whatsoever. Respiratory artifact (arrows) superimposed on posterior lungs. Little cardiac detail is seen. *B*, Same patient, same transverse level with addition of respiratory gate. Although a portion of the liver was previously in the imaged plane, it becomes visible on this image (arrow), since data are acquired during expiration only when the hemidiaphragm and liver are at their highest level in the chest. *C*, Same patient, same level, with both cardiac and respiratory gating (spin echo 30/1000). The additional cardiac detail is striking.

depending on respiratory rate and *TR*. The use of concomitant cardiac gating may multiply this time by an additional factor.

Improvements in image quality are greatest with short *TR*'s. Ehman et al.[9] showed significant differences in the calculated *T1*'s of organs imaged while gating but without "spin conditioning." If the MR unit pulses only during the time that the MR gate is opened, protons will be exposed to varying *TR*'s between "gate-open" intervals, allowing an alteration in the degree of longitudinal relaxation occuring between trains of pulses during which data are acquired. On the other hand, if the rf pulses continue unabated through those portions of the respiratory cycle when data is not being acquired, the protons are allowed the same degree of longitudinal relaxation for each pulse, whether or not the data acquisition gate is open. Values obtained for *T1* without "spin conditioning" are shortened significantly (Fig. 26–4).

Cardiac Motion and Blood Flow

The heart causes objectionable motion artifacts not only by its own movement but also by transmitted pulsations to the diaphragm and upper abdominal organs and by pulsation of the pulmonary arteries and major systemic arteries. In addition, approximately 45 percent of the lung by weight is blood. This blood is constantly flowing, which, in turn, diminishes the amount of signal offered back from a plane or volume of interest.

Flow in the pulmonary vasculature differs with distance from the heart. More rapid and unidirectional pulsatile flow is present centrally in the chest.[11] However, the more peripheral capillary bed exhibits a much slower and more random pattern of flow.

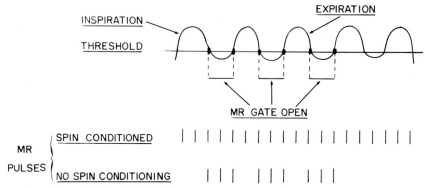

Figure 26–4. Use of a respiratory gate limits the time during which the MR device will accumulate data (MR gate open). Respiratory excursions may be converted by a transducer to a slowly alternating voltage (here represented by the sinuous line). At a predetermined voltage the gate will open, allowing data accumulation. At the beginning of the next inspiration the rising voltage will disable data input to the MR computer. Ehman et al.[9] point out the need to continue pulsing through the "gate-closed" periods to maintain consistency of *TR* to which protons are exposed. If spin conditioning is not used, calculated *T1* values will be inaccurate.

Rapidity and direction of flow are important to remember when assessing the lung on MR images.

In multislice spin-echo acquisitions, attempts at overcoming cardiac action by use of ECG gating may create flow-related artifacts in some slices but not in others.

In collecting *contiguous* multiple slices, data may be acquired by the unit in two passes through the imaged volume, collecting data first on odd-numbered slices followed by the data collection on even-numbered slices. Because of this, multislice imaging with cardiac gating accumulates images at different phases of the cardiac cycle with a spatial order different from their temporal order.[12] In those slices acquired during diastole, slowly flowing blood in some vessels may be detected as a greater signal intensity, since rf "labeled" blood is not moving out of the imaging plane before collection of the echo. Slices collected during ventricular systole exhibit little to no signal from the vascular lumen owing to the rapidity with which the blood exposed to slice-selective excitation has traversed the plane of interest.

In addition, at shorter *TR*'s blood will have undergone only partial longitudinal relaxation and will emit little signal. With repeated pulses, the slowly flowing blood becomes partially saturated and signal intensity diminishes. Blood flowing into the plane of interest, having not yet been perturbed by the rf gradients, will lend itself to an enhancement of signal from the vessel lumen. This is flow rate–dependent. Once flow velocity increases to the point at which the blood is traversing the imaging plane more rapidly than the time between application of the plane-selective pulse for excitation or the selective refocusing pulse and the reading of the echo, signal intensity again begins dropping. It rises somewhat at very high velocities because of turbulence.

The reader is referred to an excellent review by Axel[13] on flow effects, including effects of dephasing due to motion of protons through gradient fields, changes elicited by selective and nonselective exciting and refocusing pulses, and direction and velocity of motion relative to the imaging plane. These changes will be most pronounced for those vessels running either perpendicular to or slightly oblique to the imaging plane. Similarly, these effects are seen best in vessels that are visible on those slices at the ends of the imaging volume and may be reversed for veins and arteries owing to the direction that the blood is flowing in each (Fig. 26–5).

Cardiac Gating. Cardiac gating may be easily accomplished on most imagers at this time. Telemetry devices that gate off the R-wave are already commercially avail-

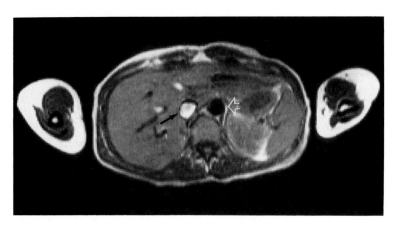

Figure 26–5. Flow-related enhancement in the inferior vena cava (closed arrow) secondary to slowly flowing blood entering tthe imaged plane. Lack of signal in aorta (open arrow) is due to the displacement of RF "tagged" blood out of the image plane because of the rapid flow in this vessel.

able. (One such unit is the Hewlett-Packard ECG Telemetry Unit [Waltham, Massachusetts], coupled to a Technicare gating module [Solon, Ohio].) ECG leads should be kept out of the volume of tissue to be imaged. In addition, the leads should be kept straight to prevent them from becoming single turn electromagnets or antennae themselves. One may acquire data in systole, diastole, or anywhere in between through the use of a physiologic delay that is programmable by the system operator, from the peak of the R-wave to the opening of the MR gate. Data acquisition time will vary depending upon the patient's heart rate, the *TR* selected, and the presence or absence of arrhythmias. The imaging system may be gated off every second or even every third heartbeat if longer *TR*'s are desired.

If one is interested in only the upper chest, consideration may be given to using a totally nongated multislice, multiecho technique, since motion is only minimal in that area and considerable savings in time may be realized by electing not to use cardiac and respiratory gating. Many patients need only cardiac gating and can be selected from the general patient population by observation. Those with very shallow respiratory movement of the rib cage and small abdominal excursions may do extremely well without respiratory gating (Fig. 26–6).

When a patient's heart rate is fortuitously at the pulse repetition rates, "pseudogating" may occur, in that slices may be acquired repeatedly at the same time following the heartbeat and flow-related enhancement may be seen if the slice is acquired during diastole (Fig. 26–7).

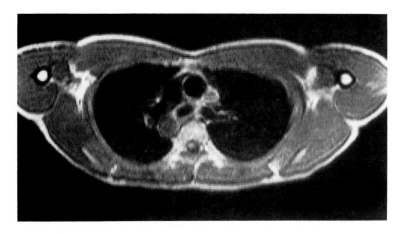

Figure 26–6. Transverse MR image of the mid-mediastinum performed without benefit of respiratory and cardiac gating.

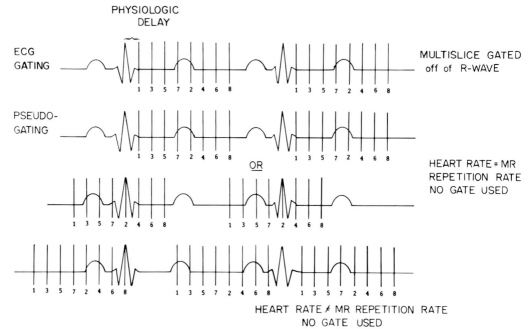

Figure 26–7. Numbered lines on ECG tracings indicate timing and spatial ordering of slices during gated and nongated multislice acquisitions. In "pseudogating," the heart rate approximates the pulse repetition rate so that slices are acquired during the same portion of each cardiac cycle. This may create flow-related artifacts on some of the slices acquired during diastole.

MOLECULAR DIFFUSION

Translational molecular self-diffusion secondary to the random thermal movement of water protons during the imaging process may become troublesome because of the measured ability of the water proton to move as much as 8 μ (longer than the length of a red blood cell) during a 30-ms period.[14] If varying slice-selective gradient pulses are used in imaging, faulty $T2$ values may be obtained from rapidly diffusing fluids.[15] It is probably more accurate to say that the distance traversed by a proton in 30 ms is only half that classically quoted, particularly when dealing with biologic systems.

Fluids within the body are somewhat restricted in their motion by membrane barriers, binding to various proteins, and the diffusion caused by concentration and temperature gradients within each tissue. Each of these would further alter in vivo displacement of resonant protons during imaging.

Clinical Imaging

As a general rule, one should try to shorten the overall examination time in an effort to diminish patient discomfort, which would result in movement during imaging. Spin-echo pulse sequences are least degraded by motion and offer the best overall technique at present.

Before imaging, a decision must be made as to the type of information one is attempting to gain from the examination.

Signal intensity on MR images is a function of $T1$, $T2$, and proton density. Given similar proton densities, those tissues with a short $T1$ have a brighter (whiter) representation of the image. Tissues with a long $T2$ also are indicated by a whiter (more intense) image. Therefore, in order to bring out *differences* in $T1$, shorter TR's (e.g.,

250 ms) should be utilized. Tissues with short *T1* (e.g., 250 ms) will show a high signal intensity, since their protons have returned to their maximum longitudinal relaxation between imaging pulses. Those with a long *T1* (e.g., 1 to 2 sec) will not have relaxed completely before the next pulse and consequently will become partially saturated. They will give off a less intense signal with subsequent pulses, thereby allowing differentiation from rapidly relaxing tissues (Fig. 26–8).

T2 relaxation is, for the most part, much shorter than *T1* relaxation, so that *differences* in *T2* are not well brought out by changes in *TR*. Alteration in the echo time *TE*, by increments of 30 ms (30, 60, 90, 120 ms *TE*'s) will enhance the differences in *T2* relaxation present within the tissues (Fig. 26–9). A tissue with a long *T2* should become brighter on the later echoes at a given *TR*. Unfortunately, increasing *T2*, decreasing *T1*, and increasing proton density may work antagonistically in the final image to mask a given lesion. This points up the importance of using multiple pulse sequences (such as *TE* 30/*TR* 500, *TE* 60/*TR* 500, along with *TE* 30/*TR* 1500, *TE* 60/*TR* 1500) in searching the chest for pathology.

If high spatial resolution is sought, long *TR*'s will be needed to increase the signal-to-noise (S/N) ratio. This is particularly true in defining the limits of mediastinal tumors and the presence or absence of infiltration of mediastinal fat or vessels by that tumor.

Increased contrast resolution, on the other hand, is best obtained with shorter *TR*'s and varying *TE*'s. These techniques heighten the differences between normal structures with short *T1*'s, such as mediastinal or hilar fat, and tumors, which tend toward longer *T1*'s and *T2*'s. The slowly relaxing tumor will undergo partial saturation at short *TR* and exhibit diminished signal intensity, in contradistinction to rapidly relaxing fat or normal parenchyma, which has had the opportunity between pulses to regain more or all of its longitudinal relaxation.

The center of the volume of interest of the patient should be placed as close to the center of the body coil as possible. The vast majority of patients in whom MRI of the chest is to be performed will require multislice data acquisition with cardiac gating. A rapid sagittal or coronal localization slice, requiring approximately two minutes, is best utilized to assure total coverage of the areas of interest. This allows the system operator to calculate the optimum offsets for each plane so that the first or last slices are at the expected limits of the volume of tissue to be imaged.

In spin-echo acquisitions, a 90 degree pulse at time (t) = 0 is followed by a 180 degree pulse at time 15 ms. The echo elicited is acquired over tens of milliseconds centered around the peak of the spin echo *TE* (30 ms). From the initial perturbing pulse,

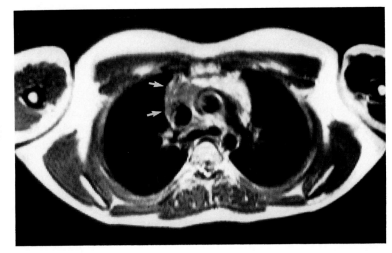

Figure 26–8. Patient with mediastinal Hodgkin's disease (arrows). Tumor tissue is easily discriminated from normal mediastinal fat owing to its long *T1*. Spin-echo image 30/500.

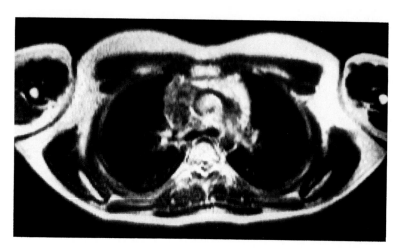

Figure 26–9. Same patient as in Figure 26–8. Spin-echo image 60/500.

the remainder of the repetition time is spent allowing the perturbed protons to undergo a degree of longitudinal relaxation predetermined by the examiner depending upon the degree of contrast and spatial resolution desired and the tissues being imaged. Since the vast majority of the *TR* is consumed by "waiting" or "idle time," the MR unit can be used to obtain information from some other slice or slices to better utilize its time. Serial slices are, therefore, excited, rephased, and read in the time remaining before the first slice is due to be read again. The number of slices that can be accumulated on a multislice study during a given *TR* can be ascertained by dividing the *TR* in milliseconds by the *TE* (e.g., 30 ms) + 15 ms. Using a shorter *TR* or a longer *TE*, or both, will considerably reduce the available time for acquisition of these additional slices.

Secondly, if one selects a multislice, multiecho sequence, in which additional refocusing 180 degree pulses are used to read echoes of substances with longer *T2*'s, the number of slices possible for a given *TR* is determined by dividing the *TR* in milliseconds by the longest echo time *TEn* + 15 ms.

As *TR* becomes shorter and *TE* longer the advantage of multislice imaging disappears. This is not only because short *TR*'s and long *TE*'s both offer poor signal-to-noise but also because the number of slices obtainable during one acquisition decreases, requiring multiple repetitions of the acquisition process to fill in the intervening anatomy. In those cases, the S/N advantages of volume acquisition techniques become more important. If the *TR* becomes short enough and the *TE* long enough to necessitate repeating the acquisition four or more times to collect the desired slices, volume acquisition should be contemplated.[12]

The maximum number of slices obtainable for a given *TR* should be one's goal, in order to shorten overall imaging time. The next parameter to decide is the slice thickness. Volume averaging in MR is equally as important as in CT. However, studies that are not respiratory gated will average a greater volume than the thickness of the slice, as tissues move through the slice plane throughout the various phases of respiration and in all three planes (craniocaudad, mediolateral, and anterioposterior). Respiratory gating usually diminishes this polydirectional averaging. Slice thicknesses of 0.75, 1.0, and 1.5 cm are now available. In the lung, 1.0 cm slices seem to be the best alternative.

Slices may be contiguous or separated by nonimaged tissue volumes of varying thickness. If contiguous slices are not available, interleaved series of slices may be obtained to fill in the "blank" areas. These then may be rearranged for display to show sequential anatomy on hard copy.

To improve the S/N ratio, increasing the number of pulse sequences per buffer (averaging repeated measurements of each data line) may be used; it should be noted, however, that this also increases data acquisition time, which creates a longer interval during which patient motion may occur.

The number of echoes available in a multiecho series may vary from one machine to another (one to eight). However, it should be noted that the later spin echoes will suffer from increasing image degradation secondary to poor S/N ratio, since the signal from most tissues with shorter $T2$'s will have died away before acquisition of the remaining spin echo.

The imaging plane to be used will depend upon the type of information sought. Transverse slices seem to be best for separating hilar lymphadenopathy from nearby vasculature. Sagittal images offer excellent detail in the work-up of mediastinal masses, as do coronal images.[16] Both transverse and coronal slices offer excellent cardiac anatomy if properly gated (Fig. 26–10).

IMAGING CONTRAINDICATIONS

Uncooperative patients are not the only persons considered to be poor MR candidates. Individuals with cardiac pacemakers would be at considerable risk not only in the bore of the imager but also within the fringing fields extending out around these

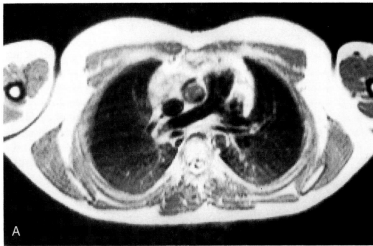

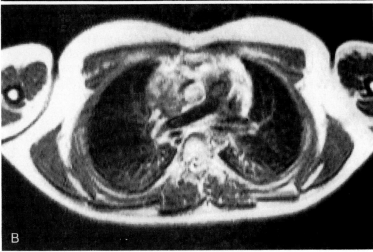

Figure 26–10. *A,* Same patient as in Figures 26–8 and 26–9. Spin echo 30/500. *B,* Spin echo 60/500. Some image degradation is noted on the second echo, owing to lower signal/noise ratio.

systems for considerable distances. These distances depend upon field strength and system design. Particularly sensitive are reprogrammable pacemakers now in general use.

Patients having vascular clips on intracranial vessels or aneurysms may be endangered by torquing forces in these clips while being moved through the main field, depending upon the metal alloy from which the clips are manufactured. Similarly, vascular clips used in coronary artery bypass grafting and sternal suture wires used to close sternal splitting thoracotomies may degrade the image, depending upon their composition.[17] Many metal prosthetic heart valves have shown no apparent torque or malfunction in the MR environment.[18]

Small cochlear implants and other prosthetic devices (including false teeth) need to be sought for by questioning every patient. Some policy may be established on an institution-by-institution basis as to the advisability of exposing these people to these high magnetic fields.

CLINICAL UTILITY

Although in its infancy, chest MRI already has many uses, with many more potential applications merely awaiting the systematic collection of reproducible data. By beginning in the airway lumen and progressing through the layers of the lung, this will allow grouping of pathologic states that can be addressed by this technique. A caution is in order here, lest the reader assume that published *T1* and *T2* values are at present diagnostic. Absolute values for *T1* and *T2* in tumors, parenchymal infiltrative diseases, and alveolar filling processes are field strength–dependent and show considerable overlap even on a given MR system.[19] While it is generally true that tumors have long *T1*'s and *T2*'s, insufficient experience exists to allow unqualified proclamation of benignancy or malignancy on the basis of these values from any individual case. Possibly, as we gain more experience and learn more about the MR process we may be able to more precisely dissect the signals from lesions for information concerning biochemical markers or identifiable cellular characteristics.

Promising new techniques, such as multispectral analysis of the MR image information using satellite image processing programs, may aid in such differentiation in the near future.[5]

AIRWAYS AND PARENCHYMA

Within the airway, mucous plugs are easily identified owing to their high signal intensity, particularly in the midlung and lung periphery. CT cannot differentiate a mucous plug within a bronchus from vessels, whereas the absence of MR signal from vascular lumen easily differentiates vessel from plug.[20]

Endobronchial neoplasms with airway narrowing are also easily detected, as is transbronchial infiltration by tumor.

Because of the low inherent signal intensity returned from the lung, loss of parenchyma in bullous disease is more difficult to detect and may be discerned only by compression of adjacent parenchyma and with long repetition times.

Only the combined walls of the bronchi and vessels can be seen centrally in the lung, since the air and flowing blood leave each devoid of signal within their lumen. The trachea is most easily evaluated using coronal and sagittal images and may be included in its entirety on approximately three contiguous coronal images because of its slightly posterior course as it passes inferiorly into the chest (Fig. 26–11).[16]

Disease states causing alveolar filling will obviously significantly increase signal

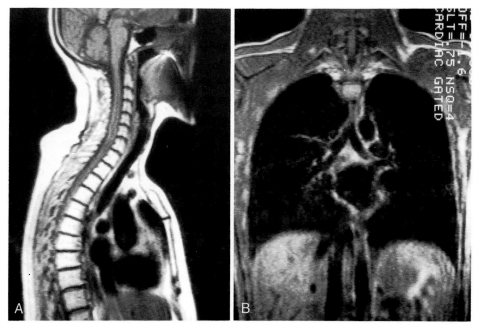

Figure 26–11. *A*, Tracheal evaluation is assisted by use of sagittal plane. Airway is visible from nasopharynx to carina. Note syrinx in cervical spinal cord. *B*, Coronal imaging may also be quite useful in tracheal assessment.

intensity from the lung (Fig. 26–12), even to the point of intensity equivalent to that of other solid organs (hepatization). Although blood and pus may be rather close in their relaxation times, several other substances causing consolidation can be differentiated. In alveolar proteinosis, for example, the material that accumulates within the alveoli has a lipid content that may approach 50 percent. Although not yet proven, its *T1* might be expected to be appreciably shorter than that of blood. Similarly, the fatty content present intra- and extracellularly in lipoid pneumonia may also be detectable. Hemosiderin deposition in alveolar macrophages and pulmonary interstitium may, if of sufficient severity, act in a manner similar to hepatic hemosiderosis.[21,22]

Atelectasis of lung will cause a marked increase in signal intensity owing to the exclusion of air from the voxel.

With changes in alveolar epithelial integrity, flooding of the alveoli with blood and proteinaceous fluid may be followed by formation of hyaline membranes within the air sacs. Investigation is now being directed toward the mechanics of development and

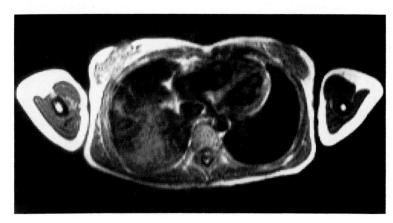

Figure 26–12. Pulmonary parenchymal consolidation in a patient with obstructive pneumonitis from a more centrally placed endobronchial lesion.

resolution of hyaline membranes in both infants with hyaline membrane disease and older individuals with adult respiratory distress syndrome.

Interstitial fibrosis has been shown to produce an alteration in *T1* of the lung. This potentially allows a means of assessing the presence and severity of idiopathic pulmonary fibrosis or the inhalational pneumoconioses and also potential separability in oncology patients of (1) pulmonary fibrosis from chemotherapeutic agents, (2) leukemic or metastatic infiltrates, (3) pulmonary hemorrhage, or (4) opportunistic infections.

Granulomatous processes in the lung have been studied in some measure by Ross et al.[19] The authors point out that there is extensive overlap in their relaxation values in a group of patients with sarcoidosis, limiting its value in this area. Confirmatory studies, possibly at a higher field strength, may be of further value.

Vascular

The search for the "ideal" noninvasive test for pulmonary embolism naturally would turn to MRI. Central large emboli can indeed be detected as high signal intensity clot in a lumen normally void of signal.[23] However, more peripherally placed and smaller emboli are less reproducibly diagnosed and may reveal their presence only by less specific changes in the lung surrounding or peripheral to an embolus, such as parenchymal hemorrhage or atelectasis.[24] Although digital subtraction angiography may add somewhat to the diagnosis of pulmonary embolus in the near future, cut film pulmonary angiography remains the diagnostic gold standard for now. Thrombosis of pulmonary veins can be diagnosed in a like fashion if centrally placed near the left atrium. Arteriovenous malformations may reveal their true nature because of the rapid blood flow through them, leaving multiple void vascular channels therein.

Neoplasms

Peripheral lung nodules are at present best studied using CT. Volume averaging, suboptimal respiratory gating, the inability to reliably detect calcifications within the lesion, and the wide overlap of reported *T1*'s and *T2*'s in these lesions leaves much to be desired toward confident classification by means of MR (Fig. 26–13).

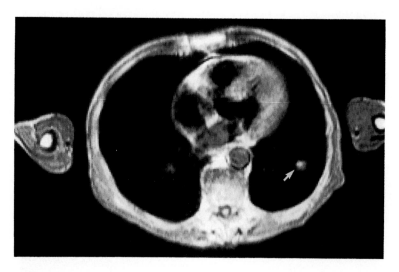

Figure 26–13. Solitary pulmonary nodule exhibiting areas of different relaxation behavior.

MR may offer better discrimination in the handling of patients with pulmonary neoplasm in the staging and post-therapeutic decision-making process. To cite the latter first, MR may be of inestimable value in the patient in whom recurrence of tumors must be differentiated from pulmonary fibrosis or atelectasis from therapy, and in separating all of this from associated pleural effusions and normal lung. Skill at dissecting these various tissues will come only with facility in the use of multiple pulse sequences to heighten *T1* and *T2* differences in the images and with a firm understanding of values to be expected on a given MR unit.

For staging malignant neoplasms in the lung, MR currently has the capacity to noninvasively discriminate nodes from mediastinal and hilar fat if the patient is examined with both a short and a long *TR* with at least two echo times approximately 30 ms apart, and a knowledge of the normal position of soft tissue collections in the hilar areas.[25] This can all be done without the use of the contrast agents needed in CT. Pretherapy radiation planning can take advantage of the sagittal, coronal, and transverse anatomic sections without the loss of resolution of reformatted images in CT. MR retains its spatial resolution in any plane.

Pleura

Pleural effusions may have a wide range of relaxation times owing to the variable nature of the fluid (Fig. 26–14). A chylous effusion with a high fat content will have a significantly shorter *T1* than a serous transudate of low protein content. Blood, pus, exudates, and transudates may all be misinterpreted if longer *TR*'s are not included in the evaluation of a patient. If sufficient relaxation time is not permitted between pulses, little to no signal may be returned from the fluid, blending in nicely with the lung so that it is missed entirely.

Subpleural fat deposits have a short *T1* and are easily differentiated from pleural tumor deposits and pleural plaques.

Fistulous tracts, carcinomatous involvement of chest wall (particularly if partial chest wall resection is contemplated), and primary chest wall tumors may all be clearly mapped by the MR process as well as with CT.

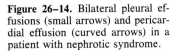

Figure 26–14. Bilateral pleural effusions (small arrows) and pericardial effusion (curved arrows) in a patient with nephrotic syndrome.

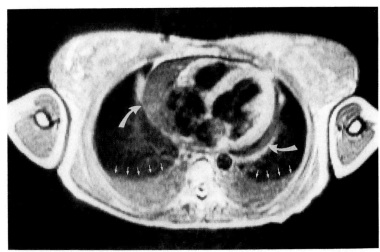

Research and Future Directions

The information previously available from a region-of-interest cursor was limited to signal intensity in arbitrary units scaled to the highest and lowest intensities within a slice, or *T1* and *T2* values for some machines. In an organ such as the lung, the cursor at any given location encompasses multiple substances, each having relaxation behavior different from the others. It has been shown that multiple *T1* calculations performed at varying inversion times and repetition times may be used to determine the percentages of each substance present within that cursor provided that the cursor area remains constant throughout the study.[6]

This information coupled with spin density and magnitude images collected simultaneously and multislice imaging may be used to glean both quantitative and qualitative information on compartmentalized fluids within the lung. Thus, four-dimensional representations of physiologic processes (craniad-caudad, medial-lateral, most dependent–least dependent, and time-dependent) may be mapped noninvasively in the lung, offering more accurate delineation than can be obtained by use of muiltiple indicator dilution curves, biopsy techniques, or even post-mortem samples.

As surface coil development and higher field strength magnets progress, "metabolic" imaging and spectra will allow us to peer into biochemical processes "on the fly."

Studies now under way are aimed at assessing fetal lung maturity in utero. Correlation with amniotic fluid samples obtained at amniocentesis, including L/S ratios as well as *T1* and *T2* values, may allow prediction of those infants who will do well out of the uterine environment—and do so without invasive procedures.

Use of high-frequency ventilators at frequencies of 1 to 1800 breaths per minute allows the study of the lung without significant motion or the development of atelectasis.[3,8]

All these techniques, coupled with a better understanding of the course and nature of changes in relaxation behavior in various normal and pathologic states, will offer us better differentiation of things that go "white in the night."

References

1. West TB (ed): Regional Differences in the Lung. New York, Academic Press, 1977.
2. Hirasina JD, Gorin AB: Effect of prolonged recumbency on pulmonary blood volume in normal humans. Appl Phys Respir Envir Exer Physiol *50*(5):950, 1981.
3. Carroll FE, Loyd JE, Nolop KB, Collins JC: MR imaging parameters in the study of lung water. A preliminary investigation. Invest Radiol *19*(5):S50, 1984.
4. Brigham KL, Parker RE, Roseli R, Hobson J, Harris TR: Exchange of macromolecules in the pulmonary microcirculation. Ann NY Acad Sci *384*:246, 1982.
5. Vannier MW, Butterfield RL, Jordan D, Murphy WA, Levitt RG, Gado M: Multispectral analysis of magnetic resonance images. Radiology *154*:221, 1985.
6. Carroll E, Dean G, Collins J, Roos C, Mitchell M, Holburn G: MR quantitation of dissimilar concentrically compartmentalized fluids using a single region-of-interest cursor. Radiology *153*P:308, 1984.
7. Schultz CL, Alfidi RJ, Nelson AD, Kopiwoda SY, Clampitt ME: Effect of motion on two-dimensional Fourier transformation magnetic resonance images. Radiology *152*:117, 1984.
8. Hedlund L, Deitz I, Lischko JM, Herfkens R, Hautzinger D, Effman E, Putman C. A high frequency jet ventilator for NMR imaging. Invest Radiol *19*(5):542, 1984.
9. Ehman RL, McNamara MT, Pallack M, Hricak H, Higgins CB: Magnetic resonance imaging with respiratory gating: Techniques and advantages. AJR *143*:1175, 1984.
10. Runge V, Clanton J, Partain CL, James AE: Respiratory gating in MRI at 0.5 tesla. Radiology *151*:521, 1984.
11. Milnor WR: Pulsatile blood flow. N Engl J Med *287*(1):27, 1972.
12. Teslacon Operator's Manual. Software Release C. Preliminary Version. Solon, Ohio, Technicare Corporation, 1984.
13. Axel L: Blood flow effects in magnetic resonance imaging. A review. AJR *143*:1157, 1984.

14. Wesbey GE, Moseley ME, Ehman RL: Translational molecular self-diffusion in magnetic resonance imaging. II. Measurement of the self-diffusion coefficient. Invest Radiol *19*:491, 1984.
15. Wesbey GE, Moseley ME, Ehman RL: Translational molecular self-diffusion in magnetic resonance imaging. Effects on observed spin-spin relaxation. Invest Radiol *19*:484, 1984.
16. O'Donovan PB, Ross JS, Sivak ED, O'Donnel JK, Meaney TF: Magnetic resonance imaging of the thorax: the advantages of coronal and sagittal planes. AJA *143*:1183, 1984.
17. Mechlin M, Thickman D, Kressel HY, Gefter W, Joseph P: Magnetic resonance imaging of postoperative patients with metallic implants. AJA *143*:1281, 1984.
18. Soulen RL, Budinger TF, Higgins CB: Safety of prosthetic heart values in MR imaging. (Abstr.) Radiology *153*(P)88, 1984.
19. Ross J, O'Donovan PB, Novoa R, Mehta A, Buonocore E, MacIntyre WJ, Golish JA, Ahmad M: Magnetic resonance of the chest: initial experience with imaging and in vivo *T1* and *T2* calculations. Radiology *152*:95, 1984.
20. Brasch RC, Gooding CA, Lallemand DP, Wesbey GE: Magnetic resonance imaging of the thorax in childhood. Works in progress. Radiology *150*:463, 1984.
21. Runge VM, Clanton JA, Smith FW, Hutchison J, Mallard J, Partain CL, James AE: Nuclear magnetic resonance of iron and copper disease states. AJR *141*:943, 1983.
22. Stark DD, Moseley ME, Bacon BR, Moss AA, Goldberg HI, Bass NM, James TL: Magnetic resonance imaging and spectroscopy on hepatic iron overload. Radiology *154*:137, 1985.
23. Moore EH, Gamsu G, Webb WR, Stulbarg MS: Pulmonary embolus: detection and followup using magnetic resonance. Radiology *153*:271, 1984.
24. Gamsu G, Hirgi M, Moore EH, Webb WR, Brito A: Experimental pulmonary emboli detected using magnetic resonance. Radiology *153*:467, 1984.
25. Webb WR, Gamsu G, Stark DD, Moore EH: Magnetic resonance imaging and abnormal pulmonary hili. Radiology *152*:89, 1984.

27

Mediastinum and Hila

W. RICHARD WEBB

In the diagnosis of chest diseases, magnetic resonance imaging appears to be most useful in the identification of mediastinal and hilar masses. This largely relates to the ease with which vessel, either normal or abnormal, and soft tissue can be distinguished. In the last three years, a number of studies have been published regarding the MR diagnosis of hilar and mediastinal lesions. These will be reviewed, with emphasis on our experience in San Francisco.

TECHNICAL CONSIDERATIONS

For our clinical studies we have employed a Diasonics MT/S system operating at 0.35 tesla. An elliptical body coil provides a pixel size of 1.7 or 2.1 mm. The operating characteristics of this scanner have been described in detail.[1,2]

Like most investigators, we routinely perform chest imaging using the spin-echo technique. Although different systems have differing imaging capabilities, most have scan sequences available similar to those we have used. With our scanner, spin-echo images can be obtained with repetition times (TR) of 0.5, 1.0, 1.5, or 2.0 sec. With each sequence, multiple images are obtained at contiguous levels, with the number of levels examined and the time required depending on the TR sequence used.[1-3] For a TR of 0.5 sec, five images are obtained at contiguous levels in a period of 4.3 minutes. With a TR of 2.0 sec, 20 images are obtained in 17 minutes.

In general, when scanning the chest, transaxial imaging is performed using two different techniques. An ECG-gated sequence (10 slice; TE 30 ms) is centered in the area of interest, usually including the upper mediastinum and hila. Depending on the subject's heart rate, the TR value will range between 0.75 and 1.0 sec, and the time required will vary from 6 to 8 minutes. This is usually followed by an ungated, 20-slice sequence (TR 2.0 sec; TE 30 and 60 ms; 17 min). If this is obtained without moving the patient or retuning the coil, T1 and T2 values can be calculated. Depending on the site and nature of the suspected abnormality, an additional ECG-gated series in the transaxial or coronal plane will often be obtained.[4-6] Gating images to the ECG can greatly improve spatial resolution and in most patients have replaced ungated images with a short TR value (TR 0.5 sec) (Fig. 27–1).[7-9]

Because of the length of time required to obtain the images, patients breathe quietly during the examination. When patients are dyspneic or cannot control their breathing, scan quality can be poor. Patients, usually are supine, with their arms positioned at their sides.

Respiratory gating of image acquisition can improve quality but also increases scan time. Clinical experience with this technique is limited.[10-12] The increased spatial resolution obtained with this technique may not justify the increase in imaging time required.

NORMAL FINDINGS

In normal subjects, most mediastinal structures visible at CT are also visible using transaxial MR (Fig. 27–1).[2,13–15] The aortic arch and its large branches are always visible on spin-echo images, with their blood-filled lumina usually producing no signal, clearly distinguished from the intense signal of mediastinal fat (Fig. 27–1). Similarly, the subclavian veins, brachiocephalic veins, and vena cava are always seen. The azygos vein or arch is visible in most patients. In areas where vessel contacts lung, the vessel wall is seen as a white stripe slightly less intense than fat. Small mediastinal veins, such as the internal mammary or superior intercostal veins, are more easily seen by MR than by CT.

The trachea, main bronchi, and bronchus intermedius are always visible but cannot be distinguished from vessels except by location. Only some segmental bronchi are clearly seen.

As with the systemic vasculature, no signal is usually recorded from the lumina of pulmonary arteries or veins (Fig. 27–1).[2,13–15] The main pulmonary artery, left and right pulmonary arteries, right interlobar pulmonary artery, right truncus anterior (right upper lobe artery), and descending left pulmonary artery are all usually seen, as are large pulmonary veins.

Normal-sized mediastinal lymph nodes, the esophagus, and the thymus gland are often visible on good-quality spin-echo images when short *TR* values are used.[3] They are intermediate in intensity, being less intense than fat and more intense than the air-filled trachea, lung, or mediastinal vessels. Also, the superior extensions of the pericardium anterior and posterior to the ascending aorta in the pretracheal space are frequently seen. Because they contain fluid that is low in protein, they appear as areas of very low intensity with both short and long *TR* and *TE* values. Thus, they can be distinguished from lymph nodes, which increase significantly in intensity from short to long *TR* values.

Flow Effects

In experimental studies of flowing blood,[16–18] it has been found that when flow occurs at a velocity greater than 10 to 15 cm, little significant MR signal results. To

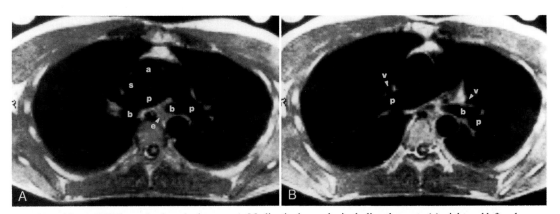

Figure 27–1. Normal ECG gated spin-echo images. *A*, Mediastinal vessels, including the aorta (a), right and left pulmonary arteries (p), and superior vena cava (s), are easily distinguished from high-intensity mediastinal fat. The air-filled right and left main bronchi (b) are also very low in intensity. The esophagus (e) is usually intermediate in intensity. *B*, At a lower level, mediastinal vessels are again clearly seen. Within the hila, bronchi (b), pulmonary arteries (p), and veins (v) are all visible, although the resolution of those structures is somewhat inferior to that of CT.

some extent, this occurs because the flowing hydrogen nuclei producing the MR signal have moved through the scan slice being imaged in the time it takes to perform the sequence of radio frequency pulses necessary to obtain the spin echo. However, blood flowing at slower velocities can result in significant signal and, in fact, can result in a more intense signal than that produced by stationary blood.[16] This generally occurs with flow rates of less than 3 cm/sec, and the intense signal is most evident with short *TR* values and on second-echo (*TE* 56 or 60 ms) images. This enhancement occurs because slowly flowing blood, entering a volume being imaged, has not been previously subjected to repeated spin-echoes and is therefore fully magnetized. It is important to note that the increased signal strength visible on second-echo images is not a result of the longer *TE* but is a feature of even-numbered (i.e., two) rather than odd-numbered numbered (i.e., one) echoes. This is termed even-echo rephasing. Although our understanding of MR flow phenomena is incomplete, further advances in the noninvasive evaluation of blood flow are likely.[16,18]

On ECG-gated images, significant signal can result from blood in the lumen of systemic and pulmonary arteries and veins, making them appear white rather than black on MR images. In particular, this occurs when vessels are imaged during diastole. Thus, this phenomenon is suspected to represent slow flow analogous to the enhancement described above. As with other flow effects, it is most evident on second-echo images. On ungated images, some signal is not uncommonly visible in the lumina of mediastinal vessels. Although it is uncertain what this signal represents, it is common enough to be of probably no consequence. It could reflect flow inhomogeneities.

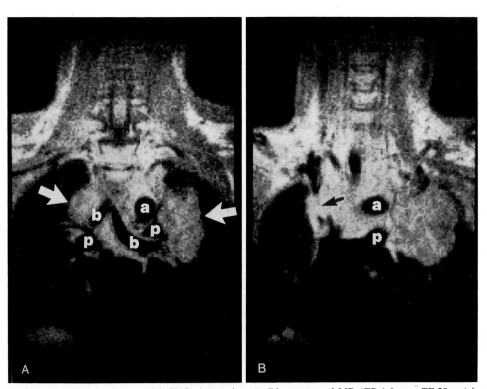

Figure 27–2. Hodgkin's disease with SVC obstruction. *A,* Direct coronal MR (*TR* 1.0 sec, *TE* 28 ms) in a patient with lymphoma and symptoms of superior vena caval obstruction. The right and left main bronchi (b), aortic arch (a), and left and right pulmonary arteries (p) are visible. Large masses (arrows) occupy the mediastinum and hila. *B,* At the level of the superior vena cava, although its proximal and distal segments are visible, its midportion (arrow) is obstructed by tumor. The aorta (a) and pulmonary artery (p) are again visible. (From Webb WR, et al: Radiology *150*:475, 1954. Used by permission.)

Vascular Lesions

A major advantage of MR imaging relative to CT is its ability to demonstrate vessels without the need for contrast agents.[16] Because of this, MR imaging has proven valuable in the diagnosis of vascular lesions involving the mediastinum. Mediastinal vascular lesions diagnosable using MR include transposition of the great arteries and other vascular anomalies as well as aortic aneurysm, dissection, and pseudoaneurysm.[19-22]

In patients with superior vena cava obstruction (Fig. 27–2) or obstruction of other great veins,[23] not only can the area of narrowing or obstruction be demonstrated but also evidence of slow flow (enhanced intraluminal signal) can sometimes be seen.

MEDIASTINAL MASS

In general, the relationship between a mediastinal mass and adjacent vessels, and vascular compression or obstruction, is better demonstrated using MR than it is with contrast-enhanced CT. This is largely a result of both the excellent mass/vessel contrast and the lack of streak artifacts on MR images.[2,14,24] On contrast-enhanced CT, streak artifacts can make the identification of small mediastinal vessels difficult.

The detection of mediastinal lymph nodes or mediastinal tumor masses using MR is based on alterations of normal anatomic contours, vascular displacement or compression, and differences in MR intensity between tumor and mediastinal fat.[2,14,24]

The differentiation of tumor from normal mediastinal fat can usually be accomplished by taking advantage of their differences in $T1$ (Fig. 27–3).[2,3,24,25] Although the $T2$ values of tumors and mediastinal fat tend to overlap, their $T1$ values are usually quite different, with fat having a much shorter $T1$. For example, in a group of patients we studied with benign and malignant mediastinal masses, $T1$ values of the masses averaged approximately 1500 ms, whereas the $T1$ values of surrounding mediastinal fat averaged slightly over 300 ms.[3] Furthermore, in every case the $T1$ value of the mass was significantly greater than the $T1$ value of adjacent mediastinal fat, measured in the same patient. Thus, if we first examine the image of a patient with a mediastinal mass obtained using a TR of 2.0 sec (an image with little $T1$ contrast), both tumor and mediastinal fat will produce an intense signal and can be difficult or impossible to distinguish (Fig. 27–3). However, if this image is compared with one obtained with a TR of 0.5, intensity differences will become apparent. Although fat remains intense because of its short $T1$, tumor, having a longer $T1$ value, decreases in intensity (Fig. 27–3). This relative decrease in intensity results in an increase in contrast between mass and fat, making detection of the mass easier. In ten patients, we measured the ratio of intensities of mediastinal mass to surrounding mediastinal fat,[3] thus providing a measurement of image contrast, with differing TR values. On the average, this ratio decreased from 0.83 with a TR of 2.0 sec (mass only slightly less intense than fat) to 0.52 with a TR of 0.5 sec (mass half as intense as fat) (Fig. 27–4). Normal lymph nodes show similar intensity changes with changing TR values.

The detection and evaluation of a mediastinal mass depends not only on the contrast between mass and fat but also on spatial resolution. In general, the spatial resolution of MR is less than that of CT, and small structures or the edges of large mediastinal masses can be more difficult to see on MR images. However, in comparison with CT, MR images obtained with a TR of 0.5 sec allow the detection of most, if not all, mediastinal lymph nodes that are borderline in size (1 to 1.5 cm) or enlarged; normal-sized nodes (less than 1 cm) visible on CT are also generally visible on MR. However, in a recent survey of MR in the evaluation and staging of bronchogenic carcinoma, we found that in two of ten patients with normal mediastinal lymph nodes proven surgically,

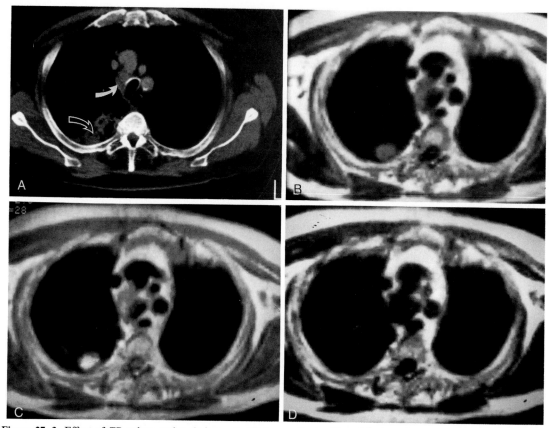

Figure 27–3. Effect of *TR* values and technique. *A*, CT in a patient with a right lung bronchogenic carcinoma (open arrow) partially obscured by bronchopulmonary lavage fluid. A paratracheal lymph node (solid arrow) involved by tumor is clearly seen. *B*, Spin-echo MR (*TR* 0.5 sec, *TE* 28 ms) at this level. The mediastinal node is much less intense than fat and is easily recognized. The lung nodule is similar to that node in intensity. *C*, Spin-echo MR (*TR* 2.0 sec, *TE* 28 ms). Both the lung nodule and the mediastinal node produce an intense signal with this long *TR*. The mediastinal lymph node is only slightly less intense than mediastinal fat. *D*, On an inversion recovery image, very sensitive to *T1* differences, the mediastinal node has decreased in intensity to such a degree that it cannot be distinguished from the trachea or mediastinal vessels. The lung nodule is no longer visible. (From Webb WR, et al: AJR *143*:723, 1984. Used by permission.)

CT was interpreted as normal and MR was interpreted as suspicious or abnormal. In these two patients, CT showed a group of two or more discrete, clearly normal-sized lymph nodes, whereas on MR the edges of the nodes could not be resolved and they were interpreted as a single, larger mass.

On the other hand, in some cases, mediastinal lymph nodes that are visible on MR are difficult to see on CT. This often occurs because streak artifacts have degraded the CT image or the node cannot be easily distinguished from a vessel on CT. On MR images obtained with a *TR* value of 2.0 sec, lymph nodes are much more difficult to detect, unless they are large.[3]

In patients with benign mediastinal lesions, values of *T1* and *T2* do not differ significantly from those of patients with malignant tumors,[2,24,25] and we have not found these values helpful in distinguishing mass lesions. However, fluid-filled or necrotic masses can be detected on the basis of long *T1* and *T2* values.[3,25] In patients with fluid-containing lesions, scans performed with long *TR* and *TE* values result in a significant increase in signal from the fluid components of the mass and can demonstrate inhomogeneities invisible with short *TR* and *TE* values. Calcification within a mediastinal mass cannot be recognized as such on MR and results in an area of low intensity.[13,23]

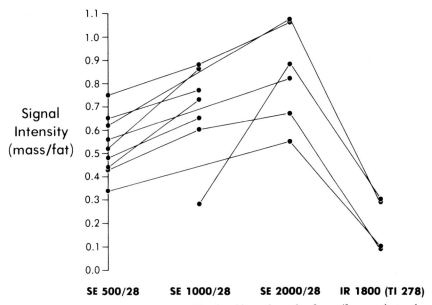

Figure 27–4. Signal intensity ratios and contrast. The signal intensity ratio of mass/fat quantitates the contrast between a mediastinal mass and surrounding fat, as visible on MR images. This has been plotted for the various techniques used in ten patients with mediastinal mass. Note that with increasing *TR*, the intensity ratio approaches 1.0; that is, mass and fat are nearly equal in intensity, and contrast decreases. With the inversion-recovery technique shown in Figure 27–3 *D*, contrast greatly increases. (From Webb WR, et al: AJR *143*:723, 1984. Used by permission.)

It has been reported that in some cases recurrent tumor can be distinguished from post-treatment radiation fibrosis by MR. In 12 patients studied by Glazer et al.[23a], post-treatment fibrosis had a low signal intensity on both *T1* and *T2* weighted images, whereas tumor showed a relative increase in intensity on *T2* weighted images. Differentiation, however, was difficult in patients who had just finished treatment or who had inflammatory disease.

HILAR MASS

The normal pulmonary hilum consists primarily of bronchi and pulmonary arteries and veins. In the interpretation of hilar CT, the diagnosis of a mass requires the differentiation of normal vasculature from abnormal soft tissue. In some locations, this differentiation can be made on anatomic grounds alone, but in other areas, mass and vessels are difficult to distinguish unless a large bolus of contrast is given, resulting in vascular opacification. In a significant number of cases, however, the degree of opacification achieved following intravenous contrast infusion is insufficient to allow a confident differentiation of mass and vessel on CT. This problem can be avoided by using MR.

Because rapidly flowing blood results in little MR signal, only the walls of pulmonary arteries and veins are visible on ungated MR or MR gated to systole.[2,13,14,24,26] Thus, MR images of the normal hilum show only the walls of bronchi and hilar vessels (see Fig. 27–1), and hilar masses should be easy to detect. For the most part, this is true. However, at several levels, small collections of tissue are present within the normal hilum, and these can cause some confusion.

In one study of the appearances of the normal hila at MR,[26] collections of soft tissue representing both fat and normal-sized nodes, large enough to be confused with an abnormally enlarged hilar lymph node (more than 1 cm in diameter), were visible in only three specific locations: on the right at the level of the bifurcation of the right pulmonary artery (Fig. 27–5A) and origin of the middle lobe bronchus, and on the left at the level of the left upper lobe bronchus (Fig. 27–5B). Otherwise, collections of soft tissue were small enough (3–5 mm) that if they were to represent lymph nodes, they would be considered normal in size.

In patients we have studied with hilar mass or lymphadenopathy resulting from lymphoma, bronchogenic carcinoma, metastasis, or inflammatory disease, MR allowed a confident diagnosis of hilar mass in each and clearly showed the relationship of mass to normal vessels and large bronchi (Fig. 27–6).[2,26] When compared with CT scans performed following the injection of a contrast bolus, MR largely confirmed the CT findings but made the diagnosis of hilar mass much easier and better showed the relationship of the mass to vessels at multiple levels (Fig. 27–7). Also, in a number of patients small but abnormally enlarged (more than 1 cm), hilar lymph nodes not clearly seen at CT were diagnosable using MR (Fig. 27–7).[26] We recently reviewed 30 patients with a hilar mass who had both contrast-enhanced CT and MR; 16 had pathologic proof of hilar mass, and 11 had pathologically proven mediastinal nodes but no hilar biopsy. Of these 30, four had a hilar node detected by MR that was not detected prospectively on CT scans. In the three who had surgery, the node was confirmed and proven to be abnormal. Also, MR is clearly superior to CT in defining a hilar mass lesion when the bolus injection of contrast is suboptimal, no contrast is given, or the mass is small. Similar results have also been reported by others.[13,14,25]

The complete radiographic evaluation of the pulmonary hilum requires the detection of bronchial abnormalities as well as hilar mass. Bronchial narrowing is commonly present in patients with bronchogenic carcinoma, and the detection of an abnormal bronchus can serve to guide transbronchoscopic biopsy procedures. Because of its better spatial resolution, CT is usually more accurate in the evaluation of bronchi (Fig. 27–7). However, MR studies performed with respiratory gating may improve the resolution of small bronchi.

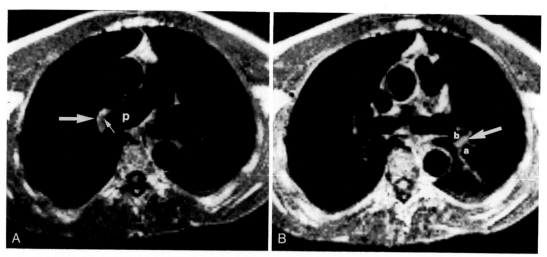

Figure 27–5. Normal hilar tissue. *A,* A spin echo image at the level of the bifurcation of the right pulmonary artery (p) into the truncus anterior or ascending branch and the interlobar or descending branch shows a collection of normal soft tissue (large arrow) in the lateral hilum. This soft tissue probably reflects both fat and normal-sized lymph nodes (small arrow). It is visible in most normal subjects. *B,* At a lower level in the same subject, tissue (arrow) is visible separating the left upper lobe bronchus (b) and the descending pulmonary artery (a). (From Webb WR, et al: *Radiology 152*:89, 1984. Used by permission.)

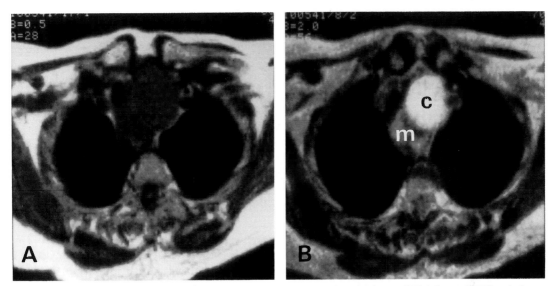

Figure 27–6. Mediastinal goiter. *A*, With a *T1* weighted technique, spin-echo image (*TR* 0.5 sec, *TE* 28 ms) shows a mediastinal mass, less intense than surrounding mediastinal fat. However, a large colloid cyst within the mass cannot be distinguished from solid components. *B*, A *T2* weighted image (*TR* 2.0 sec, *TE* 56 ms) shows a marked increase in intensity of the colloid cyst (c) relative to the solid part of the mass (m). This reflects the long *T2* of the fluid. (From Gamsu G, et al: Radiology *151*:709, 1984. Used by permission.)

It has been suggested by several authors that hilar mass and adjacent pulmonary consolidation occurring because of obstructive collapse can be distinguished on MR images. They have reported that with short *TR* values (150 to 500 ms) tumor appears more intense than distal lung disease. In three of four patients we have studied, we observed that with *TR* values of 2.0 sec, the lung consolidation appeared more intense than the hilar mass. This combination of findings suggests that the signal from lung has a *T1* longer than that of the tumor. This would be expected from fluid trapped in the obstructed lobe.

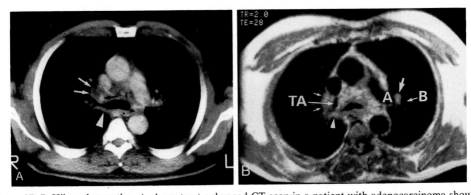

Figure 27–7. Hilar adenopathy. *A*, A contrast-enhanced CT scan in a patient with adenocarcinoma shows a right hilar mass (arrows) surrounding and narrowing the truncus anterior (black arrow). The posterior wall of the right upper lobe bronchus (arrowhead) is abnormally thickened. No definite abnormality is visible on the left. *B*, MR at the same level better shows the relationship of the right hilar mass (short arrows) to the truncus anterior (TA). Although abnormal thickening of the posterior wall of the right upper lobe bronchus (arrowhead) is also seen, the bronchus is much less clearly seen than on CT. On the left side, a lymph node (thicker arrow) can be clearly distinguished from the artery medial to it [*A*] and the bronchus (lateral to it [*B*]). (From Webb WR, et al: Radiology *152*:89, 1984. Used by permission.)

TECHNIQUE DEPENDENCE OF MR IMAGING

As was described in the discussion of the MR diagnosis of mediastinal mass, the relative signal intensities (and therefore contrast) of tissues having differing *T1* and *T2* characteristics can be altered by altering the *TR* and *TE* values used.[3,14,25] In other words, an abnormality that is visible using one technique may not be visible using another (Fig. 27–8). Because of this, it is our belief that complete MR imaging for the diagnosis of chest diseases requires the use of more than a single imaging technique. For example, although *T1* sensitive techniques (spin echo with a short *TR*, partial saturation, inversion recovery) are best for distinguishing mediastinal mass from surrounding fat, hilar masses and lung nodules are generally better seen when longer *TR* values are used (see Fig. 27–3). Such techniques, which are relatively *T1* insensitive, result in a stronger signal from the mass or nodule relative to low-intensity lung and vessels.[3]

Furthermore, because the signal strength from all tissues is increased when *TR* is lengthened, the signal/noise ratio (S/N), and therefore image quality, is better than that obtained with a short *TR*. In some patients, for example, small mediastinal or hilar structures visible when a *TR* of 2.0 sec is used, are poorly seen with a *TR* of 0.5 sec. Also, imaging with two different *TR* values is necessary if *T1* values are to be calculated. Therefore, in most patients we scan, we obtain series of images having both short (determined by ECG gating, approximately 0.5 sec) and long (2.0 sec) *TR* values.

Inversion recovery techniques that are very *T1* sensitive (*TR* 1.8 sec, *TI* 278 ms) have been of limited usefulness in diagnosing mediastinal masses. Although the contrast between mass and mediastinal fat is greatly enhanced, signal strength from the mass may be so low that the mass is difficult to distinguish from the trachea or great vessels (see Fig. 27–3*D*). Also, using such a technique the signal strength of lung nodules or masses may be so low that the mass or nodule cannot be detected.

Images with a long *TE* (56 or 60 ms) allow the detection of fluid (when compared with the shorter *TE* image) and also are important in demonstrating flow phenomena.

Sagittal and Coronal Imaging

An advantage of MR, relative to CT, is that it allows direct imaging in the sagittal or coronal plane without a degradation of spatial resolution.[4–6,14,15,25] Although direct sagittal or coronal CT can be performed, it is difficult to obtain multiple slices having a consistent relationship to one another.

In our experience, sagittal or coronal MR imaging can provide information not available on transaxial CT or MR images in some patients.[4,5] The benefits of sagittal or coronal MR are several. Structures oriented longitudinally in the sagittal or coronal plane can be imaged along their axes. Such structures include the trachea (Fig. 27–7), superior vena cava (Fig. 27–2), and aorta.[14,21] Moreover, imaging in a second plane reduces the chances of misinterpretation of findings as a result of volume averaging. This is particularly important in areas of the chest where a correct (or confident) interpretation requires the resolution of the edges of structures that lie in or near the transaxial plane. An example would be the aorticopulmonary window, in which the undersurface of the aortic arch and pulmonary artery can be difficult to clearly resolve on transaxial images or distinguish from a mass in this location (Fig. 27–9). On coronal images, the relationships of these structures can be clearly seen. Pathologic processes near the diaphragm (Fig. 27–10) or lung apices can also be better localized in some patients on sagittal or coronal images.

Lastly, images obtained in the coronal or sagittal plane quite simply provide an

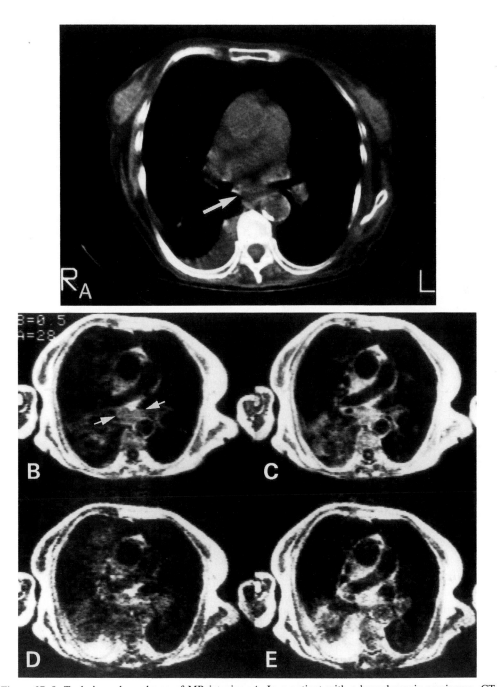

Figure 27–8. Technique dependence of MR imaging. *A*, In a patient with a bronchogenic carcinoma, CT shows subcarinal tumor (arrow) and right pleural effusion. Patchy right lower lobe consolidation was also visible using lung window settings. *B*, Spin-echo MR (*TR* 0.5 sec, *TE* 28 ms) is *T1* sensitive and clearly distinguishes mediastinal tumor (arrows) from higher intensity fat. However, the lung disease is poorly seen, and the pleural fluid is invisible. *C*, *TR* 1.0, *TE* 28 ms. With a longer *TR,* contrast between mediastinal tumor and fat decreases because of increased signal from the tumor. However, increased signal from the lung disease makes it easier to see. Improved signal/noise ratio also improves the visibility of mediastinal structures. *D*, *TR* 0.5 sec, *TE* 56 ms. Visibility of the pleural effusion is enhanced because of the *T2* sensitivity of this technique. This image, however, has the poorest signal/noise ratio and spatial resolution. *E*, *TR* 1.0 sec, *TE* 56 ms. Signal from the pleural effusion is further enhanced using this technique because of the long *T1* of fluid. The subcarinal mass cannot be distinguished from fat on this image. (From Webb WR, et al: *AJR 143*:723, 1984. Used by permission.)

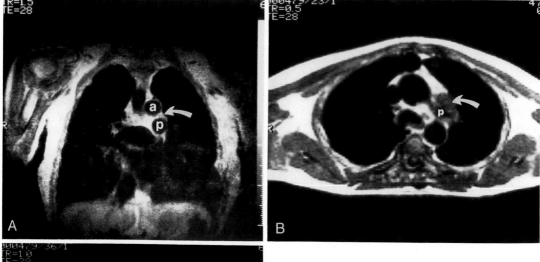

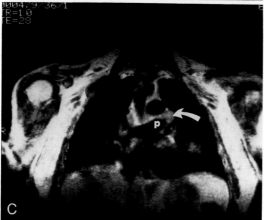

Figure 27–9. Coronal MR. *A*, Coronal MR in a normal subject at the level of the aorticopulmonary window (arrow). The aorta (a) and pulmonary artery (p) are clearly seen. *B*, MR (*TR* 0.5 sec, *TE* 28 ms) in a patient with bronchogenic carcinoma shows a mass in the aorticopulmonary window (arrow) appearing to compress or invade the left pulmonary artery (p). Also note two normal-sized lymph nodes anterior to the main bronchi. *C*, Coronal MR in the same patient as in *B* shows the mass (arrow) in the aorticopulmonary window to be above the pulmonary artery (p). The artery itself is uninvolved. (From Webb WR, et al: Radiology *153*:729, 1984. Used by permission.)

additional perspective and are often easier for clinicians unfamiliar with cross-sectional anatomy to understand and make use of.

Developing Technologies

Chemical shift imaging (hydrogen proton spectroscopy) can be performed using available MR imagers and allows the discrimination of water protons and fat protons.[27,28] Thus, images of water only and fat only can be produced and compared. The utility of this technique in studying thoracic lesions remains to be explored.

NMR spectroscopy of nuclei other than hydrogen may be of some value as well, but results remain quite preliminary. Metabolic differences between different lung cancer cell lines has been demonstrated in vitro using P-31 spectroscopy.[29]

In summary, MR can be a useful technique in evaluating mediastinal and hilar lesions. It is most advantageous in the diagnosis of mediastinal vascular lesions and hilar masses and in allowing direct sagittal and coronal imaging. MR seems to be comparable to CT in diagnosing abnormally enlarged mediastinal lymph nodes or mediastinal mass, but a precise determination of their relative value requires further study. MR is usually inferior to CT in spatial resolution. This makes the evaluation of small lymph nodes or bronchi difficult. Also, the edges of mediastinal masses are somewhat less sharply defined when MR is used.

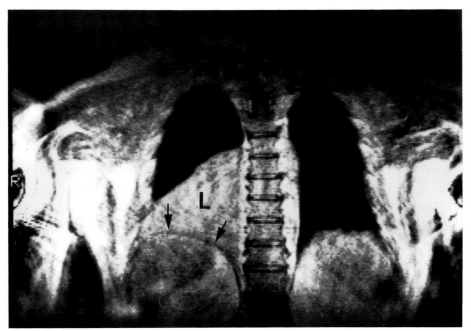

Figure 27–10. Right lower lobe collapse. In a patient with opacification of the lower right chest, coronal MR shows a consolidated right lower lobe (L) and the right hemidiaphragm (arrows). The abnormal density is clearly supradiaphragmatic. (From Webb WR, et al: Radiology *153*:729, 1984. Used by permission.)

References

1. Crooks LE, Mills CM, Davis PL, et al: Visualization of cerebral and vascular abnormalities by NMR imaging. The effects of imaging parameters on contrast. Radiology *144*:843, 1982.
2. Gamsu G, Webb WR, Sheldon P, et al: Nuclear magnetic resonance imaging of the thorax. Radiology *147*:473, 1983.
3. Webb WR, Gamsu G, Stark DD, et al: Evaluation of magnetic resonance sequences in imaging mediastinal tumors. AJR *143*:723, 1984.
4. Webb WR, Gamsu G, Crooks LE: Multisection sagittal and coronal magnetic resonance imaging of the mediastinum and hila. Work in progress. Radiology *150*:475, 1984.
5. Webb WR, Jensen BG, Gamsu G, et al: Coronal magnetic resonance imaging of the chest: Normal and abnormal. Radiology *153*:729, 1984.
6. O'Donovan PB, Ross JS, Sivak ED, et al: Magnetic resonance imaging of the thorax: The advantages of coronal and sagittal planes. AJR *143*:1183, 1984.
7. Lanzer P, Botvinick EH, Schiller NB, et al: Cardiac imaging using gated magnetic resonance. Radiology *150*:121, 1984.
8. Lieberman JM, Alfidi RJ, Nelson AD, et al: Gated magnetic resonance imaging of the normal and diseased heart. Radiology *152*:465, 1984.
9. Amparo EG, Higgins CB, Farmer D, et al: Gated MRI of cardiac and paracardiac masses: Initial experience. AJR *143*:1151, 1984.
10. Runge VM, Clanton JA, Partain CL, James AE Jr: Respiratory gating in magnetic resonance imaging at 0.5 Tesla. Radiology *151*:521, 1984.
11. Schultz CL, Alfidi RJ, Nelson AD, et al: The effect of motion on two-dimensional Fourier transformation magnetic resonance images. Radiology *152*:117, 1984.
12. Ehman RL, McNamara MT, Pollack M, et al: Magnetic resonance imaging with respiratory gating: Techniques and advantages. AJR *143*:1175, 1984.
13. Cohen AM, Creviston S, LiPuma JP, et al: NMR evaluation of hilar and mediastinal lymphadenopathy. Radiology *148*:737, 1983.
14. Cohen AM, Creviston S, LiPuma JP, et al: Nuclear magnetic resonance imaging of the mediastinum and hili: Early impressions of its efficacy. AJR *141*:1163, 1983.
15. Higgins CB, Stark DD, McNamara M, et al: Multiplane magnetic resonance imaging of the heart and major vessels: Studies in normal volunteers. AJR *142*:661, 1984.
16. Kaufman L, Crooks LE, Sheldon P, et al: The potential impact of nuclear magnetic resonance imaging on cardiovascular diagnosis. Circulation *67*:251, 1983.
17. George CR, Jacobs G, MacIntyre WS, et al: Magnetic resonance signal intensity patterns obtained from continuous and pulsatile flow models. Radiology *151*:421, 1984.

18. Axel L: Blood flow effects in magnetic resonance imaging. AJR *143*:1157, 1984.
19. Herfkens RJ, Higgins CB, Hricak H, et al: Nuclear magnetic resonance imaging of the cardiovascular system: Normal and pathologic findings. Radiology *147*:749, 1983.
20. Fletcher BD, Jacobstein MD, Nelson AD, et al: Gated magnetic resonance imaging of congenital cardiac malformations. Radiology *150*:137, 1984.
21. Moore EH, Webb WR, Verrier ED, et al: MRI of chronic post traumatic false aneurysms of the thoracic aorta. AJR *143*:1195, 1984.
22. Amparo EG, Higgins CB, Shafton EP: Demonstration of coarctation of the aorta by magnetic resonance imaging. AJR *143*:1192, 1984.
23. Farmer DW, Moore EH, Amparo E, et al: Calcific fibrosing mediastinitis: Demonstration of pulmonary vascular obstruction by magnetic resonance imaging. AJR *143*:1189, 1984.
23a. Glazer HS, Lee JKT, Levitt RG, et al: Radiation fibrosis: Differentiation from recurrent tumor by MR imaging. Work in progress. Radiology *156*:721, 1985.
24. Ross JS, O'Donovan PB, Novoa R, et al: Magnetic resonance of the chest: Initial experience with imaging and in vivo *T1* and *T2* calculations. Radiology *152*:95, 1984.
25. Gamsu G, Stark DD, Webb WR, et al: Magnetic resonance imaging of benign mediastinal masses. Radiology *151*:709, 1984.
26. Webb WR, Gamsu G, Stark DD, Moore EH: Magnetic resonance imaging of the normal and abnormal pulmonary hila. Radiology *152*:89, 1984.
27. Pykett IL, Rosen BR: Nuclear magnetic resonance: In vivo proton chemical shift imaging. Work in progress. Radiology *149*:197, 1984.
28. Dixon WT: Simple proton spectroscopic imaging. Radiology *153*:189, 1984.
29. Knop RH, Carney DN, Chen CW, Cohen JS: 31p NMR differentiation of small cell lung cancer (SCLC) and non–small cell lung cancer (NSCLC) human tumor cell lines (ab). Society of Magnetic Resonance in Medicine. New York, April 13–17, 1984.

Breast

C. LEON PARTAIN
ARTHUR C. FLEISCHER
ALAN C. WINFIELD
MADAN V. KULKARNI
SAMUEL J. DWYER, III
LARRY T. COOK

The utilization of magnetic resonance imaging in the evaluation of breast lesions has significant potential owing to the absence of known biologic hazards; the capability of thin-section, digital tomographic imaging in any plane or volume; and the capacity to provide soft tissue contrast based upon biochemical changes that are pathophysiologically specific.[1-4] Several reports have described various approaches to the evaluation of breast lesions.[5-9] One approach has utilized proton density weighted and *T1* weighted imaging at 0.3 tesla, correlated with mammography and CT.[5,6] Another approach has utilized the evaluation of the *T1* parameter in fixed pathologic surgical specimens.[7] A different approach has involved the use of fresh, unfixed tissue in evaluating mathematical models for *T2*.[8] The first report of functional *T1* images and three-dimensional images of breast lesions was also released recently.[9]

This chapter illustrates the results of breast MRI in 32 patients, ranging in age from 16 to 70 years, and ten normal volunteers. The patients were selected by virtue of clinically palpable breast masses, with clinical suspicion of malignancy supported by xeromammography and/or ultrasound. Each patient received excisional biopsy for pathologic confirmation following the MR scan. Exclusion criteria from this study included the existence of a pacemaker or prior neurosurgical procedure involving a clip in the brain. Written informed consent was obtained from each patient or volunteer.

The range of breast lesions is summarized in Table 28–1. Correlative xeromammographic images were obtained in the lateral and craniocaudal views. Mammographic ultrasound images in selected patients were obtained in the transverse and sagittal projections through the palpable lesions of interest.

TECHNIQUE

MR imaging was accomplished using 0.5 tesla superconducting magnetic resonance scanning system (Teslacon, Technicare Corporation, Solon, Ohio). For MRI of the breast a specialized breast coil was added as a minor modification of the patient couch. The breast surface coil aperture measures 16 cm × 8 cm. The patient assumes the prone position so that the breast lies in the dependent position, thus maximizing cross-sectional area for tomographic imaging. Pulse sequences include multislice tomographic imaging using spin echo 500/30 (TR = 500 ms, TE = 30 ms) imaging in the coronal,

Table 28–1. DISTRIBUTION OF PATIENTS AND NORMAL VOLUNTEERS FOR THE BREAST MRI STUDY

Category		Number
Normal		10
Abnormal		32
Carcinoma	15	
Benign masses	8	
Cyst	2	
Fibrocystic disease	5	
Fibroadenoma	2	
Total		42

sagittal, and transverse projections. In these images, fat appears to have increased intensity or to be white. Arteries, veins, and glandular tissue appear to have decreased intensity. Multiecho pulse sequences were also utilized with *TE* varying in steps of 30 ms from 30 ms to 120 ms, the *TR* being held at 1000 ms. As *TE* is increased, added *T2* weighting is provided for the MR images. In addition, inversion spin-echo pulse sequences (*IR* 450/30/1500) were utilized with *T1* weighting, including inversion time (*TI*) of 450 ms, spin-echo *TE* times varying from 30 to 120 ms, and a *TR* time of approximately 1500 ms. Further, calculated *T1* images (also called observed *T1*) were obtained and displayed in the transverse perspective, with region-of-interest analyses comparing abnormal with adjacent normal tissue.

Conventional xeromammograms were obtained using a Picker GX-600 generator and a Machlett Dynamax x-ray tube with a molybdenum target and 0.6 mm focal spot with a conventional Xerox Model 125 processor or a Phillips Mammo DIAGNOST with a molybdenum target x-ray tube and 0.2 to 0.5 mm focal spot. Lesions were identified in the craniocaudal and lateral views.

Ultrasound tomographic images were obtained for selected patients, using the water-bath breast ultrasound unit. Images were obtained in multiple planes and directions.

Postprocessing of MR images included the region-of-interest calculations, calculated *T1* images, and the computer-aided interactive process of identifying borders of lesions and the margins of breast tissue for subsequent generation of color-coded three-dimensional images in cooperation with the radiological sciences group at the University of Kansas.[10,11]

RESULTS

A wide variety of breast morphology is apparent in normal volunteers. Figure 28–1 demonstrates two adjacent 0.5 cm tomographic images of the breast in the transverse projection of an asymptomatic 55-year-old volunteer. In these images, fat has increased intensity and appears white, as do some of the connective ligaments in the subcutaneous tissue of the breast. Arteries, veins, and glandular tissue are distinguished as areas of decreased intensity. It is also significant to observe (Fig. 28–1) that maximal signal-to-noise, and hence superior imaging, is possible in the sensitive center area of the coil, although significant information is also obtained in axillary soft tissue and thoracic tissue in the region of the pectoralis muscle, rib, intercostal muscles, and sternum. These are actually physically located outside the field of view of the specialized breast coil. Also apparent is the deeper field of view allowed in comparison with x-ray mam-

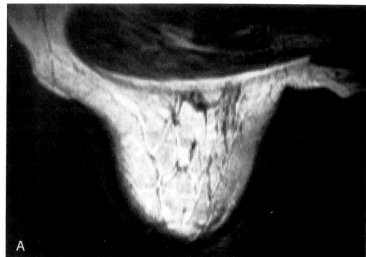

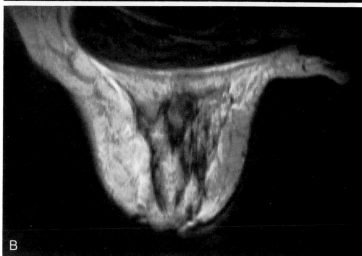

Figure 28–1. Normal volunteer. Transverse MR images using spin-echo 30/500 pulse sequence, slice thickness 0.5 cm, with breast coil. *A*, 0.5 cm below superior breast surface. *B*, 1.0 cm below superior breast surface.

mography, illustrative of the potential to visualize lesions on or approaching the thoracic wall.

Figure 28–2 demonstrates two tomographic views in the transverse, coronal, and sagittal projections. Observe that fat has increased intensity and that glandular and ductal tissue is again demonstrated by decreased intensity.

A patient with fibrocystic disease is shown in MR images (Fig. 28–3). The cysts are multiple, small, and well marginated and have decreased intensity on spin-echo 500/30 pulse sequences.

Benign solid masses of the breast are evidenced by low intensity on spin-echo 500/30 images and by well-marginated borders. A benign fibroadenoma with these characteristics is illustrated in Figure 28–4.

Several patients with malignancies have been studied, and a variety of patterns are illustrated. First, the correlation of xeromammography and MR imaging using the breast coil is illustrated (Fig. 28–5). The tumor was observed to have a significantly prolonged $T1$ (decreased intensity on this $T1$ weighted image, and increased intensity on functional $T1$ images) compared with adjacent normal fat (see Table 28–3).

One patient had both tumor and cystic disease and was evaluated with ultrasound

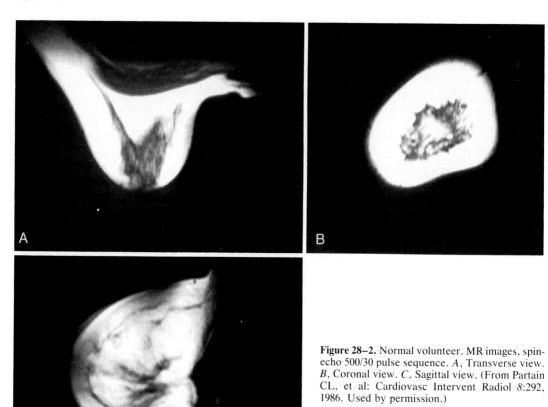

Figure 28–2. Normal volunteer. MR images, spin-echo 500/30 pulse sequence. *A*, Transverse view. *B*, Coronal view. *C*, Sagittal view. (From Partain CL, et al: Cardiovasc Intervent Radiol *8*:292, 1986. Used by permission.)

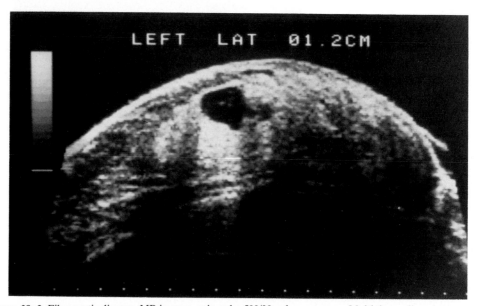

Figure 28–3. Fibrocystic disease. MR images, spin-echo 500/30 pulse sequence. Multiple small cysts are areas of decreased intensity on this pulse sequence.

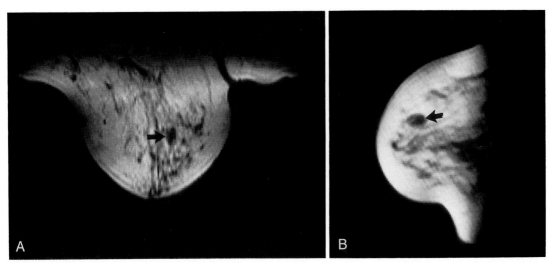

Figure 28–4. Fibroadenoma. MR image spin-echo 500/30 pulse sequence. Adenoma (arrow) indicated by well-marginated, low-intensity lesion. *A,* Transverse view. *B,* Coronal view. (From Partain CL, et al: Cardiovasc Intervent Radiol *8*:292, 1986. Used by permission.)

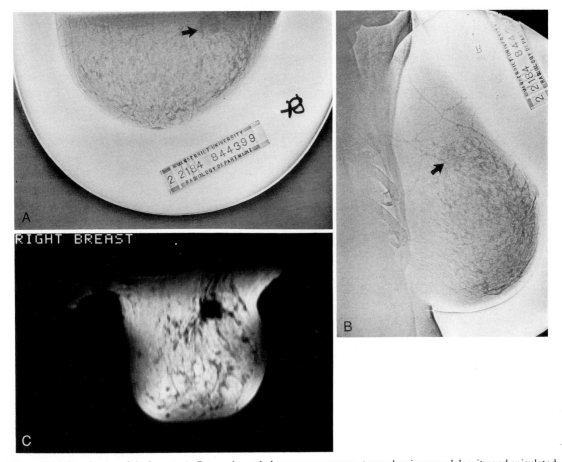

Figure 28–5. Carcinoma of the breast. *A,* On craniocaudad xeromammogram, tumor has increased density and spiculated margins (arrow). *B,* Lateral xeromammogram (arrow). *C,* Transverse spin-echo 500/30 MR image. *D,* Sagittal spin-echo 500/30 MR image. *E,* Transverse inversion spin-echo 1500/450/30 MR image. *F,* Transverse calculated *T1* (*OT1*) image. *G,* Transverse calculated *T1* image; region of interest defined within tumor. *H,* Transverse calculated *T1* image; large region of interest within fat. (From Partain CL, et al: Cardiovasc Intervent Radiol *8*:292, 1986. Used by permission.)

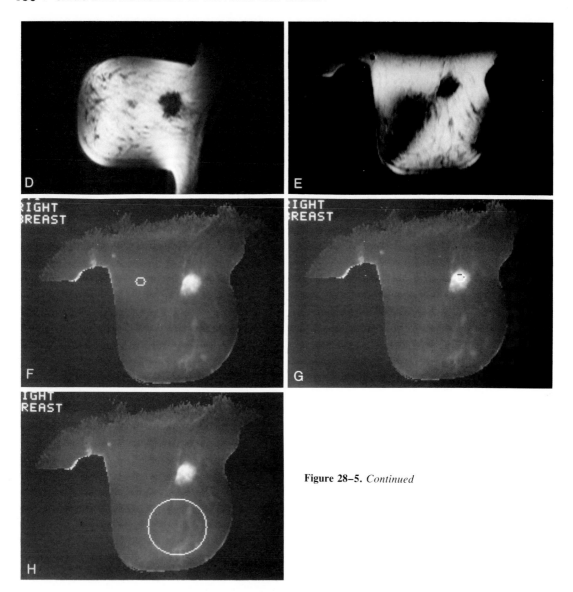

Figure 28–5. *Continued*

and magnetic resonance imaging (Fig. 28–6). These MRI scans were used as the basis for color three-dimensional imaging, in which the cyst and tumor are assigned contrasting colors. Observe that the three-dimensional evaluation and display may be taken from any viewing projection and at multiple viewing angles (Fig. 28–7), thus extending, in a summary way, the identification of mass lesions and their relationships to normal structures.

Surface coil technology provides magnification imaging and increased signal-to-noise but compromises field of view and image uniformity.

CONCLUSIONS

In our study of breast lesions using the spin-echo 500/30 pulse sequence, which yields soft tissue contrast that is a function of both the proton spin density and the *T1* parameter, four patterns have been recognized and are summarized in Table 28–2.

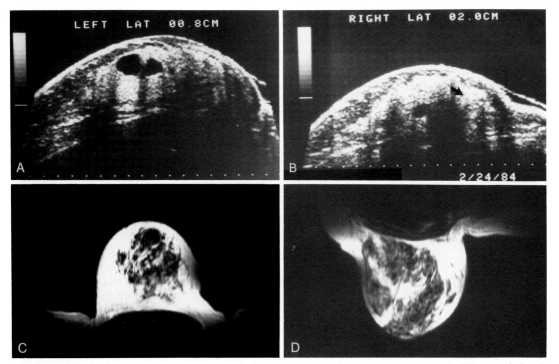

Figure 28–6. Cyst and tumor in one breast, correlating ultrasound and magnetic resonance. *A,* Ultrasound showing bilobulated cysts as echo-free areas *B,* Ultrasound showing echogenic mass lateral to cysts, suspicious for tumor. *C,* Transverse, spin-echo 500/30 MR image showing cyst as circular region of decreased intensity. *D,* Transverse, spin-echo 500/30 MR image showing mass as inhomogeneous area of relatively low intensity at lateral aspect of breast.

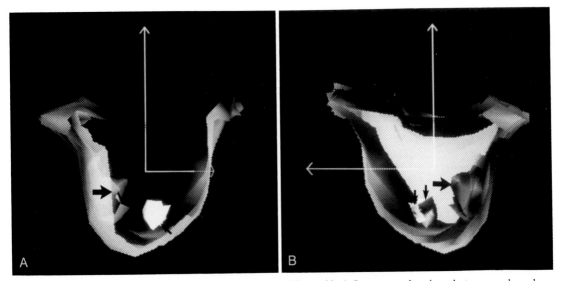

Figure 28–7. Three-dimensional image in same patient as in Figure 28–6. Image may be viewed at any angle and any direction. Arbitrary assignment of gray level in relation to normal breast structures: tumor (large arrow), and cysts (small arrows). *A,* Three-dimensional image at 30 degrees. *B,* Three-dimensional image at 180 degrees. (From Partain CL, et al: Cardiovasc Intervent Radiol *8*:292, 1986. Used by permission.)

Table 28–2. MR SCAN PARAMETERS USING BREAST COIL AND SPIN-ECHO 500/30 PULSE SEQUENCES

Pattern	Possible Significance
Increased intensity— well marginated	Cyst
Increased intensity— poorly marginated	Fibrocystic changes
Decreased intensity— well marginated	Benign masses
Decreased intensity— poorly marginated	Malignancy

These patterns include (1) areas of increased intensity that are well marginated; (2) areas of increased intensity that are poorly marginated; (3) areas of decreased intensity that are well marginated; and (4) areas of decreased intensity that are poorly marginated. Cystic lesions of the breast have, in general, tended to fall into category 1; fibrocystic changes into category 2; benign solid masses, including fibroadenoma, into category 3; and carcinoma of the breast into category 4. At this stage of our experience, we feel that it is unlikely that one pulse sequence can specifically differentiate benign from malignant lesions and have proceeded to correlate spin echo 500/30 with calculated *T1* images as a possible means of added specificity.

The results of in vivo *T1* measurements in breast lesions in our study are summarized in Table 28–3. It is observed that there is significant difference in the *T1* in a tumor in comparison to the *T1* in adjacent normal tissue, composed primarily of fat. Some overlap in *T1* values does appear to exist in *T1* measurements from adjacent tissue that is fibrocystic in nature, rendering the initial results disappointing. Hence, the evaluation of the fibrocystic breast continues to be a diagnostic challenge with regard to specific, noninvasive diagnostic work-up in suspected malignancies.

The significance of breast cancer as a serious clinical problem is indicated by the fact that 1 out of 11 women will experience this disease. Further, the availability now of a potential screening device that uses no ionizing radiation and has no known adverse effects[12–14] renders magnetic resonance imaging an exceedingly powerful and attractive technique.

The clinical potential of magnetic resonance imaging is further enhanced by virtue of the exquisite sensitivity to breast pathology and the possibility of added specificity, which may well allow malignant lesions to be distinguished from benign lesions using this technique.[15–18]

Table 28–3. T1 IN BREAST MALIGNANCIES

Category	No. Patients (p)	No. Measurements (n)	T1 in Milliseconds*	
Normal				
Fat	5	235	144	12.0
Glandular tissue	5	235	248	15.7
Abnormal				
Fibrocystic changes	5	235	315	17.7
Cyst	2	94	410	20.2
Fibroadenoma	2	94	425	20.7
Carcinoma				
In vivo	15	705	670	25.9
In vitro	5	235	509	22.6

* Average calculated *T1* using a two-point iterative algorithm and a ratio of inversion spin-echo to spin-echo procedure.

Future directions should include validation and continued improvement in in-vivo *T1* and *T2* measurements. Investigation of the analysis of the basic MR signal from breast tissue with regard to identification of parameters not previously defined, together with the conventional MR parameters of spin density, *T1*, and *T2*, should be pursued. Specific data are likely to be able to distinguish malignant from benign lesions and, possibly, have the capability of distinguishing among different types of malignancies. Further, the potential of proton chemical shift data demonstrated to be capable of distinguishing water from fat molecules may be useful in this regard.[19]

Finally, this study demonstrates the feasibility of screening palpable breast lesions based on the capability of magnetic resonance imaging to provide thin-section (2 to 5 mm) tomographic imaging at any angle through the breasts. MR can visualize with high resolution breast pathology at any location, including breast tissue adjacent to the thoracic wall (which is difficult, or impossible, to visualize in conventional mammography). It can also image axillary soft tissue and soft tissue of the sternum, pectoralis muscle, and bony thorax. The search for specificity continues based upon well-understood MR parameters and other MR measurements that are likely in the future to increase specificity in the diagnosis of breast malignancy. Future techniques should also involve high field strengths and multinuclear MR imaging and NMR spectroscopic measurements.[20,21]

Finally, this chapter and other reports[5-9] yield the following evaluation of the state of the art in breast MRI:

1. Malignant lesions are well identified in a stromal environment of mostly fatty tissue and are well characterized by *T1* weighted (SE 500/30) and calculated *T1* (*OT1*) images.

2. Malignant lesions are difficult to visualize and distinguish with a stromal tissue involving significant fibrocystic disease.

In conclusion, the utility of MRI in screening breast malignancies must await more accurate criteria that may include (1) pulse sequence optimization, (2) application of fast scan techniques (see Chapter 96), (3) contrast enhancement (see Chapters 46 to 52), (4) dynamic contrast-enhanced MRI (see Chapter 52), and (5) in vivo multinuclear NMR spectroscopy.

ACKNOWLEDGMENTS

The authors gratefully acknowledge the contributions of Margaret Moore for assistance in the preparation and editing of this manuscript; of John Bobbitt for photographic assistance; and of Jill Craig for technological assistance.

References

1. Margulis AR, Higgins CB, Kaufman L, Crooks LE: Clinical Magnetic Resonance Imaging. San Francisco, Radiology Research and Education Foundation, 1983.
2. James TL, Margulis AR: Biomedical Magnetic Resonance. San Francisco, Radiology Research and Education Foundation, 1984.
3. Partain CL, James AE, Rollo FD, Price RR: Nuclear Magnetic Resonance (NMR) Imaging. Philadelphia, WB Saunders, 1983.
4. Partain CL: Nuclear Magnetic Resonance and Correlative Imaging Modalities. New York, The Society of Nuclear Medicine, 1984.
5. El Yousef SJ, Duchesneau RH, Alfidi RJ, Haaga JR, Bryan P, LiPuma JP: Magnetic resonance imaging of the breast. Radiology *150*:761, 1984.
6. El Yousef SJ, Alfidi RJ, Duchesneau RH, et al: Initial experience with nuclear magnetic resonance of the human breast. J Comput Assist Tomogr 2:215, 1983.
7. Stelling CB, Wang PC, Lieber A, Griffen WO, Mattingly SS, Powell DE: Lexington, University of Kentucky, A.B. Chandler Medical Center. Personal communication, 1987.
8. McSweeney MB, Small WC, Cerny V, Sewell W, Powell RW, Goldstein JH: NMR discrimination of

benign and malignant human breast tissue based upon transverse relaxation (*T1*) parameters. Radiology *153*:741, 1984.

9. Partain CL, Kulkarni MV, Price RR, Fleischer AC, Page DL, et al: Magnetic resonance imaging of the breast: Functional *T1* and three-dimensional imaging. Cardiovasc Intervent Radiol *8*:292, 1986.

10. Batnitsky S, Price HI, Lee KR, Cook LT, Ritz SL, Dwyer SJ: Three dimensional computer reconstructions of brain lesions from surface contours provided by computed tomography: A prospectus. Neurosurgery *1*:1, 1982.

11. Batnitksy S, Price HI, Cook PN, Cook LT, Dwyer SJ: Three-dimensional computer reconstruction from surface contours for head CT examinations. J Comput Assist Tomogr *5*:60, 1981.

12. Budinger TF: Nuclear magnetic resonance (NMR) in vivo studies: known thresholds for health effects. J Comput Assist Tomogr *5*:800, 1981.

13. Saunders RD, Orr JS: Biological effects of NMR. *In* Partain CL, James AE, Rollo FD, Price RR (eds): Nuclear Magnetic Resonance (NMR) Imaging. Philadelphia, WB Saunders, 1983.

14. Patton JA, Lagan JE, Price RR, Stephens WH, Partain CL: NMR site planning and patient safety. *In* Partain CL (ed): Nuclear Magnetic Resonance and Correlative Imaging Modalities. New York, Society of Nuclear Medicine, 1984.

15. Bovee WMMJ, Getreuer KW, Smidt J, Lindeman J: Nuclear magnetic resonance and detection of human breast tumors. J Natl Cancer Inst *61*:53, 1978.

16. Hollis DP, Economou JS, Parks LC, Eggleston JC, Saryan LA, Czeisler JL: Nuclear magnetic resonance studies of several experimental and human malignant tumors. Cancer Res *33*:2156, 1973.

17. Medina D, Hazelwood CF, Cleveland GG, Chang DC, Spjut HJ, Moyers R: Nuclear magnetic resonance studies on human breast dysplasias and neoplasms. J Natl Cancer Inst *54*:813, 1975.

18. Ling GN, Tucker M: Nuclear magnetic resonance relaxation and rate/contrast in normal mouse and rat tissue and in cancer cells. J Natl Cancer Inst *64*:1199, 1980.

19. Pykett IL, Rose BR: Nuclear magnetic resonance: in vivo proton chemical shift imaging. Radiology *149*:197, 1983.

20. Koenig SH: Brown RD: Determinants of proton relaxation rate in tissue. Magn Reson Med *1*:347, 1984.

21. Chance B, Eleff S, Leigh JS, Barlow C, Ligetti L, Gigulai L: Phosphorus NMR: Potential application to diagnosis. *In* Partain CL, James AE, Rollo FD, Price RR (eds): Nuclear Magnetic Resonance (NMR) Imaging. Philadelphia, WB Saunders, 1983.

VI

CLINICAL EXPERIENCE: MRI OF THE ABDOMEN

29

Liver and Spleen

DAVID D. STARK

Magnetic resonance imaging (MRI) has become an established technique for diagnosis of central nervous system (CNS) disorders.[1,2] Indeed, major health insurance companies in several states now reimburse for CNS examinations. Owing to the excellence of x-ray CT in the body, the need for MRI has been more difficult to establish. The abdomen in particular has been a difficult anatomic region to study because of respiratory, cardiac, and peristaltic motion artifacts.[3–5] Moreover, no reliable gastrointestinal contrast material exists for MRI, whereas abdominal CT examinations are routinely improved by oral administration of dilute barium or iodine solutions.[6]

To date, research and development by manufacturers and educational programs by universities have emphasized CNS imaging. Despite technical limitations and initial pessimism regarding abdominal MRI, significant advances have occurred in recent years. The use of *T1* weighted spin-echo (SE) imaging techniques with short *TR*–short *TE* reduces motion artifacts, improves anatomic resolution, and obviates the need for respiratory gating. Clinical advantages achieved by using *T1* weighted versus *T2* weighted imaging techniques will be reviewed, and potential abdominal applications of paramagnetic contrast enhancement will be discussed.

The tremendous flexibility of MR imaging techniques offers the advantage of tailoring examinations to a specific clinical question. Selection of appropriate imaging techniques can dramatically improve both anatomic resolution and tissue characterization information, which determine the clinical value of abdominal MR examinations. Furthermore, economic considerations such as patient throughput and examination costs are directly affected by selection of efficient techniques.

General technical principles will be illustrated with examples of clinical applications in which MRI is likely to become a primary diagnostic modality (e.g., screening for liver metastases) as well as unique applications of MRI as a secondary diagnostic modality (e.g., for evaluation of hepatic iron overload).

ANATOMIC CONSIDERATIONS

Motion Artifacts. The principal factor limiting clinical applications of MRI in the abdomen is physiologic motion (cardiac, respiratory, and peristaltic). Respiratory or cardiac gating has been used to reduce motion artifacts.[4,5] Both methods synchronize data acquisition to physiologic signals. Cardiac gating is simplified by availability of an electronic trigger (the electrocardiographic ''R-wave'') and periodicity of the cardiac cycle.[7] Respiratory gating is much more difficult to implement and requires a mechanical linkage to convert chest wall motion into an electrical signal. Furthermore, respiratory motion is neither periodic nor constant in amplitude. As a result, only imperfect synchronization of data acquisition is possible, and this is often achieved by rejecting data from unwanted portions of the respiratory cycle (Fig. 29–1).

For most abdominal imaging applications, both cardiac and respiratory gating require unacceptable tradeoffs. Cardiac gating physiologically limits *TR* to a minimum of 500 ms (corresponding to a heart rate of 120 beats per minute) and therefore limits the selection of image contrast (i.e., limited to *T2* weighted SE techniques). On the other hand, respiratory gating allows free selection of *TR* and *TE* but requires rejection of data from portions of the respiratory cycle. For example, by accepting data from a portion of the respiratory cycle such as end-expiration, motion artifacts are reduced but imaging time is increased in direct proportion to the fractional time of the respiratory cycle that is excluded.[5] In practice, this has resulted in unacceptable increases in imaging time. Although first-generation respiratory gating has not been widely used, newer techniques have been proposed that do not sacrifice imaging time.[8]

ROPE (respiratory ordered phase encoding), COPE (centrally ordered phase encoding), and EXORCIST differ from conventional respiratory gating in that data are acquired throughout the entire respiratory cycle. These techniques are effective because pulse repetitions used for different phase-encoding steps (MR images are usually generated using 128 or 256 phase-encoding steps) are "ordered" in a way so as to reduce inconsistencies due to motion that occurs in the time interval between steps. Whereas ungated images and conventional respiratory gated images proceed in a linear fashion from 0 to 128 steps (phase angles), ordered phase encoding selects a desirable

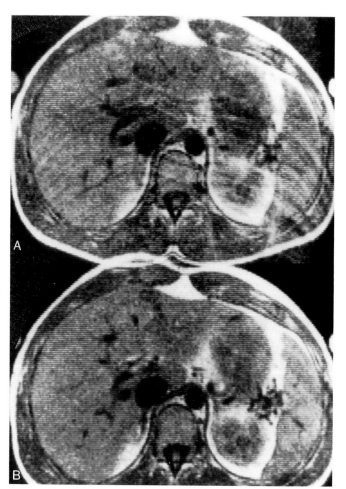

Figure 29–1. *A,* Transverse SE 500/28 image of the liver shows ghost artifacts from the high signal intensity subcutaneous fat projected across the liver and outside the patient. Anatomic resolution is decreased for small structures, such as the right adrenal gland. *B,* Respiratory gating reduces spatial misregistration of the subcutaneous fat and improves image quality. Examination time is typically increased by 50 percent. (Courtesy of Joel Blank, Ph.D., Diasonics NMR, Inc.)

phase angle for each phase of the respiratory cycle.[8] Naturally, this requires monitoring the respiratory cycle during imaging. Although imaging time is not prolonged, additional time is necessary to set up the device for monitoring respiration. Furthermore, techniques directed at respiratory motion artifacts do not reduce artifacts due to cardiac and aortic pulsations or peristalsis. Nevertheless, respiratory motion is the major contributor to abdominal ghost artifacts, and initial results with these techniques have been quite promising.

Another solution to the problem of physiologic motion has recently emerged from innovative adaptation of pulse-sequence timing parameters.[9] Motion artifacts resemble other types of image noise in that they are reduced by signal averaging. Selection of short TR spin-echo (SE) technique allows averaging of a large number of data acquisitions without prolonging imaging time. For example, using a TR of 260 ms, 18 data acquisitions can be averaged with a total imaging time of 10 minutes. On the other hand, selection of a 2000 ms TR allows averaging of only two data acquisitions with a 9 minute scan time.

Abdominal MR images obtained using short TR–short TE technique with averaging of multiple data acquisitions show dramatic reductions in motion artifacts and image noise (Fig. 29–2). Indeed, this appears to be a solution that simultaneously reduces cardiac, respiratory, and peristaltic motion artifacts. This technique results in greatly improved resolution of abdominal anatomy. The tradeoff for increased anatomic resolution using this technique is in the restriction of image contrast to tissue $T1$ differences.

Multislice Imaging. Multislice two-dimensional MR imaging techniques are time-efficient and essential for abdominal imaging.[10,11] Imaging systems that interleaf contiguous slices with minimal gaps between slices are preferred. The operator has free selection of slice thickness, typically ranging from 7 to 20 mm. It is important to note that the maximum number of slices that can be obtained with a given pulse-sequence technique is limited by TR and TE according to the formula:

$$\text{Maximum number of slices} = \frac{TR}{TE + \text{constant}}$$

$$\text{e.g., 11 slices} = \frac{500 \text{ ms}}{30 \text{ ms} + 12 \text{ ms}}$$

Where the 12 ms "constant" will vary between different imaging systems and is a function of gradient performance.

It follows from this equation that more slices can be obtained with large TR values and that the number of slices increases as TE is decreased. This formula has considerable practical importance. For example, transverse images of the liver must span a 15 cm craniocaudal distance in the average patient if the entire liver is to be included on a single study. Selection of a SE 500/30 pulse sequence allows up to 11 slices and therefore is compatible with the use of 1.5 cm thick slices to cover the entire liver. Use of $T2$ weighted imaging techniques with longer TR values may allow more slices; however, use of longer TE (180 ms or more) can become the limiting factor. Our fast spin-echo (short TR–short TE) technique permits simultaneous acquisition of 12 contiguous slices and therefore includes the entire liver in a single 10 minute examination time (Fig. 29–3).

Spatial Resolution. Volume element voxel dimensions must be selected with several tradeoffs in mind. As shown above, increasing slice thickness offers practical gains in terms of reduced examination time and increased patient throughput. We routinely use 1.5 cm slice thickness to screen the liver for focal lesions (Figs. 29–2 and 29–3). Supplemental thin-slice (0.5 to 1.0 cm) images are obtained in selected cases. Choice of

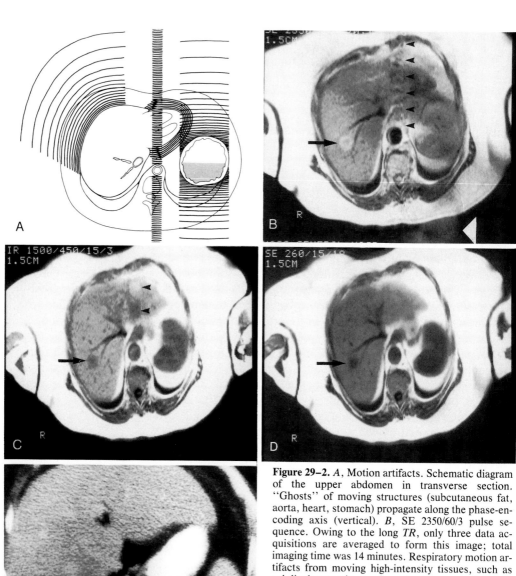

Figure 29–2. *A*, Motion artifacts. Schematic diagram of the upper abdomen in transverse section. "Ghosts" of moving structures (subcutaneous fat, aorta, heart, stomach) propagate along the phase-encoding axis (vertical). *B*, SE 2350/60/3 pulse sequence. Owing to the long *TR*, only three data acquisitions are averaged to form this image; total imaging time was 14 minutes. Respiratory motion artifacts from moving high-intensity tissues, such as subdiaphragmatic and subcutaneous fat, are projected outside the patient (large arrowhead). Artifacts due to pulsatile motion of the aorta are also seen and interfere with examination of the left hepatic lobe (small arrowheads). A high-intensity lesion (long *T2*) is seen in the right hepatic lobe (arrow). *C*, IR 1500/450/15/3 pulse sequence obtained by averaging three data acquisitions required 10 minutes of imaging time. Ghost artifacts resulting from aortic pulsations are seen overlying the left hepatic lobe (arrowheads). The right lobe lesion now has a low signal intensity (arrow) owing to its long *T1*. *D*, SE 260/15/ 18 image obtained by averaging 18 data acquisitions required an imaging time of 10 minutes. The image is less grainy (less noisy); detailed vascular anatomy is well seen. The left hepatic lobe is visualized free of motion artifacts, and the single right hepatic lobe lesion is easily identified (arrow). *E*, CT scan with bolus contrast administration missed the lesion shown by MRI. In this patient, a total of four lesions, all missed by CT, were shown by MRI.

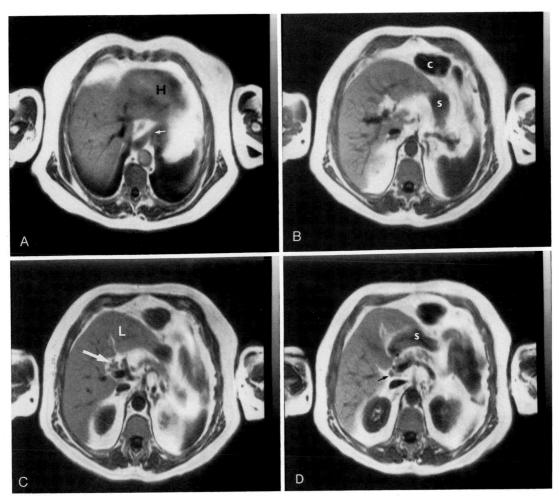

Figure 29–3. Normal abdominal anatomy obtained using a SE 260/15/18 pulse sequence; averaging of 18 data acquisitions resulted in a scan time of 10 minutes. *A*, The right hepatic vein, intrahepatic inferior vena cava, and gastroesophageal junction (arrow) are seen. Artifacts from cardiac motion, aortic pulsation, and respiratory excursions are not present. *B*, The caudate lobe of the liver is seen between the portal vein and inferior vena cava. Both the right and the left adrenal glands are visualized. Colon (c), stomach (s). *C*, Detailed anatomy of porta hepatis. The celiac, splenic, and hepatic arteries are seen. A convoluted cystic duct of intermediate signal intensity is seen (arrow) lateral to the hepatic artery and anterior to the portal vein. The falciform ligament (fat, high signal intensity) is seen to contain the ascending left portal vein (low signal intensity) and demarcates the lateral segment of the left hepatic lobe (L). *D*, The pancreatic body can be distinguished from collapsed gastric antrum (s) by delineation of the fatty retroperitoneal tissue plane and by the lower signal intensity of the gastric antrum. Lateral to the pancreatic neck, the gastroduodenal and retroduodenal arteries are seen as low signal intensity structures. The normal-sized distal common bile duct is also seen in cross section and has an intermediate signal intensity (arrow). *E*, The pancreatic head is delineated and can be distinguished from adjacent duodenum and gallbladder (arrow). The left and right renal veins and right renal artery are seen. *F*, The pancreatic head and uncinate process are distinguished from the descending duodenum (arrow). Note the left renal artery and vein. *G*, The transverse duodenum is seen as a low-intensity structure (and can be distinguished from the higher signal intensity pancreatic head on more cephalic sections). High signal intensity within the inferior vena cava (arrow) indicates that this is the bottom slice produced by a multislice imaging technique. Inflowing blood has a high signal intensity owing to its greater magnetization. *H*, SE 2000/60/3 image obtained by averaging three data acquisitions; total imaging time was 15 minutes. This *T2* weighted image corresponds to *D*. The gallbladder shows a dramatic increase in signal intensity that is due to the long *T2* relaxation time of bile. Contrast between fat and abdominal viscera is decreased. Anatomic delineation is further degraded by motion artifacts. Chemical-shift artifact is seen as a low-intensity line at interfaces between retroperitoneal fat and water-containing viscera (arrows); the opposite side shows a high signal intensity line (arrowheads). On *T1* weighted images this artifact is present but is not conspicuous.

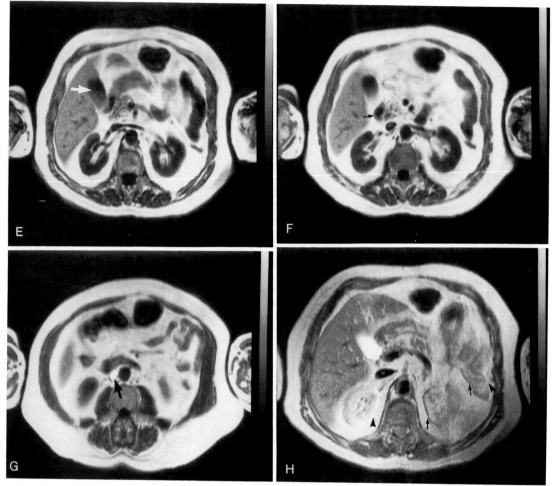

Figure 29–3. *Continued*

in-plane spatial resolution, i.e., picture element (pixel) size, requires a direct tradeoff between spatial resolution and imaging time according to the following formula:

$$\text{Exam time} = \begin{array}{c}(\text{\# of } Y\text{-lines} \\ \text{resolved})\end{array} \times \begin{array}{c}(\text{\# of} \\ \text{excitations})\end{array} \times \begin{array}{c}(\text{Pulse sequence} \\ \text{repetition time } TR)\end{array}$$

$$\text{e.g., 10 min} = 128 \times 18 \times 0.26 \text{ sec}$$

Examination time is proportional to spatial resolution along the in-plane phase-encoded dimension (Y), as resolution of each Y-line requires a separate pulse repetition (TR). Averaging of multiple data acquisitions to improve image signal-to-noise (S/N) ratio also has a direct time penalty. It should be noted that slice selection (Z-dimension for transverse images) and the in-plane frequency-encoded dimension (X-dimension for transverse images) do not have a time penalty. For most abdominal applications, MR images are obtained with 128 phase-encoded lines and 256 frequency-encoded points along each line. For a field of view that measures 46×46 cm, the resultant pixel size is 3.6×1.8 mm.

Gastrointestinal Contrast Material. Oral administration of paramagnetic compounds has been utilized in attempts to develop a bowel contrast material analogous to the radiographic agents used for CT.[6] Although paramagnetic contrast agents can be used to increase or decrease signal from the gastric lumen (or colon, following rectal administration), reliable alteration of duodenal and small bowel image signal intensity has not yet been achieved (Fig. 29–4). Orally administered paramagnetic agents have not been successful distal to the ligament of Treitz, presumably owing to changes in pH and reduced solubility or changes in ion solvation resulting from secretory and adsorptive processes in the jejunum. Unfortunately, the lack of small bowel contrast is the greatest remaining problem in abdominal MRI. Small bowel loops adjacent to the liver, pancreas, and retroperitoneal structures are easily mistaken for pathologic masses. Furthermore, peristaltic motion of bowel loops contributes to image noise and reduced anatomic resolution.

Pending availability of a reliable small bowel contrast agent, we have employed short *TR* multiple-average imaging techniques to reduce motion artifacts due to peristalsis (Figs. 29–2 and 29–3). An additional advantage of this *T1* weighted imaging technique is that the fluid-containing bowel lumen has a very low signal intensity and can often be distinguished from abdominal viscera that have higher signal intensity (Fig. 29–3*D–G*). Nonetheless, development of a reliable small bowel contrast agent will be necessary for routine use of abdominal MRI.

Surface Coils. Most examinations are performed using a circumferential "saddle" type radio frequency (rf) coil that serves as an antenna for both transmission and reception. This coil design has the advantage of a large uniform sensitive volume that allows acquisition of images with a large field of view. "Surface" coils have recently become available for clinical studies.[12] A surface coil can be placed adjacent to an anatomic region of interest to replace the receiver functions of the circumferential coil, which usually remains in use as a transmitter only (Fig. 29–5). Surface coils have the advantage of improved rf signal reception, resulting in greater image S/N levels.[13] The disadvantages of surface coils are their small field of view and the nonuniformity of their sensitive volume. As a result, signal intensity is greatest for subcutaneous fat and falls off with distance from the center of the surface coil (Fig. 29–6). This nonuniformity may interfere with comparison of tissue signal intensities and calculation of relaxation times. However, computer programs are being developed to normalize surface coil images over the field of view.

Surface coils are particularly useful for examination of superficial structures such as the cervical and lumbar spine.[12] For examination of abdominal viscera, large surface coils, 15 to 30 cm in diameter, offer significant gains in S/N and allow improved visualization of selected organs. An additional advantage of abdominal surface coil MRI is reduction of motion artifacts.[14] Signal from moving structures outside the coil's

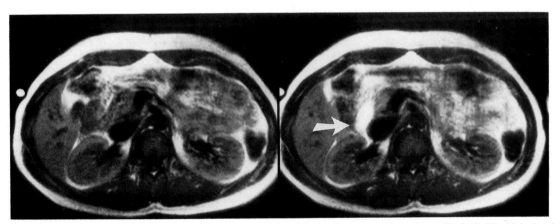

Figure 29–4. MR images of a normal volunteer before and after drinking iron-ammonium citrate (Geritol). The high signal intensity in the duodenum (arrow) is attributable to paramagnetic effects of soluble ferric ions, which shorten the *T1* relaxation time of bowel contents. (Courtesy of Dr. C. Leon Partain.)

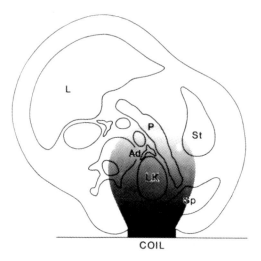

Figure 29–5. Schematic drawing of a surface coil positioned to examine the left adrenal gland. The patient is in a left posterior oblique (LPO) position. The "sensitive volume" of radio frequency (rf) signal reception is small (shaded area), permitting only a limited field of view. Signal reception falls off from tissues distant from the surface coil, as indicated by shading.

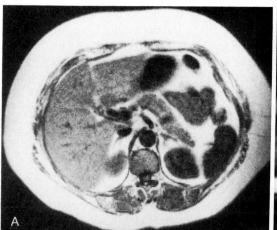

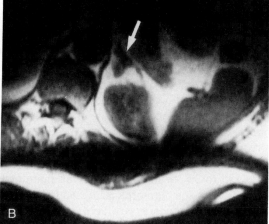

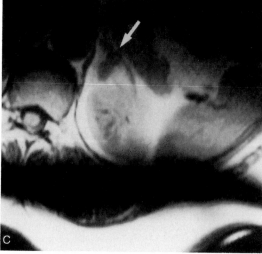

Figure 29–6. Patient with a functioning left adrenal adenoma. *A*, Transverse MR image obtained using a circumferential body coil. Pulse sequence = SE 500/30; slice thickness = 1.0 cm. *B*, Surface coil image at the same level, obtained with the same pulse sequence technique, has greater signal-to-noise (S/N) ratio and therefore can be acquired with greater spatial resolution (slice thickness 0.75 cm, pixel size 0.9 × 0.9 mm). Improved anatomic resolution now demonstrates enlargement of the medial adrenal limb (arrow). The dark band covering the left paraspinous muscle results from utilization of this prototype surface coil in both the transmit and the receive modes. *C*, Surface coil image obtained using a SE 2000/30 technique (*T2* weighted image). Note the absence of artifacts from respiratory or peristaltic motion. The bowel and liver are anterior to and outside the surface coil's field of view and therefore cannot project artifact over the retroperitoneum.

sensitive volume cannot cause image artifacts. For example, positioning a surface coil beneath the adrenal gland improves S/N for the anatomic region of interest and excludes signal from more anterior structures, such as the bowel and anterior abdominal wall. Surface-coil MR imaging of the liver has shown the potential for improved detection of small surface metastases.[13]

TISSUE CHARACTERIZATION

The ability of MRI to characterize normal and abnormal tissues is based upon the ability of specific pulse-sequence techniques to detect differences in one or more MR tissue parameter(s) as differences in signal intensity on the image gray scale (image contrast). Four distinct tissue parameters contribute to the appearance of MR images:
1. Hydrogen density
2. Motion
   A. Flow—macroscopic
   B. Diffusion—microscopic
3. Chemical shift
4. Relaxation times
   A. $T1$ = longitudinal
   B. $T2$ = transverse

Depending upon the imaging technique chosen, each parameter has a different degree of influence on image contrast. **Hydrogen density** usually has the least influence, as only fat differs significantly from other tissue (adipose tissue has approximately 50 percent greater hydrogen density than liver).[15] **Macroscopic motion** in the form of blood flow is responsible for the superb delineation of blood vessels. The contribution of diffusion to MR image contrast appears to be small but requires further study.[16]

Chemical shift, i.e., differences in resonant frequency between hydrogen nuclei chemically bound to different molecules, is relevant to abdominal imaging in two respects: First, the difference in hydrogen resonant frequency for water and fat molecules is responsible for "chemical shift artifact" on conventional MR images.[17] This artifact can be seen as a spatial misregistration along the frequency encoded axis at interfaces between water-containing viscera and fat-containing retroperitoneal adipose tissue (see Fig. 29–3H). It is important to note that lipids in cell membranes of the liver, brain, and all other organs are not "observable" by MRI and therefore do not cause artifacts or contribute to image signal intensity. In normal subjects only adipose tissue and bone marrow contain both MR-observable water and fat (in the form of triglycerides).

One clinical disorder that can be studied by chemical shift imaging is fatty infiltration of the liver.[18] Conventional MR imaging techniques have not been sensitive for detection of fatty infiltration of the liver, as they do not discriminate fat signal from water signal.[18–20] Dixon[21] has introduced a novel spectroscopic imaging technique that retains excellent anatomic resolution. This technique separates liver water signal intensity from liver fat signal intensity (Figs. 29–7 and 29–8). Although detection of fatty liver itself may be of limited clinical significance, fat-water contrast can be manipulated to improve detection of liver metastases in patients with fatty liver (Fig. 29–9A–B).[22,23]

Although pure "fat" and "water" images can be calculated using the Dixon method, the intermediary "opposed-phase" image often contains the necessary diagnostic information.[21] Phase-contrast (opposed-phase) images are generated by modifying conventional (in-phase) SE or IR techniques, resulting in images with tissue contrast dependent on both relaxation effects and chemical shift. Opposed-phase images are obtained by moving the gradient-induced spin echo 5.4 ms (at 0.6 tesla) off center with respect to the Hahn spin echo induced by the 180 degree pulse.[21] Temporal dis-

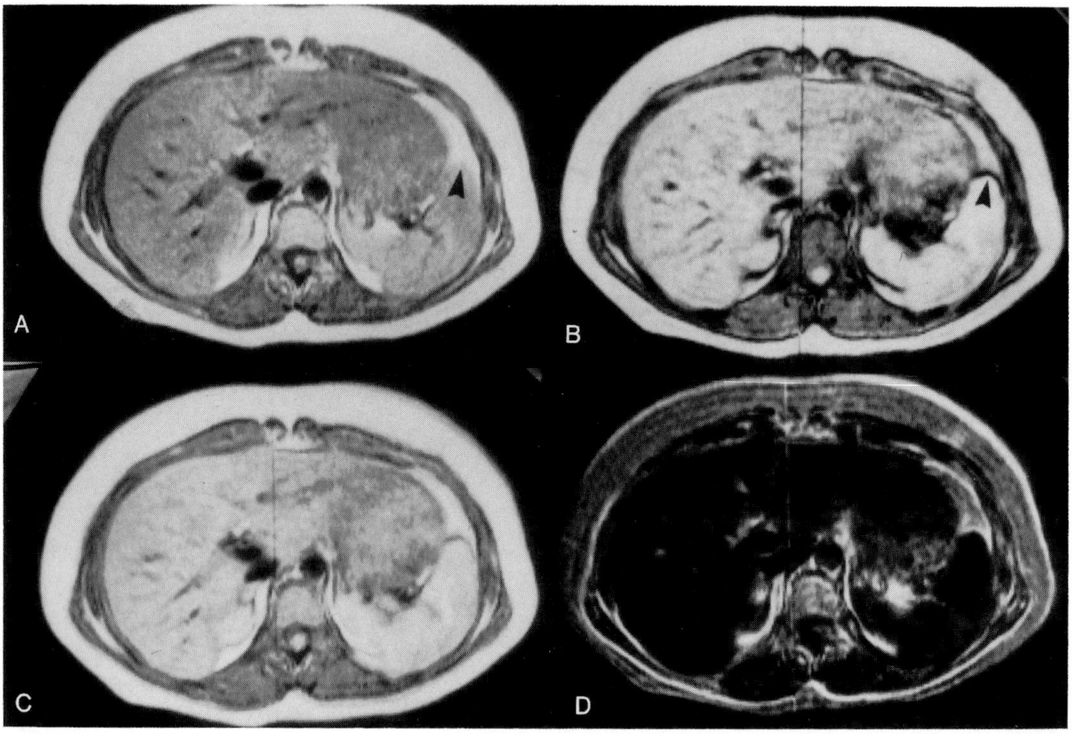

Figure 29–7. Chemical-shift imaging of the liver in a normal volunteer. *A*, Conventional "in-phase" SE 1500/30 image shows the spleen to have a slightly higher signal intensity than the liver. *B*, Phase contrast ("opposed-phase") SE 1500/30 image again shows the nonfatty spleen to have a slightly higher signal intensity than the normal, nonfatty liver. A dark band of signal intensity (arrowhead) demarcates interfaces between water-containing viscera and fat-containing adipose tissue. *C*, Calculated "water" image is derived by adding the in-phase (*A*) and opposed-phase (*B*) images. This image is similar to *A*, indicating that all the liver and spleen signal intensity is from water. *D*, Calculated "fat" image is derived by subtracting the opposed-phase image (*B*) from the in-phase image (*A*). The absence of signal from the spleen and liver indicates that neither tissue contains MR-observable fat. The ambiguous appearance of subcutaneous gas is due to magnitude reconstruction and has been explained in detail by Dixon.[21]

placement of the refocused echo by 5.4 ms corresponds to $1/[2(V_f - V_w)]$ where $V_f - V_w$ is the resonance frequency difference between fat and water protons. This resonance frequency difference is the product of the resonance frequency of the imaging system (25.1 MHz) and the chemical shift between fat and water protons expressed as parts per million (3.7 ppm). As a result of displacing the gradient and Hahn echoes by $\frac{1}{2}$ precession cycle (5.4 ms $\times$ 93 Hz), the phases of fat and water magnetization are 180 degrees opposed at the time of the gradient-induced spin echo. Therefore, in the resulting "opposed-phase" image, pixel brightness is the net difference between fat and water magnetization.[21]

MR-observable lipid, possibly triglyceride ("fatty liver"), is present in the majority of patients with liver cancer.[22,23] Since noncancerous liver tissue contains the predominant amount of observable lipid, the phase-contrast technique can improve cancer-liver contrast, thereby enhancing lesion detectability. With the use of appropriate *T2* weighted pulse sequences, MR examinations are improved by employing the phase-contrast technique. Unfortunately, as *T2* weighted phase contrast imaging of the liver requires use of long *TR* pulse sequences,[23] motion artifacts remain a problem and scan times are long.

Opposed-phase images alter cancer-liver contrast (signal difference, SD; scaled to background noise this is expressed as the signal difference–to–noise ratio, SD/N) by decreasing the signal intensity of fatty liver tissue; cancer signal intensity shows little

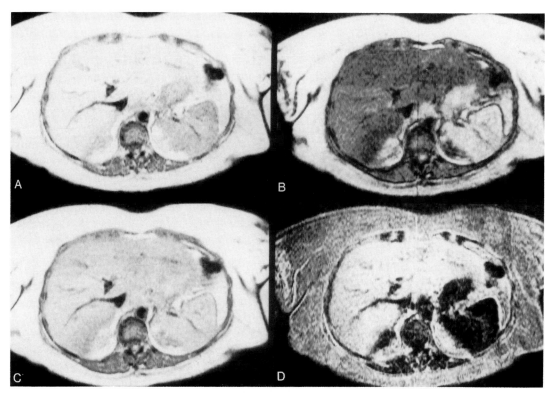

Figure 29–8. Chemical-shift imaging of the liver showing diffuse fatty change in a patient with alcoholic pancreatitis. *A*, Conventional "in-phase" SE 1500/30 image shows the liver to have a slightly greater signal intensity than the spleen. This subtle increase in intensity is due to admixture of high-intensity fat signal with the lower signal intensity of normal liver tissue. *B*, Phase-contrast "opposed-phase" SE 1500/30 image shows a dramatic decrease in signal intensity relative to the spleen. This finding is diagnostic of fatty liver. *C–D*, Calculated "water" image and "fat" image show no MR-observable fat in the spleen but considerable fat signal intensity in the liver.

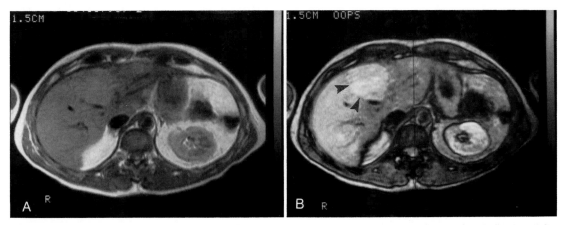

Figure 29–9. Chemical-shift and conventional MR imaging in metastatic liver cancer. *A*, Conventional "in-phase" SE 2000/30 image (*T2* weighted) shows only a subtle difference in signal intensity between the left and right hepatic lobes. *B*, Chemical-shift "phase contrast" (opposed-phase) SE 2000/30 image shows a high-intensity mass (arrowheads) consistent with metastatic cancer. Overall hepatic signal intensity is decreased owing to diffuse fatty infiltration; the metastasis does not contain MR-observable fat, and its signal intensity relative to surrounding liver is increased.

or no change. Total cancer-liver SD/N is the summation of contrast due to phase-contrast (chemical shift) effects and contrast due to conventional relaxation effects. Cancer-liver contrast is additive on *T2* weighted opposed-phase pulse sequences, as both the *T2* relaxation time difference and the MR-observable fat content difference tend to decrease liver signal intensity relative to cancer. Conversely, *T1* weighted opposed-phase pulse sequences show loss of cancer-liver contrast, as the *T1* relaxation time difference decreases cancer signal intensity and the MR-observable fat content difference decreases liver signal intensity. Although *T1* weighted pulse sequences do not benefit from the phase-contrast technique, excellent SD/N can be achieved using conventional in-phase technique by selecting optimal timing parameters to maximize contrast due to cancer-liver *T1* differences (see Fig. 29–3).[31] Furthermore, conventional *T1* weighted images compared directly with *T2* weighted (conventional or phase-contrast) images show greater cancer-liver contrast and better anatomic resolution (Fig. 29–9).[23] Therefore, when optimal *T1* weighted imaging techniques are available, *T2* weighted phase-contrast imaging should be used in a secondary, complementary fashion.

Tissue relaxation times, *T1* and *T2*, are by far the most important parameters for selection of the proper MR imaging technique. Large differences in *T1* and *T2* between normal and abnormal tissues are responsible for the superb soft tissue contrast of conventional MR images. Although both *T1* and *T2* increase in nearly all pathologic conditions, it is important to note that *T1* and *T2* have opposite effects on image signal intensity. Long *T1* relaxation times lead to decreased signal intensity, whereas long *T2* relaxation times lead to increased signal intensity. It is possible to mask pathologic increases in *T1* and *T2* by allowing both *T1* and *T2* to influence image contrast. Therefore, imaging techniques should be selected to maximize either *T1* or *T2* contrast, but not both.

LIVER CANCER DETECTION

Detection of liver metastases by MR is dependent upon both anatomic resolution and image display of differential tissue characteristics as cancer-liver contrast (signal intensity difference, SD). Anatomic resolution is a complex function of image geometry (spatial resolution) and S/N ratios. For example, decreased signal intensity or increased background noise results in a dark or grainy image with poor resolution of normal anatomic structures (Fig. 29–10*C*). Motion artifacts also degrade MR images in a complex manner. For example, respiratory motion causes blurring (reduced edge sharpness), while aortic pulsations result in "ghost" artifacts, obscuring the left hepatic lobe (see Fig. 29–2).

MR pulse-sequence performance quantitated by signal difference(SD)–to–noise (SD/N) values correlates with anatomic resolution and conspicuousness of hepatic metastases.[23] The data in Table 29–1 allow direct comparison of pulse-sequence performance and resolve previous uncertainty[24–27] in selection of MR techniques for the evaluation of hepatic metastases. Significant differences exist among the six widely available spin-echo pulse sequences. Several studies[25–27] have shown the SE 2000/60 sequence superior to the SE 2000/30 sequence for detection of hepatic metastases (Fig. 29–10*A–B*). Furthermore, it is evident that the SE 500/30 technique has superior anatomic resolution but is inferior to the SE 2000/60 technique for demonstration of metastases *when the same number of data acquisitions are used* (Figs. 29–10*B* and 29–12*A*).[25–27] However, it is inappropriate to compare an 18-minute SE 2000/60 pulse sequence (acquired by averaging four data acquisitions [acquisition = data set = buffer]) with a 4.5-minute SE 500/30 pulse sequence also obtained by averaging four

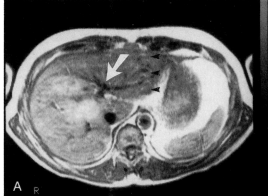
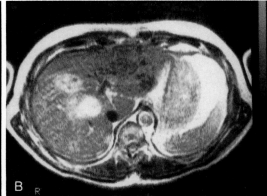
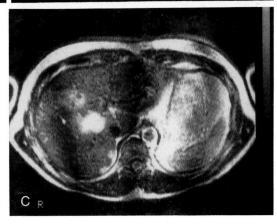

Figure 29–10. Liver metastases. *T2* weighted spin-echo images. *A*, SE 2000/30/2 acquisition (9 minute) image shows two metastases to the right hepatic lobe as poorly marginated, high-intensity lesions. The left hepatic lobe is partially obscured by motion artifacts (''ghosts'') from aortic pulsation (arrowheads). The ascending left portal vein is divided into branches supplying the medial and lateral segments (arrow). *B*, SE 2000/60/2 image. The metastases are better seen because of increased contrast with the surrounding liver. However, the image is grainy, and anatomic resolution of structures such as the left portal vein is decreased owing to a decreased signal-to-noise ratio as compared with the *TE* = 30 ms image. Aortic pulsation artifact again obscures part of the left hepatic lobe. *C*, SE 2000/90/2 image shows further increase in contrast between metastases and liver, allowing identification of additional lesions. However, a markedly decreased signal-to-noise ratio has greatly reduced anatomic resolution, and the left portal vein is obscured.

data sets. Quantitative comparison of pulse sequences requires image acquisition using identical imaging times (isotime) or standardization of noise measurements to reflect the known relationship between background noise levels and imaging time.[28,29] The data shown in Table 29–1 reflect SD/N values corrected for differences in imaging times.

T2 Weighted SE Imaging. The selection of techniques for abdominal studies has been limited to pulse sequences developed primarily for use in the CNS. Because CNS pathology is most reliably detected using *T2* weighted SE sequences, these have become widely available and manufacturers have emphasized their advantages. Consequently, the SE 2000/60 sequence was initially recommended for evaluation of hepatic metastases.[26,27]

Until recently, MR images obtained with *TE* greater than 60 ms have been unavailable or technically inadequate owing to low S/N levels and artifacts due to poor gradient performance. Improvements in gradient design now allow imaging with *TE* of 180 ms or longer.[30] Statistically significant increases in cancer-liver SD/N and improved conspicuousness of hepatic metastases are achieved when *TE* is increased from 60 ms to 90 (Fig. 29–1*C*) or 120 ms (Table 29–1).[31] These results are in agreement with a previous experience in a series of 22 patients with liver metastases in which the SE 2000/120 sequence offered the maximum cancer-liver SD/N and was superior to both *TE* = 60 and *TE* = 180.[30] The data in Table 29–1 also show that *T2* weighted SE pulse sequences should be obtained using *TR* of at least 2000 ms. This finding is explained by the long *T1* relaxation times of metastases (Table 29–2), which prevent complete recovery of longitudinal magnetization at *TR* = 1500 ms. Unfortunately, increasing *TR*

Table 29–1. CANCER-LIVER SD/N

			Rank Order of Performance	
Pulse Sequence	(N)	SD/N Magnitude	SD/N	Confidence Factor
SE 1500/30	7	1.9 ± 0.9	14	
SE 1500/60	7	3.5 ± 3.0	12	
SE 1500/90	6	5.5 ± 4.2	9	
SE 2000/30	27	2.4 ± 2.1	13	9
SE 2000/60	33	4.7 ± 3.6	10	8
SE 2000/90	27	7.5 ± 5.3	5	7
SE 2000/120	5	7.7 ± 3.4	4	
SE 2000/180	4	4.2 ± 2.0	11	
IR 1500/450/30	33	6.2 ± 3.6	8	5
IR 1500/450/18	35	7.9 ± 4.2	3	3
IR 1500/280/18	30	7.2 ± 3.7	6	2
SE 500/30	37	6.4 ± 4.1	7	6
SE 260/30	32	8.1 ± 4.6	2	4
SE 260/18	39	10.3 ± 5.2	1	1

(N) = Number of patients studied; SD/N magnitude = mean ± standard deviation of cancer-liver signal difference–to–noise ratio.
SD/N data are corrected to a standard 9-minute scan time.
Significant differences ($p < 0.05$) between cancer-liver SD/N values were as follows:
    SE 260/18 rank 1:   SD/N greater than all other sequences.
    Sequences rank 2, 3, 5, 6:   SD/N greater than sequences rank 10–14.
    Sequences rank 7, 8:   SD/N greater than sequences rank 13, 14.
Confidence factor: (mean SD/N)/(standard deviation of SD/N).
This analyis is performed for samples (N) of 27 or more; pulse sequences used on seven or fewer patients were not ranked.

and *TE* to improve *T2* contrast requires an unfavorable tradeoff of reduced signal averaging, decreased S/N, increased sensitivity to motion artifacts, and decreased anatomic resolution.

T1 Weighted IR Imaging. Studies reporting in vivo relaxation times for liver metastases and surrounding liver tissue have shown that cancer-liver *T1* differences are substantially greater than *T2* differences (Table 29–2). Theoretical analyses of image contrast that consider image noise and standardized examination times predict that *T1* weighted images should offer greater cancer-liver contrast than *T2* weighted images.[28,29] IR sequences are superior to *T2* weighted SE sequences with respect to SD/N, S/N,

Table 29–2. RELAXATION TIMES OF LIVER CANCER

		Moss et al.[25]	Schmidt et al.[27]	Stark*
T1 ms	Liver	533	350	499 ± 140
	Cancer	746	730	876 ± 334
	(increase)	40%	109%	76%
T2 ms	Liver	56	46	48 ± 11
	Cancer	68	68	78 ± 32
	(increase)	21%	49%	63%
Proton density	Liver			583 ± 151
	Cancer			606 ± 154
	(increase)			4%
	ln2			
Field strength		0.35 T	0.35 T	0.6 T

* Unpublished data; based upon 40 patients, fitting three or more spin-echo measurements for each relaxation time determination. Hydrogen density is relative on an arbitrary scale.

and resultant lesion conspicuousness (Figs. 29–10 and 29–11).[31] Reduction of *TE* to 18 ms or less improves the performance of IR sequences by increasing both SD/N and S/N over the IR 1500/450/30 sequence (see Table 29–1). Centering the 90 degree pulse of the IR sequence near the inversion or "null" point of magnetization recovery for cancer tissue (at time *TI* = 280 ms) has the negative effect of decreasing liver S/N but has the benefit of increasing cancer-liver contrast (Fig. 29–11*C*).

T1 Weighted SE Imaging. Theoretical predictions that optimized *T1* weighted sequences (short *TR*) are time-efficient and offer superior SD/N performance for tissue discrimination[28,29] have been confirmed (see Table 29–1).[31] Currently, the SE 500/30 sequence enjoys widespread use owing to its relatively high S/N and good anatomic resolution (Fig. 29–12*A*). Unfortunately, this pulse sequence is unsuitable for cancer-liver discrimination because of balanced *T1* and *T2* contrast effects that result in low image SD/N and poor lesion conspicuousness (Fig. 29–12*A*). Reducing the *TR* to 260 ms has several beneficial effects: First, *T1* weighting is increased, improving cancer-liver contrast (Fig. 29–12*B*). Second, more data acquisitions can be averaged within a standard imaging time, preserving S/N and anatomic resolution. Third, signal averaging reduces artifacts due to physiologic motion.

Reduction in *TE* complements reductions in *TR* by further increasing *T1* dependent image contrast, increasing S/N, and further reducing motion artifacts. The SE 260/18 sequence has cancer-liver SD/N values that are significantly better than all other imaging techniques evaluated to date. Furthermore, this technique has the greatest S/N values and greatest anatomic resolution.[31]

It must be noted that the "optimal" pulse sequence will vary with field strength owing to the frequency dependence of tissue *T1* relaxation times.[13–15] Additionally, image noise will behave differently in different imaging systems. Therefore, these spe-

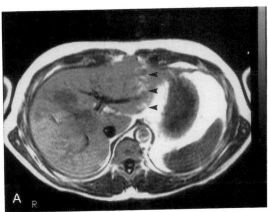
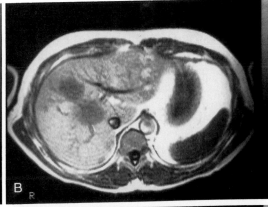
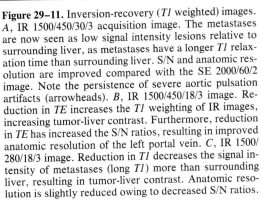
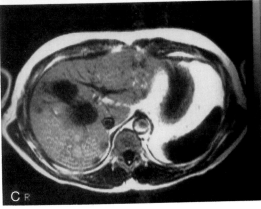

Figure 29–11. Inversion-recovery (*T1* weighted) images. *A*, IR 1500/450/30/3 acquisition image. The metastases are now seen as low signal intensity lesions relative to surrounding liver, as metastases have a longer *T1* relaxation time than surrounding liver. S/N and anatomic resolution are improved compared with the SE 2000/60/2 image. Note the persistence of severe aortic pulsation artifacts (arrowheads). *B*, IR 1500/450/18/3 image. Reduction in *TE* increases the *T1* weighting of IR images, increasing tumor-liver contrast. Furthermore, reduction in *TE* has increased the S/N ratios, resulting in improved anatomic resolution of the left portal vein. *C*, IR 1500/280/18/3 image. Reduction in *TI* decreases the signal intensity of metastases (long *T1*) more than surrounding liver, resulting in tumor-liver contrast. Anatomic resolution is slightly reduced owing to decreased S/N ratios.

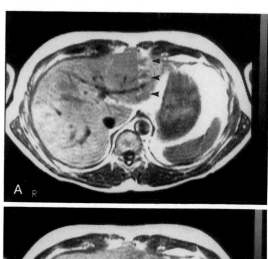
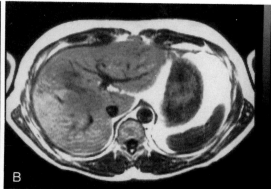
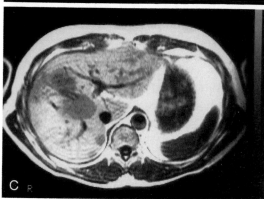

Figure 29–12. *T1* weighted spin-echo images. *A*, SE 500/30/4 (4.5 minute image). This traditional *T1* weighted sequence has poorer tumor-liver contrast than any of the *T2* weighted or IR pulse sequences. Note that the artifacts due to aortic pulsation persist (arrowheads). *B*, SE 260/30/8 (5 minute image). Reduction of *TR* allows increased signal averaging without increased examination time. Compared with the traditional SE 500/30/4 pulse sequence, tumor-liver contrast is increased, anatomic resolution of the left portal vein is improved, and motion artifacts are decreased. *C*, SE 260/18/16 (10 minute image). Reduction in *TE* further increases *T1* weighting, increasing tumor-liver contrast. Small metastases in the posterior segment of the right hepatic lobe are now easily seen. Shorter *TE* also increases the S/N ratio, improving anatomic resolution of structures such as the left portal vein. Furthermore, artifacts due to aortic pulsation are eliminated.

cific pulse-sequence recommendations are directly applicable only to Technicare 0.6 tesla systems. However, methods of pulse-sequence selection and image analysis will apply to all MR systems and, furthermore, should be generally applicable to comparative evaluations of pulse sequence performance for a variety of clinical tasks.

LIVER LESION CHARACTERIZATION

If a particular pathologic process is characterized by a unique *T1* or *T2* relaxation time, an appropriate imaging technique can be selected to display this diagnostic feature. Unfortunately, most pathologic processes nonspecifically increase both *T1* and *T2*.[19,25] Nevertheless, the ability of MR to make clinically relevant diagnoses based upon tissue-specific relaxation time differences has recently been confirmed.[30,35–37] Cavernous hemangioma of the liver is the most common benign hepatic neoplasm and is second only to liver metastases among all focal liver lesions. Cavernous hemangiomas differ from solid hepatic neoplasms in that they are essentially a fluid, a lake of slowly flowing blood. Fluids have extremely long *T1* and *T2* relaxation times and would be expected to differ significantly from solid neoplasms. We have recently shown that *T2* weighted SE images display hemangiomas as having significantly greater signal intensity than solid neoplasms.[30] Currently available MRI techniques appear to be competitive with existing CT and scintigraphic techniques for establishing a tissue-specific diagnosis of cavernous hemangioma of the liver (Fig. 29–13).

A second unique situation in which MRI can offer a tissue-specific diagnosis is pathologic iron overload.[19,37] Iron deposited in tissues in the form of ferritin, hemosiderin, or other molecular species is paramagnetic and influences tissue hydrogen

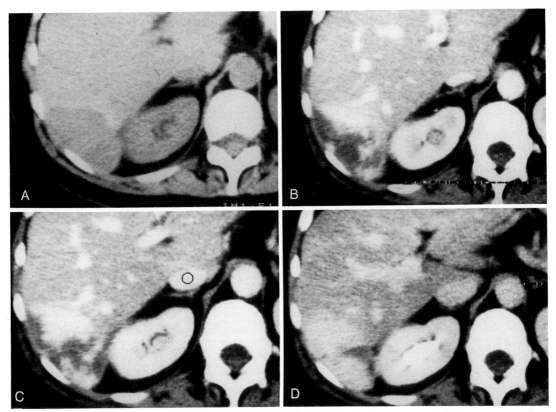

Figure 29–13. Cavernous hemangioma of the liver. *A*, CT scan without contrast shows a low-density exophytic lesion of the right hepatic lobe. *B*, Peripheral enhancement is seen during bolus contrast administration. *C*, At 60 seconds following contrast administration, further filling of the lesion is seen. *D*, Five minutes after contrast administration, near-complete filling of the lesion is seen. The lesion has higher signal intensity than adjacent liver parenchyma. This sequence of scans is considered diagnostic of cavernous hemangioma. Unfortunately, difficulty with breath holding and slice registration makes sequential visualization of small lesions difficult, and CT scans of this quality are unusual. *E*, *T1*-weighted IR 1500/450/30/4 image shows the hemangioma to have a relatively low signal intensity, indicating a long *T1* relative to adjacent liver. *F*, SE 500/30/4 image shows reduced contrast between the hemangioma and the liver. *G*, *T2*-weighted SE 2000/30/4 image shows the hemangioma to have an increased signal intensity relative to liver, indicating an increased *T2*. *H*, SE 2000/60 image shows further increase in the signal intensity of the cavernous hemangioma relative to liver (increased contrast). Motion artifacts are increased. *I*, SE 2000/120 image. The signal intensity of the cavernous hemangioma equals that of CSF in the thoracic spinal canal. The liver and even the subcutaneous fat have reduced signal intensity owing to their shorter *T2* relaxation times. *J*, SE 2000/180/4 image shows greatly reduced signal intensity from all solid tissues. The cavernous hemangioma and cerebral spinal fluid maintain a high signal intensity owing to their extremely prolonged *T2* relaxation times.

relaxation times. Endogenous iron overload predominantly shortens *T2* and is manifested on spin-echo images as decreased signal intensity (Fig. 29–14).[37] These changes can be dramatic and thus allow detection of pathologic iron overload in the liver, pancreas, and spleen. Quantitation of tissue iron levels by MRI is a subject of current research.

Paramagnetic Agents. MR contrast materials are undergoing clinical evaluations in Europe and the United States.[38–40] For example, gadolinium-DTPA is a paramagnetic ion-ligand complex that decreases both *T1* and *T2* relaxation times of nearby hydrogen nuclei. Paramagnetic contrast agents are most useful for enhancing MR image contrast when selective accumulation occurs in one of two tissues being compared. For example, Gd-DTPA has improved detectability of diverse CNS lesions by accumulating selectively in tissues with a damaged blood-brain barrier. Owing to the high concentrations of filtered Gd-DTPA in kidneys it is anticipated that this agent will be useful for delineating both functional and structural abnormalities of the genitourinary system. For

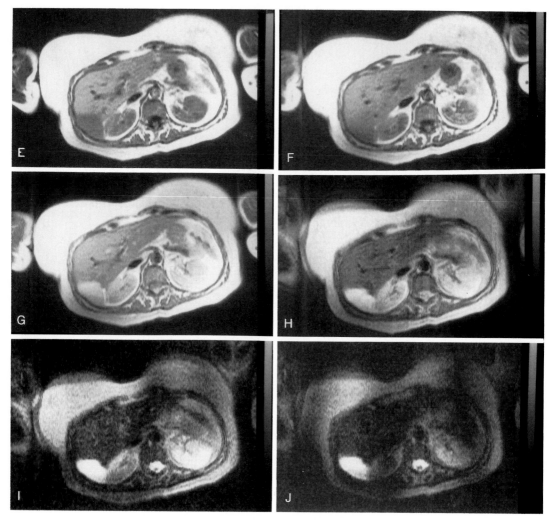

Figure 29–13. *Continued*

example, selective enhancement of functioning renal tissue is expected to increase detectability of renal neoplasms. Unfortunately, Gd-DTPA may also accumulate in tumors and, in fact, may obscure some lesions. Preliminary experience with hepatic neoplasms shows loss of tumor-liver contrast on MR images obtained following administration of Gd-DTPA.[38] It is evident that tissue-specific distribution of contrast materials is a desirable feature.

Although Gd-DTPA is distributed nonspecifically throughout the vascular and extracellular space, by analogy to iodinated (urographic) contrast agents in routine use for CT scanning some degree of tissue-specific biodistribution can be achieved. Bolus administration of Gd-DTPA favors enhancement of normal liver tissue, rather than tumor, if fast scanning techniques are employed (Fig. 29–15). Also analogous to iodine-enhanced CT scanning of liver metastases is the rim enhancement of tumors seen when Gd-DTPA is used in a similar manner.[42] One general advantage of Gd-DTPA and similar "*T1* type" paramagnetic contrast agents is the overall gain in image S/N seen during the vascular phase of agent distribution (Fig. 29–15A–B).

Tissue-Specific Contrast Agents. Paramagnetic ion complexes and nitroxides offer enormous flexibility in chemical design. For example, iron is paramagnetic and can be

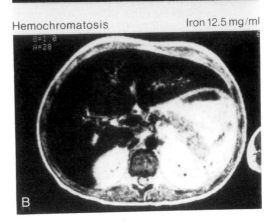

Figure 29–14. *A*, Normal child, SE 1000/28 image. The pancreas signal intensity is slightly greater than the liver, which is slightly greater than paraspinous flank muscle. *B*, Child with hemochromatosis (iron overload) secondary to repeated blood transfusions administered for treatment of thalassemia. Dramatic decrease in signal intensity of the liver relative to flank muscle is shown. Pancreatic signal intensity is also decreased; the spleen has been surgically removed.

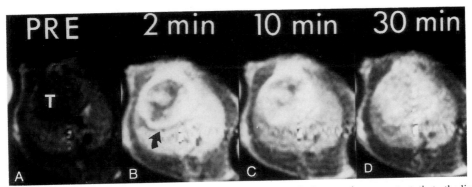

Figure 29–15. Gd-DTPA enhanced MR imaging using a rat model of adenocarcinoma metastatic to the liver. Rapid scanning at 1.4 tesla using a SE 250/15 sequence, averaging two data acquisitions for a 60-second scan time. *A*, Precontrast image. Overall image signal intensity and signal-to-noise ratios (S/N) are low. Tumor (T) is seen as a low signal intensity region because of its long *T1* relaxation time. *B–C*, Following intravenous administration of 0.2 mmol Gd-DTPA/kg, overall image S/N improves owing to generalized tissue *T1* reductions. Cancer-liver contrast (signal intensity difference [SD]) is increased. Note early rim enhancement of tumor (*B*, arrows). *D*, Delayed image at 30 minutes shows redistribution of Gd-DTPA to the tumor, reducing cancer-liver SD and obscuring the lesion.

bound to EHPG (ethylenebis-[2-hydroxyphenylglycine]), an analogue to the IDA (iminodiacetic acid) class of scintigraphic agents used for nuclear medicine studies of biliary function.[41] This prototypical tissue-specific hepatobiliary agent has shown a significant (6 percent) fraction of tissue-specific uptake and excretion by functioning hepatocytes. It is hoped that this class of agent will allow selective enhancement of functioning liver tissue and thereby improve detection of nonfunctioning hepatic neoplasms.

A novel class of particulate iron oxide MR contrast agents has recently been described.[42,43] Particulate agents show tremendous tissue specificity, as they are selectively phagocytosed by the reticuloendothelial system (RES).[43] Phagocytosis allows selective uptake of particulate materials by the liver, spleen, and bone marrow. Magnetite (Fe_3O_4) particles can be directly administered in this manner and show selective relaxation enhancement of the liver and spleen.[43,44] Magnetite particles are not taken up by tumor, which lacks reticuloendothelial cells. As a result, magnetite selectively decreases the $T2$ of normal liver, increasing tumor-liver contrast (Fig. 29–16).

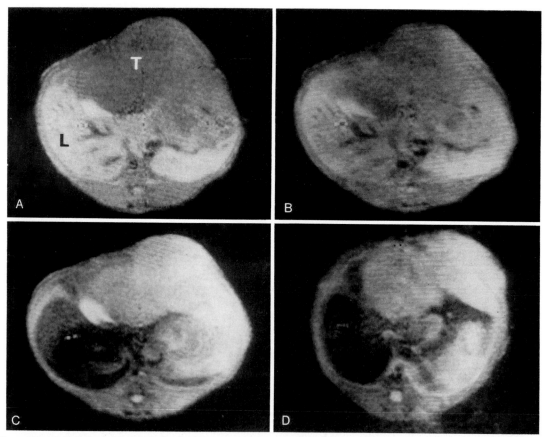

Figure 29–16. Rabbit model of metastatic liver cancer. VX2 carcinoma implanted in the left hepatic lobe. *A*, SE 260/15/16 image shows the tumor (T) as a low signal intensity region owing to its long *T1* relative to liver. Normal branching portal and hepatic veins are seen in the adjacent normal liver tissue (L). *B*, SE 500/30 image shows reduced tumor-liver contrast and reduced anatomic resolution. *C*, Following intravenous administration of magnetite particles, the SE 500/30 image shows a dramatic decrease in liver signal intensity resulting in increased tumor-liver contrast. *D*, SE 1600/60 image is heavily *T2* weighted and shows complete loss of signal from the magnetite-enhanced normal liver. Tumor has a high signal intensity and is easily seen. This image has increased noise and motion artifacts owing to the use of long *TR* and long *TE*. This animal study indicates that the *T1* weighted SE 260/15 image is superior for non–contrast enhanced imaging of liver cancer. With magnetite contrast enhancement, a slightly *T2* weighted sequence, such as the SE 500/30 sequence, is more effective for delineating tumor.

SPLEEN

The spleen is a unique immunologic organ with a large fractional blood content and relatively long $T1$ and $T2$ relaxation times. Metastatic cancer and lymphoma also have long $T1$ and $T2$ relaxation times and would be expected to have little contrast with surrounding spleen. Indeed, conventional MR imaging techniques have provided little or no useful information about the spleen (Fig. 29–17). It is hoped that paramagnetic contrast materials will be able to selectively enhance either tumors or normal splenic parenchyma and thereby allow adequate $T1$ or $T2$ contrast for tumor detection.

One potential application of splenic MRI is in detection and tissue-specific diagnosis of subcapsular hematoma.[45] Owing to the extremely long $T2$ of blood, hematoma can be distinguished from normal splenic parenchyma on $T2$ weighted images (Fig. 29–18). Blood undergoes a unique transformation, possibly paramagnetically mediated, during the first 24 to 48 hours following extravasation and deoxygenation. Bradley has suggested that the decreased $T1$ of hemorrhagic fluid collections is due to accumulation of methemoglobin, a paramagnetic degradation product of hemoglobin.[46] We have confirmed that methemoglobin levels in subcapsular splenic hematoma can increase from 0 to 70 percent during the first 72 hours.[47] This rise in paramagnetic methemoglobin levels is associated with shortening of $T1$, observable by spectrometer measurements in vitro or increase in signal intensity on $T1$ weighted images in vivo. Older hematomas undergo a complex evolution characterized by cellular sedimentation (visible on MR images as a "hematocrit" effect) and subsequent aggregation of a central clot (which has a shorter $T2$ than the surrounding liquid) (Fig. 29–18).

In summary, clinical applications of magnetic resonance imaging have been described for every organ in the body. As we learn more about the unique potential of this diagnostic modality, some applications will become routine, whereas others will remain research techniques. Owing to complex interactions between multiple biologic parameters and technical features unique to first-generation MR imaging systems, it is far too early to determine what the ultimate clinical value of MRI will be. Our recent results indicate that abdominal MRI has major clinical value for the evaluation of focal liver disease; with additional technical developments MRI is likely to have a significant role in the clinical evaluation of other abdominal organs.

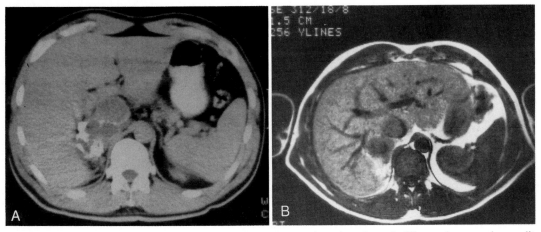

Figure 29–17. Renal cell carcinoma (right kidney, not shown) metastatic to the spleen. *A*, CT scan shows no abnormality. *B*, MR image, SE 330/18, shows a focal lesion in the spleen. Invasion of the inferior vena cava is also seen. Splenic metastases are rarely seen this well.

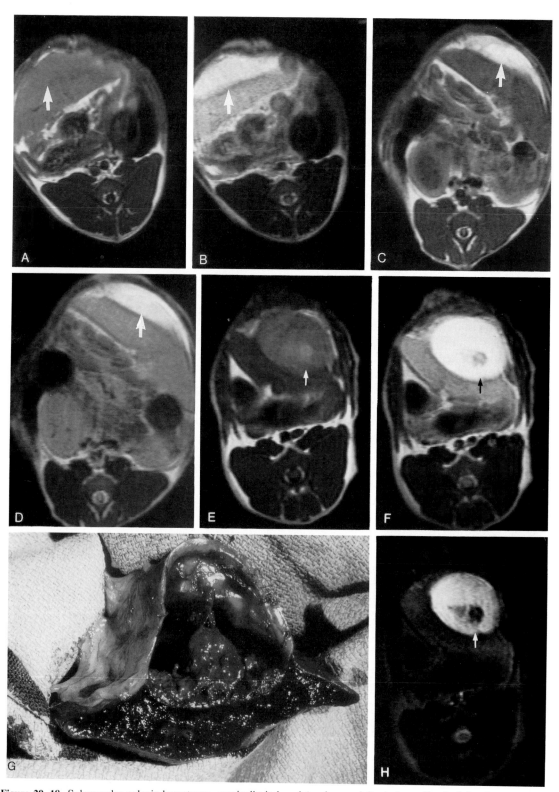

Figure 29–18. Subcapsular splenic hematoma, surgically induced (canine model). *A*, Immediately following trauma to the spleen, the SE 500/30 image shows a bulge in the splenic contour (arrow). *B*, Simultaneously obtained SE 2000/60 image shows the subcapsular hematoma as increased signal intensity (arrow) relative to the adjacent normal spleen. *C*, Forty-eight hours after hematoma formation, a dramatic increase in signal intensity is seen on the SE 500/30 image

Legend continues on opposite page

References

1. Steinberg EP, Cohen AB: Nuclear Magnetic Resonance Imaging Technology: A Clinical, Industrial, and Policy Analysis. Washington, DC, US Congress, Office of Technology Assessment, OTA-HCS-27, September 1984.
2. diMonda R: NMR—Issues for 1985 and Beyond. Hospital Technology Series; Guideline Report 4:3,4. Chicago, American Hospital Association, Division of Technology Management and Policy, 1985.
3. Buonocore E, Borkowski GP, Pavlicek W, Ngo F: NMR imaging of the abdomen: Technical considerations. AJR *141*:1171, 1983.
4. Schultz CL, Alfidi RJ, Nelson AD, Kopiwoda SY, Clampitt ME: The effect of motion on two-dimensional Fourier transformation magnetic resonance images. Radiology *152*:117, 1984.
5. Ehman RL, McNamara MT, Pallack M, Hricak H, Higgins CB: Magnetic resonance imaging with respiratory gating: Techniques and advantages. AJR *143*:1175, 1984.
6. Wesbey GE, Brasch RC, Engelstad BL, et al: Nuclear magnetic resonance contrast enhancement study of the gastrointestinal tract of rats and a human volunteer using nontoxic oral iron solutions. Radiology *149*:175, 1983.
7. Lanzer P, Botvinick EH, Schiller NB, et al: Cardiac imaging using gated magnetic resonance. Radiology *150*:121, 1984.
8. Glover G: Physiological motion and gating in MRI. Presented at the 3rd Annual Meeting of the Society for Magnetic Resonance Imaging, San Diego, March 1985.
9. Stark DD, Ferrucci JT Jr: Technical and clinical progress in MRI of the abdomen. Diagn Imag 7(11):118, 1985.
10. Crooks LE, Ortendahl DA, Kaufman L, et al: Clinical efficiency of nuclear magnetic resonance imaging. Radiology *146*:123, 1983.
11. Kneeland JB, Knowles RJR, Cahill PT: Multi-section multi-echo pulse magnetic resonance techniques: Optimization in a clinical setting. Radiology *155*:159, 1985.
12. Edelman RE, Shoukimas GM, Stark DD, et al: High-resolution surface-coil imaging of lumbar disk disease. AJR *144*:1123, 1985.
13. Edelman RE, McFarland E, Stark DD, et al: High resolution surface coil magnetic resonance imaging of abdominal viscera: I—Theory, technique and initial results. Radiology *157*:425, 1985.
14. White M, Edelman RR, Stark DD, et al: High resolution surface coil magnetic resonance imaging of abdominal viscera: II—The adrenal glands. Radiology *157*:431, 1985.
15. Ehman RL, Kjos BO, Hricak H, Brasch RC, Higgins CB: Relative intensity of abdominal organs in MR images. J Comput Assist Tomogr 9(2):315, 1985.
16. Wesbey GE, Moseley ME, Ehman RL: Translational molecular self-diffusion in magnetic resonance imaging. I. Effects on observed spin-spin relaxation. Invest Radiol *19*:484, 1984.
17. Babcock EE, Brateman L, Weinreb JC, Horner SD, Nunnally RL: Edge artifacts in MR images: Chemical shift effect. J Comput Assist Tomogr 9(2):252, 1985.
18. Lee JKT, Dixon WT, Ling D, Levitt RG, Murphy WA Jr: Fatty infiltration of the liver: Demonstration by proton spectroscopic imaging. Preliminary observations. Radiology *153*:195, 1984.
19. Stark DD, Bass NM, Moss AA, et al: Nuclear magnetic resonance imaging of experimentally induced liver disease. Radiology *148*:743, 1983.
20. Stark DD, Goldberg HI, Moss AA, Bass NM: Chronic liver disease: Evaluation by magnetic resonance. Radiology *150*:149, 1984.
21. Dixon WT: Simple proton spectroscopic imaging. Radiology *153*:189, 1984.
22. Lee JKT, Heiken JP, Dixon WT: Detection of hepatic metastases by proton spectroscopic imaging. Work in progress. Radiology *156*:429, 1985.
23. Stark DD, Wittenberg J, Middleton MS, Ferrucci JT Jr: Liver metastasis: detection by phase contrast MR imaging. Radiology *158*:327, 1986.
24. Doyle FH, Pennock JM, Banks LM, et al: Nuclear magnetic resonance imaging of the liver: initial experience. AJR *138*:193, 1982.

(arrow). *D*, At 48 hours the SE 2000/60 image is unchanged. The striking increase in hematoma signal intensity on the relatively *T1* weighted SE 500/30 image indicates evolution of a decreased *T1* relaxation time of the hematoma (arrow). During the first 48 hours of evolution, hematoma methemoglobin levels increased from zero to 40 percent of total hemoglobin. Methemoglobin is known to be paramagnetic and may account for the rapid and dramatic evolution of the MR appearance of hematoma on *T1* weighted images. *E–F*, Sixteen days following formation, the hematoma has dramatically increased in size and shows evidence of increased *T1* (less intense on *T1* weighted images than the 48-hour hematoma) and increased *T2* (more intense than earlier hematomas on *T2* weighted images). These findings all suggest influx of water into the hematoma, possibly mediated by the osmotic effect of hemoglobin degradation. A central area of high signal intensity is seen on the SE 500/30 image (arrow), consistent with a focal area of short *T1*. The SE 2000/60 image shows this area as a low signal intensity region, consistent with short *T2*. These MR findings suggest that this focal area within the hematoma contains a higher concentration of paramagnetic material, shortening both *T1* and *T2*. *G*, Pathologic specimen of the hematoma confirms the fluid nature of the large, high-intensity region of the hematoma. Methemoglobin content measured 70 percent of total hemoglobin. The central region of short *T1* and *T2* seen in *E* and *F*, respectively, is seen to be a central clot. *H*, A heavily *T2* weighted SE 2000/180 image delineates the full extent of this central short *T2* clot (arrow) surrounded by a higher signal intensity fluid of much longer *T2*.

25. Moss AA, Goldberg HI, Stark DD, et al: Hepatic tumors: Magnetic resonance and CT appearance. Radiology *150*:141, 1984.
26. Heiken JP, Lee JKT, Glazer HS, Ling D: Hepatic metastases studied with MR and CT. Radiology *156*:423, 1985.
27. Schmidt HC, Tscholakoff D, Hricak H, Higgins CB: MR image contrast and relaxation times of solid tumors in the chest, abdomen, and pelvis. J Comput Assist Tomogr *9*(4):738, 1985.
28. Wehrli FW, MacFall JR, Glover GH, Grigsby N: The dependence of nuclear magnetic resonance (NMR) image contrast on intrinsic and pulse sequence timing parameters. Magn Reson Imag *2*:3, 1984.
29. Hendrick RE, Nelson TR, Hendee WR: Optimizing tissue contrast in magnetic resonance imaging. Magn Reson Imag *2*:193, 1984.
30. Stark DD, Felder RC, Wittenberg J: Magnetic resonance imaging of cavernous hemangioma of the liver: Tissue-specific characterization. AJR *145*:213, 1985.
31. Stark DD, Wittenberg J, Edelman RR, et al: Detection of hepatic metastases by magnetic resonance: analysis of pulse sequence performance. Radiology *159*:365, 1986.
32. Bottomley PA, Foster TH, Argersinger RE, Pfeifer LM: A review of normal tissue hydrogen NMR relaxation times and relaxation mechanisms from 1–100 MHz: dependence on tissue type, NMR frequency, temperature, species, excision, and age. Med Phys *11*(4):425, 1984.
33. Fullerton GD, Cameron IL, Ord VA: Frequency dependence of magnetic resonance spin-lattice relaxation of protons in biological materials. Radiology *151*:135, 1984.
34. Johnson GA, Herfkens RJ, Brown MA: Tissue relaxation time: In vivo field dependence. Radiology *156*:805, 1985.
35. Glazer GM, Aisen AM, Francis IR, et al: Hepatic cavernous hemangioma: magnetic resonance imaging. Radiology *155*:417, 1985.
36. Ohtomo K, Itai Y, Furui S, et al: Hepatic tumors: differentiation by transverse relaxation time ($T2$) of magnetic resonance imaging. Radiology *155*:421, 1985.
37. Stark DD, Moseley ME, Bacon BR, et al: Magnetic resonance imaging and spectroscopy of hepatic iron overload. Radiology *154*:137, 1985.
38. Carr DH, Brown J, Bydder GM: Gadolinium-DTPA as a contrast agent in MRI: Initial clinical experience in 20 patients. AJR *143*:215, 1984.
39. Runge VM, Clanton JA, Herzer WA, et al: Intravascular contrast agents suitable for magnetic resonance imaging. Radiology *153*:171, 1984.
40. Weinmann HJ, Brasch RC, Press WR, Wesbey GE: Characteristics of gadolinium-DTPA complex: a potential NMR contrast agent. AJR *142*:619, 1984.
41. Lauffer RB, Greif WL, Stark DD, et al: Iron-EHPG as an hepatobiliary MR contrast agent: initial imaging and biodistribution studies. J Comput Assist Tomogr *9*(3):431, 1985.
42. Saini S, Stark DD, Ferrucci JT Jr: Gd-DTPA enhanced dynamic MR scanning of liver cancer. Presented before Society of Gastrointestinal Radiology, Acapulco, January 1986.
43. Wolf GL, Burnett KR, Goldstein EJ, Joseph PM: Contrast agents for magnetic resonance imaging. *In* Kressel H (ed): Magnetic Resonance Annual. New York, Raven Press, 1985, pp 231–266.
44. Saini S, Widder D, Stark DD, et al: Reticuloendothelial contrast agents for enhanced MRI detection of liver tumors. Poster, Presented at the Society of Magnetic Resonance in Medicine, Fourth Annual Meeting, London, August 19, 1985.
45. Moss AA, Stark DD, Margulis AR: Liver, gallbladder, alimentary tube, spleen, peritoneal cavity, and pancreas. *In* Margulis AR, Higgins CB, Kaufman L, Crooks LE (eds): Clinical Magnetic Resonance Imaging. San Francisco, Radiology Research and Education Foundation, 1984, pp 185–207.
46. Bradley WG, Schmidt PG: Effect of methemoglobin formation on the MR appearance of subarachnoid hemorrhage. Radiology *156*:99, 1985.
47. Saini S, Stark DD, Hahn P: MRI of the liver. *In* Bradley WG, Stark DD (eds): Magnetic Resonance Imaging. St. Louis, CV Mosby, 1987.

30

Gastrointestinal Tract

ALBERT TEDESCHI
ALAN J. KAUFMAN
ROBERT W. TARR
C. LEON PARTAIN

Contrast examinations, endoscopy, and colonoscopy are the usual procedures of choice for the initial evaluation of alimentary tract disorders. Recently, computed tomography (CT) has received attention in the initial evaluation of gastrointestinal pathology.[1-8] Although experience with magnetic resonance imaging (MRI) has been anecdotal, it has contributed to the diagnostic work-up. The ability of MRI to image in the sagittal, axial, and coronal as well as nonorthogonal planes, can be helpful in delineating the manifestations of disease processes. The postoperative CT evaluation of patients with metal prostheses and surgical clips has been described as less than optimal.[9-11] In a review of ten postsurgical patients with metallic implants in the abdomen and pelvis, MRI was suggested as a valuable adjunctive technique in the assessment of these individuals.[12] Digestive tract MRI is in its initial stages of development. Improvement in technology will naturally reduce limitations associated with motion artifacts. As with other imaging modalities of the gastrointestinal tract, contrast material may be essential. Various paramagnetic agents and other contrast agents are being investigated. These agents must be nontoxic, stable, and not absorbed. With further experimentation and development of the suitable contrast agents and with continued investigations of the diverse pathologic processes within the digestive tract, MRI will progressively enrich, complement, and perhaps in some cases surpass our current diagnostic capabilities.

Figure 30–1 illustrates a normal abdomen scanned with a spin-echo sequence of 500/32 (pre- and postrespiratory gating and intravenous glucagon administration). Scanning was performed with 1 cm thick sections. On the non–respiratory gated image, ghost artifact is seen anterior to the abdominal wall. The transverse colon is not well visualized, nor are the adjacent intra-abdominal structures. Following the intravascular administration of 1 mg of glucagon, image detail is improved with respiratory gating. The haustral pattern within the transverse colon is well visualized. Edge detail is also enhanced within the abdomen. The techniques and advantages of respiratory gating and glucagon administration have been mentioned in previous chapters as well as by several investigators.[14-20] Figure 30–2 also was obtained with respiratory gating. The body and tail of the pancreas are well visualized, as are the edges of the spleen and liver. The vessels in the upper abdomen, including the splenic vein, superior and inferior mesenteric arteries and inferior vena cava (IVC), can be clearly seen because of the signal void that occurs in flowing blood.

Investigators have reported on the use of oral contrast media to improve imaging of the alimentary tract (see Chapter 48). Mineral oil, CO_2, oral gadolinium-DTPA (Gd-DTPA), and magnetite in the form of albumin microspheres or as particulate iron oxide

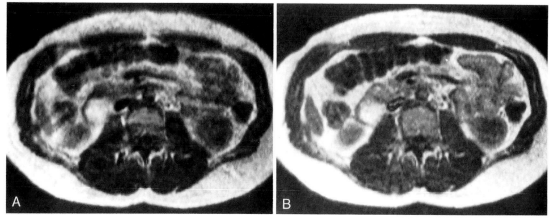

Figure 30–1. Normal midabdomen. *A*, Transverse image through the midabdomen with a pulse sequence of SE 32/500. Ghost artifacts are seen anterior to the abdominal wall, and anatomic detail within the abdomen is poorly visualized. *B*, Following the administration of glucagon and with respiratory gating, resolution is improved in the midabdomen. Haustral folds are well seen in the transverse colon. This image shows a marked improvement in diagnostic quality.

have all been used to enhance the distinction between the gastrointestinal structures and adjacent abdominal viscera.[21–26] Magnetite albumin microspheres, in suspension, administered orally appear to have a greater magnetic moment than other paramagnetic contrast agents. The magnetite microspheres demonstrate decreased *T1* and *T2* signal intensity within bowel, and preliminary animal studies suggest encouraging results. Magnetite, when administered as particulate iron oxide, is appealing in that it does not appear to be associated with signal distortion from retroperitoneal structures or from peristaltic motion. Oral Gd-DTPA also has been suggested as an effective contrast

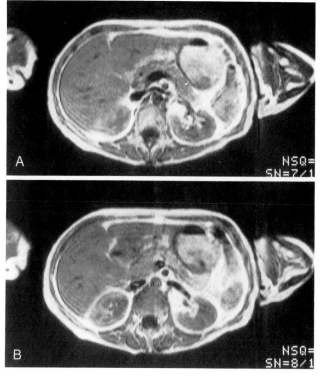

Figure 30–2. Normal abdomen. *A*, Normal *T1* sequence. SE 32/600 image of the upper abdomen with respiratory gating shows the splenic vein, with the body of pancreas anteriorly. Also well seen are the gastric fundus, left kidney, aorta, and IVC. *B*, One cm caudad, the head of the pancreas and gastric antrum are identified. Also seen with improved resolution are the inferior vena cava, aorta, SMA, and inferior mesenteric vein.

agent for gastrointestinal contrast enhancement. However, there is a biphasic signal intensity effect, which appears to be related to its dilution in bowel while in transit. Ferric ammonium citrate (180 ml of 1 mM concentration), when injected approximately 15 minutes before imaging, pacifies the proximal small bowel well. One disadvantage of ferric ammonium citrate is that, like Gd-DTPA, the high-intensity signal of the intraluminal contents on $T1$ weighted sequences may not be easily separated from retroperitoneal fat.

When the esophagus is filled with fluid or gas, it can be well seen on MRI in the axial and coronal planes. Figure 30–3 demonstrates a distal esophageal carcinoma that is extending into the cardia of the stomach. There is diffuse thickening of the esophageal wall and proximal stomach. Esophageal carcinoma can extend to nearby structures as well as to adjacent lymph nodes, as the esophagus has no serosal layer. CT has been reported to be a useful modality in determining local spread of disease as well as metastatic involvement of the liver and adrenal. Magnetic resonance imaging has demonstrated an ability to evaluate extraesophageal spread of disease; however, experience is limited. With further refinement of technique, it also may become a useful adjunct in the staging of esophageal carcinoma. Figure 30–4 demonstrates mediastinal lymphadenopathy that is compressing the midesophagus. In this sagittal image, air is seen within the proximal and distal esophagus. An esophageal duplication cyst was recently described in the literature.[27] In this case, MRI provided specific information about the nature of the fluid in this cyst that was not obtainable by other imaging methods. On $T1$ weighted images the esophageal duplication cyst demonstrated relatively high signal intensity, which was postulated to be secondary to a combination of cellular inflammatory debris and hemorrhagic fluid in this patient with an acute presentation.

The fundus of the stomach is well seen with an oral positive contrast agent. The distal stomach is often better delineated with a negative contrast agent, such as CO_2. Figure 30–5 presents images of a patient with esophageal carcinoma status post gastric pull-through procedure. Positive contrast agent is seen within the gastric conduit. Multiple areas of decreased signal intensity, which represent spinal metastatic deposits, are seen within the thoracic and lumbar spine. Also well seen are ascites and a right renal cyst. The hepatic veins and superior vena cava are enlarged as a result of compression by the gastric conduit (Fig. 30–5B). Often a coronal view is helpful in identifying the position and extent of abnormal masses in the upper abdomen, including, in particular, their relationship to the hepatic veins, IVC, portal vein, and aorta.

Multiple tubular serpiginous areas of signal void are present in the region of the gastric fundus and distal esophagus (Fig. 30–6). This represents a case of esophageal

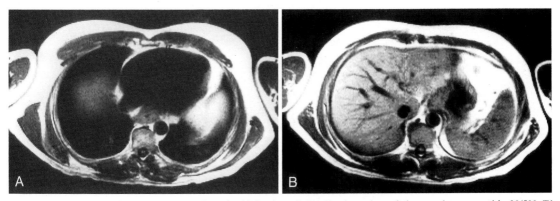

Figure 30–3. Esophageal carcinoma. *A*, There is thickening of the distal portion of the esophagus on this 30/500 *T1* weighted image. *B*, Approximately 2 cm caudad there is thickening of the gastric cardia, representing extension of esophageal carcinoma into the proximal portion of the stomach.

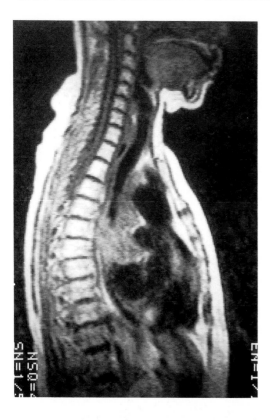

Figure 30–4. SE 32/500 sequence demonstrates intermediate *T1* signal intensity within the mediastinum, consistent with the patient's diagnosis of lymphoma. The adenopathy is seen to extend posteriorly and to compress the midportion of the esophagus. Also well seen is the trachea to the level of the tracheal bifurcation and the left atrium just anterior to the distal esophagus. Adenopathy (with intermediate *T1* intensity) in the thorax is usually better contrasted with mediastinal fat, which has increased *T1* signal intensity.

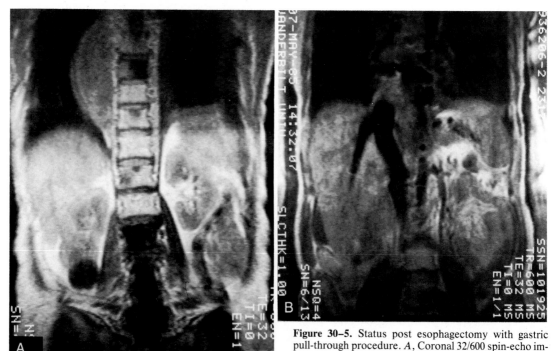

Figure 30–5. Status post esophagectomy with gastric pull-through procedure. *A,* Coronal 32/600 spin-echo images demonstrate the gastric remnant in the right paravertebral region. Also seen is a cyst in the inferior pole of the right kidney. Multiple areas of decreased *T1* signal intensity within the thoracolumbar spine represent metastatic deposits from the patient's esophageal carcinoma. *B,* Hepatic vein and inferior vena cava are enlarged owing to compression by the gastric pull-through procedure. Also noted is ascites lateral to the right lobe of liver.

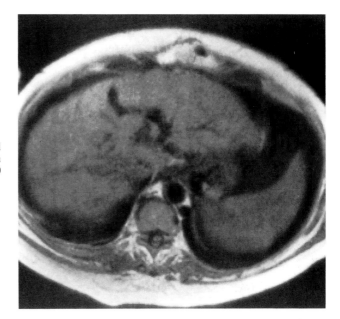

Figure 30–6. Esophageal varices. Multiple small tubular serpiginous areas of signal void are seen in the region of the gastric cardia. SE 32/500 sequence.

and gastric varices in a patient with portal hypertension secondary to liver cirrhosis. A patent umbilical vein is visualized in the anterior abdominal wall as an area of signal void secondary to high-velocity flow. Also well seen is ascitic fluid in the upper abdomen. Figure 30–7 shows a patent splenic-renal shunt as well as ascites in a patient with hepatic cirrhosis and portal hypertension. Well seen are the aorta and inferior vena cava in this coronal section. With MRI it is possible to establish the direction of flow in the portal or umbilical vein in patients with portal hypertension and hepatic cirrhosis.

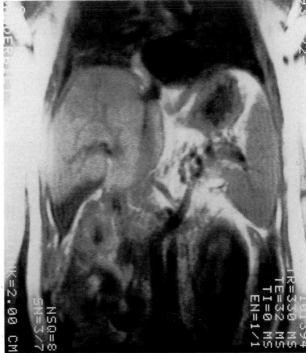

Figure 30–7. Splenorenal shunt. A coronal 32/350 image of the upper abdomen demonstrates a splenorenal shunt. The origin and insertion of the splenic vein postoperatively are well visualized, as are the aorta and inferior vena cava. A fluid collection seen inferior to the right lobe of liver represents ascites.

A retrocardiac "mass" (Fig. 30–8) represents a sliding hiatal hernia. The hernia possesses intermediate signal intensity compared with adjacent soft tissue structures.

Often the distal stomach and antrum are not well visualized or delineated unless distended by CO_2. Glucagon has also been reported to facilitate the imaging of the stomach and proximal small bowel by reducing the peristaltic motion of bowel. In Figure 30–9 a mass is seen within the antrum of the stomach that is of intermediate signal activity on a 32/600 spin-echo sequence. The mass is well marginated in its relationship to the liver and the lumen of the stomach, which has been opacified with a dilute oral contrast agent. Focal wall thickening is the most frequent finding in a gastric adenocarcinoma, which is the most common type of primary malignancy of the stomach. Endoscopy and barium examination are the procedures of choice to initially evaluate the stomach. However, MR may play a role in the detection of metastatic deposits to liver, adrenal, and adjacent lymph nodes in cases of gastric malignancies. Additionally, MR scanning of the pelvis may detect ovarian metastatic disease (Krukenberg tumors).

MR can be useful in detecting and characterizing fluid collections within the abdomen. Figure 30–10 demonstrates air within multiple dilated loops of large and small bowel within the abdomen. This patient had an adynamic ileus secondary to recent surgery. Also well seen is ascites within the lateral abdominal compartment. MR has provided useful information as to the position of abdominal fluid collections and is able to clearly distinguish these collections from surrounding normal tissues. Bilomas and hemorrhagic renal cysts as well as subacute and chronic hemorrhagic collections within the abdomen are better seen on MR than on CT.[28-30] Inflammatory collections within the abdomen demonstrate increased *T1* signal intensity relative to transudates, which have longer *T1* relaxation times. This correlates with the protein content of the fluid and relative relaxation times.

Little attention has been directed to the MR appearance of inflammatory bowel disease. Figure 30–11 demonstrates an area of increased *T2* signal intensity in the left lower quadrant in a patient with Crohn's disease. The increased *T1* and *T2* relaxation times are demonstrated by relatively decreased signal intensity on the *T1* weighted sequence and increased *T2* signal intensity on the 45/90/2000 sequence. While barium examination and endoscopy remain the procedures of choice in the initial evaluation of patients with inflammatory bowel disease, the role of MRI has yet to be established. Increased signal intensity within the bowel wall on *T2* weighted pulse sequences, as well as increased signal intensity within the adjacent mesentery on *T1* weighted images, may prove to be a sensitive parameter in the MR detection of inflammatory changes. Figure 30–12 represents *T1* and *T2* weighted sequences in a patient with Crohn's disease

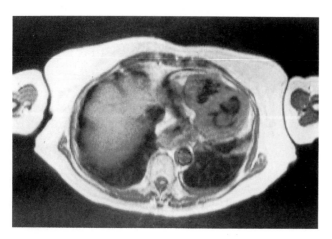

Figure 30–8. Sliding hiatal hernia. SE 30/500 images reveal thickened distal esophagus with patent esophageal lumen. This represents a sliding esophageal hernia. The inferior aspects of the right and left ventricles are seen anterior and lateral to the hiatal hernia. A small area of discoid atelectasis also is seen in the left lung base.

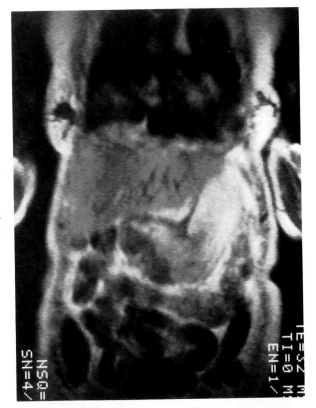

Figure 30–9. Gastric carcinoma. SE 32/600 coronal images of the abdomen reveal a large mass in the inferior aspect of the gastric antrum. The mass is of intermediate signal intensity and represents a gastric carcinoma. This lesion is well delineated in relation to the liver and other abdominal structures. In the inferior abdomen, multiple air-filled loops of bowel are well visualized.

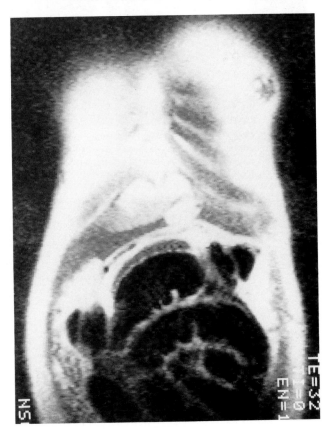

Figure 30–10. SE 32/500 images of the abdomen reveal multiple dilated loops of large and small bowel within the anterior abdomen. This represents a postsurgical paralytic ileus. Also well seen is ascites in the right upper quadrant and along the right lateral abdominal wall.

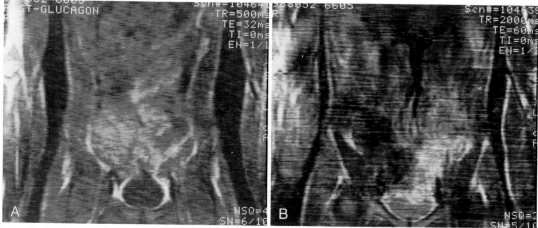

Figure 30–11. Crohn's disease. *A*, SE 32/500 *T1* weighted image reveals two fixed loops of bowel in the left lower quadrant, representing distal descending colon and an adjacent loop of jejunum. *B*, A SE 60/2000 *T2* sequence reveals increased *T2* signal intensity in the left lower quadrant. This represents an inflammatory response in bowel and adjacent mesentery from recurrent Crohn's disease.

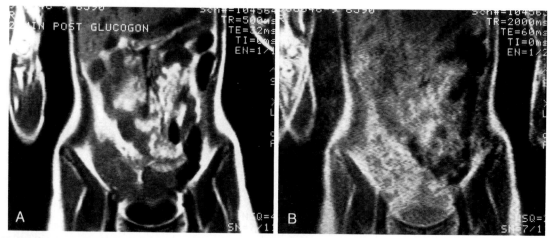

Figure 30–12. Crohn's disease. *A*, SE 32/500 image (postglucagon) reveals a mass of intermediate signal activity in the right lower quadrant. Adjacent bowel loops are displaced superiorly and medially. *B*, A 60/2000 *T2* weighted coronal image reveals increased *T2* signal intensity in the right lower quadrant corresponding to mesenteric edema and inflammation involving the terminal ileum in a patient with known Crohn's disease.

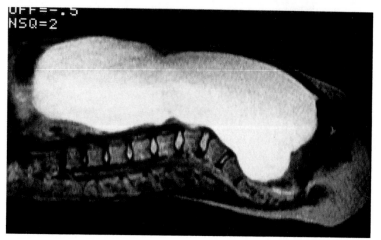

Figure 30–13. Mesenteric cyst. A sagittal 45/2000 *T2* sequence demonstrates a large, partially bilobed mass filling the entire abdomen and pelvic cavity. This mass extended from the xyphoid to the pubic symphysis. The mass had a short *T1* as well as a long *T2* relaxation time and was of uniform signal intensity. At surgery this mass was found to be a mesenteric cyst. The short *T1* and long *T2* relaxation times of the fluid reflect the high protein content of the cyst.

of the terminal ileum. Increased signal activity is seen within the region of the terminal ileum as well as within the adjacent mesentery.

A huge mass with short *T1* and long *T2* relaxation time is revealed within the abdomen and pelvis of a child (Fig. 30–13). This represents a mesenteric cyst. The sagittal plane obtained in this patient well delineates the extent of the lesion. The increased *T2* signal identified in this case represents increased protein content within the cyst.

In Figure 30–14 there is increased *T2* signal intensity within the lateral portion of the right pelvis. This is of intermediate signal intensity on the *T1* weighted sequence. This represented an iliacus muscle abscess that extended inferiorly along the medial femoral compartment. The margins of the abscess within the pelvis are well delineated on this coronal section. Also identified is decreased *T1* signal intensity within the proximal right femoral head, which represented osteonecrosis secondary to osteomyelitis. MRI has been helpful in accurately identifying the location as well as the size of intraabdominal abscess collections. MR, however, does have its limitations when the abscess collection is adjacent to retroperitoneal fat or fluid-filled non-opacified bowel loops. The most common MR finding for abscess collections has been abnormal areas of decreased signal intensity on *T1* weighted images. The abscess collections show a relative increase in signal intensity on *T2* weighted acquisitions. The collections usually appear to be heterogeneous in character and can often be distinguished from adjacent normal musculature.[31]

The MR appearance of extracranial and intracranial hematomas has been described by several investigators.[32–38] Hematomas in the abdomen appear to be better visualized with MR than with CT because of the paramagnetic effects of iron. Recent studies of 14 patients with hematomas within the musculoskeletal system, abdominal viscera, and retroperitoneum revealed temporal variations in signal intensity that were slightly different from that previously observed with intracranial hematomas.[32–34] Intra-abdominal hematomas appeared initially isointense relative to muscle on *T1* weighted sequences and became more intense at approximately seven days. Acute hematomas demonstrated relatively increased signal intensity on *T2* weighted images. At times, these signal characteristics make the differentiation of acute intra-abdominal hematomas from abscess

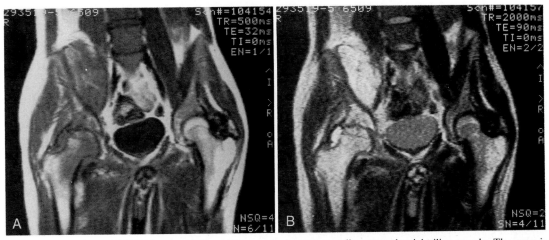

Figure 30–14. *A*, Coronal 32/500 images of the pelvis reveal a large mass adjacent to the right iliac muscle. The mass is of intermediate signal intensity. *B*, On *T2* weighted sequences, SE 90/2000, the mass demonstrates increased signal intensity that is heterogeneous. This mass extended inferiorly along the medial aspect of the proximal right femur. At laparotomy this collection proved to be an abscess adjacent to the iliac muscle that extended inferiorly along the medial aspect of the right hip. Also note on the *T1* weighted sequence the decreased signal activity in the right femoral head and neck. This represented osteonecrosis secondary to osteomyelitis.

or solid tumor difficult. The concentric ring sign has been described as being useful in identifying duodenal hematomas as well as other intra-abdominal hematomas.[35] The concentric ring sign has been described as a ring of decreased $T2$ signal intensity surrounding the hematoma, which is of increased $T2$ signal intensity. Although duodenal hematomas are uncommon, they may present as an intramural mass with complete or partial obstruction. They have been observed more frequently in children and young adult males and are usually related to blunt abdominal trauma.

The changes in bowel infarction and ischemia have been recently reported.[39] Mortality from bowel infarction is high and is often attributed to delayed diagnosis. Clinical, laboratory, and standard radiographic studies are often equivocal and nonspecific. Figure 30–15 (SE 120/2000) is an example of bowel infarction in the rabbit model. The areas of bowel infarction in this axial image demonstrate a two- to threefold increase in signal intensity compared with normal bowel. In addition, in this study, graded areas of increased signal intensity were demonstrated that correlated pathologically with areas of ischemic change without total infarction. The relative merits of magnetic resonance imaging in bowel infarction have not yet been assessed sufficiently to gauge its possible impact in clinical practice. MRI may prove to be the most sensitive modality in the evaluation of small bowel ischemia.

In conclusion, magnetic resonance imaging is still in its developmental stages, especially with respect to the evaluation of digestive tract abnormalities. With continued research and investigation, MRI will no doubt supply the radiologist and clinician with essential diagnostic information. There is great potential for high-sensitivity imaging and earlier diagnosis, with resultant improvement in prognosis in a diverse group of gastrointestinal disorders.

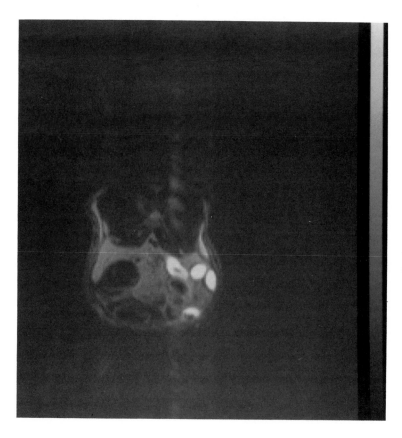

Figure 30–15. Bowel infarction. SE 120/2000 transverse image through the midabdomen. Study performed 45 minutes after surgical ligation of the ileocolic artery and its segmental branches. Note increased signal intensity in the bowel wall of loops of distal ileum and ascending colon. This is a reflection of bowel wall edema and early infarction.

References

1. Balfe DM, Koehler RE, Karstaedt N, Stanley RJ, Sagel SS: Computed tomography of gastric neoplasms. Radiology *140*:431, 1981.
2. Clark KE, Foley WD, Lawson TL, Berland LL, Maddison FE: CT evaluation of esophageal and upper abdominal varices. J Comput Assist Tomogr *4*:510, 1980.
3. Kressel HY, Callen PW, Montagne JP, Korobkin M, Goldberg HI, Moss AA, Arger PH, Margulis AR: Computed tomography evaluation of disorders affecting the alimentary tract. Radiology *129*:451, 1978.
4. Lee JKT, Stanley RJ, Sagel SS, Levitt RG, McClennan BL: CT appearance of the pelvis after abdominal peritoneal resection for rectal carcinoma. Radiology *141*:739, 1981.
5. Mayes JB, Zornoza J: Computed tomography of colon carcinoma. AJR *135*:45, 1980.
6. Moss AA, Margulis AR, Schnyder P, Theoni RF: A uniform CT based staging system for malignant neoplasms of the alimentary tube. AJR *136*:1251, 1981.
7. Moss AA, Schnyder P, Candargis G, Margulis AR: Computed tomography of benign and malignant gastric abnormalities. J Clin Gastroenterol *2*:401, 1980.
8. Theoni RF, Moss AA, Schnyder P, Margulis AR: Detection and staging of primary rectal and rectal sigmoid cancers by computed tomography. Radiology *141*:135, 1981.
9. Marks WM, Callen PW: CT in evaluation of patients with surgical clips. Surg Gynecol Obstet *151*:557, 1980.
10. Faxe AW, Doppman JL, Brennan MF: Use of titanium surgical clips to avoid artifacts seen on CT. Arch Surg *117*:978, 1982.
11. Glover GH, Pelc NJ: An algorithm for the reduction of metallic clip artifacts in CT reconstruction. Med Physics *8*:799, 1981.
12. Mechlin M, Thickman D, Kressel HY, et al: MRI of postoperative patients with metallic implants. AJR *143*:1281, 1984.
13. Steiner RE, Bydder GM: NMR in gastroenterology. Clin Gastroenterol *13*:265, 1984.
14. Prato FS, Nicholson RL, King M, Knill RL, Reese L, Wilkins K: Abolition of respiratory movement markedly improved in NMR images of the thorax and upper abdomen. Magn Reson Med *1*:227, 1984.
15. Runge VM, Clanton JA, Partain CL, James AE: Respiratory gating in magnetic resonance imaging at 0.5 tesla. Radiology *151*:521, 1984.
16. Ehman RL, McNamarra MT, Pallack M, Hricak H, Higgins CB: Magnetic resonance imaging with respiratory gating: techniques and advantages. AJR *143*:1175, 1984.
17. Groch MW, Turner DA, Clark JW: Respiratory gating device for MR imaging. Radiology *153*(P):98, 1984.
18. Lewis CE, Prato FS, Drost DJ: Comparison of respiratory triggering and gating techniques: the removal of respiratory imaging artifacts in MRI. Radiology *160*:803, 1986.
19. Wood ML, Henkelman RM: MR image artifacts from periodic motion. Med Physics *12*:143, 1985.
20. Axel L, Charles C, Kressel HY, Summers R, Kundel HL: Respiratory effects in two dimensional Fourier transform MR imaging. Radiology *157*(P):296, 1985.
21. Runge VM, Stewart RG, Clanton JA, et al: Work in progress: potential oral and intravenous paramagnetic NMR contrast agents. Radiology *147*:789, 1983.
22. Wesbey GE, Brasch RC, Englestadt B, et al: Nuclear magnetic resonance contrast enhancement: study of the gastrointestinal tracts of rats and a human volunteer using non-toxic oral iron solutions. Radiology *149*:175, 1983.
23. Wolf GL, Burnett KR, Goldstein EJ, Joseph PM: Contrast agents for magnetic resonance imaging. *In* Kressel HY (ed): Magnetic Resonance Annual. New York, Raven Press, 1985, pp 235–266.
24. Barnhart JL, Hegenauer J, Bakan GA, Witt BL, Bakan DA: Orally administered manganese gastrointestinal uptake and potential for MRI contrast of the GI tract. Proceedings, Society of Magnetic Resonance in Medicine, August 1986, pp 1520–1521.
25. Hahn PF, Saini S, Stark DD, Ferrucci JT: Particulate iron oxide (magnetite) as a gastrointestinal contrast agent for magnetic resonance imaging. Proceedings, Society of Magnetic Resonance in Medicine, August 1986, p 1537.
26. Kornmesser W, Hamm B, Laniado M, Claub W: First clinical use of gadolinium DTPA for gastrointestinal contrast enhancement. Proceedings, Society of Magnetic Resonance in Medicine, August 1986, pp 1522–1523.
27. Lupetin AR, Dass N: MRI appearance of esophageal duplication cyst. Gastrointest Radiol *12*:7, 1987.
28. Wall SD, Hricak H, Bailey RK, Kerlan HI, et al: MRI of pathologic abdominal fluid collections. J Comput Assist Tomogr *10*(5):746, 1986.
29. Terrier F, Risel D, Tajaunen H, et al: MRI of body fluid collection. J Comput Assist Tomogr *10*(6):953, 1986.
30. Cohen JM, Weinreb JC, Maravilla KR: Fluid collections in the intraperitoneal and extraperitoneal spaces: comparison of MRI and CT. Radiology *155*:705, 1985.
31. Wall SD, Fisher MR, Amparo EG, Hricak H, Higgins CB: Magnetic resonance imaging in the evaluation of abscesses. AJR *144*:1217, 1985.
32. Gomori JN, Grossman RI, Goldberg HI, Zimmerman RA, Bilaniuk LT: Intracranial hematomas: imaging by high field MR. Radiology *157*:87, 1985.
33. Swenson SJ, Keller PL, Berquist TH, McCleod RA, Stephens DH: Magnetic resonance imaging of hemorrhage. AJR *145*:921, 1985.
34. Unger EC, Glazer HS, Lee JKT, Ling D: MRI of extracranial hematomas: preliminary observations. AJR *146*:403, 1986.

35. Hahn PF, Stark DD, Vici LG, Ferrucci JT: The ring sign in MR imaging of duodenal hematoma. Radiology *159*:279, 1986.
36. Bradley WG, Schmidt PF: Effect of methemoglobin formation on the MR appearance of subarachnoid hemorrhage. Radiology *156*:99, 1985.
37. Brown JJ, VanSonnenberg E, Gerber KH, Stritch G, Wittisch GR, Slutsky RA: Magnetic resonance relaxation times of percutaneously obtained normal and abnormal body fluids. Radiology *154*:727, 1985.
38. Hahn PF, Saini S, Stark DD, Papanicolaou N, Ferrucci JT: Intraabdominal hematoma: the concentric ring sign in MR imaging. AJR *148*:115, 1987.
39. Tarr RW, Kaufman AJ, Holburn GE, Wilson RB, Brury H, Holscher M, Partain CL, James AE: Magnetic resonance imaging of bowel infarction in the rabbit model. Proceedings, Society of Magnetic Resonance in Medicine, August 1986, p 1238.

31

Kidneys and Retroperitoneum

SNEHAL D. MEHTA
MADAN V. KULKARNI
PONNADA NARAYANA
C. LEON PARTAIN

Magnetic resonance imaging (MRI) is the latest and potentially most effective modality for noninvasive imaging of the kidneys and the retroperitoneum. Over a short time, MRI has made rapid strides in imaging of the brain and spinal cord as well as of the cardiovascular system.[1-11] It offers tremendous potential in imaging of the chest and abdomen[12-15] and, even at this early stage, compares quite favorably with computed tomography (CT) and ultrasound in display of anatomy and detection of disease processes. Compared with CT, MRI has the advantage of superior soft tissue contrast and ability to image in multiple planes. Also, vascular structures are imaged without contrast administration. Tissue characterization is a promising possibility for the future.

The largely unexplored area of magnetic resonance spectroscopy can provide information about various intracellular metabolites and their relative concentrations by identifying their characteristic peaks due to chemical shift.[16,17] For example, various organic and inorganic phosphate metabolites of ATP can be identified using P-31 nuclei. Similarly, intracellular pH in kidneys and other organs has been determined.[18] In kidneys and in renal transplants, various processes such as ischemia, hypotension, and rejection can be studied to get better insight into the basic metabolic pathway most affected. It has also been shown that tumors have slightly different intermediary metabolic pathways compared with normal tissues. Although rapid strides are being made, routine magnetic resonance spectroscopy in humans is still a few years away from practical utility.

Another exciting development involves paramagnetic contrast agents,[8] which by their presence alter the $T1$ and $T2$ relaxation times and hence the tissue contrast, which is inherently superior in MRI as compared with other imaging modalities. This topic is covered in detail in Chapters 46 to 52.

The current disadvantages of MR imaging include degradation of image quality because of respiratory and cardiac motion; inability to visualize areas of calcification; and, in abdominal imaging, lack of a suitable gastrointestinal contrast agent.

MRI, unlike CT, does not use ionizing radiation, can differentiate vascular structures from surrounding soft tissues without the use of intravenous contrast, and has intrinsically superior tissue contrast. Unlike gray-scale ultrasonography, it does not depend so much on operator expertise and cannot display real-time images. However, MRI shares with sonography the advantages of safety and the capacity for unlimited imaging planes. Thus, it combines certain advantages of computed tomography and sonographic imaging parameters.

NORMAL ANATOMY

MR can clearly display normal retroperitoneal and renal anatomy in multiple planes.[12-14,19-22] In axial image, similar to other imaging planes, kidneys can be seen contrasted against perinephric fat. On spin-echo (SE) images, the abundant retroperitoneal adipose tissue appears bright secondary to high signal intensity due to its short *T1* relaxation time. Gerota's fascia is not always seen in normal individuals but, when seen, appears as a thin line of low signal intensity separating the perirenal and pararenal adipose tissue.[21,22]

The renal capsule is usually not visualized. However, owing to the chemical shift phenomenon, a low-intensity curvilinear artifact at the periphery of the kidney may be mistaken for the renal capsule. That it is an artifact caused by chemical shift can be inferred from its characteristic pattern of low signal intensity on one side and higher signal intensity on the other side of the renal outline (Fig. 31–1).

The renal cortex can be easily differentiated from the medulla on spin-echo images (Fig. 31–2). The cortex has a higher signal intensity than the medulla. On images with a short *TE* (echo time) and *TR* (repetition time) interval, tissue differences due to varying *T1* relaxation times are accentuated. The medulla has a longer *T1* relaxation time than that of the renal cortex and appears as a lower signal intensity on short *TE/TR* pulse sequences, such as the spin-echo (SE 30/500) image. The renal sinus has brighter signal intensity than that of the renal cortex owing to renal sinus fat. Normal blood vessels appear as low intensity signal in the renal hilum as a result of flowing blood.

On spin-echo technique the pelvicalyceal system, when seen, appears dark because of its low signal intensity. This is secondary to the very long *T1* and *T2* relaxation parameters of urine. When the *TE* and *TR* are prolonged, as in *T2* weighted images, the appearance changes from dark to low-level gray signal intensity.[46] It is important to note that while both blood vessels and renal collecting systems appear as low signal intensity, the mechanisms for their similar appearances are different. In case of blood vessels, owing to rapid flow there is no time for recovery of magnetization in that

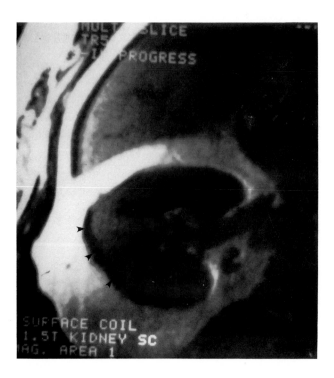

Figure 31–1. Surface coil image of the kidney: spin echo technique at 1.5 tesla field strength. Note curvilinear low-intensity band along the lateral margin of the kidney (arrowheads) due to chemical shift. Also note bright signal intensity along the medial border, which is also an artifact caused by the same phenomenon.

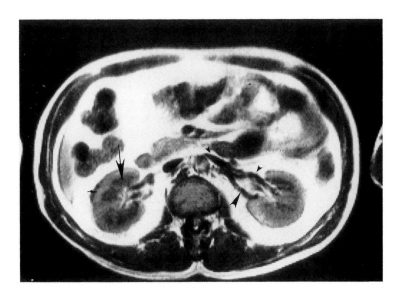

Figure 31–2. Axial spin-echo (SE) image of normal kidneys obtained at *TE/TR* = 30/500 ms. Left renal vein (small arrowheads) is seen anterior to the left renal artery (large arrowhead). Vascular structures have virtually no signal intensity compared with the renal parenchyma. This pulse sequence best demonstrates the difference in signal intensity of the renal cortex (long arrow) and of the medulla (short arrow). The relatively lower signal intensity of the medulla is due to its increased water content, and hence longer *T1* relaxation time, compared with the renal cortex.

particular imaging plane, resulting in lack of signal.[38,47] The renal collecting system, best seen with increasing diuresis,[46] appears dark because of the very long *T1* and *T2* parameters of water, the major component of urine.

The renal vein lies anteriorly in relation to the renal artery and can be traced back to the inferior vena cava. In axial planes, similar to CT, the left renal vein is seen coursing between the aorta and the superior mesenteric artery (Fig. 31–3). Origins of renal arteries can be seen on axial images (Fig. 31–4), although at times they are better seen in coronal or oblique coronal planes. The ability of MR to image in multiple planes, including nonorthogonal[48] planes, is useful in evaluating major vessels and their pathology, such as tumor thrombus extension in the inferior vena cava and abdominal aortic aneurysms.

The major vessels also can be clearly seen in the retroperitoneum and do not show any internal signal; they can be easily separated from retroperitoneal lymph nodes, which have different signal intensity. The psoas muscles as well as the paraspinous

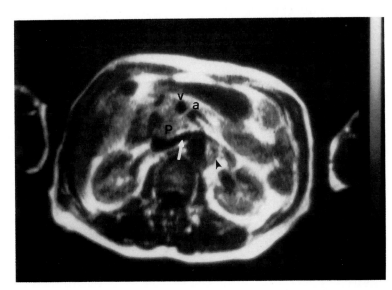

Figure 31–3. Spin echo transverse image displays the left renal vein (arrow) coursing between the SMA (a) and the aorta. Superior mesenteric vein (v) and the uncinate process of the pancreas (P) are also clearly visualized. An enlarged left para-aortic lymph node is seen (arrowhead) and has intermediate signal intensity.

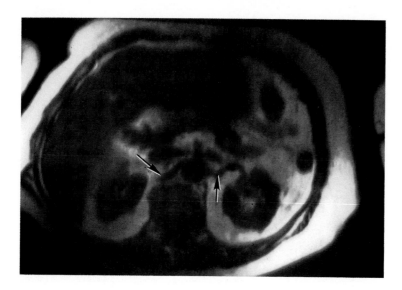

Figure 31–4. Origins of both renal arteries are clearly demonstrated (arrows). The origins of the superior mesenteric artery, left renal vein, and inferior vena cava are also noted.

muscles exhibit intermediate signal intensity on spin-echo sequences owing to their moderately long *T1* and short *T2* relaxation times.

The corticomedullary differentiation, seen very well with spin-echo technique using short *TR* interval, is even more marked on inversion recovery (IR) pulse sequence.[22] However, owing to overall lower signal strength the images are poorer in quality. Again, on inversion recovery the renal sinus and perinephric fat have bright signal, whereas the blood vessels and collecting system appear as areas of decreased signal intensity. The corticomedullary differentiation decreases as the *TR* interval is increased and is almost completely lost with *T2* weighted images (Fig. 31–5).

IMAGING TECHNIQUES

The transverse or coronal view is the preferred plane for screening patients with suspected renal or retroperitoneal pathology. Previous experience with CT has improved our knowledge of axial anatomy significantly. Evaluation of the kidney and retroperitoneal spaces is excellent on transverse sections. But MR has the additional benefits of multiplanar imaging, in which relationships of abdominal masses are seen better on sagittal and coronal planes. These two planes also image major blood vessels

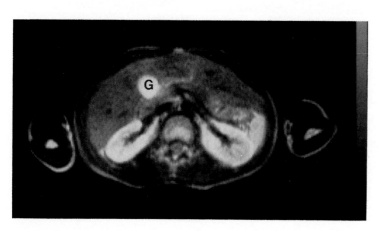

Figure 31–5. *T2* weighted image showing very bright signal due to long *T2* relaxation times of the bile in the gallbladder (G). Note the loss of distinction between the cortex and the medulla compared with a *T1* weighted image (Fig. 31–2). Liver has intermediate signal intensity.

along their long axis, which is helpful in determining tumor or thrombus extension in major vessels or in determining the limits of an aneurysm.

For screening renal and retroperitoneal anatomy, axial spin-echo images with relatively short *TE* or *TR* parameters (SE 30/500) are obtained. These are relatively *T1* weighted images and provide excellent contrast between retroperitoneal fat (bright signal), blood vessels (usually no signal), and abdominal viscera (intermediate signal). Although respiratory gating frequently improves image quality, it is not necessary in the evaluation of the kidney and retroperitoneum on a routine basis. Similarly, oral contrast agents, such as ferrous gluconate and Geritol, are not routinely used for the renal and retroperitoneal MR examinations. The respiratory gating devices may be necessary if the initial MR studies show marked image degradation due to respiratory artifacts. Oral contrast is used to identify stomach and duodenum in patients who, on initial acquisition, demonstrate peripancreatic masses or absence of significant fat planes between the abdominal viscera.

The initial screening series is followed by axial spin-echo images with long *TE* and *TR* (i.e., SE 60/2000 or SE 120/2000) sequences. Use of multislice-multiecho technique offers at least two series with different *TE* times, without increasing data acquisition times. After these sequences, additional imaging planes are acquired depending upon the renal or retroperitoneal pathology. For the evaluation of vascular extension of renal tumor, the coronal plane is preferred, whereas the sagittal plane is utilized to determine the origin of an unusual mass lesion, (i.e., kidney, adrenal, or liver). Occasionally, nonorthogonal images are obtained to study the origins of the renal artery from the aorta. *T1* weighted sagittal or coronal images (i.e., SE 30/5090) are used to delineate an anatomic lesion such as a renal mass or an abdominal aortic aneurysm. Sequences with long *TR* (i.e., SE 30/2000 and SE 60/2000) are useful in determining vascular extension from tumor and are also sometimes valuable in differentiating tumor thrombus from blood clot.[49]

When using multislice or multislice-multiecho techniques, it is essential to remember that MR blood flow principles, such as even-echo rephasing and so forth, must be considered during image interpretation.[47] Similarly, chemical shift artifacts are dependent on pulse sequences as well as field strength and need to be identified according to the individual equipment.

The MR imaging protocols are determined by the available equipment, software limitations, and disease processes. Small lesions, such as adrenal aldosteronoma and renal arteriovenous malformation, may require the use of surface coils. The time factor is important not only for cost effectiveness but also for patient comfort. We strongly recommend the use of at least two and possibly three pulse sequences in characterizing the renal or retroperitoneal pathology.

RENAL MASSES

MRI compares favorably with contrast-enhanced CT in its ability to discriminate between cystic and solid renal masses.[22,23] It also shows characteristic signal intensities in the presence of hemorrhagic and infected cysts, which are distinctly different when compared with simple cysts.[19-24]

On spin-echo pulse sequences with short *TR* interval (SE 30/500) simple renal cysts are seen as areas of homogeneous low-level signal intensity; the cyst is sharply marginated from surrounding renal parenchyma (Fig. 31–6). The cyst wall is usually not visualized. The fluid content in the simple renal cyst has long *T1* and *T2* relaxation characteristics. As either the *TE* or the *TR* interval increases, the signal intensity from the fluid within the cyst starts increasing and becomes brighter with images using long

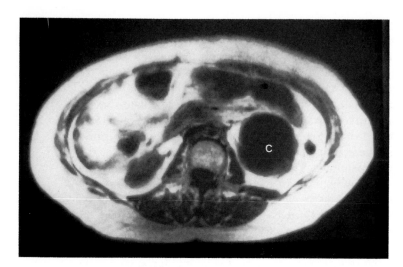

Figure 31–6. Simple renal cyst (C) arising from the lower pole of the left kidney has low signal intensity owing to the long $T1$ and $T2$ relaxation characteristics of the cyst fluid. (Spin echo 30/500.)

TE and *TR*. Inversion recovery sequences reveal low signal from the cyst fluid owing to longer *T1* values of clear cyst fluid (Fig. 31–7).

The ability to distinguish between simple and hemorrhagic renal cysts is very useful in the evaluation of patients with acute flank pain. Hemorrhagic cysts (Fig. 31–8) in a patient with polycystic renal disease have high signal intensity on SE sequences with short *TE* and *TR* intervals. This is probably due to the short *T1* relaxation times of hemorrhage within the cyst. These lesions also demonstrate bright signal on *T2* weighted images. Signal intensities depend upon the stage of resolution of the hemorrhage. The age of the hemorrhage can be judged from the degree of brightness of the signal.[21] The reported strong association of neoplasms suggests that all hemorrhagic cysts be aspirated. The ability of MRI to differentiate simple from hemorrhagic cysts is very valuable in this regard.

MR is useful in the diagnosis and follow-up of patients with acute polycystic kidney disease and in those on long-term dialysis who have multiple cysts presenting with flank pain. MRI permits coronal imaging, which gives a better appreciation of the location of a hemorrhagic cyst in the presence of multiple cysts and when cyst aspiration is contemplated.

Neoplasms

Malignant renal tumors account for 2 to 3 percent of all neoplasms,[25,26] with renal cell carcinoma (hypernephroma) accounting for 85 percent of all kidney tumors.[26] It is most frequently encountered in the sixth decade and is two to three times more prevalent in males than in females. A review of 890 cases of renal cell carcinoma by Noronha et al.[27] showed a significant increase in number of patients in the 42 to 49 year group. Clinically, the classic triad of hematuria, pain, and flank mass is seen in only 20 percent of the patients, whereas about one third manifest metastatic spread at the time of diagnosis.

Accurate staging is crucial at the time of diagnosis, as it has profound implications on method of treatment, prognosis, and survival. Patients with tumor confined to kidney (Stage I) or perinephric space (Stage II) as well as those with tumor thrombus extension to the renal vein or inferior vena cava (Stage IIIA) have a 60 to 70 percent five-year survival rate when treated with radical nephrectomy. On the other hand, those who experience local recurrence, which most likely represents persistence of malignancy in regional lymph nodes, have an 86 percent mortality rate at the end of one year.

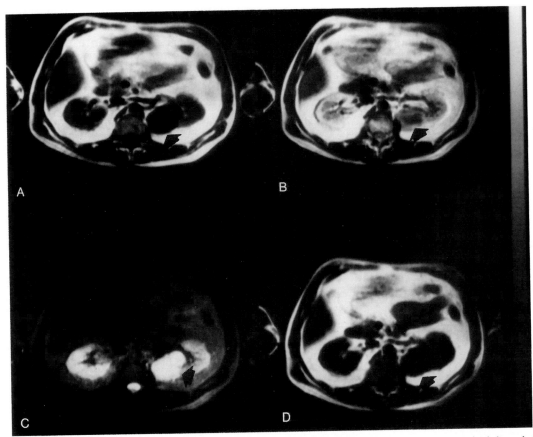

Figure 31–7. A simple cyst of the left kidney (arrows) is illustrated with different pulse sequences acquired through the same axial plane. *A*, The cyst has a low signal intensity in this spin-echo 30/500 image. Increasing the pulse sequences to 60/1000 ms (*B*) and 120/2000 ms (*C*) shows increasing signal intensity due to the long *T2* values of clear cyst fluid. *D*, Inversion recovery demonstrates low signal intensity due to long *T1* values. (From Kulkarni MV, et al: J Comput Assist Tomogr 5:861, 1984. Used by permission.)

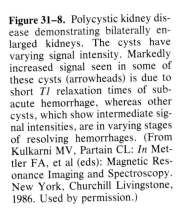

Figure 31–8. Polycystic kidney disease demonstrating bilaterally enlarged kidneys. The cysts have varying signal intensity. Markedly increased signal seen in some of these cysts (arrowheads) is due to short *T1* relaxation times of subacute hemorrhage, whereas other cysts, which show intermediate signal intensities, are in varying stages of resolving hemorrhages. (From Kulkarni MV, Partain CL: *In* Mettler FA, et al (eds): Magnetic Resonance Imaging and Spectroscopy. New York, Churchill Livingstone, 1986. Used by permission.)

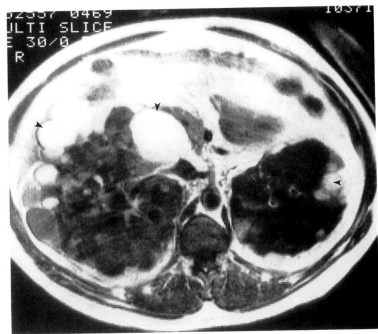

MRI appears to be superior to other imaging techniques in the diagnosis and precise staging of renal cell carcinoma.[29] Intravenous pyelography is still the most common initial examination used to search for suspected renal masses. Since the advent of computed tomography[25,30,31] and ultrasonography,[35] the accuracy in diagnosis of renal masses has improved significantly. These modalities not only distinguish cystic from solid masses but also provide information about local extension, regional nodal metastasis, and venous extension of tumor thrombus.

MRI, owing to its multiplanar imaging capability, is better suited than CT to correctly determine the organ of origin of a retroperitoneal mass. Also, the tumor thrombus extension is better visualized, even in intrarenal venous radicles, and sluggish blood flow in vessels due to mass effect can be differentiated from actual tumor thrombi.[22,29,49]

On MRI, solid renal tumors (Fig. 31–9) are easily separated from surrounding renal parenchyma.[19–24,29,30,34] Tumor signal varies from hypo- to hyperintense in comparison with renal parenchymal signal intensity, and both *T1* and *T2* relaxation times are higher when compared with normal renal parenchyma. Areas of inhomogeneity noted in the tumor mass correspond to areas of tumor necrosis and hemorrhage. A low-intensity band surrounding the tumor mass is shown to be due to a pseudocapsule[34] and may be similar to the "hypernephroma halo" seen on angiography. Owing to the fibrous tissue in the capsule, the signal intensity is low in both *T1* and *T2* weighted images. In contrast to CT, areas of calcification are poorly visualized because of the absence of signal from them.

Poor visualization or nonvisualization of soft tissue calcifications on MRI is one of its drawbacks and has been described.[21] This paucity of signal from areas of calcification results from the low density of mobile protons in the calcification matrix. Larger areas of calcification are poorly visualized, and smaller calcific deposits and stones are not seen. It has been suggested that visualization of calcium may be related to the age of the calcification.[53] An immature area of calcification may give low-level intensity signal because of the high percentage of water molecules within it, whereas mature calcifications with much smaller percentages of water molecules may give no signal at all.

The absence of signal from areas of calcification in itself can be useful to indirectly indicate their presence, since this characteristic absence or persistent low-intensity signal is noted with all pulse sequences. This would distinguish calcifications from fluid collections, which would exhibit some increase in signal intensity with prolongation of

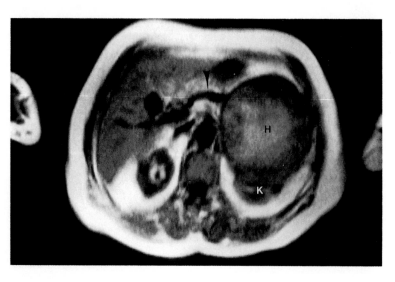

Figure 31–9. Hypernephroma (H) arising from the anterior aspect of the left kidney (K) and elevating the splenic vein, which is well defined because of the lack of signal within it. The tumor mass has increased signal intensity in the center as the result of tumor necrosis. This area of necrosis appeared brighter on SE 60/1000 sequence owing to its relatively longer *T2* relaxation time. (From Kulkarni MV et al. *In* Peterson SB et al (eds): An Introduction to Biomedical Nuclear Magnetic Resonance. New York, Georg Thieme Verlag, 1985. Used by permission.)

TE and *TR* intervals on spin-echo images. Dense fibrous tissue similarly has low density of mobile protons and is difficult to distinguish from calcification deposits.

Use of the intravenous paramagnetic contrast agent Gd-DTPA has been shown to produce a marked decrease in *T1* and *T2* relaxation values of renal parenchyma and urine. There is an increased signal intensity in low concentrations of Gd-DTPA but decreased signal intensity with higher concentrations. Hypernephroma has shown increased signal intensity, and the tumor margin has been better defined.[19] Paramagnetic contrast agents, such as Gd-DTPA, may be a helpful adjunct in MR imaging and may play a role similar to that of conventional iodinated contrast agents in radiographic evaluation of the kidney.

Tumor extension beyond the renal capsule and into the perinephric fat can be accurately judged on MRI, and the presence of retroperitoneal adenopathy[29,42] is also demonstrated.

MR is extremely sensitive in recognizing extension of tumor thrombus into the renal vein and inferior vena cava. Unlike CT, this is achieved without the use of intravenous contrast administration or ionizing radiation. Intrarenal vessels are also well seen; imaging of tumor thrombus within larger intrarenal venous radicles is possible (as it is not with CT), thereby offering more accurate staging in such instances. When presented with a retroperitoneal mass, MRI with its direct multiplane imaging capability is superior to CT in correctly identifying the origin of the mass and separating adrenal masses and retroperitoneal tumors from masses of renal origin.

Pulse sequences using a long *TR* and a long *TE* are more useful in delineating normal kidney from renal tumors, whereas pulse sequences using a short *TR* and a short *TE* present the best contrast between the tumor and surrounding fat. Thus, in the staging and detection of tumors, a sequence using a short *TE* and a short *TR*, such as SE 30/500, and one utilizing a long *TR* and a long *TE*, such as a *T2* weighted image, are useful. According to Hricak et al., inversion recovery (IR) images did not add any significant information in a study of seven cases of renal cell carcinoma.[46]

MRI can be useful in patients in whom there is a high clinical suspicion of a renal cell carcinoma despite a normal intravenous urogram (IVU), which can miss exophytic masses or those along the anterior and posterior aspects of the kidneys. By use of different pulse sequences, small contrast differences can be enhanced; supplementing axial images with coronal and sagittal imaging can enhance our ability to define the tumor extension and vascular involvement.

Among other kidney masses, angiomyolipoma (Fig. 31–10) is a benign fatty tumor that is commonly encountered in the young to middle-aged. With the advent of computed tomography it is increasingly discovered incidentally, and it has a characteristic appearance on CT.[51] It is a hamartoma composed of varying proportions of lipomatous,

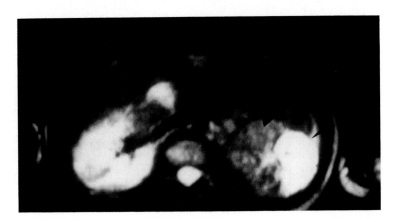

Figure 31–10. Angiomyolipoma of the left kidney. This *T2* weighted image obtained with spin-echo 120/2000 pulse sequence demonstrates the hamartomas as an inhomogeneous area of intermediate signal intensity (arrow). The region of brightened signal intensity (arrowhead) was probably secondary to hemorrhagic infarction of the portion of the angiomyolipoma following embolization.

myomatous, and angiomatous elements and most commonly presents clinically with flank pain due to tumor hemorrhage. On MRI these lesions demonstrate high signal intensity similar to that of subcutaneous fat, regardless of the *TR* and *TE* used.[52]

Other commonly encountered solid renal tumors include benign adenoma (oncocytoma), renal lymphoma, Wilms' tumor (Fig. 31–11) and metastasis. In evaluating Wilms' tumor in infants and children, because of the paucity of intra-abdominal fat there is poor definition of tissue planes; better soft tissue contrast with MR may provide an edge over CT.[33] A case of Wilms' tumor has been described in which MRI showed invasion of posterior pararenal fat that was missed on CT.[21] On the pulse sequences currently in use, these tumors demonstrate signal intensities varying from hypo- to hyperintense compared with normal renal parenchyma and as such do not have a characteristic appearance.

The MR appearance of papillary renal cell carcinoma has been described[39]; although most renal cell carcinomas have higher *T1* and *T2* values when compared with renal cortex, occasionally a tumor such as this papillary carcinoma[30] may demonstrate lower *T1* and *T2* values as seen by decreased signal intensity on a *T2* weighted image (Fig. 31–12).

Renal Hilum

MRI can readily detect pelvicaliectasis. Normal ureter is not commonly seen, but a dilated ureter can be traced along its course. Hydronephrosis is seen as decreased signal intensity in renal calyces and pelvis on spin-echo images with short *TE* and *TR* (Fig. 31–13). This is accompanied by loss of normal corticomedullary contrast in the presence of obstructive hydronephrosis and is seen with both SE and IR sequences.[20] MRI, like contrast-enhanced CT and ultrasonography, can differentiate parapelvic cyst from renal sinus lipomatosis. This is because of the marked difference in relaxation parameters between fat (short *T1*) in sinus lipomatosis and fluid (long *T1*) in parapelvic cysts. However, parapelvic cysts may be mistaken for hydronephrosis. MRI has the

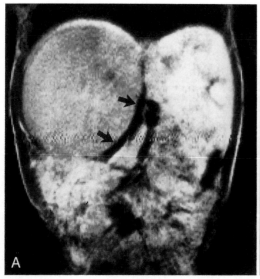
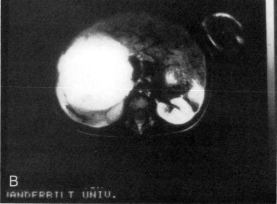

Figure 31–11. *A*, Coronal spin-echo 30/500 image reveals a large Wilms' tumor displacing and compressing the inferior vena cava (IVC) (arrows). At surgery, there was no evidence of invasion of the IVC by the tumor. *B*, *T2* weighted axial image demonstrates increase in signal intensity of the tumor mass due to its prolonged *T2* relaxation time. (From Kulkarni MV et al: J Nucl Med *26*:944, 1985. Used by permission.)

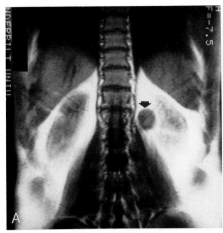

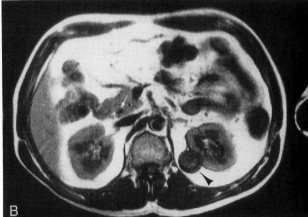

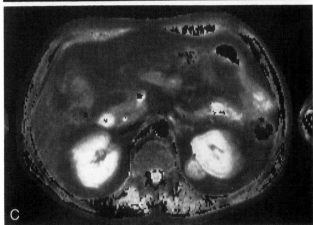

Figure 31–12. *A*, Coronal spin-echo 30/500 image demonstrating an exophytic papillary cell carcinoma arising from the medial aspect of the left kidney (arrow). *B*, Axial spin-echo image shows the mass (arrowhead), which has slightly decreased signal intensity compared with the renal cortex. The corticomedullary differentiation is well seen. The common bile duct (white arrow) is well seen within the head of the pancreas. *C*, *T2* weighted image from a multiecho sequence demonstrates decreased signal intensity within the mass compared with normal kidney, indicating a short *T2* value. This is uncommon, as most renal cell carcinomas have prolonged *T2* values (From Kulkarni MV et al: J Comput Assist Tomogr 8:861, 1984. Used by permission.)

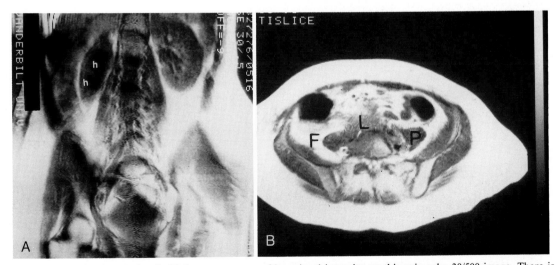

Figure 31–13. *A*, Hydronephrosis (h) is seen as areas of low signal intensity on this spin-echo 30/500 image. There is also evidence of parenchymal loss when compared with a normal left kidney. *B*, Retroperitoneal lymphadenopathy (L) from carcinoma of the uterine cervix. P = Psoas muscle; F = retroperitoneal fat. (From Kulkarni MV et al: RadioGraphics 5(4):621, 1985.

ability to further characterize the fluid within the dilated collecting system (Fig. 31–14). Presence of a subcapsular or perinephric hematoma would appear as a mass, with the signal intensity depending on the stage of hemorrhage resolution (Fig. 31–15).

The presence of renal artery aneurysms and arteriovenous malformation (AVM) is diagnosed by MRI,[54] as these lesions exhibit absence of signal in the AVM together with a dilated renal vein. Rapidly flowing blood shows absent signal, whereas slowly flowing blood shows high signal intensity on spin-echo images.

The MR appearance of renal abscess is similar to that of solid renal tumors and appears as an inhomogeneous mass of lower intensity compared with renal parenchyma. Thickening of Gerota's fascia and extension of the inflammatory process in perinephric fat can sometimes be appreciated as decreased signal intensity, although malignancy can also mimic this appearance.

Xanthogranulomatous pyelonephritis (Fig. 31–16) is a chronic inflammatory process that may involve the entire kidney or occur focally. It is always associated with renal calculi and is seen predominantly in diabetic persons. On sonography and intravenous pyelogram, a nonfunctioning kidney with calculi and hydronephrosis is noted. On MRI[21,40] an enlarged kidney with a dilated collecting system is evident. The affected renal parenchyma has higher than normal signal intensity as it is replaced by lipid-laden macrophages (xanthoma cells), whereas the purulent material in the dilated collecting system gives it a signal intensity that is higher than that of normal urine. Also, on inversion recovery, the affected renal parenchyma has a different signal intensity compared with retroperitoneal fat; this may differentiate between two types of lipid tissue.[21]

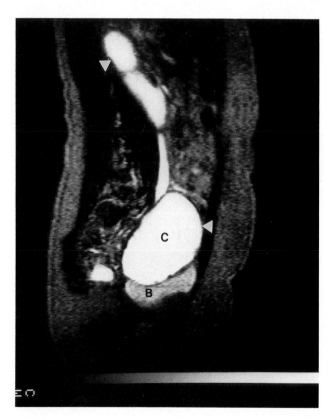

Figure 31–14. Sagittal spin-echo 120/2000 image showing a benign hemorrhagic ovarian cyst (C) along with hydroureter and hydronephrosis. Note that the signal intensity of the collecting system and the ureter is similar to that of the cystic mass (arrowheads). These signal intensities are different from that of the urine in the bladder (B) on this *T2* weighted image. This was due to an abnormal communication between the ureter and the hemorrhagic cyst, with reflux of its contents into the ureter.

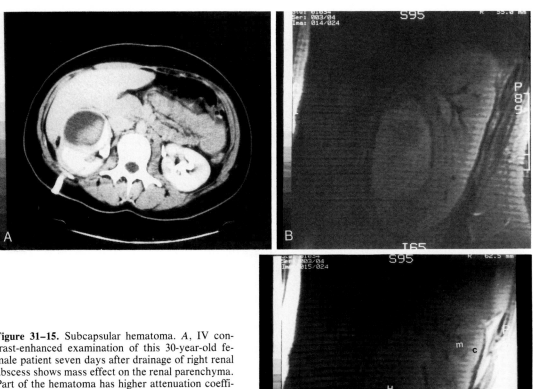

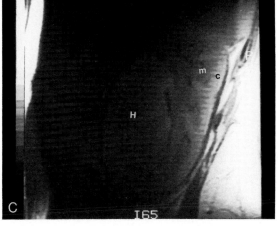

Figure 31–15. Subcapsular hematoma. *A*, IV contrast-enhanced examination of this 30-year-old female patient seven days after drainage of right renal abscess shows mass effect on the renal parenchyma. Part of the hematoma has higher attenuation coefficients because of hemoconcentration. *B*, Coronal surface coil image at 1.5 tesla shows subcapsular mass that demonstrates decreased intensity in the area corresponding to the area of increased attenuation on CT. Also note the thickening of the capsule as well as visualization of intervening vessels. *C*, Another image demonstrates the differentiation of the medulla from the renal cortex. H = Hematoma; c = cortex; m = medulla.

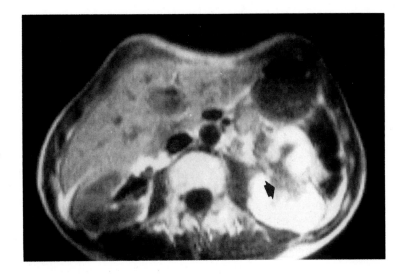

Figure 31–16. Xanthogranulomatous pyelonephritis. Spin echo 30/500 image shows abnormal signal intensity of left kidney compared with the right kidney. The left kidney is replaced with fat. Also note dilated collecting system with signal intensity that is higher than that of normal urine owing to its purulent content (arrow).

Renal Parenchymal Disease

On spin-echo images, Hricak and coworkers first noted loss of normal signal intensity difference between the cortex and medulla in renal parenchymal disease, such as chronic glomerulonephritis. Renal parenchymal thickness is decreased, and there is increased renal sinus fat deposition. Also, the intensity of renal cortex, which is normally similar to that of liver, is less than hepatic signal intensity.[20,21] In normal individuals the corticomedullary differentiation is easily visualized on spin-echo images with short *TR* and *TE* intervals; with prolonged *TR* and *TE* intervals this contrast decreases and is virtually nonexistent on *T2* weighted images. This differentiation also depends on the state of hydration and is better visualized on well-hydrated normal subjects. Loss of normal corticomedullary contrast is also noted in the presence of hydronephrosis in renal transplant rejections as well as after extracorporeal shockwave lithotripsy.

In the case of glycogen storage disease, Hricak and colleagues have described enlarged kidneys bilaterally with much greater than normal intensity of renal cortex compared with adjacent liver on spin-echo images.[20]

Renal Transplants

Renal transplantation is being performed increasingly and is the current treatment of choice for the long-term management of chronic renal failure patients.

Radionuclide imaging[60] and sonography[58-60] are well-established imaging techniques in evaluating renal transplants. Experience with MRI is limited at this stage.[21,44,64] There are indications that in cases in which initial investigations with established modalities, such as ultrasound imaging and Doppler evaluation as well as radionuclide imaging, are difficult for technical reasons or disagree with clinical findings, MRI would be the study of choice.[45]

Because of the pelvic location, MRI of renal transplant is only minimally degraded by respiratory and peristaltic motion artifacts. There is also the advantage of multiplanar imaging, which shows the relationships of peritransplant fluid collections, urinary bladder, and allograft to better advantage.

Unlike computed tomography, there is no need for intravenous contrast administration, which, in renal transplant patients with poor renal function, should be avoided. With the advent of surface-coil imaging, the superficial location of the renal transplant in the iliac fossa makes it possible to image with improved spatial resolution by magnification techniques and better signal-to-noise ratio as compared with body-coil imaging.[61]

In the immediate post-transplantation period, deteriorating renal function and decreasing urinary output may be due to various conditions such as acute tubular necrosis (ATN), rejection, cyclosporine toxicity, and obstructive uropathy. MRI can also demonstrate hydronephrosis and peritransplant fluid collections.

Imaging parameters and morphologic features seen on renal transplants are similar to those of native kidneys. Spin-echo technique with short *TR* and *TE* intervals (*TR* 500 ms, *TE* 30 ms) gives a *T1* weighted image and shows the corticomedullary differentiation to best advantage. In normal renal transplants, cortex has higher signal intensity than medulla, with a sharp corticomedullary boundary. Spin-echo technique also gives better spatial resolution as compared with inversion recovery techniques, although both have demonstrated the loss of signal intensity difference of cortex to medulla in renal transplant rejection.

In acute rejection, there is loss of corticomedullary contrast differentiation, due to prolongation of *T1* relaxation time of the cortex, which is thought to be due to cortical edema.[62] This was the most sensitive finding on MR evaluation of rejecting renal transplants[45,64]; it helps differentiate rejection from cyclosporine toxicity, in which case there is preservation of normal cortical intensity with normal morphologic features.

Associated findings on MRI in rejecting transplants include increase in size, globular shape, loss of renal sinus fat, peritransplant fluid collections, and sometimes pelvicaliectasis, which may be a manifestation of associated ureteric rejection with decreased peristalsis.

There is similar decrease in cortical intensity with ATN; preliminary findings question how useful MR would be in differentiating ATN from acute rejection.[43]

Chronic rejection similarly has a decrease in cortical intensity on *T1* weighted images. The renal allograft is smaller, unlike acute rejection, which is accompanied by enlargement and globular shape of the renal transplant.

Peritransplant fluid collections can be further characterized with demonstration of higher signal intensity on *T1* weighted images in cases of perirenal abscesses and hematomas and separating them from lymphoceles and urinomas.[44,45]

Retroperitoneum

As described earlier, high intensity signal of retroperitoneal fat combined with absence of signal from vascular structures and minimal image degradation caused by physiologic motion artifacts make magnetic resonance imaging an attractive modality in evaluation of the retroperitoneum.

Adrenal glands are seen as intermediate-intensity structures surrounded by high-intensity fat on spin-echo images. MR imaging of adrenals is discussed in Chapter 32.

Retroperitoneal lymph nodes have slightly less intense signal compared with psoas muscles and are outlined by surrounding high intensity (Fig. 31–17). As with CT, enlarged lymph nodes are considered abnormal when greater than 1 cm in diameter. Retrocrural nodes larger than 6 mm are considered abnormal. MRI compares favorably to CT in correctly diagnosing retroperitoneal adenopathy (Fig. 31–18). Although lack of a suitable gastrointestinal contrast agent is a drawback, the advantages of MRI include absence of ionizing radiation and no need for intravenous contrast. MRI may surpass CT in detecting recurrent adenopathy in patients with multiple surgical clips creating significant artifacts.

Owing to their orientation the aorta and inferior vena cava can be better imaged along their course on coronal and sagittal scans.

The abdominal aorta and its major branches are clearly delineated, including renal

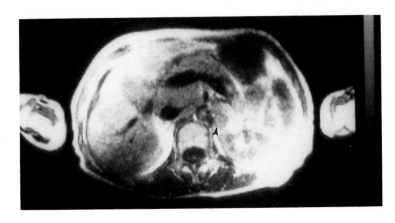

Figure 31–17. Retrocaval and enlarged left para-aortic lymph node is noted (arrowhead) in a patient with carcinoma of the breast. Lymph nodes have different signal intensity as compared with the retroperitoneal vessels and are easily recognized.

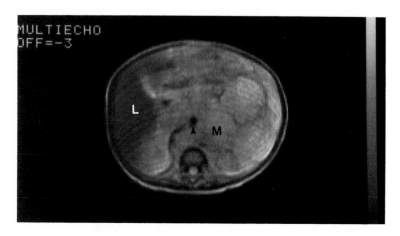

Figure 31–18. Metastatic retroperitoneal neuroblastoma (M) on *T2* weighted image demonstrates abdominal aorta (arrowhead) displaced by the lymph node mass. Liver (L) has lower signal intensity on *T2* weighted images compared with the lymphadenopathy. Also, respiratory artifacts are seen as multiple parallel lines in this nongated image. (From Kulkarni MV et al. Pediatr Clin North Am *32*:1509, 1985. Used by permission.)

arteries and their origins (see Fig. 31–4). In normal young individuals, on transverse axial images, the abdominal aorta has very thin walls and, owing to rapid blood flow, demonstrates lack of intraluminal signal. Stagnant blood, blood clots, and atheromatous plaques produce low to medium gray-level signal intensities.[55] Aortic aneurysms can be accurately diagnosed, including extent, external and luminal diameters, involvement of renal arteries, and continuation into iliac vessels (Fig. 31–19).[55,56] MRI is comparable to other modalities, such as CT and ultrasonography, in accuracy of measurements of extent and size of the aneurysms. Although ultrasonography should be the screening modality of choice in persons with suspected abdominal aortic aneurysms because of its ease of performance and low cost, detection of involvement of renal artery origins and both iliac arteries may be suboptimal owing to overlying bowel gas. CT, although

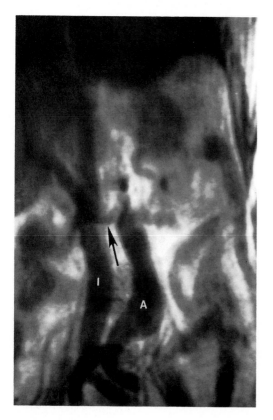

Figure 31–19. Abdominal aortic aneurysm (A) is well visualized on this spin-echo coronal image. Its dimensions and extent are better appreciated on a coronal image. The right renal artery (arrow) is well depicted. The aneurysm is infrarenal and does not extend into the aortic bifurcation. I = IVC.

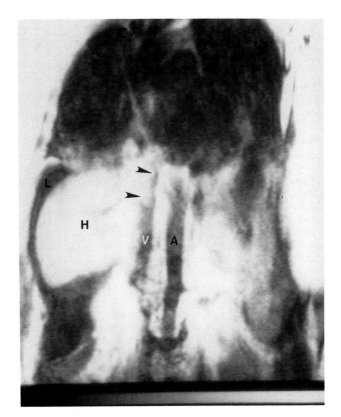

Figure 31–20. Coronal spin-echo 30/500 image shows a large high signal intensity mass (H) arising from the right lobe of the liver. Note the tumor extension (arrowheads) into the inferior vena cava. Also compare the intensity of the hepatocellular carcinoma (H) with that of the normal liver (L). A = Abdominal aorta.

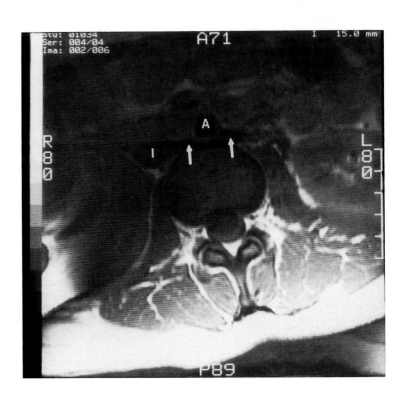

Figure 31–21. Surface coil spin-echo image shows a tubular low-intensity structure continuous with the inferior vena cava and posterior to the abdominal aorta as an incidental finding. I = Inferior vena cava; A = abdominal aorta. Arrows point to retroaortic left renal veins.

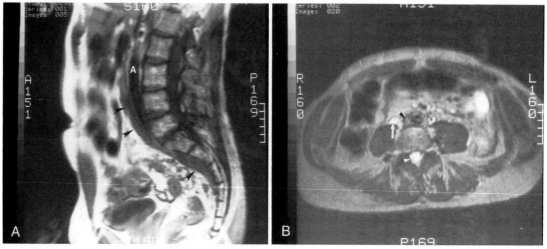

Figure 31–22. Retroperitoneal fibrosis. *A*, Sagittal spin-echo 20/800 image showing an abnormal soft tissue of intermediate signal intensity in the retroperitoneum. It extends from just about the level of bifurcation into the presacral region (arrowheads). Distal abdominal aorta is also visualized (A). *B*, Axial *T2* weighted image shows an abnormal thickened tissue surrounding the abdominal aorta, having signal intensity intermediate between that of the psoas muscles and that of the subcutaneous fat. This persistently low signal intensity tissue represents fibrous tissue and is consistent with retroperitoneal fibrosis. Also note right hydroureter (arrow), seen as bright signal intensity owing to prolonged *T2* relaxation time of the urine. The urine has signal intensity similar to that of the CSF within the spinal canal (white arrowhead). Intraluminal signal is noted within the attenuated inferior vena cava (black arrowhead). Sluggish flow is consistent with involvement in the process of retroperitoneal fibrosis.

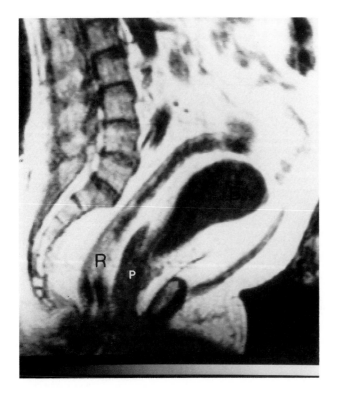

Figure 31–23. Retroperitoneal lipomatosis. Sagittal SE 30/500 image in a patient with retroperitoneal lipomatosis demonstrates increased amount of fat deposition. The rectum (R) and bladder (B) are elevated and stretched owing to this deposition of fat. P = Prostate. (From Kulkarni MV et al: RadioGraphics *5*(4):624, 1985. Used by permission.)

more accurate than sonography, involves use of intravenous contrast agents and ionizing radiation. Aortic dissections are well visualized with MRI. Intimal flap and false and true lumen as well as origins of celiac, superior mesenteric, and renal arteries from true or false lumen are correctly predicted. The false lumen, owing to very slow flow in it, has intraluminal signal and can be differentiated from true lumen, which has characteristically absent signal on spin-echo images.[57]

Inferior vena cava and renal veins and retroperitoneal venous collaterals, when present, are clearly visualized on MRI. Distinction of intraluminal thrombus from slow flow due to venous compression has been shown by Hricak and associates.[49] Slow flow demonstrates increase in intraluminal intensity on second-echo image as a result of even-echo rephasing phenomena. Extension of tumor thrombus (Fig. 31–20) and bland venous thrombus can be accurately diagnosed. Sagittal images are particularly helpful. Various developmental venous anomalies, such as retroaortic left renal vein (Fig. 31–21) and azygos continuation with interruption of inferior vena cava, can be diagnosed in a noninvasive manner.[50]

Other retroperitoneal processes, such as retroperitoneal and perinephric hematoma[37] as well as retroperitoneal fibrosis (Fig. 31–22)[41] and retroperitoneal lipomatosis (Fig. 31–23), not only are diagnosed but also their extent, their effect on major vessels, and postoperative evaluation are possible in a noninvasive fashion.

In conclusion, magnetic resonance imaging has made rapid strides in the evaluation of kidneys and retroperitoneum in a relatively short time. It offers superior tissue contrast and multiple imaging planes without the use of ionizing radiation or intravenous contrast administration. Owing to different pulse sequences, various tissues are more correctly characterized. Spectroscopy and chemical-shift imaging offer future scope of metabolic and physiologic imaging capabilities, especially in a dynamic organ such as the kidney. Surface coils offer better resolution in evaluating renal transplants and other superficial structures.

ACKNOWLEDGMENT

The authors express appreciation to Adlene Rehfeld, Anna Miller, and Diane McNamara for the preparation and editing of this manuscript, as well as to Jay Johnson and John Bobbitt for photography.

References

1. Alfidi RJ, Haaga JR, El Yousef SF, et al: Preliminary experimental results in humans and animals with superconducting whole body nuclear magnetic scanner. Radiology *143*:175, 1982.
2. Bydder GM, Steiner RE, Young TR, et al: Clinical NMR imaging of the brain, 160 cases. AJR *139*:215, 1982.
3. Lanzer P, Botvinick EH, Schiller NB, et al: Cardiac imaging using gated magnetic resonance. Radiology *150*:121, 1984.
4. Runge VM, Price AC, Kirshner MS, et al: The evaluation of multiple sclerosis by magnetic resonance imaging. The current state. AJR *143*:1015, 1984.
5. James AE, Partain CL, Holland IN, et al: Nuclear magnetic resonance imaging. AJR *138*:201, 1981.
6. Bradley WG Jr, Waluch V, Yadley RA, Wycoff RR: Comparison of CT and MR in 600 patients with disease of the brain and central spinal cord. Radiology *152*:695, 1984.
7. Araki T, Inouye T, Suzuki H, et al: Magnetic resonance of brain tumors: measurement of T1. Radiology *150*:95, 1984.
8. Runge VM, Clanton JA, Lukehart CM, et al: Paramagnetic agents for contrast enhanced NMR imaging: A review. AJR *141*:1209, 1983.
9. Brant-Zawadzki M, Norman D, Crooks LE, et al: Magnetic resonance imaging of the brain: The optimal screening technique. Radiology *152*:71, 1984.
10. Modic MT, Weinstein MA, Pavlicek W, et al: Nuclear magnetic resonance imaging of the spine. Radiology *148*:757, 1983.
11. Edelman RR: High resolution surface coil imaging of lumbar disc disease. AJR *144*:1122, 1985.

12. Buonocore E, Borkowski GP, Pavlicek W, et al: NMR imaging of the abdomen: technical considerations. AJR *141*:1171, 1983.
13. Hawkes RC, Holland GN, Moore WS, et al: Nuclear magnetic resonance (NMR) tomography of the normal abdomen. J Comput Assist Tomogr *5*(5):613, 1981.
14. Kulkarni MV, Partain CL, Tishler JM, et al: Magnetic resonance imaging of the abdomen. *In* Peterson SB et al (eds): An Introduction to Biomedical Nuclear Magnetic Resonance. New York, Georg Thieme, 1985.
15. Gamsu G, Webb WR, Sheldon P, et al: Nuclear magnetic resonance imaging of the thorax. Radiology *147*:473, 1983.
16. Gadian DG: Introduction to principles and instrumentation of metabolic magnetic resonance: *In* Peterson SB et al (eds): An Introduction to Biomedical Nuclear Magnetic Resonance. New York, Georg Thieme, 1985.
17. Wong GG, Ross BD: Applications of phosphorous nuclear magnetic resonance to problems of renal physiology and metabolism. Mineral Electrolyte Metab *9*:282, 1983.
18. Weiner NW, Adam WR: Magnetic resonance spectroscopy for evaluation of renal function. Semin Urol *3*:34, 1985.
19. Leung AW, Bydder GM, Steiner RE, et al: Magnetic resonance imaging of the kidneys. AJR *143*:1215, 1984.
20. Hricak H, Crooks L, Sheldon P, Kaufman L: Nuclear magnetic resonance imaging of the kidney. Radiology *146*:425, 1983.
21. LiPuma J: Magnetic resonance imaging of the kidney. Radiol Clin North Am *22*:925, 1984.
22. Hricak H, Moon K: Kidneys and adrenal glands. *In* Clinical Magnetic Resonance Imaging. San Francisco, Radiology Research and Educational Foundation, 1983.
23. Smith FW, Hutchison JMS, Mallard JR, et al: Renal cyst or tumor? Differentiation by whole-body nuclear magnetic resonance imaging. Diagn Imag *50*:61, 1981.
24. Kulkarni MV, Sandler MP, Shaff MI, Partain CL, James AE, et al: Clinical magnetic resonance imaging with nuclear medicine correlation. J Nucl Med *26*:944, 1985.
25. McClennan BL, Balfe DM: Oncologic imaging: kidney and ureter. Int J Radiat Oncol Biol Phys *9*:1683, 1983.
26. Sufrin G, Murphy GP: Renal adenocarcinoma. Urol *30*:129, 1980.
27. Noronha RFX, Johnson DE, Guinee VF, Borlase BC: Changing patterns in age distribution of renal cell carcinoma patients. Urology *13*:12, 1979.
28. Patel NP, Lavengood RW: Renal cell carcinoma: natural history and results of treatment. J Urol *13*:12, 1979.
29. Hricak H, Demas BE, Williams RD, et al: Magnetic resonance imaging in the diagnosis and staging of renal and perirenal neoplasms. Radiology *154*:709, 1985.
30. Kulkarni MV, Shaff MI, Winfield AC, Partain CL, James AE, et al: Evaluation of renal masses by MR imaging. J Comput Assist Tomogr *8*(5):861, 1984.
31. Lang EK: Comparison of dynamic and conventional computed tomography, angiography and ultrasonography in the staging of renal cell carcinoma. Cancer *54*:2205, 1984.
32. Merten DF, Kirks DR: Diagnostic imaging of pediatric abdominal masses. Pediatr Clin North Am *32*:1397, 1985.
33. Kulkarni MV, Kirschner SG, Heller RM, et al: Magnetic resonance imaging in pediatrics. Pediatr Clin North Am *32*(6):1509, 1985.
34. Hricak H, Crooks L, Sheldon P, Kaufman L: Nuclear magnetic resonance imaging of the kidney: Renal masses. Radiology *147*:765, 1983.
35. Maklad NF, Chuang VP, Doust BD, Cho KJ, Curran JE: Ultrasound characterization of solid renal lesions: echographic, angiographic and pathologic correlation. Radiology *123*:733, 1977.
36. Weyman PJ, McClennan BL, Stanley RJ, Levitt RG, Sagel SS: Comparison of computed tomography and angiography in the evaluation of renal cell carcinoma. Radiology *137*:417, 1980.
37. Mastrodomenico L, Korobkin M, Silverman PM, Dunnick NR: Case report: Perinephric hemorrhage from metastatic carcinoma to the kidney. J Comput Assist Tomogr *7*:727, 1983.
38. Bradley WG, Waluch V, Lai KS, et al: The appearance of rapidly flowing blood on magnetic resonance images. AJR *143*:1167, 1984.
39. Herman SD, Friedman AC, Siegelbaum M, Ramachandani P, Radecki PD: Magnetic resonance imaging of papillary renal cell carcinoma. Urol Radiol *7*:168, 1985.
40. Hadley MD, Nichols DM, Smith FW: Nuclear magnetic resonance tomographic imaging in xanthogranulomatous pyelonephritis. J Urol *127*:301, 1982.
41. Hricak H, Higgins CB, Williams RD: Nuclear magnetic resonance imaging in retroperitoneal fibrosis. AJR *141*:35, 1983.
42. Ellis JH, Blies, JR, Kenyon KK, Donohue JP, et al: Comparison of NMR and CT imaging in the evaluation of metastatic retroperitoneal lymphadenopathy from testicular carcinoma. J Comput Assist Tomogr *8*(4):709, 1984.
43. Terrier F, Hricak H, Revel D, Alpers C, Feduska NJ, et al: Magnetic resonance imaging in the diagnosis of acute renal allograft rejection and its differentiation from acute tubular necrosis. Experimental study in the dog. Invest Radiol *20*:617, 1985.
44. Geisinger MD, Risius B, Jordan ML, Zelch MG, et al: Magnetic resonance imaging of renal transplants. AJR *143*:1229, 1984.
45. Hricak H, Terrier F, Demas BE: Renal allografts: evaluation by MR imaging. Radiology *159*:435, 1986.

46. Hricak H, Newhouse JH: MR imaging of the kidney. Radiol Clin North Am 22:287, 1984.
47. Bradley WG Jr, Waluch V: Blood flow: Magnetic resonance imaging. Radiology 154:443, 1985.
48. Kulkarni MV, Mehta SD, Price RR, Partain CL, et al: Techniques of non-orthogonal magnetic resonance imaging and its clinical applications. J Magn Reson Imag 5:39, 1987.
49. Hricak H, Amparo E, Fisher MR, Crook L, Higgins CB: Abdominal venous system: assessment using MR. Radiology 156:415, 1985.
50. Fisher MR, Hricak H, Higgins CB: Magnetic resonance imaging of developmental venous anomalies. AJR 145:705, 1985.
51. Freidman AC, Hartman DS, Sherman J, et al: Computed tomography of abdominal fatty masses. Radiology 139:415, 1981.
52. Dooms GC, Hricak H, Sollitto RA, Higgins CB: Lipomatous tumors and tumors with fatty component: MR imaging potential and comparison of MR and CT results. Radiology 157:479, 1985.
53. Steiger D, Miraldi FD, Haagu JR, et al: Soft tissue calcifications in NMR scans. Presented at the 69th Annual Meeting of the Radiological Society of North America, Chicago, November 1983.
54. Amparo E, Higgins CB, Hricak H: Primary diagnosis of abdominal arteriovenous fistula by MR imaging. J Comput Assist Tomogr 8(6):1140, 1984.
55. Lee Joseph KT, Ling D, Heiken JP, et al: Magnetic resonance imaging of abdominal aortic aneurysms. Radiology 143:1197, 1984.
56. Amparo EG, Hoddick WK, Hricak H, et al: Comparison of magnetic resonance imaging and ultrasonography in the evaluation of abdominal aortic aneurysms. Radiology 154:451, 1985.
57. Amparo EG, Higgins CB, Hricak H, Sollitto R: Aortic dissection: magnetic resonance imaging. Radiology 155:399, 1985.
58. Maklad NF, Wright C, Rosenthal S: Gray scale ultrasonic appearance of renal transplant rejection. Radiology 131:711, 1979.
59. Fleischer A, Hricak H, McDonell R, et al: Sonographic evaluation of patients with renal transplants: a review. CRC Crit Rev Diagn Imag 18:197, 1982.
60. Singh A, Cohen W: Renal allograft rejection: sonography and scintigraphy. AJR 135:73, 1980.
61. Kulkarni MV, Patton JA, Price RR: Technical considerations for the use of surface coils in MRI. AJR 147:373, 1986.
62. Todd L, Perez J, Guillermo E, et al: In vivo T1 relaxation times in transplanted kidneys of human subjects. Physiol Chem Phys 15:27, 1983.
63. Baumgartner BR, Nelson RC, Bernardino ME, et al: MR imaging of renal transplants. AJR 147:949, 1986.
64. Halasz NA: Commentary: Differential diagnosis of renal transplant rejection: Is MR imaging the answer? AJR 147:954, 1986.

32

Adrenal Glands

THEO H. M. FALKE
MARTIN P. SANDLER
BERT TE STRAKE
MAX SHAFF
ARNOUD P. VAN SETERS

The introduction of both functional and anatomic radiographic techniques, and their rapid technical evolution, have resulted in significant improvement in the localization of adrenal gland disorders over the past decade.[1-6] Computed tomography (CT) has been one of the most significant advances among the different modalities.[5-9] It is generally agreed that with the current generation of CT scanners, CT should be used as the initial screening procedure to visualize adrenal gland pathology.[2,4,7-9] Radiologic techniques, including venous sampling and adrenal scintigraphy, are both invasive and often too time-consuming for initial screening procedures and should be reserved for localization of functioning adrenal tumors when CT findings are equivocal.[2,5-12]

Magnetic resonance imaging (MRI) is a potential modality for the evaluation of adrenal gland disorders. The MRI findings in adrenal gland disorders have been previously described.[13-19] Advantages of MRI include the absence of radiation hazard, superior contrast, and the capacity for direct multiplanar image acquisition. In addition, MRI provides new image parameters, the potentials of which have yet to be explored. At present the advantages compared with CT are negated by the reduced anatomic resolution caused by respiratory motion and the limited accuracy of quantitative data. It can be expected that further technical improvements will resolve some of the disadvantages of MRI and will have a positive influence on its use in adrenal gland disease.

In this chapter we will review what is currently known about MRI of the adrenals and point out some of its potential uses. Examples of MRI findings in various conditions of the adrenal glands will be demonstrated. The role of MRI as an alternative to radionuclide studies and invasive radiologic techniques when CT findings are equivocal will be discussed.

TECHNIQUE

Forty patients with various adrenal gland disorders (Table 32–1) were evaluated at two institutions using a 0.5 tesla superconductive MR scanner (Teslacon-Vanderbilt/Gyroscan S-Leiden). Most images were obtained with two multislice sequences (Table 32–2). The first sequence had a short TR interpulse time and provided the best anatomic information. The second sequence consisted of a multiecho technique with a long TR and was used primarily to obtain $T2$ information on the abnormality. In some cases, additional inversion recovery (IR) ($T1$ 400/TR 1600/TE 30–50) sequences or multiecho

Table 32–1. PATIENT DISTRIBUTION

Hyperplasia	10
Macronodular hyperplasia	2
Adenoma (>1.5 cm)	13
Microadenoma	1
Cyst	3
Pheochromocytoma	17
Metastasis	9
Carcinoma	2
Neuroblastoma	1
Lipoma	1
Miscellaneous	4

Table 32–2. PULSE SEQUENCES

SE short *TR* (single echo)
TR 150–500
TE 30–50

SE long *TR* (multiple echo)
TR 1500–3000
TE 30–50/60–100

(ME) sequences with more than two echoes were performed to optimize *T1* and *T2* information. The image parameters used are summarized in Table 32–3.

The area of interest was imaged in the transverse plane, using additional sagittal or coronal slices in selected cases. The area of interest was defined on an initial sagittal scout view. The slice thickness and distance between slices were adjusted to the size of the pathology under observation. Total examination time varied from 30 minutes to one hour, depending on matrix size and the number of collections desired.

ANATOMY

Each adrenal gland lies in the perinephric space and is firmly attached to Gerota's fascia by fibrous bands. The glands are flat triangular (right) or crescent-shaped (left) organs. Their position in the retroperitoneum and relationship to surrounding structures can be evaluated with MRI using different slice orientations. The configuration of the adrenals shows considerable variation on cross-sectional imaging depending on the slice orientation and level of sectioning.

Right Adrenal

The right adrenal is situated above the upper pole of the right kidney, posterior to the inferior vena cava, with short venous branches draining the gland (Fig. 32–1).

Table 32–3. IMAGING PARAMETERS IN MRI

Multislice
Slice thickness 0.5–1 cm
Slice distance 0.5–2 cm
Acquisition matrix
Gyroscan 256 × 256
Teslacon 128 × 256
Total imaging time 30–60 min
Number of buffers 2

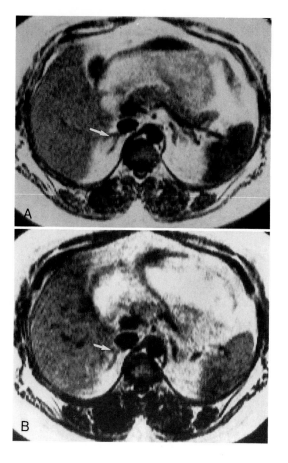

Figure 32–1. Normal upper abdomen. *A*, Transverse MRI, SE 500/30, slice thickness 0.5 cm; normal adrenal (arrow). *B*, Transverse MRI, SE 2000/60, slice thickness 1 cm; normal adrenal (arrow).

In transverse plane, MRI depicts the right gland most commonly as a linear or inverted V shape. The axis of the gland runs parallel to the crus of the diaphragm. The tail and head of the gland are approximately in the same sagittal plane through the axis. As a consequence, the longitudinal axis of the gland is almost completely imaged on a single sagittal slice (Fig. 32–2). With this slice orientation the adrenal shows a dorsal curvature or "bow" configuration. Separation of the adrenal from the right lobe of the liver and identification of the limbs on sagittal slices are usually not possible. The wings of the right adrenals are best visualized on transverse or coronal images. The shapes observed in the coronal images (Fig. 32–3) are more or less identical to the shapes found for transverse planes.

Left Adrenal

The left adrenal is situated medial to the kidney above the left renal vein (Fig. 32–4). The gland is bordered anteriorly by the splenic vessels and is most often visualized at the level of the pancreatic tail. The shape of the left adrenal most frequently is depicted as an inverted V or Y on the transverse images. Sagittal slices through the left gland produce a "bow" configuration similar to that of the right gland. Configurations found on coronal images are the inverted V and Y.

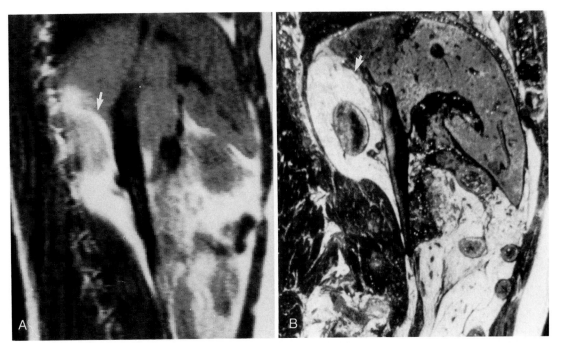

Figure 32–2. Normal abdomen. *A*, Sagittal MRI, SE 500/30; adrenal gland (arrow). *B*, Sagittal cadaveric slice corresponding to *A*; adrenal gland (arrow). (From Falke THM, et al: RadioGraphics 7(2):343, 1987. Used by permission.)

SIGNAL INTENSITY

Adrenal glands have a moderate signal intensity (SI) similar to the signal intensity of liver parenchyma on short *TR* sequences (see Fig. 32–1). Because of the poor anatomic resolution, it is difficult to discriminate adrenal cortex from adrenal medulla in the head of the adrenal gland with certainty on long *TE/TR* sequences. Similarly, spin-

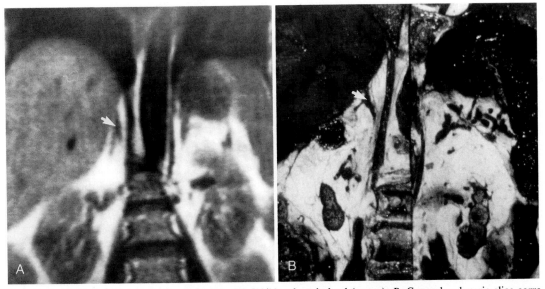

Figure 32–3. Normal abdomen. *A*, Coronal MRI, SE 500/30; adrenal gland (arrow). *B*, Coronal cadaveric slice corresponding to *A*; adrenal gland (arrow). (From Falke THM, et al: RadioGraphics 7(2):343, 1987. Used by permission.)

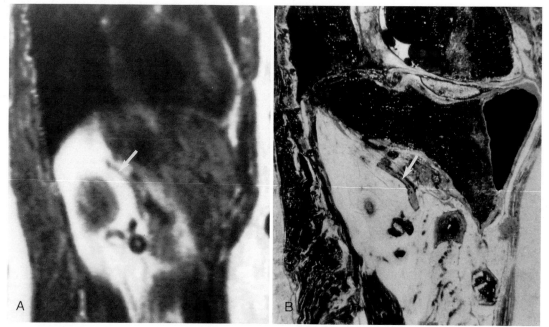

Figure 32–4. Normal abdomen. *A*, Sagittal MRI, SE 400/30; left renal vein (arrow). *B*, Sagittal cadaveric slice corresponding to *A*; left renal vein (arrow). (From Falke THM, et al: RadioGraphics *7*(2):343, 1987. Used by permission.)

echo (SE) sequences with a short *TR* could not differentiate adrenal cortex from adrenal medulla.

IMAGE OPTIMIZATION

Adrenal gland imaging can be improved in several ways, including respiratory gating (Fig. 32–5), surface coils (Fig. 32–6), thin slices (Fig. 32–7), oral contrast (Figs. 32–1 and 32–8), and fast acquisition techniques (see Chapter 96).

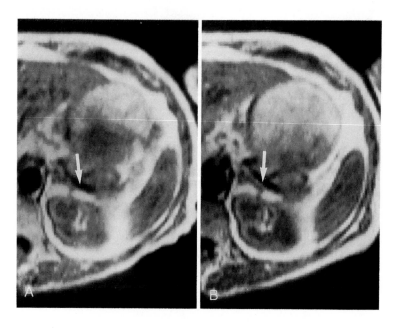

Figure 32–5. Normal abdomen. *A*, Transverse MRI, SE 500/30, without respiratory gating; adrenal gland (arrow). *B*, Transverse MRI, SE 500/30, with respiratory gating; adrenal gland (arrow).

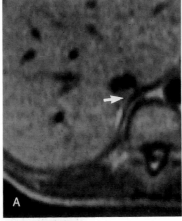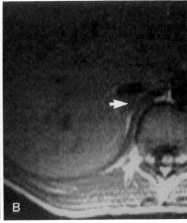

Figure 32–6. Surface coil imaging of adrenal gland. *A*, SE 500/32. Lesion demonstrates medium signal intensity slightly lower than adjacent liver; adrenal gland (arrow). *B*, SE 500/32 with surface coil. Lesion demonstrates superior anatomic resolution; adrenal gland (arrow).

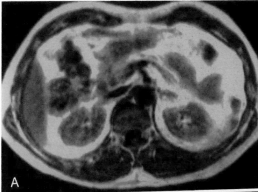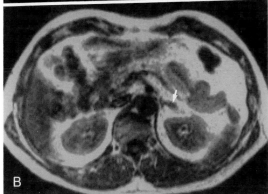

Figure 32–7. Adrenal adenoma. *A*, Transverse MRI, SE 500/32, slice thickness 1 cm. *B*, Transverse MRI, SE 500/32, slice thickness 0.5 cm. Adenoma (arrow) better visualized than in *A*. (From Falke THM, et al: RadioGraphics 7(2):343 1987. Used by permission.)

Figure 32–8. Normal coronal abdomen. Stomach enhanced with oral administration of ferrogluconate (black arrow). Improved delineation of adrenal is demonstrated (white arrow).

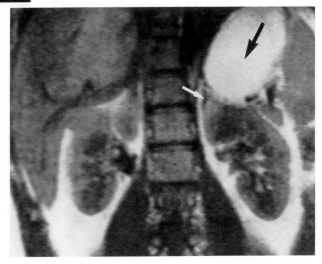

PATHOLOGY

Cushing's Syndrome

Clinical symptoms in Cushing's syndrome result from continued exposure to elevated plasma cortisol levels and include Cushing habitus, hirsutism, hypertension, diabetes mellitus, and osteoporosis.[21] The diagnosis is confirmed by elevated cortisol levels and sustained cortisol values following low-dose dexamethasone suppression. The syndrome may be produced by adrenal cortical hyperplasia in response to increased ACTH plasma levels (70 percent), adrenal adenoma (20 percent), or adrenal carcinoma (10 percent). Biochemical studies, including determination of ACTH levels and response to high-dose dexamethasone, can be used to separate adrenal neoplasias from ACTH-dependent Cushing's syndrome, including pituitary Cushing's syndrome and ectopic ACTH-producing tumors. As adrenal tumors in Cushing's syndrome are usually large,[7-10] MRI is capable of localizing most of these neoplasms prior to surgery (Fig. 32–9).

The diagnosis of hyperplasia can be suggested when gross enlargement or nodular changes are present (Fig. 32–10). Several authors have suggested that MRI is capable of differentiating the higher intensity hypertrophic adrenal cortex from the lower intensity adrenal medulla.[14] Variation in pulse sequences in our patients revealed no significant change in signal intensity, and a possible increased visibility of the corticomedullary junction was not observed. However, accurate observations in this respect are hampered by image degradation with long *TE* sequences caused by respiratory motion and chemical-shift artifacts. Our observations correspond to previous studies[16]

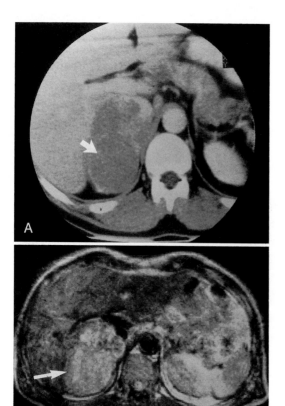

Figure 32–9. Patient with severe Cushing's syndrome, right adrenal carcinoma. *A*, X-ray CT; adrenal tumor (arrow). *B*, Transverse MRI, SE 1500/50. Adrenal tumor demonstrates increased intensity secondary to *T2* weighting; adrenal tumor (arrow).

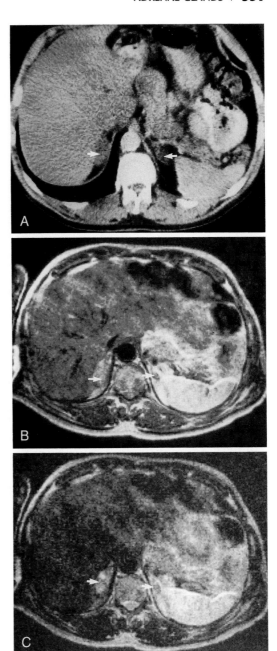

Figure 32–10. Patient with ACTH-dependent macronodular hyperplasia. *A*, CT; bilateral nodular enlargement (arrows). *B*, Transverse MRI, SE 500/50. Note moderately increased signal intensity of adrenal nodules bilaterally (arrows). *C*, Transverse MRI, SE 2000/50. Note further increase in signal intensity compared with intensity of liver secondary to increased *T2* weighting (arrows).

in which adrenal hyperplasia has been seen as increased thickness of the gland in comparison with the thickness of the ipsilateral crus of the diaphragm.

At this stage we consider MRI to be of limited additional value to CT in Cushing's syndrome. Further technical improvement will have to demonstrate whether MRI is capable of detecting cortical hyperplasia at an earlier stage than CT.

Primary Hyperaldosteronism

Primary hyperaldosteronism is a clinical syndrome that is characterized by excessive production of aldosterone and low plasma renin levels. The diagnosis is usually

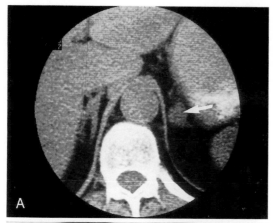

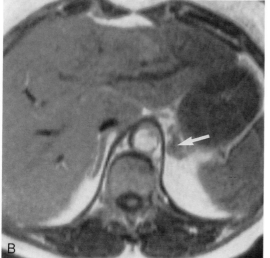

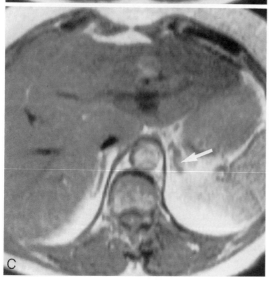

Figure 32–11. Patient with primary hyperaldosteronism. *A*, CT demonstrates mass lesion on left (arrow). *B*, Transverse MRI, SE 500/30. Left adrenal mass (arrow) demonstrates moderate increase in signal intensity. *C*, Transverse MRI, SE 2000/300. Note further increase in signal intensity of the adrenal nodule in comparison with remainder of adrenal gland (arrow). (From Falke THM, et al: J Comput Assist Tomogr *10*(2):242, 1986. Used by permission.)

suspected when hypertension and hypokalemia are present. Symptoms are related to high blood pressure and also include episodic weakness, paresthesias, transient paralysis, and tetany.[22]

The biochemical profile of the patient suggests the diagnosis, and saline suppression tests provide an indication as to whether the patient has hyperplasia (70 percent) or adrenal adenoma (30 percent).[16] Adrenal carcinoma producing primary hyperaldosteronoma has been reported but is extremely rare.[24]

The main role of radiologic investigation in the evaluation of patients with primary hyperaldosteronism is the detection of an adenoma, since only patients with primary hyperaldosteronism caused by adenomas can be cured by surgery. The chance of missing a microadenoma with CT varies from 10 to 30 percent.[6,7] Most of the lesions missed by CT are usually less than 1.2 cm in diameter. The limitation of CT in detecting these very small lesions may necessitate venous sampling or radionuclide studies when CT results are equivocal.[5-8]

MRI has the potential to detect adenomas based on contour distortion of the adrenals (Figs. 32–6, 32–7, 32–11, and 32–12).[18] In addition, aldosteronomas on MRI have a slightly increased signal intensity on long *TR/TE* sequences (Figs. 32–11 and 32–12) compared with the signal intensity of the remaining gland. This capability represents an advantage over CT in cases in which adenomas are too small to be depicted by contour abnormality alone.[2,5,7-9,12,23] However, the present limited anatomic resolution of MRI will probably negate the advantage of superior contrast resolution for most of these lesions.

As in CT, hyperplasia in primary hyperaldosteronism can be detected on MRI when gland enlargement is present.

At this stage we do not consider MRI the method of choice in the evaluation of primary hyperaldosteronism. Its alternative role to radionuclide studies and invasive radiologic techniques when CT is equivocal is limited by low anatomic resolution. However, MRI may be useful if there is a need to confirm the presence of an aldosteronoma found on CT.

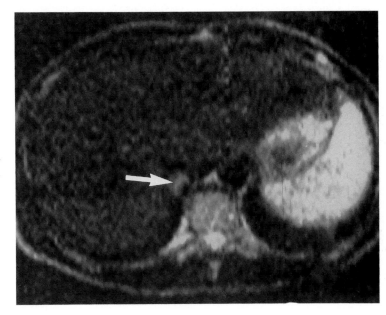

Figure 32–12. Aldosteronoma. Transverse MRI, SE 2000/120. Tumor nodule demonstrates increased intensity (arrow).

Virilizing States

Virilizing syndromes result from excessive androgen production. Clinical symptoms are related to the onset of the disease, genetic sex, and severity of the hormonal disturbance. The clinical picture may include (intrauterine) virilization, change of phenotypic sex, and (pseudo) pubertas praecox. Etiologies include congenital adrenal hyperplasia (CAH), adrenal tumor, and extra-adrenal pathology such as genital tumors and Stein-Leventhal syndrome.

Adrenal tumors causing virilizing syndromes are usually large and therefore detectable on MRI. In CAH there is usually gross enlargement that is also easily detected on MRI (Fig. 32–13). As in other endocrine disorders with adrenal hyperplasia due to chronic exposure to elevated ACTH levels, MRI was not able to detect an abnormal change in signal intensity.

Since virilization is often a childhood disease, MRI may be preferable in this group of patients to exclude a possible tumor.

Nonhyperfunctioning Adenoma

Nonhyperfunctioning adenomas are detected on CT in 0.6 percent of routine upper abdominal studies.[33–35] When an incidental mass is found, CT cannot reliably distinguish between a nonhyperfunctioning adenoma and metastasis despite the use of predictive indices such as size, configuration, and enhancement pattern of the lesion.[36,37]

Nonhyperfunctioning adenomas on MRI have a low signal intensity on SE sequences with a short *TR*, and a moderate or low signal intensity on SE sequences with a long *TR*.[18,38] However, adenomas may show necrosis, hemorrhage, and cystic changes, in which case SI observations can be equal to metastasis, pheochromocytomas, or cysts.[39]

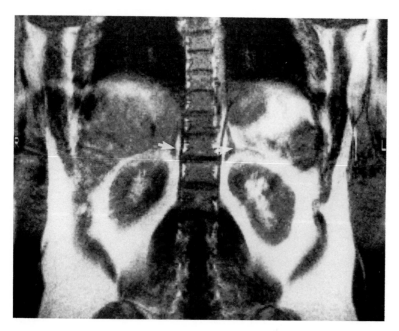

Figure 32–13. Congenital adrenocortical hyperplasia. Coronal MRI, SE 500/30. Note bilateral enlargement of adrenal gland (arrows).

Most of the incidental adenomas have a signal intensity equal (90 percent) to the signal intensity of the liver (Fig. 32–14), whereas most other adrenal masses, including metastasis, have a signal intensity that is higher than the signal intensity of the liver (Figs. 32–15 and 32–16). These results suggest that MRI may be useful to noninvasively distinguish between nonhyperfunctioning adenomas and metastatic disease in cases of an incidental silent adrenal mass. However, since overlap in signal intensity between benign and malignant masses does occur, a presumably benign silent mass has to be monitored by follow-up studies over a period of time to exclude the possibility of a low-signal metastasis.[18]

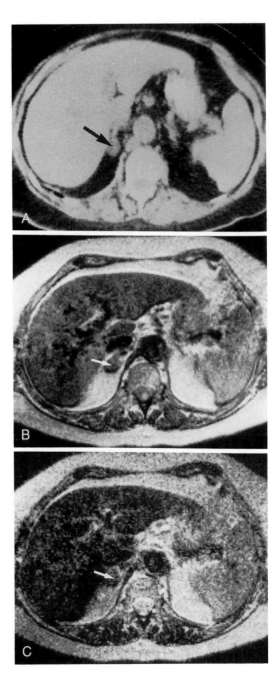

Figure 32–14. Nonfunctioning adenoma. *A*, CT demonstrates lesion in right adrenal (arrow). *B*, Transverse MRI, SE 1500/50. Adrenal mass has the same intensity as the liver (arrow). *C*, Transverse MRI, SE 1500/100. Lesion is again isointense in comparison with liver (arrow).

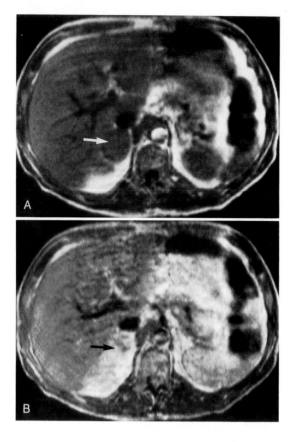

Figure 32–15. Right adrenal metastasis from lung cancer. *A*, Transverse MRI, SE 500/32. Metastatic lesion demonstrates signal intensity equal to liver (arrow). *B*, Transverse MRI, SE 2000/60. Metastatic lesion demonstrates intensity greater than liver (arrow).

Metastasis

The adrenals are a common site for hematogenous metastatic disease. Adrenal metastases are usually clinically silent and seldom cause hypoadrenalism due to parenchymal destruction.[41] On MRI, metastases usually present as masses of increased intensity *T1* and *T2* weighted images (Figs. 32–16 and 32–17). On SE sequences with a short *TR* or on IR sequences the signal intensity is lower than the signal intensity of the normal liver. On SE sequences with a long *TR/TE*, metastases have a signal intensity equal to (15 percent) or higher than (85 percent) the signal intensity of the liver (Figs. 32–15 and 32–17). In the case of necrosis, further increase in signal intensity may be observed.[15] Although the signal intensity characteristics may be of some use in differentiating metastasis from nonfunctioning adenomas, in patients with a known primary tumor CT or ultrasound-guided biopsy is required if a definitive diagnosis is critical to patient management.[42] When patients with primary malignancies of the lung or kidney are staged with MRI, we believe that imaging (as in CT) should include the adrenal area to detect possible metastatic spread (Fig. 32–15).[43]

Adrenal Carcinoma

Adrenocortical carcinomas are extremely rare and often slow-growing. Most patients with an adrenal carcinoma present with a large mass and upper abdominal symptoms. About 50 percent of the tumors produce endocrine symptoms. In those cases atrophy of the contralateral adrenal may be found, especially if cortisol secretion is

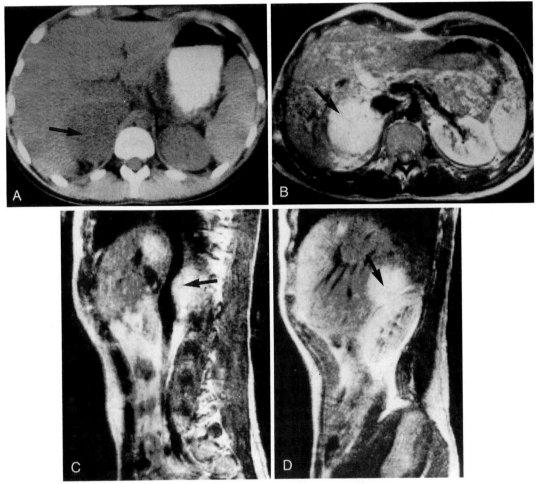

Figure 32–16. Right adrenal metastatic melanoma. *A*, CT demonstrates large mass with density less than liver (arrow). *B*, Transverse MRI, SE 1500/50. Signal intensity increased in comparison with liver (arrow). *C*, Sagittal MRI, SE 1500/ 50. Tumor impressing posteriorly on inferior vena cava (arrow). *D*, Sagittal MRI, SE 1500/50. Note relationship of tumor to right kidney (arrow).

excessive. Since 80 percent of tumors are detected on plain film or IVP, MRI is not likely to be used for tumor detection. Most adrenocortical carcinomas have a low signal intensity on short *TR* sequences and an increased signal intensity on long *TR/TE* sequences (see Fig. 32–9). Because of their size, adrenal carcinomas are difficult to evaluate on CT with regard to origin and relationship to surrounding structures.[7] The availability of direct multiplanar image acquisition with MRI is helpful in such cases. MRI may also be helpful to distinguish postoperative fibrosis from recurrent tumor in this group of patients; this distinction is frequently a problem on CT, especially when baseline scans are not available.[44]

Cysts

The most common adrenal cysts are pseudocysts and lymphangiectatic cysts. Cysts may present in any size and in most instances are unilateral. On MRI an uncomplicated cyst has a negative signal on IR sequences and a low signal intensity on SE sequences with a short *TR*. On sequences with a long *TR/TE* the lesions have a more or less bright

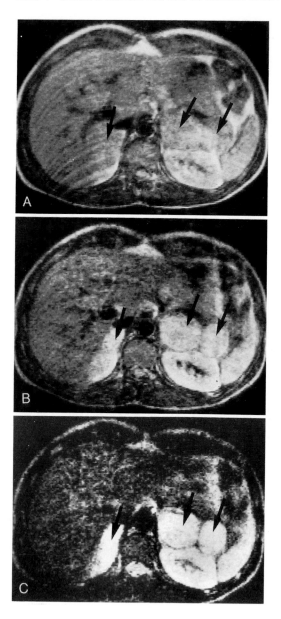

Figure 32–17. Patient with multiple endocrine neoplasia II syndrome and bilateral pheochromocytomas. *A*, Transverse MRI, SE 500/50. Lesions demonstrate equal intensity to liver (arrows). *B*, Transverse MRI, SE 1500/50. Tumors demonstrate increased intensity to liver (arrows). *C*, Transverse MRI, SE 1500/100. Note further increase in signal intensity (arrows).

signal intensity depending on the protein content (Fig. 32–18). When hemorrhage occurs in a cyst, characteristically a bright signal intensity is observed on short *TR* sequences (Fig. 32–19). The appearance of a hemorrhagic cyst has been described for other anatomic regions, and MRI proved to be useful to detect complication of a cyst in a noninvasive way—information not readily available with either CT or sonography.[45]

Myelolipoma

Adrenal myelolipoma is a rare condition. Usually, myelolipomas have an increased SI on both short and long *TR* sequences. The irregular shape and inhomogeneity of the mass as well as the isointensity of retroperitoneal fat on later echoes separate myelolipomas from hemorrhagic cysts.[39]

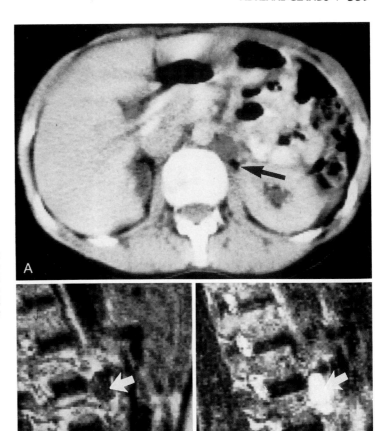

Figure 32–18. Patient with small left adrenal cyst. *A*, CT demonstrates decreased density (arrow). *B*, Sagittal MRI, SE 1500/50. Signal intensity is decreased (arrow). *C*, Sagittal MRI, SE 1500/100. Note increase in intensity (arrow).

Pheochromocytoma

Patients with pheochromocytoma usually present with episodic or sustained hypertension and elevated levels of catecholamines or their metabolites in blood and urine.[26,27] Occasionally symptoms and biochemical findings are absent (especially in multiple endocrine neoplasia [MEN] syndrome).

Pheochromocytomas originate from chromaffin cell nests along the autonomic ganglia chain or chromaffin bodies such as the adrenal medulla or organ of Zuckerkandl. In adults 90 percent of the pheochromocytomas are located in one adrenal gland, and 10 percent occur bilaterally. Most ectopic pheochromocytomas are located in the abdomen (9 percent). Unusual locations include the chest (1 percent) and urinary bladder (1 percent). In children and patients with associated neurocristopathies (MEN, neurofibromatosis) the incidence of bilateral or ectopic location is higher. As the masses are usually larger than 3 cm in diameter and predominantly located in the adrenals, MRI will be capable of detecting most of these lesions.[26,27]

Pheochromocytomas have a moderate signal intensity on SE sequences with a

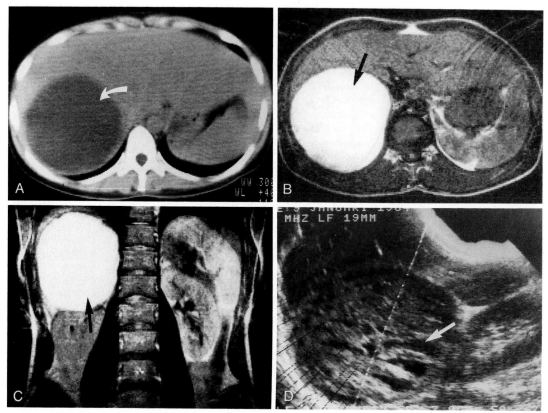

Figure 32–19. Patient with large right adrenal hemorrhagic cyst. *A*, CT demonstrates large low-density mass (arrow). *B*, Transverse MRI, SE 500/30. Lesion demonstrates increased intensity (arrow). *C*, Coronal MRI, SE 1800/500. Cyst demonstrates increased intensity (arrow). *D*, Longitudinal ultrasound. Cyst demonstrates complex echo pattern (arrow).

short *TR*, a low signal intensity on IR sequences, and a considerably increased signal intensity on SE sequences with a long *TR/TE* (see Figs. 32–17 and 32–20).[17,18] In the presence of hemorrhagic cystic degeneration, increased SI may also be observed on short *TR* sequences.[39] The signal intensity on long *TR* sequences is consistently higher than the signal intensity of adenomas regardless of the size of the pheochromocytoma (Fig. 32–20). The high signal intensity on *T2* weighted sequences provides an excellent means to delineate tumors from surrounding structures, including major vessels.

In complex cases, including extra-adrenal location, small and multiple lesions in MEN syndrome, and recurrent tumor or metastatic spread, CT findings may be negative.[28,29] A relatively new radionuclide imaging procedure, iodine-131 metaiodobenzylguanide scanning (I-131-MIBG), is valuable in this group of patients.[30] However, the results of this test have to be confirmed by an imaging technique to eliminate both false positive and false negative results.[30–32]

The combination of optimal plane selection and superior contrast (Fig. 32–20*D*) with MRI as compared with CT may be useful in detecting and localizing pheochromocytomas in complex cases in which CT is equivocal. The bright signal intensity on long *TR/TE* sequences is useful to differentiate pheochromocytomas from nonhyperfunctioning adenomas in hypertensive patients when clinical findings are less straightforward.[18,39] In addition, MRI may be useful to identify unsuspected pheochromocytomas prior to biopsy[48] in patients with an incidental adrenal mass.

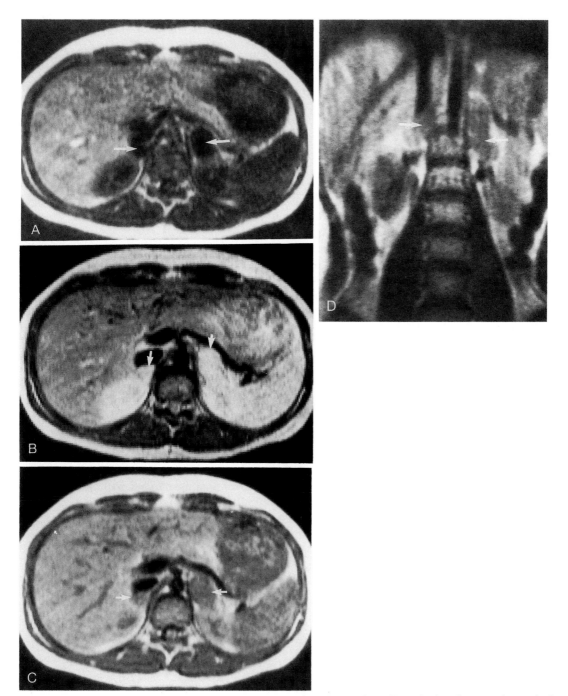

Figure 32–20. Bilateral pheochromocytomas. *A*, Transverse MRI, SE 500/30. Bilateral adrenal tumors (arrows). *B*, Transverse MRI, SE 2000/90. Note increase in signal intensity in adrenal tumors (arrows). *C*, Transverse MRI, IR 1800/400/30. Note lesions with decreased signal intensity compared with liver (arrows). *D*, Coronal MRI, IR 1800/400/300. Bilateral adrenal tumors demonstrate decreased signal intensity compared with liver (arrows). (From Falke THM, et al: J Comput Assist Tomogr *10*(2):242, 1986. Used by permission.)

Neuroblastoma

Neuroblastoma is a common tumor in children less than five years old (80 percent). Prognosis depends on the onset of the disease but is usually poor after the neonatal period. The tumors arise in neural crest cells and are found in a variety of locations. The adrenal medulla or adjacent retroperitoneum account for 50 to 80 percent of the tumors. Clinical symptoms may vary and are related to the rapid growth of the neoplasm and its secretory products.[46]

MR imaging in these patients has several advantages over other modalities because it is noninvasive and does not require ionizing radiation. Superior contrast and optimal plane selection are useful to delineate tumor extent in relation to surrounding structures and vessels as an aid in predicting resectability and in detecting recurrence of tumor. The use of MRI to monitor chemotherapy or radiotherapy treatment of neuroblastomas has been suggested.[47]

On SE sequences with a short TR, the tumors have a moderate signal intensity equal to the signal intensity of liver parenchyma. On SE sequences with a long TR/TE, the signal intensity is brighter than the signal intensity of the liver (Fig. 32–21).

In conclusion, MRI is capable of identifying most adrenal abnormalities previously detected by CT. At this stage the overall accuracy of MRI in adrenal disease as compared with other imaging modalities is not known. In our experience MRI is capable of overcoming some limitations of CT in adrenal disease. MRI has a greater specificity for mass lesions and may be useful to differentiate nonhyperfunctioning adenomas from metastases and pheochromocytomas. However, overlap between nonhyperfunctioning adenomas, functioning adenomas, and metastases has been documented,[18] and actual accuracy of MRI in this respect has to be established in a large prospective evaluation. MRI has the potential to detect aldosteronomas by increased SI in addition to contour distortion. It is unlikely at present that MRI will replace functional or invasive radiologic techniques in most equivocal CT cases. Further technical developments and the use of intravenous contrast agents may have a positive influence on the role of MRI in adrenal disease. Although MRI is capable of detecting adrenal pathology, there are numerous disadvantages to its use as the initial imaging modality in the evaluation of patients with adrenal disease. The disadvantages include long examination times, low anatomic resolution due to respiratory motion, and the inability to adequately visualize calcifications. In addition, the interference between metal hardware and magnetic fields and the necessity for patient cooperation exclude a number of individuals from examination.

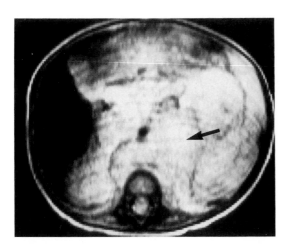

Figure 32–21. Patient with neuroblastoma. Transverse MRI, SE 1800/60. Notice increased intensity in tumor (arrow).

MRI might be preferred as the initial study when exposure to radiation is considered a relative contraindication, for instance, in children and pregnant women, when reaction to intravenous contrast agents is expected and contrast optimization is essential, and in postoperative patients when metallic clips degrade the CT image. MRI is helpful in the assessment and origin of large lesions through anatomic definition in various planes and aids in predicting tumor resectability. MRI provides useful information when hemorrhage is suspected, for instance, in a pre-existing cyst. MRI may be helpful to detect recurrent tumor and differentiate it from postoperative fibrosis. In addition, the high signal intensity of pheochromocytomas on *T2* weighted sequences may be beneficial when MRI is used in complex pheochromocytoma cases. In such cases MRI is useful to (1) confirm extra-adrenal location or recurrent tumor suspected on radionuclide (I-131-MIBG) studies; (2) detect small and multiple lesions associated with neurocristopathies such as MEN II syndrome; (3) differentiate nonfunctioning adenomas from pheochromocytomas in hypertensive patients; and (4) exclude a pheochromocytoma in patients with an incidental mass prior to percutaneous adrenal biopsy.

References

1. Beierwaltes WH, Lieberman LM, Ansari AN, Nishiyama H: Visualization of human adrenal glands in vivo by scintillation scanning. JAMA *216*:275, 1971.
2. Guerin CK, Wahner WH, Gorman CA, Carpenter PC, Sheedy PI II: Computed tomographic scanning versus radioisotope imaging in adrenocortical diagnosis. Am J Med *75*:653, 1983.
3. Karstaedt N, Sagel SS, Stanley RJ, Melson GL, Levill RG: Computed tomography of the adrenal gland. Radiology *129*:723, 1978.
4. Abrams HL, Siegelmann SS, Adams DF, et al: Computed tomography versus ultrasound of the adrenal gland: A prospective study. Radiology *143*:121, 1982.
5. Dunnick NR, Doppman JL, Mills SR, Sill JR: Preoperative diagnosis and localization of aldosteronomas by measurement of corticosteroid in adrenal venous blood. Radiology *133*:331, 1979.
6. Geisinger MA, Zelch MG, Bravo EL, Risius BF, O'Donovan PB, Borkowski GP: Primary hyperaldosteronism: Comparison of CT, adrenal venography and venous sampling. AJR *141*:299, 1983.
7. Moss AA: Computed tomography of the adrenal glands. *In* Moss AA, Gamsu G, Genant HU: Computed Tomography of the Body. Philadelphia, WB Saunders, 1983, pp 837–876.
8. Sheedy F III, Mattery RR, Stephens DH, Van Heerden JA, Sheps SG: The adrenal glands. *In* Haaga JR, Alfidi RJ (eds): Computed Tomography of the Whole Body. Vol. II. St. Louis, CV Mosby, 1983, pp 681–705.
9. Kenney PJ, Berlow ME, Ellis DA: Current imaging of adrenal masses. RadioGraphics *4*(5):743, 1984.
10. Falke THM, te Strake L, van Seters AP: CT of the adrenal glands: Adenoma or hyperplasia (Scientific Exhibit), 518. Radiology (special edition) *153*(3):358, 1984.
11. Gross MD, Shapiro B, Thrall JH, Freitas JE, Beierwaltes WH: The scintigraphic imaging of endocrine organs. Endocr Rev *5*(2):221, 1984.
12. Bernardino ME, Walther MM, Philips VM, Graham SP Jr, Sewell CW, Gedgandas-McClees K, Baumgartner BR, Torres WE, Erwin BC: CT-guided adrenal biopsy: Accuracy, safety and indications. AJR *144*:67, 1985.
13. Moon KL, Hricak H, Crooks LE, Gooding EA, Moss AA, Englestad BL, Kaufman L: Nuclear magnetic resonance of the adrenal glands: A preliminary report. Radiology *147*:155, 1983.
14. Schultz U, Haaga JR, Fletcher BD, Alfidi KJ, Schultz MA: Magnetic resonance imaging of the adrenal glands: A comparison with CT. AJR *143*:1235, 1984.
15. Reinig JW, Doppman JL, Dwyer AJ, Johnson AR, Knop RH: Adrenal masses: differentiation by MRI, Radiology *158*:81, 1986.
16. Davis PL, Hricak H, Bradley WG Jr: Magnetic resonance imaging of the adrenal glands. Radiol Clin North Am *22*(4):891, 1984.
17. Fink IJ, Reinig JW, Dwyer JA, Doppman JL, Linehan WM, Keiser HR: MR imaging of pheochromocytomas. J Comput Assist Tomogr *9*(3):454, 1985.
18. Falke THM, te Strake L, Shaff MI, Sandler MP, et al: MRI of the adrenals: Correlative imaging with CT. J Comput Assist Tomogr *10*(2):242, 1986.
19. Glazer SM, Woolsen FS, Borrello J, Franci JR, et al: Adrenal tissue characterization using MR imaging, Radiology *158*:73, 1986.
20. Wilms G, Baert A, Marchal G, Godderis P: Computed tomography of the normal adrenal glands: Correlative study with autopsy specimens. J Comput Assist Tomogr *3*(4):467, 1979.
21. Besser GM, Edwards CRW: Cushing's syndrome. Clin Endocrinol *1*:451, 1972.
22. Naville AM, O'Hara MJ: The Human Adrenal Cortex Pathology and Biology: An Integrated Approach. Monograph. Heidelberg, Springer-Verlag, 1982.

23. Page DL, Hough A, DeLellis R: Tumors of the adrenal. AFIP, Washington, DC, 1986.
24. Kidd GS, Hofeldt FD: Pure primary hyperaldosteronism due to adrenal cortical carcinoma. Am J Med 76:1132, 1984.
25. Falke THM, van Seters AP, et al: CT in untreated adults with congenital adrenal hyperplasia (CAH) Clin Radiol. In press.
26. Thomas JL, Bernadino ME, et al: CT of pheochromocytoma. AJR 135:477, 1980.
27. Blickman JG, Falke THM: Radiology of pheochromocytoma: impact of modern imaging on surgical management. J Radiol. In press.
28. Kadir S, Robertson D: Pitfalls in the diagnosis of extra adrenal phaeochromocytoma. Cardiovasc Intervent Radiol 4:99, 1981.
29. Felson B, Wiot JF: The MEN syndromes. Semin Roentgenol 20:1, 1985.
30. Francis IR, Slazer GM, Shapiro B, Sisson JC, Gross BH: Complementary roles of CT and 131I-MIBG scintigraphy in diagnosing pheochromocytoma. AJR 141:719, 1983.
31. Chatel GF, Tellyer JL, Charbonell B (letter 1); Ackery D, Tippet P, Marley A, Weynhove C (letter 2): False positive diagnosis of pheochromocytoma with I^{131} M-iodobenzyl-guanide scintigraphy. Lancet 31 1, (8379):733, 1984.
32. Brown MJ, Fuller RW, Lavender JP: False diagnosis of bilateral pheochromocytoma by iodine-131–labelled meta-iodobenzylguanicine (MIBG). Lancet 7 1 (8367):56, 1984.
33. Siegelman SS, Fishman EK, Gatewood OMB, Goldman SM: CT of the adrenal gland. Contemp Issues Comput Tomogr 3:223, 1984.
34. Glazer HS, Weyman PJ, Sagel SS, Leitt KG, McClennan BL: Non-functioning adrenal masses: Incidental discovery on CT. AJR 139:81, 1982.
35. Mitnick JS, Bosniak MA, Meglibaw AJ, Naidich DP: Non-functioning adrenal masses: adenomas discovered incidentally on CT. Radiology 148:495, 1983.
36. Hussain S, Belldegrun A, Seltzer SE, Richie JP, Gittes RF, Abrams HL: Differentiation of malignant from benign adrenal masses: Predictive indices on CT. AJR 144:61, 1985.
37. Oliver TW Jr, Bernadino ME, Miller JI, Mansour K, Greene D, Davis WA: Isolated adrenal masses in non small-cell bronchogenic carcinoma. Radiology 153:217, 1984.
38. Reinig JW, Doppman JL, Dwyer AJ, Johnson AR, Knop RM: Distinction between adrenal adenomas and metastasis using MR imaging. J Comput Assist Tomogr 9(5):898, 1985.
39. Falke THM, te Strake L, Sandler MP, Shaff MI, van Seters AP, Partain CL, James AE Jr: Scientific Exhibit RSNA 85. RadioGraphics 7(2):343, 1987.
40. Wolfman NT, Karstaedt N, Albertson D, Bechtold RE: MR imaging of the adrenal glands at 0.15 Tesla. Society of Magnetic Resonance in Medicine. Fourth Annual Meeting. London, August 19–23, 1985.
41. Meyer JE, Halperin EC, Levene SR, Stomper PC: Adrenal insufficiency secondary to metastatic lung carcinoma: CT aided diagnosis. J Comput Assist Tomogr 7(6):1107, 1983.
42. Montali G, Solbiati L, Bossi MC, DePra L, Di Donna A, Ravelto C: Sonographically guided fine-needle aspiration biopsy of adrenal masses. AJR 143:1081, 1984.
43. Sandler MA, Pearlberg JL, Madrazo BC, Sitschlag UF, Gross SC: Computed tomographic evaluation of the adrenal gland in the preoperative assessment of bronchogenic carcinoma. Radiology 145:733, 1982.
44. Floryn J, Falke THM, et al: Computed tomography of the adrenals. Diagn Imag 49:273, 1980.
45. Wilcos DM, Weinreb JC, Lesh P: MR imaging of a hemorrhagic hepatic cyst in a patient with polycystic liver disease. J Comput Assist Tomogr 9(2):183, 1985.
46. Robbins SL, Cotran RS: The endocrine system; adrenal medulla. In Robbins SL, Cotran RS (eds): Pathologic Basis of Disease. Philadelphia, WB Saunders, 1979, pp 1402–1407.
47. Cohen MD, Weetman R, Provisor A, et al: Magnetic resonance imaging of neuroblastoma with a 0.15 T magnet. AJR 143:1241, 1984.
48. Casola G, Nicolet V, van Sonnenberg E, Withers C, Bretagnolle M, Saba RM, Bret PM: Unsuspected pheochromocytoma: Risk of blood-pressure alterations during percutaneous adrenal biopsy. Radiology 159:733, 1986.

VII

CLINICAL EXPERIENCE: MRI OF THE PELVIS

33

Prostate and Urinary Bladder

MADELEINE R. FISHER
HEDVIG HRICAK
BERNIE J. SAKS

Computed tomography and sonography markedly improved demonstration of the prostate gland and urinary bladder. Recently, the value of magnetic resonance imaging (MRI) for analysis of normal and pathologic conditions in the male and female pelvis has been described.[1-3] This chapter describes present experience with MRI of the prostate gland and urinary bladder, including anatomic considerations, technical considerations, and the potential of MR in various benign and malignant entities affecting these organs.

PROSTATE

Normal Anatomy

The prostate gland, enclosed in a dense fascial sheath, lies behind the symphysis pubis. The approximate prostate size is 4 cm wide, 2 cm anteroposteriorly, and 3 cm long.[3] Anterior to the prostate is a venous network called the prostatic plexus, into which the dorsal vein of the penis drains. This plexus is continuous around the sides of the prostate, with large veins located between the bladder and prostate, and communicates with the vesical plexus.[4] The prostatic plexus is seen with high signal intensity on MR images using the long repetition (TR) and echo delay (TE) times (TR = 2.0 sec; TE = 60 ms).

The anatomic description of the prostate gland has evolved as further investigations have been performed. Earlier work,[5] based on fetal and newborn prostate glands, divided the gland into lobes. More recent studies[6] showed that the morphologic appearance of the adult prostate gland does not demonstrate lobes but rather well-delineated zones (regions). The peripheral zone constitutes approximately 75 percent of the gland; the central zone occupies 20 percent. The remaining 5 percent of the gland is the transitional zone. This distinction is clinically important, as the peripheral zone is the primary site of origin of prostatic carcinoma. The transitional zone is the site of origin of benign prostatic hyperplasia.[2] Although the transitional zone contains glandular tissue histologically similar to that of the peripheral zone, anatomic separation is possible, as the transitional zone is adjacent to the periprostatic sphincter.

Optimum Spin-Echo Technique and Imaging Planes

The zones of the normal prostate gland in young men can be delineated using the spin-echo (SE) imaging technique, utilizing a long TR and TE. In young subjects there is differentiation between the peripheral and central zones on the longer *TR/TE* images. On the shorter *TR/TE* images the prostate is visualized with a homogeneous medium-signal intensity, whereas on the longer *TR/TE* images the central zone has lower signal intensity than the surrounding peripheral zone. This may be related to differences in *T2* relaxation times between the two regions, since the difference in *T1* is negligible. It is postulated that closely packed glands and muscle bundles within the central zone, and the resultant shortening of *T2*, may account for the lower signal intensity observed within the central zone.

Periprostatic structures are clearly delineated from the prostatic parenchyma on images obtained with a *TR* of 1.0 sec or greater (Fig. 33–1). The surrounding levator ani muscles are of lower signal intensity than the prostatic parenchyma, and this difference is further accentuated with longer *TR* and *TE* (Fig. 33–1). On the sagittal image, because of the differences in MR tissue properties, the bladder base is clearly separable from the dome of the prostate gland, even though a fat plane between the two is not present (Fig. 33–2). The relationship of the prostate gland to the symphysis pubis is well delineated (Figs. 33–1 and 33–2). Fat in the retropubic-preprostatic space of Retzius is seen with high signal intensity. An anterior fibromuscular band, seen with low signal intensity, covers the anterolateral surface of the prostate, allowing distinction between the prostate and preprostatic space. Occasionally, the periprostatic venous plexus is visualized, particularly on the long *TR* and long *TE*, anteriorly on the sagittal image or on the lateral aspect of the prostate on the transverse and coronal images. Delineation between the rectum and prostate is possible because of the superb soft tissue contrast provided by MR, allowing depiction of Denonvilliers' fascia. The fascia has lower intensity than both the rectal wall and the prostate gland, and its low intensity is further accentuated on the second spin-echo image. Between the dome of the prostate and rectum, a small amount of subperitoneal fat is present, allowing differentiation between the two structures in this region.

MR, a modality capable of direct multiplanar imaging, is invaluable in assessment of the prostate gland. All three planes—transverse, coronal, and sagittal—clearly display the prostate. Each plane has its own merits for evaluation of the prostate. The transverse plane allows assessment of the gland and its relationship to the seminal vesicles; it also complements other planes in the demonstration of the levator ani and obturator internus muscles and preprostatic space as well as relationship to the rectum. However, the transverse axis provides limited information about the relationship of

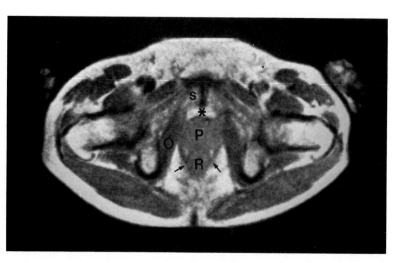

Figure 33–1. *TR* = 1.0 sec, *TE* = 28 ms. Normal prostate gland (P) is of homogeneous intermediate signal intensity on this sequence. Note the levator ani muscles (arrows) symmetric around the gland and rectum (R). Obturator internus muscle (0). Symphysis pubis (S). Preprostatic fat (*).

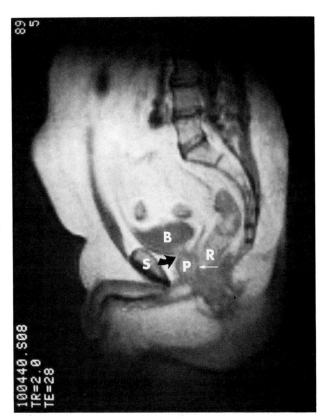

Figure 33–2. *TR* 2.0, *TE* 28 ms. Sagittal image demonstrates the bladder (B) separable from the prostate gland (P). The anterior fibromuscular band (black curved arrow), of low signal intensity, covers the anterolateral surface of the prostate. Denonvilliers' fascia (white arrow), of low signal intensity, separates the rectum (R) from the prostate. Symphysis pubis (S).

the prostate to the bladder base. The coronal plane clearly delineates the prostate zones and optimally displays the relationship of the prostate to the levator ani muscles and pelvic side walls (Fig. 33–3). The sagittal plane is beneficial for evaluating the interface between the prostate and bladder base, for defining the region of the prostatic urethra, for demonstrating the anterior fibromuscular band that separates the prostate from the preprostatic space, and for demonstrating the relationship of the prostate to the rectum.

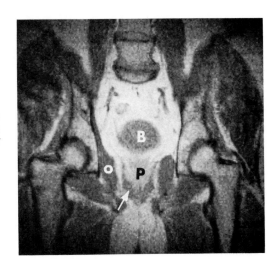

Figure 33–3. *TR* = 2.0 sec, *TE* = 28 ms. Coronal image of the prostate delineates the relationship of the prostate (P) to the levator ani muscles (arrow). Obturator internus (o). Bladder (B).

Pathology

Three main pathologic processes affect the prostate gland: inflammation, benign nodular hyperplasia, and neoplastic tumors. Benign nodular hyperplasia is the most common of these entities.[7]

BENIGN PATHOLOGY

Benign prostatic hyperplasia has a variable MR appearance, depending on the sequence utilized and whether the condition is diffuse or nodular. Diffuse enlargement ranges from a homogeneous low-intensity signal with a short repetition time to a medium-high intensity with a long repetition time; it often has similar signal intensity to that of the normal prostate gland (Fig. 33–4).[1,8] Nodular hyperplasia demonstrates similar intensity changes but involves the gland more focally. Evaluation of this abnormality with MR, utilizing its multiplanar capabilities, allows accurate volumetric measurement of the gland, displays the intravesicular portion of the hyperplastic nodule, and demonstrates its effect on the bladder neck. Knowledge of the intravesicular extension of the gland is important prior to surgical planning. Sagittal imaging demonstrates the lobularity of the posterior and intravesicular portions of the gland. This plane is particularly useful for evaluation of the bladder trigonum, where thickening or mucosal congestion secondary to bladder outlet obstruction from prostatic enlargement is well visualized. The anterior fibromuscular band of the prostate, best seen on sagittal images, retains its slight concave configuration regardless of the degree of prostatic hyperplasia. Thickening of the surgical pseudocapsule surrounding the adenomatous tissue on the *T2* weighted image is delineated on any imaging plane but is not visualized in all cases.

Limited experience with other benign entities has shown a variable pattern with acute and chronic prostatitis. Acute prostatitis may focally or diffusely involve the prostate and is usually secondary to a suppurative inflammation by a pyogenic organism. Chronic prostatitis is characterized by a persistent infection with neutrophilic infiltration as well as destruction and fibroblastic proliferation. On MRI, prostatitis may be seen as diffuse involvement of the peripheral lobes, depicted with increased signal

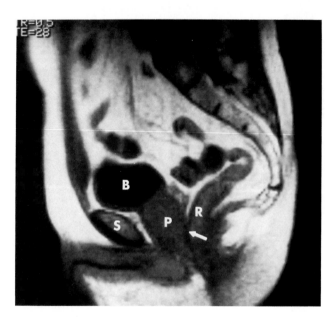

Figure 33–4. *TR* = 0.5 sec, *TE* = 28 ms. Benign prostatic hyperplasia (sagittal image) demonstrates an enlarged prostate gland (P) with homogeneous intermediate signal intensity when shortened *TR* is used. Symphysis (S). Bladder (B). Rectum (R). Denonvilliers' fascia (arrow).

intensity on the *T2* weighted image.[9] Adenomas and granulomatous lesions have been seen as localized processes with high signal intensity on long *TR* images.

MALIGNANT PATHOLOGY

A simple screening modality for prostatic carcinoma detection is not available. Reliance on the rectal examination for both diagnosis and staging may result in errors. While MRI is a highly sensitive modality for the depiction of an abnormality, it is still nonspecific.[1,8,9] Prostatic carcinoma is seen optimally on a long *TR/TE* image as areas of inhomogeneous increased or decreased signal intensity within the gland (Fig. 33–5). Localization of the carcinoma to the gland and the determination of periprostatic extension are areas of ongoing research. MRI, although not specific, is an important staging modality. Multiplanar imaging is a major benefit of MR compared with other techniques. It offers the potential of improved detection of bladder base and seminal vesicle involvement and, in the rare cases of posterior extension of prostatic carcinoma, involvement of the rectum. Accurate staging is essential for planning appropriate therapy. MRI is accurate in Stage B through Stage D prostatic disease. While other benign entities may cause similar intensity changes within the prostate, MR evaluation should always be conducted in conjunction with prostate biopsy. Stages B1 and B2 are seen as high signal intensity masses confined to the gland. Several manifestations of Stage C disease are observed. Periprostatic spread is seen as obliteration of the pseudocapsule; abnormal signal intensity within the periprostatic fat, with or without invasion of the levator ani muscles, as manifested by high signal intensity within the muscle; enlargement and abnormal intensity of the seminal vesicles when invaded; and abnormal intensity within the bladder and urethra when involved. Stage D1 is manifested as abnormally enlarged pelvic lymph nodes, and Stage D2 as abnormal intensity within the pelvic bones or other distant metastases.

An important feature of MR evaluation of the prostate is its sensitivity for detection of pathologic conditions while they are confined to the gland. At the current stage of

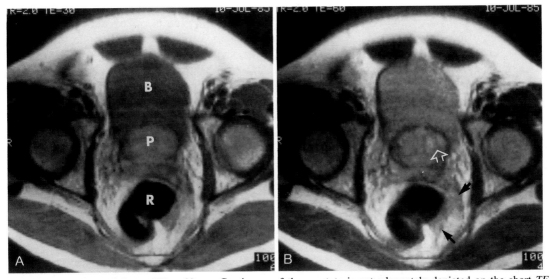

Figure 33–5. *A, TR* = 2.0 sec, *TE* = 30 ms. Carcinoma of the prostate is not adequately depicted on the short *TE* sequence. Bladder (B). Prostate (P). Rectum (R). *B, TR* = 2.0 sec, *TE* = 60 ms. On the long *TR* sequence, areas of increased signal intensity (open arrow) are visualized in the peripheral lobes and extend extracapsularly into the left levator ani muscle (closed arrows). Though the increased signal intensity in the prostate is not specific for carcinoma, this finding, together with levator ani thickening, is highly suspicious for a neoplastic or, less likely, an inflammatory process.

development, differentiation of benign from malignant lesions is not possible either by visual intensity differences or by determination of relaxation characteristics. Another essential feature of MRI is its ability to improve the accuracy of staging prostatic carcinoma as a result of its superior soft tissue contrast and capability of multiplanar imaging.

BLADDER

Normal Anatomy

The urinary bladder is a hollow muscular organ located below the peritoneum on the anterior part of the pelvic floor behind the symphysis pubis. It is bounded on each side by the obturator internus muscles laterally and by the levator ani muscles caudally. In the male the posterolateral aspect of the base is in contact with the seminal vesicles. Medial to each seminal vesicle the base is in contact with the ampulla of the ductus deferens of the same side. In the female the base is loosely attached to the anterior wall of the cervix and vagina. The normal bladder wall, when distended, measures approximately 2 mm. The ability to identify the different regions of the bladder wall is clinically important, as different pathologies are prone to affect certain portions of the bladder. The trigonum is the initial site of bladder wall hypertrophy with bladder neck obstruction. Initially, there is thickening of the bladder wall due to hypertrophy of the smooth muscle; with progressive hypertrophy, individual muscle bundles enlarge and produce trabeculation of the entire bladder wall. The overlying mucosa may be normal, but, more commonly, urinary stasis leads to bladder inflammation.[7] Transitional cell carcinomas occur most frequently on the lateral walls and trigone,[10] while adenocarcinoma usually occurs in the dome and trigone but may involve the anterior, posterior, and lateral walls.[10]

Optimum Spin-Echo Technique and Imaging Planes

The optimum spin-echo sequence for delineating the normal bladder wall and eccentric or concentric bladder wall hypertrophy is a long *TR* (2.0 sec) and long *TE* (56 ms) (Fig. 33–6). This can be explained on the basis of the intrinsic relaxation times of urine and smooth muscle. Both urine and smooth muscle have relatively long *T1* relaxation times and thus do not allow full recovery of magnetization between successive excitations. As a result, each is seen with a low signal intensity on a short *TR* (0.5 sec). The difference in the *T2* relaxation times between urine and smooth muscle is marked. On the long *TE* (56 ms), particularly when combined with long *TR*, the difference between the *T2* relaxation times (and, to a lesser degree, the difference between *T1* values) allowed separation of the bladder wall from urine. The *T2* differences are particularly well seen on the multiple-echo sequence with *TE*'s of up to 140 ms (Fig. 33–7). In this imaging sequence, the bladder wall is imaged with a very low intensity because of its short *T2* relaxation time relative to urine. The normal low-intensity bladder wall should be distinguished from the low-intensity line at the bladder edge, which is caused by the chemical-shift difference between the resonant frequency of the hydrogen nuclei of urine (water) and fat.[11] The chemical-shift artifact is recognized as a dark band along the lateral wall of the bladder on one side and a bright band along the lateral wall on the opposite side on the transverse image (Fig. 33–8). On the sagittal plane, the chemical-shift artifact is seen along the base and dome of the bladder of anterior and posterior walls depending upon the direction of the pregnancy encoding gradient. Knowledge of the appearance of this artifact prevents a diagnostic error in bladder anatomy or pathology. With our device, owing to the direction of the read-out

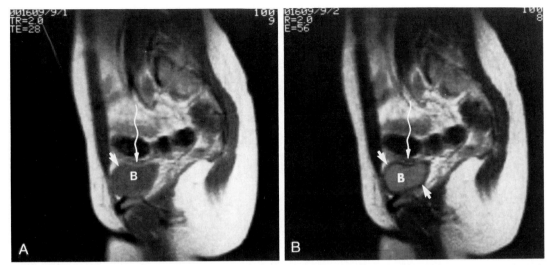

Figure 33–6. Normal bladder wall. *A, TR* = 2.0 sec, *TE* = 28 ms. The bladder wall is imaged with medium signal intensity (straight arrow) and is difficult to differentiate from lower intensity urine within the urinary bladder (B). Peritoneum (long wavy arrow). *B, TR* = 2.0 sec, *TE* = 56 ms. With longer *TE*, the bladder wall shows relative decreases in signal intensity (straight arrows), while the urine within the bladder (B) is relatively increased in signal intensity. Peritoneum (long wavy arrow).

gradient, the bright-band artifact is seen along the left lateral wall of the bladder on the transverse image and along the bladder dome on the sagittal image when the patient is in the supine position, head first.

The normal bladder wall, though seen well in all planes, demonstrates the region of the base or dome best in the sagittal plane. In the coronal plane, the bladder dome is well seen, but there is indistinctness between bladder base and prostate or urethral tissue. The normal bladder is seen whether the bladder is collapsed or distended. However, evaluation of bladder wall thickening requires bladder distention.

Pathology

BENIGN PATHOLOGY

Bladder wall hypertrophy is best seen with long *TR* (2 sec) and *TE* (56 ms) sequences (Fig. 33–9). On images obtained with a short *TE* and a short *TR*, the interface

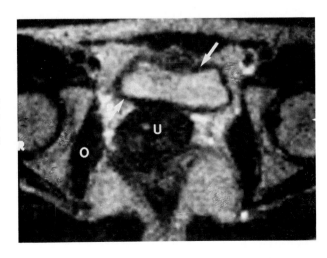

Figure 33–7. *TR* = 2.0 sec, *TE* 112 ms. Display of the bladder wall (white arrows) is even more pronounced with the longer *TE* image. Owing to decrease in S/N level the image is very noisy. Uterus (U). Obturator internus (O).

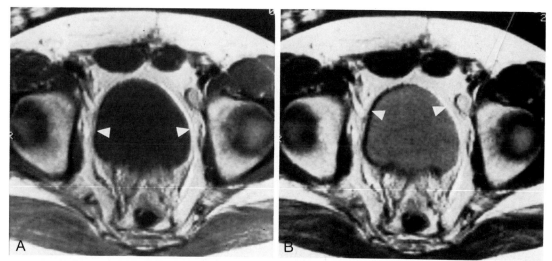

Figure 33–8. Chemical-shift artifact; normal bladder. *A, TR* = 2.0 sec, *TE* = 30 ms. *B, TR* = 2.0 sec, *TE* = 60 ms. The chemical-shift artifact results in a dark narrow band edge along the right lateral aspect of the bladder, and a white band edge (white arrowheads) along the left lateral aspect of the bladder. This is secondary to the chemical shift separation of 3 parts per million between fat and water. Application of the read-out gradient in the transverse imaging plane from right to left accounts for the dark band along the right and the bright band along the left.

between a possibly hypertrophied bladder wall and urine cannot always be distinguished. The signal intensity of the thickened wall is similar to that of a normal bladder wall.

In bladder outlet obstruction, mucosal congestion is occasionally demonstrated within the region of the bladder base. Mucosal congestion is imaged with high signal intensity on a long *TR* (2 sec) (*TE* = 28 and 56 ms). The congested area, imaged with high signal intensity, is separable from the lower signal intensity of the uninvolved bladder muscle (Fig. 33–10). With further prolongation of *TE*, the contrast between the muscle and congestion is even more pronounced, but signal-to-noise level decreases, resulting in decreased image-resolving power.

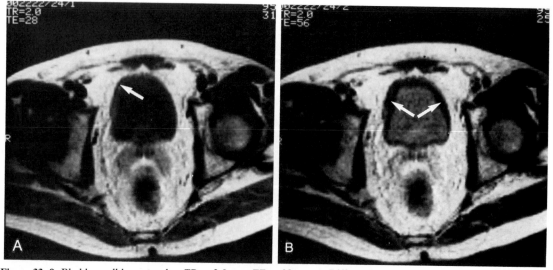

Figure 33–9. Bladder wall hypertrophy. *TR* = 2.0 sec, *TE* = 28 ms. *A*, Differentiation of the bladder wall (arrow) from urine is difficult. *B, TR* = 2.0 sec, *TE* = 56 ms. On the longer *TE*, the hypertrophied bladder wall (arrows) imaged with low intensity is clearly seen.

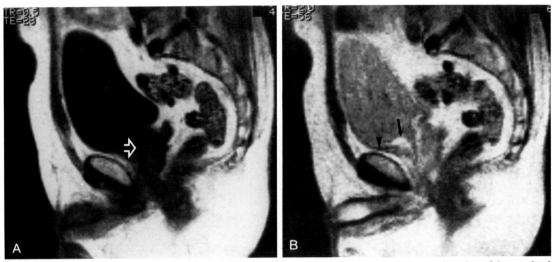

Figure 33–10. Status post TURP; congestion at the bladder base. *A, TR* = 0.5 sec, *TE* = 28 ms. Dilatation of the proximal prostatic urethra (open arrow) is secondary to TURP. There is thickening of the bladder neck. *B, TR* = 2.0 sec, *TE* = 56 ms. With longer *TE*, there is better delineation of congestion (arrow), which shows further relative increase in signal intensity as compared with lower intensity bladder wall muscle (arrowhead).

A variable appearance is found in postradiation cystitis. High signal intensity in the region of the mucosa has been noted in some cases, even though others fail to demonstrate discernible changes.

Inflammation and congestion cause prolongation of both the *T1* and the *T2* relaxation times of the bladder wall, but these values remain less than those of urine. Bladder congestion and inflammation are best seen with a long *TE* and a long *TR*.

Early studies have shown that with MR[12,13] mucosal congestion of the bladder and inflammation of the bladder wall can be differentiated from the normal bladder wall and from concentric or eccentric bladder wall hypertrophy. Based only on MR signal intensity variations, however, congestion and inflammation cannot be distinguished from each other.

MALIGNANT PATHOLOGY

Morphologic evaluation of malignant bladder tumors includes analysis of size, site, and pattern of tumor growth. Tumors are classified into four growth patterns: in situ (noninvasive), papillary, combined papillary and infiltrating, or infiltrating. (Fig. 33–11). MRI tumor staging can utilize the Tumor, Nodes, and Metastases (TNM) system for bladder neoplasms (Table 33–1)(Fig. 33–12).[14] The criteria used for MR tumor

Table 33–1. TNM CLASSIFICATION OF BLADDER CARCINOMAS

TNM System	Description
TIS	In situ
T1	Involves mucosa and submucosa
T2	Invasion of superficial muscle layer
T3a	Invasion of deep muscle layer
T3b	Perivesical extension
T4a	Extension to perivesical organs and rectum
T4b	Extension to pelvic side wall and distant metastases
N	Lymph node metastases
M	Distant metastases

PATTERNS OF TUMOR GROWTH
URINARY BLADDER

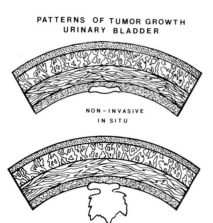

NON-INVASIVE
IN SITU

PAPILLARY

Figure 33–11. Patterns of tumor growth.

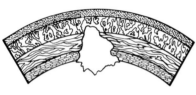

PAPILLARY & INFILTRATING

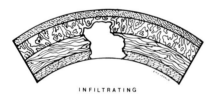

INFILTRATING

staging can be further clarified as follows: TIS are those too small for current resolution. Stage T1–T2 tumors are those confined to bladder wall with normal outer bladder wall seen as a low-intensity stripe. Stage T3a may be gross tumor involvement of bladder wall, seen as high signal intensity extending through the bladder wall but not into the perivesical fat; the remaining uninvolved bladder wall, seen as a low-intensity line, may or may not be present. Stage T3b is seen as transmural extension of the tumor with involvement of perivesical fat but not involving contiguous structures. Disruption of the normal bladder wall has to be seen in two imaging planes (transverse and sagittal). If bladder wall disruption is seen in only one plane, it is attributed to technical artifact. Stage T4 tumors demonstrate abnormal signal intensity extending to the contiguous pelvic organs (such as seminal vesicles, prostate, and rectum), suggesting invasion. For Stages T1, T2, and T3a, the ability to delineate the remaining normal bladder wall as a low-intensity rim between the tumor and perivesical fat is the main MR requirement. The presence of enlarged lymph nodes should be assessed.

Transverse images in most cases provide adequate anatomic display of tumor site and extent when the tumor is located in the anterolateral or posterolateral walls. When the tumor is located at the bladder base (Fig. 33–13) or dome, additional sagittal images are needed for optimal tumor detection and delineation of perivesical extension. Sagittal images are also needed for bladder tumors involving the posterolateral aspect of the bladder. In these types, the transverse image may falsely suggest transmural and perivesical extension, while sagittal images show an intact bladder wall. For evaluation of tumor extension to adjacent organs (i.e., symphysis pubis, prostate, or rectum) sagittal

TMN STAGING CLASSIFICATION OF BLADDER CARCINOMA

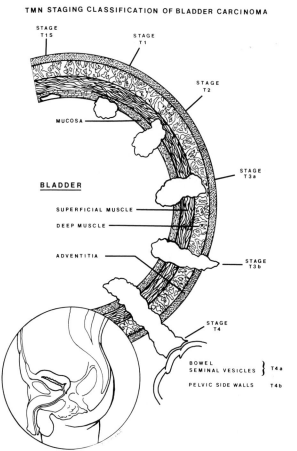

Figure 33–12. TNM system of staging bladder carcinoma.

images are necessary. The transverse plane is optimal for delineating seminal vesicle involvement.

The difference in signal intensity between the tumor and the surrounding structures allows tumor detection in both the nondistended and the distended bladders.

Several SE sequences are necessary to optimally evaluate bladder carcinomas. The papillary component of a carcinoma (Fig. 33–14) is well seen on a short *TE* (28 ms) and a *TR* of 1.0 sec or greater. The higher signal intensity of urine on the long *TR/TE* sequence may obscure the papillary extent of the carcinoma (Fig. 33–14C). For evaluation of an infiltrating component of tumor, a long *TR* and *TE* is necessary (Fig. 33–15). This SE combination is optimal for delineating the transmural infiltrating extent of the tumor and for differentiating the tumor, seen with high signal intensity, from the uninvolved bladder wall, seen with low signal intensity. Utilization of multiecho (5 *TE*'s) sequences allows even better delineation of the bladder wall on longer *TE*'s of 112 or 140 ms. Visualization of the low-intensity line, representing the uninvolved bladder wall between the tumor and perivesical fat, is an important determinant in MRI staging, specifically in differentiating between tumor Stages T2 and T3b (Fig. 33–15). A short *TR* (0.5 or 1.0 sec) is best for assessing perivesical extension of the neoplasm into the surrounding adipose tissue. With a short *TR*, the tumor has a medium signal intensity in contrast to the adipose tissue imaged with a high signal intensity. A short *TR* and *TE* sequence is optimal for lymph node detection.[15,16]

Normal bladder anatomy and pathology are clearly displayed by magnetic resonance. The normal and hypertrophied bladder walls have a unique MRI appearance

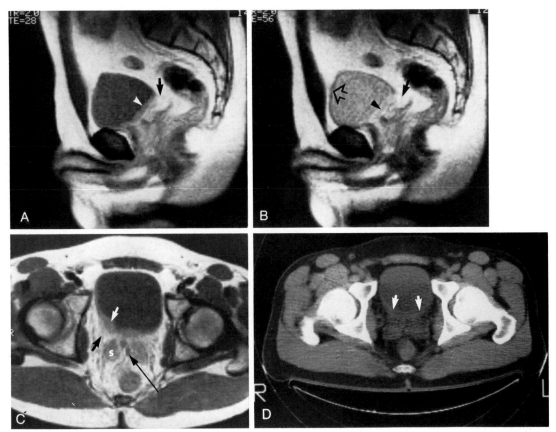

Figure 33–13. Transitional cell carcinoma, Stage T3b: infiltrating and papillary tumor growth. *A, TR* = 2.0 sec, *TE* = 28 ms. A tumor (white arrowhead) is seen at the bladder base and appears to extend into the perivesical region (black arrow). *B, TR* = 2.0 sec, *TE* = 56 ms. Image obtained with a longer *TE* demonstrates tumor (arrowhead) infiltrating through the entire width of the bladder wall (black arrow). There is disruption of the low-intensity rim of the normal bladder (open arrow). *C, TR* = 1.5 sec, *TE* = 28 ms. Transverse image in the same patient demonstrates the tumor in the right posterolateral aspect of the bladder (white arrow). Perivesical extension (short black arrow) is seen. Normal seminal vesicle (s). Ductus deferens (long arrow). *D,* Non–contrast enhanced transverse CT scan through the same region as the MR transverse image shows thickened posterior bladder wall (white arrows). Whether the tumor was confined to the bladder wall or extended into the perivesical fat could not be determined.

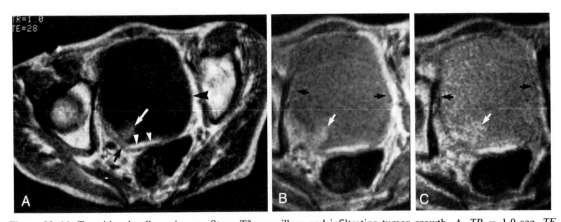

Figure 33–14. Transitional cell carcinoma, Stage T3a; papillary and infiltrating tumor growth. *A, TR* = 1.0 sec, *TE* = 28 ms. The papillary component of the tumor (white arrow) is optimally visualized because of the contrast difference between tumor and urine. In the region of the tumor the outer portion of the bladder wall (black arrow) is visualized, while urine–normal bladder wall contrast interface (black arrowhead) is not sufficient for differentiation. The small white arrowheads denote congestion of the posterior bladder wall. *B, TR* = 2.0 sec, *TE* = 28 ms. *C, TR* = 2.0 sec, *TE* = 56 ms. Increasing *TR* and *TE* (*C*) causes almost complete obliteration of the extent of the papillary tumor (white arrow). On this sequence, the normal bladder wall, seen with a low signal intensity, is well defined (black arrows).

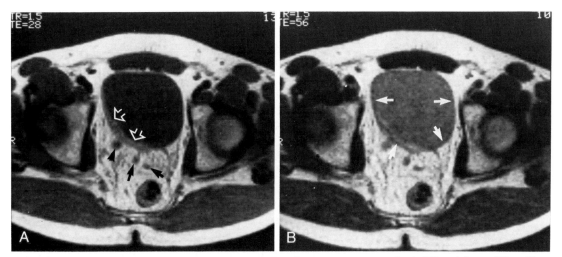

Figure 33–15. Transitional cell carcinoma, Stage T3a: infiltrating type tumor growth. *A, TR* = 1.5 sec, *TE* = 28 ms. Bladder carcinoma (open arrow) is seen along the right posterolateral bladder wall. On this sequence, the luminal component of the tumor is well seen, but assessment of bladder wall infiltration is difficult. No perivesical extension is seen. Dilated right ureter (black arrowhead). Ducti deferens (black arrows). *B, TR* = 1.5 sec, *TE* = 56 ms. The remaining intact bladder wall (white arrows) is visualized as an outer low-intensity rim at the site of tumor invasion.

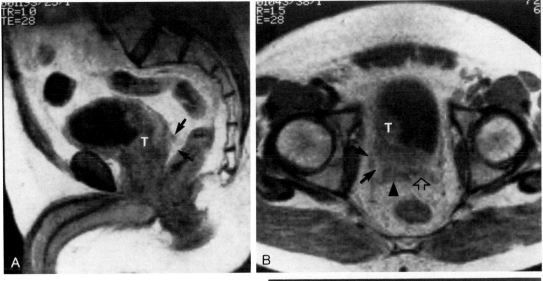

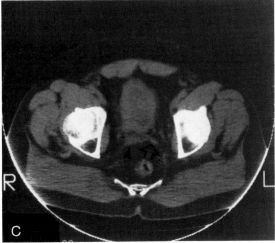

Figure 33–16. Transitional cell carcinoma, stage T4; papillary and infiltrating tumor growth. *A, TR* = 1.0 sec, *TE* = 28 ms. Sagittal image demonstrates the bladder carcinoma (T) arising in the posterior aspect of the bladder base. Perivesical extension (arrows) is well displayed on this sequence. *B, TR* = 1.5 sec, *TE* = 28 ms. Transverse image demonstrates the intraluminal extent of the tumor (T). The tumor extends into the perivesical fat, obliterating the fat plane between the bladder and right seminal vesicle (arrows). The right seminal vesicle (arrowhead) is invaded. Normal left seminal vesicle (open arrow). *C,* Non–contrast enhanced CT section through the same level as the transverse MR image (see Fig. 33–7*B*). The thickening of the bladder wall is nonspecific and can be secondary to a nondistended bladder or to a bladder carcinoma. Asymmetry between right (arrowhead) and left (open arrow) seminal vesicle is seen.

clearly distinguishable from any other bladder pathology.[12] Utilizing relaxation values only, because of large standard deviations, bladder congestion and bladder tumors cannot be differentiated.[13] Based upon the characteristic symmetrical location of bladder congestion, it usually can be distinguished from bladder neoplasms. However, a localized inflammatory process cannot be differentiated from bladder tumors, as they cause prolongation of *T1* and *T2* relaxation times and both may cause asymmetric abnormalities of the bladder wall. Tumor size (when greater than 1.5 cm), tumor site, and pattern of tumor growth do not affect neoplasm depiction by MRI. While tumor depiction by MRI is accurate for initial diagnosis of bladder carcinoma, biopsy is necessary. Besides improved detection, the primary value of MRI is in staging bladder neoplasms. MRI currently is unable to differentiate tumor Stage T1 from Stage T2. However, tumor Stage T2 should be distinguishable from Stage T3a if extension into the deep muscle involves the entire bladder wall. Subtle involvement of the deep musculature is not discernible at this time. Importantly, Stages T2 and T3a should be distinguished from Stage T3b. Stage T4 (Fig. 33–16), with local involvement of adjacent structures, is detected by MRI, but metastases, particularly to the peritoneal cavities, are more difficult to diagnose.

MRI appears to be an excellent modality for depicting bladder pathology and for differentiating normal or hypertrophied bladder wall from other bladder diseases. The main advantage of MRI lies in its ability to improve the detection and staging of bladder neoplasms.

References

1. Hricak H, Williams RD, Spring DB, Moon KL, Hedgcock MW, Watson RA, Crooks LE: Anatomy and pathology of the male pelvis by magnetic resonance imaging. AJR *141*:1101, 1983.
2. Hricak H, Alpers C, Crooks LE, Sheldon PE: Magnetic resonance imaging of the female pelvis: initial experience. AJR *141*:1119, 1983.
3. Bryan PJ, Butler HE, Lipuma JP, Haagas JR, El Yousef SJ, Resnick MI, Cohen AM, Malviya VK, Nelson AI, Clampitt M, Alfidi RJ, Cohen J, Morrison SC: NMR scanning of the pelvis: initial experience with a 0.3T system. AJR *141*:1111, 1983.
4. Harrison RG: The urogenital system. *In* Romanes GJ (ed): Cunningham's Textbook of Anatomy. London, Oxford University Press, 1972, pp 514–520, 532–534.
5. Lonsley OS: The development of the human prostate gland with reference to the development of other structures at the neck of the urinary bladder. Am J Anat *13*:229, 1912.
6. McNeal JE: The prostate gland: morphology and pathology. Monogram *4*:3, 1983.
7. Robbins SL: Pathologic Basis of Disease. Philadelphia, WB Saunders, 1974, pp 1166–1167, 1190–1197.
8. Poon P, McCallum RW, Henkelman MM, et al: Magnetic resonance imaging of the prostate. Radiology *154*:143, 1985.
9. Buonocore E, Hesemann C, Pavlicek W, Montie JE: Clinical and in vitro magnetic resonance imaging of prostate carcinoma. AJR *143*:1267, 1984
10. Ney C, Friedenberg R: Radiographic Atlas of the Genitourinary System. Philadelphia, JB Lippincott, 1981, pp 1478–1479.
11. Babcock EE, Brateman L, Weinreb JC, Hornre DS, Nunnally RL: Edge artifacts in MR images. Chemical shift effect. J Comput Assist Tomogr *9*:252, 1985.
12. Fisher MR, Hricak H: MR of the urinary bladder: normal and benign pathology. Radiology *157*:467, 1985.
13. Fisher MR, Hricak H: Magnetic resonance imaging of the urinary bladder: Neoplasm Part II. *157*: 471, 1985.
14. American Joint Committee on Staging and End-Results Reporting Manual for Staging of Cancer. Chicago, AJC, 1978.
15. Dooms GC, Hricak H, Crooks LE, Higgins CB: Magnetic resonance imaging of the lymph nodes: comparison with CT. Radiology *153*:719, 1984.
16. Lee JRT, Heiken JP, Ling D, et al: Magnetic resonance imaging of abdominal and pelvic lymphadenopathy. Radiology *153*:181, 1984.

34

Female Pelvis

MADAN V. KULKARNI
LEO F. DROLSHAGEN III

Noninvasive imaging techniques for the female pelvis have recently been significantly improved and extended. Developments in computed tomography (CT) and ultrasound have dramatically improved the ability to diagnose female pelvic disorders. Tomographic display of anatomy enhances identification of the disease process and also facilitates detection of the extent of disease. Magnetic resonance (MR) currently demonstrates considerable potential in pelvic imaging. Unfortunately, labored respiratory motion, when present, degrades MR image quality to a larger extent than with CT or ultrasound. The spatial resolution of MR in the pelvis is also slightly inferior to ultrasound or CT, although intravenous glucagon and bowel preparation may improve image quality by reducing artifact secondary to bowel peristalsis.[1] In view of this drawback, the basic advantage of MR imaging is its improved soft tissue contrast and multiplanar imaging. Tissue characterization of most pelvic pathology is difficult with current proton imaging systems, but remains an area of future development.

Although CT has improved the ability to diagnose pelvic pathology, it still has limitations in certain disorders. Computed tomography is limited in its assessment of the bladder base or peritoneal or mesenteric spread from ovarian tumors.[2,3] and in detection of abnormal pelvic and retroperitoneal nodes. Superior soft tissue contrast[4] and excellent demonstration of the pelvic organs using multiplanar imaging are major advantages of MR over CT in diagnosing pelvic disorders. In addition, the absence of ionizing radiation with MR may prove beneficial in the future, especially in younger patients who require long-term follow-up.

NORMAL ANATOMY

Magnetic resonance imaging has the ability to depict pelvic anatomy not only in the axial plane, similar to CT, but also in the coronal, sagittal, and nonorthogonal planes. Respiratory motion does not greatly affect the quality of MR images of the pelvis in most patients.[5] Excellent images of the pelvis can, therefore, be obtained with anatomic detail comparable to that of CT but with the advantage of better visualization of pelvic structures in nonaxial planes.[6]

The contrast in MR depends on the pulse sequence employed. The relative contrast between the tissues depends on whether the sequences are relatively weighted in proton density, *T1*, or *T2* relaxation times. Pelvic fat has a stronger signal and appears brighter (increased intensity) than the pelvic organs (Fig. 34–1) and musculature in most of the pulse sequences utilized.[7] The levator ani muscles of the pelvic floor have decreased signal intensity and are well seen on the coronal plane. The levator ani consist of the medial pubococcygeus, which surrounds and encases the urethra, vagina, and rectum

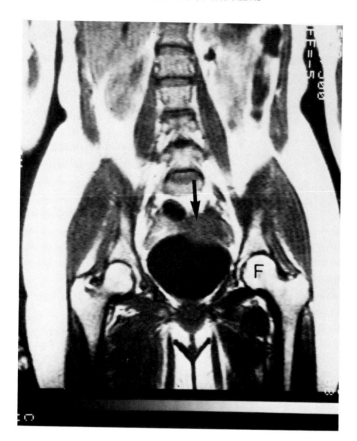

Figure 34–1. Coronal MR image (SE 30/500) of the uterus (arrow), superior to the bladder (B). Bone marrow fat (F) has bright signal intensity, while levator ani (L) muscles have decreased signal intensity.

(Fig. 34–2); the lateral iliococcygeus; and the posterior triangular sacrococcygeus muscle.[8] The paired triangular piriformis muscles are flattened against the posterior pelvis, covering the greater sciatic notch and lying posterior to the ovaries. The obturator internus, a fan-shaped muscle, covers the lateral pelvic wall. At the midlevel of the obturator muscles are the obturator lymph nodes.[8]

The vagina, a muscular canal 5 to 7 cm in length extending from the uterus to the vestibule, runs in the midline in a plane parallel to the lower sacrum and meets the cervix at a 45 to 90 degree angle.[9,10] The vagina has a lower signal intensity than the uterus and is well seen on sagittal and coronal planes. Frequently a thin layer of fat is seen between the vagina and the bladder and between the vagina and the rectum.

The cervix has anterior and posterior lips, with the anterior shorter than the posterior. The cervix has three different areas of signal intensity on MRI.[4] As first described

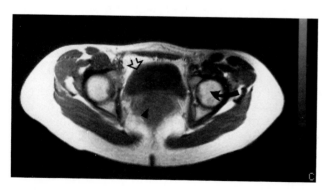

Figure 34–2. Transverse SE 30/500 image of normal female pelvis. Subcutaneous and parametrial fat has a bright signal owing to its short *T1* relaxation times on this sequence with relatively short *TE* and *TR* parameters. Bone marrow (curved arrow) has a relatively increased signal, while urine in the bladder (open arrow) has decreased signal intensity because of its long *T1* relaxation times. Uterus (arrowhead) has uniform signal. Different areas of endometrium and myometrium cannot be identified on this sequence.

by Hricak,[4] in sequences with long echo delay time (*TE*) and pulse repetition time (*TR*), there is high signal intensity from the central cervical mucus; a wide band of low signal intensity, probably from the glandular and the stromal elements; and an outer area of medium signal intensity, the muscular layer. Even late in pregnancy, the cervix is seen well with MR, an advantage over ultrasound.[11] Frequently on sequences with long *TE* and *TR* parameters, three separate zones of signal intensity are identified within the normal uterus. The innermost area of bright signal represents the endometrium. An intermediate zone of decreased signal intensity, previously referred to as stratum basale,[4] and the outer layer of intermediate signal intensity from the myometrium are also seen (Fig. 34–3). In a recent report the imtermediate zone was seen in in vitro imaging of the uterine specimen and was thought to represent the innermost portion of the myometrium.[12] The fallopian tubes, musculomembranous structures 7 to 14 cm in length, are seen in the free edge of the broad ligament. The intramural portion is 1.5 to 3.0 cm in length and is sometimes identified in coronal and transverse imaging. The isthmus and the ampullary portions run either obliquely or in a tortuous manner and normally are difficult to identify on MR.

The ovaries are attached posteriorly to the broad ligament by the meso-ovaria, which also supply the support to the blood vessels that enter the hilum of the ovary. The postpubertal ovary measures 2.5 to 5.0 cm in greatest length.[13] The ovary has low to intermediate signal intensity on pulse sequences with short *TE* and *TR* parameters. With increasing *TE* and *TR* parameters the relative signal intensity from ovaries increases and may be more intense than the pelvic fat.[7] During the follicular phase, follicles 1 cm or greater in diameter can be detected with MR. These cysts have increased signal intensity on *T2* weighted sequences.

The urinary bladder, anterior to the uterus, has long *T1* and *T2* relaxation times because of its primary component, urine. On sequences with short *TE* and *TR*, there is decreased signal from the bladder, contrasted by a thin layer of fat, which has a bright signal on these pulse sequences. Increasing *T2* weighting in the images increases relative signal intensity from the urine, and, with pulse sequences with very long *TE* and *TR* parameters (i.e., SE 120/2000), the bladder has greater signal intensity than the surrounding fat. The rectum is posterior to the uterus and is surrounded by perirectal fat. The signal intensity from the rectum depends on the presence of gas, which has

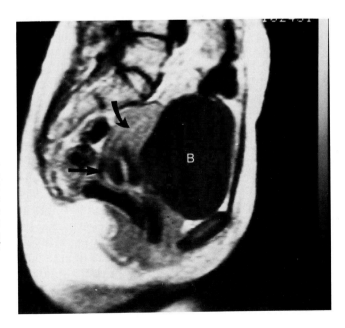

Figure 34–3. Sagittal SE 60/2000 image of the normal uterus. Cervix has decreased signal intensity (arrow). Endometrium has increased signal (curved arrow), which is probably dependent on the menstrual phase. An area of decreased signal intensity is seen between the bright signal of endometrium and the intermediate signal from myometrium and is referred to as the junctional zone. This junctional zone most likely represents the innermost layer of myometrium. Bladder (B).

markedly decreased signal, whereas fecal contents have varying degrees of signal intensity.

Pelvic lymph nodes, located in chains along the iliac vessels and medial to the obturator muscles, have longer *T2* relaxation times than does the pelvic musculature. Blood vessels are clearly distinguishable from lymph nodes and usually have markedly decreased signal because of flow.

IMAGING TECHNIQUES

Since the use of multiple sequences and imaging planes improves the ability of MRI to detect disease but also increases the imaging time, it is essential to plan the imaging planes and the pulse sequences in advance, to reduce imaging times, improve patient comfort, and achieve cost-effectiveness. We have developed protocols to keep the imaging times within an hour for a routine MR study of the female pelvis.

The anatomic images are performed in the transverse plane using spin-echo (SE) sequences with short *TE* and *TR* parameters. These sequences are relatively *T1* weighted and provide excellent contrast between retroperitoneal fat and abdominal and pelvic organs. The transverse plane anatomy is easier to understand because of previous CT experience. In addition, sagittal images are obtained using SE sequences with short *TE* and *TR* as well as relatively *T2* weighted images, with long *TE* and *TR* parameters. This protocol is used as a screening procedure and is modified, if necessary, according to the individual clinical situation. As a result of the availability of multislice-multiecho sequences, the *T2* weighted sequences are acquired with spin-echo technique with at least two *TE* values, to obtain different contrast without increasing imaging time (e.g., *TE/TR* 45/2000 and *TR* 90/2000). In evaluating myometrial invasion by endometrial carcinoma, thinner tomographic sections are utilized. Occasionally after evaluating initial images, additional pulse sequences or different imaging planes are acquired for superior definition of the abnormality.

UTERUS

The size of the uterus changes significantly during life. The normal uterus demonstrates three areas of different signal intensity on *T2* weighted images (Fig. 34–3).

The size of the endometrium changes during the proliferative and secretive phases of the menstrual cycle. This change in size is not observed in patients who take oral contraceptives.[14] The uterus is also smaller in patients taking oral contraceptives. Benign uterine leiomyomas are frequently identified as contour abnormalities of the uterus (Fig. 34–4). In our experience, uncomplicated leiomyomas have decreased or similar signal intensities compared with the uterus. Frequently these neoplasms are seen as a focal area of decreased signal compared with myometrium (Fig. 34–5), but many times leiomyomas involve the uterus diffusely (Fig. 34–6) and cause generalized uterine enlargement. Occasionally, marked decrease in signal intensity is noted in the leiomyomas on all pulse sequences without obvious calcification on the radiographs. The relative signal intensity probably depends on the amount of fibrous tissue and calcification. Hyaline degeneration within leiomyomas has also been demonstrated as a cause of marked decrease in signal intensity.[12] In general, leiomyomas have decreased signal intensity compared with myometrium,[15] but the presence of necrotic foci may cause increased signal in the center of the lesion on *T2* weighted images, owing to the prolonged *T2* relaxation times of these necrotic areas. Occasionally areas of mixed signal intensity are noted in large leiomyomas (Fig. 34–6C), probably as the result of necrosis

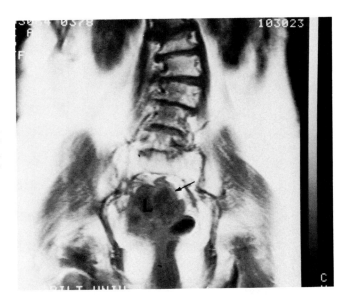

Figure 34–4. Markedly irregular and enlarged uterus with leiomyomas (L). On SE 30/500 image the leiomyomas have decreased signal compared with the normal smooth muscle of the myometrium (arrow).

or degenerative changes. Varying signal intensities can be seen within multiple leiomyomas in the same patient[16] as well as in different patients. Since leiomyomas may undergo degenerative hemorrhagic necrosis and may develop calcifications, the signal intensity in these lesions varies on all pulse sequences.

Endometrial carcinoma can be effectively imaged with MR. Normal endometrium on *T2* weighted sequences has increased signal intensity compared with adjacent myo-

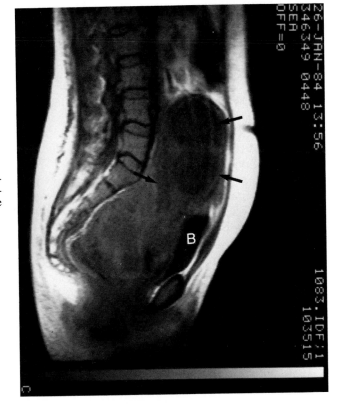

Figure 34–5. Enlarged uterus with fibroids (arrows) compressing bladder (B). Two large pedunculated leiomyomas are seen superior to the bladder.

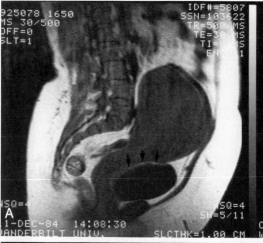

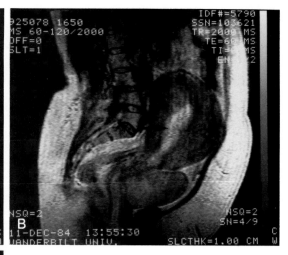

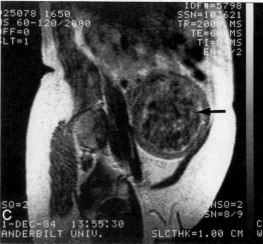

Figure 34–6. Diffuse uterine enlargement due to leiomyomas. *A*, On SE 30/500 the myometrium and endometrium cannot be separated. A thin fat plane (arrows) is identified between uterus and bladder. *B*, On SE 60/2000 the endometrium has bright signal intensity and the myometrium has an irregular shape. Also note that the endometrium is thickened (arrow). *C*, Large leiomyoma (arrow) with inhomogeneous signal on SE 60/2000 is seen on the parasagittal plane.

metrium. Small endometrial carcinomas are seen as an increase in the size of the endometrium (Fig. 34–7), but this finding is not characteristic of malignancy, since benign hypertrophy of the endometrium also demonstrates a bright signal on *T2* weighted images (see Fig. 34–6*B*). MRI in patients with endometrial carcinoma, however, can be useful in determining myometrial invasion.[17] Often the *T1* values of an endometrial carcinoma are not significantly different from those of the smooth muscle of the myometrium,[16] and on sequences with short *TE* and *TR* parameters it is difficult to separate carcinoma from myometrium. The presence of hemorrhagic changes within the tumor can shorten its *T1* relaxation times, and these tumors will then have increased signal on *T1* as well as *T2* weighted sequences (Fig. 34–8). In general, pulse sequences with long *TE* and *TR* parameters are useful in determining the extent of myometrial invasion, since the increased signal of the endometrial carcinoma is well contrasted with the markedly decreased signal of the myometrium and junctional zone (Fig. 34–9).

Magnetic resonance imaging not only detects the myometrial involvement but also may be useful in determining extrauterine spread (Fig. 34–9). In a single case comparison with 0.15 tesla MR unit, CT was considered superior in the diagnosis of endometrial carcinoma.[18] In a recent series, MR using a 0.6 telsa unit was found to be superior to CT for localization of uterine malignancy within pelvic viscera.[17] The value of MR, however, will not be known until further experience is obtained with a larger series of patients, utilizing the current generation of higher field strength magnets.

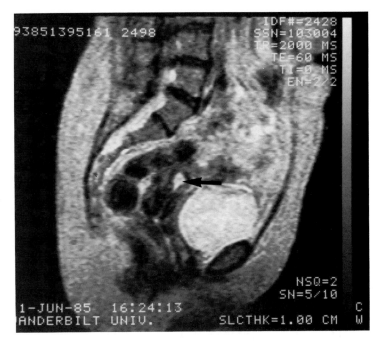

Figure 34–7. Small endometrial carcinoma at the fundus of the uterus. The plane between the tumor and the adjacent myometrium is preserved, and endometrium (arrow) and two separate zones of myometrium are identified in this *T2* weighted image (SE 120/2000).

Sagittal images with MR are certainly useful in determining myometrial invasion, and we are currently comparing MR with ultrasound in the staging of endometrial carcinoma. Preliminary results suggest that when a tumor invades deeply into the myometrium, the intermediate low signal intensity zone is abridged or indistinct.

Magnetic resonance imaging also provides valuable information in the diagnosis of cervical carcinoma. The tumor's relationship to the urinary bladder (Fig. 34–10*B*) and rectum can be accurately assessed with MR. Secondary effects, such as cervical stenosis and hematometra, are well demonstrated with MR (Fig. 34–10*A*). Magnetic resonance imaging is also useful in detecting ureteral obstruction and lymph node and skeletal metastases.[19] On sequences with short *TE* and *TR* parameters most cervical carcinomas have intermediate signal intensity (Fig. 34–11), but varying signal intensity

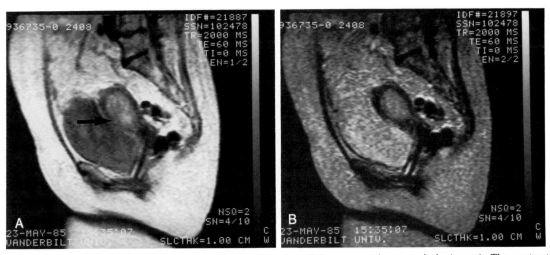

Figure 34–8. Large endometrial carcinoma with local invasion of the myometrium anteriorly (arrow). The contrast between the bladder and retroperitoneal fat is best seen on SE 60/2000 while that between the tumor and myometrium is seen on SE 120/2000 (*B*).

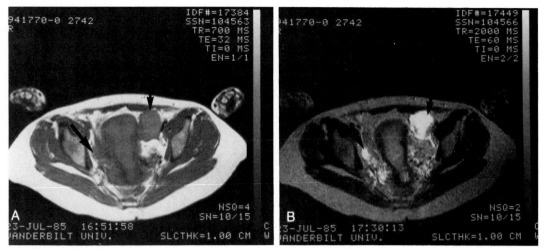

Figure 34–9. Enlargement of the uterus with endometrial carcinoma. Enlargement of the endometrial thickness is also demonstrated. Bilateral ovarian metastases (arrows) have increased signal intensities on SE 32/700 (*A*) and SE 120/2000 (*B*) sequences when compared with muscle. Also note loss of distinct margin between the fundus of the uterus and the endometrial carcinoma. Partial volume averaging could lead to similar findings and could be prevented by imaging with the use of additional planes and/or thinner sections.

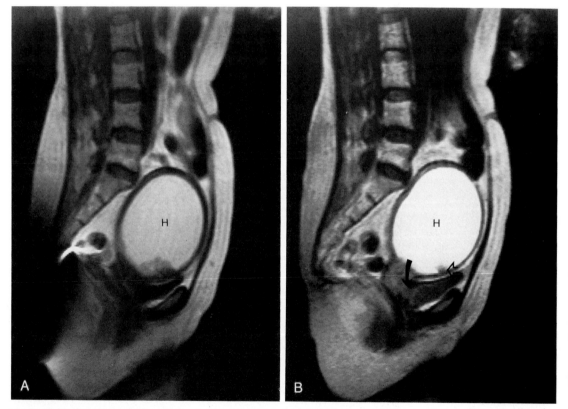

Figure 34–10. Carcinoma of the uterine cervix causing cervical stenosis and hematometra (H). *A*, Short *T1* relaxation times of the blood lead to bright signal from hematometra on SE 30/500. *B*, Carcinoma of the cervix (curved arrow) is seen invading posterior wall of the urinary bladder on SE 60/2000. Small tumor focus in the lower part of the uterus is also identified (open arrow).

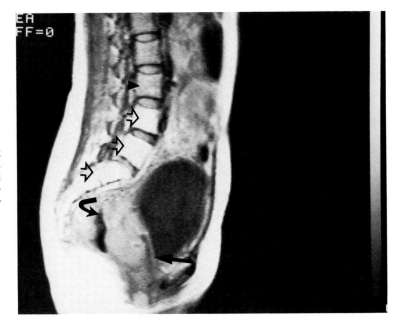

Figure 34–11. Displacement of the vagina (straight arrow) and the rectum (curved arrow) by recurrent carcinoma of the cervix. Fatty replacement of the marrow following radiation therapy leads to shortened *T1* relaxation times and bright signal on SE 30/500 sequence (open arrows) compared with normal marrow (arrowhead).

has been observed in cervical carcinoma.[20] Large recurrent tumors, however, have areas of necrosis that usually have decreased signal intensity on *T1* weighted images (Fig. 34–12). Since fat within the parametria has a bright signal on these pulse sequences, *T1* weighted images are useful in demonstrating pelvic sidewall extension (Fig. 34–12). In our experience, sagittal images are very useful in detecting extension of cervical carcinoma to the bladder and vagina. Similar findings also have been reported by Bies et al.[18]

Posthysterectomy changes are easily demonstrated by MR. Magnetic resonance is also useful in detecting various tissue components in some of the rare malignant uterine tumors (Fig. 34–13). Although signal intensity for benign and malignant tumors is not characteristic for the tumor histology, MR can be helpful in staging these unusual uterine tumors.

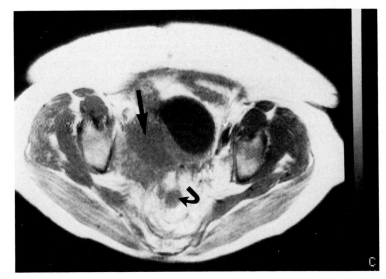

Figure 34–12. Recurrent carcinoma of the cervix with central area of tumor necrosis (arrow) and parametrial involvement reaching the right pelvic wall. Small tumor nodule (curved arrow) in the perirectal fat is identified.

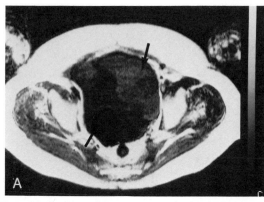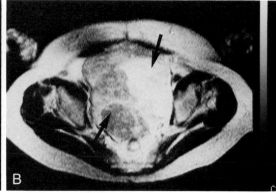

Figure 34–13. Large leiomyosarcoma is shown with areas of varying signal intensity due to different tissue elements within the tumor. Inversion-recovery image (*A*) demonstrates area of relatively decreased and intermediate signal intensities (arrows), while SE 60/1000 image (*B*) shows intermediate and increased signal in these tissue elements.

OVARIES

Normal ovaries are infrequently seen with MR and have intermediate signal intensity on *T1* weighted sequences. It is sometimes difficult to differentiate small bowel loops from normal ovaries because of the similar signal intensity of these structures. On sequences with longer *TE* and *TR* parameters, ovaries may become brighter than the surrounding pelvic fat.[17]

Benign ovarian cysts have varying signal intensities on pulse sequences with short *TE* and *TR* parameters. Simple cysts have relatively long *T1* and *T2* relaxation times and hence have decreased signal intensity on *T1* weighted sequences (Fig. 34–14) and increased signal on *T2* weighted sequences. The signal intensity depends on the contents of the cyst. The presence of hemorrhage or increased protein within the cyst shortens the *T1* relaxation times and produces an intermediate signal intensity on sequences with short *TE* and *TR* values (Fig. 34–15).

MR has demonstrated its ability to characterize fluids within the cyst on the basis of signal intensity. Although it does not often help in histopathologic diagnosis, MR occasionally suggests the correct histology on the basis of *T1* and *T2* parameters and may help in diagnosing cyst extension (Fig. 34–16). Endometriomas have long *T2* relaxation times, but the signal intensity has been variable on *T1* weighted images, depending on the hemorrhagic content.[16] Dermoid tumors of the ovaries may also have variable signal intensity because of their tissue contents, but fat within the dermoid tumors has a bright signal intensity on *T1* weighted sequences.[16] In a series of 12 patients with pelvic dermoid, only 33 percent showed the pathognomonic triple-intensity pattern secondary to the combined presence of fat, fluid, and bony components.[21]

Ovarian malignant tumors are well studied with MR. Utilization of multiple pulse sequences is necessary to image ovarian tumors.[19] Although large masses are detected with MR on sequences with relatively short *TE* and *TR* values, *T2* weighted sequences are useful in determining whether the tumor arises from the ovary or the uterus (Fig. 34–17). These sequences are also beneficial in determining tumor extension to the other pelvic organs (Fig. 34–18). The solid and cystic components of the neoplasms can also be differentiated on the basis of signal intensities.[22]

MR has been a useful modality in the staging of ovarian carcinoma, especially in the detection of ascites and periaortic lymphadenopathy. Although MR occasionally can detect omental, peritoneal, or mesenteric metastases (Fig. 34–19) and pelvic lymphadenopathy, early experience indicates that MR has a lower sensitivity than CT in

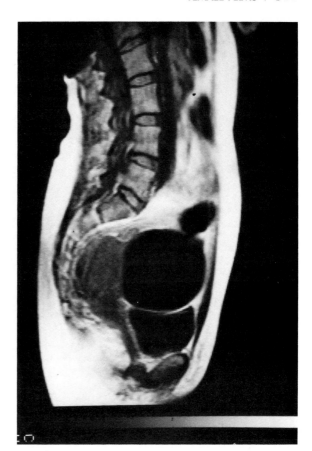

Figure 34–14. Simple serous cystadenoma has similar signal intensity as urine on SE 30/500 sequence.

detecting these lesions. This is partly due to the slightly inferior spatial resolution of MR and to respiratory motion artifact, but the major disadvantage with MR is the lack of an adequate contrast agent for small bowel.

Magnetic resonance imaging is also useful in demonstrating large mesenteric cysts (Fig. 34–20) and pelvic inflammatory disease (Fig. 34–21). The signal intensities for these disorders are not characteristic for the abnormalities, and the most important role for MR is in determining the extent of the disease process. The advantages of MR over CT scan in these situations are its superior soft tissue contrast and multiplanar imaging capabilities.

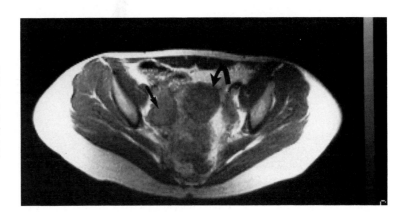

Figure 34–15. Benign ovarian cyst (straight arrow) has similar signal intensity as uterus (curved arrow). Signal intensity from an ovarian cyst depends on the content of the cyst. The presence of protein or cholesterol will decrease the $T1$ relaxation times and affect the signal intensity.

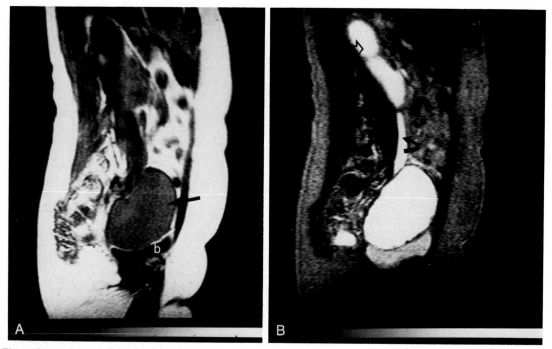

Figure 34–16. Intermediate signal intensity in a hemorrhagic cyst adenoma on SE 30/500 sequence (*A*). The recurrent tumor (arrow) was seen separate from the bladder (b). Tumor extension into the collecting system of left kidney was documented on *T2* weighted SE 120/2000 sequence (*B*), since the contents of the ureter (curved arrow) and kidney (open arrow) demonstrated similar signal intensity as the hemorrhagic cystadenoma rather than urine, as in hydronephrosis.

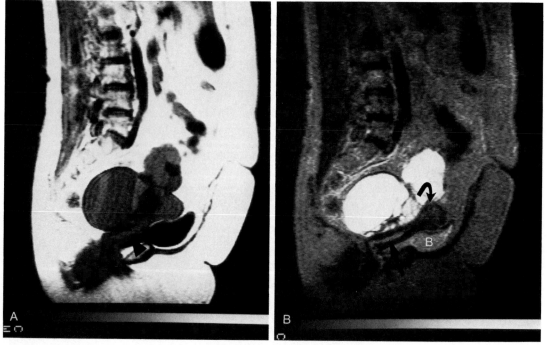

Figure 34–17. Multiloculated masses seen in the pelvis of this patient with bilateral serous cystadenocarcinoma are difficult to separate from the uterus (arrowhead) on SE 30/500 (*A*). On SE 120/2000 (*B*), multiple cysts are identified separate from the uterus (curved arrow). Endometrial polyp (arrow) is shown in the endocervix. B, Bladder.

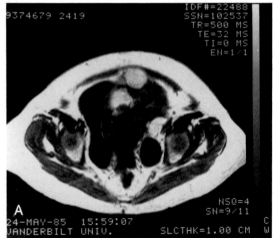
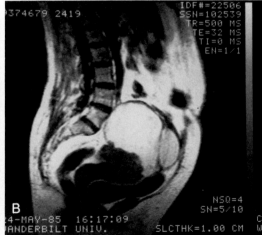

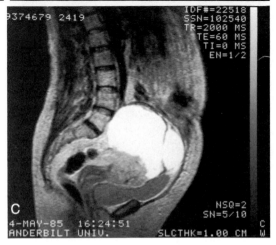

Figure 34–18. Papillary cystadenocarcinoma demonstrates areas of intermediate and increased signal intensity on SE 30/500 transverse (*A*) and sagittal (*B*) images. The area of bright signal probably represents either hemorrhage within the cyst or increased protein content. Although the majority of the pelvic mass appears to be extrauterine, the involvement of the myometrium is seen on SE 60/2000 sagittal (*C*) image.

BLADDER

Early reports[23] have shown MR to be sensitive in the detection and staging of bladder neoplasms, except for carcinoma in situ. MR was shown to be accurate in the evaluation of depth of invasion of the bladder wall. Bladder neoplasms, like bladder inflammation, cause increased *T1* and *T2* relaxation times, so biopsy is necessary for the initial diagnosis. Currently, MRI is unable to distinguish tumor Stage *T1* from *T2*, but Stages *T2* and *T3A* are differentiated from *T3B*.[23]

A short *TE* pulse sequence with *TR* of 1.0 to 2.0 sec is used to identify papillary components of bladder neoplasms, and longer *TE* pulse sequences are valuable in identifying invasion (disruption) of the bladder wall. Transverse planes can display site and extent of tumor as well as invasion of adjacent uterus and cervix. Sagittal planes are used to evaluate tumors of the posterior and posterolateral walls and base of the bladder. Inflammatory changes in the bladder are similar to neoplastic changes, with increased *T1* and *T2* best delineated on long *TE* and *TR*. Distention of the bladder aids in the diagnosis of both inflammatory and neoplastic changes.

OBSTETRICS

Magnetic resonance has also been utilized in imaging of the gravid uterus.[24–26] In the case of oligohydramnios (Fig. 34–22), when fetal motion is minimal, the depiction

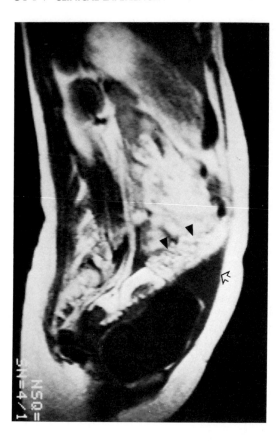

Figure 34–19. Massive ascites (open arrow) and evidence of omental and peritoneal metastasis from ovarian cystadeno-carcinoma are seen (arrowheads).

of fetal anatomy is excellent. Fetal motion is primarily limited to extremities during the third trimester,[27] and imaging patients in the third trimester results in minimal fetal motion artifacts. In patients with hydramnios the MR imaging quality is degraded because of fetal motion. Sagittal MR images have been found to be more useful in the past,[27] but the fetal anatomic display obviously depends on the fetal intrauterine position. *T1* weighted images can be acquired in a short time and do provide contrast

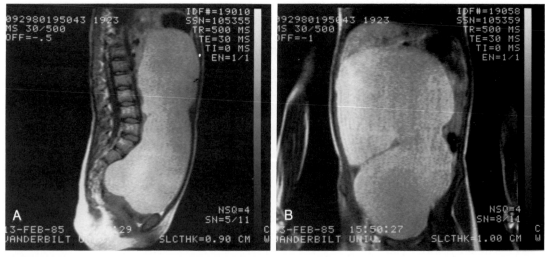

Figure 34–20. Massive mesenteric cyst demonstrates bright signal on SE 30/500 sagittal (*A*) and coronal (*B*) images.

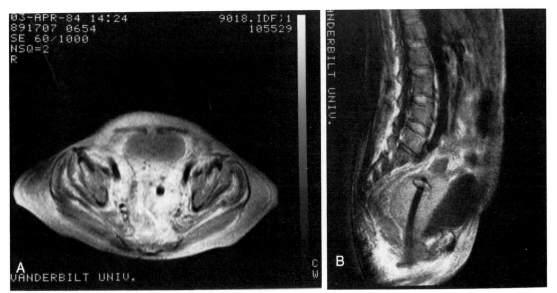

Figure 34–21. A large pelvic abscess with drainage tube (*A*) seen posterior to the urinary bladder and uterus (*B*). On transverse image, the inflammatory mass has nondistinct margins and areas of varying signal intensity.

between amniotic fluid and fetal parts, but the *T2* weighted images provide superior contrast between the fetal organs.

The signal intensities from the individual fetal organs are, in general, similar to those seen in adult organ systems. Fetal fat has increased signal intensity, whereas fetal muscles have decreased signal intensity, on *T1* weighted images. Kidneys, on the other hand, have bright signal intensity on *T2* weighted sequences (Fig. 34–22). Unlike adult lungs, the fetal lungs have increased signal intensity on *T1* as well as on *T2* weighted sequences, since the lungs do not contain air. Although mature fetal lungs have a signal intensity similar to that of liver on *T1* weighted images, on the *T2* weighted sequences the lungs have brighter signal compared with the liver. This may be related to surfactant, which is a phospholipid and alters the relaxation character of fetal lung water.[26] The placenta is well seen on all pulse sequences and has markedly increased

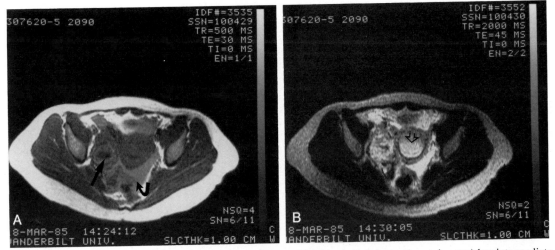

Figure 34–22. Ruptured ectopic pregnancy (straight arrow). *A*, Blood in the cul-de-sac (curved arrow) has intermediate signal intensity on SE 30/500 sequence. *B*, On SE 90/2000, however, this blood demonstrates markedly increased signal intensity. Residual reaction within the uterus also has increased signal intensity (open arrow) on *T2* weighted sequence.

signal intensity on *T2* weighted images. Because of its excellent ability to see placenta, MR may become useful in detecting placental pathology. The relationship of the placenta to the cervical os can be determined by MR.[11] MR imaging is also useful in depicting the changes in the uterine cervix during pregnancy.

Although MR is sparingly used in normal pregnancy, there are more data available about its use in complicated gestations with fetal or maternal diseases. Because of its lower costs and real-time capabilities, ultrasound is probably a preferred modality in these cases, but MR can delineate fetal anatomy superiorly in situations such as oligohydramnios, in which ultrasound is limited by lack of amniotic fluid. MR also has better soft tissue contrast, and, using multiple sequences, it can characterize fluids (Fig. 34–23) better than ultrasound. Since there is no ionizing radiation involved, MR can be used as a screening modality[28] before invasive radiographic procedures are undertaken.

Although MR does not involve ionizing radiation, the biologic hazards of MR on a developing fetus are as yet unknown. Hence, MR evaluation of the pregnancy should be approached with caution. In the first trimester of pregnancy during the period of organogenesis, MR should be utilized with extreme care. Currently, MR imaging in obstetrics is limited to patients with fetal or maternal abnormalities. MR has also been used in pregnancies that were terminated before completion of gestation. Further experience will determine the biohazards and will decide the role of MR in the evaluation of pregnancy.

In summary, magnetic resonance imaging is currently being used at multiple centers in the evaluation of female pelvic disorders. The prolonged imaging times involved in MR frequently generate significant respiratory motion artifacts in the visualization of the upper abdomen. Since the pelvis is relatively free of respiratory motion, MR imaging in this region has shown encouraging results. Soft tissue contrast using MR is superior to that obtained with CT. MR also has an advantage of multiplanar imaging and can evaluate many pelvic organs along their long axis. This has resulted in superior evaluation of the bladder, rectum, and uterus, especially in determining tumor spread in these areas. Use of multiple pulse sequences is also recommended to obtain optimum contrast between the tissues under evaluation. For example, parametrial extension of endometrial cancer is frequently better diagnosed on *T1* weighted sequences. Con-

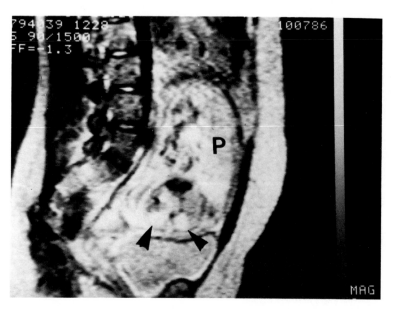

Figure 34–23. Intrauterine pregnancy in a patient with oligohydramnios. *T2* weighted images demonstrate fetal kidneys (arrowheads) and placenta (P).

versely, *T2* weighted images will better demonstrate the different zones of the endometrium and myometrium and may better assess invasion of the myometrium by an endometrial carcinoma.

Although MR has shown its excellent imaging quality, it faces tremendous competition from the conventional imaging modalities, such as CT and ultrasound. These conventional modalities have slightly superior spatial resolution compared with MR. But the major advantage for ultrasound is its real-time capabilities. Ultrasound is also cheap and portable, does not involve ionizing radiation, and is not affected by patient or fetal motion. Some of these advantages of ultrasound may be difficult for MR to overcome in the future. CT, on the other hand, can demonstrate calcification better than MR, but its major advantage in our experience is the use of small bowel contrast agent. This is particularly true in patients with sparse intra-abdominal fat. CT diagnosis is also supported by significant past experience, but our experience with MR is also increasing at a rapid pace.

With current technological developments, the spatial resolution of MR is approaching that of CT. Some of the surface-coil technology has shown better demonstration of deeper abdominal structures such as pancreas,[29] and similar techniques can be utilized to improve spatial resolution in deeper pelvic structures. Paramagnetic contrast agents will be used in the future as small bowel contrast agents. The significant advantage of MR over conventional imaging techniques may be spectroscopy. Using localization technique, P-31 or H1 in vitro spectra from deeper pelvic structures may be derived to provide biochemical information.[25] This may improve diagnosis or aid in monitoring therapy. Further research and experience are needed for this exciting technique.

Thus MR has shown its potential utility in imaging the female pelvis and, with further technological improvements, may demonstrate additional applications in the future.

References

1. Winkler ML, Hricak H: Pelvic imaging with MR: Technique for improvement. Radiology *158*(3):848, 1985.
2. Denkhaus H, Diekopf W, Grabbe E, et al: Comparative study of suprapubic sonography and computed tomography for staging of prostatic carcinoma. Urol Radiol *5*:1, 1983.
3. Brenner DE, Shaff MI, James HW, et al: An evaluation of the accuracy of CT in patients with ovarian carcinoma prior to second look laparotomy. Obstet Gynecol *65*:7145, 1985.
4. Hricak H: Pelvis. *In* Mangulis AR et al (eds): Clinical Magnetic Resonance Imaging. San Francisco, Radiology Research and Education Foundation, University of California, 1983.
5. Kulkarni MV, Partain CL, Tishler JM, et al: Magnetic resonance imaging of the abdomen. *In* Peterson SB et al (eds): An Introduction to Biomedical Nuclear Magnetic Resonance. New York, Georg Thieme, 1985.
6. Bryan PJ, Butter HE, LiPuma JP, et al: Magnetic resonance imaging of the pelvis. Radiol Clin North Am *22*(4):897, 1984.
7. Hricak H, Alpens C, Crooks LE, Sheldon PE: Magnetic resonance imaging of the pelvis; initial experience. AJR *141*:119, 1983.
8. Krantz KE: Anatomy of the female reproductive system. *In* Benson RC (ed): Current Obstetric and Gynecologic Diagnosis and Treatment. Los Altos, Lange Medical Publications, 1984.
9. Dentsch AL, Gosink BB: Normal female pelvis anatomy. Semin Roentgenol *17*(4):241, 1982.
10. Meschan I: The genital system. *In* Meschan I (ed): Anatomy Basic to Radiology. Philadelphia, WB Saunders, 1975.
11. McCarthy SM, Stark DD, Filly RA, et al: Obstetrical magnetic resonance imaging: Maternal anatomy. Radiology *154*:421, 1985.
12. Lee JK, Gersell DJ, Balfe DM, et al: The uterus: In vitro MR anatomic correlation of normal and abnormal specimens. Radiology *157*:175, 1985.
13. Zenyn S: Comparison of pelvic ultrasonography and pneumography for ovarian size. J Clin Ultrasound *2*:331, 1974.
14. McCarthy S, Tauber C, Gore J: Magnetic resonance imaging in female pelvic anatomy during the menstrual cycle and with oral contraception. Magn Reson Imag *4*(2):136, 1986.

15. Schmidt HC, Tscholakoff D, Hricak H, et al: MR image contrast and relaxation times of solid tumors in the chest, abdomen and pelvis. J Comput Assist Tomogr 9(A):738, 1985.
16. Butler H, Bryan PI, LiPuma JP, et al: Magnetic resonance imaging of the abnormal female pelvis. AJR *143*:1259, 1984.
17. Fishman MC, Stein HL, Lovecchio JL: Predicting depth of invasion of endometrial cancer by MRI. Magn Reson Imag 4(2):134, 1986.
18. Bies JR, Ellis JH, Kopecky KK, et al: Assessment of primary gynecological malignancies. Comparison of 0.15 T resistive MRI with CT. AJR *143*:1249, 1984.
19. Kulkarni MV, Shaff MI, Carter MM, et al: Magnetic resonance imaging of the pelvis. RadioGraphics 5(4):611, 1985.
20. Fishman MC, Stein HL, Lovecchio JL: Staging of carcinoma of the cervix by MRI. Magn Reson Imag 4(2):134, 1986.
21. Lupetin AR, Dash N, Beckman I, Linetsky L: Magnetic resonance appearance of the pelvic dermoid. Magn Reson Imag 4(2):135, 1986.
22. Kulkarni MV, Shaff MI, Brenner DE, et al: Magnetic resonance imaging of the gynecological masses. Presented to Association of University Radiologists, Nashville, 1985.
23. Fisher MR, Hricak H, Tanagho EA: Urinary bladder MR imaging. Part II. Neoplasm. Radiology *157*:471, 1985.
24. Johnson IR, Symonds EM, Kean DM, et al: Imaging the pregnant human uterus with nuclear magnetic resonance. Am J Obstet Gynecol *148*:1136, 1984.
25. Weinreb JC, Lowe TW, Santos-Ramos R, et al: Magnetic resonance imaging in obstetric diagnosis. Radiology *154*:157, 1985.
26. McCarthy SM, Filly RA, Stark DD, et al: Obstetrical magnetic resonance imaging: fetal anatomy. Radiology *154*:427, 1985.
27. Cohen JHM, Weinreb JC, Lowe TW, et al: MR imaging of a viable full term abdominal pregnancy. AJR *145*:407, 1985.
28. Kulkarni MV, Burks DD, Price AC, et al: Diagnosis of spinal arteriovenous malformation in a pregnant patient by MR imaging. J Comput Assist Tomogr 9(1):171, 1985.
29. Simeone JF, Edelman RR, Stark DD, et al: Surface coil MR imaging of abdominal viscera. Part III. Pancreas. Radiology *157*:437, 1985.
30. Narayana PA, Delayre JL: Localization methods in magnetic resonance. *In* Partain CL et al (eds): Magnetic Resonance Imaging, 2nd ed. Philadelphia, WB Saunders, 1988.

35

Obstetric Problems

Any discussion of imaging modalities to evaluate obstetric problems must begin with ultrasound. Real-time sonography is currently the premier imaging technique in obstetrics. It is accurate, safe, available, and inexpensive and has real-time capabilities.

MRI, on the other hand, is not widely available, is relatively expensive, and does not at present have real-time capabilities with good spatial resolution. Furthermore, its safety and accuracy have not yet been thoroughly evaluated. In view of these facts, one might legitimately ask, "Why bother with obstetric MRI?" There are at least three answers to this question:

1. *Ultrasound has some inherent limitations.* Contrast on ultrasound images is dependent upon differences in acoustical impedance between tissues. Generally, this single parameter is used to depict anatomic and pathologic features. Unfortunately, pathologic or immature tissues may have acoustical impedances that are identical to those of normal mature structures. For example, fetal lung maturity cannot be routinely assessed with ultrasound. Ultrasound may also be limited by interference from skeletal, fatty, or gas-filled structures. As a result, it is not uncommon for ultrasound to provide a suboptimal evaluation of the fetus in obese patients. This also means that pelvic masses in pregnant women may be obscured by overlying gas-filled loops of bowel or the gestational uterus itself. Finally, ultrasound imaging of deeper pelvic structures is dependent upon the presence of an acoustical window, such as the urinary bladder, and amniotic fluid.

2. *MRI can potentially provide information not available with ultrasound.* Like ultrasound, MRI is noninvasive, involves no ionizing radiation, and can provide images in multiple orthogonal planes. However, unlike ultrasound, MR images are not limited by interference from skeletal, fatty, or gas-filled structures, and imaging of deep pelvic structures is not dependent upon the presence of an acoustical window. MRI provides superb contrast resolution between different soft tissues. The contrast is dependent upon tissue characteristics (i.e., *T1, T2*, proton density, and flow) that may bring out features not detectable with ultrasound.

3. *If in vivo, NMR spectroscopic evaluation of the fetus, amniotic fluid, or placenta is ever to become a reality, one must first be able to localize the relevant structures with MRI.*

Of course, one should always be concerned with potential adverse bioeffects from MRI on the developing fetus. Whereas there is evidence to suggest that low-dose prenatal irradiation (as little as 1 to 2 rads delivered in obstetric x-ray studies) may result in significant increases of childhood cancer,[1] there is no evidence that MRI is harmful.[2-5] Nevertheless, it is prudent to exclude pregnant women during the first trimester (unless they will subsequently undergo abortion), a policy that has been adopted by the National Radiologic Protection Board in Great Britain.[6] In general, this has been our policy as well, except in cases in which the patient and her physician believe that the potential benefits outweigh the potential risks. Currently, all pregnant patients studied with MRI at our institution must sign informed consent under a protocol approved by our Institutional Review Board. The bioeffects of MRI are discussed in more detail in Chapters 84 to 87.

TECHNICAL CONSIDERATIONS

The images presented in this chapter were obtained on a cryogenic MRI system operating at 0.35 tesla (15 MHz). The pixel size was 1.7 mm; section thickness varied between 5 and 10 mm; and gaps between contiguous sections varied between 0 and 3 mm. Images were obtained using spin-echo (SE) multislice-multiecho technique. With this technique, five to ten sections were obtained simultaneously in 4.3 minutes when a *TR* of 500 ms was selected, and 20 sections were obtained in 17 minutes for *TR* of 2000 ms. Data were acquired using either two or four excitations, and images were produced using two-dimensional Fourier transformation.

THE MATERNAL PELVIS

Uterus and Placenta

Maternal pelvic anatomy is clearly depicted with MRI (Figs. 35–1 and 35–2). The uterus is visible above the bladder, often compressing the bladder dome. The myometrium is composed of smooth muscle with a relatively long *T1* relaxation time, similar to that of skeletal muscle.[7] Therefore, on relatively *T1* weighted images, it appears with signal intensity equal to or slightly greater than skeletal muscle. The *T2* relaxation time is somewhat longer than that of skeletal muscle. Thus, with more *T2* weighting, the signal intensity increases to a greater extent than the striated muscles of the pelvic wall. Despite an increase in the collagen content of the uterus during pregnancy,[8] no change in the signal characteristics of the myometrium has been noted. As pregnancy progresses, the myometrium is stretched by the gestational sac and becomes thinned. As a result, it may not be appreciated in its entire circumference in the third trimester.[9]

With ultrasound, as many as 22 percent of all fibroids may go undetected.[10] In the gravid uterus, ultrasound is even more problematic because parts of the myometrium

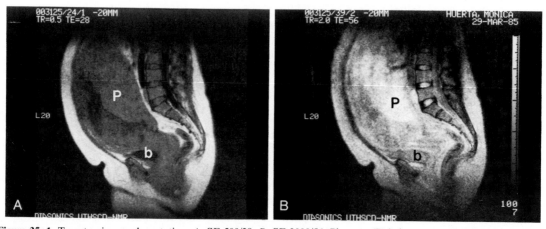

Figure 35–1. Twenty-nine week gestation. *A*, SE 500/28. *B*, SE 2000/56. Placenta (P) is homogeneous and demonstrates relative increase in signal intensity with *T2* weighting. Bladder (b).

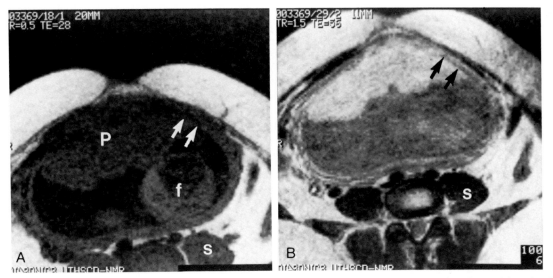

Figure 35–2. Nineteen week gestation. *A*, SE 500/28. On relatively *T1* weighted image, myometrium (arrows) has signal intensity similar to that of skeletal muscle (s). Fetus (f) is clearly outlined by dark amniotic fluid. Placenta (P). *B*, SE 1500/56. With more *T2* weighting, myometrium (arrows) has signal intensity greater than that of skeletal muscles (s). Fetus is obscured owing to motion and increased signal intensity of surrounding amniotic fluid.

may be obscured by the fetus, unusual size or location, or technical limitations. With MRI, leiomyomas are clearly visible in both the gravid and the nongravid uterus (Fig. 35–3).[11–13] Nondegenerated leiomyomas have a characteristic appearance. They are round and well circumscribed and have homogeneous low signal intensity, particularly with *T2* weighting. Degeneration within a leiomyoma cannot be reliably distinguished from sarcomatous changes at this time. MRI is probably more accurate than ultrasound for precise localization and sizing of leiomyomas. The detection of a large leiomyoma or one that impinges on the birth canal may influence the timing and mode of delivery.

In the early stages of gestation, the high signal intensity endometrium and low-intensity "junctional zone" are occasionally visible, just as in the nongravid uterus. Later, these zones are no longer appreciable.

As with ultrasound, the placenta is first seen as a focal thickening along the periphery of the gestational sac between 8 and 12 weeks (Fig. 35–4). As pregnancy pro-

Figure 35–3. Fourteen-week gestation. SE 2000/30. Nondegenerated leiomyoma (L) appears as a well-circumscribed, homogeneous, low-intensity mass. Degenerated leiomyoma (arrow) contains high signal intensity areas. Gestational sac (g).

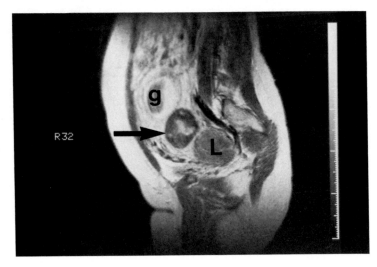

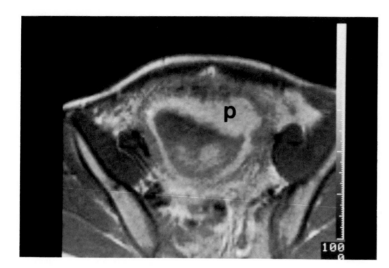

Figure 35–4. SE 2000/30. In 11-week gestation, placenta (p) is seen as a focal thickening along periphery of gestational sac.

gresses, the placenta grows and thickens.[14] On *T1* weighted images, it has a signal intensity similar to or slightly greater than myometrium (see Figs. 35–1 and 35–2). With *T2* weighting, the relative signal intensity increases substantially, a reflection of a relatively long *T2*. The placenta usually has a homogeneous appearance, and the internal architecture (i.e., chorionic plate, cotyledons, and decidua basalis) has not been appreciated with MRI. Not infrequently, vascular channels (presumably the spiral arterioles and endometrial veins that compose the subplacental complex) are visible at the placental-myometrial junction after the first trimester. Of course, physiologic placental calcifications are not visible with MRI.

The location of the placenta is readily assessable, and its relationship to the internal cervical os is clearly depicted on sagittal images.[15] Thus, MRI may be useful for distinguishing between marginal and complete placenta previa when ultrasound assessment is limited (Fig. 35–5). MRI may also prove useful for the diagnosis of abruptio placentae.

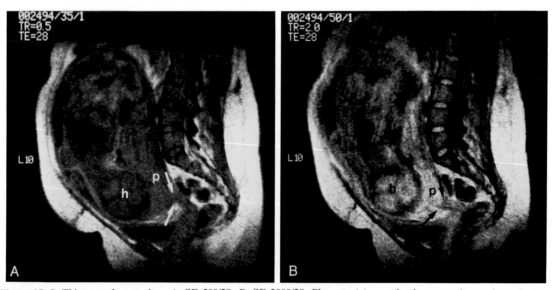

Figure 35–5. Thirty-week gestation. *A*, SE 500/28. *B*, SE 2000/28. Placenta (p) completely covers internal cervical os (arrows). Diagnosis of placenta previa was confirmed at delivery. Fetal head (h).

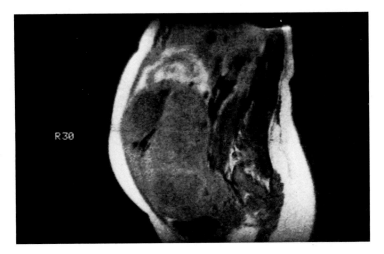

Figure 35–6. SE 500/28. Twenty-three week gestation with oligohydramnios, fetal ascites, and fetal bradycardia. Placenta is enlarged and inhomogeneous. Stillborn fetus was delivered by cesarean section, and an edematous placenta was confirmed.

Abnormal thickening or thinning of the placenta may be appreciated with MRI and may indicate the presence of a wide spectrum of pathologic processes, including nonimmune hydrops, gestational diabetes mellitus, and intrauterine growth retardation (IUGR). Occasionally, abnormal inhomogeneities are seen in the placenta in association with these conditions (Figs. 35–6 and 35–7).

Knop et al. have used nontoxic intravenous doses of $MnSo_4$ and $MnCl_2$ to enhance the placenta in monkeys.[16] This approach might provide information about regional differences in placental perfusion and metabolism.

Placental masses may be seen with MRI. An infarcted hemangioma (chorioangioma) appeared as a round mass on the fetal side of the placenta. Its signal intensity was greater than surrounding placenta on relatively *T1* and *T2* weighted images (Fig. 35–8).[13] It is not yet known whether the MRI appearance of a placental hemangioma is characteristic, as are hepatic hemangiomas.

There have also been several reports of molar pregnancies visualized on MRI.[17,18] The vesicular nature of the moles was depicted, and there was a clear separation between molar tissue and uterine wall (Fig. 35–9). These preliminary reports raise the possibility of detecting invasive gestational trophoblastic disease (chorioadenoma destruens) with MRI.

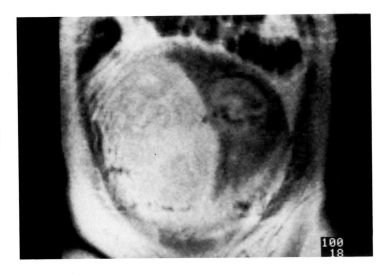

Figure 35–7. Twenty-four week gestation with Rh isoimmunization. SE 1500/28. Placenta is bulky and inhomogeneous.

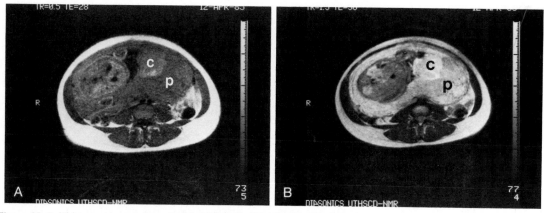

Figure 35–8. Thirty-week gestation. *A*, SE 500/28. *B*, SE 1500/56. Chorioangioma (c) has signal intensity greater than adjacent placenta (p). (From Weinreb JC, et al: Radiology *154*:717, 1986. Used by permission.)

Cervix

The positions of the internal and external cervical os are apparent on sagittal MR images. The relationship of the cervix to the placenta, lower uterine segment, and presenting fetal parts superiorly and the vagina inferiorly is apparent on these images. As with ultrasound, the length and orientation of the cervix depend on the degree of bladder filling. Unlike ultrasound, the degree of bladder distention has no effect on the ability to visualize the cervix.[9] The three cervical zones that are routinely imaged in a nonpregnant patient are also seen in pregnancy, particularly on *T2* weighted images (Fig. 35–10). The middle zone demonstrates low signal with *T1* and *T2* weighting, probably reflecting the high collagen content of cervical stroma. The central zone, which represents cervical mucus and glandular tissue, has high signal on *T1* and *T2* weighted images, reflecting its relatively short *T1* and long *T2* relaxation times. A third outer zone is variably visible. During the latter part of pregnancy, the cervix softens and begins to efface and dilate. This "ripening" process is reflected in a shortening

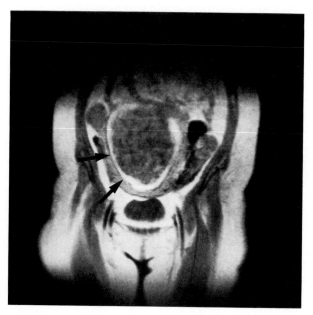

Figure 35–9. SE 1000/28. Hydatidiform mole at 18 weeks. The vesicular molar tissue is surrounded by high-intensity hemorrhagic material (arrows). There is a clear separation between molar tissue and the uterine wall.

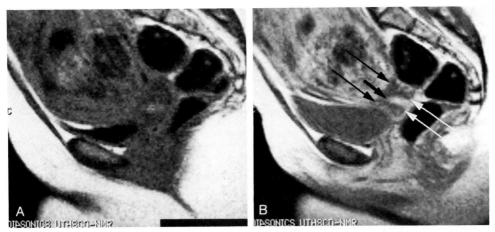

Figure 35–10. Twenty-eight week gestation. *A*, SE 500/28. *B*, 1500/28. Three cervical zones are discernible on the more *T*2 weighted image (*B*). Intermediate-intensity outer zone (long black arrows) represents muscle. Low-intensity middle zone (long white arrows) represents stroma. High-intensity central zone (short black arrow) represents mucus and glandular tissue.

and widening of the cervical lumen on MR images and is associated with a loosening of collagen fibrils within the cervix caused by increases in proteoglycan content and hydration.[9] With more experience, the ability to observe physiologic changes in the cervix may become useful to predict the outcome of induced labor and to evaluate abnormalities of cervical function, such as slow cervimetric progress, dystocia, and incompetence.

Adnexa

The normal ovaries are not routinely visible with MRI in the pregnant patient. However, normal physiologic cysts (e.g., corpus luteum) may be visible if they are not too small and if their signal characteristics permit them to be differentiated from other pelvic structures.

The discovery of an adnexal mass in a pregnant patient presents a difficult dilemma to the clinician. The size, origin, and etiology of the mass as well as the stage of gestation are all taken into account in order to arrive at the appropriate therapeutic approach. The obstetrician is reluctant to expose the fetus to ionizing radiation for diagnostic purposes. Thus, ultrasound has been widely used in this situation. Sonolucent adnexal masses are usually corpus luteum cysts, and conservative management is indicated. However, echogenic masses coexistent with pregnancy may represent a variety of benign and malignant conditions.[19] Furthermore, in the presence of a gravid uterus, overlying bowel gas, or obesity, an adnexal mass may be difficult to detect or evaluate with ultrasound. MR may be useful as a secondary imaging modality in this situation. A nonhemorrhagic corpus luteum cyst or other physiologic cyst can be differentiated from endometriomas, solid tumors, and hemorrhagic cysts.[12,13] Typically, corpus luteum cysts are rounded, smooth-walled structures with long relaxation times similar to "simple" fluid (Fig. 35–11). An increase in the size of these cysts as pregnancy progresses supports the diagnosis of a corpus luteum cyst, since the natural history of such cysts is to enlarge during the first trimester before diminishing.[20] Occasionally, they persist into the later stages of pregnancy and may attain huge proportions—so-called giant corpus luteum cysts (Fig. 35–12). Nevertheless, they will still maintain their typical MRI appearance. This knowledge may help the obstetrician select the

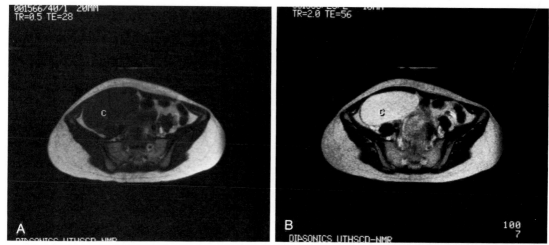

Figure 35–11. Fourteen-week gestation. *A*, SE 500/28. *B*, SE 2000/56. Corpus luteal cyst (c) is rounded, has smooth thin wall, and has signal characteristics similar to these of simple fluid. (From Weinreb JC, et al: Radiology *154*:717, 1986. Used by permission.)

appropriate therapy, as other adnexal masses (with the possible exceptions of serous cystadenomas or adenocarcinomas) are unlikely to have this appearance.

Other Structures

Within the extrauterine pelvic soft tissues, numerous dilated venous channels, including ovarian veins, are seen (Fig. 35–13). This appearance reflects normal physiologic changes as well as dilated collaterals due to impeded venous return via the inferior vena cava (which is compressed by the gravid uterus with the patient in the supine position).

MRI clearly depicts soft tissue and bony landmarks in the pelvis. Thus, sagittal and transaxial MR images can be used to accurately measure maternal pelvic dimensions, obtaining traditional pelvimetric measurements without employing ionizing radiation (Fig. 35–14).[17,21] This capability may be helpful in the evaluation of soft tissue dystocia and obstructed labor.

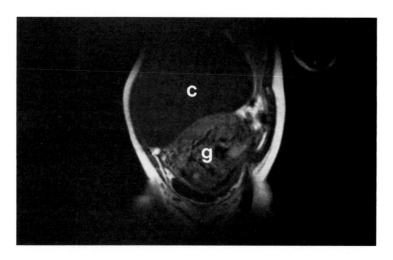

Figure 35–12. SE 500/28. "Giant" corpus luteal cyst (c) and 27-week gestation (g).

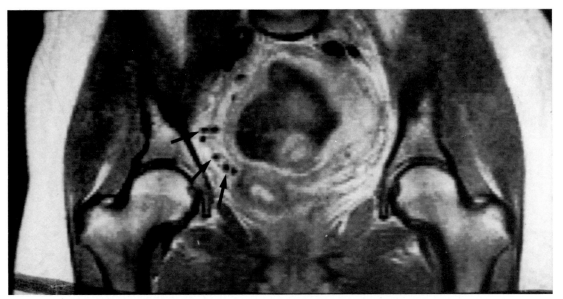

Figure 35–13. Thirteen-week gestation. SE 500/28. Numerous dilated venous channels (arrows) in the pelvic soft tissues reflect normal physiologic changes. (From Weinreb JC, et al: Radiology *157*:715, 1985. Used by permission.)

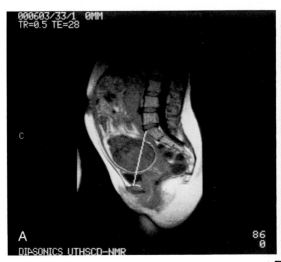

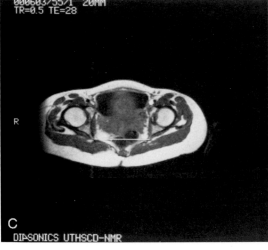

Figure 35–14. SE 500/28. Pelvimetry by MRI in 31-week gestation. Fetus is in vertex presentation. *A*, Anteroposterior pelvic inlet diameter is measured from symphysis pubis to sacral promontory on midline sagittal image. *B*, Transverse pelvic inlet diameter is measured at widest point. *C*, Transverse midpelvis diameter is the distance between ischial spines.

THE FETUS

Accurate diagnosis of suspected fetal anomalies is crucial, since some defects may be amenable to in utero correction whereas others may suggest the possibility of early delivery or pregnancy termination by abortion. Sonography has revolutionized the prenatal diagnosis of fetal anomalies. However, an alternative prenatal technique to improve diagnostic accuracy may be important when (1) the sonographic abnormality is definite but the diagnosis is uncertain; (2) the sonographic abnormality is questionable; and (3) the ultrasound study is limited owing to technical factors. Amniocentesis, amniography, and fetoscopy may be useful, but they are invasive and cannot diagnose all structural malformations. CT has occasionally aided in in utero diagnosis,[22-24] but its utility in this context has been severely limited because it utilizes ionizing radiation, has relatively poor soft tissue contrast resolution, and provides images in only one plane. MRI suffers from none of these limitations. Thus, it could potentially become a secondary noninvasive imaging modality for the evaluation of the fetus.

The first steps toward evaluating the use of MRI for fetal diagnosis have been to determine the optimal MR imaging techniques and those structures that can be depicted with current MR imaging systems.

The appropriate pulse sequences and planes for fetal imaging have not been well established and will depend to a certain extent upon the reasons for the evaluation. Both *T1* and *T2* weighted spin-echo sequences offer advantages for fetal imaging.[25] Compared with longer *TR*'s, images obtained with relatively short *TR*'s may result in less image degradation from fetal motion because of the relatively decreased time the motion can occur while the image is being produced (Fig. 35–15). *T1* weighting offers the additional advantage of producing pictures in which the fetus is clearly outlined, owing to natural contrast between the dark amniotic fluid and high-intensity fetal fat. On the other hand, *T2* weighting may improve delineation of the brain and lung (Figs. 35–16 and 35–17). Spin-echo techniques with longer repetition times also allow acquisition of a large number of anatomic sections so that the entire fetus can be observed in a single imaging sequence. Little information is available about the utility of inversion recovery sequences in this context.

Not surprisingly, preliminary investigations indicate that fetal anatomy is better delineated as gestational age increases. However, even in advanced stages of gestation, many fetal structures have not been routinely imaged.[25] There are several reasons for

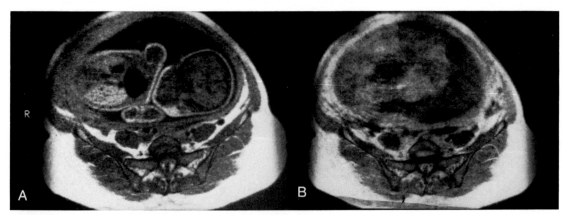

Figure 35–15. Thirty-five week gestation. *A*, SE 500/28. *T1* weighted image with relatively short *TR* shows good fetal anatomic detail. *B*, SE 1500/28. With longer *TR* (and longer imaging time), fetal anatomic detail is degraded by fetal motion. (From Weinreb JC, et al: Radiology *157*:715, 1985. Used by permission.)

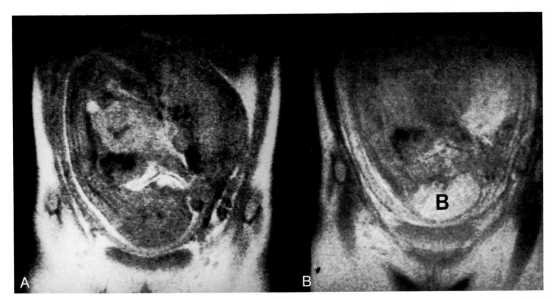

Figure 35–16. Thirty-one week gestation with oligohydramnios and minimal fetal motion. *A*, SE 500/28. *B*, SE 1500/56. The fetal brain (B) is better delineated on the more *T2* weighted image. (From Weinreb JC, et al: Radiology *157*:715, 1985. Used by permission.)

these results:

1. Fetal motion is a major culprit and causes image unsharpness and "ghosts" in the phase-encoding direction.

2. Although McCarthy et al.[15] have stated that normal fetal anatomy is seen best on sagittal images of the maternal pelvis, the ability to visualize only in planes that are parallel or perpendicular to the maternal long axis may be inadequate for in utero imaging. Fetal position may not be aligned with any of the maternal axes, and it may be difficult to mentally reconstruct the anatomy from nonorthogonal cross sections. The ability to image in any desired axis as one does with ultrasound will be helpful.

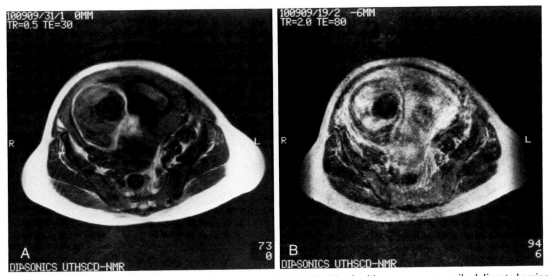

Figure 35–17. Thirty-two week gestation. *A*, SE 500/30. *B*, SE 2000/80. The fetal lungs are more easily delineated owing to a relative increase in signal intensity on the more *T2* weighted image. The low-intensity structure surrounded by fluid-filled lungs is the heart.

3. Many fetal structures are extremely small and may not attain a size that is within the spatial resolution limits of current MRI systems.

4. Contrast differences between adjacent but dissimilar tissues may not be large enough to permit discrimination with MRI in the fetus.

In spite of all these limitations, many fetal structures become routinely visible in the third trimester, and, occasionally, fetal anatomy is exquisitely displayed.

Central Nervous System

The fetal head has been discernible after the twentieth week of gestation in almost every instance. After the twenty-fifth week, much of the architecture of the head can be seen, especially the cerebral hemispheres, the ventricles, and the eyes (Fig. 35–18). The posterior fossa–cerebellum, midbrain, brainstem–craniocervical junction, and cisterna have been depicted less frequently.[25]

Gray/white matter differentiation has not been observed in the fetal brain in utero. This is not surprising, as most myelination occurs during the first year of life. It appears that the fetal brain has a longer *T1* relaxation time than the mature brain, possibly owing to a greater water and lower protein content.[15] The fetal brain also has a relatively prolonged *T2* relaxation time and thus demonstrates a relative increase in signal intensity on *T2* weighted images.[25]

Several fetal cerebral abnormalities have been imaged with MRI, including anencephaly, hydrocephalus, holoprosencephaly, Dandy-Walker cyst, and autolysis (Figs.

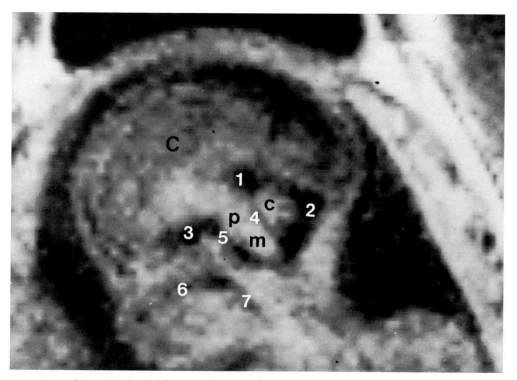

Figure 35–18. SE 500/28. Sagittal fetal head at 28 weeks. Cerebrum (C), cerebellum (c), pons (p), medulla (m), superior cerebellar cistern (1), cisterna magna (2), suprasellar cistern (3), fourth ventricle (4), prepontine cistern (5), nasopharynx (6), oropharynx (7). (From Weinreb JC, et al: Radiology *157*:715, 1985. Used by permission.)

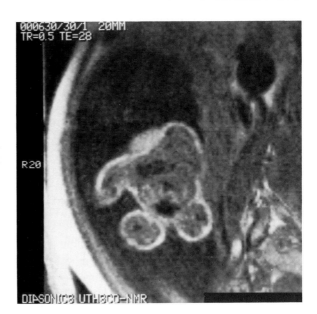

Figure 35–19. SE 500/28. Polyhydramnios and anencephaly in 29-week gestation. (From Weinreb JC, et al: Radiology *154*:157, 1985. Used by permission.)

35–19 and 35–20).[17,26,27] These preliminary results suggest that MRI may have a role in the evaluation of the fetal brain.

Some portion of the vertebral column and spinal cord is usually visible (Fig. 35–21), but it is unlikely that such fragmented bits of information would be of much clinical value.[25] Occasionally, the entire spine can be seen on a single sagittal image of the fetus (Fig. 35–22).

Cardiovascular System

The fetal heart has been visible after 15 weeks and is always seen after 25 weeks (Figs. 35–17 and 35–23).[25] This is unquestionably due to the contrast with surrounding tissues provided by the flow-void phenomenon caused by flowing blood within the

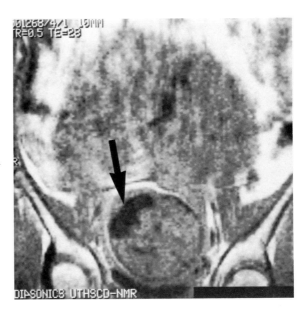

Figure 35–20. SE 500/28. Thirty-five week gestation. Symmetric low-intensity region (arrow) in posterior fossa of fetal head represents a Dandy-Walker cyst.

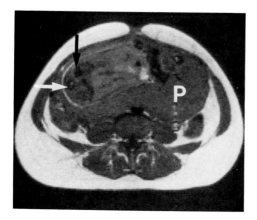

Figure 35–21. SE 500/28. Thirty-week gestation with Potter syndrome oligohydramnios. Transaxial section through fetal body shows fetal spine (white arrow). Low-intensity structure (black arrow) arising from the posterior aspect of a fetal kidney could be either a renal cyst or a dilated calyx. Placenta (P). (From Weinreb JC, et al: Radiology *154:*157, 1985. Used by permission.)

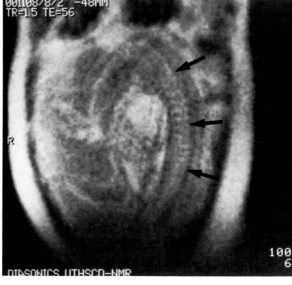

Figure 35–22. SE 1500/56. Thirty-one week fetus in vertex presentation. Almost entire spinal column (arrows) is visible on a single sagittal image.

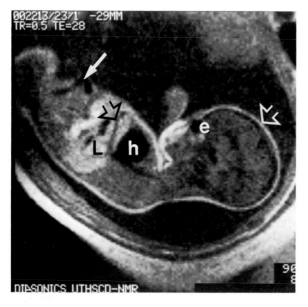

Figure 35–23. SE 500/28. Thirty-four week fetus. Heart (h), eye (e), liver (L), intrahepatic vessels (open black arrow), umbilical vessels (white arrow), and subcutaneous fat (open white arrow). (From Weinreb JC, et al: Radiology *157:*715, 1985. Used by permission.)

heart. Frequently, the interventricular septum is discernible, although the four chambers have only occasionally been resolved. The ability to depict discrete fetal cardiac chambers without ECG gating is probably due to the very small excursions of the cardiac wall when the heart rate is rapid, as in a normal fetus.[28] Major vascular structures, such as the aorta, inferior vena cava, and pulmonary vessels, have only occasionally been visible despite the flow-void phenomenon, probably secondary to their small size (Fig. 35–24).[25]

Lungs

The fluid-filled lungs are often visible and are contrasted with the vascular structures centrally and the liver inferiorly (see Fig. 35–17). Pulmonary tissue demonstrates low signal with $T1$ weighting and an increased signal intensity with increased $T2$ weighting, indicating relatively prolonged $T1$ and $T2$ relaxation times.[15] This is typical of tissues with large amounts of "simple" fluid.

Fetal lung maturation begins around 24 weeks with the production of surfactant.[28] Like other lipid-containing materials, surfactant may alter the relaxation characteristics of fetal lung water. It is possible that the MR characteristics of fetal lung may provide clues to lung maturity. This possibility has not yet been thoroughly researched. Since the decision to deliver a fetus often depends on pulmonary maturity, the availability of an accurate noninvasive test of fetal pulmonary maturity would be of tremendous clinical utility.

Liver and Spleen

The liver is almost always visible in the last trimester of gestation and occupies most of the upper abdomen (Fig. 35–25).[25] Early in gestation, the liver is difficult to identify not only because of its size but also perhaps because the cellular composition of the liver is different in the young fetus. Initially, the liver is primarily an erythropoietic organ, and at midgestation a large part consists of hematopoietic cells. Later,

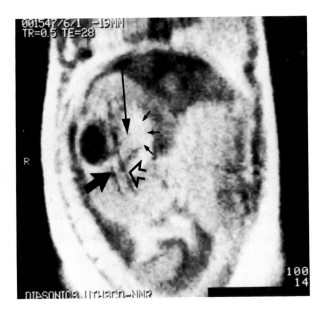

Figure 25–24. SE 1000/28. Coronal image of 28-week fetus shows inferior vena cava (closed arrow), aorta (open arrow), left renal artery (long arrow), and left kidney (small arrows). Low-intensity structure in right renal fossa represents fluid-filled obstructed right kidney. (From Weinreb JC, et al: Radiology *157*:715, 1985. Used by permission.)

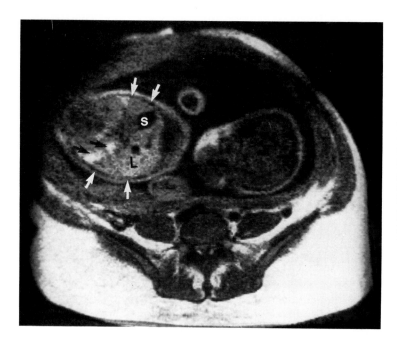

Figure 35–25. Thirty-four week gestation. SE 500/28. Coronal image through fetal body demonstrates liver (L), fluid-filled stomach (s), high signal intensity areas in abdomen (black arrows), and low-intensity muscle (white arrows) internal to high-intensity subcutaneous fat. (From Weinreb JC, et al: Radiology *157*:715, 1985. Used by permission.)

the erythropoietic function decreases markedly. By term, the proportion is less than 2 percent of the total cell population. Similarly, the chemical composition of the hepatocytes changes with gestational age. Glycogen stores are low early in gestation and accumulate toward term.[30] Measurements of liver *T1* show a steady decline throughout gestation,[31] and thus the liver demonstrates a relative increase in signal intensity as pregnancy progresses. In some cases, the hepatic venous anatomy is apparent (see Fig. 35–23).[25] Therefore, the fetal liver may also be an organ that is amenable to in utero analysis with MR techniques. The fetal spleen has not yet been assessed with MRI.

Gastrointestinal Tract

The fluid-containing stomach is sometimes seen as a low-intensity structure in the fetal left upper quadrant on *T1* weighted images (Fig. 35–25). Discrete loops of bowel are not usually discerned (see under Musculoskeletal System).

Kidneys

The fetal kidneys have rarely been identified, even late in gestation. This is probably due to the relative paucity of surrounding contrasting fat. However, fetal renal cysts and hydronephrosis may be visible (see Figs. 35–21 and 35–24).[27] If the fetal bladder is distended with urine, it is seen as a low-intensity pelvic structure on relatively *T1* weighted images (Fig. 35–26) and increases in signal intensity with more *T2* weighting.[15]

Musculoskeletal System

After 26 weeks, both upper and lower extremities can be seen (at least in part) in most fetuses (Fig. 35–26).[25] On *T1* weighed images, muscle demonstrates low signal

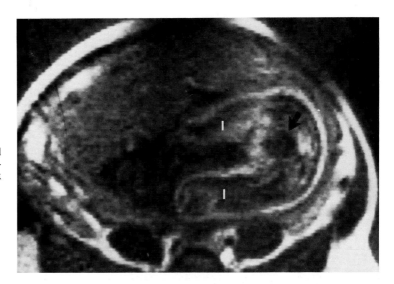

Figure 35–26. SE 500/28. Urine-filled fetal bladder (arrow) and lower extremities (l) are pictured in 36-week fetus.

intensity (relatively long *T1* and short *T2*) in contrast with subcutaneous high-intensity fat (short *T1*, intermediate *T2*) (Fig. 35–27). Definition of individual muscle groups is usually precluded by motion and absence of tissue fat planes. As in the adult, cortical bone exhibits low signal intensity, whereas cancellous bone demonstrates a moderate to high signal intensity. Epiphyseal cartilage is occasionally visible and has medium signal intensity.[15]

High-intensity subcutaneous fat is usually not visible in the first and middle trimesters (Fig. 35–28).[25] This finding is consistent with the fact that subcutaneous fat storage commences at around 27 weeks.[32] In the last trimester, relatively *T1* weighted spin-echo pulse sequences permit clear discrimination between high-intensity subcutaneous fat and adjacent low-intensity amniotic fluid and skeletal muscle (see Figs. 35–23 and 35–25). It has been suggested that quantitation of subcutaneous scalp and facial fat may be a means of diagnosing IUGR,[33] but this may prove to be very difficult in practice. IUGR increases perinatal morbidity and mortality and is associated with long-term

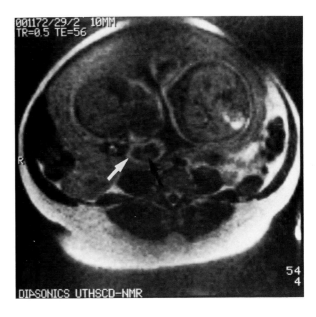

Figure 35–27. Thirty-nine week fetus. SE 500/28. Cross section of upper extremity shows low-intensity muscle surrounded by high-intensity muscle surrounded by high-intensity fat (black arrow). Cancellous bone (white arrow) demonstrates intermediate signal.

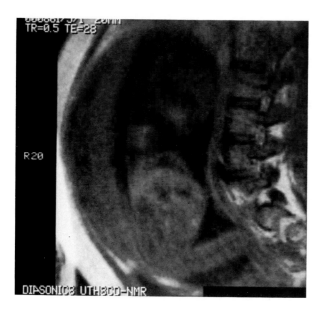

Figure 35–28. SE 500/28. Normal 24-week fetus has no discernible high-intensity subcutaneous fat.

neurologic impairment. Sonography has been the best test for diagnosis of IUGR in utero; however, overdiagnosis is common, and there is no reliable method for distinguishing IUGR fetuses from normal fetuses. At best, the diagnosis of IUGR is based upon fetal weight, birth weight and size, and physical evidence of soft tissue wasting. Thus, reduced soft tissue mass may be an early pathogenic factor in IUGR.[34] One study has demonstrated good correlation between birth weight and fetal subcutaneous fat thickness in normal fetuses and those of diabetic mothers.[31] There is another finding on MR images that may to be related to fat storage.[25] After the thirtieth week, multiple 3 to 10 mm high signal intensity areas appear in the fetal abdomen and pelvis on both *T1* and *T2* weighted spin-echo images (see Fig. 35–25). The origin of these high signal intensity areas is not yet known, but their appearance late in pregnancy and their similarity to fat may indicate the accumulation of adipose tissue in the fetal abdomen. If so, they may be useful as additional evidence for the in utero diagnosis of IUGR. Another possibility is that these areas represent normal gastrointestinal tract accumulations of mucin-containing meconium.

A thin, low-intensity rim is visible surrounding the fetal abdomen but internal to subcutaneous fat on both *T1* and *T2* weighted images in many last-trimester fetuses (Figs. 35–25 and 35–29). This region probably represents muscle (relatively long *T1* and short *T2*) and should not be confused with ascites (long *T1* and *T2*) (Fig. 35–30).[25]

Amniotic Fluid

Amniotic fluid has long relaxation times similar to other "simple" biologic fluids. Therefore, on *T1* weighted images, the extremely low signal intensity fluid can act as a natural contrast agent to outline the fetus and placenta.[15,25,35] With more *T2* weighting, amniotic fluid and placenta demonstrate increases in signal intensity, and it becomes more difficult to separate them from the fetus. We have not noted any changes in the appearance of amniotic fluid during pregnancy other than normal physiologic changes in quantity.

Since the low-intensity amniotic fluid contrasts with the fetus and placenta on *T1* weighted images, the quantity of amniotic fluid can be assessed in a manner similar to

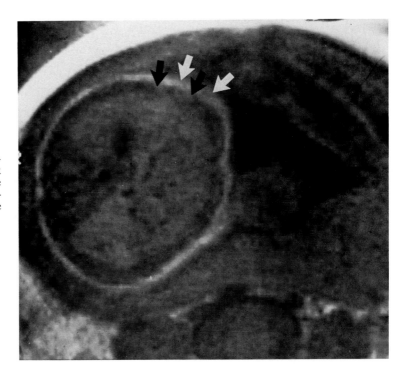

Figure 35–29. SE 500/28. Transaxial image through liver in 35-week fetus shows low-intensity muscle (black arrows) internal to high-intensity subcutaneous fat (white arrows).

ultrasound. Oligohydramnios and polyhydramnios are readily apparent (Fig. 35–31). Qualitative assessment of amniotic fluid, including in vivo measurement of *T1* and *T2* relaxation times, has not proved useful at this time.

Amniotic fluid can be considered an extension of fetal extracellular fluid in the first half of gestation. Later, it reflects fetal renal function. Thus, spectroscopic evaluation of amniotic fluid may provide clues to fetal status. Using high-resolution proton NMR spectroscopy, a number of physiologically relevant compounds have been observed in amniotic fluid obtained via amniocentesis. Some of these compounds have been implicated in fetal distress. For example, estimates of meconium concentration

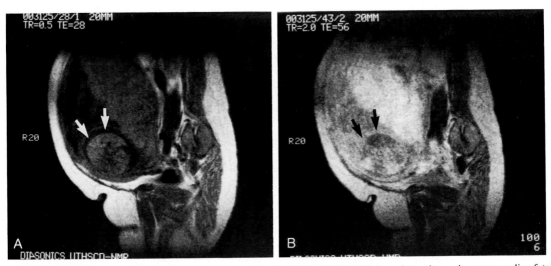

Figure 35–30. Twenty-nine week fetus with ascites. *A*, SE 500/28. *B*, SE 2000/56. Low-intensity ascites surrounding fetal abdomen (arrows) on relatively *T1* weighted image (*A*) demonstrates a relative increase in intensity with *T2* weighting (*B*).

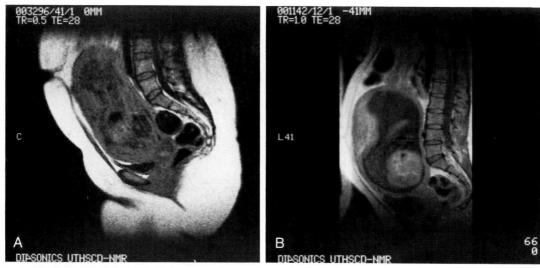

Figure 35–31. *A*, SE 500/28. Twenty-eight week gestation with oligohydramnios due to fetal renal dysplasia. *B*, SE 1000/28. Twenty-seven week gestation with polyhydramnios.

obtained from measured *T2* values may be useful as an indication of fetal distress.[36,37] Other measured compounds have been related to CNS disorders and fetal acidosis.[38] Thus, this technique offers the potential for useful in vivo analysis of amniotic fluid.

In conclusion it is unlikely that MRI will replace ultrasound as the primary obstetric imaging modality in the near future.[39] Ultrasound has a proven record of accuracy and safety in addition to its easy access, low cost, and real-time capability. At its present state of development, MR imaging of many fetal structures is often unsatisfactory and probably of limited value, particularly in the first two trimesters. Nevertheless, MRI may ultimately prove useful in obstetric diagnosis because it is not invasive, involves no ionizing radiation, and can provide images with excellent soft tissue contrast in multiple orthogonal planes. Unlike ultrasound, interference by skeletal, fatty, or gas-filled maternal structures is not a problem with MRI. Moreover, the use of tissue characteristics other than acoustic impedance may bring out anatomic and pathologic features not detectable with ultrasound.

Preliminary experience indicates that MRI may have a future role in the following obstetric scenarios:

1. Providing crucial information in pregnant patients with medical or surgical conditions that would ordinarily require ionizing radiation for diagnosis.

2. Providing important data about fetal anomalies, growth, and development when sonographic evaluation is equivocal or limited by oligohydramnios or maternal obesity.

3. Demonstrating maternal pelvic structures when ultrasound is unsuccessful owing to overlying bowel gas or obesity.

4. Obtaining pelvimetry without x-rays.

5. Estimating meconium concentration in amniotic fluid in vivo.

6. Diagnosing intrauterine growth retardation.

7. Confirming placenta previa in equivocal ultrasound cases.

8. Assessing fetal lung maturity.

9. Investigating placental insufficiency.

10. Evaluating abnormalities of cervical function, such as slow cervimetric progress, failure of ripening, dystocia, incompetence, and response to drugs.

More experience and improved imaging and spectroscopic capabilities are necessary before the potential benefits of obstetric MRI can be reasonably weighed against the potential risks.

References

1. Harvey EB, Boice JD, Honeyman M, Flannery JT: Prenatal x-ray exposure and childhood cancer in twins. N Engl J Med *312*:541, 1985.
2. Budinger TF: Nuclear magnetic resonance (NMR) in vivo studies: known thresholds for health effects. J Comput Assist Tomogr 5(6):800, 1981.
3. Schwartz JL, Crooks LE: NMR imaging produces no observable mutations or cytotoxicity in mammalian cells. AJR *139*:583, 1982.
4. Geard CR, Osmak RS, Hall EJ, Simon HE, Maudsley AA, Hilal SK: Magnetic resonance and ionizing radiation: a comparative evaluation in vitro of oncogenic and genotoxic potential. Radiology *152*:199, 1984.
5. Wolff S, James TL, Young GB, Margulis AR, Bodycote J, Afzal V: Magnetic resonance imaging: absence of in vitro cytogenetic damage. Radiology *155*:163, 1985.
6. Advice on acceptable limits of exposure to nuclear magnetic resonance clinical imaging. Radiography *50*:220, 1984.
7. Hricak H, Alpers C, Crooks LE, Sheldon PE: Magnetic resonance imaging of the female pelvis: initial experience. AJR *141*:1119, 1983.
8. Harkness MLR, Harkness RD: The collagen content of the reproductive tract of the rat during pregnancy and lactation. J Physiol *123*:492, 1954.
9. McCarthy SN, Stark DD, Filly RA, Callen PW, Hricak H, Higgins CB: Obstetrical magnetic resonance imaging: maternal anatomy. Radiology *154*:421, 1985.
10. Gross BH, Silver TM, Jaffe MH: Sonographic features of uterine leiomyomas: analysis of 41 proven cases. J Ultrasound Med 2:401, 1983.
11. Hamlin DJ, Pettersson H, Fitzsimmons J, Morgan LS: MR imaging of uterine leiomyomas and their complications. J Comput Assist Tomogr 9(5):902, 1985.
12. Hricak H, Lacey C, Shriock E: Gynecologic masses: value of magnetic resonance imaging. Am J Obstet Gynecol *153*(1):31, 1985.
13. Weinreb JC, et al: Pelvic masses in pregnant patients. MR and US imaging. Radiology *154*:717, 1986.
14. Hoddick WK, Mahony BS, Callen PW, Filly RA: Placental thickness. J Ultrasound Med 4:479, 1985.
15. McCarthy SM, Filly RA, Stark DD, et al: Obstetrical magnetic resonance imaging: fetal anatomy. Radiology *154*:427, 1985.
16. Knop RH, Mattison DR, Kay HH, et al: MR placental and fetal imaging: placental contrast enhancement following Mn^{++} infusion in primates and rats. RSNA Scientific Program, Washington, DC, November 1984.
17. Weinreb JC, Lowe TW, Santos-Ramos R, Cunningham FG, Parkey R: Magnetic resonance imaging in obstetric diagnosis. Radiology *154*:157, 1985.
18. Powell M, Buckley J, Worthington BS, Symonds EM: Case study: the features of molar pregnancy as shown by magnetic resonance imaging. Book of Abstracts for Society of Magnetic Resonance in Medicine, Fourth Annual Meeting, London, August 1985, p 241.
19. Pennes DR, Bowerman RA, Silver TM: Echogenic adnexal masses associated with first trimester pregnancy: sonographic appearance and clinical significance. J Clin Ultrasound *13*:391, 1985.
20. Miller EI, Thoms RH, Applegate JW: Persistent corpus luteum cyst of pregnancy. Sonographic evaluation of cause of third trimester bleeding. J Clin Ultrasound 6:187, 1978.
21. Stark DD, McCarthy SM, Filly RA, Parer JT, Hricak H, Callen PW: Pelvimetry by magnetic resonance imaging. AJR *144*:947, 1985.
22. Magarik DE, Dunne MG, Weksberg AP: CT appearance of intrauterine pregnancy. J Comput Assist Tomogr 8(3):469, 1984.
23. Lee LL, McGahan JP: Case report: combined use of ultrasound and computed tomography in evaluation of intraabdominal pregnancy and fetal demise. J Comput Assist Tomogr 8(4):770, 1984.
24. Siegel HA, Seltzer SE, Miller S: Prenatal computed tomography: are there indications? J Comput Assist Tomogr 8(5):871, 1984.
25. Weinreb JC, Lowe T, Cohen JM, Kutler M: Human fetal anatomy: MR imaging. Radiology *157*:715, 1985.
26. Thickman D, Mintz M, Mennuti M, Kressel HY: MR imaging of cerebral abnormalities in utero. J Comput Assist Tomogr 8(6):1058, 1984.
27. McCarthy SM, Filly RA, Stark DD, Callen EW, Golbus MS, Hricak H: Magnetic resonance imaging of fetal anomalies in utero: early experience. AJR *145*:677, 1985.
28. McCarthy S, Stark DD, Higgins CB: Case report: demonstration of the fetal cardiovascular system by MR imaging. J Comput Assist Tomogr 8(6):1168, 1984.
29. Possmayer F: The perinatal lung. *In* Jones C (ed): The Biochemical Development of the Fetus and Neonate. Amsterdam; Elsevier Biomedical Press, 1982, pp 287–328.
30. Jones C: The development of metabolism in the fetal liver. *In* Jones C (ed): The Biochemical Development of the Fetus and Neonate. Amsterdam, Elsevier Biomedical Press, 1982, pp 249–277.

31. Smith FW: Magnetic resonance imaging of human pregnancy. Book of Abstracts for Society of Magnetic Resonance in Medicine, Fourth Annual Meeting, London, August 1985, pp 214–215.
32. England MA: Color Atlas of Life Before Birth: Normal Fetal Development. Chicago, Year Book Medical Publishers, 1983.
33. Stark DD, McCarthy SM, Filly RA, Callen PW, Hricak H, Parer JT: Intrauterine growth retardation: evaluation by magnetic resonance. Radiology *155*:425, 1985.
34. Deter RL, Hadlock FP, Harrist RB: Evaluation of normal fetal growth and the detection of intrauterine growth retardation. *In* Callen PW (ed): Ultrasonography in Obstetrical Gynecology. Philadelphia, WB Saunders, 1982, pp 113–140.
35. Foster MA, Knight CH, Rimmington JE, Mallard JR: Fetal imaging by nuclear magnetic resonance: a study in goats. Radiology *149*:193, 1983.
36. Borcard B, Hiltbrand E, Magnin P, et al: Estimating meconium (fetal feces) concentration in human amniotic fluid by nuclear magnetic resonance. Physiol Chem Phys *14*:189, 1982.
37. Bene GJ: The NMR proton relaxation in biological fluids: a good way to identify precisely healthy or pathological states. 1st Ann Symp, Sanita. *19*(1):121, 1983.
38. Gillies RJ, Powell DA, Nelson TR, Shrader M, Manchester D, Henry GM: High resolution proton NMR spectroscopy of human amniotic fluid. Book of Abstracts for Society of Magnetic Resonance in Medicine, Fourth Annual Meeting, London, August 1985, pp 789–790.
39. Lowe TW, Weinreb J, Santos-Ramos R, Cunningham FG: Magnetic resonance imaging in human pregnancy. Obstet Gynecol *66*(5):629, 1985.

VIII

CLINICAL EXPERIENCE: MRI OF THE VASCULAR AND MUSCULOSKELETAL SYSTEMS

36

Blood Flow in MR Imaging

RONALD R. PRICE
DAVID R. PICKENS
THEODORE H. M. FALKE

The statement is frequently made that rapidly flowing blood produces no signal in MR images. Unfortunately, this is an oversimplification, and, in fact, the MR intensity of flowing blood depends upon many factors. These include pulse sequence timing parameters (*TR/TE*), flow orientation, physiologic gating, echo number, and multislice or single-slice technique—plus the fact that the effects of all of these are interdependent.[1,2] Generally, flow effects manifest themselves in standard spin-echo sequences as changes in image signal intensity relative to stationary spins. These changes in intensity can be either an increase or a decrease in signal strength. In addition to these changes, flow-induced image displacement artifacts are frequently present.

EXAMPLES OF FLOW EFFECTS

In an ungated spin-echo image of rapid arterial blood flow, the intensity is usually decreased relative to the surrounding tissues (Fig. 36–1). In some cases, however, it has been found that arterial flow can also yield enhanced signal strength. This is demonstrated in Figure 36–2, in which coincidental synchronization between the cardiac cycle and the repetition period (*TR*) occurred, causing enhanced signal strengths in the carotid arteries. Figure 36–2 also illustrates position displacement artifacts, in which ghost images (arrow) of the carotids appear outside the body. Such displacement artifacts are always along the phase-encoding direction in 2-DFT images and result from flow interference that moves nuclei to a y-position different from its original phase-encoded position.

Even-echo enhancement is a technique that can frequently be used to assess flow in slow-flow conditions and, in particular, to assess venous flow. It refers to a phenomenon in which slow-flowing blood that flows along a linear gradient will exhibit enhanced signal strength on even-numbered echo images in a multiecho sequence. The phenomenon, which will be discussed in more detail later, is the result of variations in the ability of the 180 degree echo pulses to rephase flowing spins. Even-echo enhancement occurs primarily either in slowly flowing venous blood or in ECG-gated arterial flow, when imaging is carried out in relatively slow-flow portions of the cardiac cycle.

Figure 36–3 illustrates the even-echo enhancement effect in an image of a vascular malformation in the brain. The pulse sequence was an ungated 32–64/500 spin-echo sequence. In the first echo image (32/500) (Fig. 36–3*A*), the malformation demonstrates a reduced signal strength relative to the brain tissue on the first echo and an enhanced signal strength on the second echo (64/500) (Fig. 36–3*B*).

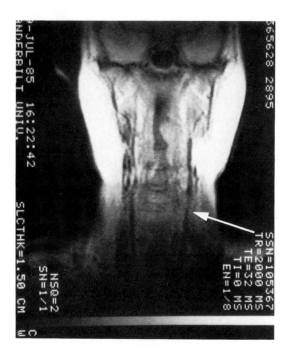

Figure 36–1. Ungated spin-echo (32/2000) coronal section image of the carotid artery (arrow), exhibiting reduced signal strength relative to surrounding tissues.

Nonflowing blood will generally exhibit an increased signal strength and will not be dependent upon echo number. A patient with an occluded right carotid artery (Fig. 36–4A) shows an increased signal in the carotid relative to the normal contralateral side. The occlusion was verified by carotid arteriography (Fig. 36–4B), which showed a complete occlusion of the carotid just distal to the bifurcation.

Complicated signal patterns related to flow are also encountered when multislice sequences are used (Fig. 36–5). Slices located at the flow entrance of the imaging volume will often exhibit enhancement for slow-flow conditions (either from venous flow or from slow arterial flow found during ECG gating). Figure 36–5A shows increased signal in the aorta when ECG gating is used and the slice is the first slice in the imaging

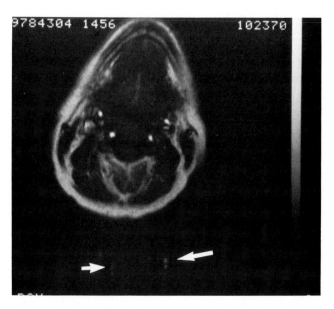

Figure 36–2. Ungated spin-echo (32/1000) transverse section image through the neck of a normal volunteer. Arteries appear enhanced in signal strength owing to coincidental synchronization with cardiac cycle. Ghost images (arrows) of the arteries appear outside the body because of interference with the phase-encoding gradient.

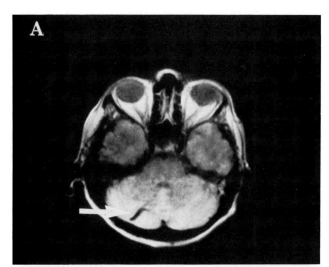

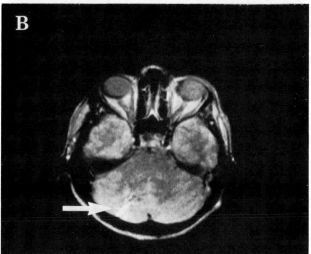

Figure 36–3. Even-echo enhancement in a two-echo (32–64/500) spin-echo sequence. *A*, Vascular anomaly appears dark on echo number one (32/500). *B*, Second echo (64/500) shows the presence of flow by its enhanced signal strength relative to the surrounding tissues.

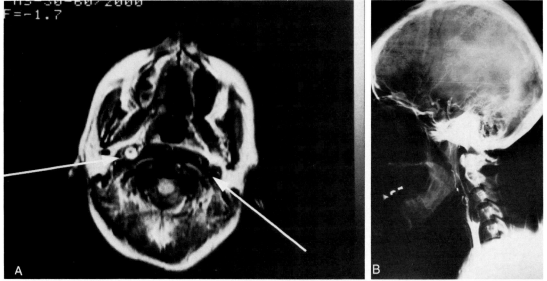

Figure 36–4. *A*, Occluded right carotid artery (left arrow) appears bright relative to the normal-flow left artery (right arrow). *B*, Carotid arteriogram shows stenosis of right carotid artery just distal to bifurcation.

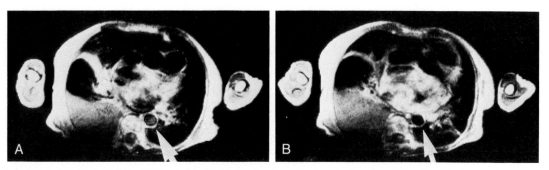

Figure 36–5. Flow effects in multislice sequences are generally related to the location of the slice relative to the entrance of the blood into the image volume. *A*, In an ECG-gated study, the first slice shows enhancement in the aorta (arrow). *B*, A lower slice shows no signal within the aorta.

volume. Figure 36–5*B* is the second slice in the multislice sequence and is located approximately 1 cm from slice number one. In the second slice the intensity in the aorta is essentially zero.

FLOW IMAGING

The study of flow artifacts has led to the investigation of a variety of different MR flow-imaging techniques, and two general approaches to MR angiography have been developed. These can be roughly categorized as "time-of-flight" and "phase-encoding" techniques. In each of these approaches, subtraction methods are used to produce an image of vascular structures similar to that of digital subtraction angiography. The images to be subtracted consist of one in which flow effects have been compensated and another in which no flow compensation was used.[3–5]

The "time-of-flight" or "washout" technique relies upon the effect of flow through a selected slice to replace the partially saturated nuclei with varying amounts of nuclei at equilibrium. The replacement rate depends directly upon the flow velocity and slice thickness. The flow replacement of nuclei in a selected slice leads to enhanced signal strength at the low velocities usually found in venous flow (Fig. 36–6) and has been

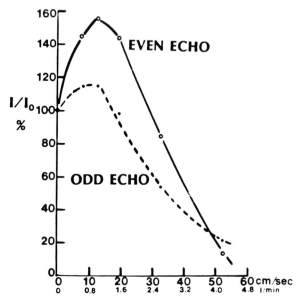

Figure 36–6. Plot of the signal strength as a fraction of the nonflowing signal strength for odd (30 ms) and even (60 ms) echoes. The sequence was a 30–60/500 spin echo. Coronal images of a continuous flow phantom and flow velocities ranging from 0–53 cm/sec were used. Note the enhancement and the unrelated phenomenon of even-echo rephasing, which causes relatively larger signals in even echoes than in odd echoes at all velocities. (The crossover of the two curves at high velocities is not considered statistically significant.)

referred to in the literature as paradoxical enhancement. This enhancement is followed by a monotonic decrease in signal with increased velocity. Fast imaging techniques utilize these effects to produce compensated and uncompensated images, in essence by producing a slow-motion or stop-action image in which a paradoxical enhancement effect is created in rapid arterial flow (see Chapter 96). ECG gating can also be used to further enhance those effects by imaging in the systolic and diastolic flow portions of the cardiac cycle. A number of investigators have reported on washout flow effects in MRI.[6-13] In addition, an excellent review of the effects of flow on MR image intensity as a function of pulse sequence has been published.[14]

Phase-encoding techniques measure phase shifts resulting from motion along a field gradient. The theoretical development of this technique along with preliminary results has been reported by Moran and others.[15-31] Flow-compensated images that correct for the flow-related phase shifts are produced by adding compensating gradients or rf pulses to conventional imaging sequences.

The two-dimensional Fourier transform (2-DFT) imaging technique used by most MRI instruments is inherently a phase-sensitive image reconstruction method that uses phase shifts (relative to a reference phase) resulting from applied field gradients to provide spatial information. Phase shifts resulting from flow along a gradient can be shown to be directly related to the velocity of motion along the gradient direction (Fig. 36–7). Pulse sequences designed specifically for flow compensation use either ''balanced'' gradient pulses or paired rf pulses to ensure that there is no net phase shift for spins that flow with a constant velocity.

In Figure 36–7 the additional balanced gradients for flow compensation are shown as dashed lines in the G_X direction. Aside from these negative gradient pulses, the imaging sequence is identical to a conventional 2-DFT imaging sequence. The phases of the transverse magnetization for spins of constant velocity (V) are shown for imaging sequences both with and without the added gradient pulses. It should be noted that, for balance, the gradient pulses should be applied in a negative sense if applied on either side of the inverting 180 degree pulse. The same effect can be achieved by applying a bipolar (both positive and negative lobes) on one side of the 180 degree pulse (Fig. 36–8). In tracing the phase angle, it is noted that the phase is inverted at each reversal of the gradients as well as being reversed following the 180 degree pulse. In the absence of the balanced gradients, the spins have gained a net phase shift (phase

Figure 36–7. Flow information is encoded into the MR image by adding to the conventional 2-DFT imaging sequence negative-gradient pulses (dashed lines) in the desired flow-sensitive direction (x). If pulses of the same polarity are used, they should be placed bracketing the 180 degree pulse. Spins with constant flow velocity will accumulate a net phase shift in the transverse magnetization ($\Delta\phi$) at the time of data sampling that is proportional to the velocity. Phase angle of zero at the time of the echo produces an enhanced signal.

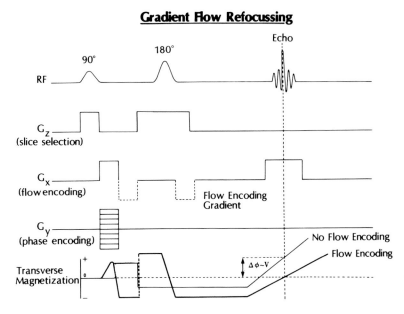

Bipolar Encoding Method

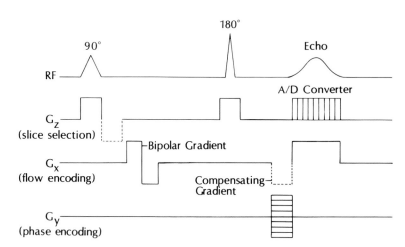

Figure 36–8. An alternative approach of balanced gradients to the method shown in Figure 36–7 is to use a bipolar pulse in the flow-encoding direction that is placed prior to the 180 degree pulse. The effect of the two methods will be identical. Additional compensating gradients (dashed lines) are added in the slice selection and read-out directions to correct for phase shifts caused by slice selection and read-out gradients. These image-compensating gradients are not purposely flow-sensitive gradients.

angle not equal to zero) at the time of the echo. The phase shift can be shown to be proportional to the velocity. The image acquired with the balanced gradients will be the flow-compensated image for the subtraction pair and will exhibit an enhanced signal. It should also be noted that flow compensation occurs for spins of constant velocities regardless of velocity magnitude.

If the flow-encoding gradient strength and time are chosen to yield a phase shift of less than 180 degrees for the highest velocity, then the phase-shift difference alone is adequate to yield flow information. If the phase shift is too great, multiple images with different gradient strengths will be needed to unravel the redundant phase-shift values. This technique can, in principle, be used to determine the flow vector in the space of any picture element by repeating the imaging procedure with the encoding gradient oriented along all three orthogonal axes. However, the major disadvantage of this approach is the required scan time, which increases linearly with the number of applied flow-encoding gradient steps.

In our laboratory we have explored the feasibility of producing images of vascular structures presented in an x-ray angiographic format using conventional MRI pulse sequences. Specifically, we have investigated the use of flow-encoding in-plane flow, which results from the application of the frequency-encoding gradient during a 2-DFT multiecho imaging sequence.

In these experiments we have used thick-section slices to minimize curvature effects and branch flow projecting out of the selected plane. In addition, we used ECG gating to restrict imaging to relatively slow-flow conditions during diastole and near-diastole.

Measurements were carried out with a 0.5 tesla MRI system; calibrations were performed using a continuous-flow phantom consisting of a DC pump operating from an enclosed reservoir of 50 percent concentration of 1,2 propanediol and water. (The 50 percent concentration of 1,2 propanediol has a *T1* of approximately 700 ms and a *T2* of approximately 115 ms and was chosen to simulate blood.) The pump was attached to a loop of $\frac{1}{2}$ inch Tygon tubing approximately 30 feet in length. A loop of the tubing was placed in the system's 25 cm diameter head coil and imaged at flow velocities ranging from 0 to 30 cm/sec with multiecho spin-echo pulse sequences. The sequence presented in this work used an eight-echo sequence of *TE* values from 30 to 240 ms and a *TR* of 500 ms. Measurements in human volunteers used identical pulse sequences (30/500) but were also ECG-gated in order to minimize the maximum velocity that would be encountered.

EVEN–ODD ECHO DIFFERENCE IMAGES

In a manner similar to balanced gradients, paired 180 degree rf pulses used in multiecho sequences can be used to produce flow-compensated images. Specifically, at the time of the second echo (and at all even echoes), all spins with constant velocity will rephase at the time of the echo to yield an enhanced signal relative to the first echo. This effect is frequently called even-echo rephasing.

The effect of even-echo rephasing was first reported in 1954 by Carr and Purcell[19] and more recently described for MR imaging by Bradley and Walach.[28,29] The effect is manifested in MR imaging as a difference in signal amplitude between the odd- and even-numbered echo images in a spin-echo experiment when there is motion along a magnetic field gradient. For in-plane flow, images that yield an angiographic type image format, the flow encoding is induced by motion along the frequency encoding or "read-out" gradient. In this orientation, the flow is orthogonal to both the phase-encoding and the slice-selection gradient. Similar even-echo enhancement effects can be seen in transverse sections, where flow encoding is induced by flow along the slice-selection gradient. The degree of signal reduction is the result of incomplete rephasing following the 180 degree rephasing pulse.

To understand even-echo rephasing, one must begin with the Larmor equation

$$\omega = \gamma \bar{B} \tag{1}$$

where ω is the resonance precessional frequency, γ is the gyromagnetic ratio, and $\bar{B}$ is the applied external magnetic field. From the definition of ω, we can determine the angular change ($d\phi$) that will result in the time interval (dt).

$$\omega = \frac{d\phi}{dt} = \gamma \bar{B} \tag{2}$$

The quantity ϕ is identified as the phase angle.

If we assume that the constant $\bar{B}$ field is replaced with a field gradient along the x-axis and that there is constant motion of the spin group with velocity (V) along that gradient, we can then rewrite the field that the spin group will experience in terms of its velocity and time.

$\bar{B} = B_0 + kx$, k is the gradient strength, and $x = Vt$.

Therefore, $\bar{B} = B_0 + kVt$.

If we then rewrite the phase angle equation in terms of this field,

$$d\phi = \gamma(B_0 + kVt)\,dt \tag{3}$$

By integration over time, we can determine the total accumulated phase angle for any spin group with velocity V. In a spin-echo pulse equation, the integration must take into account that the phase angle is inverted after each 180 degree pulse.

$$d\phi = \gamma B_0\,dt + \gamma KVt\,dt \tag{4}$$

$$\int_{t1}^{t2} d\phi = \gamma B_0 t \Big|_{t1}^{t2} + \tfrac{1}{2}\gamma KVt^2 \Big|_{t1}^{t2}, \text{ at the echo} \tag{5}$$

$$\Delta\phi = \tfrac{1}{2}\gamma KVt^2 \tag{6}$$

A graphic representation of the integration is shown (Fig. 36–9) following two 180 degree pulses at 15 and 45 ms. It should be noted that the phase angle remains non-zero at the time of the first echo at 30 ms and is identically zero at the time of the second echo. This same result can be demonstrated to be true of all odd and even echoes by further integration. An inspection of the properties of the phase-angle equation will also show that the incomplete rephasing on the odd echoes is a result of the quadratic term. It should also be noted that for nonflowing spin group ($V = 0$), complete

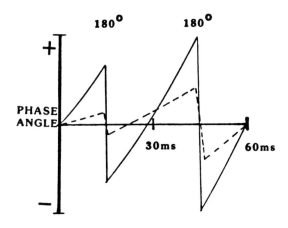

Figure 36–9. Plot of the phase angle of two different spin groups (slow [dashed line] and fast [solid line]) as a function of time. Following the 180 degree pulse at 15 ms, the spins are rotated to produce a negative phase angle. For non-flowing spins, the phase angle of all spins will return to zero (in phase) at the center of the echo (30 ms). At the first echo, flowing spins do not properly rephase and have a non-zero phase angle that results in a reduced signal strength. Owing to the quadratic nature of the phase angle evaluation function, spins moving along a linear gradient will come into phase on even-numbered echoes (non-zero phase angle).

rephasing occurs on all echoes. The result of complete rephasing on the even echoes is to yield a relatively larger signal in those picture elements in which flow is present than would be observed on the odd-numbered echoes. ("Relatively larger" should be emphasized, since T2 decay is also present and needs to be accounted for.) This effect is demonstrated in Figure 36–6, in which the spin-echo amplitude expressed as a percent of the nonflowing intensity is plotted for 30 ms (odd) and 60 ms (even) echo pulse sequences. Figure 36–10 demonstrates the technique for compensation for the T2 decay using exponential extrapolation with a four-echo pulse sequence.

With the knowledge that our system produced even-echo enhancement owing to the flow encoding of the frequency-encoding gradient, we proceeded to perform a preliminary calibration using the continuous-flow phantom. We made measurements of the flow phantom in both transverse and coronal planes. Since our goal is, in part, to produce an image similar to that of conventional angiography, we chose to first explore the calibration of the coronal section images. In coronal section images the

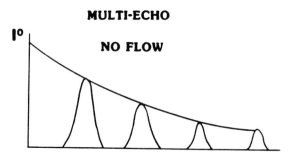

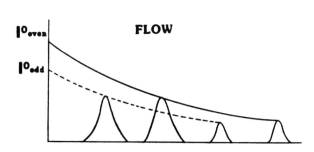

Figure 36–10. Comparison of multiecho signal decay in no-flow (top) and flow (bottom) conditions. For stationary spins, multiecho signal strength will decay at the modified T2 rates, with the even echoes decaying more slowly. Exponential extrapolation of each picture element is used to produce new images at t = 0 so that time differences between the two echoes are eliminated. The extrapolated odd and even echo images are then subtracted to yield a flow image. Nonflowing image components should subtract away, leaving only flowing structures.

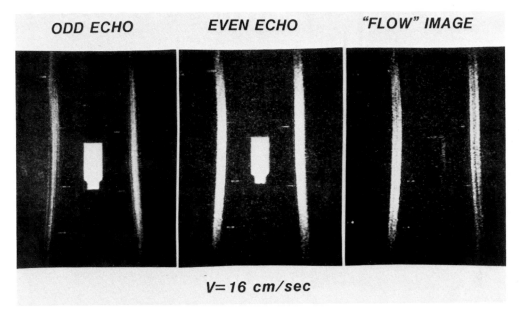

Figure 36–11. Examples of even-odd difference technique in a continuous-flow phantom. The vial in the center of the two tubes contains the same contrast material and provides a stationary reference. The enhancement of the signal strength in the tubes on the even echo relative to the odd echo should be noted. Note the absence of the nonflowing vial in the flow image following subtraction.

blood is flowing in the plane of the slice so that less paradoxical enhancement is observed as compared with transverse slices. In transverse imaging, spins flowing in from planes on either side of the selected plane have not seen a previous 90 degree pulse. This is true only for the extreme ends of the sensitive volume when coronal sections are used.

The "flow" image (Fig. 36–11) was generated by first exponentially extrapolating both the odd (30-90-150-210 ms) echoes and the even (60-120-180-240 ms) echoes back to time zero and then subtracting the extrapolated odd-echo image from the extrapolated even-echo image. The even-echo image is the flow-compensated image. In the flow image, the stationary vial is subtracted away while the flowing material remains.

The long tail on the curves in Figure 36–6 is due primarily to the fact that the velocity profile contains very slow velocity components at the edge of the tubes (vessels) and thus continues to contribute signal even at very high mean velocities.

Preliminary results with even–odd echo difference imaging in a normal volunteer (Figs. 36–12 and 36–13) have been encouraging. Flow images of the abdominal aorta at the level of the bifurcation have been created both at end-diastole (10 ms delay from R-wave) and at a time 250 ms later. The calculated flow images clearly demonstrate increased lumen size and an associated increased signal at 250 ms (near end-systole). A relatively constant signal and lumen size is observed in the vena cava lying adjacent to the aorta. Figure 36–12 is a coronal section, and Figure 36–13 is a sagittal section.

Transverse imaging was also explored at the level of the heart to measure aortic flow and to image cardiac chamber function (Fig. 36–14). These preliminary results indicate that cardiac chamber volume may be determined by this method.

PHASE ANGLE IMAGES

As mentioned earlier, conventional 2-DFT imaging sequences yield phase-encoded flow information, provided that phase-angle redundancies are kept from occurring.

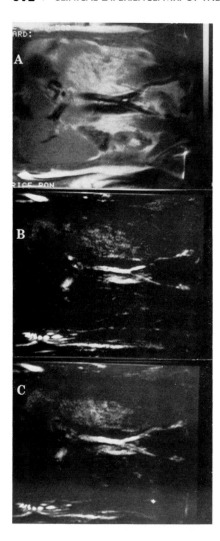

Figure 36–12. ECG-gated images of the abdominal aorta (coronal section). *A*, Conventional SE 60/500 image taken at near-systole. *B*, Even-odd difference flow image taken at near-diastole. *C*, Even-odd difference flow image taken at near-systole. Note increased intensity and lumen size in *C* relative to *B*.

Direct phase-angle images can be used in conjunction with the even–odd difference images to yield flow direction as well as flow magnitude. The phase-angle image also has the advantage in that it is not a subtraction image and as such is not subject to subtraction artifacts.

To prevent phase redundancies we have used short echo times (20 to 30 ms), relatively small gradients, and ECG gating to produce slow-flow conditions. For a well-tuned system, all nonmoving portions of the body should yield a constant phase angle. Moving portions should yield a non-zero phase angle, with the magnitude of the angle proportional to the flow velocity. An example of a phase-angle image is shown in Figure 36–15 along with the conventional SE (30/500) image.

In conclusion, flow phenomena in MR imaging have been a source of both concern and encouragement—concern in the sense of unexplained image artifacts, and encouragement in the sense of having the potential of measuring blood flow in a completely noninvasive manner.

At the present time, flow imaging remains an experimental laboratory procedure and as yet is not ready for routine clinical use. Preliminary results in patients and volunteers, however, are very encouraging and help us project that high-quality, quantitative flow images will soon be available as part of routine imaging protocols.

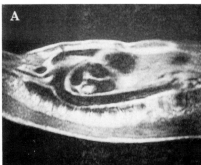

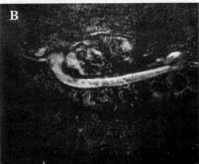

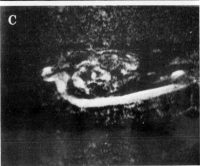

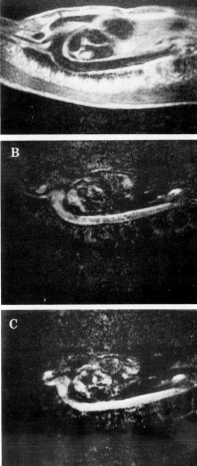

Figure 36–13. ECG-gated images of the aorta (sagittal section). *A*, Conventional SE 30/500 image taken at near-diastole. *B*, Even-echo difference flow image taken near the diastolic phase of the cardiac cycle. *C*, Flow image taken near cardiac systole.

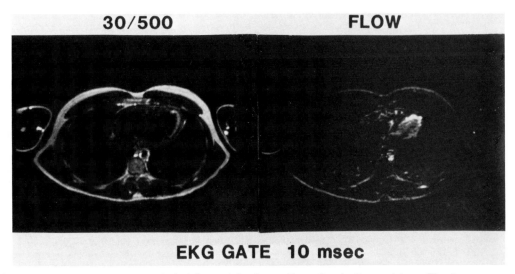

Figure 36–14. ECG-gated image through the left ventricle taken at 10 ms after the R-wave trigger. Flow image shows enhancement of left ventricular cavity and aorta.

SE 30/500   PHASE ANGLE

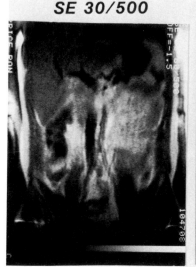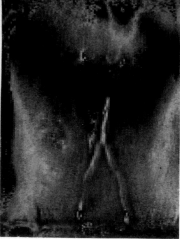

GATE 10msec

Figure 36–15. Phase-angle image of the abdominal aorta, vena cava, and hepatic vesels. Aorta is enhanced because of increased phase shift (larger phase angle) as a result of blood flow. Image nonuniformity is due to imperfect rephasing of the echo at the time of data sampling, resulting from nonuniform rf fields and from incomplete application of compensation gradients.

References

1. Wood ML, Henkelman RM: MR image artifacts from periodic motion. Med Phys *12*(2):143, 1985.
2. Perman WH, Moran PR, Moran RA, Bernstein MA: Artifacts from pulsatile flow in MR imaging. J Comput Assist Tomogr *10*(3):473, 1986.
3. Bryant DJ, Payne JA, Firmin DN, Longmore DB: Measurement of flow with NMR imaging using a gradient pulse and phase difference technique. J Comput Assist Tomogr *8*(4):588, 1984.
4. Weeden VJ, Meuli RA, Edelman RR, et al: Projective imaging of pulsatile flow with magnetic resonance. Science *230*:946, 1985.
5. Weeden VJ, Rosen BR, Baxton R, Brady TJ: Projective MRI angiography and quantitative flow-volume densitometry. Magn Reson Med *3*:226, 1986.
6. George CR, Jacobs G, et al: Magnetic resonance signal intensity patterns obtained from continuous pulsatile flow models. Radiology *151*:421, 1984.
7. Halbach RE, et al: The NMR blood flowmeter design. Med Phys *8*:444, 1984.
8. Garroway AN: Velocity measurements in flowing fluids by NMR. J Phys D: Appl Phys *7*:1159, 1974.
9. Kaufmann L, Crooks LE, et al: Evaluation of NMR imaging for detection and quantification of obstructions in vessels. Invest Radiol *17*:554, 1982.
10. Crooks L, et al: Quantification of obstructions in vessels by NMR. IEEE Trans Nucl Sci NS-*29*:1181, 1982.
11. Grant JP, Back C: NMR rheotomography: feasibility and clinical potential. Med Phys *9*(2):188, 1982.
12. Wehrli FW, et al: Approaches to in-plane and out-of-plane flow imaging. Noninvas Med Imag *1*:127, 1984.
13. Singer JR, Crooks LE: Science *221*:654, 1983.
14. Axel L: Review: Blood flow effects in magnetic resonance imaging. AJR *143*:1157, 1984.
15. Moran PR: A flow velocity zeugmatographic interlace for NMR imaging in humans. Magn Reson Imag *1*:197, 1982.
16. Moran PR: Evaluation of the phase-modulation method for true flow imaging by NMR. Radiology *149*(P) 206, 1983.
17. Wehrli FW, et al: Visualization and quantification of flow by NMR in phantoms and in the normal brain and neck. Radiology *149*(P):205, 1983.
18. Lent AH, et al: Flow-velocity imaging by NMR. Radiology *149*(P):237, 1983.
19. Carr HV, Purcell EM: Effects of diffusion of free precision in NMR experiments. Phys Rev *94*(3):630, 1954.
20. O'Donnell M: NMR blood flow imaging using multiecho, phase contrast sequences. Med Phys *12*(1):59, 1985.
21. Redpath TW, Norris DG: A new method of NMR flow imaging. Phys Med Biol *29*(7):891, 1984.
22. O'Donnell M, et al: Multiple-echo blood flow imaging using phase contrast (abstract). *In* Proceedings of the Third Annual Meeting of the Society of Magnetic Resonance in Medicine, 1984, pp 561–562.
23. Smith LS, et al: Cardiac gated flow measurement in NMR imaging (abstract). *In* Proceedings of the Third Annual Meeting of the Society of Magnetic Resonance in Medicine, 1984, pp 690–691.

24. Feinberg DA, et al: Fluid velocity vector components imaged by multiple-spin-echo MRI (abstract). *In* Proceedings of the Third Annual Meeting of the Society of Magnetic Resonance in Medicine, 1984, pp 229–230.
25. Norris C: Phase encoded NMR flow imaging (abstract). *In* Proceedings of the Third Annual Meeting of the Society of Magnetic Resonance in Medicine, 1984, pp 559–560.
26. Wedeen V, et al: MR velocity imaging by phase display (abstract). *In* Proceedings of the Third Annual Meeting of the Society of Magnetic Resonance in Medicine, 1984, pp 742–743.
27. Wendt RE, et al: NMR pulse sequence for rapid imaging of flow (abstract). *In* Proceedings of the Third Annual Meeting of the Society of Magnetic Resonance in Medicine, 1984, pp 749–750.
28. Walach V, Bradley WG: NMR even-echo rephasing in slow laminar flow. J Comp Assist Tomogr *8*:594, 1984.
29. Bradley WG, Walach V: Blood flow: magnetic resonance imaging. Radiology *154*:443, 1985.
30. Moran PR, et al: Verification and evaluation of internal flow and motion. Radiology *154*:433, 1985.
31. Singer JR: NMR diffusion and flow measurements and an introduction to spin phase graphing. J Phys E *11*:281, 1978.

37

Musculoskeletal System

MADAN V. KULKARNI
E. PAUL NANCE, JR.
JOHN H. HARRIS, JR.

The musculoskeletal system is one of the areas of greatest clinical application for magnetic resonance imaging (MRI). Although cortical bone does not provide adequate MR signal, the bone marrow, because of its normal fat content, provides a comparatively strong signal.[1,2] The multiplanar imaging capabilities of MR allow evaluation of extremities in their long axis. Nonorthogonal imaging as used in cardiac MRI[3] is useful in evaluating structures, such as cruciate ligaments, that are not in orthogonal planes. Magnetic resonance imaging has demonstrated superior soft tissue contrast compared with conventional radiographic techniques.[4]

TECHNIQUES OF IMAGING

Over the past few years, there has been gradual improvement in the imaging techniques of MR. Developments in surface-coil technology have improved the ability to evaluate small structures such as cruciate ligaments and the intervertebral disc.[5] The improved signal-to-noise (S/N) ratio offered by surface coils can be effectively utilized to decrease slice thickness without degrading image quality and, hence, reduction in partial volume effects. Similarly, this gain in S/N is used to improve spatial resolution by decreasing pixel size.

The imaging techniques applied to the musculoskeletal system depend on the part of the body being examined as well as on the pathology under consideration. The evaluation of the pelvis requires a larger diameter radio frequency (rf) coil, whereas the lower thigh and leg are studied using smaller diameter coils (i.e., head coil). The use of a smaller coil improves the spatial resolution but also decreases the field of view.

Occasionally, after an area of abnormality such as an osteogenic sarcoma has been initially examined with a smaller-diameter coil, further evaluation using a larger coil is necessary to determine the extent of soft tissue and marrow involvement. Surface coils should be used whenever possible, especially when pathology is limited to a relatively small area of the body, such as the traumatized knee or a suspected lumbar disc herniation.

The contrast in MR imaging depends on the pulse sequences utilized, and therefore at least two, and preferably three, pulse sequences are recommended. Optimum contrast between multiple structures or tissues cannot be obtained on a single pulse sequence. Multislice-multiecho techniques are useful in this situation because they significantly reduce imaging times. Since MR allows the use of multiple imaging planes, it is necessary to determine the plane of imaging in advance of the study. Use of at least two imaging planes in the visualization of bone tumors and infections is recommended. Imaging along the long axis of the extremities determines the craniocaudal extent of the abnormality, while axial imaging demonstrates lateral spread. Although this approach usually requires data acquisition on two or more occasions and hence increases imaging time, proper advance planning can significantly streamline the procedure.

Prolonged MR imaging times may require sedation of infants and young children. Patients with intracranial vascular clips and cardiac pacemakers currently are not imaged with MR because the strong magnetic field may displace the metallic vascular clips[6] and the rf applied during the imaging procedure may interfere with the pacemaker mechanism.[7] Ferromagnetic clothing accessories and prostheses may cause artifacts. The heating effects of changing magnetic fields and rf fields on small metallic implants have been described previously.[8] Proper screening precautions, such as removal of jewelry and metallic clothing objects (belt buckle, hairpins), are necessary to prevent artifacts in the image.[9]

NORMAL MR ANATOMY

The MR signal that generates the image is dependent not only on the proton density but also on other parameters, including $T1$ and $T2$ relaxation times.[10] The relaxation times provide the major contribution to the contrast in MR images. These, in turn, are dependent upon the physical and chemical composition of the tissues. Cortical bone produces minimal signal intensity on all pulse sequences because of the lack of mobile protons in the cortical bone, whereas fat has a bright signal on $T1$ weighted images owing to its shorter $T1$ relaxation time (Fig. 37–1). Bone marrow, because of its high

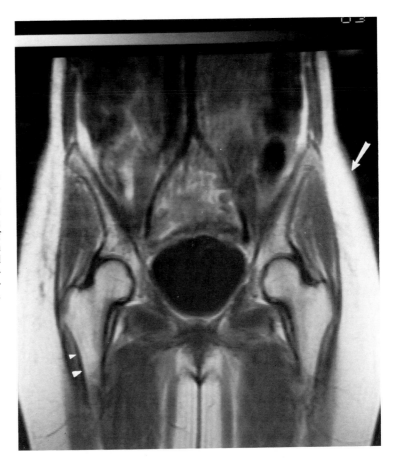

Figure 37–1. Coronal MR image of the pelvis using SE 30/500 sequence. Subcutaneous fat (arrow) has bright signal owing to shorter $T1$ relaxation times of fat. Bone marrow also has increased signal intensity because of its relative high fat content. Urine in the bladder has a markedly decreased signal because of its long $T1$ relaxation times. Cortical bone (arrowheads) has decreased signal intensity.

fat content, has increased signal intensity on *T1* weighted sequences, while clear fluids, such as CSF, have decreased signal intensity because of their long *T1* relaxation times.

Normal muscle has decreased signal intensity compared with fat on both *T1* and *T2* weighted images; therefore, fascial planes between the muscle bundles are well seen on *T1* weighted sequences. Fibrous tissue, on the other hand, has relatively decreased signal intensity compared with fat on all pulse sequences.

NEOPLASMS

As in radiographic imaging, the MR evaluation of benign and malignant neoplasms depends on many different clinical and imaging features. The patient's age and sex and the location of the lesion are important parameters. The presence or absence of calcification within the lesion is a significant radiographic feature. Figure 37–2 illustrates an epiphyseal lesion in the proximal femur of a 12-year-old patient. The location of the lesion is typical of a chondroblastoma. The coronal MR image helps in the evaluation of the lesion and its relationship with the hip joint. Magnetic resonance imaging also demonstrates expansion of the bone effectively (Fig. 37–3). Benign neoplasms usually have long *T2* relaxation times, and the contrast between the lesion and the bone marrow is best demonstrated with pulse sequences with long echo delay (*TE*) and pulse repetition times (*TR*). The signal intensity on *T1* weighted sequences depends on the nature of the contents of the lesion (Fig. 37–4). High protein content or blood within the lesion usually demonstrates relatively short *T1* relaxation times, resulting in increased signal intensity on *T1* weighted sequences (see Fig. 37–3). The signal intensity from the lesion depends on the presence of hemorrhage secondary to pathologic fracture or biopsy. These factors must be considered before one attempts to characterize the contents of a bone lesion. When imaging is performed in two planes perpendicular to each other, the anterior posterior craniocaudal and lateral extent of the abnormality can be determined accurately (Fig. 37–5).

Currently, it is not possible to differentiate all benign bone lesions on the basis of signal intensity on *T1* and *T2* weighted images. Although MR does not establish the histopathologic diagnosis, it may be useful in determining soft tissue or joint extension. This feature of MR has been helpful in surgical management of these lesions.

MR is extremely useful in the evaluation of malignant neoplasms of the muscu-

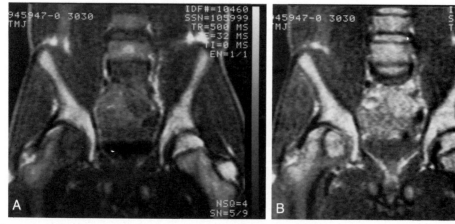

Figure 37–2. Chondroblastoma arising in the right capital femoral epiphysis has decreased signal intensity on SE 32/500 (*A*) and increased signal intensity on SE 45/2000 (*B*). Normal femoral epiphysis and the greater trochanter epiphysis have relatively increased signal intensity compared with bone marrow on both sequences.

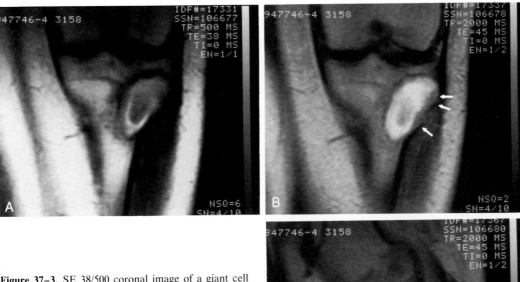

Figure 37–3. SE 38/500 coronal image of a giant cell tumor. *A*, The peripheral portion of the lesion has a relatively increased signal, suggesting relatively shorter *T1* relaxation times of that portion of the tumor. *B* and *C*, *T2* weighted images demonstrate longer *T2* relaxation times in the periphery and relatively shorter *T2* relaxation times near the center. Also note cortical expansion laterally (*B*, arrows). The line separating the epiphysis and metaphysis is seen.

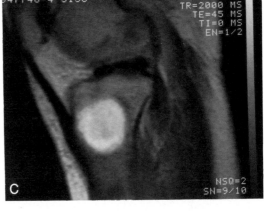

loskeletal system. The techniques of MR imaging of the malignant neoplasms are similar to those of benign neoplasms. Currently, computed tomography (CT) is used to determine soft tissue extension of malignant skeletal tumors. MRI is also useful in determining soft tissue involvement and has some advantages over CT. It has superior soft tissue contrast,[4] and imaging can be performed in multiple planes; reconstruction techniques to obtain multiple planes, as in CT, are not necessary. Spin-echo images with relatively short *TE* and *TR* parameters (*T1* weighted) frequently demonstrate contrast between tumor and bone marrow (Fig. 37–6), since tumors frequently have long *T1* relaxation times. The *T1* sequences is not adequate to differentiate tumor extension in the muscle. *T2* weighted sequences (i.e., long *TE* and *TR*) should be used for this purpose, since tumors have longer *T2* relaxation times compared with muscle

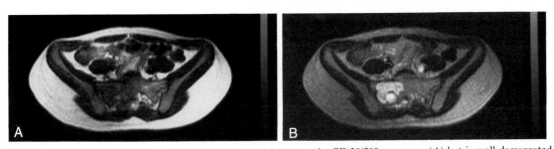

Figure 37–4. Aneurysmal bone cyst is rather difficult to detect on the SE 30/500 sequence (*A*) but is well demarcated on the SE 45/2000 sequence (*B*) obtained in a transverse plane.

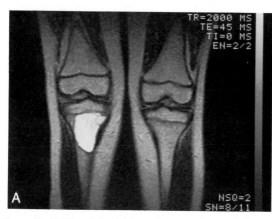 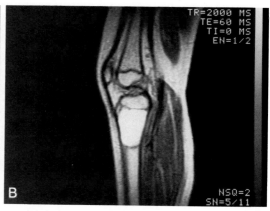

Figure 37–5. *T2* weighted images in coronal (*A*) and sagittal (*B*) planes demonstrate excellent contrast between bone marrow and lesion and between bone marrow and muscle. With the use of two different planes, the extent of the lesion is better defined. There is no evidence of extension into the epiphysis or extraskeletal soft tissue.

(Fig. 37–7). Similarly, excellent contrast between extraskeletal extension of the tumor and the subcutaneous fat has been demonstrated using MR.[11]

While large areas of calcification or ossification are identified with MR, since they produce decreased signal intensity (Fig. 37–6) on *T1* as well as on *T2* weighted sequences,[12] small areas of calcification may not be detected. This inability to detect small areas of calcification, ossification, or sclerosis with MR is one of its major drawbacks and probably decreases its specificity of histologic diagnosis. CT, on the other hand, is excellent in detecting calcification, ossification, and the thin rims of cortical

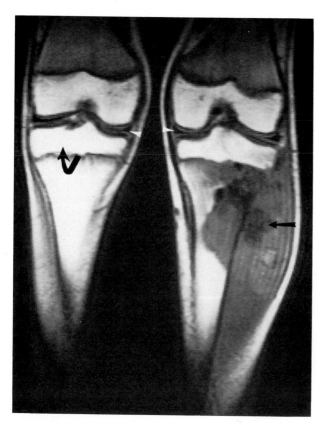

Figure 37–6. Osteogenic sarcoma on SE 30/500 image demonstrates excellent contrast between tumor and marrow. The extension into the muscle was seen better on a *T2* weighted sequence. Large areas of calcification are demonstrated (arrow). Meniscus (arrowheads) and epiphysis (curved arrow) are also noted.

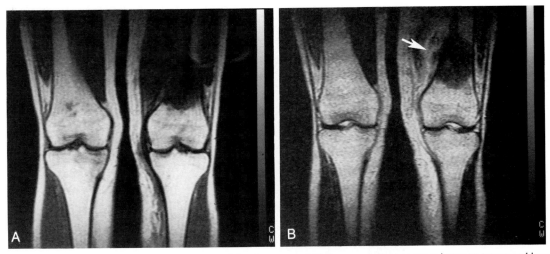

Figure 37–7. Large osteogenic sarcoma on *T1* weighted sequence (*A*) shows excellent contrast between tumor and bone marrow. Extension of the tumor into the muscle is not seen on the *T1* weighted image but is well documented on the *T2* weighted sequence (*B*). This is because tumor and edema (arrow) have marked increase of signal, whereas muscle continues to show decreased signal intensity on the *T2* weighted image.

bone in expansile lesions; pathologic fractures also are better seen with CT than with MR. With use of surface-coil technology, the spatial resolution with MR can be further improved,[13] and the lesions will be better defined. With current-generation surface coils the spatial resolution of MR approaches that of CT. Although the signal intensity changes on *T1* and *T2* weighted images are currently nonspecific for tumor histology, evaluation of larger series of cases is necessary to establish the role of MR in histologic diagnosis. Chemical-shift imaging may be useful in determining tumor metabolism.[14] Until these advantages are utilized, the major advantage of MR is its superior soft tissue contrast and consequent excellent determination of the extent of skeletal tumors. The information obtained with MR should be considered complementary to that obtained from plain film and CT studies.

Magnetic resonance has also proved to be valuable in the diagnosis of soft tissue tumors.[15] Longer *T2* relaxation times of tumor and edema provide MR contrast between tumor and normal muscle (Fig. 37–8). MRI can also be used to determine the involve-

Figure 37–8. Surface-coil sagittal image of a recurrent fibrous histiocytoma anterior to the humerus. The clinical question of involvement of the bone can be answered by using high resolution on surface coil images, as the tumor (arrow) is seen separate from the cortical bone (curved arrow) and the bone marrow (open arrow). The slice thickness is 7 mm.

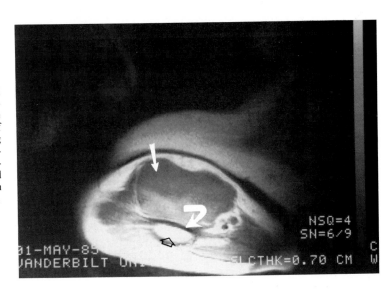

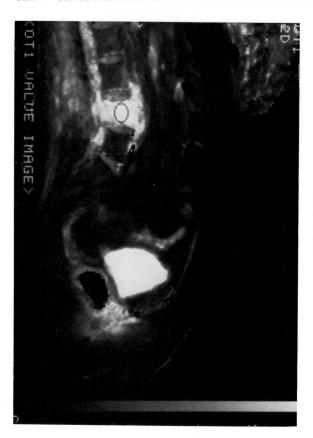

Figure 37–9. Calculated *T1* value image in a patient with metastatic renal cell carcinoma in the third lumbar vertebra. The *T1* value in the metastatic lesion is 898 ms, while bone marrow in the normal vertebral body is approximately 300 ms.

ment of cortical bone and bone marrow by primary muscle tumors, and the technique will be helpful in planning surgical treatment.

The role of MR in skeletal metastasis is currently being evaluated. Since metastatic disease frequently starts within the marrow, MR can demonstrate these lesions as an abnormal signal within the marrow (Fig. 37–9). Radionuclide (RN) studies are more sensitive than other radiographic procedures in detecting bony metastasis; however, MR can demonstrate bone marrow involvement before the osseous changes are detected on a radiography. In a few instances, skeletal metastatic lesions not detected by RN bone scans have been demonstrated by MR. The RN study should still be used as a screening procedure, since evaluation of the entire skeleton by MR is tedious, uncomfortable for the patient, and probably not cost-beneficial.

INFECTION

Since MR demonstrates strong signal from the bone marrow, it is extremely valuable in the detection of inflammatory processes involving the musculoskeletal system. The associated edema causes an increase in mobile hydrogen atoms within the marrow. This results in longer *T1* and *T2* relaxation times from the areas of infection, which contrasts with the relatively shorter *T1* and *T2* relaxation times from the normal bone marrow. While inflammation of the marrow causes increased signal compared with the normal marrow on *T2* weighted sequences, the opposite occurs in disc infection, in which the normal bright signal from the disc is lost (Fig. 37–10). Multiplanar MR imaging is useful in demonstrating the extent of the infection, and it provides distinction of the abnormality from the surrounding normal structures (Fig. 37–11). Use of multiple pulse

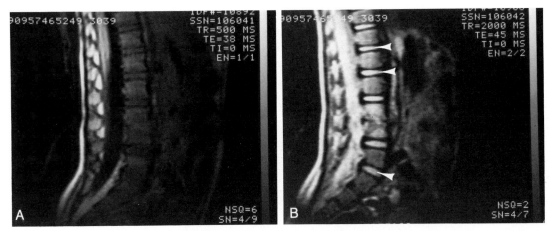

Figure 37–10. Sagittal *T1* weighted image (*A*) in a patient with disc infection fails to demonstrate significant abnormality, but *T2* weighted sequence (*B*) demonstrates loss of normal water and architecture of nucleus pulposus at L3–4. Normal discs (arrowheads) have increased signal on this pulse sequence (SE 45/2000). A slight increased signal is also noted in the L3 and L4 vertebral bodies, probably indicating the extension of inflammation and/or edema in the marrow.

sequences may be necessary to demonstrate adequate contrast between the inflammatory processes and surrounding normal tissues (Figs. 37–10 and 37–11). Associated abscesses can also be demonstrated with MR (Fig. 37–12).

Compared with the conventional radiographic procedures, MR and RN studies are both more sensitive in the detection of early osteomyelitis.[16] Current work with animal models has demonstrated similar sensitivity using MR and RN studies in surgically induced osteomyelitis in rabbits.[17] In a recent series, MR proved excellent in the diagnosis of vertebral osteomyelitis, and it was at least as accurate and sensitive as RN scanning.[18] Further work based upon larger series is needed to establish the respective roles of MR and RN studies in osteomyelitis. Magnetic resonance, like RN studies, is nonspecific for osteomyelitis, since abnormal *T1* and *T2* relaxation times are seen in neoplastic, traumatic, and other noninfective inflammatory disorders.

MRI has been used in the evaluation of inflammatory disorders of joints, such as rheumatoid arthritis.[19] The soft tissue pannus associated with C1–C2 dislocation in

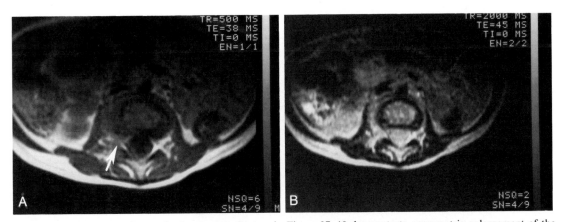

Figure 37–11. Transverse images in the same patient as in Figure 37–10 demonstrate asymmetric enlargement of the right psoas muscle. On the *T1* weighted image (*A*) there is obliteration of the epidural fat and fat in the intervertebral foramina on the right (arrow). The normal bright signal of fat, caused by its short *T1* relaxation time, is lost. The extension of the inflammatory process into the right psoas muscle is demonstrated superiorly on the SE 90/2000 sequence (*B*). On this surface-coil *T2* weighted sequence, there is markedly decreased contrast between fat and inflammatory process, which was best seen on the *T1* weighted sequence.

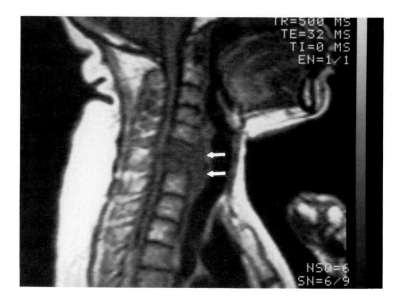

Figure 37–12. Vertebral TB osteomyelitis with abscess formation demonstrates deviation of the cord posteriorly as well as extension of the abscess (arrows) in the retropharyngeal space.

rheumatoid arthritis and its relationship to the spinal cord can be demonstrated using MR (Fig. 37–13). The inflammatory changes seen in the synovium of patients with hemophiliac arthropathy have been described previously.[20]

TRAUMA

The role of MR in acute skeletal trauma has not been adequately studied. The encroachment on the spinal subarachnoid space and the cord from vertebral body fracture can be evaluated with MR in multiple planes (Fig. 37–14). Because MR may be unable to detect small calcifications, small bone fragments are better seen with CT. However, the effects of vertebral fracture upon the cord, such as contusion, edema, and traumatic syringomyelia, can be demonstrated better with MR than with other imaging modalities.

Magnetic resonance has also proved to be useful in acute joint trauma.[21] The

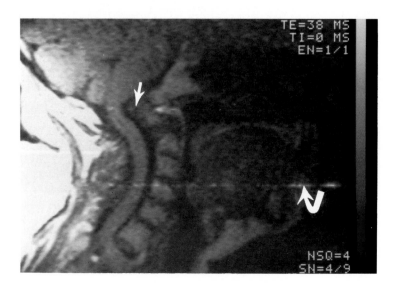

Figure 37–13. Granulation tissue (arrow) from rheumatoid arthritis is deviating brainstem and cervical cord posteriorly. Artifact from rf interference (curved arrow) is shown.

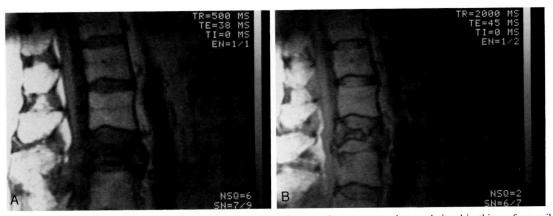

Figure 37–14. *T1* weighted image (*A*) in an old compression fracture demonstrates abnormal signal in this surface-coil image. The preservation of the discs and the extradural compression of the spinal subarachnoid space is seen superiorly on SE 45/2000 sequence (*B*).

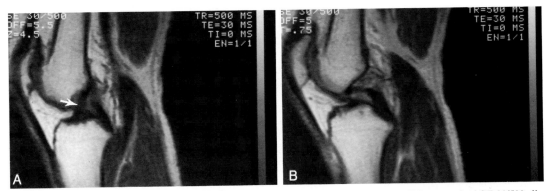

Figure 37–15. *A,* Normal anterior (arrow) and posterior cruciate ligaments are seen on a 7.5 mm sagittal SE 30/500 slice. Posterior cruciate ligament is not seen in its entirety owing to its oblique path and rotation of the knee in this head-coil image. *B,* The anterior cruciate ligament is absent in the other knee owing to old trauma, and only the posterior cruciate ligament is identified.

Figure 37–16. Surface-coil imaging of a knee in acute trauma demonstrates absence of the anterior cruciate ligament. The posterior cruciate ligament is seen in its entirety in this 3 mm thick slice, since the image is acquired in an oblique sagittal plane by changing gradient angles electronically. In addition to spatial resolution, it is improved by decreasing pixel size to approximately 0.7 mm by a decreasing field of view. Acute hemarthrosis (arrows) is demonstrated by abnormal signal between patella and femur.

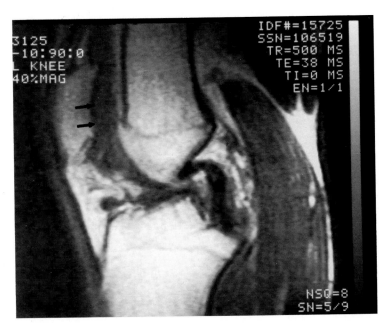

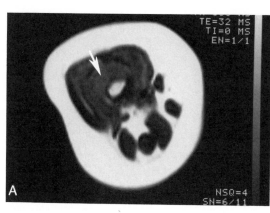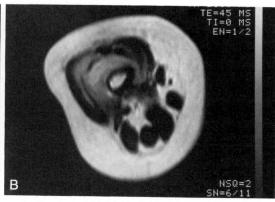

Figure 37–17. Transverse 32/500 images in a patient with acute swelling of the left thigh. The patient was on chemotherapy. SE 32/500 sequence (*A*) demonstrates slight increase in signal intensity (arrow) anterolateral to the femur, but this acute bleed has best contrast on the *T2* weighted sequence (*B*) with surrounding normal muscle. Acute hemorrhage is best demonstrated on *T2* sequences.

cruciate ligaments (Fig. 37–15) and their tears can be demonstrated using surface coils and very thin sections (Fig. 37–16). Associated hemarthrosis and collateral ligament injuries have been demonstrated.[21] Large meniscal tears have been detected with MR,[21] but the detection of smaller tears requires the use of surface coils and ultrathin tomographic sections. These studies are currently under way, and comparative studies will be useful in defining the role of MRI compared with invasive procedures such as arthrography and arthroscopy.

Magnetic resonance is useful in the diagnosis of hemorrhage and its precise localization (Fig. 37–17). Based upon its MR characteristics, hemorrhage can be further characterized according to its stage, i.e., acute, subacute, or chronic.[20] This technique can be used as a noninvasive method for patient follow-up.

VASCULAR DISORDERS

One of the earliest diagnostic uses of MR in the musculoskeletal system was in the diagnosis of avascular necrosis (AVN). Because the bone marrow is so clearly

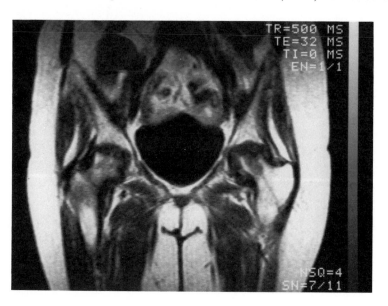

Figure 37–18. Bilateral AVN of the femoral head is seen on SE 32/500 sequence. Tract of the core biopsy is seen on the left. Normal femoral heads are demonstrated in Figure 37–1.

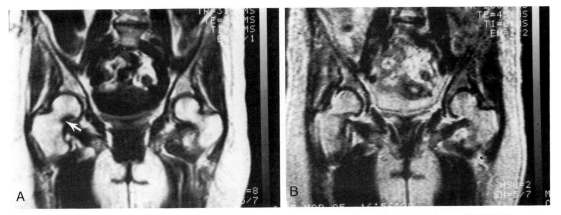

Figure 37–19. Decreased signal intensity of the inferomedial aspect of femoral neck (arrow) is seen on SE 30/315 sequence (*A*) in a patient suspected of having AVN. *T2* weighted image (*B*) demonstrates increased signal in this region, suggesting relatively longer *T1* and *T2* relaxation times. The radiograph of the hip was normal, while radionuclide bone scan showed a slight increase in RN accumulation. The MR findings were attributed to insufficiency fracture in this patient with chronic renal failure.

depicted by MR, it is a very sensitive indicator of the presence of AVN.[15,17,22] Areas of AVN produce decreased signal compared with normal marrow on *T1* weighted images (Fig. 37–18). Current experience suggests that MR is far superior to conventional radiography in the early detection of AVN. MR should be compared with RN bone scanning because of its high sensitivity in detecting AVN. Although lesion detectability in AVN is superior with both MR and RN studies, their respective roles in this diagnosis have yet to be determined.

Magnetic resonance also has superior sensitivity in the demonstration of insufficiency fractures, sometimes seen with chronic renal failure (Fig. 37–19) and in bone infarctions associated with long-term steroid use. Since MR is a unique imaging tool for the bone marrow, some of the abnormalities seen in MR have not been confirmed by the other imaging modalities.

As with AVN, the diagnosis of Legg-Perthes disease is readily made with MR (Fig. 37–20). Because of its superior sensitivity in detecting Legg-Perthes disease, the MR

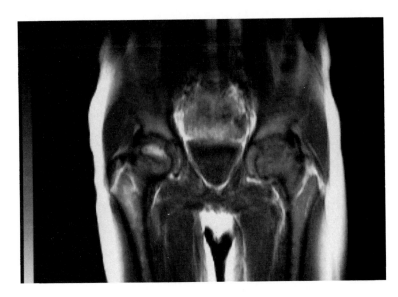

Figure 37–20. Distortion of the left femoral head and increase in size of the femoral neck are seen in patients with Legg-Calvé-Perthes disease. Right proximal capital femoral epiphysis is normal.

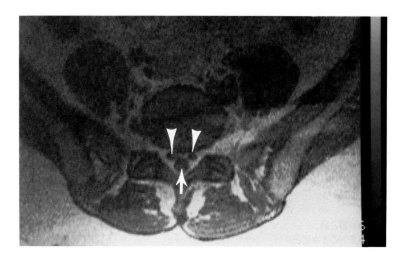

Figure 37–21. Angled transverse view with image parallel to the L5–S1 disc plane demonstrates normal disc and cauda equina (arrow). Nerve roots (arrowheads) and epidural fat have bright signal on this *T1* weighted surface-coil image.

examination should include both hips, since the condition is bilateral in 10 percent of the cases.

DISC DISEASE

Magnetic resonance imaging of the spine is described in Chapters 17 and 18. The development of surface-coil technology has made a tremendous contribution to the evaluation of disc disease using MR. The normal disc not only can be imaged in the transverse plane (Fig. 37–21), similar to CT, but also direct sagittal and parasagittal anatomy display with improved resolution is available with MR (Fig. 37–22) as com-

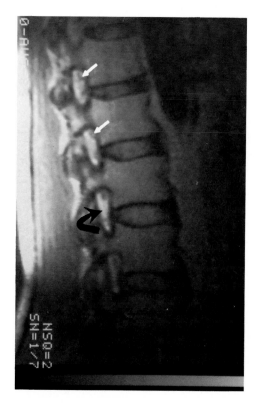

Figure 37–22. Normal parasagittal anatomy is seen in this image with bright signal from the fat (curved arrow) around the nerve roots (arrows). Disc anulus is well contrasted against the fat in the intervertebral foramen.

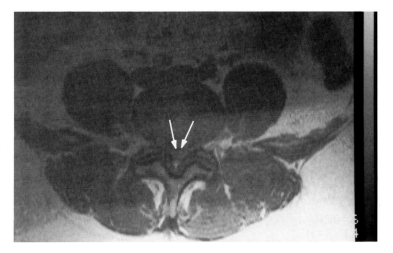

Figure 37–23. Angled transverse *T1* weighted image demonstrates disc herniation (arrows) in the middle and slightly to the left of the midline. The contrast between herniated disc and CSF is poor on this SE 38/750 sequence.

pared with the reformatted CT images. Disc herniation can been seen in the transverse (Fig. 37–23) and in the sagittal planes (Fig. 37–24). The information obtained in disc disease by MR is comparable to that obtained by CT and myelography. MRI can be performed on an outpatient basis, minimizing the cost of diagnosis on these patients and at the same time eleminating patient discomfort and potential complications of myelography. Further studies with high-resolution MR are necessary to establish the roles of MR and of CT and myelography in the evaluation of disc disease.

MISCELLANEOUS DISORDERS

The detection and characterization of the subchondral cysts of hemophiliac arthropathy with MR is superior to that of other imaging modalities (Fig. 37–25). MR is also useful in the detection of the periarticular abnormalities of hemophilia. Joint effusions and subchondral cysts in degenerative arthritis are well seen with MR. Use of MR has also been documented in disease processes such as congenital dislocation of

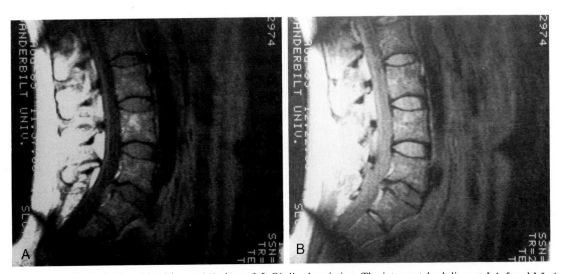

Figure 37–24. Sagittal *T1* weighted image (*A*) shows L5–S1 disc herniation. The intervertebral discs at L4–5 and L3–4 are normal. The extradural defect is best seen on the relatively *T2* weighted sequence (*B*).

the hips, cavernous hemangioma,[15] and leukemia.[1] Investigations are currently under way in multiple centers to evaluate the exact role of MR in musculoskeletal disorders and its importance relative to other imaging modalities.

In conclusion, magnetic resonance is currently used in the evaluation of multiple musculoskeletal disorders. Although cortical bone does not provide adequate signal for MR imaging, the bone marrow has a strong signal. The ability to utilize signal from bone marrow with MR is unique, and although bone marrow can be imaged using CT and RN studies, neither has been very successful in detecting changes early in disease processes. Since many disease processes involve marrow before they affect cortical bone, it is logical to expect MR to be more sensitive than conventional radiography and RN in detecting these disorders. Recent investigations have reported this finding.[23] Similar findings are seen with marrow infarctions, but more experience is needed using all imaging modalities in detection of disease processes presenting as abnormality of marrow in early stages.

As in radionuclide imaging, the advantage of improved sensitivity with MR is partially offset by its current lack of specificity. The other major disadvantage of MR is its failure to detect small foci of calcification, since, from past experience, the detection of calcification enhances the specificity of diagnosis not only in musculoskeletal but also in other organ systems. The initial promise of in vivo measurements of $T1$ and $T2$ relaxation times in differentiating neoplastic versus inflammatory, or benign versus malignant, disorders has yet to be realized. Our early experience in measuring in vivo $T1$ relaxation times has been disappointing. With development of paramagnetic contrast agents and the possibility of chemical-shift imaging using P-31 spectra, the specificity of MR could be further improved. Initial results of in vivo spectroscopy in the evaluation of muscular dystrophy are encouraging.[24]

The major advantages of MR in the musculoskeletal system are markedly improved soft tissue contrast and multiplanar imaging. With the use of surface-coil imaging, the spatial resolution of MR should approach that seen with CT scanning. Multiplanar tomographic imaging and improved soft tissue contrast, combined with improved spatial

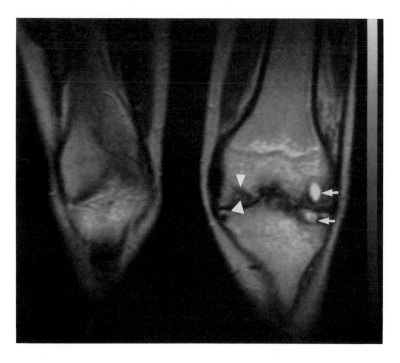

Figure 37–25. Subchondral cysts with hemorrhage or fluid have an increased signal on $T2$ weighted sequence (arrows), whereas cysts with fibrosis (arrowheads) have decreased signal intensity.

resolution of surface coils, may allow MR to be used as a screening procedure in the evaluation of spine and joint diseases. These same advantages also apply to the role of MR in determining the extent of malignant and inflammatory processes. Thus, MR has demonstrated its current role in the diagnosis of musculoskeletal disorders. With further development in technology, it will surely play a primary or complementary role in multiple disease processes.

ACKNOWLEDGMENTS

The authors gratefully acknowledge Ms. Sue Orkin, Ms. Holly Pelton, and Ms. Millicent Williams for editorial help, and Ms. Debbie Freeland for technical assistance.

References

1. Cohen MD, Klattle EC, Boehner R, et al: Magnetic resonance imaging of bone marrow diseases in children. Radiology *155*:715, 1984.
2. Fletcher BE, Scoles DV, Nelson AD: Osteomyelitis in children: Detection by magnetic resonance. Radiology *150*:57, 1984.
3. Kulkarni MV, Mazer M, Waddil WB, et al: Role of non-orthogonal images in cardiac magnetic resonance imaging. Association of University Radiologists, 33rd Annual Meeting, Nashville, 1985.
4. Moon KL, Genant HK, Helms CA, Chafetz NI, Crooks LE, Kaufman L: Musculoskeletal applications of magnetic resonance. Radiology *147*:161, 1983.
5. Edelman RR, Shoukimas GM, Stark DD, et al: High resolution surface coil imaging of lumbar disc disease. AJR *144*:1123, 1985.
6. New PF, Rosen BR, Brady TJ, et al: Potential of artifacts of ferromagnetic and non-ferromagnetic surgical and dental materials and devices in nuclear magnetic resonance imaging. Radiology *147*:139, 1983.
7. Pavlicek W, Geisenger M, Castle L, Borkowski CP, Meaney R, Beam BL, Gallagher JH: The effects of nuclear magnetic resonance on patients with cardiac pacemakers. Radiology *147*:149, 1983.
8. Davis PL, Crooks R, Arakawa L, McKee R, Kaufman L, Margulis AR: Potential hazards in NMR imaging: Heating effects of changing magnetic fields and RF fields on small metallic implants. AJR *137*:857, 1981.
9. Kulkarni MV, Patton JA: Techniques, pitfalls and artifacts in magnetic resonance imaging. *In* Mettler FA, Muroff LA, Kulkarni MV (eds): Clinical NMR. New York, Churchill Livingstone, 1986.
10. Partain CL, Price RR, Patton JA, et al: Overview of nuclear magnetic resonance imaging: Physical principles, clinical potentials, and interrelationship with radionuclide and other imaging modalities. *In* Partain CL (ed): Nuclear Magnetic Resonance and Correlative Imaging Modalities. New York, Society of Nuclear Medicine, 1984.
11. Brady TJ, Gebhart MC, Pykett IL, et al: Nuclear magnetic resonance imaging of forearms in healthy volunteers and patients with giant cell tumors of bone. Radiology *144*:549, 1982.
12. Kulkarni MV, Partain CL, Sandler MP, et al: Magnetic resonance imaging: Skeletal applications. JAMA. In press.
13. Kulkarni MV, Patton JA, Price RR: Surface coils: optimization of techniques and clinical applications. AJR *147*:373, 1986.
14. Nidecker AC, Muller S, Ane WP, et al: Extremity bone tumors: evaluation of P-31 magnetic resonance spectroscopy. Radiology *157*:167, 1985.
15. Moon KL, Genant HK, Helms CA, Chafez NI, Crooks LE, Kaufman L: Musculoskeletal applications of nuclear magnetic resonance. Radiology *147*:161, 1983.
16. Kulkarni MV, Sandler MP, Shaff MI, Jones J, Patton JA, Partain CL, James AE, Jr: Clinical magnetic resonance imaging with nuclear medicine correlation. J Nucl Med *26*:944, 1985.
17. Dickinson CZ, Kulkarni MV, Sandler MP, Partain CL, James AE, Jr: Diagnosis of osteomyelitis using multiple modalities. Gallium 67, Indium III labeled granulocytes and magnetic resonance imaging. Proceedings of the Society of Nuclear Medicine, 32nd Annual Meeting, Houston, 1985.
18. Modic MT, Feiglin DH, Piraino DW, Boumphrey F, Weinstein MA, Duchesneau PM, Rehm SA: Vertebral osteomyelitis: assessment using magnetic resonance. Radiology *157*:157, 1985.
19. Modic MT, Weinstein MA, Pavlicek W, Boumphrey F, Starnes D, Duchesneau PM: Magnetic resonance imaging of the cervical spine. AJR *144*:1129, 1983.
20. Kulkarni MV, Kaye JJ, Green NE, Piatt BM, Burks DD, Janco RL, Nance EP: Magnetic resonance imaging of the knee in hemophiliac arthropathy. Proceedings of the 69th Annual Meeting of Scientific Assembly of the Radiological Society of North America, Washington, DC, November 1984.
21. Li KC, Henkelman, Poon PY, Rubenstein J: Magnetic resonance imaging of the normal knee. J Comput Assist Tomogr *8*(6):1147, 1985.

22. Margulis AR: Overview: Current status of clinical magnetic resonance imaging. RadioGraphics *4*:76, 1984.
23. Markisz JA, Kazan E, Knowles RJ, Bottger BA, Shalen JP, Cahill PT: Role of MR imaging in the diagnosis and evaluation of bone disease: Comparison with bone scan, CT and radiographic study. Proceedings of the 70th annual Meetings and Scientific Assembly of the Radiological Society of North America, Chicago, November 1985.
24. Narayana PA, Delayre JA, Misra LK: *In vivo* 31P NMR studies of avian dystrophic muscles. Magn Reson Med. In press.

38

Primary Malignant Bone Tumors*

J. L. BLOEM
R. G. BLUEMM
A. H. M. TAMINIAU
A. T. VAN OOSTEROM
T. H. M. FALKE
J. DOORNBOS

Primary malignant bone tumors, despite the low incidence, are an important entity because they affect mainly young individuals, and the disease has a major influence on life expectancy and quality of remaining life. Treatment has been improved considerably by effective chemotherapy and by modern operative techniques that often allow reconstructive and limb-saving procedures instead of amputation or exarticulation.[1,10–14,17,20,23–25,27,28,31,32,35]

In addition to excluding disseminated disease, three diagnostic procedures are essential for effective treatment:

1. *Tissue characterization.* It is initially made by plain radiographs and always histologically verified by needle or open biopsy prior to therapy. At present, specific preoperative diagnosis is based on conventional radiographs. New imaging techniques, including CT, have not improved specificity.[13,20,23] Since a correct histologic diagnosis is mandatory, a biopsy is always taken. A new modality, in this case MRI, must be competitive not only with plain radiographs but also with biopsy. MRI is limited in its ability to make an accurate specific diagnosis based on quantitative data.[36] As will be shown, MRI is sometimes able to make a specific diagnosis, but this is exceptional.

2. *Local tumor staging.* Especially in patients in whom resection and reconstruction is considered, accurate preoperative tumor staging is essential.[18,24,35] Local tumor staging is the major application of MRI.[3–6] Reconstructive, limb-saving procedures can be performed only when the surgeon is informed in detail about the intra- and extraosseous extension of tumor growth.[3] Because this is a problem only in primary malignant tumors, our discussion will exclude benign and secondary tumors. The accuracy of MRI in staging these tumors, as compared with existing modalities such as CT and angiography, will be discussed.

3. *Monitoring of preoperative chemotherapy.* This is important in order to determine the effect of a certain chemotherapeutic regime and to select the proper time for surgery.[28,33] The purpose of this chapter is to evaluate the potential place of MRI in the diagnostic management of patients with primary malignant bone tumors. Large tumors, depending on their histology, often are initially treated by chemotherapy followed by surgery or radiation therapy.[29] MRI is tested for its ability to monitor the effect of chemotherapy, indicating whether prolongation or cessation of chemotherapy

* Study supported by The Netherlands Cancer Foundation; Grant IKW 8589.

will be of benefit to the patient. Timing of surgery, following chemotherapy, may be facilitated by MRI.[3]

MATERIAL AND METHODS

This report is based on 80 MRI examinations in 53 patients. All patients had primary malignant bone tumors (Table 38–1) and, with the exception of those with chordoma and non-Hodgkin lymphoma, were operated upon. The surgical specimen was used as the gold standard to evaluate the diagnostic preoperative procedures, including MRI (53 patients), CT (53 patients), angiography (12 patients), and Tc–bone scan (16 patients). The prospective data were available for statistical analysis in 24 patients (Table 38–2). Unless otherwise stated, data refer to this prospectively evaluated group.

The group was subdivided into three major anatomic areas: the knee (11 patients), pelvis (6 patients), and shoulder region (6 patients). In one patient the tumor was located in the toe. For each area, tumor extension into bone marrow, cortex, fat, neurovascular bundle, and muscle compartments was predicted. Patients were examined with a 0.15 tesla Philips resistive system (7 patients) or a 0.5 tesla Philips Gyroscan (46 patients).

$T1$ weighted sequences were made by the use of IR (TI 400, TR 1400, TE 50) for the 0.15 tesla resistive system or with SE technique (TR 250–600 ms, TE 30 ms) for the 0.5 tesla system. $T2$ weighted sequences were made by SE technique with long TR and TE (TR 1000–3000 ms, TE 50–200 ms). Gadolinium-DTPA (Gd-DTPA) enhanced studies were performed following intravenous injection of 0.1 to 0.2 mmol Gd per kg of body weight with SE technique TR 250–600 ms and fast field echo (FFE) imaging. Slice thickness is 10 mm for the body coil and 5 or 10 mm for surface coils.[15]

MRI CHARACTERISTICS AND SPECIFICITY

Like most pathologic tissues, primary malignant bone tumors have prolonged $T1$ and $T2$ relaxation times.[4,9,19,36] Therefore, osteolytic tumors have a relatively high signal intensity on $T2$ weighted images and a relatively low signal intensity on $T1$ weighted images (Fig. 38–1, Table 38–3).[3] Because of their low spin density and short $T2$ relaxation time, osteosclerotic components or calcifications within the tumor have a low signal intensity on both $T1$ and $T2$ weighted images (Fig. 38–2, Table 38–3). Small calcifications detected by plain radiographs or CT often cannot be detected by MRI. Necrosis within a tumor can be identified because $T1$ and $T2$ relaxation times are even longer than those of viable tumor (Fig. 38–1).

Edema surrounding a tumor can be diagnosed because it is located outside the pseudocapsule and therefore has fading margins, whereas tumor often has a distinct interface with reactive changes or normal tissue due to this pseudocapsule (Fig. 38–3). Another feature of edema is the slightly different $T2$ relaxation time, allowing differentiation from tumor to be made by looking at signal intensity on a multiple-echo sequence.[4,6]

Table 38–1. MRI OF PRIMARY MALIGNANT BONE TUMOR

53 Patients Undergoing 80 MRI Examinations	
13 osteosarcoma	2 chordoma
17 Ewing sarcoma	1 clear cell sarcoma
9 chondrosarcoma	1 giant cell tumor
3 fibrosarcoma	1 synovial sarcoma
2 non-Hodgkin lymphoma	

Table 38–2. PROSPECTIVE DATA ON 24 PATIENTS WITH PRIMARY BONE MALIGNANCIES

Statistical Analysis (N = 24)

6 osteosarcoma
5 Ewing sarcoma
9 chondrosarcoma
3 fibrosarcoma
1 clear cell sarcoma

Table 38–3. SIGNAL INTENSITY (SI) OF TUMOR RELATIVE TO SI OF BONE MARROW
(N = 23)

	High	Low
T1 weighted:		
Osteolytic tumor	2	12
Sclerotic tumor	—	9
T2 weighted:		
Osteolytic tumor	14	—
Sclerotic tumor	—	9

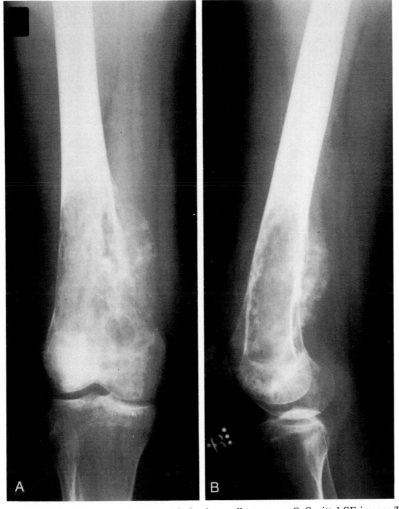

Figure 38–1. *A–B,* Radiograph shows large osteolytic clear cell sarcoma. *C,* Sagittal SE image; *TR* 250, *TE* 30. Bone marrow involvement is conspicuously well shown on this relatively *T1* weighted image owing to high contrast between the low signal intensity of the tumor and the high signal intensity of normal bone marrow.

Illustration continued on following page

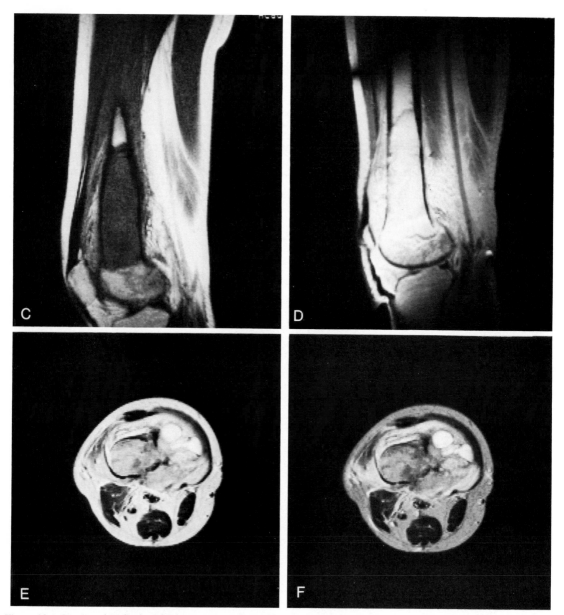

Figure 38-1 *Continued D*, Sagittal SE image; *TR* 1650, *TE* 50. On this relatively *T2* weighted image, the tumor has a high signal intensity, almost identical to that of normal bone marrow. Therefore, marrow involvement is difficult to ascertain with this pulse sequence. *E–F*, Transverse SE images; *TR* 1700, *TE* 50 (*E*) and 100 (*F*). The two areas of necrosis have an even higher signal intensity than viable tumor tissue. (From Bloem JL, et al: RadioGraphics 5:853, 1985. Used by permission.)

In certain cases MRI has limited specificity. The inhomogeneity of the tumor, consisting of viable tumor with different histologic components, necrosis, hemorrhage, and reactive changes, makes it impossible to differentiate histologic types via relaxation times.[30,36] Only three tumors may have a characteristic MRI appearance:

1. *Osteosclerotic osteosarcoma.* Although MRI does not provide more information than plain radiographs do, it can demonstrate the typical sclerotic part of the tumor as a signal void on a combination of *T1* and *T2* weighted images (Fig. 38–2).

2. *Telangiectatic osteosarcoma.* The blood-filled cavity of this tumor may result in areas of high signal intensity on *T1* and *T2* weighted images. This combination sug-

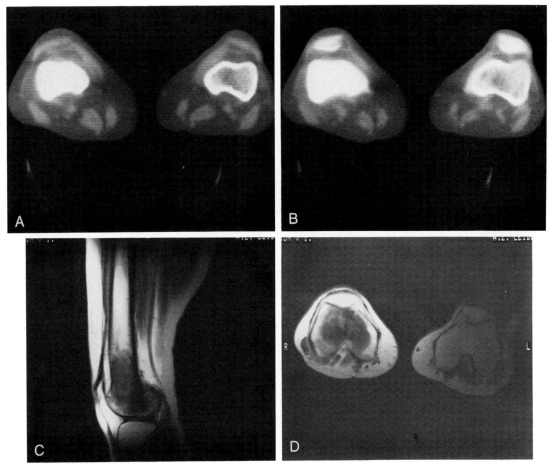

Figure 38–2. Sclerotic osteosarcoma of the distal femur. *A–B*, On CT, the osteosarcoma has the same density as cortical bone. Although no obvious soft tissue extension is seen, involvement of the cortex cannot be excluded. *C*, Sagittal SE image; *TR* 700, *TE* 30. Low signal intensity of tumor demonstrates marrow involvement. Tumor traverses the growth plate. Black line of cortex seems to be intact. *D–F*, Transverse SE images; *TR* 1800, *TE* 50. Heterogeneous low signal intensity of sclerotic tumor is easily differentiated from still lower signal intensity of cortex. *G*, Surgical specimen cut in coronal plane. Cortex was not involved by tumor. (From Bloem JL, et al: RadioGraphics 5:853, 1985. Used by permission.) *Illustration continued on following page*

gests the presence of blood and should bring to mind the diagnosis of telangiectatic osteosarcoma (Fig. 38–4).[2,3] Differential diagnosis includes massive hemorrhage in any other tumor type or benign aneurysmal bone cyst.

3. *Cartilaginous tumor.* The combination of an increased signal intensity relative to fat on *T2* weighted images and the lobulated appearance indicates the presence of noncalcified cartilage (Fig. 38–5). As in telangiectatic osteosarcoma, MRI was often the only modality making a correct histologic diagnosis. Although MRI can diagnose a noncalcified cartilage-containing tumor, it cannot differentiate between chondroma and chondrosarcoma.

LOCAL TUMOR STAGING

Because each anatomic region presents its own specific problems in staging tumors, a subdivision was made in three main areas: the knee, the pelvis, and the shoulder region.

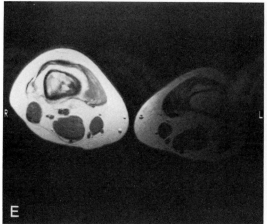

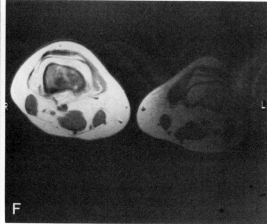

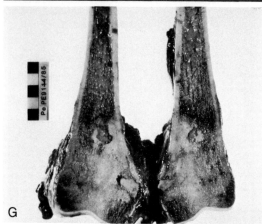

Figure 38–2 *Continued*

Intraosseous Staging

BONE MARROW INVOLVEMENT

Definition of bone marrow involvement is essential in determining the level of amputation or resection. Conventional modalities have some disadvantages.

Radiograph. Bone marrow is not visualized. Only advanced disease in epiphyseal and metaphyseal areas can be detected when bone trabeculae are destroyed.

CT Scan. The transverse imaging plane is a disadvantage in defining tumor extending in a longitudinal plane.[3,6,21,36] A second major disadvantage is the beam-hardening artifact. This is a more serious problem here than in a general CT population because patients with primary malignant bone tumors are usually young people with a high amount of calcium in their bones. Again, destruction of trabeculae is the most important sign.[36]

Tc–Bone Scan. This modality offers the advantage of the ideal imaging plane. However, reactive changes, and especially tumor-related hyperemic osteoporosis, result in increased uptake that is indistinguishable from increased uptake due to presence of tumor.[3] CT and plain radiographs are also unable to diagnose this hyperemic osteopororis (Fig. 38–6).[3]

Magnetic Resonance Imaging. MRI offers some crucial advantages. It is a tomographic modality used in the ideal imaging plane. For extremities, a plane through the long axis of a long bone is chosen—either sagittal or coronal. Sometimes a little

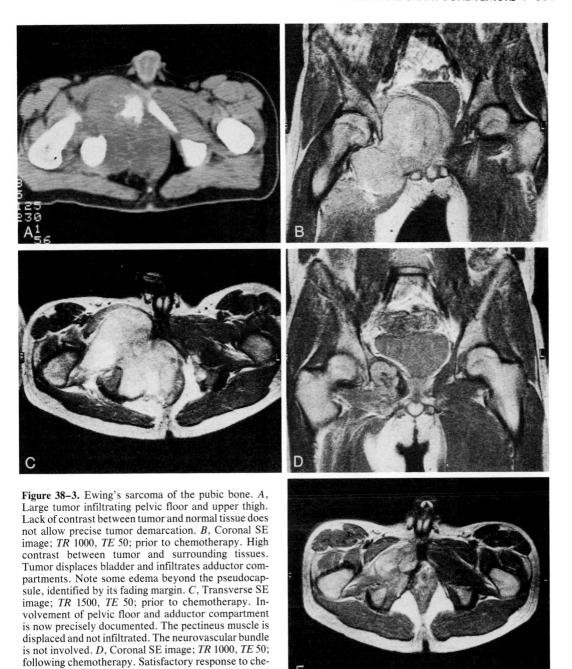

Figure 38–3. Ewing's sarcoma of the pubic bone. *A*, Large tumor infiltrating pelvic floor and upper thigh. Lack of contrast between tumor and normal tissue does not allow precise tumor demarcation. *B*, Coronal SE image; *TR* 1000, *TE* 50; prior to chemotherapy. High contrast between tumor and surrounding tissues. Tumor displaces bladder and infiltrates adductor compartments. Note some edema beyond the pseudocapsule, identified by its fading margin. *C*, Transverse SE image; *TR* 1500, *TE* 50; prior to chemotherapy. Involvement of pelvic floor and adductor compartment is now precisely documented. The pectineus muscle is displaced and not infiltrated. The neurovascular bundle is not involved. *D*, Coronal SE image; *TR* 1000, *TE* 50; following chemotherapy. Satisfactory response to chemotherapy indicated by decrease in tumor volume and signal intensity. *E*, Transverse SE image; *TR* 1500, *TE* 50; following chemotherapy. Decrease in signal intensity is partly caused by calcifications. Owing to decrease in tumor volume, the pectineus muscle is now in its normal position. (From Bloem JL, et al: RadioGraphics 5:853, 1985. Used by permission.)

angulation is needed. Use of surface coils and 5 mm thick slices produces high spatial resolution.[15]

For optimal contrast, *T1* weighted sequences are used because contrast between the low signal intensity of tumor and the high signal intensity of normal bone marrow is highest (see Fig. 38–1).[3,12] Because of the high fat content of bone marrow, normal bone marrow can be directly visualized by MRI and will have, on both *T1* and *T2*

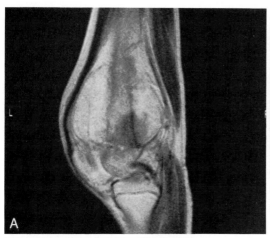
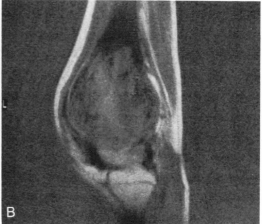
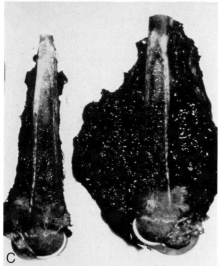

Figure 38–4. Telangiectatic osteosarcoma of the femur. *A*, Sagittal SE image; *TR* 1000, *TE* 50, 0.15 tesla. The osseous part of the tumor as well as the soft tissue extension has a high signal intensity. The femoral artery is displaced posteriorly. The low signal intensity area on the posterior side of the metaphysis represents an osteosclerotic component. *B*, Sagittal IR image; *TI* 400, *TR* 1400, *TE* 50. The central part of the tumor has a relative high signal intensity, indicating short *TI* relaxation time consistent with blood. *C*, Sagittal sliced surgical specimen. Telangiectatic osteosarcoma with large blood-filled cavity and sclerotic component on the posterior side of the metaphysis. (From Bloem JL, et al: RadioGraphics 5:853, 1985. Used by permission.)

weighted sequences, a high signal intensity (see Fig. 38–1). MRI is superior to Tc–bone scanning because tumor-related hyperemic osteoporosis is not depicted on MRI and is therefore not a source of false positive readings (Fig. 38–6).[3] In Tc–bone scanning the difference between predicted tumor length and the real length can be several centimeters in some patients.

The correlation coefficients of CT and MRI by pathologic examination on intraosseous tumor length do not differ among the three anatomic areas. The correlation coefficients for all areas together demonstrate that MRI (correlation coefficient = 0.997, n = 23) is significantly better than CT (correlation coefficient = 0.950) for defining intramedullary tumor extent.

CORTICAL INVOLVEMENT

Destruction of cortical bone is no diagnostic problem, since it can be evaluated on plain radiographs combined with tomography and CT scan. Identical to calcifications, normal cortical bone, because of low spin density and a short *T2* relaxation time, has a low signal intensity on *T1* and *T2* weighted images.

Invasion of cortex by tumor is best shown on *T2* weighted images as a disruption

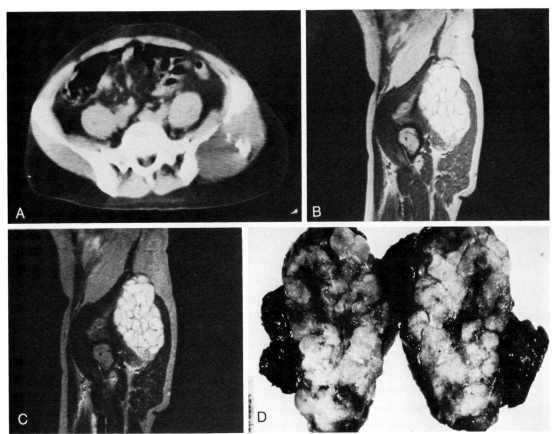

Figure 38–5. *A*, CT scan of chondrosarcoma located in iliac bone and gluteus muscle compartment. *B–C*, Sagittal SE images; *TR* 2700, *TE* 50 (*B*) and 100 (*C*). Lobulated high signal intensity tumor on *T2* weighted images typical of noncalcified cartilage. *D*, Surgical specimen, cut in the sagittal plane, again shows the typical lobulated appearance. (From Bloem JL, et al: RadioGraphics 5:853, 1985. Used by permission.)

of the cortical line and replacement of cortex by high signal intensity of tumor (Figs. 38–7 and 38–8). To evaluate the accuracy of MRI in diagnosis of cortical involvement, cortical bone was divided into four quadrants. In 23 patients 54 quadrants were involved by tumor; the other 38 quadrants were normal. MRI made only one false positive and one false negative diagnosis; CT made five false positive and four false negative diagnoses. MRI is slightly better than CT because the signal intensity of osteosclerotic tumor is still a little brighter than the low signal intensity of normal cortex (see Fig. 38–2). The high density of osteosclerotic tumor and cortex often make them indistinguishable on CT.

Extraosseous Staging

Soft tissue extension in relation to joints, large vessels, and nerves is best evaluated on *T2* weighted images.[3,34] On the *T2* weighted images, contrast between the high signal intensity of tumor and the intermediate to low signal intensity of muscle is optimal (see Figs. 38–1 and 38–8). Contrast between tumor and fat is suboptimal on *T2* weighted images.[3,5,36] If it is important to have a distinct tumor-fat interface in a certain area, *T1* weighted sequences are needed to produce high-contrast images.[3] The transverse plane is usually the most informative for definition of soft tissue extension. Depending

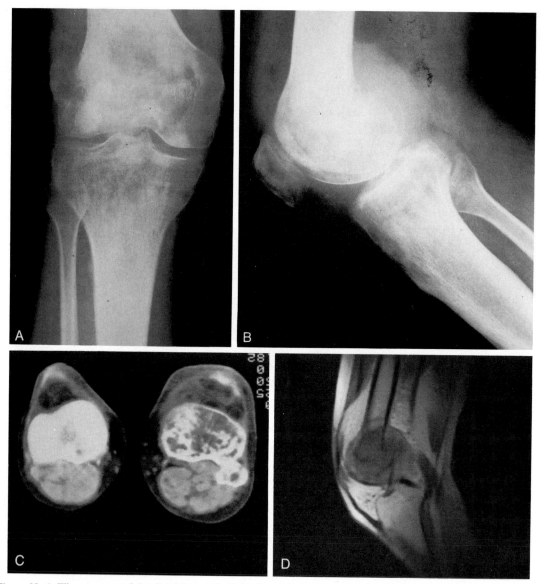

Figure 38–6. Fibrosarcoma of the distal femur. *A–B*, Radiograph shows permeative destruction in the femur caused by tumor. The osteolysis in the tibia can be explained by osteoporosis or tumor. *C*, Osteolytic destruction in the tibia visualized by CT. CT cannot differentiate osteoporosis from tumor. *D*, Sagittal SE image; *TR* 630, *TE* 30; following intravenous administration of GD-DTPA. High signal intensity of tumor located in distal femur is due to enhancement with Gd-DTPA. The anterior cruciate ligament inserts in the tumor. The tibia epiphysis and metaphysis have a normal signal intensity, indicating osteoporosis. This suggests that the abnormality seen on radiographs and CT is caused by osteoporosis, which was confirmed at surgery. (From Bloem JL, et al: RadioGraphics 5:853, 1985. Used by permission.)

on the evaluation of the transverse series and the questions of the surgeon, additional images in sagittal, coronal, or oblique planes are made.

INVOLVEMENT OF MUSCULAR COMPARTMENTS

Muscle Compartments of the Knee. This anatomic area was prospectively evaluated in 11 patients. Muscle compartments were subdivided into eight different units. Twenty compartments were involved by tumor; 68 compartments were not involved. CT made

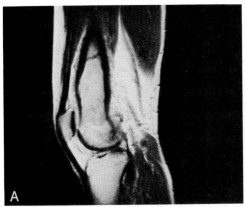
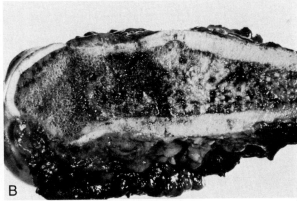

Figure 38–7. Chondrosarcoma of distal femur. *A*, Sagittal SE image; *TR* 1500, *TE* 50. High signal intensity tumor invades anterior cortex. This chondrosarcoma does not display the lobulated appearance. *B*, Surgical specimen cut in the sagittal plane. Tumor invaded cortical bone anteriorly. No soft tissue extension was present. (From Bloem JL, et al: Radio-Graphics 5:853, 1985. Used by permission.)

no false positive diagnoses and four false negative diagnoses. MRI did not make false positive or negative diagnoses (see Fig. 38–8).

Muscle Compartments of the Pelvis. This anatomic area was prospectively evaluated in six patients. Muscle compartments were subdivided into 17 units; 23 compartments were involved by tumor, and 79 compartments were not involved (see Figs. 38–3 and 38–5). CT made four false positive and nine false negative diagnoses. MRI made no false positive and four false negative diagnoses. All four false negative diagnoses by MRI were made in one patient with a Ewing sarcoma. Prior to chemotherapy, the piriform, quadrate, inferior, and superior gemelli muscles were involved by tumor. Following chemotherapy and preoperatively these muscles had a normal appearance on CT and MRI (Fig. 38–9). At pathologic examination, however, these muscles still contained some residual tumor.

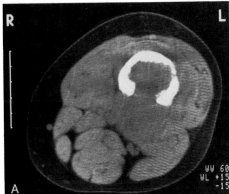
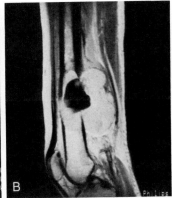
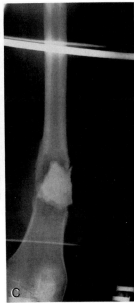

Figure 38–8. Fibrosarcoma of distal femur. *A*, CT scan demonstrates osteolytic tumor with cortical destruction. Although soft tissue extension is seen, precise definition of posterior soft tissue extension is difficult owing to absence of contrast. *B*, Sagittal SE image; *TR* 1050, *TE* 50. Lobulated high signal intensity tumor infiltrates anterior cortex and posterior muscle compartment. The femoral artery is displaced backward. Codman's triangle (elevated periosteum) is seen superior to the tumor. The absence of signal intensity in the center is caused by methacrylate cement, which was left in place following biopsy. *C*, Radiograph taken after biopsy shows fracture and methacrylate cement, which was used to stop the bleeding. (From Bloem JL, et al: RadioGraphics 5:853, 1985. Used by permission.)

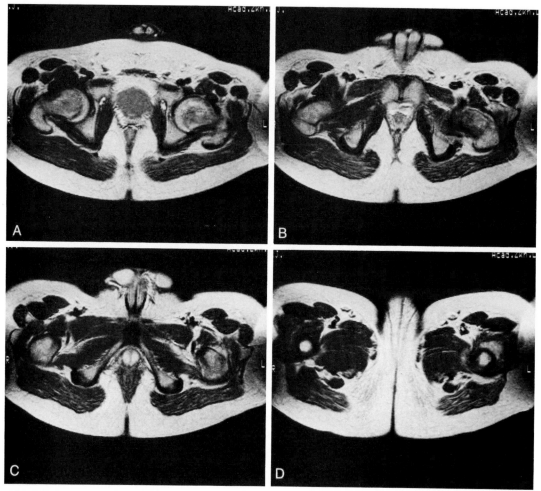

Figure 38–9. Ewing's sarcoma following chemotherapy. *A–C*, Contiguous transverse slices, SE *TR* 1350, *TE* 50. The quadrate and superior gemelli muscles were interpreted as being normal. On closer inspection, however, subtle residual changes are seen at the level of the insertion on the femur. This area contained tumor on pathologic examination. *D*, At the level inferior to the minor trochanter, residual tumor is seen medial and lateral to the femur. (From Bloem JL, et al: RadioGraphics 5:853, 1985. Used by permission.)

Muscle Compartments of the Shoulder Region. Six patients are included in this group. Muscle compartments were subdivided into nine units; 7 compartments were involved, 47 compartments were not involved by tumor. CT made three false positive diagnoses and one false negative diagnosis. MRI made one false positive diagnosis and no false negative diagnoses (Fig. 38–10).

Conclusions. The number of patients in the prospective study is too limited to draw final statistically significant conclusions. A few conclusions, however, can be made.

There do not seem to be differences between the three anatomic areas: knee, pelvis, and shoulder. The prospective study combined with the retrospective analysis of our cases indicates that MRI is more accurate than CT in staging soft tissue extension when *T2* weighted sequences are used.[3–6,36]

Access to preoperative staging modalities was evaluated by asking the staff of orthopedic surgeons how they felt MRI compared with CT with respect to soft tissue extension in the prospectively evaluated group of 24 patients. MRI was believed to be superior to CT in 17 cases and equal to CT in 7 cases. CT was never found to be superior to MRI. The most important advantages for the orthopedic surgeon are the

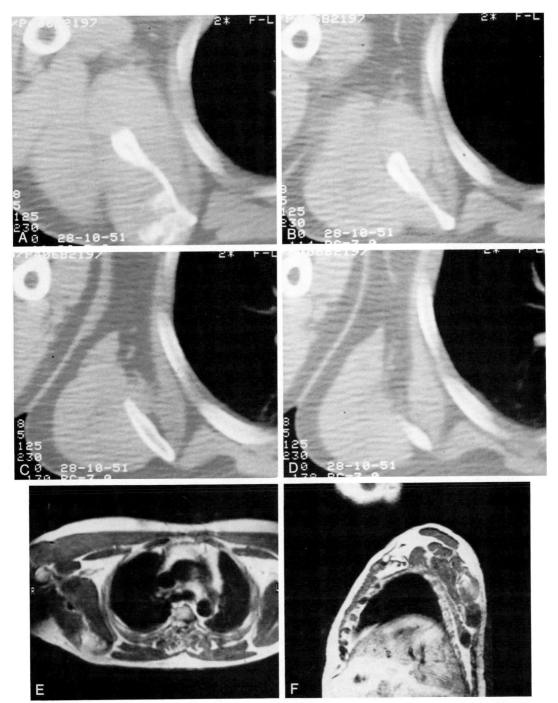

Figure 38–10. Partly calcified chondrosarcoma of the scapula. *A–D,* The calcified tumor is easily depicted on CT, but CT fails to clarify the relation of tumor to the teres major muscle. *E,* Transverse SE image; *TR* 1500, *TE* 50. Tumor invades infraspinatus muscle. *F,* Sagittal SE image; *TR* 1000, *TE* 50. Normal teres major muscle is identified. Tumor invades only infraspinatus muscle. (From Bloem JL, et al: RadioGraphics 5:853, 1985. Used by permission.)

superior contrast resolution between tumor and normal muscle compartments on MRI and the display of tumor anatomy in any desired plane.

VASCULAR INVOLVEMENT

The relation of tumor and neurovascular bundle is easily evaluated on *T2* weighted images because normal flow in a vessel results in low or absent signal intensity, the so-called flow-void phenomenon (Figs. 38–4, 38–8, 38–11, and 38–12).[26] The lumen of the vessel may have a higher signal intensity owing to paradoxical enhancement, or even echo rephasing or turbulence with slow flow caused by compression.[2,6]

Of 12 patients prospectively evaluated by CT, angiography, and MRI, only two had their neurovascular bundles (knee region) involved by tumor. Only one false negative diagnosis was made by CT, which predicted a normal femoral artery. MRI and angiography did not make any errors. The figures of this small group of patients do not suggest large differences in accuracy between MRI, CT, and angiography. All three modalities were unable to differentiate an intimate contact between tumor and vessel from early infiltrative growth in a given case of fixation of tumor to the neurovascular bundle (Figs 38–11 to 38–13). MRI and CT can diagnose only noninvolvement of the neurovascular bundle or possibly, in a given case, obvious involvement of the neurovascular bundle. Retrospective analysis of our total group of patients suggests that CT and MRI provide more information than angiography because large vessels are,

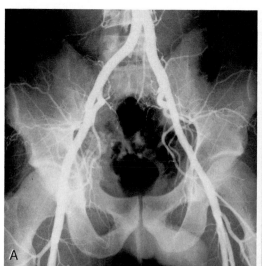

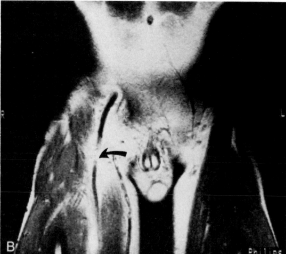

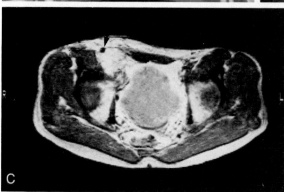

Figure 38–11. Chondrosarcoma of the pelvis. *A*, Tumor calcifications are seen medial to the acetabulum, projecting over the internal iliac artery. The external iliac in the femoral artery is displaced laterally. *B*, Coronal SE image; *TR* 1500, *TE* 50. At the level of the tumor (high signal intensity) the iliac artery is leaving the imaging plane (arrow). The iliac artery superior to the tumor and the femoral artery inferior to the tumor are in the imaging plane, indicating displacement of the femoral artery by tumor. *C*, Transverse SE image; *TR* 1500, *TE* 50. Calcified tumor originating from the pubic bone has a low signal intensity; the noncalcified cartilage has a high signal intensity. The femoral artery is only displaced anteriorly and is not encased by tumor (arrow). (From Bloem JL, et al: RadioGraphics 5:853, 1985. Used by permission.)

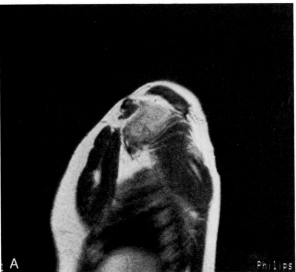
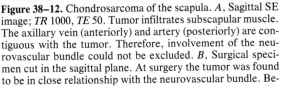
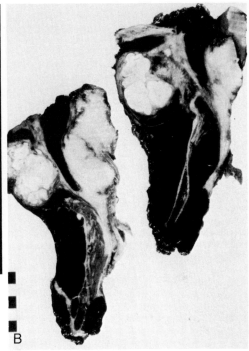

Figure 38–12. Chondrosarcoma of the scapula. *A*, Sagittal SE image; *TR* 1000, *TE* 50. Tumor infiltrates subscapular muscle. The axillary vein (anteriorly) and artery (posteriorly) are contiguous with the tumor. Therefore, involvement of the neurovascular bundle could not be excluded. *B*, Surgical specimen cut in the sagittal plane. At surgery the tumor was found to be in close relationship with the neurovascular bundle. Because the tumor was not fixed to the neurovascular bundle, a resection could be performed. (From Bloem JL, et al: RadioGraphics 5:853, 1985. Used by permission.)

especially with MRI, visualized in relation to the tumor. Angiography seldom produces additional information and thus is rarely indicated as a staging procedure.

Because of superior contrast and optimal imaging planes, especially sagittal and sometimes coronal planes, MRI is, as the only modality that does not need iodinated contrast material, the ideal staging modality for the orthopedic surgeon. The surgeons were of opinion that MRI was superior to CT in 10 patients and equal to CT in 14 cases, and never was CT found to be superior to MRI.

JOINT INVOLVEMENT

Joint involvement is more accurately demonstrated on *T2* weighted images than on CT, because the articular surfaces are often parallel to the axial CT plane (see Fig. 38–4). For the knee and hip, coronal and sagittal images are most informative. The shoulder joint is best evaluated on a combination of transverse planes and slices made sagittal or oblique sagittal perpendicular to the glenoid.[22] Joint effusion with or without hemorrhage, often a secondary sign of a contaminated joint, is well seen on *T1* and *T2* weighted images (see Fig. 38–4).

CHEMOTHERAPY

In eight patients the effect of chemotherapy was monitored by CT and MRI. Two or three CT and MRI examinations were performed prior to chemotherapy and, following chemotherapy, prior to surgery. Pathology includes osteosarcoma (three patients), Ewing sarcoma (four patients), clear cell sarcoma (one patient), and fibrosar-

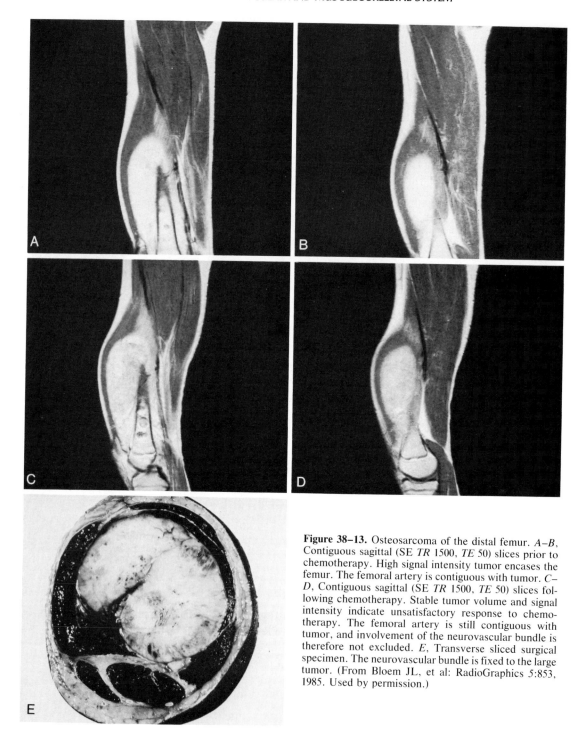

Figure 38–13. Osteosarcoma of the distal femur. *A–B,* Contiguous sagittal (SE *TR* 1500, *TE* 50) slices prior to chemotherapy. High signal intensity tumor encases the femur. The femoral artery is contiguous with tumor. *C–D,* Contiguous sagittal (SE *TR* 1500, *TE* 50) slices following chemotherapy. Stable tumor volume and signal intensity indicate unsatisfactory response to chemotherapy. The femoral artery is still contiguous with tumor, and involvement of the neurovascular bundle is therefore not excluded. *E,* Transverse sliced surgical specimen. The neurovascular bundle is fixed to the large tumor. (From Bloem JL, et al: RadioGraphics *5:*853, 1985. Used by permission.)

coma (one patient). Two tumors, one osteosarcoma and one Ewing sarcoma, did not respond and had a larger stable tumor volume in a given case. In these two patients the signal intensity did not change on *T2* weighted images (Fig. 38–13).

In the six patients in whom tumor volume decreased following chemotherapy, a change of signal intensity was observed (Figs. 38–4 and 38–14). In four patients a decrease of signal intensity on *T2* weighted sequences occurred probably because of

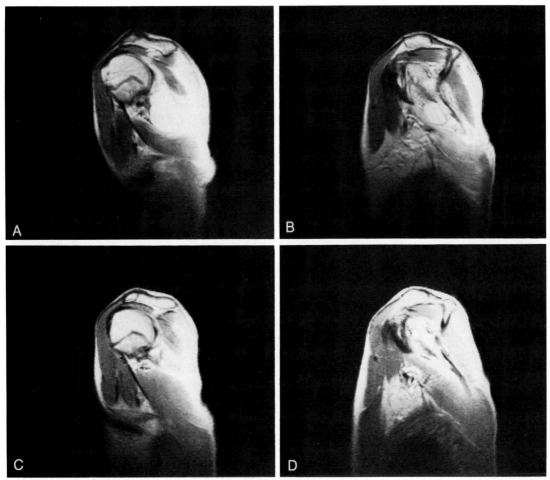

Figure 38–14. Fibrosarcoma of the scapula. *A–B*, Contiguous sagittal slices prior to chemotherapy; SE *TR* 1950, *TE* 50. Tumor extends into axillary fossa and displaces subscapular and teres major muscles. *C–D*, Contiguous sagittal slices following chemotherapy; SE *TR* 1950, *TE* 50. Satisfactory response to chemotherapy. Only minor residual changes are seen. The axillary fossa is now free of tumor. (From Bloem JL, et al: RadioGraphics 5:853, 1985. Used by permission.)

calcifications, dehydration, and fibrosis. In two patients a high increase in signal intensity was seen, caused by necrosis and hemorrhage in the tumor (see Fig. 38–1). These changes of signal intensity can occur earlier than decrease of tumor volume.[3] Accumulation of cis-platinum within the tumor influences the relaxation times only slightly, and this cannot account for the observed changes following chemotherapy.[3]

Although more research is needed in this field, these preliminary results suggest that MRI can monitor chemotherapy by looking at signal intensity of the tumor and changes of tumor volume. Because changes of signal intensity and therefore relaxation times, especially *T2*, reflect early changes within the tumor, this may be useful to indicate early response to chemotherapy.

NEW DEVELOPMENTS

Gadolinium-DTPA enhanced conventional and dynamic (FFE) MRI of primary malignant bone tumors is an area of current development. In neuroradiology the use of a paramagnetic chelate, such as Gd-DTPA, has proved to be safe and to extend the diagnostic capabilities of MRI.[16] Therefore, it was of interest to gain experience concerning the relative merits of administering this contrast agent intravenously in patients with primary malignant bone tumors.[7]

Methods. SE *TR* 500–600/*TE* 30 images pre- and 5 minutes post contrast following 0.1 to 0.2 mmol per kg body weight intravenous administration of Gd-DTPA were compared to *T2* weighted dual-echo SE scans. In eight cases we performed dynamic MRI by applying so-called fast field echo imaging (FFE)[8] (see also Chapter 42). A programmable sequence of up to 16 slices, 10 to 15 mm thick, with a matrix size of 128 × 128 was used. The minimal time interval between two fast scans was 0.15 sec-

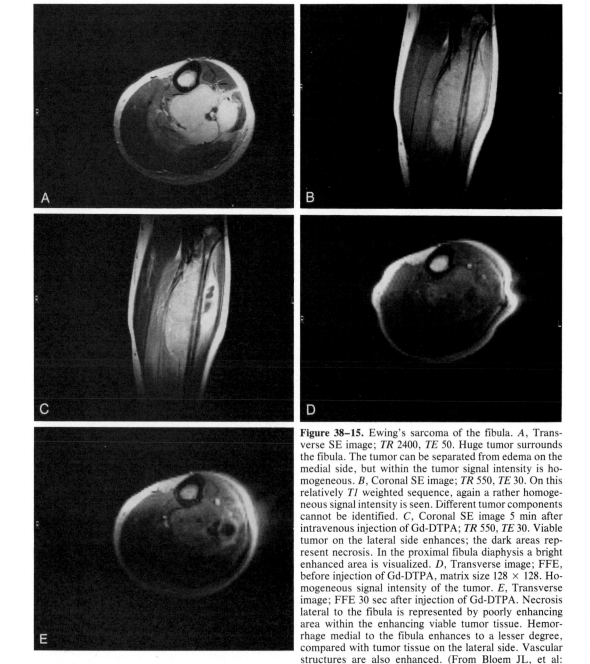

Figure 38–15. Ewing's sarcoma of the fibula. *A*, Transverse SE image; *TR* 2400, *TE* 50. Huge tumor surrounds the fibula. The tumor can be separated from edema on the medial side, but within the tumor signal intensity is homogeneous. *B*, Coronal SE image; *TR* 550, *TE* 30. On this relatively *T1* weighted sequence, again a rather homogeneous signal intensity is seen. Different tumor components cannot be identified. *C*, Coronal SE image 5 min after intravenous injection of Gd-DTPA; *TR* 550, *TE* 30. Viable tumor on the lateral side enhances; the dark areas represent necrosis. In the proximal fibula diaphysis a bright enhanced area is visualized. *D*, Transverse image; FFE, before injection of Gd-DTPA, matrix size 128 × 128. Homogeneous signal intensity of the tumor. *E*, Transverse image; FFE 30 sec after injection of Gd-DTPA. Necrosis lateral to the fibula is represented by poorly enhancing area within the enhancing viable tumor tissue. Hemorrhage medial to the fibula enhances to a lesser degree, compared with tumor tissue on the lateral side. Vascular structures are also enhanced. (From Bloem JL, et al: RadioGraphics 5:853, 1985. Used by permission.)

onds. Thus a dynamic imaging sequence, monitoring the first three to four minutes following the bolus injection of Gd-DTPA, can be obtained (Fig. 38–15).

Preliminary Results. Gd-DTPA enhances viable tumor, resulting in a high signal intensity on $T1$ weighted images owing to a shortened $T1$ relaxation time (Figs. 38–15 and 38–16).[16] In all 12 tumors examined with Gd-DTPA, a relative increase of signal intensity of 40 to 180 percent has been found as compared with nonenhanced $T1$ weighted images. This enhancement of viable tumor adds dynamic information that

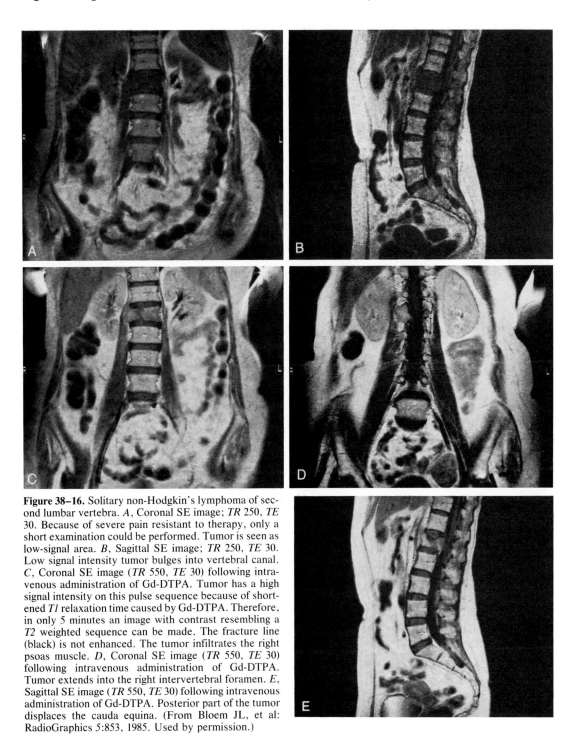

Figure 38–16. Solitary non-Hodgkin's lymphoma of second lumbar vertebra. *A*, Coronal SE image; *TR* 250, *TE* 30. Because of severe pain resistant to therapy, only a short examination could be performed. Tumor is seen as low-signal area. *B*, Sagittal SE image; *TR* 250, *TE* 30. Low signal intensity tumor bulges into vertebral canal. *C*, Coronal SE image (*TR* 550, *TE* 30) following intravenous administration of Gd-DTPA. Tumor has a high signal intensity on this pulse sequence because of shortened *T1* relaxation time caused by Gd-DTPA. Therefore, in only 5 minutes an image with contrast resembling a *T2* weighted sequence can be made. The fracture line (black) is not enhanced. The tumor infiltrates the right psoas muscle. *D*, Coronal SE image (*TR* 550, *TE* 30) following intravenous administration of Gd-DTPA. Tumor extends into the right intervertebral foramen. *E*, Sagittal SE image (*TR* 550, *TE* 30) following intravenous administration of Gd-DTPA. Posterior part of the tumor displaces the cauda equina. (From Bloem JL, et al: RadioGraphics 5:853, 1985. Used by permission.)

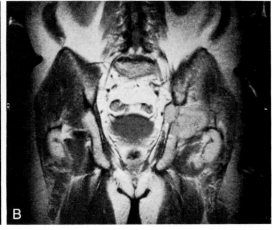

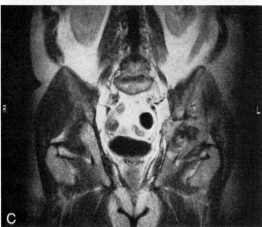

Figure 38–17. Osteosarcoma of the pelvis with large cartilaginous part. *A*, Coronal SE image; *TR* 550, *TE* 30; matrix size 128 × 128. Low signal intensity of the tumor. Differentiation of the two main histologic components of the tumor is not possible. *B*, Coronal SE image; *TR* 1400, *TE* 50. On this more *T2* weighted image, the tumor has a homogeneous high signal intensity. Again, no differentiation between the two histologic components of the tumor can be made. *C*, Coronal SE image (*TR* 550, *TE* 30) following intravenous administration of Gd-DTPA. Two minutes after injection, the bladder is not yet filled with Gd-DTPA. The periphery of the tumor, consisting of osteosarcomatous tissue, has a high signal intensity owing to Gd-DTPA uptake. The central cartilaginous part is not enhanced. Thus, the two components can be identified because of different enhancement patterns. (From Bloem JL, et al: RadioGraphics 5:853, 1985. Used by permission.)

may be able to differentiate certain histologic tumor components (Fig. 38–17). In contrast to the situation with brain tumors, Gd-DTPA seems to accumulate to a lesser degree in perifocal edema.[16] Gd-DTPA enhanced MRI may thus surpass CT in providing information on tumor perfusion, facilitating both tumor staging and determination of the proper site for biopsy.[7]

An additional advantage of conventional Gd-DTPA enhanced imaging, and especially of Gd-DTPA enhanced FFE imaging, is the ability to obtain images that contain *T2* information resulting in high signal intensity of tumor, using short (*TR* 600, *TE* 30 or FFE) pulse sequences. Because of the consequent high S/N ratio, a surface coil is not necessary (see Fig. 38–16). These two factors shorten examination time considerably, which may be advantageous in scanning moving objects, such as the thoracic wall. The examination time for patients who are experiencing severe pain can be reduced to a minimum (see Fig. 38–16).

IMPACT OF MRI ON MANAGEMENT OF PATIENTS WITH PRIMARY MALIGNANT BONE TUMORS

From a radiologic standpoint MRI should be the first procedure in local staging of primary malignant bone tumors because it is the only procedure without side effects (i.e., noninvasive, noniodinated contrast material) and provides the greatest information on intra- and extraosseous tumor extension. CT and angiography together yield less information. In the total work-up other diagnostic procedures, such as plain radiograph and Tc–bone scan, lung tomography, and CT scan of the chest, are, of course, still mandatory for diagnosis of disseminated disease.

An obvious but important question, in addition to the above-mentioned radiologic opinion, is, "How important is MRI for the orthopedic surgeon in planning and executing therapeutic strategies?"

On the question of how surgeons felt that MRI influenced therapy, the following answers were given: MRI was superior to CT in 12 patients; MRI was never found to be inferior to CT. MRI was found to be superior to angiography in all 12 cases in which angiography was performed. For defining intramedullary extension, MRI was superior to Tc–bone scan in 13 patients and was equal to Tc–bone scan in 11 patients. Never was Tc–bone scan superior to MRI. In this group of 24 patients, one exarticulation and four amputations were performed. In 19 patients, resections with reconstructive procedures were performed. Thirteen patients were treated with chemotherapy prior to operation.

The results of retrospective and prospective analysis and the figures of the questionnaire suggest that MRI is the superior modality in local staging of patients with primary malignant bone tumors.[3,36] In addition, access to this information for the orthopedic surgeon is higher with MRI than with any other modality. The introduction of MRI as the first diagnostic procedure in staging primary malignant bone tumors is also beneficial to the patient because it is fast, noninvasive, and comfortable compared with the combination of CT and angiography.

In our group of patients, claustrophobia was a minor problem (1 percent). A larger problem, often mistaken for claustrophobia, is pain, which may be severe enough to obstruct the examination seriously. These patients can be helped by shortening the examination time with the aid of intravenous administration of Gd-DTPA.

ACKNOWLEDGMENTS

The authors wish to thank J. Stolk, Ph.D.; L. Papapoulou, M.D.; W. van der Eyken, M.D.; and S. de Lange, M.D., for their valuable assistance, and Mrs. F. H. Noorderijk for preparing the manuscript. Gd-DTPA was kindly supplied by Schering.

References

1. Apple JS, Martinez S, Nelson PA, Rosenberg ER, Harrelson JM, Bowie JD. Sonographic correlation in extremity soft tissue masses. Noninvas Med Imag *1*:75, 1984.
2. Berquist TH: Magnetic resonance imaging—preliminary experience in orthopedic radiology. Magn Reson Imag *2*:41, 1984.
3. Bloem JL, Falke THM, Taminiau AHM, Van Oosterom AT, Steiner RM, Overbosch EH, Ziedses des Plantes BG Jr: Magnetic resonance imaging of primary malignant bone tumors. RadioGraphics *5*(6):853, 1985.
4. Bloem JL, Bluemm RG, Falke THM, Taminiau AHM, Van Oosterom AT, Doornbos J: MR imaging in staging primary malignant bone tumors (SS). Radiology *157*(P):110, 1985.
5. Bloem JL, Bluemm RG, Falke THM, Taminiau AHM, Van Oosterom AT: MR imaging in staging primary malignant bone tumors: prospective study (SE). Radiology *157*(P):363, 1985.
6. Bloem JL, Falke THM, Taminiau AHM, Van Oosterom AT, Doornbos J: Magnetic resonance imaging of primary malignant bone tumors. Proceedings, European Society of Magnetic Resonance in Medicine and Biology (ed: Dr. M.-A. Hopf), 1985; pp 208–219.
7. Bluemm RG, Bloem JL, Doornbos J, Claus W, Taminiau AHM, Van Oosterom AT: Gadolinium DTPA–enhanced MR imaging of malignant bone tumors: initial experience (WIP). Radiology *157*(P):341, 1985.
8. Bluemm RG, Doornbos J, Van der Meulen P, Cuppen J, Claus W: First clinical results of fast field echo (FFE) MR imaging: a very fast imaging technique (WIP). Radiology *157*(P):335, 1985.
9. Brady TJ, Gebhardt MC, Pykett IL, et al: Imaging of forearms in healthy volunteers and patients with giant cell tumor of bone. Radiology *144*:549, 1982.
10. Brady TJ, Rosen BR, Pykett IL, McGuire MH, Mankin HJ, Rosenthal DI: NMR imaging of leg tumors. Radiology *149*:181, 1983.

11. Campbell CJ: Place of resection in the management of primary bone tumors. Can J Surg 6:518, 1977.
12. Cohen MD, Klatte EC, Baehner R, Smith JA, Martin-Simmerman P, et al: Magnetic resonance imaging of bone marrow disease in children. Radiology 151:715, 1984.
13. De Santos LA, Goldstein HM, Murray JA, Wallace S: Computed tomography in the evaluation of musculoskeletal neoplasms. Radiology 131:431, 1979.
14. Destouet JM, Gilula LA, Murphy WA: Computed tomography of long-bone osteosarcoma. Radiology 131:439, 1979.
15. Doornbos J, Grimbergen HAA, Booijen PE, Te Strake L, Bloem JL, Vielvoye GJ, Boskamp E: Application of anatomically shaped surface coils in MRI at 0.5 T. Magn Reson Med 3:270, 1986.
16. Felix R, Schorner W, Laniado M, Niendorf H, Claussen C, Fiegler W, Speck U: Brain tumors: MR imaging with gadolinium-DTPA. Radiology 156:681, 1985.
17. Fortner JG, Kim DK, Shin MH: Limb preserving vascular surgery for malignant tumors of the lower extremity. Arch Surg 112:391, 1977.
18. Genant HK, Cann CE, Dalinka MK, De Smet AA, Henrix R: Musculoskeletal radiology. Invest Radiol 19:530, 1984.
19. Goldsmith M, Koutcher JA, Damadian R: NMR in cancer XIII. Application of the NMR malignancy index to human mammary tumors. Br J Cancer 38:547, 1978.
20. Heelan RT, Caird Watson R, Smith J: Computed tomography of lower extremity tumors. AJR 132:933, 1979.
21. Jones ET, Kuhns LR, Arbor A: Pitfalls in the use of computed tomography for musculoskeletal tumors in children. J Bone Joint Surg 63a(8):1297, 1981.
22. Kieft G, Bloem JL, Obermann WO, Rosing P, Verbout A: Normal shoulder: MR imaging. Radiology 159:741, 1986.
23. Levine E, Lee KR, Neff JR, Maklad NF, Robeson RG, Preston DF: Comparison of computed tomography and other imaging modalities in the evaluation of musculoskeletal tumors. Radiology 131:431, 1979.
24. Lukens JA, McLeod RA, Sim FH: Computed tomographic evaluation of primary osseous malignant neoplasms. AJR 139:45, 1982.
25. Miller TR: Surgical management of malignant bone tumors. Can J Surg 20:513, 1977.
26. Mills CM, Brant-Zawadzki M, Crooks LE, et al: Nuclear magnetic resonance: principles of blood flow imaging. AJR 142:165, 1984.
27. Moon KL, Genant HK, Helms CA, Chafetz NI, Crooks LE, Kaufman L: Musculoskeletal applications of nuclear magnetic resonance. Radiology 147:161, 1983.
28. Morton DL, Eilber FR, Townsend CM, Grant TT, Mirra J, Weisdenburger TH: Limb salvage from a multidisciplinary treatment approach for the skeletal and soft tissue sarcomas of the extremity. Ann Surg 184:268, 1976.
29. Ramsey RG, Zacharias CE: MR imaging of the spine after radiation therapy: easily recognizable effects. AJR 144:1131, 1985.
30. Reiser M, Rupp N, Biehl Th, Allgayer B, Heller HJ, Lukas P, Fink U: MR in the diagnosis of bone tumours. Eur J Radiol 5:1, 1985.
31. Rosen G, Surwasirikul S, Kwon C, Tan C, Wu SJ, Beattie EJ, Murphy ML: High dose methotrexate with citrovorum factor–rescue Adriamycin in childhood osteogenic sarcoma. Cancer 33:1151, 1975
32. Simon MA, Enneking WF: The management of soft tissue sarcomas of the extremities. J Bone Joint Surg (A) 58:317, 1976.
33. Smith J, Heelan RT, Huvos AG, Caparros B, Rosen G, et al: Radiographic changes in primary osteogenic sarcoma following intensive chemotherapy: radiological-pathological correlation in 63 patients. Radiology 143:355, 1983.
34. Weekes RG, Berquist TH, McLeod RA, Zimmer WD: Magnetic resonance imaging of soft-tissue tumors: comparison with computed tomography. Magn Reson Imag 3:345, 1985.
35. Yiu-Chiu V, Chiu L: Multiple imaging modalities in the evaluation of musculoskeletal masses. J Comput Assist Tomogr 6:201, 1982.
36. Zimmer WD, Berquist TH, McLeod RA, et al: Bone tumors: Magnetic resonance imaging versus computed tomography. Radiology 155:709, 1985.

IX

CLINICAL EXPERIENCE: SPECIAL APPLICATIONS OF MRI AND GUIDELINES

39

Practical Pediatric MRI

BRIAN D. FELLMETH
RICHARD M. HELLER
C. LEON PARTAIN

Magnetic resonance imaging (MRI) in children is an ideal imaging modality for selected clinical problems.[1] Initial enthusiasm for pediatric MRI was restrained because of the requirement for prolonged scanning times with perfect immobility. This concern is rapidly disappearing owing to the recent development of fast scan techniques (see also Chapter 96).[69,70] We recommend the following sedation scheme, which was devised by Dr. Robert Kaufman and his colleagues at the Cincinnati Children's Hospital.

1. Under the age of ten weeks—drugs usually not needed. A feeding just prior to the scan and a quiet, darkened scanning environment will usually provide the desired result.

2. Under the age of two years—chloral hydrate, 50 mg per kg. Supplement 25 to 50 mg/kg orally PRN.

3. Older child—intravenous pentobarbital (Nembutal), 2 mg per kg. Add as necessary to maximum dosage of 9 or 10 mg per kg. Fentanyl, 1 μg per kg titrated (IV), in addition to Nembutal, is used to put the child to sleep when the sedation is not adequate.

4. Older child alternative—intramuscular Nembutal 6 mg per kg under 15 kg, 5 mg per kg over 15 kg. This is useful when there is no concern about the timing of sedation and is especially useful if oral contrast is needed.

With sedation of the child, monitoring of vital signs becomes a very important function. At the beginning of our pediatric MRI experience we simply placed on the precordium an inverted paper cup that was observed to rise and fall as the patient breathed. At the present time, a pneumatic tube system is used for respiratory monitoring and also for respiratory gating. Doppler probes can be used to record blood pressure and heart rate.

PRACTICAL TECHNICAL CONSIDERATIONS

A useful principle to employ is that image resolution can be improved by utilization of the smallest coil into which the anatomic part will fit. For example, the extremities of a child can always be studied in a head coil, and, with smaller children, the head coil can be utilized to study the chest and abdomen.

Resolution of thoracic and upper abdominal structures is improved with respiratory gating, and studies of the heart require cardiac gating.

Prior to initiating the scan, the plain radiographs, CT, any contrast studies, or any nuclear medicine procedures are reviewed, and a clear-cut objective of the MRI study is decided upon. We have found that without such prior planning the studies tend to become interminable.

CLINICAL RESULTS

The following is a survey, organized by anatomic region, of our clinical results at Vanderbilt Children's Medical Center. We have emphasized cases in which MRI made a major or unique contribution to the diagnostic evaluation. Pediatric CNS disease is included, and additional information on pediatric neuro-MRI can be found in the general CNS discussions. Cardiac MRI is not addressed, as a detailed discussion can be found in Chapters 23, 24, 25 and 80.

Head

MRI has had its major impact in pediatrics through imaging CNS disease, as in adult medicine. In fact, when compared with CT, MRI is particularly advantageous for evaluating children. Most childhood brain tumors occur in the posterior fossa, where CT is weak. The tumors that are sometimes missed by MRI, such as meningioma, acoustic neuroma, and pituitary adenoma, are rare in children. Further, the absence of ionizing radiation is especially welcome for the young patient.

IMAGING STRATEGY

While CT of the head can run efficiently on autopilot using present protocols, MRI requires constant physician supervision to assure that the optimal sequences are performed and that precious instrument time is not wasted on low-yield collections. Good MRI practice requires that all brain abnormalities be imaged with both *T1* and *T2* weighted sequences and at least two planes be used for a complete study. The *T1* weighted image is required to detect fat or subacute hemorrhage within a tumor as bright areas,[2] and it usually provides the best demonstration of the relationship between an abnormality and the adjacent CSF spaces (cisterns and ventricles).[3] It may also resolve tumor from adjacent brain edema, both of which may be equally bright on *T2* sequences.

T2 weighted sequences take longer to perform and are noisier, but they have exquisite sensitivity and are needed to detect subtle lesions that may be missed on *T1* or proton-density images.[4,5]

Sequence Selection

At Vanderbilt Medical Center, we have found the following strategy to be a reasonable compromise between maximizing throughput and performing adequate studies. All initial studies begin with a 15-slice, 9 mm multiecho axial collection covering the area from the odontoid to the vertex. Two echoes are collected simultaneously: 32/3000 and 64/3000 (or 100/3000). This collection takes about 15 minutes. The first echo (32/3000) is a balanced image with a mixture of *T1*, *T2*, and proton density contrast with good anatomic detail. The second echo (64/3000 or 100/3000) provides the high sensitivity of *T2* weighting. The MRI physician then immediately reviews the images. If they are normal, additional sequences have a low yield and the study is thus terminated. (*Exception:* If there is strong evidence of temporal lobe disease, a coronal, heavy *T2* image through the temporal lobes will be required in addition.)

When an abnormality is detected on the initial sequences, one of two strategies is employed to fulfill the foregoing criteria. If the abnormality is complex and heterogeneous, an axial inversion-recovery sequence is performed for strong *T1* weighting and excellent anatomic detail. A sequence in a second plane is then collected. The coronal plane is selected for supratentorial lesions, whereas the sagittal plane is better for infratentorial lesions. The pulse sequence selected is the one that best demonstrates the abnormality on the axial slices. Typically, this is a triple echo (for very strong $T2$ weighting), five-slice sequence confined to the abnormal area, but a moderately $T1$ weighted spin-echo sequence (e.g., 32/500) is much faster and can be used if the inversion-recovery sequence showed that $T1$ contrast depicted the pathology well. In the case of complex, puzzling lesions or lesions that will require complex surgery, the third plane is imaged as well.

The alternative strategy is much quicker and is used when the abnormality is relatively simple (i.e., a small, homogeneous mass). After the initial two-echo scanning sequences, the second plane is imaged with the rapid, moderately $T1$ weighted 32/500 sequence. This saves considerable time by providing the $T1$ information and a second plane simultaneously. These two strategies are summarized in Table 39–1.

For follow-up scans, the strategy is different. The most recent MRI study is reviewed, and the plane and sequence that best demonstrates the abnormality is repeated exactly. Occasionally, it is necessary to repeat more than one plane or sequence. It is very difficult to interpret subtle interval changes unless the sequence is repeated exactly.

Special Considerations in Infant Brains. Two changes occur in the developing brain that affect the appearance of $T1$ weighted images of young children. First, after birth, there is a gradual shortening of the $T1$ of both gray and white matter as the brain matures. This is probably due to the increased water content of neonatal brain tissue.[6,7] Dubowitz et al.[8] have recommended lengthening the TR and TI when performing inversion-recovery collections in young children in order to compensate for this effect.

While the $T1$'s of both gray and white matter are shortening with age, they also change with respect to each other. In the normal adult, a strong $T1$ image shows clear contrast between gray and white matter, with the latter more intense. This is presumably due to the increased lipid content of myelinated white matter, which lengthens the $T1$. The unmyelinated newborn brain has a different $T1$ appearance, with the white matter tracts hypointense to gray matter.[7,8] As myelination proceeds, the white matter will

Table 39–1. SEQUENCES USED TO CHARACTERIZE A PEDIATRIC HEAD ABNORMALITY

	Collection Number	Plane	Sequence	Weighting
Complex lesion (approx 90 min)	1	Axial	32/3000, 64/3000 Multiecho	Balanced, $T2$
	2	Axial	32/400/1800 Inversion recovery*	Strong $T1$
	3	Coronal (if supratentorial)	Triple echo	Strong $T2$
		or Sagittal (if infratentorial)	or 32/500 Spin echo	$T1$
	4	Third plane (if needed)	(Fastest sequence that shows lesion)	
Simple lesion (approx. 30 min)	1	Axial	32/3000, 64/3000 Multiecho	Balanced, $T2$
	2	Coronal (if supratentorial) or Sagittal (if infratentorial)	32/500 Spin echo	$T1$

* TI and TR values are lengthened in very young children.[8]

progress through an isointense stage to assume the adult pattern. This process begins in the internal capsule, where increased *T1* signal becomes visible as early as age two weeks. The corpus callosum and periventricular white matter are visually myelinated by age one year, and the process is virtually complete by age two years, when cortical radiations become bright.[6-8] It is possible for an infant under age two years to have central white matter hyperintense to gray matter with immature cortical white matter hypointense to gray matter, and this appearance should not be mistaken for disease. This phenomenon is less apparent on *T2* weighted images, in which normal gray matter has slightly greater intensity at all ages.[6,9]

Illustrative Cases

We have selected cases that demonstrate the special advantages of MRI vis-à-vis CT of the head.

Tumors

Most brain tumors encountered in the pediatric population have the same general signal characteristics, with both long *T1* and long *T2* relaxation.[4,10] MRI is exquisitely sensitive to tumor detection, which approaches 100 percent if good-quality *T2* images are obtained.[11] Sensitivity is superior to that of CT,[5] but it is not yet clear whether MRI will offer enough specificity to make "tissue diagnoses."

Figure 39–1 is a typical example. The patient is a 10-year-old with new seizures and cranial neuropathies. A CT scan failed to detect an abnormality in the brainstem even with double-dose contrast enhancement (Fig. 39–1A). On MRI (Fig. 39–1B–D) the tumor, a pontine glioma, is obvious. The *T2* image (Fig. 39–1B) shows the extent of the tumor most clearly, while the *T1* images (Fig. 39–1C–D) best demonstrates the relationship of the tumor to the fourth ventricle.

In inoperable tumors, MRI is ideally suited to monitor the effects of chemotherapy and radiation. Figure 39–2 documents an excellent response to therapy on another brainstem glioma. Should the appearance of the tumor not improve, MRI provides adequate evidence for abandoning the therapy and substituting another regimen.

Figures 39–1 and 39–2 show the value of sagittal images for infratentorial lesions. Figure 39–3 is a typical example of a supratentorial mass that is best appreciated in the coronal plane. This is a chiasm glioma in a child with neurofibromatosis. The coronal slice (Fig. 39–3C) defines the relationship of the mass to the suprasellar cistern and the lateral ventricles, localizing it to the chiasm. MRI is efficacious in evaluating the optic nerves and chiasm.[12,13]

Two frequent limitations of CT are the inability to distinguish tumor from adjacent brain edema and recurrent tumor from postsurgical or radiation changes. Edematous brain exhibits long *T1* and *T2* values, which unfortunately mimic tumor and makes this distinction also difficult on MRI. However, by careful study of multiple pulse sequences, tumors can often be convincingly separated from edema. In Figure 39–3C, for example, tumor and adjacent edema are difficult to separate on the *T2* image, where they both appear bright. The *T1* image (Fig. 39–3A) clearly shows the tumor as a well-defined hypointense mass, whereas the edematous brain is isointense to normal brain and is easily separated.

Postoperative scarring and radiation also appear as areas of lengthened *T2*. The shape of the increased signal area and the pattern of mass effect can be used to help differentiate these from recurrent tumor. Recurrent tumor in a postoperative ependymoma patient (Fig. 39–4) was strongly suspected because of the mass effect and the fact that the bulk of the *T2* signal was located away from the area of surgical manipulation.

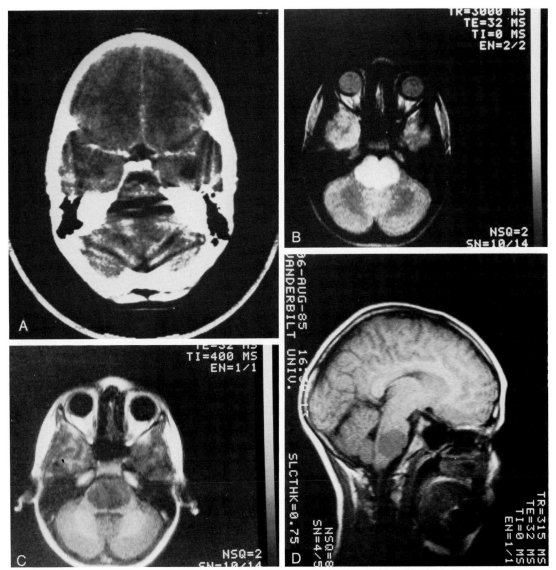

Figure 39–1. Pontine glioma. *A*, Double-dose contrast-enhanced (2 ml per kg) CT slice through the level of petrous ridges shows no obvious abnormality, but the pons is obscured by bone artifact. *B*, *T2* weighted (64/3000) and MR slice through approximately the same level shows a large area of abnormal high *T2* signal corresponding to a bulky pontine glioma. *C*, Heavily *T1* weighted inversion-recovery scan (32/400/1800) at the same level again depicts the tumor, this time as a low-intensity region. Distortion of the fourth ventricle is evident. *D*, *T1* weighted (32/315) midline sagittal sequence shows the expansile pontine tumor, again depicted as of low intensity owing to the *T1* weighting.

Another weakness in the MRI evaluation of tumors is the potential inability to identify cystic components. Cysts also image like solid tumors with long *T1* and *T2*. CT is thus superior to MRI with respect to this distinction. In the future, gadolinium enhancement may help MRI sort out these difficulties (see Chapter 12).

INFLAMMATORY DISEASE

Areas of inflammation contain edema and thus increased tissue water and prolonged *T2* relaxation. This makes *T2* weighted images sensitive for detecting areas of infection.[14]

Figure 39–5 is an example of a subdural empyema, proven by tap. Bilateral frontal

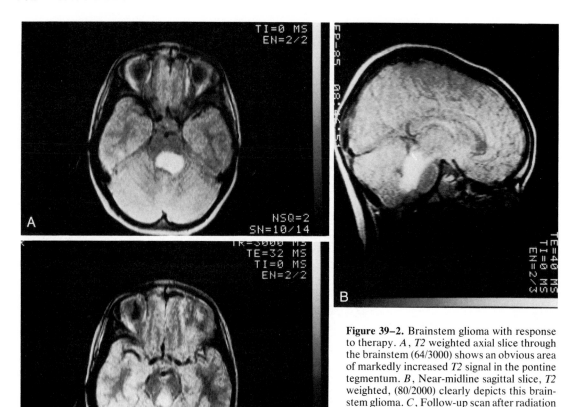

Figure 39–2. Brainstem glioma with response to therapy. *A*, *T2* weighted axial slice through the brainstem (64/3000) shows an obvious area of markedly increased *T2* signal in the pontine tegmentum. *B*, Near-midline sagittal slice, *T2* weighted, (80/2000) clearly depicts this brainstem glioma. *C*, Follow-up scan after radiation and chemotherapy nine months later shows considerable shrinkage of the lesion, indicating a good response to therapy.

subdural collections are seen in this febrile child with lethargy and meningeal signs. Note the striking increase in *T1*, and especially *T2*, relaxation. The coronal *T2* image (Fig. 39–5*B*) demonstrates the collections best and documents that they have a longer *T2* than CSF in the lateral ventricles. Noninfected chronic subdural hematomas have a similar *T2* appearance but usually exhibit a short (bright) *T1*.[15–17] Thus, *T1* images are useful to help distinguish chronic subdural hematomas (short *T1*) from subdural empyemas (long *T1*). Small collections located high over the convexity may be impossible to appreciate on CT but are obvious on coronal *T2* images, and such a case has been described.[18]

The studies in Figure 39–6 were performed because of a suspicion of intracranial abscess complicating frontal sinusitis. The enhanced CT scan (Fig. 39–6*A*) through the inferior frontal lobes suggests a small area of curvilinear dural enhancement surrounding an epidural mass. Interpretation of the CT in this area is difficult, however, because of partial-volume bone artifact from the undulating bony plate beneath. The MRI (Fig. 39–6*B*), being free of this bone artifact, gives unequivocal evidence of an epidural abscess adjacent to the inflamed frontal sinus. The thickened dura appears as a relatively hypointense band between the abscess and brain. Intra-axial abscesses would have a similar *T2* appearance with a high-intensity core, a lower intensity thick capsule, and adjacent brain edema.[14]

MRI is extremely sensitive for detecting inflammation in the paranasal sinuses and mastoid air cells. These structures are normally air-filled and appear black as complete

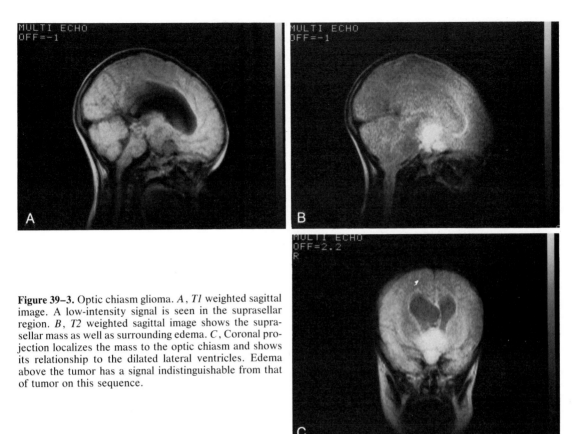

Figure 39–3. Optic chiasm glioma. *A*, *T1* weighted sagittal image. A low-intensity signal is seen in the suprasellar region. *B*, *T2* weighted sagittal image shows the suprasellar mass as well as surrounding edema. *C*, Coronal projection localizes the mass to the optic chiasm and shows its relationship to the dilated lateral ventricles. Edema above the tumor has a signal indistinguishable from that of tumor on this sequence.

signal voids (air contains very few protons). This makes it very easy to recognize inflammation with its associated bright *T2* signal. In Figure 39–7, changes of mastoiditis and maxillary sinusitis are obvious. Sphenoid sinusitis, a potentially serious infection, can be seen just as easily. These diagnoses can be difficult to make in young children on plain films.

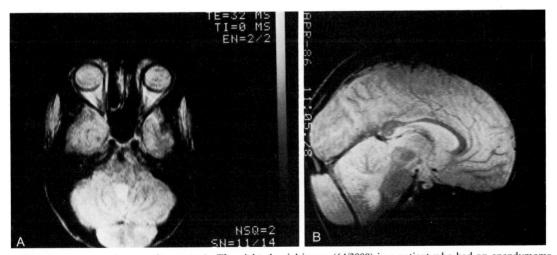

Figure 39–4. Postoperative ependymoma. *A*, *T2* weighted axial image (64/3000) in a patient who had an ependymoma excised nine months previously. *B*, Midline sagittal *T2* weighted image (96/2000) in the same patient. An area of markedly increased *T2* signal is seen just inferior to the fourth ventricle, corresponding to recurrence of the ependymoma.

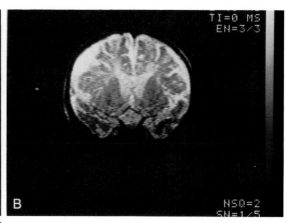

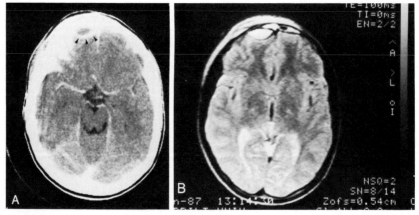

Figure 39–5. Subdural empyema. A, Axial T2 weighted image (64/3000) shows high T2 signal emanating from bilateral frontal subdural collections. B, Coronal T2 image (120/2000) shows the collections to better advantage. They are much brighter than CSF in the lateral ventricles. C, Inversion-recovery axial image (32/410/1800) shows a slow T1 relaxation. This is an important differential point between empyema and chronic subdural effusion.

Viral encephalitis has been a difficult diagnosis to make without biopsy. CT and nuclear medicine brain scan have been helpful but lack high sensitivity and specificity. MRI would be expected to be sensitive to the brain inflammation on T2 weighted sequences, and cases in which MRI has contributed to the diagnosis have been reported.[14,19,20]

Figure 39–6. Frontal epidural abscess. A, Contrast-enhanced CT scan just above the orbits. There is a suggestion of low-density epidural mass with curvilinear dural enhancement (arrowheads). It is difficult to distinguish this from partial volume averaging of the right orbital roof. B, T2 weighted (100/3000) sequence at the same level clearly demonstrates an epidural collection of very high T2 signal. Adjacent inflammatory change in the upper aspect of the frontal sinus is also seen.

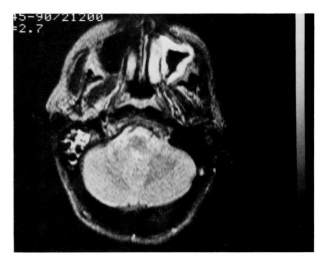

Figure 39–7. Sinusitis and mastoiditis. *T2* weighted (90/2100) axial slice shows high *T2* signal originating from the right petrous air cells. Obvious changes of left maxillary sinusitis are also noted.

HYDROCEPHALUS

Ventricular dilatation is evaluated equally well by CT and MRI. The only advantage of MRI is that it is more likely to identify a cause for the hydrocephalus, such as an Arnold-Chiari malformation, aqueductal stenosis, or a posterior fossa tumor.[15] CT is adequate for follow-up of hydrocephalus of known cause.

Reports have appeared claiming that high-pressure hydrocephalus can be distinguished from low-pressure hydrocephalus by the presence of periventricular high *T2* signal in the former.[5,21] In our experience, this sign is unreliable, being neither sensitive nor specific for high pressure.

CONGENITAL MALFORMATIONS

MRI is superb for demonstrating congenital brain malformations, and a specific diagnosis can usually be made. *T1* images are best owing to their good anatomic resolution and high contrast between CSF and brain.

The most common significant anomaly is the Arnold-Chiari malformation. This is actually a broad spectrum of hindbrain dysplasia that is sometimes classified into three types. Type I involves various degrees of cerebellar tonsil protrusion below the foramen magnum, with occasional coexisting hydrocephalus or syrinx. This can be identified on a *T1* sagittal image by comparing the position of the inferior cerebellar tip to the bone marrow in the dens and the posterior C1 arch. Mild cerebellar protrusion is now found so commonly in asymptomatic adults by MRI that it probably should be considered a normal variant rather than a true anomaly if there are no associated abnormalities.

Chiari Type II malformations are more complex and have a very high association with other anomalies. The medulla and pons are displaced inferiorly, and the fourth ventricle is elongated into a tubular configuration. Upward herniation of the superior vermis also occurs as the cerebellum appears "squeezed out" of the small bony posterior fossa (Fig. 39–8). Spinal meningocele or meningomyelocele and hydrocephalus are almost invariably present. Syringomyelia is occasionally present as well.

Chiari Type III malformations are rare. They are characterized by downward cerebellar herniation into a cervical meningocele. The Dandy-Walker malformation and Dandy-Walker variant involve vermian agenesis or hypoplasia with massive dilatation and distortion of the forth ventricle and/or the cisterna magna.

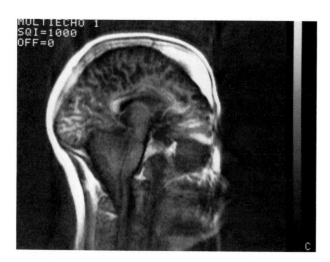

Figure 39–8. Arnold-Chiari malformation Type II. Note the cerebellar tonsils extending far below the foramen magnum. Note also tubulation of the fourth ventricle and a slight kink at the cervico-medullary junction.

Aqueductal stenosis is a relatively common cause of hydrocephalus. Axial images will show dilatation of the third and lateral ventricles with a normal fourth ventricle. The diagnosis is confirmed with *T1*, midline sagittal sequences that show obliteration of the dark aqueduct signal.[22]

Agenesis of the corpus callosum is the most important supratentorial anomaly. This is recognized on coronal or sagittal *T1* MR images by the absence of a corpus callosum, upward displacement of the roof of the third ventricle, and lateral displacement of the lateral ventricles. Sagittal slices easily distinguish the partial from the complete forms, which is difficult with CT.[18,23] In partial agenesis, the posterior portion of the corpus callosum is intact, with a variable-sized defect involving the anterior portion. A very detailed discussion of the MRI appearance of this malformation can be found in the work of Atlas et al.[24]

Porencephalic and congenital arachnoid cysts will generate signals similar to CSF on all sequences and are thus easy to identify. Encephaloceles are well demonstrated, and their contents can be accurately analyzed.

TRAUMA

The important findings in head trauma are depressed skull fracture, base of skull fracture, intra- or extra-axial hemorrhage, cerebral contusion, and increased intracranial pressure from edema. With the possible exception of mild cerebral contusion, CT is equal or superior to MRI for all of these. Sedation is undesirable, so the risk of motion artifact is high. Further, monitoring and ventilatory support are more awkward in the MRI setting. For these reasons, CT remains the study of choice for acute head trauma.[25]

MISCELLANEOUS

One of the unexpected properties of MRI is that rapidly flowing blood generates no signal on any sequence, giving excellent visualization of patent blood vessels as black flow voids. In adults, this can be used to detect occluded arteries. This feature can also be useful in pediatrics, as it provides a tool for detecting dural sinus thrombosis.

Figure 39–9 is from a markedly dehydrated five-year-old with papilledema and lethargy. Strong signal is seen within the superior sagittal sinus on multiple sequences and two planes. This is diagnostic of superior sagittal sinus thrombosis. However,

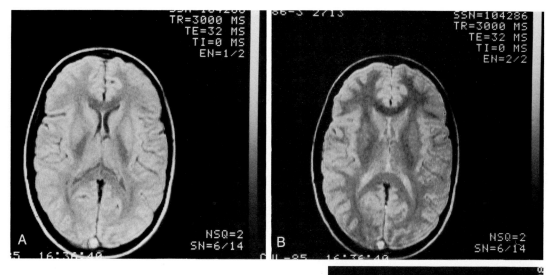

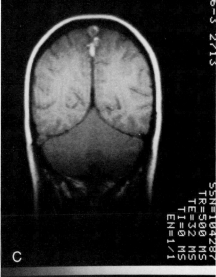

Figure 39–9. Superior sagittal sinus thrombosis. *A–B*, Two echoes of a multiecho sequence (32/3000 and 64/3000) show a strong signal emanating from the posterior portion of the superior sagittal sinus. The fact that this is seen on both images eliminates odd-even rephasing as an explanation for this signal. *C*, *T1* weighted coronal image (32/500) confirms the markedly abnormal signal emanating from the superior sagittal sinus. When this signal is seen on all sequential echoes of a multiecho sequence and is consistent in different planes 90 degrees apart, sagittal sinus thrombosis can be confidently diagnosed.

normal-flowing venous blood can sometimes generate spurious signals, mimicking thrombosis. When such signals are seen only on alternate echoes of a multiecho sequence, this is an artifact known as odd-even rephasing.[26] Short *TR* sequences are susceptible to a similar artifactual signal, flow-related enhancement.[27] This is caused by blood excited in previously pulsed slices flowing into the slice being collected, where it relaxes to generate a signal. True thrombosis can be easily distinguished from these artifacts if the signal is consistently present on multiple sequences and multiple planes.[27,28]

Brain imaging of children with long-standing seizure disorders is usually a fruitless endeavor.[18] However, an occasional low-grade glioma, area of gliosis, or other indolent mass lesion not seen on CT will be detected by MR imaging.[29] Figure 39–10 illustrates such a case, in which a subtle area of increased *T2* signal in the medial temporal lobe corresponds in location to an EEG focus. This presumably represents mesial temporal sclerosis, a brain disease of unknown etiology, in which patches of disorganized, scarred cortex serve as a seizure focus. MR is the only imaging modality capable of documenting this lesion.

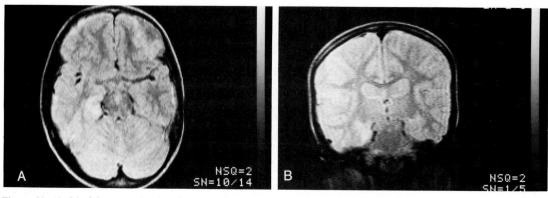

Figure 39–10. Mesial temporal sclerosis. *A*, Axial *T2* weighted image (64/3000) in a four-year-old with temporal lobe seizures. A vague area of increased *T2* signal is seen emanating from the medial portion of the right temporal lobe. *B*, These findings are confirmed on a *T2* weighted (80/2000) coronal scan through the temporal lobes.

SUMMARY

We have specifically chosen cases that capitalize on the advantages of MRI over CT over a wide spectrum of pediatric brain disease. These advantages are (1) absence of bone artifact (Figs. 39–1, 39–2, 39–4, 39–6, and 39–8); (2) increased contrast between normal and abnormal brain (Figs. 39–1 to 39–4, 39–6, 39–7, 39–9, and 39–10); and (3) ability to choose nonaxial planes (Figs. 39–1 to 39–5, and 39–8). For complex tumors, MR and CT should be considered complementary rather than competitive. For example, Figure 39–11 shows the MRI and CT of a complex oligodendroglioma arising near the floor of the third ventricle. The MR alone is confusing, as the dark areas could represent large blood vessels or calcifications. The CT clearly demonstrates the extent of the calcifications, but it alone provides an inferior anatomic characterization.

Although the inability to detect calcification is a weakness of MRI, it clearly detects more abnormalities than CT and characterizes them better. Because of these advantages, MRI should now be the initial imaging procedure of choice for all suspected childhood intracranial disease, with the exception of head trauma.

Spine

MRI competes with myelography and, to a lesser extent, with CT in evaluating pediatric spinal disease. Although the new myelographic contrast agents have improved patient safety and comfort, pediatric myelography remains a difficult examination to perform, requiring hospitalization, radiation exposure and, possibly, general anesthesia and a significant radiation dose. Furthermore, only MRI provides information about the cord itself rather than imaging it as a filling defect. Spine MRI is diagnostically contributory, if not definitive, in a wide variety of spine diseases[30] and has been shown to influence patient treatment in 70 percent of sequential patients scanned.[31]

IMAGING STRATEGY

T1 and *T2* images are very complementary in the spine, and both are needed for all studies. Table 39–2 lists the *T1* and *T2* signal characteristics of structures imaged in the spine and can be used to predict which sequence type will provide the better contrast between adjacent structures.

T1 images provide the best contrast between cord and CSF and best demonstrate

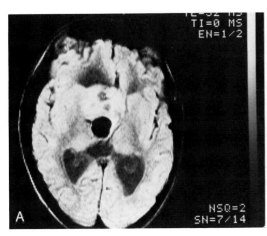 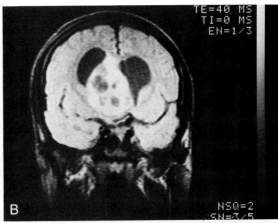

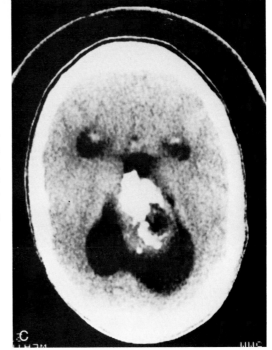

Figure 39–11. Heavily calcified oligodendroglioma: complementary MR and CT studies. *A*, Balanced axial MR image (32/3000) shows a bulky, heterogeneous tumor with areas of signal void. *B*, Balanced coronal MR image (40/3000) through the same tumor. This plane shows the anatomy best, suggesting that the origin is near the floor of the third ventricle with superior extension between the leaves of the septum pellucidum. Origin from the sella is excluded. *C*, Nonenhanced CT at the same level as *A*. This proves that the MR signal void represents calcification.

Table 39–2. APPROXIMATE INTENSITY LEVELS OF TISSUES IMAGED WITH SPINE MRI

Tissue	T1	T2
Cortical bone	Black	Black
Vertebral body	Bright	Intermediate
Bone metastasis	Dark	Intermediate
Nucleus pulposus	Intermediate	Bright
Anulus fibrosus	Intermediate	Dark
Epidural fat or lipoma	Very bright	Bright
CSF	Dark	Bright
Syrinx cavity	Dark	Bright
Normal spinal cord	Intermediate	Bright
Abnormal* spinal cord	Intermediate	Very bright
Hematoma	Bright	Bright to dark

* Intramedullary tumor or edema.

intramedullary fluid collections. They are also exquisitely sensitive for infiltrating processes in the bone marrow, such as metastatic disease or osteomyelitis. However, the outer margins of the subarachnoid space are indistinct because CSF, cortical bone, and spinal ligaments are all dark. Thus, these images are poor for epidural masses.

On *T2* images, normal cord and surrounding CSF are about equally bright. The cord may vanish into a bright cast of the subarachnoid space. Epidural masses are best seen on these sequences.[30] Cord pathology becomes visible because it is usually brighter than both normal cord and CSF.[32] Abnormalities of the intervertebral discs are also best seen with *T2* weighting.

The sagittal plane is ideal in the spine, since a relatively large area can be covered in one collection. Axial slices may help characterize an abnormality but are not needed routinely. In patients with scoliosis and minimal kyphosis or lordosis, coronal or tilted coronal scans may be useful.

In very young patients who will fit, we use the head coil. Otherwise, surface coils are always used. The coil is centered close to the level of clinical interest for the initial *T1* and *T2* sagittal scans. The upper and lower extent of all detected abnormalities are studied, if necessary, by repeating the collections after moving the coils to overlapping fields.

PULSE SEQUENCE SELECTION

We begin with three sagittal, 5 mm thick spin-echo collections: 38/500, 45/2000, and 90/2000 for *T1*, balanced, and *T2* weighting, respectively. The latter two are collected simultaneously as a multiecho sequence. These are usually adequate, but axial imaging is sometimes required to clarify the findings. The 38/500 spin-echo sequence provides enough *T1* weighting to easily separate cord from CSF, so that we never have to use inversion recovery.

TUMORS

MRI is very sensitive in detecting tumors originating from all four spinal compartments: osseous, extradural, intradural, and intramedullary.[30,32–35] By combining information from *T1* and *T2* images, the compartment of origin is usually easily identified. After plain films, MRI is now the procedure of choice for suspected spinal tumors.[4,32,33,35]

Intramedullary tumors appear the same as brainstem tumors: bright on *T2* images and iso- to hypointense on *T1* images (see Figs. 39–1 and 39–2). *T2* images will demonstrate the tumor mass, while *T1* images will show cord expansion and possibly the tumor itself. The scans occasionally fail to demonstrate tumor-related intramedullary cysts.[36]

Intradural, extramedullary tumors are best appreciated on *T1* images when they appear as filling defects in the dark CSF column.[35] Displacement of the cord may be appreciated. In contrast, extradural masses are best appreciated with *T2* weighting (Fig. 39–12), which better delineates the outer margin of the subarachnoid space.[32] Metastatic deposits in the bony spine are seen best with *T1* weighting, which offers maximal contrast between very bright bone marrow and intermediate-intensity tumor.[30]

INTRAMEDULLARY FLUID COLLECTIONS

Intramedullary fluid can be caused by hydromyelia, syringomyelia, or cystic glial tumor. All three have the same nonspecific myelographic appearance. Hydromyelia is dilatation of the central spinal canal and is usually caused by a Chiari malformation.

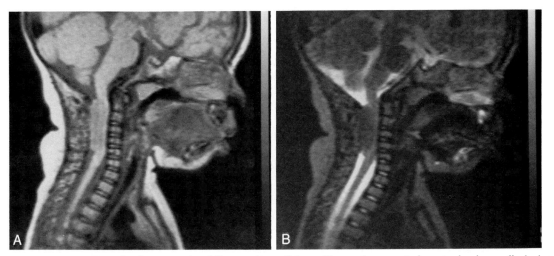

Figure 39–12. *A–B*, Extradural mass: eosinophilic granuloma. Balanced image shows posterior extradural mass displacing the cervical spinal cord anteriorly.

Thus, if a fluid cavity is seen in the cord, the brainstem should be scanned to exclude this condition. Syringomyelia is a generic term for any fluid collection within the cord but outside the central canal (some classify hydromyelia as a type of syringomyelia). Etiologies include idiopathic, post-traumatic, deriving from old hematoma, and tumor-related. MRI is reliable in determining whether a tumor is causing the syrinx.[37,38]

The MRI appearances of syringomyelia and hydromyelia are identical with current technology. *T1* images are best, showing the low-intensity fluid cavity surrounded by a thin, smooth rim of cord (Fig. 39–13). The role of *T2* images is to exclude an underlying tumor.[4,37,38] Cystic tumors have irregular borders and heterogeneous signal intensity,[38] but there are insufficient data at present to determine if MRI can reliably distinguish benign syrinx from a cystic tumor.

Figure 39–13. Large idiopathic cervicothoracic syrinx. *T1* weighted image (30/315). Note the very large, low-intensity cavity surrounded by a thin rim of cord. There is no evidence of tumor or a Chiari malformation.

SPINE ANOMALIES

Spinal dysraphism is a broad spectrum of myelodysplasia that can occur as an overt lesion, such as meningomyelocele, or an occult derangement with a normal bony spine, such as tethered cord or diastematomyelia.

MRI is effective for analyzing the contents of a meningomyelocele. *T1* sagittal images show neural tissue either entering the defect or passing alongside unmolested (Fig. 39–14).

Tethered cord or diastematomyelia can occur with or without visible bony anomalies. *T1* images can accurately locate the conus and establish or exclude tether in children with evidence of cord dysfunction and normal plain films.[33,39,40] Coronal images may help locate the conus when the initial sagittal images are equivocal.[40] Associated lipomas are easy to detect because of very bright *T1* relaxation.[33]

Diastematomyelia is a form of spinal dysraphism characterized by division of the cord into two limbs. A cartilaginous or bony septum may be between the limbs. Associated tether, lipoma, or syrinx is common. MRI characterizes all these findings well except for the septum[41] (unless bright marrow is present). Thus, this disorder can be evaluated with a combination of MRI and uncontrasted CT (to image the septum), avoiding an intrathecal contrast injection. Anomalies of the vertebral bodies may or may not have associated cord lesions. MRI is a good screening examination in this situation. Figure 39–15 shows a hemivertebra where MRI excluded a major cord abnormality.

INFECTION

Accurate imaging is needed for suspected disc space infections and spinal osteomyelitis in order to restrict invasive needle aspirations in patients likely to have infection. MRI has excellent sensitivity and specificity for infection in these areas, having an accuracy of 94 percent compared with 73 percent for plain films.[42] The findings in disc space infection are characteristic: loss of the bright disc *T1* signal, with decreased *T1* signal from the marrow of adjacent vertebral bodies (Fig. 39–16).[42,43] *T2* images may show bright paraspinal tissue, representing induration or abscess (Fig. 39–17). The disc will appear distorted and may be hypo-, iso-, or hyperintense to the normal discs. Similarly, affected marrow may have *T2* intensity above or below that of the

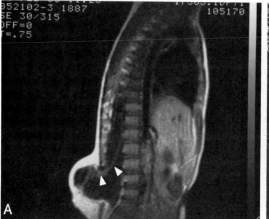 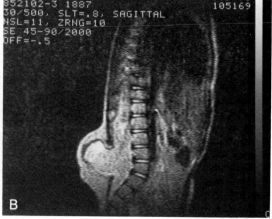

Figure 39–14. Large lumbosacral meningomyelocele. *A*, *T1* weighted (30/315) sagittal image shows the pocket filled with dark CSF. No fat is present. The spinal cord is seen entering the pocket (arrowheads). *B*, *T2* weighted image loses the contrast between cord and CSF.

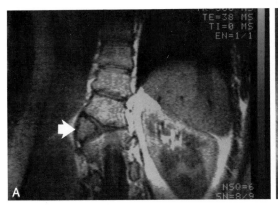 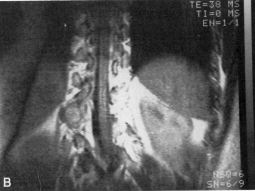

Figure 39–15. Hemivertebra. *A*, *T1* weighted (38/500) coronal slice showing the hemivertebra (arrow). *B*, Slice posterior to *A*, showing the cord appearing to be normal at the level of the hemivertebra.

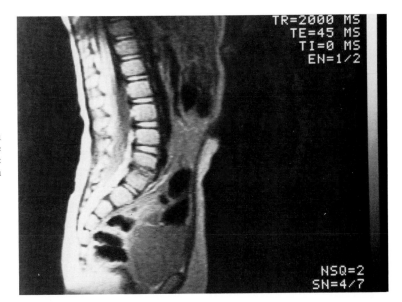

Figure 39–16. Disc space infection at L4–5. Balanced sagittal image shows loss of *T1* signal from the disc and indistinct end-plates on both sides of the disc.

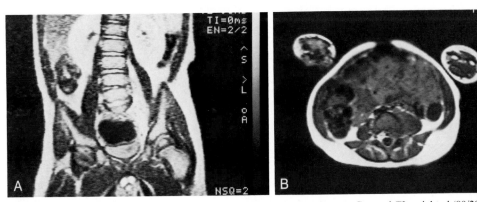

Figure 39–17. Disc space infection at L4–5 with paraspinal inflammation. *A*, Coronal *T2* weighted (90/2000) slice shows normal *T2* brightness but distortion of the L4–5 disc signal. The left psoas muscle is in spasm, causing splinting of the spine. There is a marked increase in the *T2* signal of the medial left psoas, indicating inflammation. *B*, Axial *T1* image (32/506) near the infected disc level shows that the left medial psoas is of low *T1* intensity, confirming paraspinal inflammation and excluding fat deposition.

normal marrow. Coronal and axial *T2* images are best for showing paraspinal changes (Fig. 39–17).

MRI is ideal for follow-up after antibiotic therapy. Figure 39–18 shows the loss of abnormally bright *T2* signal in an infection after treatment.

TRAUMA

Myelography is relatively undesirable in the child with a potentially unstable spine fracture because manipulation and, possibly, general anesthesia may be needed for a good study.

Unlike the case with head trauma, we have found MRI to be extremely helpful in evaluation of spine trauma. Although the configuration of fractured bony fragments is poorly seen, compression of the dural sac is accurately assessed using *T2* images, and spinal cord contusion is detected as a zone of increased *T2* signal (Figs. 39–19 and 39–20).[44] Epidural hematomas are clearly seen (Fig. 39–20*B*). *T1* or balanced images depict the anatomy and malalignment best (Fig 39–20*B*). MRI is the only imaging modality capable of detecting cord contusion. Follow-up scans are valuable to detect complications such as syringomyelia, atrophy, or osteomyelitis. CT is safe and provides excellent information about bone fragments but is virtually restricted to the axial plane (making assessment of alignment difficult) and provides little information about the cord.

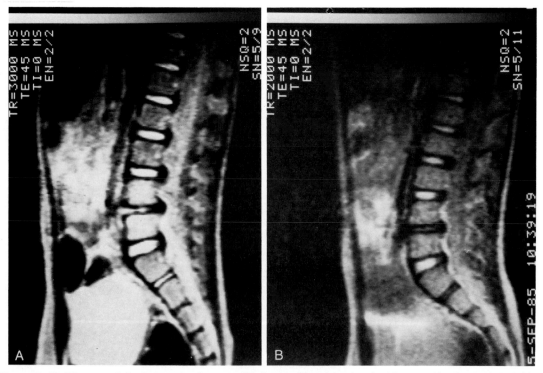

Figure 39–18. Disc space infection, pre- and post antibiotics. *A*, *T2* weighted sagittal image (45/3000) show the typical changes of infection at L4–5, with irregularity of the disc signal. There is also an abnormally bright *T2* signal from the entire L4 and L5 vertebral bodies. *B*, Same sequence after therapy. The bright disc signal has "burned out," leaving a degenerated, dim disc. The marrow signal has returned to normal.

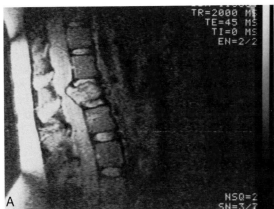
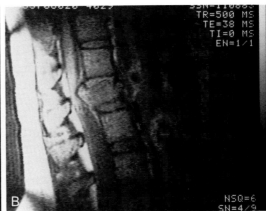

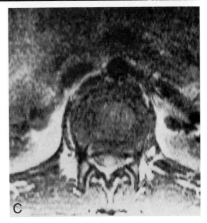

Figure 39–19. L1 compression fracture with conus contusion. *A*, Midline sagittal *T2* weighted image (90/2000) through the thoracolumbar spine. There is an acute compression fracture of L1, with retropulsion of fragments and marked narrowing of the subarachnoid space. The conus cannot be distinguished from CSF on this sequence. *B*, *T1* weighted sequence (38/500) through the same area shows compression at the tip of the conus and slightly increased signal, indicating contusion of the cord at the lowermost point. *C*, Balanced axial image (45/1000) shows the retropulsed fragment that has narrowed the spinal canal at this level.

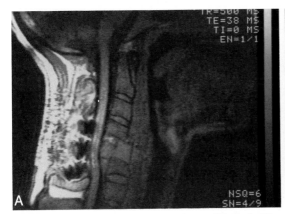
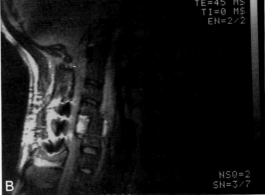

Figure 39–20. Acute fracture dislocation at C4–5. *A*, *T1* sagittal image (38/500) shows the 50 percent dislocation and deviation of the cord around the fracture. *B*, *T2* image (90/2000) shows a bright epidural collection representing hematoma. The dural sac is narrowed, but adequate space for the cord is present. There is no evidence of cord contusion.

Chest

LUNG

The utility of magnetic resonance imaging for evaluation of pediatric pulmonary parenchymal disease has not been determined at this time. In fact, the pediatric lung is one of the least studied organs, and the application of MRI technology has not been evaluated to the extent that it has in other regions of the body.[45] It has been suggested that without cardiac or respiratory gating MR does not offer a significant advantage over contrast-enhanced CT.[46] Furthermore, *T1* and *T2* measurements do not appear to predict the type of tissue from which the signal is emanating. The literature indicates that there is significant overlap in *T1* and *T2* values in lung pathology.[45]

At Vanderbilt University Hospital we have employed respiratory gating on a routine basis.[46] Our initial scans are *T1* weighted to optimally demonstrate anatomy. We have found that the coronal plane is especially helpful because it corresponds to the image that we are accustomed to viewing on a conventional radiograph. Axial slices are obtained as well as sagittal or oblique images, when indicated. *T2* weighted images are collected also in at least one plane.

MR and CT have been found to be roughly equivalent in overall sensitivity for detecting intrapulmonary masses.[47] CT is superior for small masses close to the pleura or nodules close to each other because of increased spatial resolution,[47] but MRI is superior for nodules near blood vessels.[47,48] MRI's inability to detect calcification is a definite disadvantage in the lungs.

MRI may have a role in cystic fibrosis, in which it can distinguish impacted bronchi from normal vessels[48,49] and detect peribronchial inflammation.[49]

MEDIASTINUM

In the mediastinum, MRI offers an advantage over x-ray CT in that the major blood vessels are easily identified and the thymus is clearly seen (Fig. 39–21). Contrast between vascular and nonvascular structures is excellent because flowing blood produces no signal and appears black. *T1* spin-echo images (short *TE*, short *TR*) are usually best in the mediastinum because they provide the best contrast between normal mediastinal

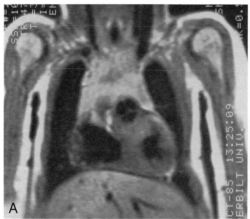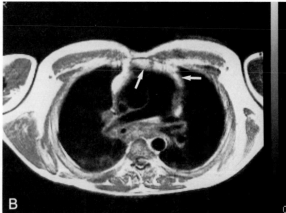

Figure 39–21. Normal thymus in two children. *A*, Gated *T1* weighted (38/475) coronal slice through mediastinum in a four-year-old. Note the thymus appearing draped over the base of the heart. The borders are smooth and concave. The signal is bright, indicating fat content in this *T1* image. *B*, Ungated axial *T1* weighted (30/500) slice through the great vessels in a 16-year-old. The thymus is the thin rim of bright tissue anterior to the great vessels (arrows). It has been nearly replaced by fat (compare signal intensity with the subcutaneous fat).

fat and abnormal masses,[48,50] have a better signal-to-noise ratio, and are quickest to collect, allowing more scanning time for multiple planes. However, the *T2* character-istics of an abnormality should be assessed in at least one plane.

For evaluation of the mediastinum, sagittal, coronal, and axial images are obtained and supplemented by *T2* images in the plane that demonstrates the pathology best.[51] We have found that the thymus routinely has smooth margins and appears draped over nondisplaced mediastinal structures. This can be contrasted to the appearance of lym-phoma (Fig. 39–22), which has a lumpy appearance in which adjacent mediastinal structures are displaced.[48,50,52,53]

A discussion of the advantages and disadvantages of MRI of the chest has to include the following concepts. First, MR imaging has a great capability to discriminate tissues of different composition, to identify the heart and vessels and their abnormalities with-out use of contrast materials, and to demonstrate well those areas where partial-volume effect may limit the applicability of x-ray CT. In our review of the experience at Van-derbilt University Children's Hospital we have not been able to document that MR imaging offers a major incremental advantage over x-ray CT in the context of recog-nition of a specific pathologic entity. The main use of MR in the pediatric chest relates to mediastinal problems, including the differentiation of normal thymus from a me-diastinal mass, the differentiation of enlarged lymph nodes from hilar blood vessels, and the identification of displaced blood vessels by mediastinal masses.

Abdomen

ALIMENTARY CANAL

Efforts in bowel imaging have been hampered by peristaltic motion and abundant, interfering, bright *T2* fat. MRI can detect areas of bowel inflammation and may even-tually become useful for Crohn's disease and ulcerative colitis (see Chapter 30). Another potential use is to depict the anatomy of children with choledochal cysts.[54] We found MRI helpful in a newborn with anal atresia (Fig. 39–23).

The use of oral iron-containing materials, such as Geritol or iron-rich vitamins, has been suggested as a bowel contrast agent, but the effects on relaxation are unpre-

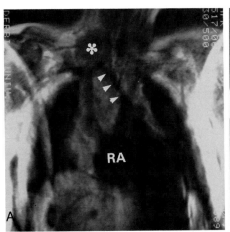
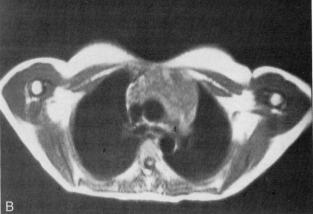

Figure 39–22. Lymphoma. *A*, Ungated *T1* weighted (30/500) coronal image through anterior mediastinum. A bulky, low signal intensity mass is seen between the base of the heart and the thoracic inlet. The brachiocephalic artery is draped and displaced to the left (arrowheads). The SVC appears encased. RA, Right atrium. * = Supraclavicular adenopathy. Note the motion degradation of the image from lack of gating. *B*, Axial *T1* weighted slice just below the aortic arch in a different patient. A bulky, low-intensity mass has convex borders and displaces the ascending aorta and SVC posteriorly.

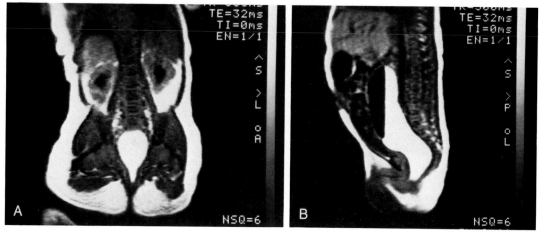

Figure 39–23. High type anal atresia in a two-day-old male. Meconium in the colon has a very bright *TI* signal, providing excellent contrast of the bowel lumen. *A*, Coronal *TI* (32/500) image shows the dilated rectum ending abruptly above the levator sling. *B*, Sagittal midline *TI* (32/500) image confirms the findings. No fistula into the collapsed bladder is seen. There is an air-meconium level in the left colon.

dictable.[1] We have found that intravenous glucagon may decrease bowel motion artifact.

SOLID ORGANS

MRI is at least as sensitive as CT for detecting hepatic mass lesions,[55] but it has failed thus far to provide additional specificity.[56] All abnormalities look about the same: long *T1*, long *T2*.[55] Figure 39–24 demonstrates a hepatic abscess that was equally obvious on CT. MRI has the potential to specifically diagnose portal vein thrombosis or hepatic vein thrombosis (Budd-Chiari syndrome).[57] Hemochromatosis also has specific changes, with very low *T2* signal.[58] MRI is capable of demonstrating adrenal masses (Fig. 39–25) but has no particular advantage over CT except perhaps in children with very little perinephric fat. No clear role for MRI has yet emerged for splenic or pancreatic disease.

URINARY TRACT

MRI is extremely helpful for evaluating Wilms' tumor and differentiating it from neuroblastoma.[59] The extent of invasion of blood vessels and adjacent organs is ac-

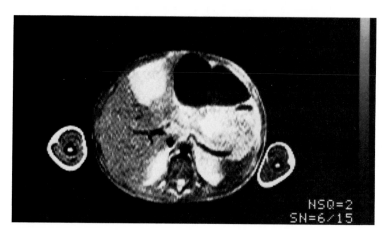

Figure 39–24. Liver abscess in a five-year-old with chronic granulomatous disease of childhood. Balanced (45/2000) image shows a well-defined, very bright *T2* collection in the left lobe.

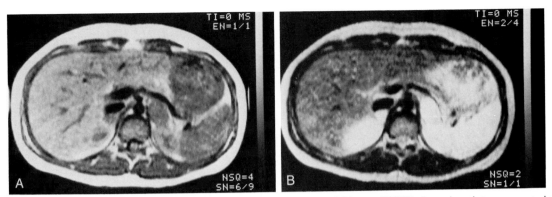

Figure 39–25. Bilateral pheochromocytomas in a ten-year-old. *A*, *T1* axial image (32/500) shows hypointense masses in both adrenals. The right is directly posterior to the caval flow void, and the left is behind the splenic artery flow void. *B*, On a *T2* sequence (64/2000), the tumors become hyperintense.

curately depicted.[59–61] Figure 39–26 shows a bulky Wilms' tumor from the left upper pole. Invasion of the left renal vein and cava is clearly seen. This patient went to surgery on the basis of this study alone, avoiding a contrast cavogram.

Except for solid tumors, ultrasound remains the imaging method of choice for renal disease, with MRI offering little additional information.[62]

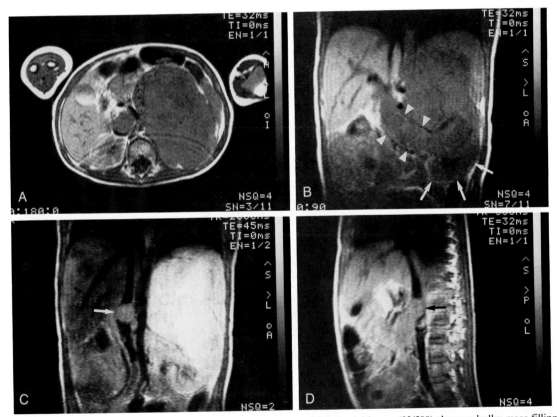

Figure 39–26. Bulky Wilms' tumor with caval invasion. *A*, *T1* weighted axial image (32/500) shows a bulky mass filling the left upper quadrant. *B*, Coronal image confirms renal origin. A relatively normal lower pole of left kidney (arrows) is seen displaced by the mass. The left renal vein is expanded and packed with tumor (arrowheads). *C*, Coronal balanced image (45/2000) posterior to *B*. Tumor is seen within the infrahepatic cava (arrow). *D*, Sagittal *T1* (32/500) image again shows tumor extending into infrahepatic cava (arrow).

Bone and Soft Tissues

TUMORS

MRI has a limited but important role in the evaluation of musculoskeletal tumors. It cannot make a specific diagnosis or even reliably distinguish benign from malignant tumors.[63]

Plain films remain the best method for narrowing the differential diagnosis. While CT can identify matrix calcification to suggest a cartilaginous tumor, MRI is unreliable for this purpose.[63] Furthermore, osteomyelitis can simulate bone malignancy closely on MRI.[63]

MRI's role is to evaluate the extent of bone marrow and soft tissue involvement in lesions that appear malignant on plain films. The superior bone marrow and soft tissue contrast can provide crucial information for tumor staging, surgical planning, and judging response to therapy.

As *T1* weighting increases, normal bone marrow becomes brighter and tumor-contaminated marrow becomes darker. Thus, the extent of marrow involvement is best appreciated as coronal *T1* images through long bones (Fig. 39–27). Tumor–to–bone marrow contrast is poor on *T2* images, where both appear bright. Conversely, *T2* images provide the best contrast between tumor and soft tissue. Although both are dark on *T1*, tumor brightens with *T2* weighting to a much greater extent than muscle. Thus, soft tissue extension is best demonstrated with axial *T2* slices. The most efficient strategy for studying a suspected long bone malignancy is a coronal *T1* collection and an axial *T2* collection.

MRI was found to be as good as or better than CT for demonstrating extent of marrow involvement in 98 percent, and as good or better for soft tissue involvement in 100 percent, of a wide variety of bone tumors.[74]

In addition to evaluating primary bone tumors, MRI is sensitive for detection of metastatic lesions or leukemic infiltration. These appear as dark areas within the bright marrow on *T1* images.[64] Because a skeletal MRI survey is impractical, radioisotope bone scan remains the procedure of choice for screening the skeleton for metastatic lesions.

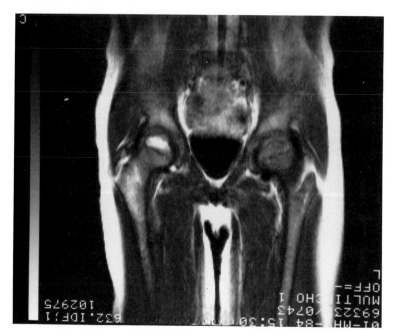

Figure 39–27. Legg-Perthes disease (left). Coronal *T1* image shows normal bright marrow signal from the right femoral epiphysis but markedly decreased signal on the left.

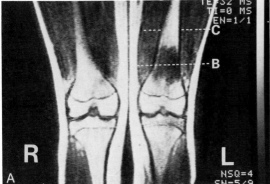
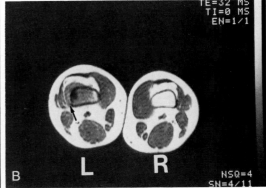
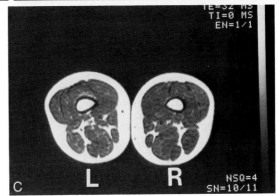

Figure 39–28. Osteogenic sarcoma, left distal femoral metaphyses. *A*, Coronal *T1* image (32/500) shows marked decrease in signal from metaphyseal marrow as a result of tumor infiltration. The epiphysis and growth plate are not involved. *B*, Axial *T1* slice at level indicated. Abnormal marrow is demonstrated in cross section. A soft tissue component is seen displacing the prepatellar fat anteriorly (arrow). *C*, Axial marrow *T1* slice more proximally is normal at this level, but a sliver of tumor in the soft tissues is seen anterior to the femur.

AVASCULAR NECROSIS

MRI is probably the procedure of choice for diagnosing Legg-Perthes disease. Its sensitivity and specificity is superior to that of plain films, CT, and bone scanning.[65,66] A single coronal *T1* collection through both hips constitutes an adequate evaluation. This takes only about six minutes on most instruments.

Avascular necrosis is easily recognized as diminished *T1* intensity on *T1* to the femoral epiphyseal marrow signal (Fig. 39–28). The opposite hip or the femoral neck marrow can serve as controls. Complications of avascular necrosis can also be seen. Deformity of the femoral head becomes apparent at about the same time as on the plain film. Early subchondral fractures appear as linear lucencies in the diminished epiphyseal signal. MRI does not detect these quite as well as CT.[67]

INFECTION

As discussed earlier, MRI has a significant role in spinal infection. The situation is less clear in the long bones. Early work has been encouraging, showing decrease of marrow *T1* signal while plain films were still normal.[68] However, we see no advantage of MRI over nuclear medicine studies, in which the bone scan is sensitive and the gallium scan is specific.

References

1. Cohen MD: Pediatric Magnetic Resonance Imaging. Philadelphia, WB Saunders, 1986.
2. Gomori JM, Grossman RI, Goldberg HI, Zimmerman RA, Bilaniuk LT: Intracranial hematomas: Imaging by high field MR. Radiology *157*:87, 1985.
3. Pennock JM, Bydder GM, Dubowitz LM, Johnson MA: Magnetic resonance imaging of the brain in children. Magn Reson Imag *4*:1, 1986.

4. Kucharczyk W, Brant-Zawadzki M, Sobel D, Edwards MB, Kelly WM, Norman D, Newton TH: Central nervous system tumors in children: Detection by magnetic resonance imaging. Radiology 155:131, 1985.
5. Bradley WG Jr, Waluch V, Yadley RA, Wycoff RR: Comparison of CT and MR in 400 patients with suspected disease of the brain and cervical spinal cord. Radiology 152:695, 1984.
6. Johnson MA, Pennock JM, Bydder GM, Steiner RE, Thomas DJ, Hayward R, Bryant DR, Payne JA, Levene MI, Whitelaw A, et al: Clinical NMR imaging of the brain in children: Normal and neurologic disease. AJR 141:1005, 1983.
7. Holland BA, Haas DK, Norman D, Brant-Zawadzki M, Newton TH: MRI of normal brain maturation. AJNR 7:201, 1986.
8. Dubowitz LM, Pennock JM, Johnson MA, Bydder GM: High resolution magnetic resonance imaging of the brain in children. Clin Radiol 37:113, 1986.
9. Darwin RH, Drayer BP, Reiderer SJ, Wang HZ, MacFall JR: T2 estimates in health and diseased brain tissue: A comparison using various MR pulse sequences. Radiology 160:375, 1986.
10. Zimmerman RA, Bilaniuk LT: Applications of magnetic resonance imaging in diseases of the pediatric central nervous system. Magn Reson Imag 4:11, 1986.
11. Packer RJ, Batnitzky S, Cohen ME: Magnetic resonance imaging in the evaluation of intracranial tumors of childhood. Cancer 56:1767, 1985.
12. Daniels DL, Herflgens RJ, Gager WE, Meyer GA, Koehler PR, Williams AL, Haughton VM: Magnetic resonance imaging of the optic nerve and chiasm. Radiology 152:79, 1984.
13. Albert A, Lee BCP, Deck MDF: MRI of the optic chiasm and optic pathways. AJNR 7:255, 1986.
14. Davidson HD, Steiner RE: Magnetic resonance imaging in infections of the central nervous system. AJNR 6:499, 1985.
15. Sipponen JT, Sipponen RE, Sivula AS: Chronic subdural hematoma demonstration by magnetic resonance. Radiology 150:79, 1984.
16. Moon KL Jr, Brant-Zawadzki M, Pitts LH, Mills CM: Magnetic resonance imaging of CT isodense subdural hematomas. AJNR 5:319, 1984.
17. Han JS, Kaufman RJ, Alfidi RJ, Yeung HN, Benson JE, Haaga JR, El Yousef SJ, Clampitt ME, Bonstelle CT, Huss R: Head trauma evaluated by magnetic resonance and computed tomography: A comparison. Radiology 150:71, 1984.
18. Han JS, Benson JE, Kaufman B, Rekate HL, Alfidi RJ, Huss RG, Sacco D, Yoon US, Morrison SC: MR imaging of pediatric cerebral abnormalities. J Comput Assist Tomogr 9:103, 1985.
19. Brandt-Zawadzki M, Davis PL, Crooks LE, Mills CM, Norman D, Newton TH, Sheldon P, Kaufman L: NMR demonstration of cerebral abnormalities: Comparison with CT. AJNR 4:117, 1983.
20. Tarr RW, Edwards KM, Kessler RM, Kulkarni MV: MRI of mumps encephalitis: Comparison with CT evaluation. Pediatr Radiology 17:59, 1987.
21. Randell CP, Collins A, Young IR, Haywood R, Thomas DJ, McDonnell MJ, Orr JS, Bydder JM, Stiener RE: Nuclear magnetic resonance imaging of posterior fossa tumors. AJNR 4:127, 1983.
22. Novetsky GJ, Berlin L: Aqueductal stenosis: Demonstration by MR imaging. J Comput Assist Tomogr 8:1170, 1984.
23. Davidson HD, Abraham R, Steiner RD: Agenesis of the corpus callosum: Magnetic resonance imaging. Radiology 155:371, 1985.
24. Atlas SW, Zimmerman RA, Bilaniuk LT, Rorke L, Hackney DB, Goldberg HI, Grossman RI: Corpus callosum and limbic system neuroanatomic MR evaluation of developmental anomalies. Radiology 1609:355, 1986.
25. Hanigan WC, Wright SM, Wright RM: Clinical utility of magnetic resonance imaging in pediatric neurosurgical patients. J Pediatr 103:522, 1986.
26. Bradley WG, Waluch V: Blood flow magnetic resonance imaging. Radiology 154:443, 1985.
27. McMurdo SK Jr, Brant-Zawadzki M, Bradley WG Jr, Chang GY, Berg BO: Dural sinus thrombosis: Study using intermediate field strength MR imaging. Radiology 161:83, 1986.
28. Macchi PJ, Grossman RI, Gomori JM, Goldberg HI, Bilaniuk LT: High field MR imaging of cerebral venous thrombosis. J Comput Assist Tomogr 10:10, 1986.
29. Laster DW, Penry JK, Moody DR, Ball MR, Witcofski RL, Riela AR: Chronic seizure disorder: Contribution of MR imaging when CT is normal. AJNR 6:177, 1985.
30. Berger PE, Atkinson D, Wilson WJ, Wiltse L: High resolution surface coil magnetic resonance imaging of the spine: Normal and pathologic anatomy. RadioGraphics 4:573, 1986.
31. Franken EA, Berbaum KS, Dunn V, Smith WL, Ehrhardt JC, Levitz GS, Breckenridge RE: Impact of MR imaging on clinical diagnosis and management: A prospective study. Radiology 161:377, 1986.
32. Hyman RA, Edwards JH, Vacirca SJ, Stein HL: 0.6 T MR imaging of the cervical spine: Multislice and multiecho techniques. AJR 6:229, 1985.
33. Packer RJ, Zimmerman RA, Sutton LN, Bilaniuk LT, Bruce DA, Schut L: Magnetic resonance imaging of spinal cord disease of childhood. Pediatrics 78:251, 1986.
34. Chiro GD, Doppman JL, Dwyer AJ, Patronas NJ, Knop RH, Bairamian D, Vermess M, Oldfield EH: Tumors and arteriovenous malformations of the spinal cord: Assessment using MR. Radiology 156:689, 1985.
35. Scotti G, Scialfa G, Colombo N, Landoni L: MR imaging of intradural extramedullary tumors of the cervical spine. J Comput Assist Tomogr 9:1037, 1985.
36. Goy AM, Pinto RS, Raghavendra BN, Epstein FJ, Kricheff II: Intramedullary spinal cord tumors: MR imaging, with emphasis on associated cysts. Radiology 161:381, 1986.

37. Kokmen E, Marsh WR, Baker HL: Magnetic resonance imaging in syringomyelia. Neurosurgery *17*:267, 1985.
38. Lee BCP, Zimmerman RD, Manning JJ, Deck MDF: MR imaging of syringomyelia and hydromyelia. AJNR *6*:221, 1985.
39. Roos RAC, Vielvoye GJ, Voormolen JHC, Peters ACB: Magnetic resonance imaging in occult spinal dysraphism. Pediatr Radiol *16*:412, 1986.
40. Barnes PD, Lester PD, Yamanashi WS, Prince JR: MRI in infants and children with spinal dysraphism. AJR *147*:339, 1986.
41. Han JS, Benson JE, Kaufman B, Rekate HL, Alfidi RJ, Bohlman HH, Kaufman B: Demonstration of diastematomyelia and associated abnormalities with MR imaging. AJNR *6*:215, 1985.
42. Modic MT, Feiglin DH, Piraino DW, Boumphrey F, Weinstein MA, Duchesneau PM, Rehm S: Vertebral osteomyelitis: Assessment using MR. Radiology *157*:157, 1985.
43. Modic MT, Pavlicek W, Weinstein MA, Boumphrey F, Ngo F, Hardy R, Duchesneau PM: Magnetic resonance imaging of intervertebral disk disease. Radiology *152*:103, 1984.
44. Hackney DB, Asato R, Sci DM, Joseph PM, Carvlin MJ, McGrath JT, Grossman TI, Kassab EA, Desimone D: Hemorrhage and edema in acute spinal cord compression: Demonstration by MR imaging. Radiology *161*:387, 1986.
45. Ross JS, O'Donovan PB, Novoa R, Mehta A, et al: Magnetic resonance of the chest. Initial experience with imaging and in vivo T1 and T2 calculations. Radiology *152*:95, 1984.
46. Runge VM, Clanton JA, Partain CL, James AE: Respiratory gating in magnetic resonance imaging at 0.5 tesla. Radiology *151*:521, 1984.
47. Muller NL, Gamsu G, Webb WR: Pulmonary nodules: Detection using magnetic resonance and computed tomography. Radiology *155*:687, 1985.
48. Brasch RC, Gooding CA, Lallemand DP, Wesbey GE: Magnetic resonance imaging of the thorax in childhood. Radiology *150*:463, 1984.
49. Gooding CA, Lallemand DP, Brasch RC, Wesbey GE, David B: Magnetic resonance imaging in cystic fibrosis. Pediatrics *105*:383, 1984.
50. Dooms GC, Hricak H, Crooks LE, Higgins CB: Magnetic resonance imaging of the lymph nodes: Comparison with CT. Radiology *153*:719, 1984.
51. Webb KR, Gamsu G, Crooks LE: Multisection sagittal and coronal magnetic resonance imaging of the mediastinum and hila. Radiology *150*:475, 1984.
52. Cohen AM, Creviston S, LiPuma JP, Bryan PJ, Haaga JR, Alfidi RJ: NMR evaluation of hilar and mediastinal lymphadenopathy. Radiology *148*:739, 1983.
53. Gamsu G, Stark DD, Webb WR, Moore EH, Sheldon PE: Magnetic resonance imaging of benign mediastinal masses. Radiology *151*:709, 1984.
54. Alexander MC, Haage JR: MR imaging of a choledochal cyst. J Comput Assist Tomogr *92*:357, 1985.
55. Ferrucci JR: MR imaging of the liver. AJR *147*:1103, 1986.
56. Weinreb JC, Cohen JM, Armstrong E, Smith T: Imaging the pediatric liver: MRI and CT. AJR *147*:785, 1986.
57. Murphy FB, Steinberg HV, Shires GT, Martin LG, Bernadino ME: The Budd-Chiari syndrome: A review. AJR *147*:9, 1986.
58. Stark DD, Moseley ME, Bacon BR, Moss AA, Goldberg HI, Bass NM, James TI: Magnetic resonance imaging and spectroscopy of hepatic iron overload. Radiology *154*:137, 1985.
59. Cohen MD, Weetman RM, Provisor AJ, Grosfeld JL, West KW, Cory DA, Smith JA, McGuire W: Efficacy of magnetic resonance imaging in 139 children with tumors. Arch Surg *121*:522, 1986.
60. Kangarloo J, Dietrich RB, Ehrlich RM, Boechat MI, Feig SA: Magnetic resonance imaging of Wilms' tumor. Urology *28*:203, 1986.
61. Belt TG, Cohen MD, Smith JA, Cory DA, McKenna S, Weetman R: MRI of Wilms' tumor: Promise as the primary imaging method. AJR *146*:955, 1986.
62. Dietrich RB, Kangarloo H: Kidneys in infants and children: evaluation with MR. Radiology *159*:215, 1986.
63. Zimmer WD, Berquist TH, McLeod RA, Sim FH, Pritchard DJ, Shives TC, Wold LE, May GR: Bone tumors Magnetic resonance imaging versus computed tomography. Radiology *155*:709, 1985.
64. Cohen MD, Klatte E, Baehner R, Smith JA, Martin-Zimmerman P, Carr BE, et al: Magnetic resonance imaging of bone marrow disease in children. Radiology *151*:715, 1984.
65. Scoles PV, Yoon YS, Makley JT, Kalamchi A: Nuclear magnetic resonance imaging in Legg-Calvé-Perthes disease. J Bone Joint Surg *66*:1357, 1984.
66. Mitchell MD, Kundel HL, Steinberg ME, Kressel HY, Alavi A, Axel L: Avascular necrosis of the hip: Comparison of MR, CT and scintigraphy. AJR *147*:67, 1986.
67. Mitchell DG, Kressel HY, Arger PH, Dalinka M, Spritzer CE, Steinberg ME: Avascular necrosis of the femoral head: Morphologic assessment by MR imaging with CT correlation. Radiology *161*:739, 1986.
68. Fletcher BD, Scoles PV, Nelson AD: Osteomyelitis in children: Detection by magnetic resonance. Radiology *150*:57, 1984.
69. Haacke EM, Bearden FH, Clayton JR, Linga NR: Reduction of MR imaging time by the hybrid fast scan technique. Radiology *158*:521, 1986.
70. Haage A, Frahm J, Matthaei D, et al: FLASH imaging: rapid NMR imaging using low flip angle pulses. J Magn Reson *67*:258, 1986.

40

Surface Coil Imaging of the Spine

D. BALERIAUX
E. BOSKAMP
C. SEGEBARTH

In standard MR imaging, a single coil is used both for excitation of the spin system and for detection of the nuclear signal. The coil is then usually shaped so as to optimize rf homogeneity over its sensitive volume. Thus, a uniform excitation and detection sensitivity is obtained over the regions to be imaged.

Assuming that the object extends in the image plane's principal directions over a distance L, the field of view to be selected will thus equal this distance. And, if ultimately a spatial resolution ΔL is desired in the image plane, the number of measurements to be performed with a standard imaging technique will be given by $L/\Delta L$, in the simplifying additional assumption that the overall signal-to-noise ratio does not require any signal averaging.

One is often interested, however, in the examination of a small region in the image plane, extending over no more than a fraction of the object's extension L. The acquisition of data leading to an image with spatial resolution ΔL and field of view L then represents a considerable waste of time. Conversely, for a given total acquisition time, one would prefer to image only the region of interest, with increased spatial resolution. This is what has triggered the development of surface coils, which perfectly satisfy these requirements when the region of interest is located near the body surface.

Indeed, with surface coils the sensitivity to the nuclear signal is deliberately made strongly nonuniform. It is optimized to tissue near the coil (there is a good magnetic coupling between coil and nearby spins) and decreases rapidly with distance (consequently, the thermal noise superimposed on the nuclear signal is reduced, as tissues well beyond the sensitive region of the surface antenna no longer contribute to the overall noise of the measurement). Thus the field of view may be selected to much lower values, with a concomitant reduction of the minimal acquisition time at constant spatial resolution, or with a concomitant increase in spatial resolution at constant total acquisition time.

MATERIALS AND METHODS

With our imager (a Philips Gyroscan S15), surface coils are used in a double-coil configuration, the surface coil serving as detection coil and the rf excitation being applied through one of the standard rf coils (the body coil). This double-coil configuration has the advantage that, within the sensitive volume of the excitation coil, the rf pulses tilt the magnetization over identical angles.

Some problems may arise from the magnetic coupling between the two coils, however. During the excitation phase, currents may be induced in the surface coil, thus destroying the rf pulse homogeneity. And during the detection phase, the noise generated in the body coil may lower the signal-to-noise ratio of the measurement. One approach to avoid these pitfalls consists in the reduction of the magnetic coupling between the two coils. This is cumbersome and ineffective, however: It would force one to reorient the excitation coil at any change in the detection coil position (performed when proceeding to the examination of another body region).

In our system, the current intensities, induced in the surface coil during the excitation phase, are minimized through the maximizing, at that time, of the surface coil's impedance. Practically, this is realized by gating a reverse voltage over varicaps connected in parallel with the surface coil. The surface coil is thus detuned to higher frequencies during the pulse. During the detection phase, mutual induction between the two coils is minimized by increasing the excitation coil impedance. This is realized by gating a forward bias voltage over a diode bridge, connected in parallel with the excitation coil.[2]

The surface coil used for the thoracolumbar spinal examinations has been designed so as to provide a sensitive volume extending in one direction over 40 cm. A thin rectangular copper layer is deposited on a flexible support, so that a perfect match between coil and spine can be obtained, providing optimal magnetic coupling with the region of interest.

This surface coil may also be used for cervical spine examinations. Generally, though, we prefer to image the cervical spine with the head coil, which has been saddle-shaped so as to allow the imaging of the spine extending as low as T3 or T4. With respect to the surface coil, the head coil generally provides better quality images of the craniovertebral junction, at which level it is important to demonstrate associated malformations, if any.

The choice of the optimal pulse sequences obviously does not depend on the coil configuration. The only parameters affecting the selection of the pulse timings are the relaxation times and proton densities characterizing the tissues (neglecting the effects of flow and diffusion). When these are known, the contrast-to-noise ratio between tissues can be predicted and maximized for any pulse sequence.

When imaging the spine, contrast between CSF and normal CNS tissues very often has to be optimized. We have made use of published values[15] of the NMR parameters characterizing these tissues at 0.5 tesla (the field strength at which our imager is currently operating to plot the contrast curves relating the contrast-to-noise ratio between CSF and white or gray matter to the timing of the pulse sequences available (multiple-echo, spin echo, and inversion recovery, with echo delay time fixed initially at 50 ms and, more recently, at 50, 30, or 21 ms). We thus have been able to conclude that, at constant total acquisition time, the contrast-to-noise ratio between CSF and white or gray matter is optimal, in the case of a single-echo SE sequence, for a repetition time (TR) of about 400 ms. However, with this sequence, the CSF appears dark and iso-intense to the dural sac and the adjacent ligamental and bony structures, which one often would like to be able to distinguish from the CSF. Since, with the current NMR imaging techniques, the latter structures never give rise to observable signal intensity, we have been led to select, on the basis of the contrast curves, a second spin-echo sequence, leading this time to a reversed contrast between CSF and cerebral matter. This contrast behavior is obtained when using much longer repetition times in combination with longer echo-delay times.

The lack of published NMR parameters characterizing the different pathologic states of CNS tissues, besides the fact that our imager did not provide reliable $T1$ and $T2$ images until very recently, has forced us to a much more pragmatic approach when deciding upon the sequences preferable to use in case of suspected medullary pathologies. We apply the two sequences discussed earlier for these types of examinations, considering that the short *TR* sequence will provide images with predominant *T1* weighted contrasts, whereas the multiple-echo long *TR* sequence will provide *T2* weighted contrasts.

To stay within reasonable total acquisition times, we thus image the spine with two different pulse sequences, taking two averages in both cases, and imaging on a 256 × 256 matrix. The short *TR* sequence (*TR* = 400 ms) requires a total acquisition time of 3.4 minutes, whereas the multiple-echo long *TR* sequence (*TR* = 2000 ms) requires 17 minutes, in the case of single-slice imaging. We label the latter sequence as "myelographic," as it provides contrasts similar to those observed with hydrosoluble myelography. Analogous contrast patterns can be obtained with the inversion-recovery sequence. But, currently, we did not optimize the interpulse delays for this pulse sequence.

The current protocol being routinely used for spine imaging starts with a quick transverse scan (*TR* = 250 ms, 128 × 256 matrix), the result of which is used for the localization of the eventual sagittal slices. This localization scan is followed by a multiple-slice scan, imaging five adjacent slices, with the short repetition time of 450 ms. The third (median) slice is centered on the spine at the level of measurement of the previous transverse scan. Slice thickness is 5 mm, a compromise based on the conflicting requirements derived from signal-to-noise ratio, which one desires to optimize, and the partial-volume effects, which one aims to reduce. Total imaging time of this acquisition procedure is around eight minutes (as the slices are adjacent, our imager acquires data in two separate "packages," grouping nonadjacent slices). Finally, the long *TR* scan is performed (17 minutes total acquisition time) to obtain the image of a single 5 mm thick sagittal slice, displaying the reversed contrast between spine and CSF.* And, when considered useful to the diagnosis, additional coronal, transverse, or oblique cuts are subsequently imaged.

CLINICAL RESULTS

Our clinical experience with surface-coil imaging of the spine dates from July 1984, when we examined patients at the Philips factory, in Best. Since December 1984, the Gyroscan S15 imager has been fully operational at Erasme Hospital, allowing us to perform the spine examinations on a more frequent and regular basis. As of July 1985, we had performed more than 200 spinal cord examinations, of which about 50 percent included imaging of the thoracolumbar region with a surface coil.

Normal Anatomy

The short *TR* pulse sequences provide excellent delineation of the spinal cord (Fig. 40–1*A*). Signal intensity of the spinal cord is superior to that of the adjacent spinal fluid, which appears isointense with the dura and the adjacent cortical bony structures. Hence, the "perimedullary space" appears much larger than it is in reality. Fat gives rise to high-intensity signals on *T1* weighted images, leading to easily recognizable epidural fat and ligamentum flavum. Intervertebral discs and the adjacent vertebral bodies are the source of comparable low-intensity signals.

---

* Following a recent suggestion,[6] we have appreciably reduced the artifacts due to CSF pulsation by ECG triggering the data acquisition (we skip one or two cardiac cycles out of every two or three). None of the figures in this chapter has benefited from this improvement, inasmuch as they were obtained prior to implementation of the technique.

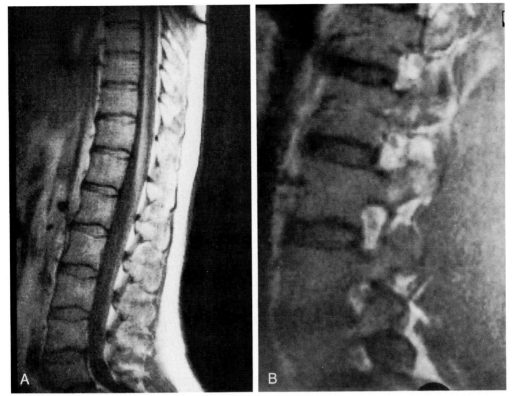

Figure 40–1. *A*, normal surface coil image of the lower thoracic spine and lumbar region. Short *TR* spin-echo pulse sequence. Good visualization of the normal conus medullaris. *B*, Parasagittal lumbar cut at the level of neural foramina. Nerve roots and surrounding vascular structures are well seen.

The long *TR*, multiple-echo pulse sequences provide the "myelographic" images (see Fig. 40–10*B*). CSF appears bright and is clearly differentiated from the dura and cortical bone, always of low signal intensity. This results in a precise delineation of the subarachnoid space. Contrast between spinal cord and CSF is enhanced for echo delays in the range of 150 to 200 ms. The spinal cord then provides low signal intensity, in contrast to the CSF, characterized by much longer *T2* values. The intervertebral discs appear brighter than the adjacent vertebral bodies. Often, a line of low signal intensity can be recognized within the normal disc, presumably corresponding to the central nucleus pulposus.

Pathologic Findings

Prior to the advent of MRI, spinal cord visualization could be considered to present a very difficult challenge to the neuroradiologist. A high number of x-ray examinations were required, including aggressive procedures such as myelography and myelo–computed tomography, which often led to an incomplete depiction of the disease. MRI provided, for the first time, an excellent quality and complete image of the spinal cord and spinal canal content.[3,7,9–14] We consider it of predominant importance in the spinal cord examination. MRI equally readily depicts disc and bony lesions,[4,8] but we limit the spinal MRI examinations mainly to the spinal cord diseases.

INTRAMEDULLARY LESIONS

Hydro- and Syringomyelia. Thirty percent of our surface-coil examinations revealed the presence of hydro- or syringomyelia (Figs. 40–2 to 40–4), the diagnosis of which has often been confirmed by complementary transverse cuts (Fig 40–3*C*). We fully support the idea that MRI is the optimal imaging modality for the diagnosis of syringomyelia.[5,17] Moreover, the ease of performance and the innocuousness of the examination allow elegant postoperative controls, usually not performed in the pre–MRI era. Seventeen percent of the detected lesions appeared to be of traumatic origin (Fig. 40–3): This suggests a general underestimation of the occurrence of this disease.

In two cases, extensive syringomyelia could be attributed to arachnoiditis (Fig. 40–4). This type of lesion is generally impossible to disclose by myelography and often difficult to image on delayed myelo-CT. It has rarely been reported in the literature,[1,15] most likely as a result of the diagnostic difficulty.

Intramedullary cavities are well visualized on short *TR* images. They appear as sharply delineated, low-density areas. Often we have observed that the hydromyelia and syringomyelia extend to the whole spinal cord, ending in a V-shape within the conus medullaris (see Fig. 40–2*A*).

On *T2* weighted images, surprisingly, the syrinx often remains a low-intensity area, usually when it is large (Fig. 40–4*B*). This could arise from the transmission of the cardiac pulses to the fluid within the cavity. In other cases, the syrinx appears bright on the "myelographic" views (see Fig. 40–10*B*).

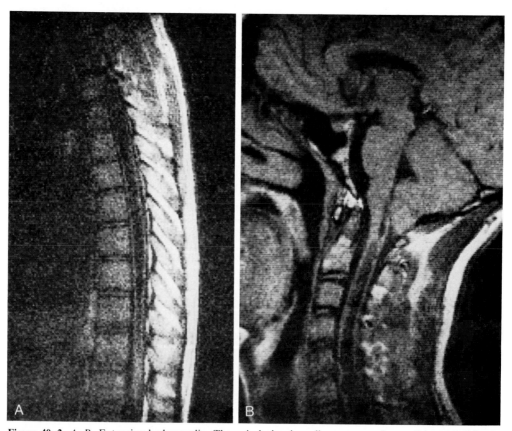

Figure 40–2. *A–B*, Extensive hydromyelia. Thoracic lesion is well seen on surface coil image, while the cervical status has been explored by standard head coil. The communication between intramedullar cavity and lower fourth ventricle is well demonstrated, as is the Chiari malformation.

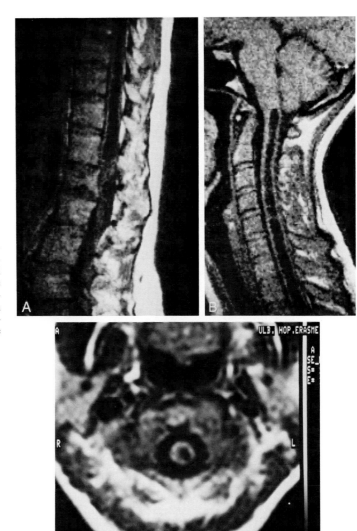

Figure 40–3. *A,* Post-traumatic syringomyelia. Fracture of T11, producing medullar lesion of the conus and an associated ascending cavity. *B,* Head coil image showing the extension up to the bulbar region without apparent communication with fourth ventricle. *C,* Slightly eccentric location of the syrinx is best shown on the transverse image.

INTRAMEDULLARY TUMORS

MR examination of spinal cord tumors appears to be extremely valuable. On short *TR* images, the spinal cord enlargement is clearly demonstrated (Fig. 40–5*A*). Associated cystic components, frequently observed, appear as well-delineated hyposignal areas. Some tumors, moreover, present ill-defined hyposignal areas, most likely of increased *T1,* as is often encountered with brain tumors.

With the long *TR* pulse sequence, the high intensity of the tumor tissue provides a clear delineation of the tumor infiltration (Fig. 40–5*B*). However, no specific signal disturbances have yet been associated with the histologic findings. MRI appears to be superior to myelography in that it provides on a single scan the total extent of the lesion, that it clearly indicates the presence of cystic components, and, above all, that it in no way affects the patient's neurologic condition. Intramedullary hemangioblastoma and angioma appear as hyposignal, spherical, often very small, sharply delineated areas in combination with similar hypersignal zones. This signal behavior is analogous to what is observed with cerebral AV malformations.

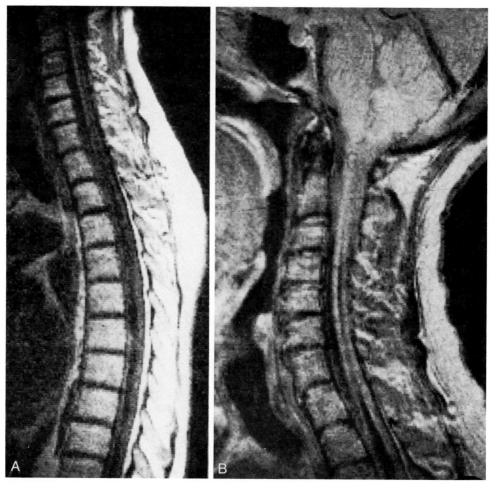

Figure 40–4. *A*, Syringomyelia secondary to tuberculous arachnoiditis. The cavitation is well seen, and the subarachnoid space appears completely obstructed by material isointense with the normal spinal tissue at the thoracic level. *B*, Upper syrinx. Note the hypointense aspect resulting from the use of the long *TR* spin-echo sequence.

On three occasions we have observed hematomyelia. On short *TR* images (Fig. 40–6) the shape of the cord was normal, but within the medulla a small hypersignal area could be detected. The location of this area was in perfect concordance with the clinical symptoms. We did not apply the long *TR* pulse sequences to these patients, considering that their condition was too poor for a long examination time to be imposed.

EXTRAMEDULLARY INTRACANALAR TUMORS

Neuromas. Neuromas are difficult to detect. On short *TR* images (Fig. 40–7), their signal intensity is very similar to that of the adjacent spinal cord, whereas with the long *TR* sequence, they are only slightly hypersignal with respect to the adjacent normal tissue.

Lipomas. Intracanalar lipomas are readily and exquisitely depicted on the short *TR* images (Fig. 40–8), as a result of the short *T1* of fatty issue. The bright signal associated to this pathology provides one of the rare true specific diagnoses of MRI.

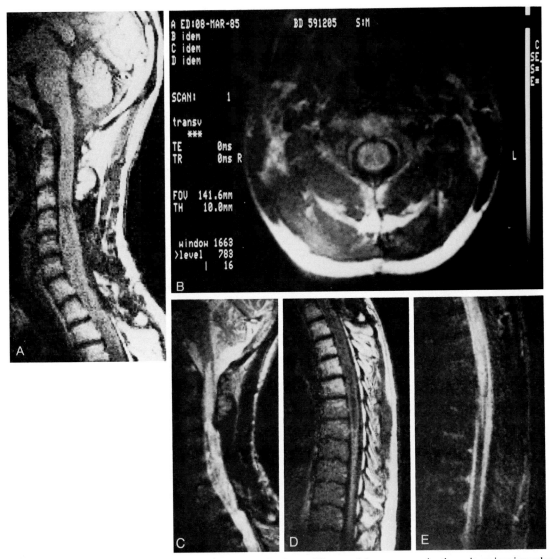

Figure 40-5. Recurrence of an extensive ependymoma. *A*, Surface coil image of the upper cervicothoracic region: irregular enlargement of the medulla. Ill-defined, low-intensity areas within the spinal cord, equally well shown on transverse sections (*B*). *C*, Same cut as *A* but with use of longer *TR* sequence. Extension of the tumor within the upper spinal cord is better demonstrated. *D–E*, Thoracic extension of the same tumor depicted with short (*D*) and long (*E*) *TR* sequences. Cystic components are clearly demonstrated at midthoracic level.

Meningiomas. Similar signal intensity is associated with meningioma and normal medulla (Fig. 40-9), with both of the pulse sequences used. With the myelographic technique, the lesion is perfectly delineated within the hypersignal subarachnoid space.

Epidural Tumors

We have imaged metastatic lesions, Hodgkin's disease, and one hemangiopericytoma. The extradural location as well as the precise extent of the lesions was best demonstrated on short *TR* images. No specific signal intensity could be linked to the histologic findings.

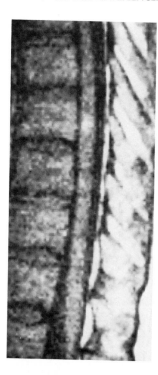

Figure 40–6. Hematomyelia at T6 level: small hypersignal area on short *TR* sequence.

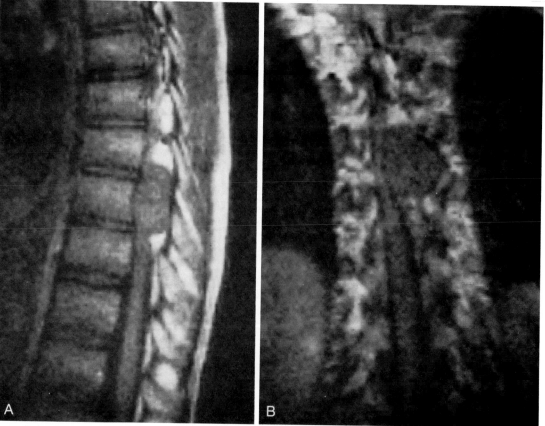

Figure 40–7. Midthoracic neuroma. Tumoral signal is very similar to that of the normal spinal cord, on short *TR* images. *A*, Parasagittal cut. *B*, Coronal cut.

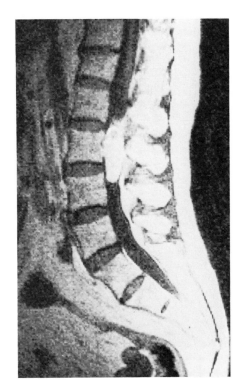

Figure 40–8. Lumbar lipoma: bright signal within the sharply outlined tumor on short *TR* image.

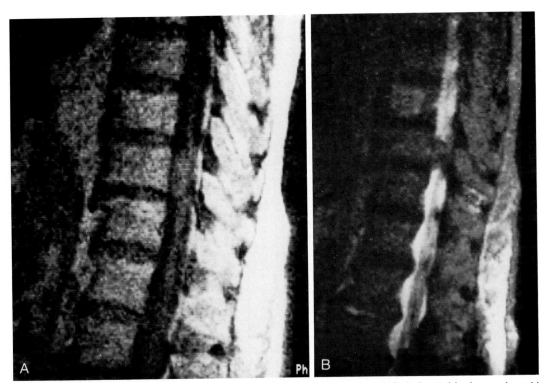

Figure 40–9. Thoracic meningioma. *A*, Short *TR* image. The isosignal tumor is anteriorly located in the canal, pushing the medulla backward. *B*, Long *TR* image. The tumor appears to be of low signal intensity and is sharply delineated from the hyperintense CSF.

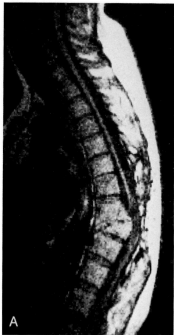

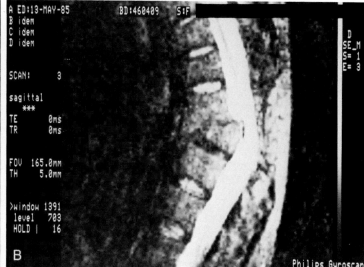

Figure 40–10. Secondary narrow thoracic spinal canal, due to traumatic lesion of the T7–8 vertebrae. Spinal cord compression with associated small secondary syringomyelia above and below the fracture site. *A*, Short *TR* image. *B*, Long *TR* image optimally demonstrates the subarachnoid space impairment.

MEDULLARY COMPRESSION OF EXTRINSIC NONTUMORAL ORIGIN

The narrowing of the spinal canal due to bony lesions (polyarthritis, Morquio's disease, fracture, degenerative diseases, dorsal disc herniation) and the associated medullary compression are extremely well seen on MRI. Both the short (Fig. 40–10*A*) and the long *TR* (Fig. 40–10*B*) techniques appear valuable to demonstrate cord compression and subarachnoid space impairment.

In conclusion, MRI with surface coils provides a unique and powerful imaging modality for the spinal cord. The high signal-to-noise ratio and the adequate spatial resolution allow accurate diagnosis of several spinal cord lesions, including syringomyelia, medullary tumors, extramedullary intracanalar tumors, and extrinsic cord compressions. Some limitations still remain, mainly related to the patient's anatomic configuration (scoliosis). In these cases, the multiplanar approach of MRI allows one to extract useful diagnostic information nevertheless.

References

1. Barnett HJM: Syringomyelia associated with spinal arachnoiditis localised to the spinal canal. *In* Barnett HJM, Foster JB, Hudgson P (eds). Major Problems in Neurology: Syringomyelia. Philadelphia, WB Saunders, 1973, pp. 245–258.
2. Boskamp EB: Improved surface coil imaging by decoupling of the excitation coil and receiver coil in MR tomography. Radiology *157*:449, 1985.
3. Brant-Zawadzki M, Norman D, Mills C: Nuclear magnetic resonance imaging of the spinal cord. *In* Genant HK, Helms CA, Chafetz NI (eds): Spine Update 1984. San Francisco, Radiology Research and Education Foundation, 1983, pp 383–390.
4. Chafetz NI, Genant HK, Moon KL, et al: Recognition of lumbar disk herniation with NMR. AJNR *5*:23, 1984.
5. DeLaPaz RL, Brady TJ, Buonanno FS, et al: Nuclear magnetic resonance (NMR) imaging of Arnold-Chiari type 1 malformation with hydromelia. J Comput Assist Tomogr 7:126, 1983.
6. Enzmann DR, Rubin JB: Using CSF gating to obtain T2 information from the spinal cord. Proc 5th Annual Meeting SMRM 1986, pp 5–6.

7. Han JS, Benson JE, Yoon YS: Magnetic resonance imaging in the spinal column and craniovertebral junction. Radiol Clin North Am *22*(4):805, 1984.
8. Han JS, Kaufman B, EL Yousef SJ, et al: NMR imaging of the spine. AJNR *141*:1137, 1983.
9. Modic MT, Hardy RW, Weinstein MA, et al: Nuclear magnetic resonance of the spine: Clinical potential and limitation. Neurosurgery *15*(4):583, 1984.
10. Modic MT, Weinstein MA: Nuclear magnetic resonance of the spine. Br Med Bull *40*(2):183, 1984.
11. Modic MT, Pavlicek W, Weinstein MA, et al: Nuclear magnetic resonance of intervertebral disc disease: Clinical and pulse sequence considerations. Radiology *152*:103, 1984.
12. Modic MT, Weinstein MA, Pavlicek W, et al: Magnetic resonance imaging of the cervical spine: Technical and clinical observations. AJR *141*:1129, 1983.
13. Modic MT, Weinstein MA, Pavlicek W, et al: Nuclear magnetic resonance imaging of the spine. Radiology *148*:757, 1983.
14. Norman D, Mills CM, Brant-Zawadzki M, et al: Magnetic resonance imaging of the spinal cord and canal: Potentials and limitations. AJNR *5*:9, 1984.
15. Simmon JD, Newton TH: Arachnoiditis. *In* Newton TH, Potts DG (eds): Computed Tomography of the Spine and Spinal Cord. San Anselmo, California, Clavadel Press, 1983.
16. Wehrli FW, et al: The dependence of nuclear magnetic resonance (NMR) image contrast on intrinsic and pulse sequence timing parameters. Magn Reson Imag *2*:3, 1984.
17. Yeates A, Brant-Zawadzki M, Norman D, et al: Nuclear magnetic resonance imaging of syringomyelia. AJNR *4*:234, 1983.

41

MRI at Low Field Strength

FRANCIS W. SMITH

Considerable controversy surrounds the question of which is the "best" field strength for magnetic resonance imaging (MRI). There is no doubt that the superb spatial resolution afforded by high field strength, superconductive magnets gives an excellent display of human anatomy. However, this high spatial resolution is not always necessary for MR images to be diagnostically useful, since much useful work has been performed at low field strengths.

MRI instruments based on magnets whose field strengths vary from 0.02 to 2.0 tesla are available for clinical use at the present time. For the purposes of this chapter, low field is considered to be that below 0.1 tesla. Considerable experience with MRI systems operating at 0.02, 0.04, and 0.08 tesla has been published, and there are even reports of work using the earth's magnetic field (0.00005 tesla) alone to image in vitro and to make in vivo $T2$ measurements of blood and amniotic fluid.[1,2]

The main advantage to working at higher field strength is the resultant stronger NMR signal and better signal-to-noise ratio that can be achieved with high spatial resolution imaging. Images made at lower field strength may have less spatial resolution but usually have greater contrast resolution between different tissues. This is because the differences in $T1$ relaxation time between different tissues are more accurately measured at low field strength and are more widely separated below 0.01 tesla, beginning to overlap above 0.1 tesla.[3] $T2$ relaxation times, however, are not as dependent upon field strength and therefore of Lamor frequency, being more dependent upon tissue type.[4] Because the characteristic $T1$ and $T2$ measurements can be accurately quantified at low field strength, the unique ability to observe water and its relationship to different tissues in disease states, which is available with MRI, can best be exploited at low field strength. While it is important that high-resolution instruments be used for the investigation of areas where excellent anatomic detail is required, it is also important to research the full capability of MRI in order to understand the mechanisms for what is being seen in any given image. It is likely that a significant contribution to our better understanding of MRI will come from work performed at low magnetic field strength.

Probably more important than the strength of the magnet used for imaging is the homogeneity of its field. The best images are produced from the most homogeneous fields using well-shimmed magnets and accurately tuned gradient, transmit, and receive coils. The main reason for low-field imaging's being less popular than it might have been is that all the available low-field systems were developed either as university-based experiments or as commercial ventures with a relatively low budget. As a result, many of the software methods for image acquisition and display have not been developed. If multiple-acquisition buffers were averaged and the image matrix increased from 128 $\times$ 128 to 256 $\times$ 256, there is no reason why images of significantly improved spatial resolution could not be made. All the imaging techniques—partial saturation, spin density, spin echo, and inversion recovery—can be employed at low field, making these instruments as versatile as the higher field strength ones.

The lowest field strength MRI system to be used clinically is a 0.02 tesla system developed in Finland. This system employs an 0.02 tesla resistive magnet and the two-dimensional fast Fourier transformation method of imaging. Data acquisition can be carried out by both the spin-echo and the inversion-recovery techniques, using a 128 × 256 pixel imaging matrix. The final image is displayed by a 256 × 256 matrix. The system has been designed as a small, cost-effective instrument that can be installed in existing accommodation, such as the emergency department of a hospital, with a minimum of site preparation. Single- and multislice imaging is possible in the axial, sagittal, and coronal planes. Using sequences that can be performed in four minutes, both inversion recovery (*TR* = 1000, *TI* = 200, *TE* = 70 [Fig. 41–1]) and spin echo (*TR* = 2000, *TE* = 160), this system is claimed to be as clinically useful as x-ray CT performed with either EMI CT 1010 or Somatom DR 2.[5] With shorter spin-echo sequences the basic anatomy of the spine and pelvis is displayed (Fig. 41–2).

In 1980 the development of the 0.04 tesla (1.7 MHz) instrument designed and built at the University of Aberdeen had reached the stage at which the body images were of sufficient quality to commence clinical trials (Fig. 41–3). Throughout 1981 new developments improved image display, especially the interpolation of the 128 × 128 data acquisition matrix to 256 × 256 to the point at which small vessels, such as the superior mesenteric artery, could be seen (Figs. 41–4 and 41–5). Images of the brain were initially very poor but still of sufficient quality to demonstrate gross pathology by virtue of the good contrast resolution between normal and abnormal tissue.[6] Although the system had not been designed for this purpose, when a series of brain images are studied it can be appreciated how improvements in acquisition and display improve the image. Figure 41–6 shows an axial section of a normal brain using a 64 × 64 image acquisition matrix displayed by 128 × 128; Figure 41–7 is another normal brain study acquired using a 128 × 128 data acquisition matrix displayed by 256 × 256. Further improvement is achieved by the use of a specialized receiver coil placed around the head (Fig. 41–8) and doubling of the field strength to 0.08 tesla (3.4 MHz). There is an increase in spatial resolution but a decrease in contrast resolution, clearly seen in Figure 41–9 when compared with Figure 41–8.

The 0.04 imager built in the Department of Bio-Medical Physics and Bio-Engineering at the University of Aberdeen is based on a four-coil, air-cored resistive magnet. The spin-warp method of imaging is used as well as a fixed-pulse sequence consisting of read-out pulses every 1000 ms with alternate read-out pulses preceded by inversion.

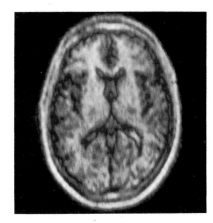

Figure 41–1. Inversion recovery image (*TR* = 1000 ms, *TI* = 200 ms, *TE* = 70 ms) of a normal brain made with a 0.02 tesla system. (Acutscan, Instrumentarium Corporation, Helsinki, Finland.)

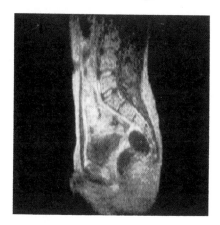

Figure 41–2. Spin-echo ($TR = 250$ ms, $TE = 40$ ms) sagittal section of lumbar spine and pelvis made with a 0.02 tesla system. (Acutscan, Instrumentarium Corporation, Helsinki, Finland.)

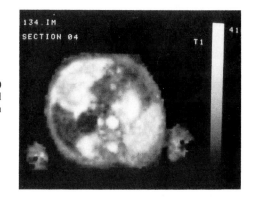

Figure 41–3. Calculated *T1* image made at 0.04 tesla ($TR = 1000$ ms, $TI = 200$ ms); 64 × 64 pixel data acquisition matrix displayed by a 128 × 128 matrix. A large cholangiocarcinoma (white) is seen in the liver (dark gray).

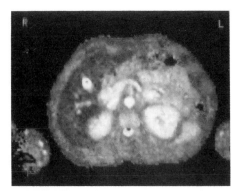

Figure 41–4. Calculated *T1* image made at 0.04 tesla ($TR = 1000$ ms, $TI = 200$ ms); 128 × 128 data acquisition matrix displayed by a 256 × 256 matrix. Normal upper abdomen at the level of the superior mesenteric artery.

Figure 41–5. Calculated *T1* image of a hepatoma in the left lobe of the liver, made with a 0.04 tesla instrument using the same parameters as in Figure 41–4.

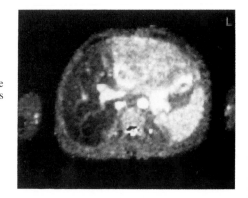

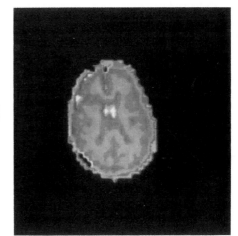

Figure 41–6. Calculated *T1* image of normal brain, made at 0.04 tesla using a *TR* of 1000 ms and *TI* of 200 ms, with a 64 × 64 acquisition matrix displayed by a 128 × 128 pixel matrix.

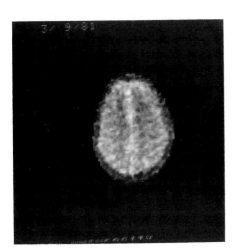

Figure 41–7. Calculated *T1* image of normal brain, made at 0.04 tesla using *TR* = 1000 and *TI* = 200 ms, with a 128 × 128 acquisition matrix displayed by a 256 × 256 matrix.

Figure 41–8. Calculated *T1* image of normal brain made at 0.04 tesla using a head coil and a 128 × 128 data acquisition matrix displayed by a 256 × 256 matrix (*TR* = 1000, *TI* = 200).

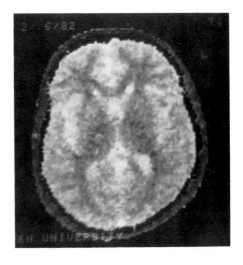

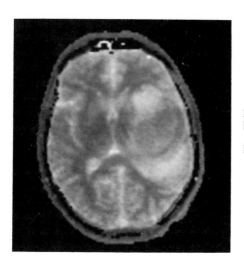

Figure 41–9. Calculated *T1* image of brain made at 0.08 tesla using a head coil and a 128 × 128 data acquisition matrix displayed by a 256 × 256 pixel matrix (*TR* = 1000, *TI* = 200). Three-week-old cerebral hemorrhage is present in right hemisphere.

The inversion is accomplished by adiabatic fast passage with continuous delay of 200 ms. In other words, the pulse sequence consists of interleafed saturation-recovery (*S1*) and inversion-recovery (*S2*) sequences (*TR* = 1000, *TI* = 200). Initially, the *S1* and *S2* data are Fourier-transformed into two 128 × 128 element arrays before being interpolated into 256 × 256 arrays for display on a visual display unit. The acquisition time for each section is collected in 4 min, 16 sec. The data can be displayed in a number of ways. Four types of image are produced: inversion recovery; proton density; a difference image that is calculated by subtracting *S2* from *S1*, giving a *T1* weighted image; and a calculated *T1* image. The *T1* value for each pixel of this image is calculated from the formula $T1 = 200/\ln (2 \times S_1) (S_1 - S_2)$. The details of this system are fully described elsewhere.[7–11]

This 0.04 tesla instrument was used in clinical practice from mid-1980 until the end of 1982 in over 1000 patients to demonstrate the potential of nuclear magnetic resonance as a safe, noninvasive imaging technique and to show that the *T1* contrast between different tissues was sufficient to accurately diagnose both benign and malignant disease. It was also used to show that on measuring the *T1* relaxation time of tissues most diseases had a characteristic relaxation time, but that unfortunately these values overlapped and that there were no pathognomonic diagnostic values for any one disease.

In the first patient studied, a 66-year-old man with an inoperable carcinoma of the esophagus and hepatic metastases, it was possible to demonstrate malignancy in vivo as having a longer than normal *T1* relaxation time. Both the primary tumor and the hepatic metastases were clearly seen as well as metastatic disease in the vertebral bodies, which had hitherto not been suspected but was subsequently confirmed by radionuclide bone scan.[12] It is interesting that this case demonstrated the ability of MRI to show disease of bone, a fact that was not fully appreciated until two to three years later, when the advent of surface coils produced high spatial resolution images of the musculoskeletal system. The potential for imaging the skeletal system has always been evident at low field strength, where the good contrast resolution between normal and abnormal tissues, based on differences in *T1* relaxation time, has been diagnostically useful.[13–16]

Because of the usefulness of the 0.04 tesla instrument, a larger 0.08 tesla system was developed and has been in use in the Aberdeen Royal Infirmary since the beginning of 1983. Since this time, more than 3500 patients have been studied. The 0.08 tesla instrument differs from the 0.04 tesla system in its magnet strength and the versatility

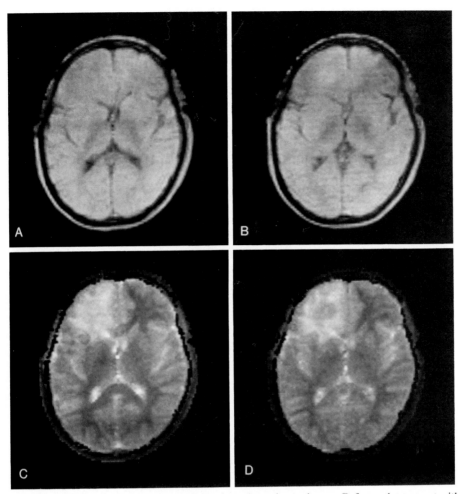

Figure 41–10. Left frontal metastasis from primary bronchogenic carcinoma. Before enhancement with gadolinium-DTPA (*A, C, E, G, I*). After enhancement (*B, D, F, H, J*). *A–B*, Proton density. *C–D*, Calculated *TI*.
Illustration continued on the following page

of its software. The same basic imaging pulse sequence is employed with the additional ability to vary the *TI* from between 50 to 450 ms.

The improved spatial resolution, together with the ability to display calculated *TI* and inversion-recovery images using different *TI* intervals, has proved this instrument to be a valuable diagnostic system. The appearances of the brain using different *TI* values at a *TR* of 1000 ms are shown in Figure 41–10, and those in the abdomen are shown in Figure 41–11. Saturation-recovery (Fig. 41–12) and spin-echo images (Fig. 41–13) may also be made at 0.08 tesla and, as can be seen, appear very similar to those made at higher field strength.

CLINICAL APPLICATIONS

Central Nervous System

As indicated earlier, the 0.04 tesla instrument was not designed primarily to image the brain but as a whole-body system. The early brain images made without the use of a head-coil receiver were adequate, by virtue of their good contrast resolution, to

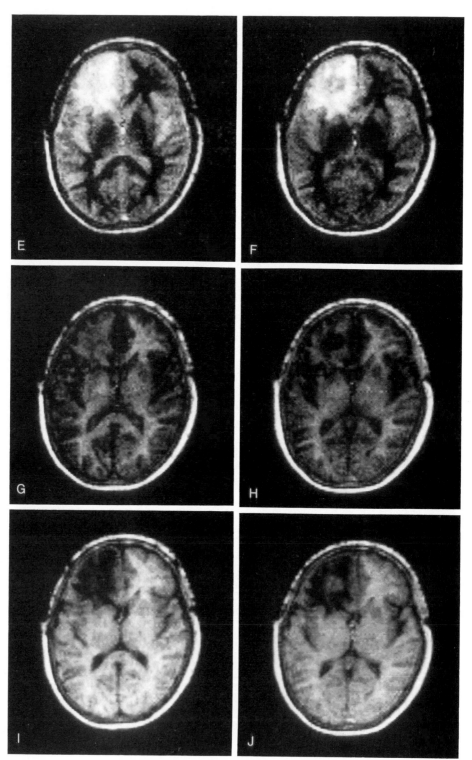

Figure 41–10 *Continued E–F*, Inversion recovery *TI* = 200 ms. *G–H*, Inversion recovery *TI* = 300 ms. *I–J*, Inversion recovery *TI* = 400 ms. The effects of changing *TI* are well demonstrated, as is the effect of shortening relaxation time in the tumor to increase the contrast between tumor and surrounding edema.

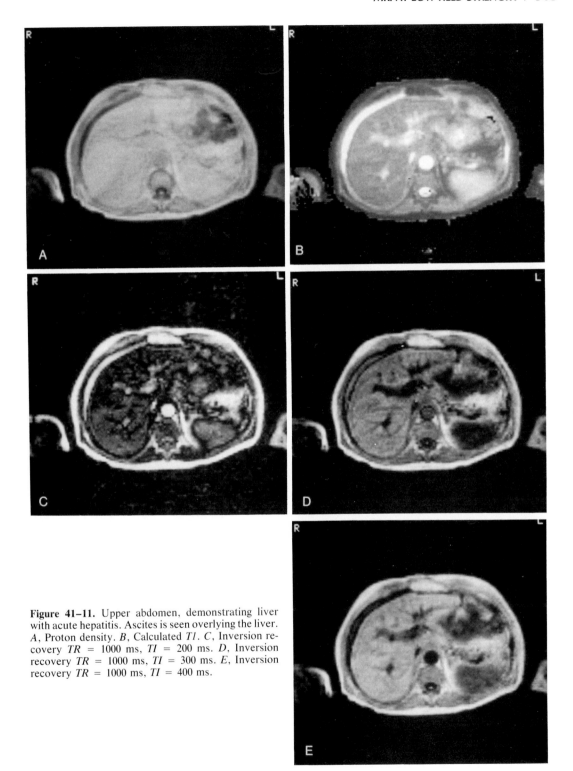

Figure 41–11. Upper abdomen, demonstrating liver with acute hepatitis. Ascites is seen overlying the liver. *A*, Proton density. *B*, Calculated *T1*. *C*, Inversion recovery *TR* = 1000 ms, *TI* = 200 ms. *D*, Inversion recovery *TR* = 1000 ms, *TI* = 300 ms. *E*, Inversion recovery *TR* = 1000 ms, *TI* = 400 ms.

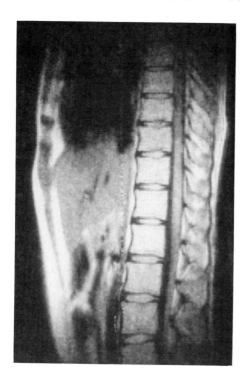

Figure 41–12. Midline sagittal section of a normal lumbar spine. Saturation recovery image *TR* 500/20. (M&D Technology, Aberdeen, Scotland.)

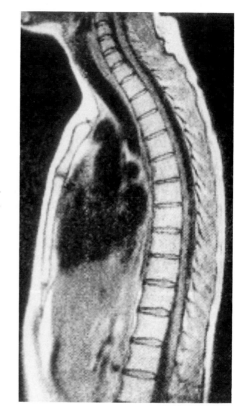

Figure 41–13. Mid-line sagittal section of normal dorsal spine. Spin-echo *TR* = 1000 ms, *TE* = 80 ms. (M&D Technology, Aberdeen, Scotland.)

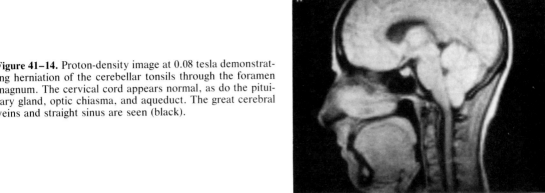

Figure 41–14. Proton-density image at 0.08 tesla demonstrating herniation of the cerebellar tonsils through the foramen magnum. The cervical cord appears normal, as do the pituitary gland, optic chiasma, and aqueduct. The great cerebral veins and straight sinus are seen (black).

demonstrate gross pathology such as primary and secondary tumors, infarction, and hemorrhage.[6,17] The development of a head coil improved the images significantly (see Fig. 41–8) and demonstrated the potential of NMR for the study of white matter disease and disease in the posterior fossa. With the development of the 0.08 tesla instrument came the ability to visualize coronal and sagittal sections as well as conventional axial ones, and it soon became evident that MRI was the method of choice for the investigation of the cerebellum, brainstem, cervical cord, and base of the skull. Although the images lack the fine detail of higher field strength images, all the important midline brain structures are clearly identified: the pituitary gland, optic chiasma, aqueduct, and great cerebral veins (Fig. 41–14). In the Arnold-Chiari malformation, herniation of the cerebellar tonsils is easily seen in the sagittal plane, and syringomyelia of the cervical cord can be diagnosed (Fig. 41–15) even when very small (Fig. 41–16).

As with the higher field instruments, it is possible to display large extracanalicular acoustic neuromas (Fig. 41–17) and tiny intracanalicular ones as well (Fig. 41–18).

As would be expected, tumors, infarcts, and hemorrhage are best displayed using calculated *T1* and inversion-recovery images and may be seen when no space-occupying effect is present (Fig. 41–19). Above the tentorium, the strong contrast between tumor and normal brain compensates for the lower spatial resolution. The same difficulties exist in discriminating between edema and some tumors as exist at high field strength. It may be that paramagnetic contrast agents will help in this area. Gadolinium-DTPA

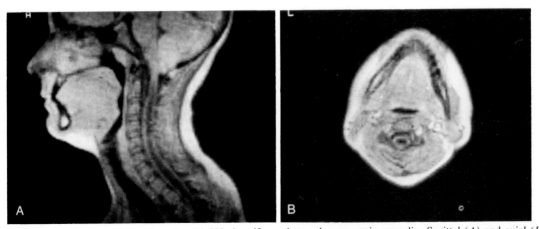

Figure 41–15. Proton-density image. Arnold-Chiari malformation and gross syringomyelia. Sagittal (*A*) and axial (*B*) sections.

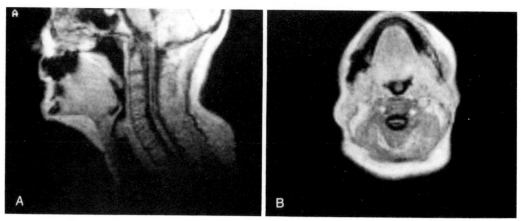

Figure 41–16. Proton-density image. Small cervical cord syrinx. Sagittal (*A*) and axial (*B*) sections.

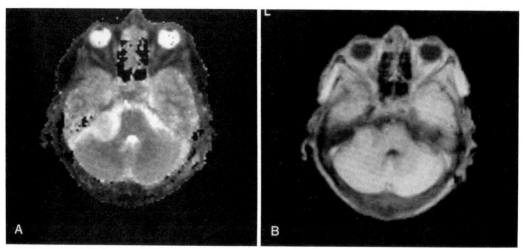

Figure 41–17. Large extracanalicular acoustic neuroma. Calculated *T1* (*A*) and proton-density (*B*) images.

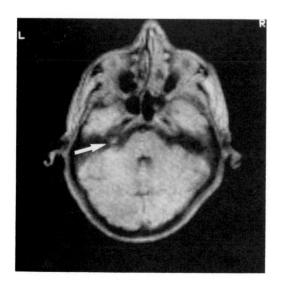

Figure 41–18. Small intracanalicular acoustic neuroma in left internal auditory canal (arrow). Proton density image made at 0.08 tesla (3.4 MHz).

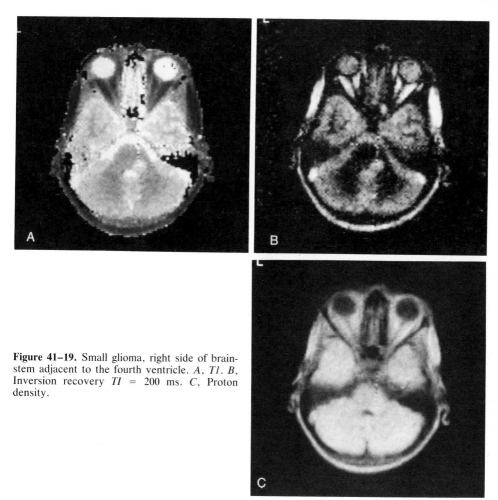

Figure 41–19. Small glioma, right side of brainstem adjacent to the fourth ventricle. *A, T1. B,* Inversion recovery *TI* = 200 ms. *C,* Proton density.

has been used, and the same effects that are seen at high field strength are seen at 0.08 tesla (see Fig. 41–10).

Difficulty has been experienced in differentiating some small early infarcts from recent hemorrhage, but less difficulty has been experienced in differentiating demyelination in multiple sclerosis from old lacuna infarcts. Old infarcts appear to have a lower proton density than normal brain and appear black on the proton-density image and white on the *T1* image. Demyelination appears gray on the proton-density and white on the *T1* image. Although these appearances are not pathognomonic of multiple sclerosis, they do serve to distinguish demyelination from infarction. Differentiation from hypertensive changes, nonspecific periventricular white matter lesions, and other causes of strong signal in white matter is difficult, and the size, shape, and distribution of lesions is helpful. Large and small subdural hemorrhage is best demonstrated using MRI. Localization of the size and extent of these hemorrhages is best achieved by the use of coronal sections with either calculated *T1* or proton-density images (Fig. 41–20).

In common with most other workers, we have found that MRI at 0.08 tesla is no better than x-ray CT for the examination of the cerebral hemispheres but far superior in the examination of the posterior fossa and cervical canal. The pituitary fossa and orbits are also better displayed using MRI. The improved signal-to-noise ratio obtained with surface coils contributes significantly to the examination of the orbits, where the

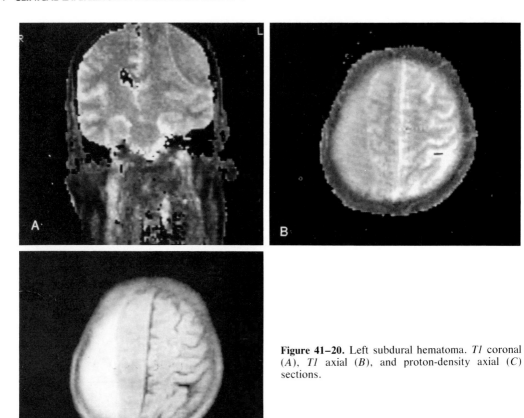

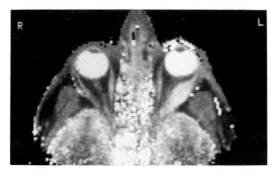

Figure 41–20. Left subdural hematoma. *T1* coronal (*A*), *T1* axial (*B*), and proton-density axial (*C*) sections.

lens and chambers of the eye can be examined and the optic nerve, ophthalmic vessels, and ocular muscles clearly seen (Fig. 41–21).[18]

Head and Neck

X-ray CT has a number of major limitations for the examination of head and neck tumors. The experience with both 0.04 and 0.08 tesla MRI systems has been good, and the method has been shown to be more sensitive and accurate in the diagnosis of tumors and infections of this region.

Figure 41–21. Calculated *T1* image of the orbits using an eyeglass-shaped surface coil to examine both orbits simultaneously. Pseudotumor (myositis) of the right lateral rectus muscle is shown.

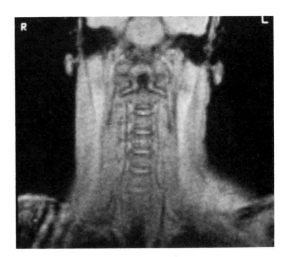

Figure 41–22. Coronal section, proton-density image of a normal neck demonstrating the vertebral bodies and vertebral arteries.

Sufficient spatial detail is available in the proton-density images to define the cervical spine and canal (Fig. 41–22) and to see the carotid and vertebral arteries. When infection is present in a vertebral body, destruction of cortical bone is recognizable if present (Fig. 41–23). The long $T1$ associated with inflammatory change, which is not usually as long as that seen in malignancy, is very evident at low field.[13] The signal seen on spin-density–proton-density images tends to be stronger in infection than in malignancy, a fact that is useful for the differentiation of the two (Figs. 41–23 and 41–24).

Evaluation of the soft tissues of the neck using 0.04 tesla has been limited to the study of the thyroid gland and the demonstration of malignant lymph nodes. In both cases the contrast between the $T1$ values of normal and abnormal tissue makes for easy tissue recognition. At 0.08 tesla the relaxation time contrast makes for recognition of diseased lymph nodes before this is evident on x-ray CT. Because inflammation, reactive hyperplasia, and malignancy all have long relaxation times it is not possible to be specific as to why a lymph node has a long relaxation time; it does, however, allow for more accurate staging of head and neck malignancy (Fig. 41–25). Tumors of the salivary glands (Fig. 41–26); naso-, oro-, and hypopharynx; tonsils; tongue; and larynx (Fig. 41–27) are all easily recognized and staged.

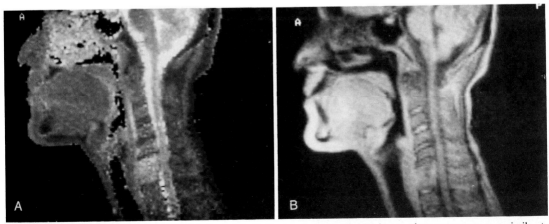

Figure 41–23. Tuberculous infection of C6–7. *A, T1. B,* Proton density. The *T1* image gives an appearance similar to that of a cervical myelogram or that seen in spin-echo imaging when a long *TE* value is used. It clearly demonstrates the narrowing of the spinal canal.

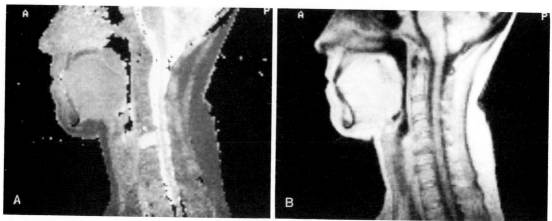

Figure 41-24. *T1* (*A*) and proton-density (*B*) images of non-Hodgkin's lymphoma of C5. Note the stronger (whiter) *T1* signal from this lymphoma than from the tuberculosis shown in Figure 41-23.

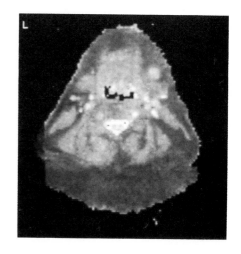

Figure 41-25. Axial *T1* image demonstrating single impalpable lymph node in right side of neck involved with carcinoma from a primary tumor of the tonsil.

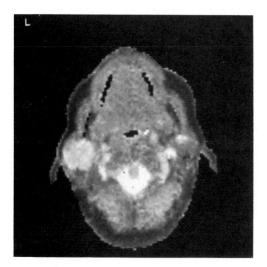

Figure 41-26. Axial *T1* image of carcinoma of the left parotid gland.

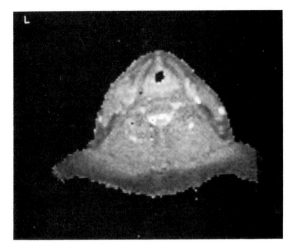

Figure 41–27. Axial *T1* image of laryngeal carcinoma with left-sided lymph node involvement.

Thorax

The most striking feature of the normal chest is the clarity with which the major blood vessels and cardiac chambers are seen without the use of contrast medium or cardiac gating (Fig. 41–28), although the images are improved by the application of cardiac gating. Blood has its own typical *T1*, which is very different from vessel walls and cardiac muscle. It appears white on the calculated *T1* image and appears as a "void" on the proton-density and inversion-recovery images. This finding has been used successfully at 0.04 tesla to differentiate vascular mediastinal masses from tumors by *T1* measurement, thereby avoiding bronchoscopy and arteriography in cases of vascular anomaly and aortic aneurysm.[9]

In common with most centers using MRI for diagnosis, we have not devoted a lot of time to the examination of the chest, believing that the potential for diagnosis demonstrated at 0.04 tesla will be better realized when cardiac and respiratory gating is employed.

Abdomen

Despite the image degradation that must be present in abdominal images made at 0.08 tesla without respiratory gating, they show a remarkable amount of anatomic detail

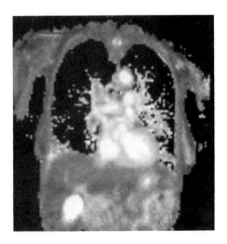

Figure 41–28. Coronal *T1* image of the chest demonstrating cardiac chambers and pulmonary vessels (white) without the use of intravenous contrast material or cardiac gating.

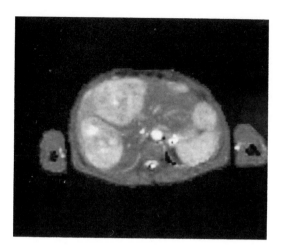

Figure 41–29. Axial *T1* image of the liver containing two large metastases from a primary adenocarcinoma of the breast.

and are as good as, if not better than, the majority of published abdominal images from higher field strength instruments. The reasons for this probably are the use of the spin-warp imaging method and the good contrast between different tissues that is present using *T1* based images. Small structures, such as the adrenal glands (see Fig. 41–11) and mesenteric vessels, are clearly visualized. This difference in *T1* was more marked at 0.04 tesla, where it appears possible to characterize disease by the recognition of certain patterns of change within the liver and by measurement of *T1*.[19] However, at 0.08 tesla the *T1* values overlap more between disease states, leading to decreased accuracy.[20] In the search for tumor, the contrast between tumor and normal liver is such that tumors are easily recognized, although it is impossible to differentiate hepatoma from metastatic adenocarcinoma (Figs. 41–29 to 41–31).

The ability to obtain sections in the coronal plane is considered to be very useful, since this view displays the abdomen in a familiar radiologic way. The ability to demonstrate the aorta and inferior vena cava in their entire length (Fig. 41–32) is useful in the diagnosis of para-aortic node enlargement and aortic disease. The long relaxation time of ascitic fluid allows for accurate localization of fluid collections in the abdomen (Fig. 41–33), although it may be difficult to differentiate ascites from intraperitoneal sepsis. A number of structures and fluids, including ascites, urine, sepsis, flowing blood, and bile, have long relaxation times and therefore appear white. Differentiation of bile within dilated bile ducts from the portal vein is accomplished by viewing both *T1* and

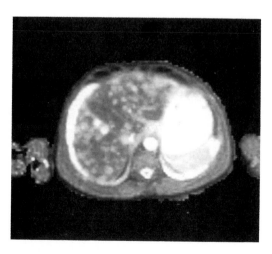

Figure 41–30. Axial *T1* image. Multiple small metastases in the liver from primary carcinoma of the pancreas. Ascitic fluid is present (white).

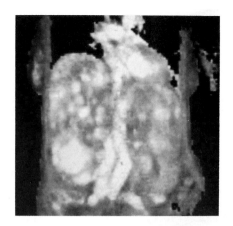

Figure 41–31. Coronal *T1* image of abdomen showing major vessels (white) and liver and peritoneum containing multiple metastases from ovarian carcinoma.

proton-density images, where bile appears white on *T1* images and black on proton density, whereas blood in the portal vein is gray on proton density (Fig. 41–34). In general, care must be taken in the interpretation of *T1* images and values. The presence of a lesion with a long *T1* is not synonymous with the presence of malignancy, as has been suggested previously.[21] In fact, many benign conditions have longer *T1* values than those found in cancers. By careful scrutiny of the entire section together with attention to the clinical history and other clinical findings, the correct diagnosis can usually be made.

The pancreas is an organ in which this problem is well demonstrated, and the earlier promise of NMR as an accurate diagnostic method at 0.04 tesla[32] has become more complex with the better resolution afforded at 0.8 tesla and above. Carcinoma of the pancreas, when associated with pancreatitis, is difficult to diagnose. It is true, however, that diagnosis of carcinoma of the pancreas and pancreatitis can be made in most cases without too much difficulty.

Pelvis

The anatomy of the pelvis is best seen on proton-density and inversion-recovery images, where the bony anatomy, muscle planes, bladder, and rectum are clearly seen. Assessment of the soft tissue organs, such as the prostate in the male (Fig. 41–35) and uterus in the female, is best made using *T1* images. Staging of bladder neoplasia is best achieved from *T1* weighted images (Fig. 41–36).

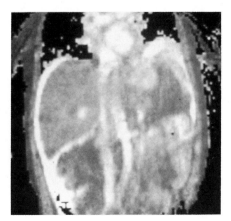

Figure 41–32. Coronal *T1* image in early cirrhosis showing major vessels, large liver, and ascitic fluid.

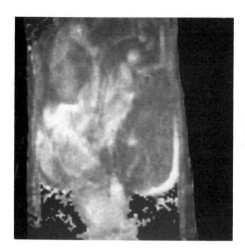

Figure 41–33. Coronal *T1* image of the abdomen showing carcinoma of the pancreas and surrounding edema and ascitic fluid. The liver appears normal.

A study of patients with prostatic enlargement, using the 0.04 tesla instrument, indicated that by the measurement of *T1*, benign hypertrophy could be differentiated from carcinoma. However, it was not possible to differentiate carcinoma from prostatitis in a number of cases because both have a long *T1*.[22] When a similar series of patients was studied using the 0.08 tesla instrument, it was found that *T1* measurement alone was not as accurate as at 0.04 tesla; however, when the improved spatial resolution was taken into account, morphologic changes were more evident and the diagnostic rate was similar.[23] This is a further example demonstrating the better sensitivity of *T1* measurement at very low field strength.

The relative lack of motion in the pelvis together with the ability to acquire sagittal, coronal, and axial sections has proved MRI to be better than ultrasound or x-ray CT in the diagnosis of endometrial carcinoma and at least as good as x-ray CT in the staging of ovarian malignancy. Using the three planes of imaging, the uterus, bladder, and rectum are localized and the origin of all pelvic masses readily recognized (Figs. 41–37 and 41–38). In the normal uterus, good contrast between normal endometrium and myometrium is seen, and in endometrial carcinoma the strong signal from tumor out-

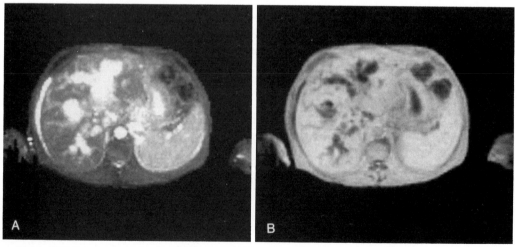

Figure 41–34. *T1* (*A*) and proton-density (*B*) images of biliary tract obstruction and dilatation due to pancreatic tumor (not shown).

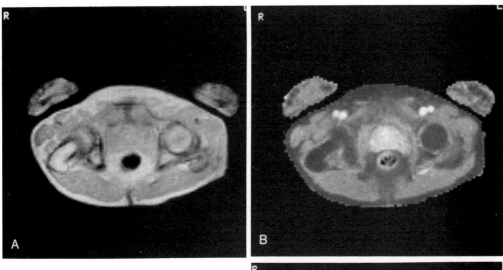

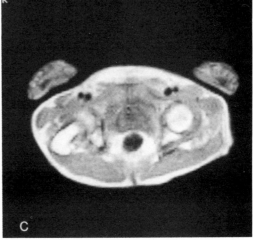

Figure 41–35. Normal pelvis at the level of the prostate. *A*, Proton density. *B*, Calculated *T1*. *C*, Inversion recovery. *TR* = 1000 ms, *TI* = 400 ms.

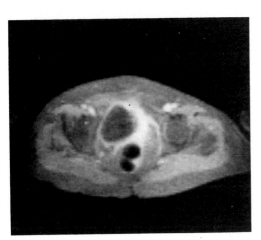

Figure 41–36. *T1* weighted image of transitional cell carcinoma of bladder (white).

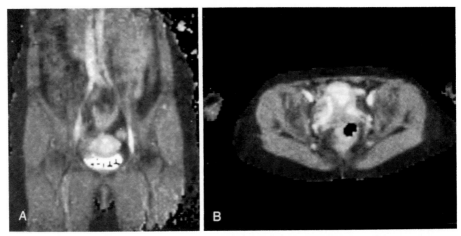

Figure 41–37. Coronal (*A*) and axial (*B*) *T1* images of endometrial carcinoma.

weighs the relative lack of spatial resolution to enable accurate staging. Normal ovaries are not readily seen except in disease, and cystic and solid tumors are recognized.

Obstetrics

The application of MRI to obstetric practice seems obvious. The technique is free from biologic hazard, and the ability to image in three planes and to study water distribution in mother and fetus provides strong incentives for developing MRI in this area. Although the NMR technique is safe for adult imaging, there has been a natural reluctance to expose the developing fetus to the technique until it has been proved safe. Currently it is accepted that fetal imaging is safe in the second and third trimesters of pregnancy, after organogenesis is complete.[24] Before this was accepted, a number of patients were examined in the first trimester by both 0.04 and 0.08 tesla instruments prior to therapeutic termination of pregnancy. The patients were imaged with MRI and ultrasound, and good correlation between measurements of fetal size and placental localization were found.[25,26] After it was agreed that second and third trimester pregnancy could be studied,[24] a series of normal pregnancies were studied at four-week

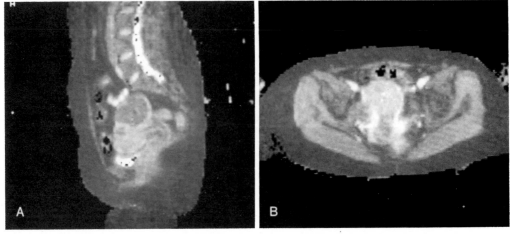

Figure 41–38. Ovarian carcinoma. *A*, Midline sagittal section. *B*, Axial section.

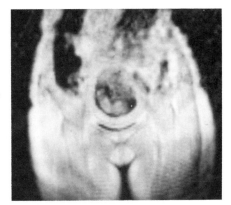

Figure 41–39. Coronal section, proton-density image of 12-week-gestation fetus.

intervals from 16 weeks' gestation to term to build up an atlas of normal development. Prior to 26 weeks the relatively large amount of amniotic fluid relative to the fetus and any fetal movement caused difficulty in seeing fetal organs. The uterus, placenta, and fetus are well seen using proton-density images, especially before 26 weeks (Figs. 41–39 and 41–40). After 26 weeks the fetal organs may be recognized (Fig. 41–41), and they become more recognizable as pregnancy progresses. With normal cephalic presentation and lie, sagittal imaging is found to be most useful for study of the fetus (Fig. 41–42). In cases of oblique and transverse lie and in midtrimester pregnancy it has been found that axial as well as sagittal imaging is important. It has also been found that fetal movement is minimized and maternal comfort enhanced by imaging the patient lying on her side (Fig. 41–43).

All the major fetal organs are demonstrable from 26 weeks and assessment of brain development is possible. Myelination of the basal ganglia has been observed, and it is believed that MRI is a good method for the study of central nervous system development.

Following the acquisition of a normal atlas of fetal development a series of patients with diabetes mellitus were studied. Good correlation between the subcutaneous fat, as measured by MRI, and birth weight was found. These measurements are most easily made from either calculated $T1$ images or inverse-recovery images made with $TR = 1000$ ms and $TI = 200$ ms.[27,28] The use of MRI to screen patients with gestational diabetes mellitus for macrosomia is advocated because of the noninvasive nature of the technique.

Placental localization is simple using MRI, and even in cases of posterior placenta,

Figure 41–40. Axial section, proton-density image of 18-week gestation fetus through fetal abdomen, demonstrating umbilical cord and anterior placenta.

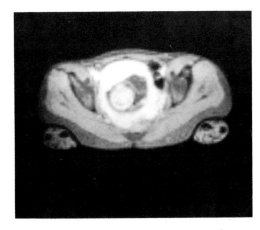

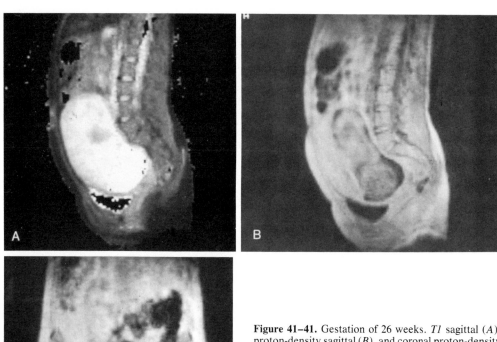

Figure 41–41. Gestation of 26 weeks. *T1* sagittal (*A*), proton-density sagittal (*B*), and coronal proton-density (*C*) images through fetal head. *A*, The fetal detail is obscured by the long relaxation time of amniotic fluid, though the liver is recognizable (dark gray). Fetal detail is best seen in proton-density images (*B* and *C*).

which may be difficult to delineate with ultrasound, the technique is proving to be useful in the diagnosis of placenta previa. Because of the relative absence of signal from cortical bone on the proton-density and inversion-recovery images it is a useful, accurate, and safe alternative to x-ray pelvimetry.

Pediatrics

After birth, brain development may be studied further using MRI. At 0.04 tesla it has been shown that MRI is useful for the investigation of a wide range of pediatric conditions, and because of its absence of ionizing radiation it should be considered the method of choice for the CT examination of children.[29] With the improved resolution available at 0.08 tesla, the technique allows for the accurate staging of such pediatric tumors as neuroblastoma.[30]

In conclusion, the images produced by the Aberdeen 0.04 and 0.08 tesla MRI systems are significantly different in appearance from most MR images produced at higher field strength. This fact does not detract from their usefulness in clinical practice. Seven years' experience in the examination of over 7500 patients testifies to their value. The difference in appearance of the images is due to the exploitation of *T1* observations, which do not overlap for different tissues at very low field strength as they do at high field—one of the reasons why spin-echo imaging is more popular than inversion-

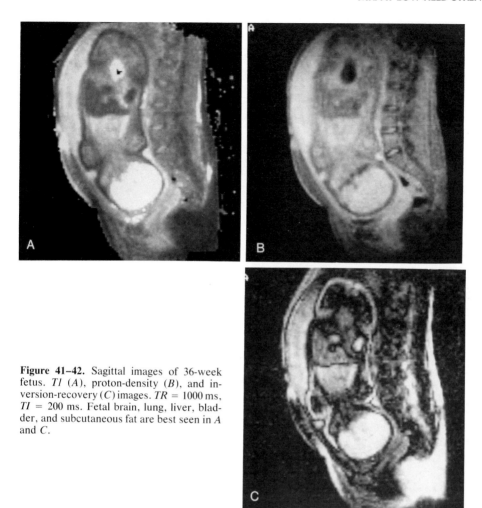

Figure 41–42. Sagittal images of 36-week fetus. *TI* (*A*), proton-density (*B*), and inversion-recovery (*C*) images. *TR* = 1000 ms, *TI* = 200 ms. Fetal brain, lung, liver, bladder, and subcutaneous fat are best seen in *A* and *C*.

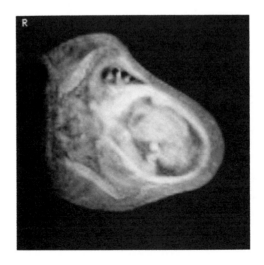

Figure 41–43. Fetus at 26–28 weeks' gestation. Proton-density image demonstrates the right lateral imaging position of mother to obtain best fetal image.

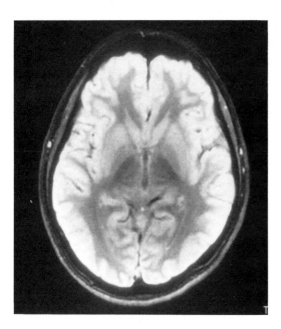

Figure 41–44. Normal brain at 0.1 tesla using a resistive system, spin-echo pulse sequence with TR = 2000 ms and TE = 21 ms. (Courtesy of Asahi Medical, Tokyo, Japan.)

recovery imaging at high fields. This ability to make good inversion-recovery and calculated $T1$ images may help in the understanding of the causes of changes seen in disease. If a reasonable amount of capital were provided to improve the final image quality of any of the low field systems, images comparable with high-field, commercially developed instruments would be possible.

Apart from the advantage of greater contrast between tissues of different $T1$ re-

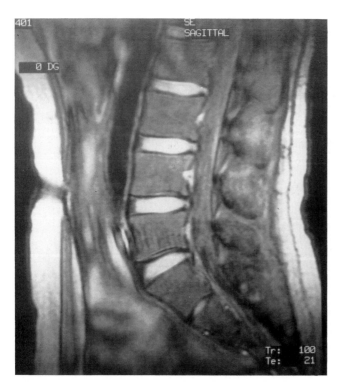

Figure 41–45. Normal lumbar spine, TR = 100 ms, TE = 21 ms. (Courtesy of Asahi Medical, Tokyo, Japan.)

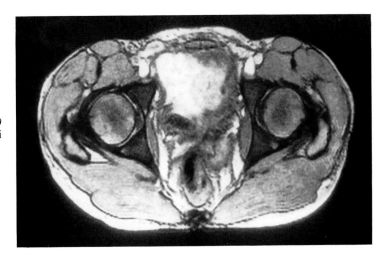

Figure 41–46. Normal pelvis, *TR = 500 ms and TE* = 21 ms. (Courtesy of Asahi Medical, Tokyo, Japan.)

laxation times, low-field MRI has a number of advantages. The capital cost is lower and room preparation is minimal as compared with that for high-field instruments. Shielding is required to protect the instrument from external radio frequency and electromagnetic interference, but this is much less than is required for the superconducting systems. No shielding is required to protect the environment because of the low field, and the 5 gauss line is no more than 3 feet from the imager at 0.08 tesla. Operating costs are similar whatever system is used, and currently (1987) our running cost per patient is less than £60 per examination.[31]

The Aberdeen MR imaging system developed in Japan by the Asahi Medicine Company functions at slightly increased field strength of 0.1 tesla and applies improved image processing techniques, which results in images with higher spatial resolution (Figs. 41–44 to 41–47).

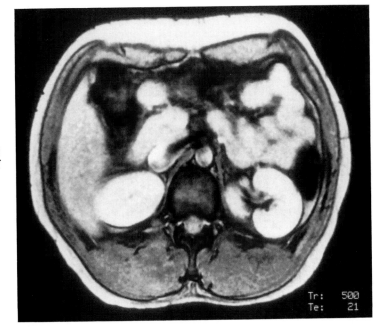

Figure 41–47. Normal abdomen, *TR* = 500 ms, *TE* = 21 ms. (Courtesy of Asahi Medical, Tokyo, Japan.)

ACKNOWLEDGMENTS

Except where otherwise acknowledged, the images used to illustrate this chapter were made with either the 0.04 tesla or the 0.08 tesla NMR imagers, designed and built in the Department of Bio-Medical Physics and Bio-Engineering at the University of Aberdeen. To Professor J. R. Mallard, Dr. J. M. S. Hutchison, and Dr. T. W. Redpath I extend my thanks for the use of these instruments.

References

1. Hiltbrand E: In-vivo measurement of T_2 in physiological fluids. *In* Hopf MA, Smith FW (eds): Progress in Nuclear Medicine, Vol 8. Magnetic Resonance in Medicine and Biology. Basel, Karger, 1984, pp 149–156.
2. Hiltbrand E, Mehier H, Farve B: Prospectives of medical applications of the protons' free precession at low field. *In* Hopf MA, Bydder GM (eds): Magnetic Resonance Imaging and Spectroscopy. Geneva, European Society of Magnetic Resonance in Medicine and Biology, 1985, pp 12–16.
3. Mather-De Vré R: Biomedical implications of the relaxation behaviour of water related to NMR imaging. Br J Radiol *57*:955, 1984.
4. Bottomley PA, Foster TH, Argersinger RE, Pfeifer LM: A review of normal tissue hydrogen NMR relaxation times and relaxation time mechanisms from 1–100 MHz: Dependence on tissue type, NMR frequency, temperature, species, excision and age. Med Phys *11*:425, 1984.
5. Sepponen RE, Sipponen JT, Sivula A: Low field (0.02 T) nuclear magnetic resonance imaging of the brain. J Comput Assist Tomogr *9*:237, 1985.
6. Smith FW: Whole body nuclear magnetic resonance imaging. Radiography *67*:297, 1981.
7. Edelstein WA, Hutchison JMS, Johnson G, Redpath TW: Spin-warp NMR imaging and applications to human whole-body imaging. Phys Med Biol *25*:751, 1980.
8. Edelstein WA, Hutchison JMS, Smith FW, Mallard JR, Johnson G, Redpath TW: Human whole-body NMR tomographic imaging: Normal sections. Br J Radiol *54*:149, 1981.
9. Hutchison JMS, Smith FW: NMR Clinical results: Aberdeen. *In* Partain CL, James AE, Rollo FD, Price RR (eds): Nuclear Magnetic Resonance (NMR) Imaging. Philadelphia, WB Saunders, 1983, pp 231–249.
10. Hutchison JMS, Edelstein WA, Johnson G: A whole-body NMR imaging machine. J Phys E *13*:947, 1980.
11. Johnson G, Hutchison JMS, Eastwood LM: Instrumentation for spin-warp imaging. J Phys E *15*:74, 1982.
12. Smith FW, Hutchison JMS, Mallard JR, Johnson G, Redpath TW, Selbie RD, Reid A, Smith CC: Oesophageal carcinoma demonstrated by whole-body nuclear magnetic resonance imaging. Br Med J *282*:510, 1981.
13. Smith FW, Runge V, Permezel M, Smith CC: Nuclear magnetic resonance (NMR) imaging in the diagnosis of spinal osteomyelitis. Magn Reson Imag *2*:53, 1984.
14. Hull RG, Rennie JAN, Eastmond CJ, Hutchison JMS, Smith FW: Nuclear magnetic resonance (NMR) tomographic imaging for popliteal cysts in rheumatoid arthritis. Ann Rheum Dis *43*:56, 1984.
15. Cherryman GR, Smith FW: NMR Scanning for skeletal tumours. Lancet *1*:1403, 1984.
16. Smith FW: Nuclear magnetic resonance (NMR) proton imaging in cancer. Eur J Cancer Clin Oncol *21*:379, 1985.
17. Smith FW: Clinical application of NMR tomographic imaging. *In* Proceedings of International Symposium on Nuclear Magnetic Resonance Imaging. Winston-Salem, Bowman Gray School of Medicine, 1982.
18. Smith FW, Cherryman GR, Singh AK, Forrester JV: Nuclear magnetic resonance tomography of the orbit at 3.4 MHz. Br J Radiol *58*:947, 1985.
19. Smith FW, Mallard JR, Reid A, Hutchison JMS: Nuclear magnetic resonance tomographic imaging in liver disease. Lancet *1*:963, 1981.
20. Cherryman GR, Smith FW, Bayliss AP, Brunt PW, Calder J, Harvey JA, Hussey JK, MacDonald AF, Mowat NAG, Robertson EM, Simpson J, Weir J: NMR in parenchymal liver disease. Proceedings of the Fourth Annual Meeting of the Society of Magnetic Resonance in Medicine, London, August 1985.
21. Damadian R: Focused NMR scanning of the intact human body by FONAR. Proceedings of International Symposium on Nuclear Magnetic Resonance Imaging. Winston-Salem, Bowman Gray School of Medicine, 1982.
22. Steyn JH, Smith FW: Nuclear magnetic resonance imaging of the prostate. Br J Urol *54*:726, 1982.
23. Smith FW, Cherryman GR, Steyn JH: A comparison of T1 measurements at 1.7 MHz and 3.4 MHz in the diagnosis of prostatic carcinoma. Magn Reson Med *2*:350, 1985.
24. The National Radiological Protection Board Ad Hoc Advisory Group on Nuclear Magnetic Resonance Clinical Imaging: Revised guidance on acceptable limits of exposure during nuclear magnetic resonance imaging. Br J Radiol *56*:974, 1983.
25. Smith FW, Adam AH, Phillips WDP: NMR imaging in pregnancy. Lancet *1*:61, 1983.
26. Smith FW, MacLennan F, Abramovich DR, MacGillivray I, Hutchison JMS: NMR imaging in human pregnancy: A preliminary study. Magn Reson Imag *2*:57, 1984.
27. Smith FW: The potential use of nuclear magnetic resonance imaging in pregnancy. J Perinat Med *13*:265, 1985.

28. Smith FW, Kent C, Abramovich DR, Sutherland HW: Nuclear magnetic resonance imaging: A new look at the fetus. Br J Obstet Gynaecol *92*:1024, 1985.
29. Smith FW: The value of NMR imaging in pediatric practice: A preliminary report. Pediatr Radiol *13*:141, 1983.
30. Smith FW, Cherryman GR, Redpath TW, Crosher G: The nuclear magnetic resonance appearances of neuroblastoma. Pediatr Radiol *15*:329, 1985.
31. Cherryman GR: Cost of operating a nuclear magnetic resonance imaging system. Br Med J. *291*:1437, 1985.
32. Smith FW, Reid A, Hutchison JMS, Mallard JR: Nuclear magnetic resonance imaging of the pancreas. Radiology *142*:677, 1982.

42

Fast, Small Flip-Angle Field Echo Imaging

R. G. BLUEMM
W. KOOPS
J. DEN BOER
J. DOORNBOS
P. VAN DIJK
P. VAN DER MEULEN
J. CUPPEN

The conventional 2D Fourier multiple-slice technique is an efficient method that is adequate for most diagnostic purposes. However, the scan time is in the order of minutes, which prohibits dynamic imaging and causes sensitivity to motion artifacts. In 1984, manufacturers of MR imaging equipment doubted whether intrinsic factors, such as the relatively long relaxation times and the detection sensitivity of MRI, would ever allow imaging speed to reach that of present-day CT scanners. It turned out that these doubts were largely unfounded.

Several methods exist for fast MR imaging with special characteristics that are advantageous or disadvantageous in different circumstances. An early method developed by Mansfield and coworkers[8] is the echo planar technique, in which an additional strong oscillating gradient is employed during sampling. In this way, an image can be formed after only one excitation. However, the spatial resolution is limited (64 × 64 matrix), the signal-to-noise (S/N) ratio is very low, and important technical and safety problems persist. Generalizations of echo planar imaging were developed by van Uijen[9] and by Haacke.[10] All these methods employ a low-frequency modulation gradient during the sampling period, which reduces the number of excitations necessary to form an image with a factor 2 to 8. The 2D multiple slice and 3D volume modes are speeded up but are still not fast enough to permit dynamic imaging. A characteristic of these methods is that the images are usually more T2 than T1 weighted, as opposed to the strong T1 weighting in fast field echo (FFE) imaging, a feature that will be discussed further on.

FFE imaging recently has been proposed by van der Meulen et al.[1] and by Haase et al.[17] This method, although still in an early stage of development, has proved to be of clinical relevance because it shortens the scan time to values in the order of seconds, a decrease with a factor of 10 or more compared with conventional MR imaging.[3]

GENERAL FEATURES OF THE FFE TECHNIQUE

FFE imaging is a very simple T1 weighted technique that is not very different from standard 2D and 3D MR imaging methods (Fig. 42–1). The conventional SE technique

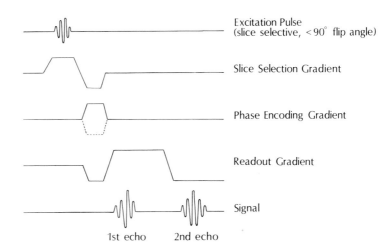

Figure 42–1. The FFE pulse sequence.

is modified by applying a flip angle α smaller than 90 degrees and by generating echoes through gradient reversal instead of 180 degree refocusing pulses. As a result, repetition times in the order of 15 to 100 ms are feasible, and at these short repetition times a sufficient S/N ratio is still achieved.

At small flip angles the magnetization settles at some intermediate value between zero and its maximum value, instead of close to zero as would be the case for 90 degree pulses (see Fig. 42–2B). The excitation pulse is a slice-selective rf pulse. As with conventional imaging, 128 or 256 signals are obtained with various degrees of phase encoding. The echoes of the signal are generated by inversion of the read-out gradient, resulting in a short TE (e.g., 10 ms; see also under "Preferred Values of TE" and "$T1/T2$ weighting") and in low energy deposits in the patient. The short TE limits the effects of inhomogeneity of the magnetic field that are not corrected by gradient reversal, as opposed to the effect of a 180 degree refocusing pulse. After signal sampling it is essential that certain spoiler gradients be used; this is to prevent interference of the residual signals with subsequent signal read-out periods, which would result in ghost images and other artifacts.

FFE Properties in Detail

A simplified analysis follows to introduce some properties of FFE images. Signal intensity will be discussed as a function of α, TR, and tissue $T1$. It will be shown that the FFE image is usually predominantly $T1$ weighted, especially with short TR and large α. The analysis neglects the fact that for TR's that are not much longer than $T2$, some order in the spin-phase distribution carries over from excitation to excitation. This effect leads to increase of signal strength, especially for long $T2$'s, depending on the exact gradient pulse shapes used, and hence a somewhat more $T2$ weighted contrast may result. This, however, is not discussed below.

The magnetization is assumed to be in equilibrium saturation all the time, either for stationary tissue or for steady flow of blood. This provides a qualitatively correct description of the typical character of the FFE image. The analysis is not adequate for a quantitative determination of image contrast in real conditions, in which equilibrium saturation does not exist from the beginning of the image acquisition and in which blood flow may be turbulent and pulsatile.

EQUILIBRIUM SATURATION

The FFE consists of a series of small-angle excitation pulses at short time intervals. The excitation pulses (α degrees spin rotation, Fig. 42–2A) convert a part of the longitudinal magnetization M in the transverse state. The rapid repetition rate of the pulses prevents the longitudinal magnetization from fully recovering its maximum value M_0. As a result, M will decrease from pulse to pulse until an equilibrium is reached. Figure 42–3 shows the time course of M during the first 20 excitations for some pulse angles. Noteworthy is the low value of M at equilibrium, especially for large α; apparently the spin system is strongly saturated by the FFE sequence.

The value of the magnetization M, once equilibrium has been reached, is

$$M/M_0 = \frac{1 - \exp(-TR/T1)}{1 - \cos \alpha \cdot \exp(-TR/T1)} \tag{1}$$

where M is expressed as a fraction of the maximum magnetization M_0 and depends on the repetition time TR, the flip angle α, and the tissue $T1$ relaxation value.

PREFERRED VALUES OF α AND TR

If the signal value for stationary tissue during the FFE acquisition is denoted as S and the magnetization as M, the following relationship holds

$$S = M \cdot \sin \alpha \cdot \exp(-TE/T2) \tag{2}$$

and it can be seen that S is proportional both to M and to $\sin \alpha$. As a consequence, S is small for large α (where M is small) as well as for small α (where $\sin \alpha$ is small). A maximum of S will be reached at some intermediate value of α. Figure 42–4 is a graphic representation of Equations (1) and (2). It shows the magnetization and the signal as a function of α for a tissue with $T1 = 500$ ms imaged with a repetition time of 35 ms. Maximum signal is obtained at $\alpha = 20$ degrees in this case (the value of α for maximum signal intensity depends on the tissue $T1$ value). However, a range of values for α can be used (e.g., a value with minimum flow artifact) without too much loss of signal. Alternatively, this means that a given value of α can be used for a range of $T1$'s.

Figure 42–5A shows the signal strength as a function of $T1$ for some values of α and for $TR = 35$ ms. One can see again that for any $T1$, a value of α exists that gives the strongest signal. Further, for all α the signal is relatively weak for long $T1$'s (Fig.

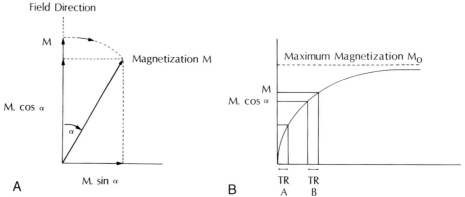

Figure 42–2. *A,* A flip angle smaller than 90 degrees results in two components of the magnetization: (1) a residual longitudinal component (M. cos α) in the field direction, and (2) a transverse component (M. sin α) that evokes the signal in the detection coil. *B,* Recovery of the magnetization. *A* corresponds to $\alpha = 90$ degrees and *B* to a smaller value of α.

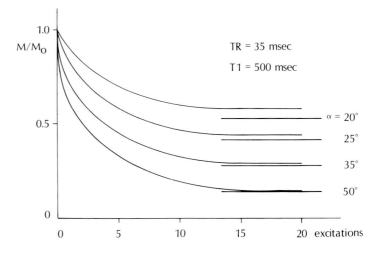

Figure 42–3. The decrease of the longitudinal magnetization M after the onset of an FFE sequence is depicted for $TR = 35$ ms, $T1 = 500$ ms, and flip angles of 20 to 50 degrees. The horizontal lines indicate equilibrium values of M reached during FFE imaging. The values of M are relative to the maximum magnetization M_0.

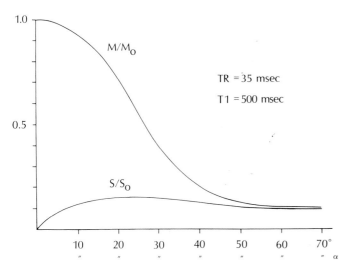

Figure 42–4. Graphic representation of Equations (1) and (2) with $TR = 35$ ms and $T1 = 500$ ms. The equilibrium values during FFE imaging of the magnetization M and the signal S are shown as a function of the flip angle. The values of S are relative to the signal S_0 obtained at magnetization M_0 and 90 degrees excitation.

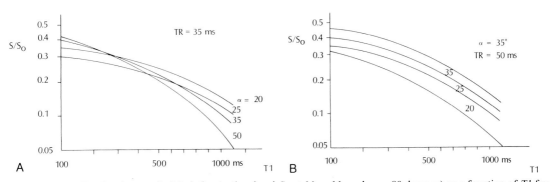

Figure 42–5. A, The signal strength S (relative to the signal S_0 at $M = M_0$ and $\alpha = 90$ degrees) as a function of $T1$ for some values of α and for $TR = 35$ ms. B, The signal strength for some values of TR and for $\alpha = 35$ degrees.

42–5*A*). In particular, for large values of α, the signal of tissues with short *T1* dominates; a small α results in somewhat more equal signal strengths from different tissues.

The choice of *TR* depends on the time resolution that is desired for the specific investigation. The signal increases with increasing *TR* (Fig. 42–5*B*) Increasing *TR* by a factor of 2 leads to less than a doubling of the signal. Therefore, to increase the signal-to-noise (S/N) ratio it might be advantageous to keep *TR* short and average a number of acquisitions.[11] This approach, of course, holds only when the echo time is kept constant, and this will set a minimum to *TR*. Closer inspection of Figure 42–5*B* demonstrates that an increase in TR leads to less emphasis on short *T1*'s. In this aspect, increasing *TR* has a similar effect as decreasing α.

PREFERRED VALUES OF TE

The FFE method, like any other field echo method, does not allow long echo times. The inhomogeneity of the magnetic field is not corrected by the field echo, and loss of signal will occur with increasing echo time because of destructive dephasing, i.e., loss of coherence of the spins in each voxel. Apart from field inhomogeneity, dephasing occurs as a result of the chemical-shift difference between fat- and water-bound spins. This dephasing is destructive only in voxels that contain both water and fat. The phenomenon can be used to generate contrasting boundaries between water and fat, the so-called ink line effect.[12] One should, however, be aware of the artifactual nature of these lines and not misinterpret them as anatomic structures. To avoid chemical-shift dephasing, the phase shift between water and fat has to be 0, 360, or 720 degrees (and so forth). The echo times *TE* hence have to be

$$TE = n \cdot \gamma \cdot B_0 \cdot \delta_{ch}$$

where *n* is an integer, γ is the gyromagnetic ratio, B_0 is the magnetic field strength, and δ_{ch} is the chemical shift. For $B_0 = 0.5$ tesla, this leads to values for *TE* of 0, 15, 30, 45 ms, and so forth. Whereas 0 ms cannot be reached for instrumental reasons and 30 ms is too long for most magnets, in practice a *TE* of 15 ms is used for in-phase imaging. Values of *TE* around 8, 22, and 36 ms give full dephasing of water and fat. Alternatively, this dephasing can be utilized for FFE chemical-shift imaging.

T1 AND *T2* WEIGHTING

For arbitrary *T1* and *T2*, the contrast type in a FFE image can be evaluated clearly with the help of displays.[13] For a given pulse sequence, the theoretical value of the

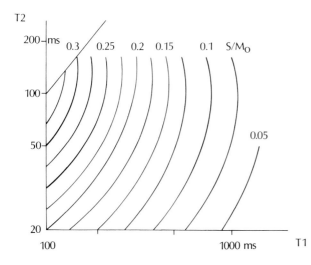

Figure 42–6. Contrast characteristics of an FFE sequence with *TR* = 35 ms, α = 35 degrees, and *TE* = 15 ms. This is an isointensity plot of signal strength in the log *T1*, log *T2* plane. The values of *S* are relative to the magnetization M_0 (the proportionality constant between *S* and M_0 is not included). The predominantly vertical orientation of the isointensity lines indicates that the image contrast is more sensitive to relative differences in *T1* than to relative differences in *T2*.

signal is then visualized in a *T1*, *T2* plot in which a set of curves connects all with equal signal strength. This has been done (Fig. 42–6) for an example of the FFE sequence. The contrast between two tissues can be read when both tissues are mapped as points in the *T1*, *T2* plane and their signal strengths estimated. Correction for proton-density differences can be easily made. Figure 42–6 illustrates the fact that the FFE image contrast is heavily *T1* dependent, especially for long *T1* values. This holds for most FFE sequences with practical values of α, *TR*, and *T1* but *T2* weighted contrasts can occur for small α and/or large *TR*. A great distance between the lines of constant signal strength indicates that for a given pair of tissues the signal difference will not be large, so that the contrast-to-noise ratio for such a pair will be limited. This is especially the case for tissue pairs with large *T1* and small *T2*.

THE SIGNAL-TO-NOISE RATIO IN PRACTICE

We tested the signal-to-noise (S/N) ratio with *TR* varying from 25 to 100 ms, corresponding to a scan time of 2 to 13 sec, and with α varying from 3 to 90 degrees. The results are listed in Table 42–1 and may be summarized as follows. (1) As expected, S/N improves with increasing *TR* as a result of the decreasing saturation effect. (2) In each series, there is a flat optimum of S/N as a function of the flip angle α (see Fig. 42–4). (3) The maximum S/N is found at α values of around 35 degrees. However, at a flip angle of 22 degrees, the S/N is still acceptable, while ghost images from vessels are significantly reduced (see Fig. 42–32). (4) A slight discrepancy is observed between the theoretical and experimental values of the optimal flip angle. The theoretical optimum for the brain is about 25 degrees (estimated from a curve like the one depicted in Fig. 42–4), whereas experimentally the maximum S/N is found at a somewhat higher value.

STEADY FLOW WITHOUT ECG TRIGGERING

A change of signal value in MR images is usually obtained when tissue has moved during the acquisition time. This is a well-known effect, observable in any type of pulse sequence. The typical example of moving tissue is flowing blood, and in this discussion that example will be addressed.

The causes for flow-induced signal changes have been described by several authors[14–16] and can be summarized as (1) flow of maximally magnetized spins into the image section (increase of signal); (2) outflow of excited spins (decrease of signal); (3) destructive dephasing of spins within one voxel as a result of the presence of different

Table 42–1. SIGNAL-TO-NOISE RATIOS IN IMAGES OF THE BRAIN*

	TR = 25	50	75	100 ms
α = 3°	3.3	3.5	4.0	3.7
5°	5.0	5.5	5.8	5.8
9°	6.9	7.8	9.3	7.8
14°	9.1	9.6	12.3	12.4
22°	10.9	13.6	14.7	16.4
35°	12.3	16.0	16.6	18.1
56°	10.3	14.7	16.3	18.1
90°	7.5	10.7	12.7	14.4

* Normalized to the S/N value of an SE 4000/30 sequence the value of which was set to 100 (128^2, no averaging). *S* was measured as the average value in a large rectangle of about 60 cm^2 at the center of the image. *N* is provided by the background signal.

Table 42–2. COMPARISON OF FFE AND SE

	FFE	**Normal SE**
Inflow	Stationary tissue has a low magnetization (strong saturation). So, signal from inflowing nonsaturated blood strongly dominates.	Stationary tissue has an intermediate magnetization. So, the signal from inflowing blood is relatively lower.
Outflow	The magnetization of outflowing blood is not disturbed and fully contributes to the signal.	The magnetization of outflowing blood is not rephased by the slice-selective 180 degree pulse.
Destructive dephasing	Dephasing of the signal of flowing blood is caused only by the preparation and the measurement gradient.	Dephasing is caused by the preparation, the measurement, and the slice-selection gradient.

velocities within the voxel (decrease of signal); and (4) difference of average phase after successive excitations because of flow velocity alterations (decrease of signal).

In FFE images, flowing blood produces a bright signal that is due to several contributions: (1) The absence of a 180 degree rf pulse for echo formation reduces saturation of upstream spins. (2) The echo formation is not slice-selective, so that excited spins flowing downstream still contribute to the signal of the selected slice. (3) The small excitation pulse angle accounts for less saturation of spins within the slice. (4) Most prominent, the high signal intensity is due to the inflow of previously unexcited spins, while stationary tissue is saturated by the rapid train of rf pulses.

As a result of these facts, the sequence is sensitive to flow and provides positive contrast for flowing spins. This observation can also be explained qualitatively by a comparison with a conventional SE sequence (Table 42–2).

A particular aspect of the enhancement of the signal by the inflow of fresh blood is related to the fact that the transition from fresh magnetization to its saturated equilibrium value is slow (see Fig. 42–3). Consequently, the excess signal arises not only from the spins that have entered the slice since the previous excitation but also from a number of earlier groups of spins.

Figure 42–7 shows a simplified theoretical prediction of signal enhancement as a function of flow velocity for some values of the flip angle α. There is a strong increase in signal intensity at low velocities, which reaches a plateau at velocities much slower

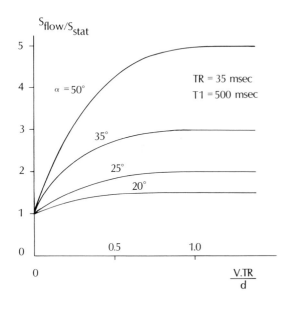

Figure 42–7. Increase of the signal with increasing flow velocity (steady flow perpendicular to the imaged slice) for $TR = 35$ ms, $T1 = 500$ ms, and some values of the flip angle. The signal strength S_{flow} is relative to the signal strength S_{stat} for stationary tissue. The velocity is relative to the velocity d/TR, which is required to cross the entire slice within one repetition time.

than necessary to replenish all blood within the slice completely between the measurements (which is the case at $v \cdot TR/d = 1$). If, for example, $\alpha = 35$ degrees, $TR = 35$ ms, $Tl = 500$ ms, and $d = 10$ mm, the signal increases by a factor 2 at a velocity of 28 mm/sec. In cardiac imaging, this is still a relatively low velocity, which means that strong signal enhancement caused by blood flow will almost always occur. As can be seen from Figure 42–7, this enhancement will be more pronounced for large flip angles and then reach a plateau at higher velocities.

With FFE imaging, destructive dephasing at high velocities occurs only in heart images, in regions where the velocity gradients are very high.

FFE IMAGING IN COMBINATION WITH ECG TRIGGERING

This technique, which will be called fast multiphase imaging (FMI), can be used beneficially for dynamic flow imaging. A diagram of the FMI sequence is shown in Figure 42–8.

The strong signals from flowing blood are also produced at high flow rates, contrary to the case for conventional SE sequences. Flow dynamics, such as turbulence or high-velocity gradients, produce new contrast in the high-intensity flow areas in images. Both phenomena give rise to irreversible dephasing or destructive phase differences for spins in the same voxel, thereby producing loss of signal and consequent dark bands or spots. This is shown in Fig. 42–9 (image 2). In this transverse slice through the ventricles the descending aorta strongly varies in brightness, with the highest intensity during the systolic flow peak. Also note the saturation of spins in the interventricular septum. The rapid-filling phase of the left ventricle produces turbulent flow and subsequent loss of signal, which is restored during the slower filling in images 14 to 16. It is remarked that the mechanisms involved in image contrast are quite different for flow within the imaged plane compared with flow perpendicular to it, the first having to deal more strongly with saturation from more excitations.

Another exciting feature of FMI is the good matching of stationary tissues in consecutive images, brought about by the aforementioned data acquisition for all phases

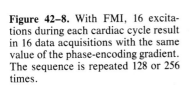

Figure 42–8. With FMI, 16 excitations during each cardiac cycle result in 16 data acquisitions with the same value of the phase-encoding gradient. The sequence is repeated 128 or 256 times.

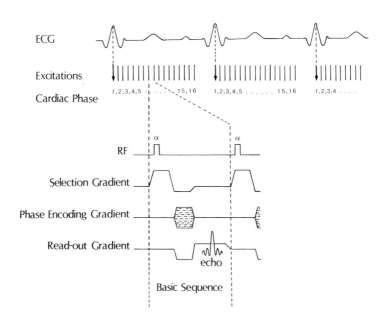

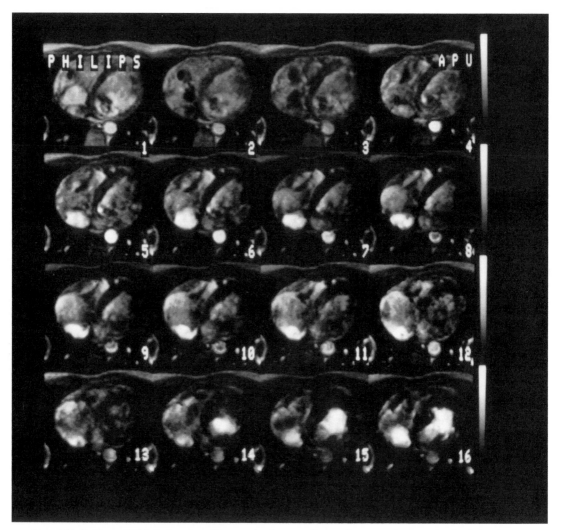

Figure 42–9. Fast multiphase imaging of a normal volunteer. Sixteen frames at the same anatomic level were made at predetermined intervals during the cardiac cycle. These anatomic sections, which can be in any orthogonal or oblique plane, may then be displayed as a movie loop.

during all heartbeats. Motion of the body during a few heartbeats will affect all images in the same way. This gives excellent subtraction possibilities of images from the same 16-image scan. This is demonstrated in Figure 42–10, in which two consecutive images from a coronal scan through the neck are subtracted to produce this vascular image of the subclavian, carotid, and vertebral arteries. The contrast for the vessels is purely from flow. Movie loops from subtracted images, e.g., subtracting the first image from all the following ones, present dynamically the evolution of flow into and out of the vessels of interest.

FAST MULTIPHASE IMAGING (FMI) OF THE HEART

The area where speed is especially desirable is cardiac imaging. Synchronization of the conventional imaging pulse sequence to the cardiac cycle has already produced impressive anatomic images but takes considerable time owing to the relatively long R-R interval and the number of heartbeats needed to image one slice in a certain heart

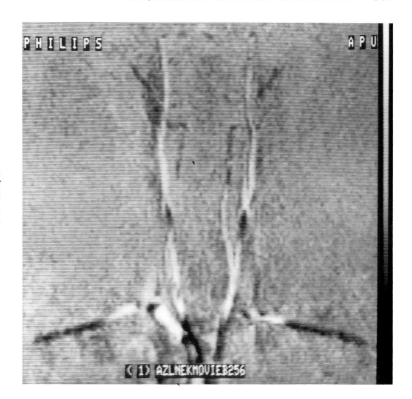

Figure 42–10. Fast multiphase imaging. Digital subtraction of two consecutive images from 16 coronal scans through the neck, resulting in a vascular image of the supra-aortic vessels.

phase. Synchronized multislice imaging produces more slices in the same time, but they are all represented in a different heart phase. Real-time imaging[4] has also been designed, but this imposes severe technical requirements on the system and so far is limited to lower spatial resolution and smaller objects. With conventional SE sequences, using a multidelay pulse program and two excitations per heartbeat, a study of one slice in 16 phases takes about 30 minutes (128×128 matrix and two averages). Movie loops from these images display the dynamic behavior of heart walls and can be used to evaluate regional wall motion and cardiac output.[5] The use of SE for anatomic imaging remains attractive because of the good delineation of heart walls against the blood-filled chambers, which produce no signal (flow void) except for the slow-flow heart phases, such as end-diastole. There is a limit, however, to the number of 90 degree excitations to be repeated during one heart cycle, mainly imposed by the saturation of heart tissue at short TR's. Waterton et al.[2] employed flip angles smaller than 90 degrees followed by a conventional 180 degree refocusing pulse.

The advent of sequences using smaller excitation pulse angles combined with gradient-reversal echoes and inherently shorter TE's considerably improved this situation, however. As has been discussed for stationary tissue, imaging of the heart with the FFE sequence is possible with very short TR while maintaining acceptable resolution and contrast. Now in one R-R interval, more than two excitations can be given, e.g., a series of 16 in 600 ms. By starting the sequence at the R wave, 16 measurements with a constant value of the preparation gradient are obtained for one slice in different phases of the cardiac cycle (see Fig. 42–8). This is repeated after every R wave with different values of the preparation gradient. After 128 or 256 cycles, images can be reconstructed for each of the 16 phases of the slice concerned. So, within a few minutes, the slice is depicted in 16 phases of the heart action. These images can be used to make a cardiac movie.

As already stated, one of the interesting properties of the FFE technique is the relatively strong signal from flowing blood. This produces even reversed contrast between the heart wall and the blood pool, the former becoming more saturated in later phases because of the higher number of excitations undergone. Thus the FFE technique may not be the sequence of choice for depicting the heart wall.

METHODS, MATERIAL, AND INITIAL CLINICAL RESULTS

FFE imaging (FFEI) with our 0.5 tesla commercial Philips Gyroscan system, located at the Radiological Department of the University Hospital of Leiden, affords images of diagnostic quality comprising relevant anatomic structures with scan times down to 2 seconds (*TR* = 15.6 ms) (Fig. 42–11). As already discussed, a variety of operator-selected parameters can be applied to achieve either a maximum of time or spatial resolution or a compromise between the two. As in "conventional" MRI, body, head, and surface coils can be used to advantage depending on the region of interest. To obtain a sufficient S/N, the slice thickness is usually chosen as 10 or 15 mm and the acquisition matrix as 128 × 128 (in the near future it will be 128 × 256).[6]

Comparison of Imaging Parameters

The following section will discuss the dependence of image quality on the acquisition matrix (128 × 128 or 256 × 256), the repetition time *TR* (20 to 100 ms), the flip angle, and 2D or 3DFT acquisition. Performing 2D acquisition with TR = 25 ms and a flip angle of 22 to 35 degrees in the region of the head (Fig. 42–12*A*–*B*) and neck, one can discriminate bright subcutaneous fat; bone marrow between the dark layers of cortical bone; air-containing sinuses; the eyeball, optic nerve, and extraocular muscles; the CSF spaces; almost featureless brain parenchyma; highlighted venous and, often, arterial vessels (see below and the section on flow); and the spinal cord and

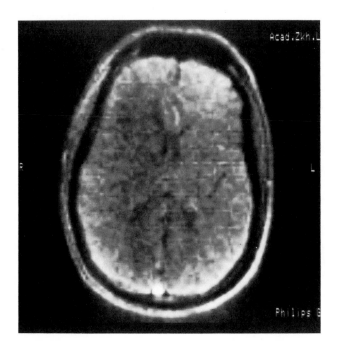

Figure 42–11. Transverse FFE 2-DFT MR scan through the head at the level of the ventricles. *TR* = 15.6 ms, α = 22 degrees, 128 × 128 matrix, 10 mm slice thickness.

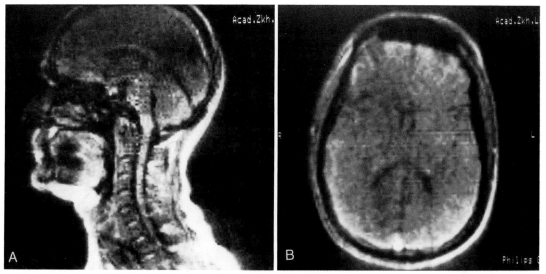

Figure 42–12. *A*, Midsagittal FFE MR scan of head and neck; *TR* = 20 ms. Spinal cord and intervertebral discs are visualized. *B*, Same level and flip angle as in Figure 42–11; *TR* = 25 ms.

intervertebral discs. These structures are usually depicted sufficiently well for positioning before a normal SE multislice set or for rough estimates of *T1*. A set of orthogonal images in the axial, coronal, and sagittal directions can be obtained under software control within 3 × 2.5 sec plus a pause of 2 × 0.15 sec. These images provide enough information to determine, for example, the angles for a double-oblique section. With a *TR* of 50 ms (Fig. 42–13) one may discriminate gyri and a subtle gray/white matter differentiation, which becomes more distinct when two to four images are averaged (Fig. 42–14). Using the same *TR*, 3D volume acquisition without averaging produces an even better delineation between the two (Fig. 42–15). When comparing the average of two *TR* = 50 ms (Fig. 42–14) with a single FID *TR* = 100 ms (Fig. 42–

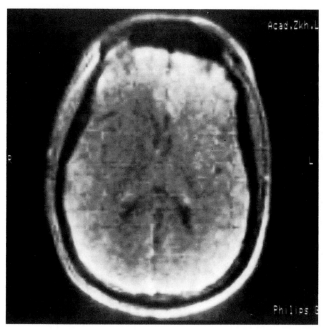

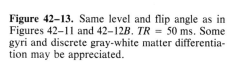

Figure 42–13. Same level and flip angle as in Figures 42–11 and 42–12*B*. *TR* = 50 ms. Some gyri and discrete gray-white matter differentiation may be appreciated.

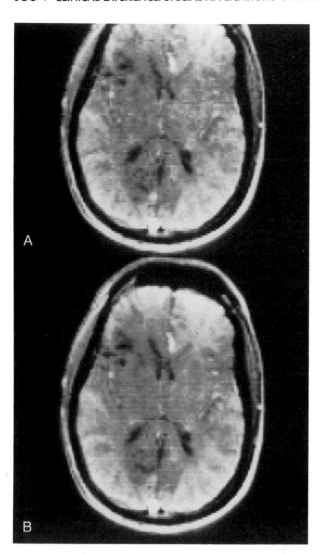

Figure 42–14. *A*, Improvement of image quality (S/N ratio) of the *TR* = 50 ms scan of Figure 42–13 by averaging two scans. *B*, Improvement by averaging four scans.

16) (both obtained at an optimal flip angle), S/N appears about 10 percent better in the averaged image. The use of a 256 × 256 instead of a 128 × 128 matrix results in a significant decrease of S/N (at *TR* = 25 and 50 ms) (Fig. 42–17), thus reducing the clinical value of single FID plain images unless S/N is increased by averaging or by applying a contrast agent. In imaging the head and neck, which are motionless objects apart from swallowing, the time resolution does not play such an important role, with the exception of dynamic imaging (see below). If high-quality images with good resolution of nonmoving objects (such as the brain) are needed, 3D FFE imaging is a good choice in terms of efficiency (Fig. 42–18) and S/N and compares favorably with normal multiple-slice technique. Theoretically, it can be shown that the S/N of a 3D FFE experiment is even better (Cuppen, personal communication). The 3D FFE method has the advantage over averaging a number of 2D FFE scans in that more slices are obtained in the same scan time with approximately the same S/N; furthermore, the slices are contiguous and can be chosen thinner. Combining 3D FFE with surface coils yields an effective means to depict finer anatomic structures in a reasonable scan time.

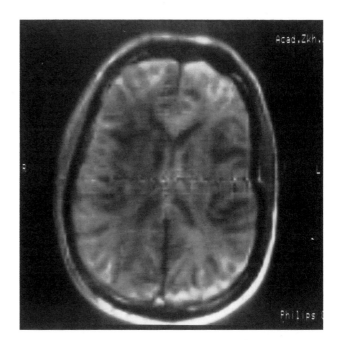

Figure 42–15. The 3-DFT, 10 mm thick, FFE MR scan (*TR* = 50 ms) exhibits the best structural resolution in comparison with the 2-DFT images in Figures 42–13 and 42–14.

Clinical Results

Mainly owing to absent or reduced saturation of flowing blood (see the section on flow), even arterial flow can be highlighted on short *TR* images. This effect is not seen at small flip angles and increases at larger values of α(35 to 90 degrees, Fig. 42–19). By careful handling of the two window settings on *TR* = 25 and 50 ms scans, we were also able to differentiate hyperintense areas of hemorrhage and fatty tumor components from other tissue (Fig. 42–20).

Physiologic motion (cardiac, respiratory, and peristaltic) is currently a limiting

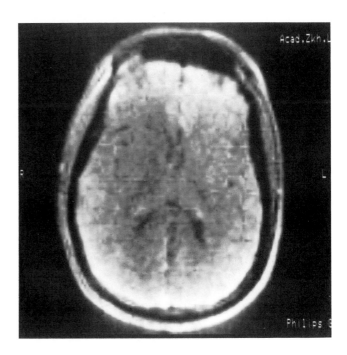

Figure 42–16. A 2-DFT FFE MR scan (*TR* = 100 ms).

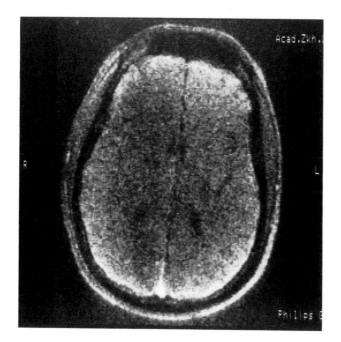

Figure 42–17. A 2-DFT FFE MR *TR* = 50 msec scan, one FID (measurement), 256 × 256 matrix. Significant decrease of S/N and C/N ratios as compared with the scan in Figure 42–13*B* obtained with a 128 × 128 matrix.

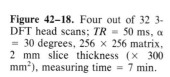

Figure 42–18. Four out of 32 3-DFT head scans; *TR* = 50 ms, α = 30 degrees, 256 × 256 matrix, 2 mm slice thickness (× 300 mm²), measuring time = 7 min.

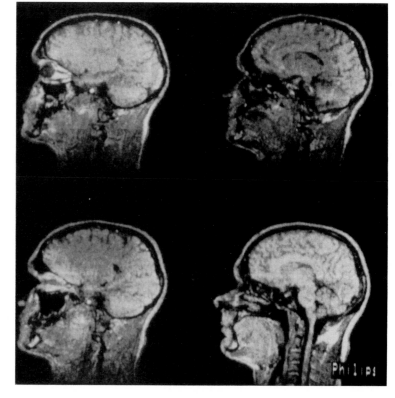

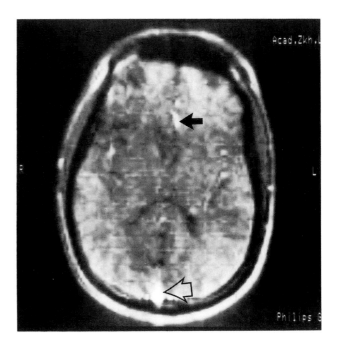

Figure 42–19. A 2-DFT FFE MR $TR = 50$ ms on FID scan, flip angle of 56 degrees. Increase of signal intensity in arterial (closed arrow) and venous (open arrow) vessels.

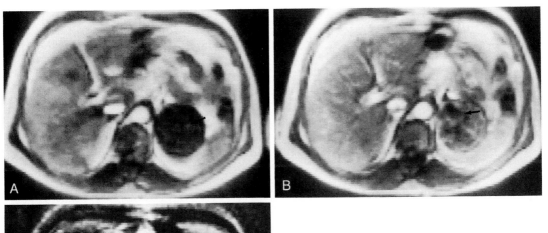

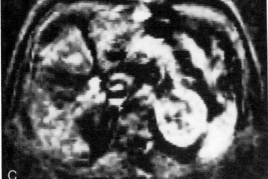

Figure 42–20. Malignant adrenal tumor. Patient was breathing normally during examination. *A*, Plain $TR = 25$ ms scan. Small hyperintense foci of hemorrhage (arrow). *B*, Demarcation of necrotic areas (arrow) about 24 sec following intravenous administration of 0.1 mmol/kg Gd-DTPA-meglumine (see also Chapters 12 and 52). *C*, Subtraction of both scans.

factor in upper abdominal imaging. As for the thoracic cage and the abdomen, FFE imaging enables MRI while the subject holds his breath, obviating the time penalty of respiratory gating.[18] Using the surface coil, major structures of the thoracic wall containing different layers of muscles, the spleen surrounded by fat, and the marrow of the ribs become visible. This is illustrated with a 8 mm thick 128 × 128 3D image (Fig. 42–21) out of a series of 15 images acquired within less than three minutes. The volunteer is permitted to take a breath between the scans.

Nonperiodic movement, such as peristalsis of the stomach or intestinum, can be almost completely frozen applying a scan time of 2.0 to 3.2 sec. Following oral administration of Gd-DTPA (1 mM) during breath-holding and without the use of spasmolytics, a 3.2 sec scan sharply outlines the contours of the stomach, including the area of the pylorus (Fig. 42–22). Notice (Fig. 42–22) the clear delineation of the stomach from retroperitoneal structures and the absence of blurring from respiratory or peristaltic motion. When applying the dynamic sequence (see below), movement due to bowel peristalsis can be registered (Fig. 42–23).

Of course, a major drawback of FFEI is its greater sensitivity to artifacts owing to the low S/N. However, as has been described in the literature,[11,23] contrast-enhancing pharmaceuticals may extend the diagnostic usefulness of MRI. The low S/N of FFEI can be improved by administering an effective intravenous paramagnetic contrast agent, such as Gd-DTPA. This chelate-meglumine complex acts as a marker of relative organ perfusion[20,21] or blood-brain barrier (BBB) disruption and has proved to be safe for clinical investigational use in more than 1000 patients.[24,25] In combination with the described time resolution of FFEI, the new diagnostic dimension of dynamic contrast-enhanced MRI becomes feasible, similar to dynamic CT.[3]

Dynamic Gd-DTPA Enhanced MRI

As indicated in the discussion of heart imaging, the implemented prototype FFEI software in our standard scanner provided us with 16 subsequent slices through the region of interest. The minimal time interval between the scans is 0.15 sec. This interval

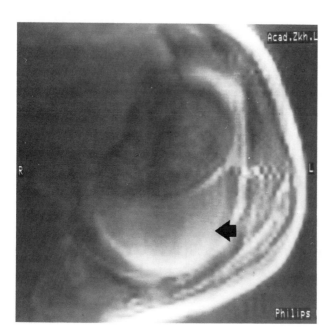

Figure 42–21. An 8 mm thick 3-DFT scan of spleen (arrow) and lateral thoracic wall performed with surface coil.

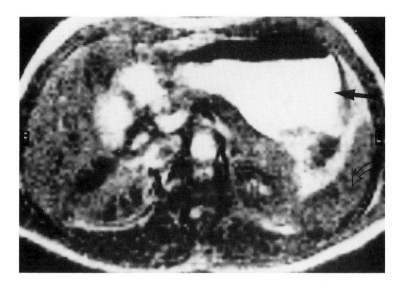

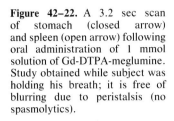

Figure 42–22. A 3.2 sec scan of stomach (closed arrow) and spleen (open arrow) following oral administration of 1 mmol solution of Gd-DTPA-meglumine. Study obtained while subject was holding his breath; it is free of blurring due to peristalsis (no spasmolytics).

can be prolonged to several seconds if the patient needs to take a breath between successive images. A *TR* between 15.6 and 25 ms is sufficient for a dynamic FFE sequence to display a contrast-enhanced lesion. To gather information about the relative merits of FFEI, the method has until now always been performed following the conventional spin-echo *T1* and *T2* weighted multislice techniques. At one level of interest, usually chosen in the transverse plane, a dynamic series is started with up to 16 subsequent scans. In general, the technical parameters used are 3.2 sec scan time (*TR* 25 ms), flip angle 40 degrees, scan time interval ranging from 0.15 sec to 6 sec (adapted to the respiratory cycle of the patient or to the expected evolution of enhancement of the suspected lesion), 128 × 128 matrix, and 10 to 15 mm slice thickness. Injection of 0.025 mmol/kg up to 0.2 mmol/kg Gd-DTPA via a 19-gauge plastic needle in the antecubital vein is followed by injection of 20 ml physiologic NaCl solution. To get *T1* information for comparison and to assess the contrast effects of Gd-DTPA, injection is started just after the measurements of the first rapid scan has been completed.

In principle, the evaluation of the series of images obtained was performed fol-

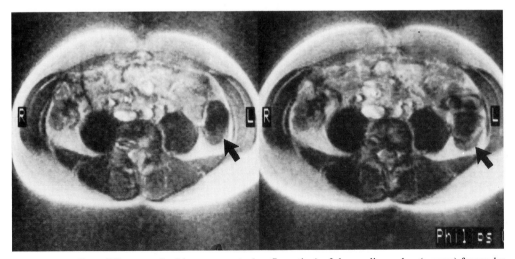

Figure 42–23. Two different peristaltic movements (configuration) of descending colon (arrows) frozen by two successive 3.2 sec FFE scans.

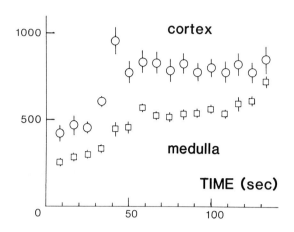

Figure 42–24. Time course of relative enhancement of signal intensity in the renal cortex and medulla of a normal kidney following bolus injection of 0.1 mmol/kg Gd-DTPA-meglumine. The subject is a 25-year-old woman.

lowing criteria analogous to those for dynamic CT: The time course of relative enhancement and the morphologic pattern were studied visually, and normal and pathologic structures were compared using identical window settings for all scans. In relevant cases, time versus signal intensity curves known to be useful for assessing relative tissue perfusion were plotted for regions of interest in normal and abnormal tissue such as renal cortex and medulla (Fig. 42–24), liver (Fig. 42–25B), tumors (Fig. 42–26), and inflammatory lesions. In addition, electronic image subtraction was available, which enabled selective highlighting of morphologic enhancement patterns (see Fig. 42–20C).

We started to use FFEI to depict the relative perfusion of the normal kidney, spleen, and liver using 0.025, 0.05, and 0.1 mmol/kg Gd-DTPA. Without ECG gating, no definitely reproducible signal enhancement could be obtained within the lumen of the aorta contrary to dynamic CT (Fig. 42–25A). As shown in Fig. 42–24, enhancement of the renal cortex begins about 10 to 20 seconds post injection (even with the lowest concentration of 0.025 mmol/kg), followed 50 to 60 seconds post injection by the parenchymal phase. Up to 110 seconds post injection, we may still see perfusional differences of cortex and medulla, followed by a rather homogeneous parenchymal plateau. The spleen increases in signal intensity (SI) shortly after the maximum SI is seen

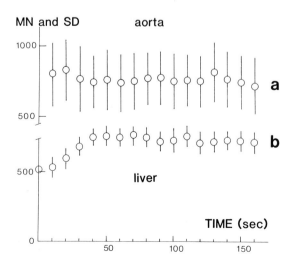

Figure 42–25. Same 25-year-old woman. A, No relative enhancement can be measured within the lumen of abdominal aorta. B, Diffuse enhancement of the liver occurs after 50 sec.

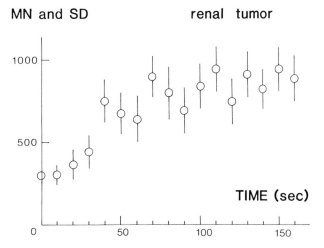

Figure 42–26. Renal cell carcinoma shown in Figure 42–29 *A–D*. Example of an enhancement curve of a vascularized (solid) component (0.1 mmol/kg Gd-DTPA-meglumine).

in the renal cortex but to a somewhat lesser degree (Fig. 42–27), followed by the liver, which appears to enhance last and is distinct only at concentrations of 0.1 mmol/kg intravenously. These normal structures, enhancing at different times, can, of course, also be displayed by image subtraction.

Until now, we were not able to examine all pathologic conditions that are especially suited for analysis by this technique. Table 42–3 lists 29 patients with known pathologies investigated at the moment of writing. These studies were performed after a period of S/N optimization of plain FFEI in normal volunteers. All lesions could be depicted by this combined approach. Paget's disease of the distal femur, metastases of the tibia from a melanoma and a hepatocellular carcinoma (all after chemotherapy), and two Stage II infarctions of the posterior fossa were better visualized on conventional *T1* weighted multislice scans five minutes after injection because of better enhancement at that time, where FFEI could not be performed according to the Schering protocol.

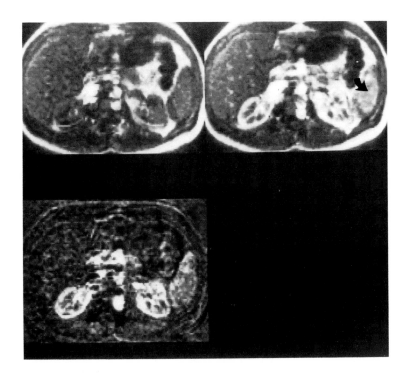

Figure 42–27. A 32-year-old volunteer. Enhancement of the spleen (arrow) is seen at the same time as the signal intensity of the renal cortex increases (0.025 mmol/kg Gd-DTPA-meglumine) (serial images top left and right). This is highlighted by subtraction (bottom). Note that the liver does not enhance at this time.

Some aspects of the clinical potential of FFEI in different parts of the body are illustrated in the following cases with pathologic conditions (selected from Table 42–3). All types of enhancement known from dynamic CT could be observed, such as diffuse, ringlike, patchy, linear, central, or none.

Cryptic vascular malformations of the brain seem to lack even-echo rephasing on conventional MRI.[26] Gd-DTPA enhanced FFEI can add diagnostic specificity within a short examination time. Figure 42–28 shows a young man with a "cryptic" vascular malformation of the lower right cerebellum that lacks distinct even-echo rephasing on a conventional multiecho SE sequence. The results of conventional MRI were nevertheless very suggestive for such a lesion. On the precontrast FFE image ($TR = 25$), flow showed up isointense despite the fact that flow in general is highlighted as bright signal intensity. (The flip angle of 35 degrees obviously was not optimal for flow detection.) About 12 seconds after administration of 0.1 mmol/kg Gd-DTPA a strong homogeneous enhancement in the somewhat serpiginous structure occurred, confirming the final diagnosis. No central perfusion defect became evident. Peripherally and unexpectedly, a constant low-intensity halo was visualized that was not as well appreciated on conventional *T1* weighted MR scans obtained five minutes after injection. This relatively less perfused region may represent steal effect or "reactive" perifocal changes, such as fibrosis. Analysis of quantitative enhancement suggested that half the dosage (0.05 mmol/kg) may be sufficient to perform this type of "MR angiotomography." In another case of cryptic malformation we were able to prove a central spotlike contrast enhancement consistent with a disruption of the blood-brain barrier. A pseudomembrane of a centrally nonenhancing extra-axial teratoma at the anterior aspect of the occipitocervical junction was visualized by 2D and 3DFT FFEI but not by angiography (photographic subtraction) and CT (beam-hardening artifacts).

FFEI also appears to be efficient in depicting different patterns of tumor perfusion and vascularity, e.g., in renal tumors. According to the literature[22] and our experience, both renal parenchyma and tumor increase in signal intensity to nearly the same extent using short *TR/TE* SE sequences five minutes after injection of Gd-DTPA. Using precontrast *T2* weighted SE sequences, these lesions can be hyper-, iso-, and hyperintense with the normal renal tissue. So far, the relatively time-consuming IR sequence 1500/400 seems to be appropriate for Gd-DTPA enhanced MRI.[22] Following the time course

Table 42–3. PATIENTS WITH Gd-DTPA ENHANCED FFE STUDY (FMI)

Pathology	Number
Renal cell carcinoma	4
Angiomyolipoma	2
Pararenal metastasis (of solid ovarian carcinoma)	1
Pheochromocytoma (bilateral with MEA II)	1
Adrenal adenoma	2
Adrenal tumors (bilateral, unknown histology)	1
Congenital adrenal hyperplasia	1
Ewing sarcoma	2
Osteosarcoma	2
Chondrosarcoma, postoperative	1
Solitary myeloma (pelvis)	1
Fibrosarcoma	1
Metastases of melanoma (tibia)	1
Paget's disease (knee)	1
Aortic aneurysm	1
Aortic dissection Type B	1
Status after heart infarction (with 1 cardiac aneurysm)	2
AVM of the brain	1
Cryptic vascular malformation	2
Posterior fossa tumor (extra-axial)	1

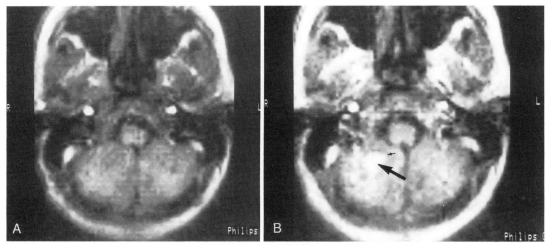

Figure 42–28. "Cryptic" vascular malformation of the right inferior cerebellum in a 24-year-old man. *A*, Plain FFE scan with a flip angle of 35 degrees did not highlight flow within lesion. *B*, Twelve sec following IV administration of 0.1 mmol/kg Gd-DTPA-meglumine, the serpiginous structure shows up (large arrow) and a relatively lesser perfused (dark) perifocal halo demarcates (small arrow).

and morphologic pattern of Gd-DTPA enhancement with the FFEI method with and without subtraction, we were able to differentiate all relevant tumor components, such as avascular (e.g., cystic) or relatively hypo- or hypervascularized regions, pseudo-capsules, and necrotic parts (Fig. 42–29*A–D*). Note the diffusion of Gd-DTPA into the cystic parts of the demonstrated renal carcinoma and the decreased signal intensity in the collecting system of the normal contralateral kidney (due to the higher Gd-DTPA concentration at this phase of excretion). Note also the image quality in comparison with the precontrast SE (2400/100) and the postcontrast SE (550/30). The described FFEI features correlated exactly with the gross specimen.

As is seen in Table 42–3, our material comprises six renal cell carcinomas of different sizes and one pararenal necrotic metastasis from a solid ovarian carcinoma. All malignancies, including their typical inherent features, were clearly depicted by Gd-DTPA enhanced FFEI. The smallest kidney tumor had a diameter of 2.5 cm and was not visible on the *T1* weighted SE postcontrast scan five minutes after injection. A solitary intra- extra-axial lipoma of one kidney enhanced, although it exhibited already high SI on the plain FFE scan. Diffuse distortion of the corticomedullary junction of both enlarged kidneys in the case of an angiolipomatosis and perfusion of obviously intact parenchyma could easily be defined by fast enhanced scans.

The four unilateral and bilateral adrenal tumors with diameters between 8 and 36 mm could be adequately classified in the same way by the evolution of their enhancement patterns. A case of an adrenal adenoma with areas of hemorrhage (see Fig. 42–20*A*) and necrosis (*B–C*) illustrate how respiratory motion can pose problems for conventional MRI even in the retroperitoneum. The fast images froze motion in this patient, who was breathing normally. Owing to the sharp delineation of the organ contours, even a small rest of normal adrenal tissue could be identified as well as appropriate subtraction performed from identical slices. Again, all findings correlated favorably with the gross specimen. The case of congenital adrenal hyperplasia examined with the body coil after intravenous administration of 0.2 mmol/kg Gd-DTPA suggests homogeneous enhancement of the diffusely enlarged cortex in the early phase and absence of nodules in the whole parenchymal phase (Fig. 42–30). These findings are encouraging as a way to further improve the examination procedure by means of adequate surface-coil technique.

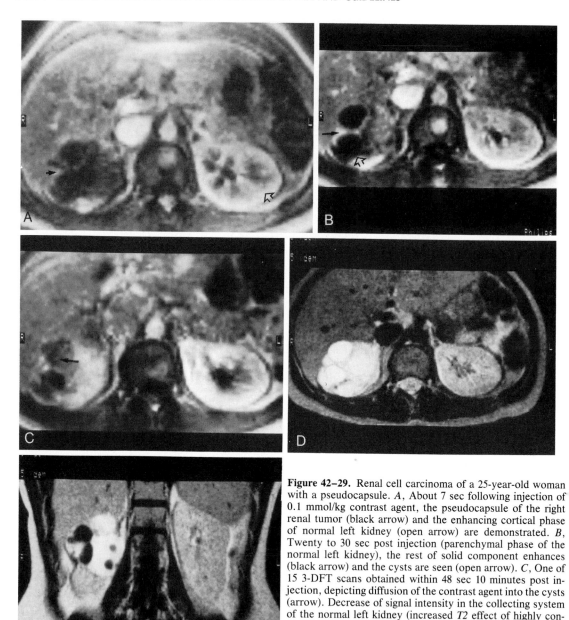

Figure 42–29. Renal cell carcinoma of a 25-year-old woman with a pseudocapsule. *A*, About 7 sec following injection of 0.1 mmol/kg contrast agent, the pseudocapsule of the right renal tumor (black arrow) and the enhancing cortical phase of normal left kidney (open arrow) are demonstrated. *B*, Twenty to 30 sec post injection (parenchymal phase of the normal left kidney), the rest of solid component enhances (black arrow) and the cysts are seen (open arrow). *C*, One of 15 3-DFT scans obtained within 48 sec 10 minutes post injection, depicting diffusion of the contrast agent into the cysts (arrow). Decrease of signal intensity in the collecting system of the normal left kidney (increased *T2* effect of highly concentrated contrast agent). *D*, SE *TR* 2400/*TE* 100 ms (precontrast). *E*, SE *TR* 550/*TE* 30 ms five minutes post injection.

In the absence of movement artifacts the technique also provides the ability to resolve the pancreas (Fig. 42–31*A*). Furthermore, the parenchyma of the pancreas enhances visually to some degree after intravenous injection of 0.1 mmol Gd-DTPA. This was confirmed by measurement of SI. Figure 42–31 shows an example of a sharply demarcated pancreatic pseudocyst in the tail. This pseudocyst possesses a distinctly longer *T1* than the anterolaterally located cyst of the left kidney. Owing to the relative absence of peristaltic motion, even the nonparamagnetically contrasted gastrointestinal tract can be well separated from the anterior contour of the pancreas. In addition, administering paramagnetic contrast agents via the oral route improves delineation of organ contours (see Fig. 42–22). Extraluminal pulsatile flow artifacts originating from

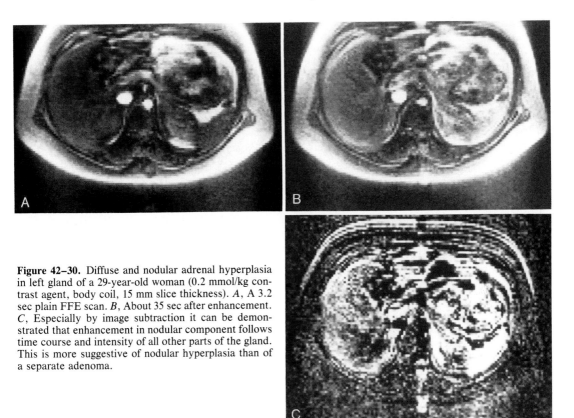

Figure 42–30. Diffuse and nodular adrenal hyperplasia in left gland of a 29-year-old woman (0.2 mmol/kg contrast agent, body coil, 15 mm slice thickness). *A*, A 3.2 sec plain FFE scan. *B*, About 35 sec after enhancement. *C*, Especially by image subtraction it can be demonstrated that enhancement in nodular component follows time course and intensity of all other parts of the gland. This is more suggestive of nodular hyperplasia than of a separate adenoma.

the aorta or other greater vessels may deteriorate (e.g., the display of the neck of the pancreas, the left liver lobe, or the vertebral body on axial scans). This is notably the case when optimal flip angles (for stationary tissue) in the order of 30 to 40 degrees are used; it can be overcome by performing an additional FFE study with smaller flip angles (see under Preferred Values of α and TR), in which the loss of S/N is still acceptable (Fig. 42–32).

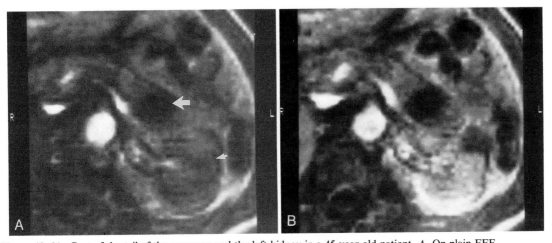

Figure 42–31. Cyst of the tail of the pancreas and the left kidney in a 45-year-old patient. *A*, On plain FFE scan, notice the longer $T1$ of the pancreatic pseudocyst (large arrow) as compared with the anteriorly located cyst of the kidney (small arrow). *B*, Enhanced scan about 42 sec following IV administration of 0.1 mmol/kg contrast agent (parenchymal phase of the otherwise normal kidney).

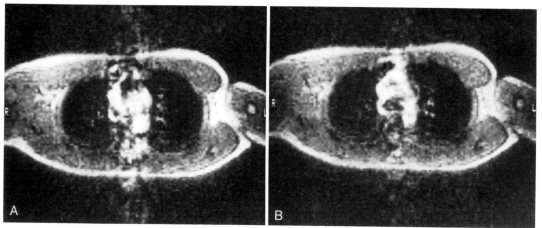

Figure 42–32. A–B, Normal volunteer. Non–ECG gated reduction of extraluminal flow artifact originating from mediastinal vessels without too much loss of S/N ratio by decreasing the flip angles. Best compromise at alpha values of Figures 42–14B and 42–22A.

Processes of the extremities, e.g., a hemorrhagic Ewing sarcoma (see Chapter 38, Fig. 38–15) are rather well delineated by contrast-enhanced FFE imaging. In this young woman with a clinical history of limb swelling one week prior to admission, the viable tumor tissue that had to be located for biopsy is seen as a ring of enhancement at the lateral aspect of the fibula about 30 seconds after injection of 0.2 mmol/kg Gd-DTPA. The orthopedic surgeon was advised to perform the biopsy at that site. The diagnosis was confirmed histologically. The necrotic part of the tumor shows up as a constant low signal intensity area with irregular and unsharp borders and absent central enhancement. The SE *TR* 2400/*TE* 50–100 ms images did not permit this discrimination of tumor from hemorrhage as distinctly.

Post-therapeutic conditions in tumors (Fig. 42–33) may be difficult to evaluate with conventional MRI. With 0.1 mmol/kg Gd-DTPA enhanced fast scans we were able to

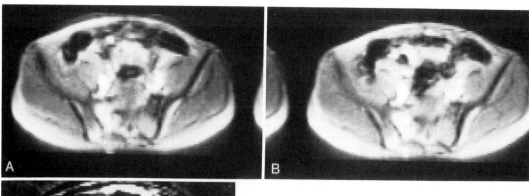

Figure 42–33. Irradiation and chemotherapy of a Ewing sarcoma of left sacroiliac joint in a 23-year-old man. A, Plain FFE scan *TR* = 50 ms. B, Enhancement about 1.5 min after IV administration of 0.1 mmol/kg contrast agent. C, Digital subtraction of the two images, highlighting "reactive" changes and the nonenhancing cyst that is located posteriorly.

determine within a very short examination time the appropriate site for rebiopsy in a young man presenting with subacute lower left back pain. (Fig. 42–33). More than one year ago a Ewing sarcoma of his left sacroiliac joint had been treated by chemotherapy and irradiation. The enhancement pattern (Fig. 42–33C), again highlighted by digital subtraction, was not characteristic for recurrence. After biopsy the cause was determined to be nonspecific granulation tissue. Serous fluid was obtained from a cyst located posteriorly that did not enhance.

Results of FMI

Although it has a somewhat inferior spatial resolution as compared with conventional SE imaging, FMI enabled, depiction of relevant features of great vessel disease, such as an intimal flap, different evolution of flow in the true and false lumens of an aortic dissection Type B (Fig. 42–34), or parietal thrombus in an aneurysm of the thoracic aorta.

Contrary to the conventional SE sequence, high-intensity flow effect adjacent to a sufficiently well-depicted aneurysm of the left heart chamber (Fig. 42–35) could easily be differentiated from parietal thrombus (in general, strongly saturated in FMI and therefore seen as a low-intensity area). Also, wall motion of the intact parts of the chamber were easily visualized. Contrary to non–ECG gated FFEI, these described pathologic changes could be highlighted by intravenous administration of 0.1 mmol/kg Gd-DTPA, resulting in visible and measurable intraluminal enhancement (subtraction of identical phases pre- and post contrast).

Our first observations using FFEI with and without contrast enhancement led us to conclude that this modality provides clinically valuable *T1* weighted images (demonstration of relevant anatomic structures, including gray and white matter in the brain and corticomedullary demarcation in the kidney, fat, hemorrhage, and differentiation of flow from calcification). Blurring effects from nonperiodic and periodic physiologic motion are reduced or completely eliminated. Although S/N drops significantly more with 2D than with 3DFT acquisition, higher S/N can be achieved nevertheless by in-

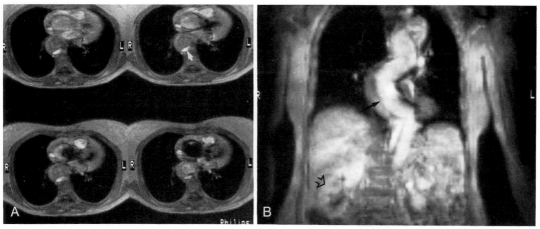

Figure 42–34. Aortic dissection, Type B, in a 65-year-old woman FMI, total measurement time about 4 min. *A*, The first four transverse sections after the R-top. The smaller true lumen shows high signal intensity (arrow) compared with the larger false lumen. Adjacent parietal thrombus appears more strongly saturated. *B*, First scan out of 16 acquired within the same examination time following IV administration of 0.1 mmol/ kg contrast agent. Signal intensity in the larger false lumen is now stronger owing to the relatively longer persistence of the paramagnetic agent in the false lumen (closed arrow). The intima flap is clearly depicted. Note also the contrast-enhanced right kidney (open arrow).

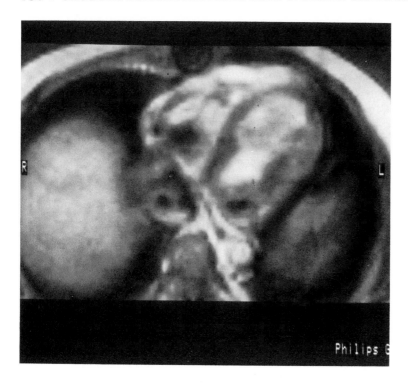

Figure 42–35. FMI of an aneurysm at the apex of the left ventricle in a 57-year-old man, first (after the R-top) out of 16 images. Intraventricularly, high flow signal intensity indicates absence of parietal thrombus.

creasing *TR*, averaging 2DFT scans, 3DFT imaging, or use of a relaxation enhancer. If this FFEI technique is supplemented by administering a paramagnetic contrast agent such as Gd-DTPA (or perhaps in the future, organ-selective contrast agents), functional information may be obtained about the integrity of the blood-brain barrier and renal perfusion. The method enables rapid, and perhaps better, characterization of tissue, including properties of vascularity, necrosis, pseudocapsules, "reactive" changes, and edema before and (perhaps even better) after chemotherapy, irradiation, and surgery, as compared with conventional MRI.

Looking at our initial results, we are impressed by the fact that Gd-DTPA enhanced FFEI provides easily interpretable images according to the principles known from dynamic CT and angiography. At the expense of somewhat lower spatial resolution, more functional information (heart wall motion, flow dynamics) is gained by FMI. A sensitive differentiation of true from false lumen in aortic dissection, wall thinning (aneurysm), and thrombus from flow effects appears to be reliably possible. This technique holds great promise for fast-flow quantification and plain MR angiography. Whether Gd-DTPA, at least in part, is an indispensable or an unnecessary adjunct awaits further investigation.

GENERAL CONSIDERATIONS

The rate of development of MRI is rapid—breakthroughs as significant as the successive generations of x-ray CT scanners may occur every half year. At present, efforts concentrate on developing faster scan techniques, such as fast Fourier[9] or RARE[28] imaging. FFEI represents the newest development. It is a very flexible and rapid technique. As supported by our initial clinical results, it holds great promise to definitely extend the versatility of MR imaging systems. Although S/N optimization by use of flip angles smaller than 90 degrees is a principle well known from spectroscopy for many years,[29] FFEI became technically and clinically available in proton-imaging systems only in May 1985. With the advent of this rapid MR pulse sequence, high-quality MR images can be recorded within two to six seconds. This is, of course, somewhat surprising. A technique such as MRI is predominantly characterized by an intrinsically weak detection sensitivity, and S/N remains the single most important criterion. The reasons that sufficient S/N is nevertheless achieved are discussed in the section on FFE properties.

Compared with "conventional" MRI, the FFEI technique shows a diminished S/N ratio; nevertheless this technique exhibits considerable advantages: (1) no image degradation due to relaxation effects (short *TE*); (2) completely arbitrary compromise between S/N, time, and spatial resolution; (3) no need for extremely rapid gradient switching; (4) low radio-frequency power deposition; (5) use in combination with superconducting magnets even at high field strength (Fig. 42–36); (6) optimum S/N per measuring time; (7) use of conventional Fourier imaging reconstruction algorithm; (8) attractive three-dimensional imaging; (9) chemical-shift imaging possible; and (10) new access to the detection of periodic and nonperiodic physiologic processes (e.g., heart cycle, perfusion of internal organs or lesions after administration of MR contrast agents).

Gd-DTPA-meglumine—in practical circumstances a *T1* contrast agent—seems to be tailored to that pulse sequence to enhance a rapid train of *T1* weighted FFE scans via the intravenous route.[31] The nonlinearity of SI with contrast concentration using Gd-DTPA and SE imaging techniques does not complicate the optimization of this pulse technique.[20] The time course of relative perfusion of organs or components of tumorous or inflammatory tissue by iodinated contrast agents—known from angiography and dynamic CT—has to be programmed in the set of fast serial MR scans before the start.

Enhanced FFEI admittedly duplicates results of dynamic CT and, unlike CT, disease of greater vessels can not be examined accordingly without use of the somewhat more time-consuming FMI (using one average in the order of four to five minutes). There are, however, potential advantages over CT that make application of this tech-

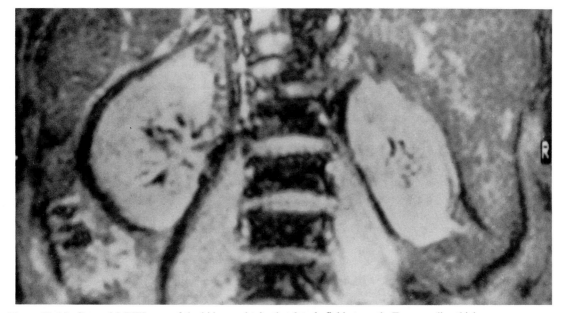

Figure 42–36. Coronal 2-DFT scan of the kidneys obtained at 2 tesla field strength. Ten mm slice thickness, *TR* = 20 ms, scan time 2.5 sec, flip angle 40 degrees, matrix 128 × 128.

nique much more attractive: (1) no radiation hazards; (2) display in any arbitrary plane, (3) 3DFT volume acquisition within a very short time and without mechanical table incrementation or heat-loading problems of x-ray tubes; (4) probably much greater diagnostic safety index (effective dose/lethal dose) than iodinated contrast agents in humans and no adverse reactions from injecting small amounts of Gd-DTPA as a bolus (see under Clinical Results); and (5) no blocking of the thyroid gland through Gd-DTPA.

Owing to the absence of beam-hardening artifacts, lesions of the bone, such as necrosis or vascular malformations (especially skull base and vault), can be evaluated dynamically. An intravenous, non–ECG gated, easily interpretable Gd-DTPA "MR angiotomography," eliminating complex flow phenomena, of aneurysms and vascular malformations in any arbitrary plane (including determination of aneurysm origin and of afferent and efferent vessel components) is a potential advantage over CT and conventional angiotomography. FFEI will facilitate evaluation of biodistribution of other gadolinium-labeled substances, e.g., Gd bound to albumin.[30] So far, our knowledge of Gd-DTPA in terms of early vascular and extracellular biodistribution is somewhat limited. This is because MR studies with conventional techniques can only be done a few minutes after intravenous administration.[19–21,23,25] Systematic in vivo studies can now easily be performed, as indicated in the section on clinical results.

To avoid confusion (and based on our experience and viewpoint), the term "dynamic contrast-enhanced MRI" should be applied only in terms of fast scan techniques, such as FFEI, that permit time resolution similar to that of dynamic CT. Faster conventional techniques using 1.5 tesla and 25.6 sec SE images[27] are a possible approach to reduce examination time but lack the time resolution of dynamic CT and FFEI.

Apart from vascular malformations of the brain, the main indication for Gd-DTPA enhanced FFEI will presumably be in the abdominal and thoracic area or when perfusion of tumors following chemotherapy or embolization as follow-up is of interest. With and without contrast enhancement, 3DFT FFEI techniques are promising in the head and neck; in mediastinal, retroperitoneal, and pelvic areas; and in the extremities.

The technical development of FFEI is in the early stages; on the basis of the initial results, software (similar to that of dynamic CT and DSA) is being adapted for clinical application.

Current efforts are directed at the potential of FFEI to obtain *T2* weighted images. Comparison of this technique to conventional *T1* and especially *T2* weighted images will possibly show that *T2* weighted conventional MRI will no longer be mandatory in many cases. However, the standard *T1*, but even more, the *T2* weighted sequences, will remain the gold standard until the definitive role of *T1* and *T2* weighted FFEI with and without contrast agent has been established in prospective studies.

FFEI provides answers to the problems cited at the beginning of this chapter. For measuring a large set of not-too-thin slices, however, the 2DFT multiple-slice method is more efficient at present. Efforts will also be directed toward developing an integrated concept of fast and conventional MRI that improves both patient throughput and diagnostic accuracy. It seems justified to state that FMI promises noninvasive dynamic flow visualization in any part of the body. In the near future, studies will focus on the possible quantitation of flow and other motion with this method. Also, multiple-slice modification is possible. Instead of measuring, for example, 32 phases of one slice in the cardiac cycle, eight phases of four different slices can be measured in order to cover a larger volume.

A minor disadvantage of FFEI is the increase in audible noise secondary to the rapid pulse sequence train. Sound protection, e.g., ear plugs for patients, may be required, especially in high-field system. Also, future design criteria may require an engineering solution to decrease the audible sound level.

References

1. van der Meulen P, Groen JP, Cuppen JJM: Very fast MR imaging by field echoes and small angle excitation. Magn Reson Imag *3*:297, 1985.
2. Waterton JC, et al: Magnetic resonance (MR) cine imaging of the human heart. Br J Radiol *58*:711, 1985.
3. Bluemm RG, Doornbos J, van der Meulen P, Cuppen J, Clauss W: First clinical results of fast field echo (FFE) MR imaging. A very fast imaging technique. RSNA Work in Progress Paper 1000. Radiology *157*P:335, 1985.
4. Rzedzian R, Doyle M, Mansfield P, Chapman B, Guilfoyle D, Coupland RE, Small P, Chrispin A: Echo planar imaging in paediatrics: real-time nuclear magnetic resonance. Ann Radiol *27*:182, 1984.
5. van Dijk P: Direct cardiac NMR imaging of heart wall and blood flow velocity. J CAT *8*:429, 1984.
6. van der Meulen P, McKinnon GC, in den Kleef JJE, Cuppen JJM: Fast field echo imaging: MR imaging with very short acquisition time. RSNA Work in Progress Paper 999. Radiology *157*P:335, 1985.
7. Edelstein WA, Hutchinson JMS, Johnson G, Redpath T: Spin warp NMR imaging and application to human whole body imaging. Phys Med Biol *25*:751, 1980.
8. Mansfield P, Pykett IL: Biological and medical imaging by NMR. J Magn Reson *29*:355, 1978.
9. van Uijen CMJ: Fast Fourier imaging. Presented at SMRM, San Francisco, 1983, p 363.
10. Haacke EM: A generalized fast scan technique for two-dimensional fourier transform imaging. Presented at SMRM, New York, 1984, pp 286–287.
11. Frahm J, Haase A, Matthaei D, Hanicke W, Merboldt KD: Flash MR imaging: from images to movies. RSNA Work in Progress Paper 426. Radiology *157*P:156, 1985.
12. Haase A, Matthaei D, Hanicke W, Frahm J: Digital subtraction MR imaging. RSNA Work in Progress Paper 915. Radiology *157*P:319, 1985.
13. Ziedses de Plantes BG, et al: Pulse sequences and contrast in magnetic resonance imaging. RadioGraphics *4*:869, 1984.
14. Moran PR, et al: Verification and evaluation of internal flow and motion. Radiology *154*:433, 1985.
15. Axel L: Blood flow effects in magnetic resonance imaging (review). Am J Roentgenol *143*:1157, 1984.
16. Ehmann RL, Felmlee JD, Houston DS, Tulsrud PR, Gray JE: Non-dispersive phase shifts caused by bulk motion and flow: Significance for clinical MR imaging. SMRM, Montreal, 1986, p 1099.
17. Haase A, Frahm J, Matthaei D, Haenicke W, Merboldt KD: Rapid images and NMR movies. Presented at SMRM, London, 1985, pp 980–981.
18. Runge VM, Clanton JA, Partain CL, James AE: Respiratory gating in magnetic resonance imaging at 0.5 tesla. Radiology *151*:521, 1984.
19. Brasch RC: Work in progress: methods of contrast enhancement for NMR imaging and potential applications. A subject review. Radiology *147*:781, 1983.
20. Runge VM, et al: Intravascular contrast agents suitable for magnetic resonance imaging. Radiology *153*:171, 1984.
21. Strich G, et al: Tissue distribution and magnetic resonance spin lattice relaxation effects of Gd-DTPA. Radiology *154*:723, 1985.
22. Laniado M, Claussen C, Schoerner W, Fiegler W, Felix R: Gd-DTPA in magnetic resonance imaging of renal tumors. Presented at SMRM, London, 1985, pp 877–878.
23. Gadian DG, et al: Gadolinium-DTPA as a contrast agent in MR imaging—theoretical projections and practical observations. J CAT *9*:242, 1985.
24. Felix R, et al: Brain tumors: MR imaging with gadolinium-DTPA. Radiology *156*:681, 1985.
25. Carr DH, et al: Gadolinium-DTPA as a contrast agent in MRI: initial clinical experience in 20 patients. AJR *143*:215, 1984.
26. Kucharczyk W, Lemme-Pleghos L, Uske A, Brant-Zawadski M, Dooms G, Norman D: Intracranial vascular malformations: MR and CT imaging. Radiology *156*:383, 1985.
27. Yoshikawa K, et al: Dynamic magnetic resonance imaging using Gd-DTPA. Presented at SMRM, London, 1985, pp 908–909.
28. Hennig J: RARE-imaging: a fast imaging method for clinical routine. Presented at SMRM, London, 1985, pp 988–989.
29. Becker ED, Ferretti JA, Gambhir PN: Selection of optimum parameters for pulse Fourier transform nuclear magnetic resonance. Anal Chem *51*:1413, 1979.
30. Grodd W: Perfusion contrast agents for MR imaging: evaluation of two paramagnetically labeled albumins. RSNA Work in Progress Paper 255, Radiology *157*P:100, 1985.
31. Bluemm RG, Doornbos J, Koops W, Bloem JL, te Strake B, van Voorthuizen AE: Gd-DTPA in fast scan techniques. Presented at the International Workshop on Contrast Agents in Magnetic Resonance Imaging, San Diego, January 17–18, 1986.

43

Sonography and MRI Correlation

ARTHUR C. FLEISCHER
THEODORE H. M. FALKE
MADAN V. KULKARNI
A. EVERETTE JAMES, JR.

This chapter will describe and illustrate both current and potential complementary clinical uses of sonography (US) and magnetic resonance imaging (MRI).

GENERAL CONSIDERATIONS

Since the clinical experience with sonography is much more extensive than that with magnetic resonance imaging, many of these areas for potential correlative imaging can be only speculative. In addition, the use of MRI has to be considered relative to the applications of computed tomography (CT). As its diagnostic efficacy relative to CT becomes established in certain areas, such as evaluation of the posterior cranial fossa, MRI may replace CT in many of its more conventional uses. US, on the other hand, does not compete directly with CT or MRI in many areas, such as in evaluation of the gallbladder and obstetric disorders.

There appears to be great potential for improving diagnostic specificity through the combined use of US and MRI. Specifically, with the increased utilization of pulsed duplex Doppler assessment of blood flow to sonographic imaging, the potential exists for expanding diagnosis into physiologic parameters. The ability of MRI to distinguish normal from abnormal tissues by their intrinsic time relaxation parameters and through the use of multiple-pulse sequences may further improve diagnosis that was previously based on depiction of abnormal anatomy by sonography.

MRI and US share a number of advantages compared with CT, primarily (1) the ability to image a region of interest in a variety of selected planes and (2) the absence of radiation hazard. In addition, both modalities may generate images with greater inherent tissue contrast than that obtained with CT, which has to rely on contour distortion or intravenous injection of contrast material for tissue contrast. MRI cannot reliably depict calcifications, which may limit its ability to detect occult carcinoma of the breast, for example.

In a practical sense, sonography is a nearly ideal initial diagnostic modality, since it is relatively inexpensive, has a high degree of patient acceptance, and does not use ionizing radiation. Sonographic units are widely available and markedly less expensive when compared with magnetic resonance scanners. Most US units are mobile and can be used in intensive care units and in labor and delivery areas. Specialized facilities are not required for sonography as they are for MRI and CT.

The resolution of currently available real-time scanners depends on the organ system examined and its location in the body. Under optimal circumstances, the resolution with 3.5 MHz transducers is in the 2 to 3 mm range, whereas with higher frequency transducers used for superficial structures, resolution of less than 1 mm can be achieved. Real-time scanning allows the operator to image an area of interest in a variety of scan planes. However, sonographic imaging of the abdomen remains limited by gas-filled bowel loops and bone. These are not detrimental to MRI.

A disadvantage of MRI is the long data acquisition time, which causes severe motion artifacts in the abdomen as a result of respiration and peristaltic movement. Examination times required for most MRI procedures are long, ranging from 45 minutes to 2 hours. Imaging of the pelvis and neck is relatively free from blurring caused by respiration. However, it is important to realize that motion artifacts may be produced by bladder wall contraction and swallowing. In addition to the high costs of MRI and complex site planning, this modality cannot be used to examine patients with metallic implants or pacemakers, or those who are severely ill. These limitations of MRI make the method less suitable than US for initial examination of the body.

The major advantage of MRI and CT over US is the excellent anatomic resolution as depicted in reproducible serial sections. MRI and CT can be more diagnostically accurate than US, especially in obese patients. When compared with sonographic images produced by sector real-time scanners, CT and MRI images provide a clear document of cross-sectional anatomy that is more readily understood by clinicians. Both CT and MRI can be performed when US is inconclusive, negative, or difficult to perform.

The remainder of this chapter will discuss and illustrate some potential areas for coordinated imaging with sonography and magnetic resonance imaging. The relative role of two-dimensional echocardiography and cardiac MRI is covered in Chapters 23 to 25. Those areas that will be discussed in this chapter include (1) evaluation of potentially malignant pelvic masses and the endometrium; (2) evaluation of endometrial carcinoma; (3) evaluation of breast masses; (4) evaluation of prostate abnormalities; (5) evaluation of thyroid abnormalities (6) evaluation of certain obstetric disorders; and (7) other potential applications.

POTENTIALLY MALIGNANT PELVIC MASSES

Sonography has proved to be an accurate modality for evaluation of adnexal masses. Computed tomography can accurately assess ovarian and uterine malignancies. MRI seems to be of equal value as CT for detection of recurrent or residual tumor.[1]

Magnetic resonance imaging has great potential in evaluation of tumor extent and involvement of surrounding structures, such as bowel and lymph nodes.[1-4] As with sonography and CT, there appears to be a great overlap in the appearance of pelvic masses, with a few exceptions. Dermoid cysts that contain a significant amount of fat have a specific appearance on all these modalities.[4] Similarly, physiologic ovarian cysts have a rather consistent appearance on US and MRI (Fig. 43-1). Outside of these two entities, there is significant overlap in the appearance of a variety of ovarian masses, such as cystadenomas, endometriomas, and hematomas (Fig. 43-2). MRI seems to be accurate in the detection of tumor invasion into surrounding structures, such as bowel and bladder, and in the detection of lymphadenopathy (Fig. 43-3). Because of its ability to image in several selected planes and to image the mass relative to other pelvic organs, such as the uterus, MRI may prove to be superior to CT in the diagnosis of certain entities.

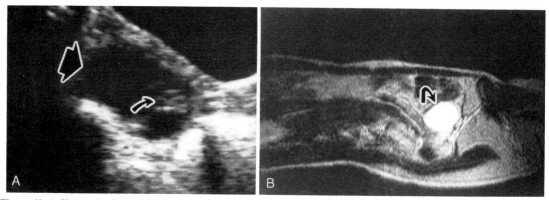

Figure 43–1. Hemorrhagic corpus luteum cyst. *A*, Magnified longitudinal real-time sonogram demonstrating hypoechoic adnexal mass (large arrow), with echogenic focus (curved arrow) representing clot. *B*, SE 2000/90 (*T2* weighted) MR image showing high-intensity signal within mass (curved arrows), that is, greater intensity than the urinary bladder.

ENDOMETRIAL CARCINOMA

Recently, the sonographic appearance of the normal endometrium has been described.[5] During menses, the endometrium appears as a thin, broken, echogenic interface. During the proliferative phase, the endometrium thickens and becomes iso- to hyperechoic. In the late proliferative and secretory phases, the endometrium becomes echoic, probably in relation to the more numerous and tortuous glands that contain inspissated secretions. A hypoechoic halo can be seen surrounding the internal echogenic layer, which seems to correspond to an increased fluid content of the hypovascular area of the inner third of the myometrium immediately beneath the basal layer of the endometrium (Fig. 43–4).

The appearance of endometrium and myometrium has been reported on magnetic resonance imaging.[3] The uterine cervix has a distinctly different appearance from that of the remainder of the corpus. This is related to the difference in consistency and glandular architecture of the cervix and corpus-fundus of the uterus, with the cervix containing more mucin than the corpus or fundus, and the corpus and fundus containing

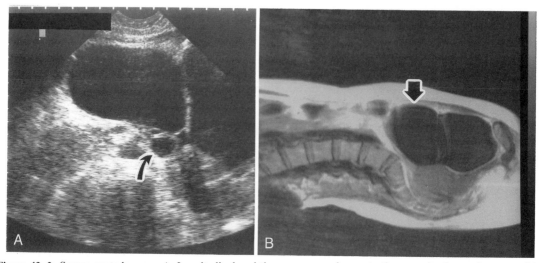

Figure 43–2. Serous cystadenoma. *A*, Longitudinal real-time sonogram demonstrating completely cystic mass arising from left ovary. An immature follicle (curved arrow) within left ovary is also identified. *B*, MR (*T1* weighted image) showing unilocular mass (arrow) superior to bladder, which has a similar intensity to urine.

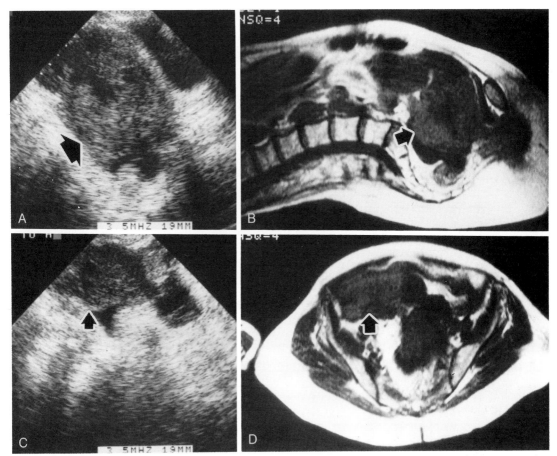

Figure 43–3. Advanced ovarian carcinoma. *A*, Longitudinal sonogram demonstrating ill-defined solid mass (arrow) superior to bladder. *B*, MR of same showing large mass (arrow) of low signal intensity. *C*, Transverse sonogram in same patient showing mass adjacent to peritoneum (arrow). *D*, MR (30/500) showing peritoneal mass (arrow).

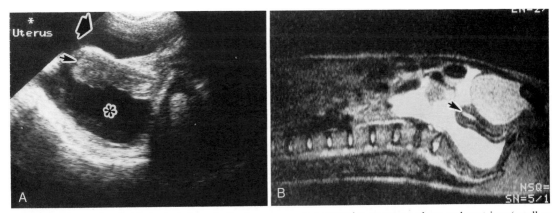

Figure 43–4. Normal endometrium. *A*, Longitudinal sonogram demonstrating secretory-phase endometrium (small arrowhead). Intraperitoneal fluid (asterisk) is present in the posterior cul-de-sac. There is a cystic mass immediately anterior to the uterus (large arrowhead). *B*, MRI (60/2000) of same patient showing intraperitoneal fluid and mass anterior to uterus. The mass has an intensity that is less than the intraperitoneal fluid. At surgery, a ruptured hemorrhagic ovarian cyst was found. Normal endometrium (arrow) appears as high-intensity area surrounded by less intense zone. This zone corresponds to the halo seen on sonography that represents the inner third of the myometrium, which is highly vascular.

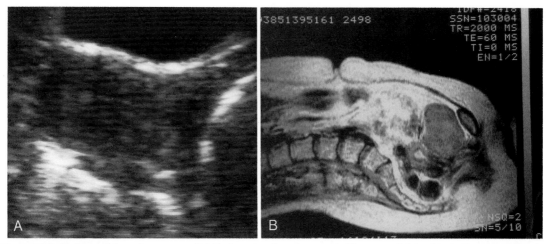

Figure 43–5. Endometrial carcinoma superficially invasive (less than one-half myometrial depth). *A*, Sonogram showing thickened endometrial interface but homogeneous myometrium. *B*, MR (60/2000) showing preserved subendometrial layer and noninvasive tumor.

the endometrium. There appears to be potential for evaluating abnormal cervices such as those encountered in patients exposed to diethylstilbestrol (DES), in whom the adenosquamous junction may be abnormal in location.

The depiction of the uterus and endometrium by MRI is independent of its position or flexion. Therefore, a severely retroflexed uterus that may be difficult to image adequately on US may be better depicted on MRI. The hypovascular layer of the myometrium appears consistently as an area of regular band, reduced signal in *T2* weighted images. Therefore, there are a variety of potential applications of MRI and US in the evaluation of uterine disorders, particularly those related to the endometrial abnormalities, and in the assessment of myometrial invasion (Figs. 43–5 and 43–6). This application may be helpful in evaluating patients with hyperplasia or low-grade tumor who do not undergo hysterectomy. Determination of the extent of tumor invasion has its greatest impact on the decision of whether or not to irradiate pelvic lymph nodes prior to hysterectomy.

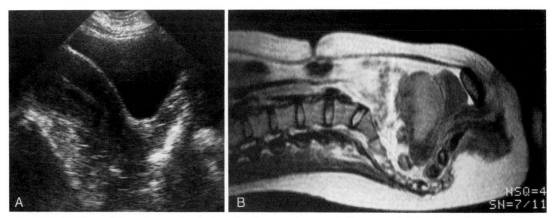

Figure 43–6. Endometrial carcinoma deeply invasive (greater than one-half myometrial depth). *A*, Sonogram showing marked irregularity of myometrium, indicating myometrial invasion up to uterine serosa. *B*, MRI (60/2000) showing deep invasion into myometrium.

BREAST

Breast sonography can be performed with a variety of scanners. These include dedicated water-path scanners or hand-held, real-time scanners. Because of the relatively inexpensive price, wide availability, and improved resolution of the equipment, hand-held, real-time scanning of the breast will probably become more extensively used than dedicated sonotomography.

The role of sonography as an adjunct to mammography in evaluation of breast diseases has been established. However, once a solid mass is depicted on sonography, it is usually not possible to distinguish benign from malignant lesions with a sufficiently high degree of confidence. Thus, a needle aspiration or excisional biopsy is indicated in most patients with a solid breast lesion. This can be performed under continuous real-time guidance with a hand-held, high-frequency transducer.

MRI has a potential role as an adjunct to mammography and sonography. For example, MRI could confirm the presence of fat lobules, which may occasionally appear as a solid mass on sonography. MRI may have an advantage over sonography in those patients with fatty breasts, since fat has a uniform signal. Although there have been some in vitro experiments to suggest a significant difference in $T1$ and $T2$ in benign and malignant breast lesions, the diagnosis of breast lesions on MRI seems to depend upon criteria similar to those used mammographically, such as the distinctiveness of borders of the mass.[9] There does not seem to be a reliable distinction in $T1$ and $T2$ in differentiating benign from malignant lesions.[9] In addition, neither MRI nor US can reliably detect microcalcifications, the basic radiographic finding in occult carcinomas. MRI has a rather thick slice (approximately 1 cm); therefore, lesions of several mil-

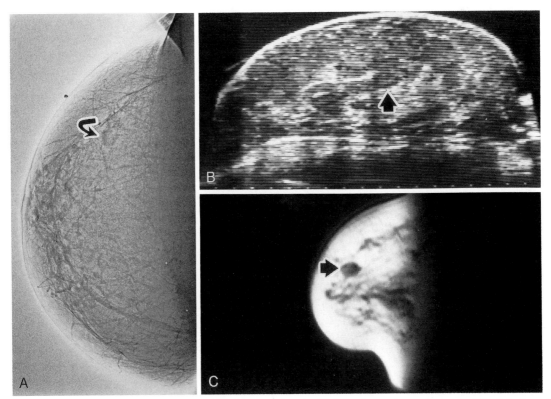

Figure 43–7. Fibroadenoma of the breast. *A*, Mammogram showing ill-defined mass (curved arrow) within fatty breast. *B*, Sonotomogram showing well-circumscribed solid mass (arrow). *C*, *T1* weighted (SE 30/200) image showing well-defined mass of low signal intensity (arrow).

limeters can be missed if they are not included in the tomographic slice. Because of the cost considerations, it is unlikely that MRI will be used as a primary means for screening. The axilla cannot be adequately imaged with specialized breast coils, and US may be more accurate in detecting abnormalities in the axilla. In general, MRI seems to have application in those cases in which both mammography and US yield equivocal findings—in other words, as one of several adjunctive modalities that can be used in the breast for improving diagnostic specificity (Fig. 43–7).

PROSTATE

Specialized US probes have been developed for evaluation of the prostate using a transrectal approach. These types of transrectal probes are introduced into the rectum covered by a condom that is filled with fluid. This allows optimal sonographic access to the prostate. The prostate can be imaged in either the longitudinal or the transverse plane. With a linear-array, real-time transducer, the prostate is imaged in a sagittal plane; with a radial scanner, moving in a circular path, the prostate may be imaged in the transverse or short-axis view. The transverse scan seems to delineate the capsule better than with a linear-array transducer.

The method of examination with the linear-array transrectal probe begins with an image in the midline of the prostate, depicting the prostatic urethra. Then the probe is rotated to the right in 10 degree intervals, and images are obtained. This process is repeated as the probe is rotated to the left. Particular attention is paid to the integrity of the borders of the prostate.

Both benign and malignant prostatic lesions as small as 2 to 3 mm can be detected.[10] The most common sonographic appearance of carcinoma is a hypoechoic focus that has smooth borders (Fig. 43–8). There does not appear to be any reliable differentiation of benign nodules from malignant ones (Fig. 43–9). Sonography can detect capsular invasion, but this is more difficult to do with a sagittally oriented scan than with an axial one.

US has an important role in guiding needle biopsy. The use of US increases the accuracy of biopsy and decreases the number of attempts needed to obtain adequate

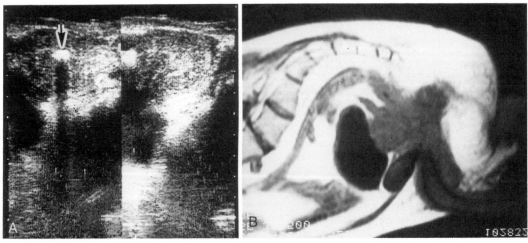

Figure 43–8. Benign prostatic hypertrophy. *A*, Transrectal sonograms of prostate. The image on the left shows an echogenic focus with shadowing (arrow). The prostate is diffusely enlarged. There are no lesions in the posterior lobes. *B*, MRI of same patient in midsagittal image (SE 30/500) showing enlarged prostate with external compression of bladder base. (Prone orientation used to match ultrasound images.)

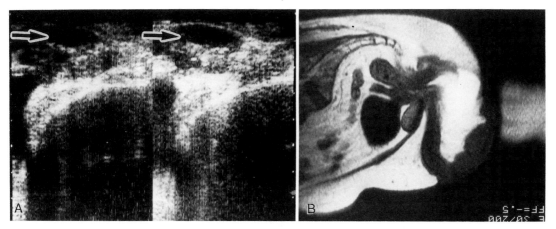

Figure 43–9. Prostatic carcinoma. *A*, Transrectal sonograms showing hypoechoic area (arrow) in posterior lobes, very suggestive of carcinoma in the posterior lobe, adjacent to the capsule. *B*, MRI of the same patient (SE 30/200) fails to show any definite abnormality. (Prone orientation used to match ultrasound images.)

material.[18] Because of its inability to reliably distinguish benign from malignant nodules, MRI may have a role complementary to prostate sonography.[11,12] However, the resolution of US is superior to that of MRI, and many lesions seen on US may not be detected on MRI. Lymphadenopathy, which is associated with malignant spread of prostatic carcinomas or extension of the tumor to other structures, may be better depicted on MRI than on US. Capsular invasion may be more apparent on MRI than with sagittally oriented transrectal US. However, there is sufficient evidence to suggest that the capsule itself can not be imaged by either MRI or US, and that the surrounding tissue that is seen on MRI is the normal, compressed tissue or surgical capsule.[17] Capsular invasion may be demonstrated on MRI by disruption of the peri-prostatic veins.

THYROID

Since the thyroid is superficially located, it can be imaged with high-frequency transducers that afford submillimeter resolution. Lesions as small as 1 to 2 mm can be reliably detected on sonography. This capability has important clinical implications, since the finding of multiple lesions reduces the likelihood that a solitary nodule is malignant. Fluid-containing lesions are typically degenerated adenomas. Sonography can evaluate the borders of a mass. A hypoechoic "halo" is typically seen around adenomas, although slow-growing neoplasms may also exhibit this finding.

Since the sonographic appearance of thyroid nodules is not specific for benign and malignant lesions, a potential for MRI evaluation of the thyroid exists based upon differences in tumor relaxation times between benign and malignant lesions (Fig. 43–10). MRI seems to be particularly useful in the evaluation of patients with substernal goiter or ectopic parathyroid in the mediastinum. Improved sensitivity over that afforded by CT is possible because of multiplanar imaging with MRI.

Sonography is an accurate modality for detection of hyperplastic parathyroid glands. Sonography may be helpful in confirming that a mass is arising from the parathyroid, since on MRI detailed anatomic evaluation usually is not possible. Perhaps with the development of specialized surface coils for evaluation of the neck, more detailed resolution of the parathyroid will be possible. Guided biopsy of the thyroid or parathyroid will not be possible on MRI, whereas US can directly visualize biopsy and aspiration procedures in real time.

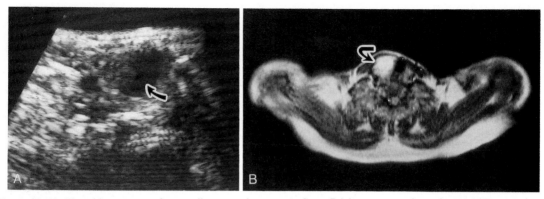

Figure 43–10. Thyroid metastases from malignant melanoma. *A,* Superficial organ scanning using 10 MHz transducer shows complex lesion (arrow) with fluid areas within the right lobe of the thyroid. This lesion was biopsied under sonographic guidance. *B,* MRI (SE 30/300), *T1* weighted, showing thyroid mass (curved arrow) with high signal intensity. *T1* relaxation confirmed by calculated 0*T1* images consisting of a hemorrhage within cyst.

CERTAIN OBSTETRIC DISORDERS

Sonography has its most important application in obstetrics. However, there are a few areas in which sonography is limited in evaluation of placental and fetal anatomy. These include imaging of the fetus when there is oligohydramnios and evaluation of possible abdominal ectopic pregnancies.[13–15] With the recent advent of duplex Doppler imaging, flow parameters within the placenta and fetus can aid in the physiologic evaluation of pregnancy. Sonography depicts anatomic changes in the placenta that occur with aging. However, the physiologic significance of these changes cannot be evaluated by imaging alone. Thus MRI and Doppler assessment may help evaluate flow disturbances in the placenta and help quantitate changes in this flow with treatment regimens that improve uteroplacental perfusion.

MRI has potential application in evaluation of hypoechoic areas surrounding the placenta that may result from retroplacental hemorrhage (Fig. 43–11). These hypoechoic retroplacental areas, which may represent abruption, can be distinguished from those related to slow flow of the basilar venous sinus complex.

MRI offers a secondary modality for documentation of abnormalities initially detected with US (Fig. 43–12). It is possible that changes in the fetal lung as it matures

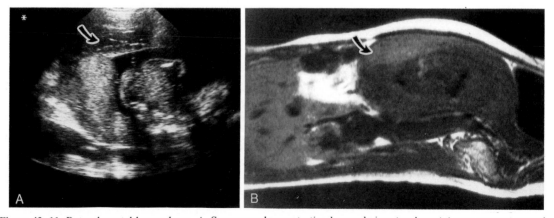

Figure 43–11. Retroplacental hemorrhage. *A,* Sonogram demonstrating hypoechoic retroplacental area (curved arrow). The fundal portion of the placenta appears normal. *B,* MRI (SE 30/500) showing area of high signal intensity (arrow) in anterior extent of placenta, compatible with hemorrhage.

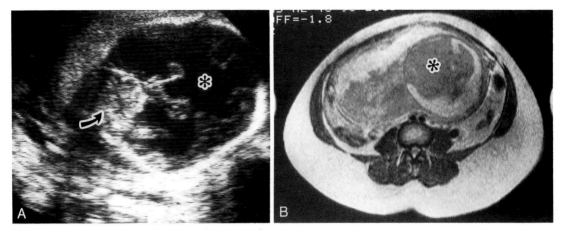

Figure 43–12. Fetus with severe ventricular dilatation. *A*, Real-time sonogram demonstrating markedly dilated internal ventricles (asterisk). The cerebellum (curved arrow) is normal. *B*, MRI (SE 45/2000) of same fetus. The fetus has moved to a more occipital posterior position. Dilated ventricles (asterisk) are again demonstrated.

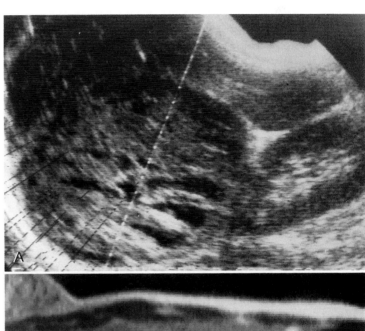

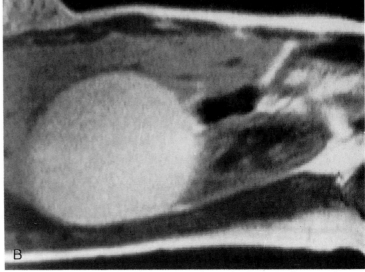

Figure 43–13. Gravid patient with adrenal hemorrhage. *A*, Longitudinal static sonogram showing large complex mass superior to the right kidney. *B*, MRI showing same mass, with increased signal intensity on this *T1* weighted image.

can be depicted by MRI.[15] The relative amount of subcutaneous fat can be depicted by MRI and may be useful in assessing the possibility of intrauterine growth retardation or macrosomia.[19]

MRI has the capability to image maternal anatomy in a more global fashion than that possible with real-time sonography.[16] It can depict the dimensions of the bony pelvis, which may afford an alternative technique for pelvimetry as performed with radiography.[20] For example, large maternal abdominal masses, such as those resulting from adrenal hemorrhage, would be depicted more reliably on MRI than on US (Fig. 43–13). The maternal spine and its contents can be imaged by MRI and not by US.

Even with these possible applications, sonography will remain the primary modality for evaluation of the uterus, fetus, and mother. The coordinated use of MRI can be envisioned only in rare circumstances when the sonographic findings are inconclusive, such as when there is suspicion of an abdominal ectopic pregnancy.

OTHER POTENTIAL APPLICATIONS

Other potential applications of MRI and US will develop as greater experience with MRI is gained. For example, MRI might be used to evaluate the renal transplant for detection of flow abnormalities associated with rejection or to fully delineate the extent of abdominal aortic aneurysms. One study suggested that MRI is more accurate than US in detecting aneurysms of the main renal arteries and common iliac arteries.[21] However, sonography is still recommended as the initial diagnostic modality for evaluation of abdominal aortic aneurysms. Duplex pulsed Doppler scanning is now being utilized and investigated as a means of early detection of flow disturbances associated with rejection. In vascular rejection, there appears to be a decrease in diastolic flow, which is a sign of increased resistance to flow. This finding is detectable prior to the deterioration found on a renal scintigram.

Carotid imaging with a specialized coil seems promising and could complement the findings encountered with duplex pulsed Doppler scanning. However, the relative simplicity and low cost continue to make sonography an attractive diagnostic modality for screening.

MRI may be helpful to further characterize masses in organs, such as liver, into infectious and neoplastic categories (Fig. 43–14). This information would be crucial in establishing the correct treatment.

In summary, there are many more potential applications that combine sonography

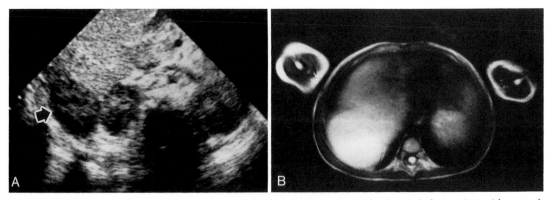

Figure 43–14. Intrahepatic abscess. *A*, Transverse real-time sonogram demonstrating hypoechoic area (arrow) in posterior segment of right hepatic lobe. *B*, MRI *T2* weighted image (SE 60/2000) of the same region, showing high-intensity area, compatible with liver abscess.

with MRI. Because of its lower cost and greater availability, sonography will remain an important initial modality for a variety of disorders. However, as further experience is gained with MRI, it is clear that there will be areas where the coordinated use of the two modalities will lead to more specific and accurate diagnoses. Currently, the main areas for coordinated use are gynecologic (ovarian and endometrial) malignancies, prostate lesions, breast masses, and certain obstetric disorders.

ACKNOWLEDGMENTS

The authors express their thanks to Drs. Gary Thieme, Deland Burks, and Snehal Mehta for their contributions to this chapter, and to Monica Harper and John Bobbitt for their assistance in manuscript preparation.

References

1. Bies JR, Ellis JH, Kopecky KK, et al: Assessment of primary gynecologic malignancies: Comparison of 0.15-T resistive MRI with CT. AJR *143*:1249, 1984.
2. Butler H, Bryan PJ, LiPuma JP, et al: Magnetic resonance imaging of abnormal female pelvis. AJR *143*:1259, 1984.
3. Hricak H, Alpert C, Crooks L, Sheldon P: Magnetic resonance imaging of the female pelvis: initial experience. AJR *141*:1119, 1983.
4. Bryan P, Butler H, LiPuma JP: NMR scaning of the pelvis: initial experience with a 0.3T system. AJR *141*:1111, 1983.
5. Fleischer A, Kalemeris G, Entman S, Machin S: Sonographic depiction of the normal and abnormal endometrium. J Ultrasound Med *5*:445, 1986.
6. El Yousef SJ, Duchesneau RH, Alfidi RJ, et al: Magnetic resonance imaging of the breast. Radiology *150*:761, 1984.
7. Stelling CB, Wang PC, Lieber A, et al: Prototype coil for magnetic resonance imaging of the breast. Radiology *154*:457, 1985.
8. McSweeny M, Small W, Cerny V, et al: Magnetic resonance imaging in the diagnosis of breast disease: use of transverse relocation. Radiology *153*: 741, 1984.
9. Partain CL, Kulkarni MV, Price RR, Fleischer AC, Page DL, Malcolm AW, Winfield AC, James AE: Magnetic resonance imaging of the breast: Functional *T1* and three dimensional imaging. Cardiovasc Intervent Radiol *8* (5–6):292, 1986.
10. Rifkin M, Kurtz A: Ultrasound of the prostate. *In* Sanders R, Hill M (eds): Ultrasound Annual 1983. New York, Raven Press, 1983, pp 95–132.
11. Poon PY, McCallum RW, Henkelman MM, et al: Magnetic resonance imaging of the prostate. Radiology *154*:143, 1985.
12. Buonocore E, Hesemann C, Pavlicek W, Montie JE: Clinical and in vitro magnetic resonance imaging of prostatic carcinoma. AJR *143*:1267, 1984.
13. Johnson IR, Symonds EM, Kean DM: Imaging the pregnant human uterus with nuclear magnetic resonance. Am J Obstet Gynecol *148*:1136, 1984.
14. Weinreb JC, Lowe TW, Santos-Ramos RS, et al: Magnetic resonance imaging in obstetric diagnosis. Radiology *154*:157, 1985.
15. McCarthy SM, Filly RA, Stark DD, et al: Obstetrical magnetic resonance imaging: fetal anatomy. Radiology *154*:427, 1985.
16. McCarthy SM, Stark DD, Filly RA, et al: Obstetrical magnetic resonance imaging: maternal anatomy. Radiology *154*:421, 1985.
17. Burks D, Lindell H, Fleischer A, MacDougal S: Sonography and MRI of the prostate. In preparation.
18. Lindell H, Burks, D, MacDougal S, Fleischer A: Digital vs. sonographically directed prostate biopsy. Urology *135*:716, 1986.
19. Stark D, McCarthy S, Filly R, et al: Intrauterine growth retardation: evaluation by magnetic resonance: work-in-progress. Radiology *155*:425, 1985.
20. Stark D, McCarthy S, Filly R, et al: Pelvimetry by magnetic resonance imaging. AJR *144*:947, 1985.
21. Flak B, Li D, Ho B, et al: Magnetic resonance imaging of aneurysms of the abdominal aorta. AJR *144*:991, 1985.

44

Overview of MRI Clinical Applications in Germany

E. ZEITLER

Since the first edition of this book,[46] industrial efforts have generated considerable technical development for the clinical use of nuclear magnetic resonance as an imaging procedure. In Germany, important progress has been achieved by Bruker GmbH, Karlsruhe, and Siemens AG, Medical Division, Erlangen. Bruker GmbH, having long experience in the area of NMR spectroscopy, supplies a large number of units for NMR spectroscopy for the investigation of anatomic specimens, for small and large animal research, and also for study of parts of the human body. Clinical experiences with MR imaging using resistive magnets were gathered in the Bruker laboratories as well as in the German Clinic of Diagnostics (GCD), Wiesbaden and at the University of Freiburg. Initial results have also been produced with a superconducting magnet with "iron self-shielding."

Siemens AG, Erlangen, first developed resistive magnets of 0.12 up to 0.20 tesla and then MR imagers with kryomagnets of 0.35, 0.5, 1.0, 1.5, 2.0, and 4.0 tesla. Investigations in patients were performed in their own laboratories. Systematic clinical examinations were assembled at the Medical University of Hanover (MUH), the Free University of Berlin, and the Ludwig-Maximilian University of Munich. Technical advancements and clinical studies are financially supported by the German Ministry of Research and Technology and the German Society of Research (GSR).

In several private radiologic practices, NMR units of different manufacturers are installed. The radiologists cooperate with university hospitals when studying patients for a wide variety of indications (Table 44–1). The University Hospitals of Cologne and Hamburg work in close cooperation with Messrs. Philips.

Whereas at the first symposium on NMR in Mayence[116] most speakers came from the United States and Great Britain, now the results of 16 German working groups are available for this chapter. Those who contributed case material are cited in Table 44–2. These working groups studied more than 4000 patients in the topographic distribution presented in Table 44–3.

The industry has mainly emphasized technical advances in improved spatial resolution, reduced investigation time, simultaneous production of multiple images, use of ECG and respiratory gating, and development of different software programs for the evaluation of special problems. The clinical research in the Federal Republic of Germany has concentrated so far on the following:

1. Development of the best quantitative investigational parameters.

2. Comparisons of computed tomography and MR imaging in the region of the brain, skull, and spinal canal were performed in Berlin, Cologne, Erlangen, Freiburg, Munich, Tübingen, Wiesbaden, and several private institutes. Studies of fewer subjects were made for the liver, pancreas, hip, and extremities.

Table 44–1. MRI UNITS IN GERMANY (FRG) (12/1/1984)

Company	Resistive	Superconducting
Siemens Factory	1	4
Siemens (delivered)	1	25(16)
Bruker Factory	1	2
Bruker (delivered)	2	2(1)
Diasonics	—	2(2)
Picker	—	6(6)
Philips	—	4(2)
Technicare	1(1)	1(1)
Elscint	—	1(1)
Total	6	46

Numbers in parentheses refer to units used in private practice.

Table 44–2. WORKING GROUPS PROVIDING CASE MATERIAL

1. Anacker, Decker, von Einsiedel, Petsch, Reiser, Rupp—München
2. Blümm—Bochum
3. Breit—Passau
4. Bücheler, Bomsdorf, Grabbe, Heinzerling, Kuhn, Kunz, Matthaei, Meyer, Röschmann—Hamburg
5. Felix, Claussen, Fiegler, Köhler, Laniado, Niendorf, Runge, Schörner, Semmler, Steiner—Berlin
6. Friedburg, Bockenheimer, Hinkelbein, Ratzel, Ströbel, Wenz—Freiburg
7. Friedmann, Beyer, Buschsieweke, Kutzim, Steinbrich—Köln
8. Frommhold, Vogt, Lutz, Bautz—Tübingen
9. Huk, Fahlbusch, Gademann, Heindel, Löffler—Erlangen
10. Hundeshagen, Becker, Hagemann, Hammer, Kotzerke, Schwarzrock, Tiffe—Hannover
11. Lissner, Baierl, Bauer, Beer, Hiemeyer, Rath, Rienmüller, Seiderer, Vogl—München
12. Pfannenstiel, Bielke, Brederhoff, Meves, Rinck—Wiesbaden
13. Rödl, Demling—Erlangen
14. Strecker—Karlsruhe
15. Zeitler Gailer, Kaiser, Oppelt, Rehm, Schuierer, Wodarz—Nürnberg

3. Development, experimental studies in animals, and clinical application of contrast media in MR imaging were performed mainly by Schering AG, Berlin, in cooperation with the Free University of Berlin, Klinikum Charlottenburg (Felix, Schörner).

4. Comparisons of MR imaging with investigative procedures made by nuclear medicine for diseases of the liver, renal transplantations, orbital diseases, and determination of the intrapulmonary water content were executed at the Medical University of Hanover.

5. Comparison of sonography with MR imaging in the liver at the University Hospitals of Erlangen and comparisons of echocardiography and CT with MR imaging of the heart and mediastinum were performed in the University Hospitals of Munich, Berlin, and Erlangen.

6. Surface coils in the diagnosis of superficial body regions are used in several institutions for the examination of the spinal canal; the vertebrae; the internal ear; the joints of the knee, shoulder, and ankle; the female breast; and in special problems as well as in other regions.

Table 44–3. STUDIES IN DIFFERENT ANATOMIC REGIONS*

Brain	2100
Spinal canal	350
Chest and heart	450
Abdomen and pelvis	750
Extremities	140
Other	250

* In ten clinics and three factories (Siemens, Bruker, Philips).

To date, five monographs have been published in German.[4,59,84,118,119] Meanwhile, many articles have appeared in German and English journals, the majority in German, presumably because they did not need to await translation.

As a result of the clinical studies so far the following results can be cited.

COMPARISON OF MR AND CT IMAGING OF THE CENTRAL NERVOUS SYSTEM*

NMR is able to produce direct sectional images of the three planes with the possibility of high-contrast resolution and a good anatomic demonstration of details. A good contrast can already be achieved at a low field strength. For the good spatial resolution required for surgical diagnosis, however, higher field strengths are necessary to obtain a sufficiently strong signal with a favorable signal-to-noise (S/N) ratio (Fig. 44-1).

A comparison of the efficacy of CT and magnetic resonance imaging can be obtained from Table 44-4.

Von Einsiedel and associates,[25] in particular, published early and thorough investigations toward more appropriate diagnosis of low-grade astrocytomas, syringomyelias, and tumors in the spinal canal (Fig. 44-2). Furthermore, more systematic studies have been performed by several groups, especially those in Berlin, Cologne, Munich, Erlangen-Nüremberg, and Wiesbaden. The results are similar to those reported in Chapters 10 to 16.

Table 44-4. COMPARISON OF EFFICACY OF CT AND MRI

Diagnosis	CT	MRI*	Additional Information by MRI
Brain tumors	+	+ +	
Tumors/edema DD	+ +	+	+
Extracerebral tumors	+	+	
Basal tumors	+	+ +	
Hypophysis tumors			
Macroadenomas	+	+ +	
Microadenomas	+ +	−	
Meningiomas	+ +	+	
Infarction	+ +	+	+
Hemorrhage, acute	+ +	+	
Hemorrhage, chronic	+	+ +	
Craniocerebral trauma, acute	+ +	−	
Contusion	+	+ +	
Multiple sclerosis	+	+ +	
Vascular anatomy	+ (CM)	+ +	
Encephalitis	+	+ +	
Temporal lobe epilepsy	+	+ +	
Brainstem process	+	+ +	
Tumors of the cerebellopontine angle	+	+ +	
Tumors of the spinal cord	+	+ +	
Syringomyelia and others	+	+ +	
Tumors of the spine	+	+ +	
Disc herniation	+ +	+	+

+ + = Very good demonstration
+ = Good demonstration
− = No demonstration or additional information
* = Without Gd-DTPA

---

* Reported by W. J. Huk, Neurosurgical University Hospital, Erlangen.

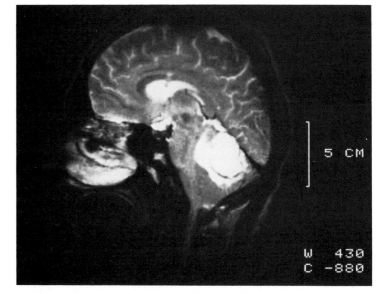

Figure 44–1. Metastatic tumor with bleeding into the cerebellum. One *T2* weighted image with a long *TE* out of a series of multiple echo images in spin-echo mode with a superconducting magnet of 1.5 tesla. Cerebrospinal fluid, edema, and bleeding into the tumor give a high signal in comparison with brain tissues.

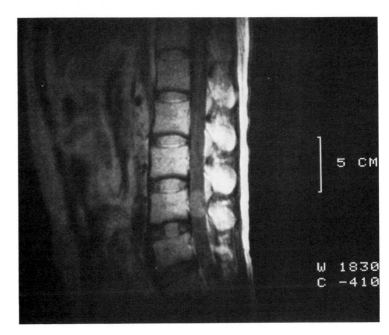

Figure 44–2. Intradural tumor in the lumbar spinal canal. Documentation with a superconducting magnet 0.35 tesla in spin-echo mode of the mid-sagittal section.

MEDIASTINAL ORGANS*

ECG gating permits a good demonstration of the heart with its cavities and boundaries, the pericardium, and the great vessels in the mediastinum without the use of contrast media, radiation, or catheter. The combination of respiratory and ECG gating improves the spatial resolution, especially at the boundary of the mediastinal organs to the diaphragm and hilum of the lung. The inner structures of the mediastinal organs, including the heart, can be visualized with a fairly good spatial resolution so that changes in the size of the ventricles and atria, in the thickness of the myocardium, and in the

---

* Reported by E. Zeitler, Diagnostic Dept., Radiological Centre, Klinikum Nürnberg.

pericardium may be shown in all three dimensions. Furthermore, changes in thickness as well as different signal intensities and flow phenomena indicate regions with disturbed contraction in the area of the ventricles. Compared with echocardiography or CT the boundaries between the heart cavities, the thickness of the myocardium in all regions, and the pericardium can be defined considerably more clearly (Fig. 44–3).

This is also valid for the anterior and posterior wall of the heart cavities and apex, which could always be accurately defined (Table 44–5). Even with the use of ECG gating, a safe topical determination of the relaxation times in the myocardium is by no means practical in vivo; at present, perhaps, a determination of *T2* relaxation time is feasible. A reliable preoperative diagnosis by MR imaging is possible for various kinds of obstructive cardiomyopathy, for the evaluation of aneurysms at the heart wall (Fig. 44–4), and for reliable proof of intracardiac thrombi.

The data for the assessment of ischemic coronary heart disease by MRI in acute myocardial infarction or chronic ischemia prior to operative and invasive procedures are currently inadequate for meaningful conclusions. First results on the use of gadolinium-DTPA in patients with ischemic myocardial disease were obtained by the Munich Working Group.[58,59]

To date, patients with acute myocardial infarction demonstrate statistically significant enhancement after Gd-DTPA injection. The first clinical results of Gd-DTPA–

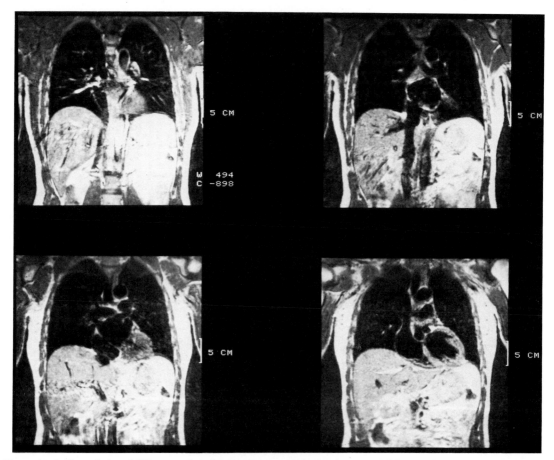

Figure 44–3. Normal chest MRI, coronal, multi-slice images. Four simultaneous ECG-gated images of the chest, demonstrating all parts of the heart, the great vessels, and the tracheobronchial system in the mediastinum. ECG-gated images demonstrating simultaneously the liver, inferior vena cava, hepatic vein, and hepatic artery. Moving artifact in the midabdomen. Flow imaging in parts of the pulmonary vascular system and intrahepatic vessels. Images with ECG- and respiratory gating with a superconducting magnet of 0.5 tesla.

Table 44–5. ACCURACY OF THE ANATOMICALLY COMPLETE DOCUMENTATION

N = 50	Axial 50	Coronal 50	Sagittal 32
Superior vena cava	–	+	–
Right atrium	+	+	+
Right ventricle	+	+	+
Ascending pulmonary artery	+	+	+
Horizontal pulmonary artery	+	+	–
Left atrium	+	+(RAO)	+
Left ventricle	+	+(RAO)	–
Ascending aorta	–	+	+
Descending aorta	–	+	+
Frontal wall	+	–	+
Side walls	+	+	–

enhanced MRI of patients with ischemic myocardial disease were obtained in Berlin and Munich.

In the mediastinal area, aortic dissections and dissecting aneurysms of the thoracic aorta can be shown axially and sagittally; the diagnosis can be ascertained by analyzing the flow phenomenon. In coronal MR tomograms, malignant lymphomas and metastases of bronchial carcinomas within the mediastinum can be discriminated from vascular structures without employing additional contrast medium. In this instance we get reliable and similar information compared with computed tomography. Endobronchial tumors can be better detected by CT. Tumor involvement in the heart and vessels is better demonstrated by MRI. The efficiency of MRI in intrapulmonary diseases cannot yet be evaluated.

The extent and localization of intracardiac thrombi and tumors can safely be depicted. Thrombi in the superior vena cava and the left atrium and ventricle have been portrayed. Hypertrophic obstructive cardiomyopathies (HOCM) can clearly be shown in order to obtain a preoperative diagnosis. Papillary muscles, tendinous fibers, and tricuspid and bicuspid aortic valves are readily distinguished in axial MR tomograms. In addition to the axial projections, coronal MR tomograms were of particular advantage. Besides X-Y-Z tomograms, paraxial sections and sections in the RAO projection are possible. The volume measurement in the left ventricle and the measurement of the myocardial thickness offer further important information.

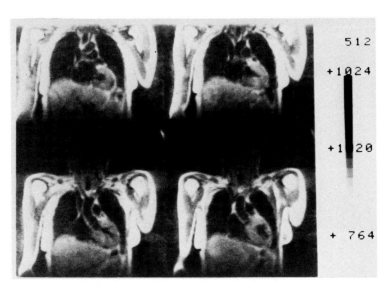

Figure 44–4. Angiographically and surgically proven asymmetric obstructive myopathy (HOCM). Four simultaneous ECG-gated MR images with 0.35 tesla imager. Slice thickness 10 mm; images 200 ms and 1 cm apart.

DIFFERENTIATION OF TISSUE

Studies of the differentiation of tissue in normal and pathologic structures have been made in the brain and in various organs by several working groups. The investigations performed at the GCD[13,14,62,66] and the University of Freiburg[30-34] are of particular interest because the constant of the *T2* relaxation time of the Carr-Purcell-Maibom-Spill spin-echo sequences has been determined. All in vivo measurements performed so far indicate, however, that the optimal method for in vivo measurements of the relaxation times has not yet been found. All measurements confirm the results of Damadian that malignant growth clearly shows a longer relaxation time than normal structures. There is, though, overlap in some diseases so that a clinical use is not yet possible. A summary of the investigative results on this topic has been published by Lissner et al.[59] and Zeitler et al.[119]

CONTRAST MEDIA IN MR IMAGING

The tolerance by humans, the excretory reaction, and the clinical efficiency of gadolinium-DTPA (Schering AG, Berlin) were systematically studied by Felix et al. in Berlin[23,24,27,56,57,93-95,97,99] In vivo examinations of subjects showed good tolerance of gadolinium-DTPA and an efficient signal influence on normal organs. Furthermore, its advantages in the diagnosis of brain tumors and in the differential diagnosis of brain tumor and brain edema as well as in some changes of disturbed blood-brain barrier have been proved. Investigations so far indicate that the concentration reaction of gadolinium-DTPA in brain tumors corresponds to that shown by iodized contrast media. These studies have to be verified by a larger collective study, with the possibility of further differentiation.

ABDOMEN AND PELVIC ORGANS

Several studies of the pelvic area have been presented that demonstrate the particularly good topographic information of various kinds of tumors in the bladder, uterus,

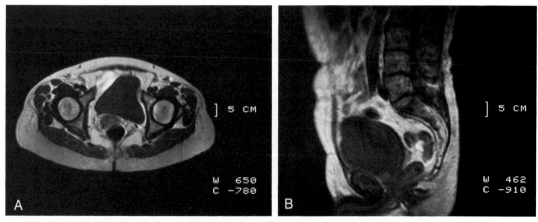

Figure 44–5. Normal anatomy, male pelvis. Axial (*A*) and midsagittal (*B*) scans of the pelvis with 1.5 tesla superconducting magnet in spin-echo mode demonstrating urinary bladder, rectum, fatty tissues, tumor on the posterior wall of the urinary bladder, bone structures of the femoral head, and inguinal vessels. On the borderline of the urinary bladder, artifacts of chemical shifting can be seen.

and ovaries (Fig. 44–5). In this respect, the reliable documentation of the boundaries of gynecologic tumors against bladder and rectum is of special value. Though various investigations in male patients with an enlarged prostate have been performed, a safe discrimination between benign and malignant changes of the prostate has not been achieved and reliable prospective studies have not yet been done.

MR investigations assessing the incompatibility of renal transplants undoubtedly produce more information than nuclear medicine examinations and ultrasound.[48]

Comparative studies performed with computed tomography, ultrasound, and MR imaging in the area of the liver show that MR imaging provides additional information on focal liver diseases. In the zone of the liver and the pancreas, the spatial resolution seems to be improved when respiratory gating is used, especially in the determination of relaxation times. To date, positive reports, including additional information compared with CT and sonography, indicate that the primary use of MRI has not yet been established. For the planning of surgery the reliable demonstration of aortic aneurysms in coronal and sagittal MR tomograms is feasible (Fig. 44–6).

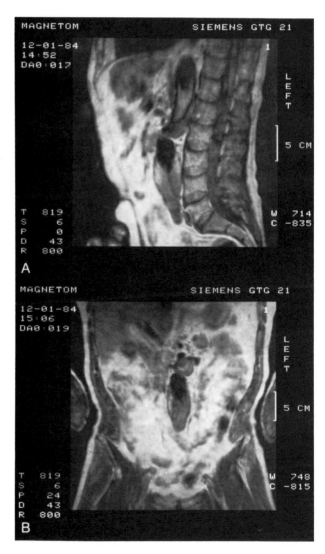

Figure 44–6. Abdominal aortic aneurysm. Sagittal (*A*) and coronal (*B*) scans in spin-echo technique with 0.35 tesla superconducting magnet in spin-echo mode without gating. Clear demonstration of the outline of an infrarenal abdominal aortic aneurysm with different components of flow imaging.

Table 44–6. LIMITS RECOMMENDED FOR STATIC AND TEMPORALLY CHANGING MAGNETIC FIELDS AS WELL AS HIGH-FREQUENCY FIELDS IN THE USE OF MAGNETIC RESONANCE TOMOGRAPHY AND IN VIVO MR SPECTROSCOPY

	NRPB (1981)*	BRH (1982)†	BGA (1983)‡	Controls Recommended to be Performed at Exceeding Values
Static magnetic field	2.5 T	2 T (whole-body and partial-body coils)	2 T (whole-body and partial-body coils)	Coronary circulation system, especially in disorders of production and management of excitation control with respect to subjective complaints
Temporally changing magnetic fields	20 T/s for circuit times of 10 ms and more	3 T/s (whole-body and partial-body coils)	Maximum current of the body 3 μA/cm^2 or field strength of 3 mV/cm for circuit times of 10 ms and more $\frac{30}{\tau}$ μA/cm^2 or $\frac{30}{\tau}$ V/cm for shorter circuit times than 10 ms (τ in ms)	Coronary circulation system, especially in disorders of stimulus production and conduction as well as epilepsy control with respect to subjective complaints
High-frequency field	Rise in temperature of 1° C	SAR = 0.4 W/kg (whole body) SAR = 2 W/kg (for each gm tissue)	SAR = 1 W/kg (whole body) SAR = 5 W/kg (partial body for each kg of tissue, including eye)	Coronary circulation system thermoregulation

* National Radiological Protection Board (UK)
† Bureau of Radiological Health (USA)
‡ Federal Department of Health Bundesgesundheitsamt (FRG)

MUSCULOSKELETAL SYSTEM

Several studies of the skeleton and soft parts show that osteonecrosis in the thigh is discernible earlier in patients undergoing therapy with cortisone when MRI is used than when x-rays or computed tomography are used. A differential diagnosis between inflammatory and tumorous diseases in the skeleton should be possible. The limitation of osteogenic and soft-part sarcomas against adjacent fasciae, vessels, and bony structures is of preoperative help. The number of accurate investigations is, however, limited.

SAFETY OF PATIENTS

The safety measures of magnetic resonance tomography have been issued by the German Ministry of Health[22] and are compared with the recommendations of the United States and Great Britain (Table 44–6).

The analysis of studies on more than 3000 patients made with various unit types shows no lesions when investigation is done with resistive and superconductive magnets. Claustrophobia that caused interruption was seen in 3 percent. It depends partly on the length of examination time. In a prospective study of 237 patients undergoing investigation of 348 organs, 18 cases of claustrophobia (7.6 percent) were encountered. Further side effects are summarized in Table 44–7. Complications in patients with pacemakers, shell splinters, metal clips, or other objects have not been reported.

In summary, because of the studies made so far in the Federal Republic of Germany and the results stated in the international literature, from January 1, 1985, MR examinations can be charged to the German Health Insurances for the following indications: brain tumors, diseases of the posterior cranial fossa, temporal lobe epilepsy, multiple sclerosis, tumors of the spinal cord, and syringomyelia. Further indications for more precise therapeutic planning, especially in cases involving the heart, mediastinum, and the pelvic organs, are still being decided.

Even taking a critical view of the potential, the prospective studies in German clinics, the use in private practice, and the cooperation between these two suggest clearly that there are indications for the application of MR imaging. Further indications can be gained by the imaging examinations used so far. Though first experiences with superficial coils and topical definition of the relaxation time have been examined with different technical facilities, and experimental P-31 spectroscopy as well as N-23 imaging is used, the results so far create no basis for a systematic clinical application. Today, MRI is, also in Germany, the most important technique besides CT for clinical use.

Table 44–7. PROSPECTIVE STUDY OF SIDE EFFECTS (N = 237 patients)

Number of Patients	Side Effect	Percent
7	Complaints about noise	3
6	Sensation of high temperature	2.5
2	Nausea	0.8
2	Measuring performance too long	0.8
2	Difficulty in swallowing	0.8
1	Sensation of coldness	0.4
1	Dyspnea	0.4
1	Headache	0.4
1	Watering eyes	0.4

References

1. Aichner F, Gerstenbrand F, Huk W, Pallua A: NMR-Tomographie in der Diagnostik der Syringohy-dromyelie. Nervenarzt 55:324, 1984.
2. Anacker H, Rupp N, Reiser M: Magnetic resonance (MR) in the diagnosis of pancreatic disease. Eur J Radiol 4:265, 1984.
3. Aue WP: Topische Kernspin-Resonanz—eine nicht-invasive Sonde für biochemische Messungen in Lebewesen. Radiologe 23:357, 1983.
4. Bauer R, Lauer O, Mörike K, Bauer U: NMR-tomographie des Kopfes—NMR Tomography of the Head. Stuttgart, Gustav Fischer Verlag, 1984.
5. Bauer M, Obermüller H, Vogl T, Lissner J: MR bei zerebraler alveolärer Echinokokkose. Digitale Bilddiagn 4:129, 1984.
6. Becker H, Schwarzrock R, Friedrich H: NMR-Untersuchungen von Hirninfarkten vor und nach extra-intrakraniellen Gefäbanastomosen. Adv Neurosurg. In press.
7. Becker H, Vogelsang H, Schwarzrock R: Vergleichende MR- und CT-Untersuchungen bei ausgewählten neuroradiologischen Fragestellungen. Fortschr Rontgenstr 142:23,1985.
8. Beer M, Rath M, Baierl P, Seiderer M: Klinische Bedeutung der Kernspin-Tomographie in der Urologie. Fortsch Med 102:891, 1984.
9. Beer M, Rath M, Baierl P, Wieland W, Seiderer M: NMR-Tomographie in der Urologie, erste klinische Ergebnisse-Verh Dtsch Ges Urol. In press.
10. Beer M, Rath M, Staehler G, Seiderer M, Bairerl P, Heywang S: NMR-Tomographie bei renalen Raum-forderungen—erste klinische Ergebnisse. Aktuel Urol. Submitted for publication.
11. Beer M, Rath M, Schüller B, Baierl P, Seiderer M: NMR-Tomographie in der Urologie. Helv Chir Acta. In press.
12. Berufsverband der Deutschen Radiologen u. Nuklearmediziner e.V., Interessengemeinschaft Computer-Tomographie e.V. (eds): Kernspintomographie—Standort—Untersuchungszeit—Jahresbetriebskosten 0.5 T Anlage supraleitender Magnet.
13. Bielke G: Pulssequenzvariationen bei der NMR-Tomographie zur optimalen Diskriminierung patholo-gischer Prozesse. In Schütz J (ed): Medizinische Physik. 1983, pp 109–114.
14. Bielke G, Meves M, Meindl S, Brückner A, von Seelen W, Rinck P, Pfannenstiel P: A systematic approach to the optimization of pulse sequences in NMR-imaging by computer simulations. In Esser PD (ed): Technology of Nuclear Magnetic Resonance. New York, Society of Nuclear Medicine, 1984.
15. Blümm RG, Spittler JF, Gehlen W, Brouwer A: NMR case study. Medicamundi 28:3, 1983.
16. Blümm RG, Brouwer A: Fallbeispiele zur neuroradiologischen Anwendung der NMR-Tomographie. Röntgenstrahlen 50:1, 1983.
17. Blümm RG, Balériaux D, Lausberg G, Brotchi J: Initial experience with MR-imaging of intracranial midline-lesions and lesions of the cervical spine at half tesla. Neurosurgery. In press.
18. Blümm RG: A case of early Legg-Perthes disease (avascular necrosis of the femoral head) demonstrated by magnetic resonance imaging. Skeletal Radiol. In press.
19. Blümm RG, Akuamoaboateng E: Technischer Stand und derzeitige Bedeutung der Kernspin-tomogra-phie bei der Diagnostik von Erkrankungen im maxillofacialen Bereich. Dtsch Z Kieferchir. In press.
20. Bomsdorf H, Buikman D, Helzel T, Kuhn MH, Kunz D, Lüdeke KM, Meyer W, Röschmann P, Tischler R, Vollmann W, Weiss H: First NMR proton images of the human head at 2 Tesla. Medicamundi 29(1):6, 1984.
21. Brederhoff J, Pfannenstiel P, Bielke G, Bieler EU, Rinck P: NMR-imaging of the human thyroid gland in comparison with radionuclide scanning and ultrasonography. In Höfer R, Bergmann H (eds.): Ra-dioaktive Isotope in Klinik und Forschung. H. Egermann Verlag, 1984, pp 321–328.
22. Empfehlungen zur Vermeidung gesundheitlicher Risiken verursacht durch magnetische und hochfre-quente eilektromagnetische Felder bei der NMR-Tomographie und In-vivo-NMR-Spektroskopie. Bun-desgesundheitsblatt 27(3):92, 1984.
23. Claussen C, Laniado M, Schörner W, Niendorf HP, Weinmann HJ, Fiegler W, Felix R: The use of gadolinium-DPTA in magnetic resonance imaging of glioblastomas and intracranial metastases. AJNR 6:669, 1985.
24. Claussen C, Laniado M, Kazner E, Schörner W, Felix R: Application of contrast agents in CT and NMR: Their potential in imaging of brain tumours. Neuroradiology 27:164, 1985.
25. von Einsiedel G, Gräfin H, Löffler W: Nuclear magnetic resonance of brain tumours unrevealed by CT. Eur J Radiol 2:226, 1982.
26. Felix R, Köhler D, Schörner W, Fiegler W: Diagnostik der Wirbelsäule mit der Magnet-Resonanz-Tomographie (MRT). Symposiumsband "Spinale Computertomograhie." In press.
27. Felix R, Laniado M, Schörner W: Bericht über die klinische Prüfung des kernspintomographischen Kontrastmittels SH L 451 an Probanden (Phase 1). In Bundesministerium für Forschung und Technologie (ed): Bonn, Kernspintomographie, 1984, pp 211–229.
28. Fiegler W, Schörner W, Felix R: Leistungsfähigkeit der Sonographie, Computertomographie, hepa-tobiliären Szintigraphie under Kernspintomographie bei Erkrankungen der Gallenblase und Gallenwege. Rontgen Bull. In press.
29. Fiegler W, Felix R, Nagel R, Schörner W, Claussen C: Die Kernspintomographie bei raumfordernden Nierenprozessen. Fortschr Rontgenstr 141:155, 1984.
30. Friedburg H, Bockenheimer ST: Klinische NMR-Tomographie mit sequentiellen T2-Bildern (Carr-Pur-cell-Spin-Echosequenzen). Radiologe 23:353, 1983.

31. Friedburg H, Ratzel D, Ströbel B, Bockenheimer ST: Dünnschicht-NMR-Imaging mit einem neuen T2-gewichteten 3-D-Verfahren. Fortsch Rontgenstr *140*(4):464, 1984.
32. Friedburg H, Post H, Crone M, Neumaier M: Messung und klinische Bedeutung der Spin-Spin-Relaxations-zeit in der NMR-Tomographie. Der Nuklearmediziner *3*(7):187, 1984.
33. Friedberg H, Wannenmacher M, Hinkelbein W: Verlaufskontrolle bei intrazerebraler Metastasierung mit NMR-Tomographie. *In* Nagel GA, Sauer R, Schreiber HW (eds): Aktuelle Onkologie 13—Hirnmetastasen, Pathophysiologie, Diagnostik, und Therapie. Munich, W Zuckschwerdt Verlag, 1983, pp 218–222.
34. Friedburg H, Wenz W, Fiebig H: Tierexperimentelle und klinissche Erfahrung mit NMR-Tomographie. Rontgenpraxis *37*:139, 1984.
35. Gademann G: NMR Tomography of a Normal Brain. Berlin, Springer Verlag, 1984.
36. Ganssen A, Löffler W, Oppelt A, Schmidt F: Kernspintomographie. Computertomographie *1*:10, 1981.
37. Habermehl A, Graul EH: Kernspinresonanz-Tomographie. Dtsch Arzteblatt *79*:17, 1982.
38. Hagemann H, Jordon K, Müller G, Tiffe HW, Schwarzrock R, Hundeshagen H: Trigger pulse generation for respiration synchronised NMR imaging (abstract). Eur J Nucl Med *9*(7): A513, 1984.
39. Heindel W, Huk W: Tissue differentiation in the area of the central nervous system with nuclear magnetic resonance tomography: first clinical experiences. Electromedica *51*:2, 1983.
40. Heinzerling J, Kuhn MH, Kunz D, Meyer W, Röschmann P, Vollmann W: Optimierung von Mebzeit und Bildqualität in der Kernspintomographie. BMFT-Broschüre "Kernspintomographie," 2. Bericht, May 1984.
41. Heller H, Petsch R, Auberger Th, Decker K, Engelmann M: Bildgebende magnetische Resonanz mit Oberflächenspulen. Jahrestag Dtsch Gesell Neuroradiol *20*:95, 1984.
42. Heller H, Petsch R, Auberger Th, Decker K: Kernspintomographie der Wirbelsäule. Fortschr Rontgenstr *142*:419, 1985.
43. Huk WJ, Gademann G: Magnetic Resonance Imaging (MRI): Method and early clinical experiences in diseases of the central nervous system. Neurosurg Rev *7*:259, 1984.
44. Huk WJ, Fahlbusch R: Nuclear magnetic resonance imaging of the region of the sella turcica. Neurosurg Rev. *8*:141, 1985.
45. Huk W, Heindl W, Deimling W, Stetter E: Nuclear magnetic resonance (NMR) tomography of the central nervous system: comparison of two imaging sequences. J Comput Assist Tomogr *7*:468, 1983.
46. Huk WJ, Löffler W: NMR Clinical Results; Erlangen. *In* Partain CL, James AE, Rollo FD, Price RR: (eds): Nuclear Magnetic Resonance (NMR) Imaging. Philadelphia, WB Saunders, 1983, pp 276–294.
47. Huk W, Heindel W: Nuclear magnetic resonance (NMR) imaging in diseases of the central nervous system: Initial results. Radiat Med *1*(2):105, 1983.
48. Hundeshagen H, Schwarzrock R, Tiffe HW: NMR-Tomographie. Klinische Studie. 2. Berichtsband "Kernspintomographie." BMFT, 1984.
49. Hundeshagen H: The present state and future of NMR-tomography. Eur J Nucl Med. In press.
50. Kaiser W, Zeitler E: Digital-Subtrahierte Magnetische Resonanz (DSMR)—Ein neues Verfahren zur Darstellung von Gefäbprozessen. Fortschr Rontgenstr *147*(5):42, 1984.
51. Kaiser W, Zeitler E: Kernspintomographie der Mamma—erste klinische Ergebnisse. 2. Kölner Symposium, 1984. Submitted for publication.
52. Köhler D, Claussen C, Schörner, W, Fiegler W, Felix R: Kontrastbeeinflussung von Hirntumoren durch Gadolinium-DPTA in der Magnetischen Resonanx-Tomographie (MRT). Electromedica. In press.
53. Kotzerke J: Die Bedeutung der Kernspintomographie für die Diagnostik raumfordernder Prozesse der Leber. Dissertation an der Medizin, Hochschule Hannover, 1985.
54. Kuhn MH: Optimierung von Meßzeit und Bildqualität in der Kernspintomographie. Projekt-Status-Bericht 1984/85 Forschung und Entwicklung im Dienste der Gesundheit.
55. Kunz D: Use of frequency modulated RF pulses in NMR imaging experiments. J Magn Reson *3*:377, 1986.
56. Laniado M, Claussen C, Schörner W, Felix R: Magnetische Resonanz Tomographie am Klinikum Charlottenburg, Berlin: Erste Ergebnisse in der Diagnostik intracranieller Tumoren mit dem Kontrastmittel Gadolinium-DPTA. Diagnostik. In press.
57. Laniado M, Weinmann HJ, Schörner W, Felix R, Speck U: First use of gadolinium-DTPA/dimeglumine in man. Physiol Chem Phys Med NMR *16*:157, 1984.
58. Lissner J: Fortschritte in der Diagnostik und ihre Bedeutung für die radiologische Praxis. Digitale Bilddiagn *4*(4):158, 1984.
59. Lissner J, Seiderer M: Klinische Kerns pintomographie, Enke-Verlag, 1987.
60. Loeffler W, Oppelt A: Physical principles of NMR tomography. Eur J Radiol *1*:338, 1981.
61. Mees K, Vogl T, Bauer M: Kernspintomographie in der HNO-Heilkunde. Z HNO-Heilkunde. In press.
62. Meves M, Bielke G, Meindl S, Pfannenstiel P, Rinck PA, Bieler EU: Klinische Erprobung und Abklärung der diagnostischen Wertigkeit der Kernspintomographie—Erfahrungen des ersten Jahres. *In* Pfannenstiel P, Meves M: (eds): Die NMR-Tomographie Klinischer Einsatz und Wirtschaftlichkeit. Stuttgart, Georg Thieme Verlag, 1984, p 20.
63. Niendorf HP, Semmler W, Schörner W: Aspekte der Anwendung bildkontrastverstärkender Substanzen in der Kernspintomographie. Der Nuklearmediziner *3*(7): 235, 1984.
64. Petsch R, Heller H, Reiser M, Decker K: Artdiagnostik mit Hilfe von Relaxationszeiten aus bildgebender magnetischer Resonanz. *In* Schmidt TH (ed): Medizinische Physik. In press.
65. Petsch R: Auswertung und Archivierung der Resonanz-Tomogramme. *In* Schopka HJ (ed): Kernspintomographie. Stuttgart, Georg Thieme Verlag, 1983, pp 181–200.

66. Pfannenstiel P, Meves M: Die NMR-Tomographie—Klinischer Einsatz und Wirtschaftlichkeit. Stuttgart, Georg Thieme Verlag, 1984.
67. Rath M, Beer M, Baierl P, Seiderer M: NMR bei Tumoren im Urogenitalbereich. Zentralbl Radiol *128*:118, 1984.
68. Reiser M, Rupp N, Stettner E: Erfahrungen bei der NMR-Tomographie des Skelettsystems. Fortschr Rontgenstr *139*(4):365, 1983.
69. Reiser M, Rupp N, Heller HJ, Allgayer B, Lukas B, Petsch R: Die Darstellung der normalen anatomischen Strukturen des Körpers durch die magnetische Resonanz (MR)-Tomographie. Der Nuklearmediziner *3*(7):165, 1984.
70. Reiser M, Rupp N, Heller HJ, Allgayer B, Lukas P, Lange J, Pfafferott K, Fink U: MR-tomography in the diagnosis of malignant soft-tissue tumours. Eur J Radiol *4*(4):288, 1984.
71. Reiser M, Rupp N, Petsch R, Heller HJ, Lukas P, Allgayer B: Die normalen anatomischen Strukturen des Körpers im MR-Tomogramm: Untersuchungen mit einem 0, 35 T supraleitenden Magneten. Teil 1: Allgemeine Abbildungscharakteristika, Hals, Herz und Mediastinum. Rontgenpraxis *37*:440, 1984.
72. Reiser M, Rupp N, Lukas P, Heller HJ, Allgayer B, Petsch R: Die normalen anatomischen Srukturen des Körpers im MR-Tomogramm: Untersuchungen mit einem 0, 35 T supraleitenden Magneten. Teil 2: Abdomen, Becken, Haltungs- und Bewegungsapparat. Rontgenpraxis *38*:11, 1985.
73. Reuther G, Huk W, Deimling M: Phaenomenologie der kernspintomographischen Blutgefässdarstellung: Möglichkeiten, Grenzen, Perspektiven. Electromedica. Submitted for publication.
74. Rinck PA, Bieler EU, Meves M, Skalej, Schütz HJ, Hornig, CR, Pfannenstiel P: CPMG-spin-echo-sequence in multiple sclerosis. Evaluation of demyelinating diseases by CPMG-spin-echo-sequence. Radiology. In press.
75. Rinck PA: Risiken und Gefahren der NMR-Tomographie. Dtsch Med Wochensch *108*:992, 1983.
76. Rödl W, Lutz H, Oppelt A: Nuclear magnetic resonance imaging in abdominal and pelvic disease—initial clinical experience in comparison with computed tomography and ultrasonography. Hepatogastroenterology *30*:37, 1983.
77. Rödl W, Nebel G: Die Kernspintomographie des Abdomens. *In*: Demling L (ed): Klinische Gastroenterologie, Vol. 1. Stuttgart, Georg Thieme Verlag, 1984.
78. Rödl W: Differential diagnosis of liver diseases with the aid of nuclear magnetic resonance imaging. *In* Diagnostic Imaging Methods in Hepatology, Falk Symposium 37. Lancaster, Massachusetts, MTP Press, 1984.
79. Rödl W: Die Kernspintomographie zur Untersuchung der Leber und ihrer Erkrankungen. Gastroenterology *23*:31, 1985.
80. Rödl W: Möglichkeiten der Gewebszuordnung im Kernspintomogramm—Formulierung der Befunde maligne, benigne, Artdiagnose, Tumor und Tumorverdacht. *In*: Workshop der Deutschen Gesellschaft für Endoskopie: Methoden der Bewertung neuer bildgebender Verfahren in der Onkologie. In press.
81. Rödl W: Differentialdiagnose von Lebererkrankungen im Kernspintomogramm. Fortschr Rontgenstr *142*:505, 1985.
82. Rödl W: Die Ganzkörper-Kernspintomographie—klinische Erfahrungen im methodischen Vergleich, Untersuchungen zu experimentellen Leberparenchymschäden. Habilitationsschrift 1984.
83. Rödl W, Nebel G, Engelhard K: Hämosuccus pancreatis—bildgebende Verfahren im Vergleich. Fortschr Rontgenstr *140*(5):531, 1984.
84. Roth K: NMR Tomographie und Spektroskopie in der Medizin. Heidelberg, Springer Verlag, 1984.
85. Roth K, Gronenborn AM: NMR-Tomographie. Chemie in unserer Zeit 2, 1982, pp 35–45.
86. Runge VM, Stewart RG, Claton JA, Jones MM, Lukehart, Ch M, Partain CL, James AE: Work in progress: potential oral and intravenous paramagnetic NMR contrast agents. Radiology *147*:789, 1983.
87. Runge V, Claussen C, Felix R, James AE (eds): Contrast agents in magnetic resonance imaging. Proceedings of an International Workshop, San Diego, January 1986. Excerpta Medica, USA, 1986.
88. Runge VM, Clanton JA, Price AC, Schörner W, Felix R, Partain CL, James AE: How contrast agents can help MRI. Diagn Imag 57, 1984.
89. Rupp N, Reiser M, Stetter E: Klinische Erfahrungen mit der NMR-Tomographie. Inn Med *10*:311, 1983.
90. Rupp H, Reiser M, Stetter E: Die klinisch-radiologische Bedeutung der verschiedenen Untersuchungsparameter in der NMR-Tomographie des Abdomens. Fortschr Rontgenstr. *139*(4):359, 1983.
91. Rupp N, Reiser M, Stetter E: The diagnostic value of morphology and relaxation times in NMR-imaging of the body. Eur J Radiol *3*:68, 1983.
92. Rupp N, Reiser M, Stetter E: NMR-Tomographie in der gastroenterologischen Diagnostik. *In* Blum AL, Ottenjann R, Siewert JR: (eds): Aktuelle Gastroenterologische Diagnostik. In press.
93. Schörner W, Felix R, Claussen C, Fiegler W, Kazner E, Niendorf HP: Kernspintomographische Diagnostik von Hirntumoren mit dem Kontrastmittel Gadolinium-DPTA. Fortschr Rontgenstr *141*:511, 1984.
94. Schörner W, Semmler W, Felix R, Laniado M, Speck U, Niendorf HP: Zur Wahl der Aufnahmesequenz in der Kontrastmittel-Kernspintomographie: Kontrastverhalten von Hirntumoren nach Gadolinium-DPTA—Anwendung bei unterschiedlichen Spin-Echo-Verfahren. Rontgenpraxis *37*:323, 1984.
95. Schörner W, Felix R, Laniado M, Lange L, Weinmann HJ, Claussen C, Fiegler W, Speck, U, Kazner E: Prüfung des kernspintomographischen Kontrastmittels Gadolinium-DPTA am Menschen: Verträglichkeit, Kontrastbeeinflussung und erste klinische Ergebnisse. Fortschr Rontgenstr *140*(5):493, 1984.
96. Schörner W, Felix R, Meencke HJ: Magnetische Resonanz Tomographie (MRT) bei Temporallappenläsionen: Eine Untersuchung von Patienten mit psychomotorischen Anfällen. Fortschr Rontgenstr *142*:282, 1985.
97. Schörner W, Kazner E, Laniado M, Sprung Chr, Felix R: Magnetic resonance tomography (MRT) of

intracranial tumours: Initial experience with the use of the contrast medium gadolinium-DPTA. Neurosurg Rev *7*:303, 1984.
98. Schörner W, Felix R, Semmler W: Kernspintomographische Diagnostik in der Gastroenterologie, eine Übersicht. Verdauungskrankheiten. In press.
99. Schörner W, Laniado M, Felix R: Erster klinischer Einsatz von Gadolinium-DPTA in der kernspintomographischen Darstellung einer parapelvinen Nierencyste. Fortschr Rontgenstr *141*:227, 1984.
100. Schuierer G, Kaiser W, Zeitler E, Raithel W, Oppelt A, von Wulfen M, Löffler W: MR-Imaging of aortic aneurysm. Ann Radiol. In press.
101. Seiderer M, Rath M, Lissner J: Untersuchungsmethode mit Zukunft: Kernspin-Tomographie. Med Klin *79*:134, 1984.
102. Seiderer M, Lissner J: Kernspin-Tomographie—ein neues diagnostisches Verfahren. Munch Med Wochenschr *126*:889, 1984.
103. Seiderer M, Rath M, Baierl P: Gefassdarstellung und Blutflussmessung in der Kernspintomographie. Proceedings des "3. Deutsch-Japan. Kongresses fur Angiologie." Submitted for publication.
104. Semmler W, Felix R: Kontraste in der Kernspintomographie. Fortschr Rontgenstr *141*(3):259, 1984.
105. Semmler W, Felix R: Der Einfluss von Kontrastmitteln auf die Grauabstufung in der Magnetischen-Resonanz-Tomographie. Fortschr Rontgenstr *142*:123, 1985.
106. Spittler JP, Blümm RG, Fritze J, Gehlen W: CT-, NMR-und neurophysiol. Befunde bei Hirnstammaffektionen. DMW. In press.
107. Steiner GF, Felix R: Wenn ein Computer mit Magnetfeldern jongliert. Physikalisch-technische Grundprinzipien der Kernspintomographie. Moku Arztl Fortb *34*(14):26, 1984.
108. Steinbrich W, Friedmann G, Beyer D, Brouwer A: Erste Erfahrungen mit der Magnetischen-Resonanz-Tomographie (MR) bei tumorösen Erkrankungen des Mediastinums und der Lungenhili. Fortschr Rontgenstr *141*:629, 1984.
109. Steinbrich W, Friedmann G, Brouwer A: NMR-Tomographie mit supraleitendem Gerät bei tumorösen Erkrankungen des Mediastinums und der Lungenhili. Rontgenstrahlen *51*:38, 1984.
110. Steinbrich W, Friedmann G, Beyer D, Brouwer A: Work in progress: MR imaging in the evaluation of neoplastic disease of the mediastinum and the pulmonary hili. Medicamundi. In press.
111. Steinbrich W, Friedmann G: Möglichkeiten dees Einsatzes der Magnetischen-Resonanz-Tomographie (MR) in der pädiatrischen Diagnostik. Ann Nestle. In press.
112. Stetter E, Oppelt A: Image quality in NMR. Proceedings of the World Congress on MP & BE *24*:10, 1982.
113. Strecker EP: Magnetische Kernresonanz. Dtsch Med Wochenschr *108*:551, 1983.
114. Unz F: Kernspintomographie: Ergebnis- und Forschungsbericht. DFVLR, 1984.
115. Vogl T, Bauer M, Seiderer M, Rath M: Kernspintomographie bei Hallervorden-Spatz-Syndrom. Digitale Bilddiagn *4*:66, 1984.
116. Vogl T, Mees K, Bauer M, Rath M: Kernspintomographie bei zervikalen Lymphknotenschwellungen. Digitale Bilddiagn *4*:132, 1984.
117. Wende S, Thelen M: Kernspin-Tomographie in der Medizin Theorie—Praxis—klinische Ergebnisse. Berlin, Springer Verlag; 1983.
118. Zeitler E, Ganssen A: Erste klinische Erfahrungen mit der Kernspintomographie. Fortschr Rontgenstr *135*:517, 1981.
119. Zeitler E, Gailer H, Ganssen A, Niendorf HP, Rehm HJ, Schuierer G, Wojtowycz M: Kernspintomographie. Köln, Deutscher Ärzte Verlag, 1984.
120. Zeitler E, Schuierer G, Wojtowycz M, Reichenberger H, Wirth, A, Stetter E, von Wulfen H: EKG-getriggerte NMR-Tomographie des Herzens. Fortschr Rontgenstr *140*(5):487, 1984.
121. Zeitler E: Assessing the mediastinum with magnetic resonance. Diagn Imag *6*(5):82, 1984.
122. Zeitler E, Kaiser W, Rogalsky W: Perspektiven der Kernspintomographie. Hamburger Ärzteblatt 11 (1984) 455–460.
123. Zeitler E, Schuierer G: Diagnosis of cardiovascular diseases with NMR imaging. *In* Hopf M-A, Smith FW (eds): Magnetic Resonance in Medicine and Biology. Vol. 8. Progress in Nuclear Medicine. Basel, S Karger 1984, pp 100–111.
124. Zeitler E: Magnetic resonance imaging—advantages at heart and vascular disease. Ann Radiol. In press.
125. Zeitler E, Kaiser W, Schuierer G, Wojtowycz M, Kunigk K, Oppelt A, Stetter E, von Wulfen H: Nuclear magnetic resonance of aneurysms and thrombi. Cardiovasc Intervent Radiol *8*:321, 1986.
126. Zeitler E: Kernspintomographie: risikoarmes Untersuchungsverfahren mit glänzender Zukunft. MoKu arztl Fortb *34*(3):20, 1984.
127. Zeitler E: Ansätze der Kernspintomographie und NMR-Spektroskopie zum medizinisch-diagnostischen Routineverfahren. Dtsch Ärzteblatt. In press.
128. Zeitler E, Kaiser W, Schuierer G, Stetter E, Oppelt A, Rogalsky W: MR-imaging of clots in the heart and vascular system. Ann Radiol. *28*:105, 1985.
129. Zeitler E: Die Wertigkeit der Kernspintomographie im Bereich des Körperstammes. 15. Tübinger Klinisch-Radiology. Seminar, 1984. In press.
130. Zeitler E: NMR-Anwendungsmöglichkeiten heute und zukünftige Aspekte in der Medizin. Biomedizinische Technik, Additional Vol 29, 1984.
131. Zeitler E, Schuierer G: NMR Clinical Results: Nuremberg. *In* Partain CL, James AE, Rollo FD, Price RR (eds): Nuclear Magnetic Resonance (NMR) Imaging. Philadelphia, WB Saunders, 1983, pp 267–275.

45

Pitfalls and Artifacts in Clinical MRI

JAMES A. PATTON
MADAN KULKARNI

There are many potential pitfalls and causes of artifacts in MRI that may present problems in the interpretation of images from routine patient procedures. The sources of artifacts must be understood and eliminated, if possible, in order that correct interpretations may be obtained. For purposes of discussion, artifacts can be grouped into three categories: those internal to the patient, those external to the patient, and those that are due to system failures or that are inherent in the data-collection and image-reconstruction techniques that are used with MRI systems.

INTERNAL SOURCES

As with most imaging modalities, patient motion degrades magnetic resonance images. It is therefore extremely important that the patient not move while data collection is in progress, a time frame of typically 1 to 20 minutes. The effect of patient motion is an overall reduction in image quality, caused by errors generated in the frequency and phase encoding of spatial information, which results in reconstructed data being placed in the wrong pixels (Fig. 45–1). Respiratory and cardiac motion can also severely degrade image quality during an MRI study (Figs. 45–2A and 45–3A). The physiologic motion in the frequency-encoding or x direction results in a blurring between the limits of excursion. The motion in the phase-encoding or y direction results in ghost structures caused by the development of a coherence between the number of gradient steps being used in the imaging procedure and the frequency of the physiologic motion, which is also periodic in nature. It has been shown that the higher the frequency of motion or the longer the time between changes in the phase encoding, the farther apart the ghosts. On the other hand, the separation is reduced by decreasing either the length of the phase-encoding gradient or the amount by which the phase-encoding gradient is incremented,[1] a fact that may be used to minimze the effects of respiratory motion in chest and abdominal imaging.

The effects of cardiac or respiratory motion can be eliminated by using physiologic gates that permit data acquisition only during a selected portion of the respiratory or cardiac cycle. Cardiac gating can be accomplished by using the ECG signal to generate an R-wave trigger, which serves as an origin for a variable time delay that can be used to select the portion of the cardiac cycle to be imaged. Respiratory gating may be accomplished using an expansion bellows coupled to a variable potentiometer and attached to the chest to monitor the excursions produced by respiration and to select the appropriate portion of the respiratory cycle to institute data collection. These techniques for "stop-action" imaging eliminate the ghost artifacts and provide high-quality images (Figs. 45–2B and 45–3B). However, images obtained with physiologic gating

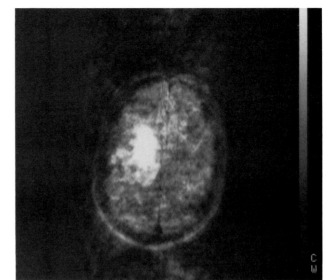

Figure 45–1. Transverse section through the brain demonstrating the effects of patient motion.

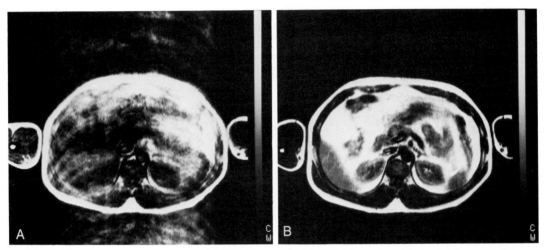

Figure 45–2. Transverse section image through the abdomen without (*A*) and with (*B*) respiratory gating.

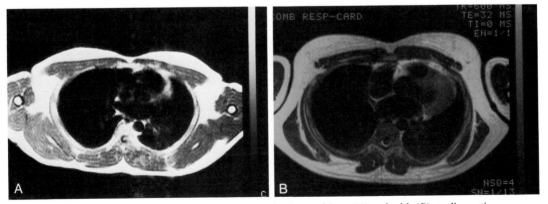

Figure 45–3. Transverse section image through the heart without (*A*) and with (*B*) cardiac gating.

require significantly longer acquisition times because data collection occurs only during a portion of the respiratory or cardiac cycle, and images of different portions of the physiologic cycles must be obtained with separate data acquisitions.

The presence of any ferromagnetic material in the imaging volume will result in a localized distortion of the image. The extent of the distortion is directly related to the amount of material present. This artifact results from the presence of the ferromagnetic material that distorts the uniformity of the magnetic field. Since spatial location in MRI

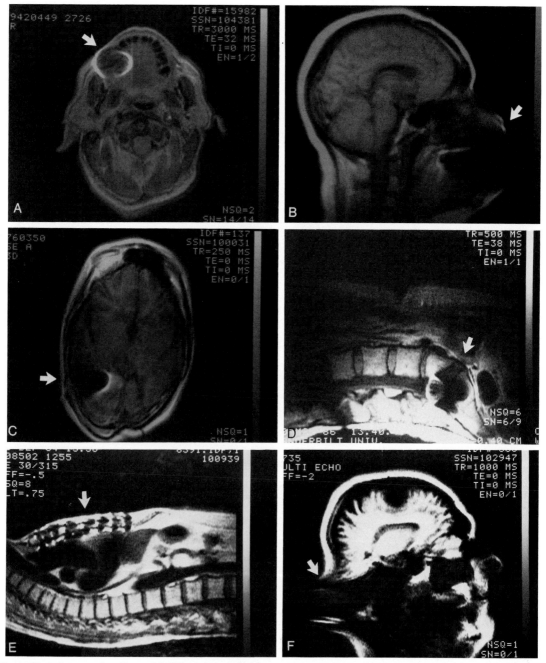

Figure 45–4. Images of patients with fillings (*A*), dental braces (*B*), ventriculoperitoneal shunts (*C*), surgical pins (*D*), surgical staples (*E*), and shrapnel (*F*), demonstrating the effects of internal ferromagnetic materials on MRI.

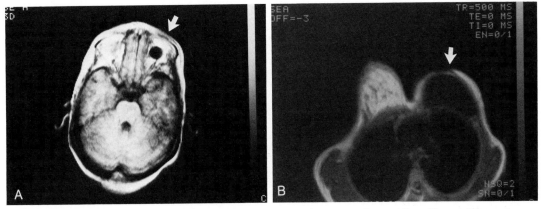

Figure 45–5. Images of patients with non–signal producing, nonferromagnetic eye (*A*) and breast (*B*) prostheses.

is determined by frequency and phase encoding, which are related to magnetic field strength, any distortion in the magnetic field will result in errors in the frequency and phase encoding of spatial information and thus produce spatial distortions in the images obtained. Possible sources of ferromagnetic materials within the body include dental work, such as fillings, braces, or bridges (Fig. 45–4*A–B*); ventriculoperitoneal shunts (Fig. 45–4*C*); and surgical clips (Fig. 45–4*D–E*). Occasionally, unusual sources of distortion, such as shrapnel (Fig. 45–4*F*), will be found.

The potential image degradation that may result from the presence of these objects, in addition to the potential harm that may result from their internal movement (such as an aneurysm clip), illustrates the importance of adequate screening of patients before the beginning of the imaging process. However, if the presence of the object is not threatening to the patient, quite often it is possible to proceed with the study. Images of diagnostic quality can be obtained if the region of interest is distal to the object, as is the case in Figure 45–4*F*. The same argument applies to surgical prostheses. However, it should be pointed out that not all prostheses are made of ferromagnetic material. The eye and breast prostheses shown in Figure 45–5, for example, do not alter the magnetic field, yield no NMR signal, and therefore do not affect image quality.

EXTERNAL SOURCES

Sources of artifacts that are external to the patient generally fall into the clothing category. All patients should be screened for jewelry, metal buttons, zippers, belt buckles, and other ferromagnetic material that may alter the uniformity of the magnetic field and distort the images obtained (Fig. 45–6*A*). For body imaging it is usually advisable to have the patient disrobe and put on a hospital gown or pajamas. Occasionally, an article such as a hairpin (Fig. 45–6*B*) will be overlooked. However, its presence is easily recognizable, and the technologist must locate and eliminate the source of the distortion before continuing the study. Another potential source of artifacts is makeup and hair oil. It has been demonstrated that some of these materials yield an NMR signal that may produce strange effects, such as the halo from the hair oil used by the patient shown in Fig. 45–7*A*. Removal of eye makeup is advisable when the orbits are being studied, in order to eliminate the presence of any external signal-producing material that may interfere with the imaging process (Fig. 45–7*B*).

Placement of ECG leads also is of importance in MRI (Fig. 45–8). Although nonferromagnetic leads are available, they should still be placed as far from the imaging

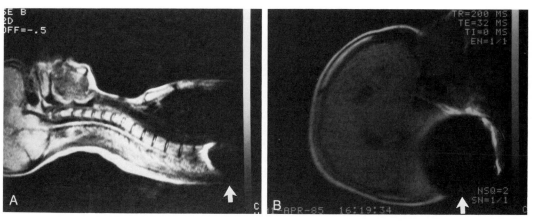

Figure 45–6. Image of a patient with a metal clothing clip (*A*) and a metal hairpin (*B*).

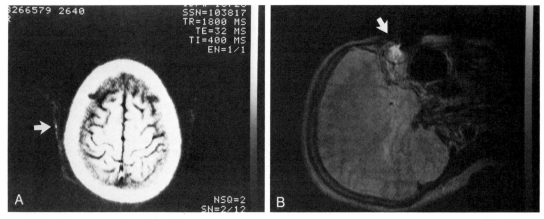

Figure 45–7. Images of patients with hair oil that yields an NMR signal (*A*) and eye makeup containing ferromagnetic material (*B*).

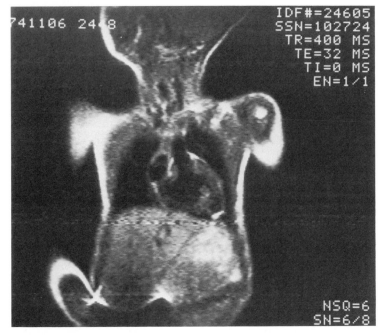

Figure 45–8. Image of a pediatric patient with ferromagnetic ECG leads in place.

volume as possible in order to eliminate the possibility of interference with the imaging process.

SYSTEM SOURCES

There are many potential sources of artifacts from malfunctions of the imaging system or simply from peculiarities of the data-acquisition and image-reconstruction process. Figure 45–9 illustrates an image wrap-around problem due to improper calibration of the phase-encoding gradients. Fig. 45–10 demonstrates two image-reconstruction problems associated with failures of the array processor. Fig. 45–11 documents a failure of the x or frequency-encoding gradient during data acquisition, resulting in all the data in the x direction being reconstructed into a narrow band.

Radio frequency (rf) interference is a potential source of problems, especially if the imaging system is not shielded from outside sources. Depending upon the frequency range of the interference, the result may be a line or band of interference that appears in the image in the y or phase-encoded direction at a specific frequency in the x or frequency-encoded direction (Fig. 45–12). If the frequency range of the interference is broad enough, the result of the interference will be an overall reduction in signal-to-noise ratio.

As described in Chapter 87, one of the most important routine quality-assurance checks is a measure of signal intensity, or signal-to-noise. The effect of reduced signal-to-noise on image quality (Fig. 45–13) is an apparent general increase in background (actually a reduction in signal intensity) and a reduction in image uniformity and resolution. When this problem appears, it is first necessary to check the tuning of the rf transmitter or the receiver and then possibly other components of the data-acquisition system, as there can be many causes of this problem.

The response of a transmitting or receiving coil is proportional to some extent to the volume of tissue within the coil owing to alterations in the capacitance and inductance of the coils. Some manufacturers have instituted either manual or automatic tuning circuitry to permit the coils to be tuned for each patient. Others provide different tuning parameters for small, medium, and large patients. The effect of improper match-

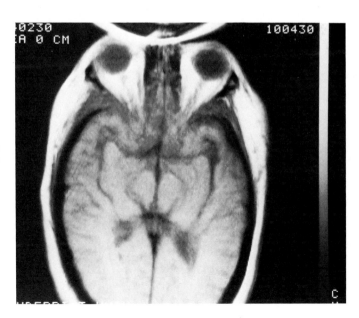

Figure 45–9. Reconstructed image with image wraparound due to improper calibration of the phase-encoding gradients.

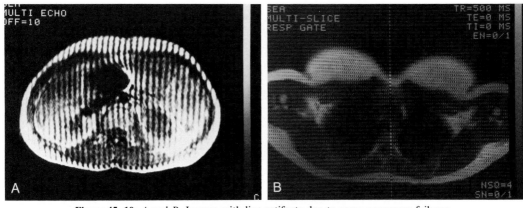

Figure 45–10. *A* and *B*, Images with line artifacts due to array processor failures.

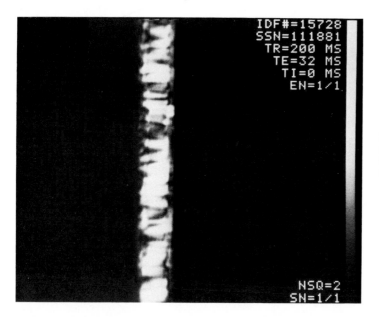

Figure 45–11. Transverse section image demonstrating a failure of the x gradient to frequency-encode data in the x direction during data acquisition.

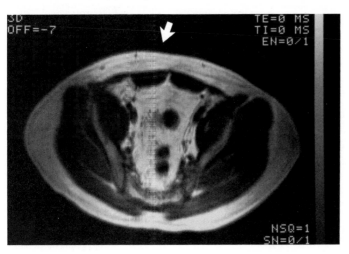

Figure 45–12. Image with radio frequency (rf) interference. See the "zipper appearance" at the arrow vertical.

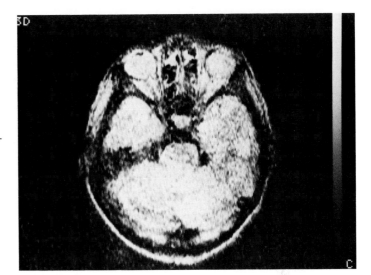

Figure 45–13. Image with reduced signal-to-noise ratio.

ing of tuning parameters to patient size is shown in Fig. 45–14 and results in an overall degradation in image quality and reduced signal-to-noise.

Early efforts at multislice, multiecho imaging provided another potential source of artifacts. This problem resulted from the need for rapidly switching gradients to collect all the data in a reasonable time. The rapidly changing magnetic field resulting from the switching of the gradients induced changes in current flow in the shim coils (Eddy currents), which altered the uniformity of the magnetic field. The net effect of this phenomenon was image nonuniformity, which became more pronounced in the longer echo images (Fig. 45–15). Considerable effort has been expended by manufacturers, and many of these problems have been eliminated by effectively isolating the gradient and shim coils.

A potential pitfall that may be encountered in MRI is the chemical-shift effect. This effect appears at sharp interfaces between fatty structures and those that are predominantly water. It is demonstrated as alternately light and dark rims around the kidney (Fig. 45–16A) at the interface of the perirenal fat and the renal parenchyma in the x

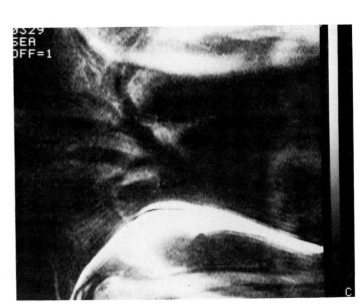

Figure 45–14. Image with improper matching of coil-tuning parameters to size of patient.

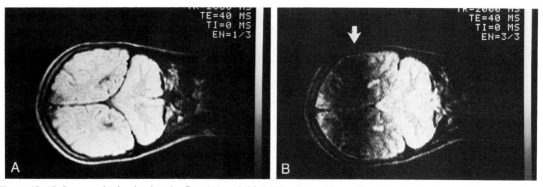

Figure 45–15. Images obtained using the first (*A*) and third (*B*) echoes. Nonuniformities in the latter echo are produced by interactions of the gradient and shim coils in a multislice/multiecho (40–120/2000) pulse sequence.

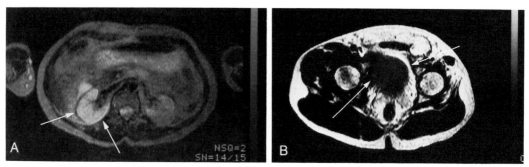

Figure 45–16. Transverse section images through the abdomen demonstrating the chemical-shift effect (black curvilinear line laterally and white line medially) around the kidneys (*A*) and bladder (*B*).

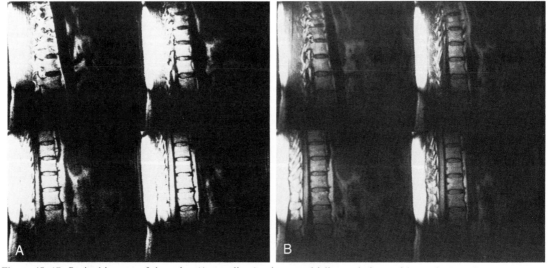

Figure 45–17. Sagittal images of the spine (4 mm slices) using a multislice technique with contiguous slices (*A*) and the same slices collected with a 1 mm spacing between adjacent slices (*B*).

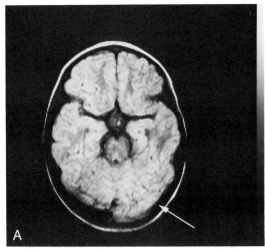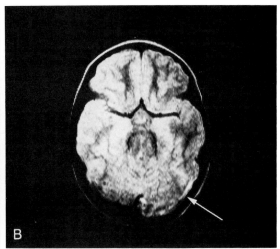

Figure 45–18. Transverse section images through the brain using a multiecho sequence. Flowing blood has diminished intensity on the odd-echo image (*A*) but increased signal intensity on the even-echo image (*B*) as the result of even-echo rephasing, a flow-related effect.

or frequency-encoding direction[2] and also at the interface of the bladder (Fig. 45–16*B*). This effect is due to the fact that water and lipid protons resonate at slightly different frequencies (3.0 to 3.5 parts per million) because of the different chemical matrices in which they reside. Since spatial position is directly related to resonant frequency, one distribution will be shifted with respect to the other in the *x* or frequency-encoded direction, resulting in alternate attenuation and enhancement (Fig. 45–16).[3] This effect becomes more pronounced at higher field strengths because the frequency difference is amplified.

Another potential source of image degradation is the cross-talk that exists in multislice techniques (Fig. 45–17*A*). When images of adjacent slices are collected simultaneously with no spacing between slices, there tends to be a slight overlap because slice thickness is not a perfect square wave but has gauss-shaped tails.[4] This effect results in a degradation of image quality. By using a small spacing between slices (i.e., 1 mm) these effects are reduced (Fig. 45–17*B*).

Flowing blood produces some interesting differences in images obtained with multiecho techniques. In odd-echo images, flowing blood has diminished signal intensity (Fig. 45–18*A*), but has increased signal intensity in even-echo images (Fig. 45–18*B*) owing to the even-echo rephasing phenomenon.[5]

As magnetic resonance imaging continues to grow, more clinical applications will probably be found. With these expanded capabilities will come more potential imaging pitfalls. Users of the technology must be constantly on the lookout for these pitfalls in order to quickly characterize and understand them, thereby minimizing their effects on image interpretation.

References

1. Wood ML, Henkelman RM: MR image artifacts from periodic motion. Med Phys *12*(2):143, 1985.
2. Hricak H, Williams RD, Moon KL, et al: NMR imaging of the kidney: renal masses. Radiology *147*:765, 1983.
3. Soila KP, Viamonte M, Starewicz, PM: Chemical shift misregistration effect in magnetic resonance imaging. Radiology *153*:819, 1984.
4. Kneeland JB, Shimakawa A, Werli FW: Effect of intersection spacing on MR image contrast and study time. Radiology *158*:819, 1986.
5. Walach V, Bradley WG: NMR even-echo rephasing in slow laminar flow. J Comput Assist Tomogr *8*:594, 1984.

X

CONTRAST MEDIA

46

Principles of Contrast-Enhanced MRI

M. F. TWEEDLE
H. G. BRITTAIN
W. C. ECKELMAN
G. T. GAUGHAN
J. J. HAGAN
P. W. WEDEKING
V. M. RUNGE

INTRODUCTION

The primer by Wolf and Popp[1] is a good place for the investigator new to this field to begin a study of relaxation phenomena as they apply to nuclear magnetic resonance (NMR), magnetic resonance imaging (MRI), and paramagnetic contrast media. It contains references to some of the basic works required for a thorough understanding of NMR. Reviews on the subject of paramagnetic contrast media have also appeared in recent years[2-4] as well as a comprehensive text on x-ray contrast media.[5] The many similarities between radiopharmaceuticals and MRI contrast agents have received relatively little notice, but that situation is changing.[6-10] Rather than reiterate the material published in these works, we will try to supplement it, demonstrating with examples, whenever possible, the principles important to the design and evaluation of new contrast agents.

Relaxation Enhancement

The following description of relaxation enhancement is a general one. The intent is to provide to the investigator new to the field enough background to follow the trends in relaxation effectiveness, which are discussed subsequently.

The parameters that govern signal intensity in each volume element (voxel) in an MR image include $T1$ and $T2$, the longitudinal and transverse relaxation times of the water protons in the tissue. In a strong magnetic field the water protons are excited when they absorb energy in the radio frequency (rf) range. In practice, the energy is offered as a microsecond pulse from an rf coil. When the pulse is turned off, the protons return to their original equilibrium state, releasing the energy as they do so. The return process is known as relaxation and is a much slower process—on the order of a second—than the rf absorption. The relaxation process is assumed to be a first-order one. That is, the rate of progress toward equilibrium is proportional to the deviation from equilibrium. Equation (1) mathematically describes a first-order relaxation process.

$$V = \exp(-t/T) \tag{1}$$

V is the magnitude of some variable directly proportional to the extent of the progress toward equilibrium, and t is the time at which V is determined. T is the relaxation time for the process. (T is the reciprocal of the rate constant for the process. It is not the half-life but is related to the half-life by T = half-life/ln 2.) In MRI the overall relaxation of the water protons is described by two related relaxation processes, represented by the $T1$ and $T2$ relaxation times. The processes represented by $T1$ and $T2$ are always related such that $T1 \geq T2$.

In the most common practice of spin-echo imaging, the relative signal intensity (SI) in each MRI image voxel is governed approximately by equation (2).

$$SI = [H]H(v) \{\exp(-TE/T2)\} \{1 - \exp(-TR/T1)\} \qquad (2)$$

where $[H]$ is the concentration of water protons in the voxel, $H(v)$ is a motion factor,[11] $T1$ and $T2$ are the relaxation times (analogous to T in Equation 1), and TE and TR are the echo-delay time and the pulse-repetition time (analogous to t in Equation 1). The imaging "pulse sequences" are protocols for applying the rf bursts and measuring the extent of the return to equilibrium, and amount to choosing TE and TR. Relaxation kinetics measurements require a waiting period between the excitation (rf pulse in MRI) and the interrogation of the system (by a second rf pulse) to determine the extent of its return to equilibrium. If protons move, governed by some $H(v)$, from one voxel to another during the relaxation experiment, it will affect the SI in both voxels.

Paramagnetic compounds, compounds containing one or more unpaired electrons, catalyze the proton relaxation of the water in which they are dissolved.[12] As a result, $T1$ and $T2$ are both decreased, and SI is affected according to Equation (2). Note that when the relaxation times are decreased, they have the opposite effect on SI; $T1$ decreases will increase SI, while $T2$ decreases will decrease SI. When paramagnetic compounds are involved in MRI, the TE and TR are usually chosen to make SI much more sensitive to $T1$ than to $T2$, so that the presence of the paramagnetic compound produces an increase in SI.

Relaxation catalysis by paramagnetic compounds is governed by a second-order rate constant called relaxivity, which describes each paramagnetic compound's ability to catalyze relaxation of bulk water protons. The longitudinal or transverse relaxivity, $^fk_1$ or $^fk_2$, of a paramagnet, P, is defined by

$$\Delta T1^{-1} = {}^fk_1[P] \qquad (3)$$

$$\Delta T2^{-1} = {}^fk_2[P] \qquad (4)$$

where the term on the left is the difference in the reciprocal of the relaxation times measured in the presence and absence of P. $[P]$ is the concentration of P in moles per liter (M) in fluids or in moles per kg tissue (m) for solid tissue (mM and mm are abbreviations for millimolar and millimolal, respectively). Relaxivities are generally not independent of the frequency, f in MHz, at which the measurement was made; f's will be omitted, however, when the discussion is for the general case.

For a first-order process the reciprocal of the relaxation time (in seconds, s) is the relaxation rate *constant* (in s^{-1}), and is often abbreviated R. The second-order rate constant, relaxivity (in $M^{-1}s^{-1}$), has also been abbreviated with R. We have chosen to use the chemist's traditional symbol, k, for the relaxivity rate constant.

$T1,2^{-1}$ are generally linear in paramagnet concentration in the range 10^{-4} to 10^{-3} M in water. Some typical experimental data are shown in Figure 46–1. The slope of this line is the relaxivity, and the intercept corresponds to the expected $T1$ of water at $[P] = 0$. The observed slopes for pure compounds are generally reproducible to within 10 percent, with most of the error coming from day-to-day variation in the instrument (IBM PC-20). Relaxivities have not been systematically measured as a function of $[P]$

RELAXIVITY OF Gd(DOTA)⁻

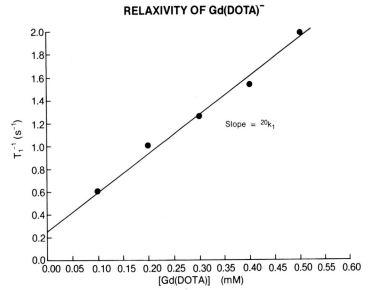

Figure 46–1. Determination of relaxivity as the slope of $T1^{-1}$ versus concentration. Relaxation times were measured at 20 MHz and 40° C on aqueous solutions of Gd(DOTA)⁻. The relaxivity, $^{20}k_1$, was 3.5 mM⁻¹s⁻¹.

in vivo, but some ex vivo determinations[13] suggest that rates may be nonlinear with [P] in some tissues. Note that at a given frequency $T1 \geq T2$, and, therefore, $k_2 \geq k_1$.

Obviously, SI is a complex function of agent, tissue, and instrument properties. To calculate the effect of relaxivity on SI we must choose constant values for some of the variables. Fixing the normal tissue relaxation times, $T1 = 0.500$ s, $T2 = 0.100$ s, and the pulse sequence, $TE = 0.030$ s, $TR = 0.500$ s, we can then use Equations (2), (3), and (4) to generate SI versus [P] curves at various values of k_1 and k_2. Figure 46–2 shows four of these curves; each curve may be taken as representing the characteristics of an individual contrast agent. The salient features are: (1) An optimum agent concentration exists, below or above which the signal intensity is diminished; (2) raising

SIGNAL INTENSITY VERSUS CONCENTRATION

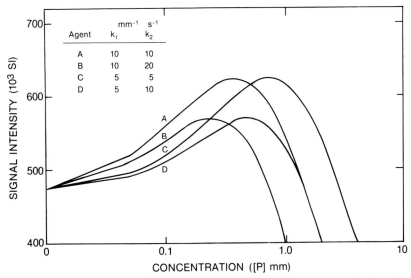

Figure 46–2. Relationship between paramagnet concentration and relative signal intensity in a tissue with $T1$ = 0.5 sec and $T2$ = 0.1 sec before adding paramagnet. The pulse sequence used was a spin-echo with TE = 0.030 sec and TR = 0.500 sec (k_1 and k_2 are in mm⁻¹s⁻¹).

k_1 with k_2 constant increases *SI;* raising k_2 with k_1 constant decreases *SI;* and (3) the maximum *SI* attained is determined by the k_2/k_1 ratio. A consequence of feature (1) is that in areas where the agent is highly concentrated, such as the urine for agents excreted via the renal route, signal intensity can approach zero. This has been observed in vivo.[14]

Features (2) and (3) suggest that it will be of interest to define, inasmuch as it is possible in such a complex milieu, the optimum agent relaxivities. From the necessary condition $T1 \geq T2$, it follows that $k_1 \leq k_2$, and highest achievable *SI* occurs when $k_2/k_1 = 1$; this maximum will occur at lowest $[P]$ when k_1 is maximum. Agent A appears, therefore, to be the best of the four in Figure 46–2. If changes of 20 percent in SI are needed in a given application, then $[P] = 10^{-4}$ *m* of agent A is sufficient to provide them. Note that the order of effectiveness of the agents in Figure 46–2 at 10^{-4} m is determined primarily by k_1 and only secondarily by k_2.

The relaxivity effects add a dimension of complexity to paramagnetic agents for MRI that does not exist for other diagnostic agents. Relaxivities are strongly affected by chemical structure, and each paramagnetic compound has a characteristic set of relaxivities. With radionuclide and iodinated x-ray agents, the gamma ray emission and x-ray absorption are nearly independent of the chemical structure of the compound containing the nuclide or the iodine. This is not to underplay the importance of chemistry in the development of radionuclide and x-ray imaging agents. Chemical structure determines the tissue distribution of the radiopharmaceutical and the acute tolerance and tissue distribution of the iodinated x-ray agent. From the chemist's point of view, however, the factors that influence a dynamic molecular property, such as the ability to catalyze relaxation, are entirely different from the largely static properties (e.g., water/lipid solubility) that influence biodistribution and toxicity. This chemical influence on the relaxivity will be further elaborated in the section on characterization of compounds.

Toxicity and Dose

Paramagnetic MRI agents are currently represented by two classes of compound, each with potential advantages and problems. On the one hand are the nitroxide free radicals,[15,16] and on the other the complexed metals.[17–22] For a given use the most important consideration in testing and comparing agents is toxicity versus dose. The dose will be proportional to the relaxivity, modified, of course, by the biodistribution, pharmacokinetics, and any metabolism that results in a molecule with different properties. Table 46–1 shows some comparison data[23] that illustrate, in large part, why gadolinium (III), Gd(III), complexes have been chosen for the initial clinical trials.

The structures of the chelating ligands and nitroxides discussed herein are included in Figure 46–3. Chelated Gd(III) appears to have the best combined toxicity and relaxivity. To this statement must be added the caveats that the field is in a relatively early stage of development and that the nitroxides, though they have lower stability and relaxivity than the metal complexes, are more easily altered synthetically. This will facilitate addressing the problems of the nitroxides and may make it relatively easy to alter their tissue distribution properties.

Gd(III) has the additional advantage of existing in only one biologically accessible oxidation state. This means that one potentially very potent toxicologic pathway is not available to Gd(III), even if the free ion is released from the chelate. Mn(II) is readily oxidized to the Mn(III), while nitroxides are easily reduced, for example, by ascorbic acid, to diamagnetic hydroxylamines. Fe exists in vivo in both its II and its III states. In addition to any toxic effects occurring as a consequence of this metabolism, the

Table 46–1. $^{20}k_1$ ($^{f}k_1$, f = 20 MHz, 39°C)
RELAXIVITY IN WATER AND ACUTE INTRAVENOUS
TOXICITY IN MICE FOR PARAMAGNETIC
COMPOUNDS

Compound	$^{20}k_1$ mM^{-1}s^{-1}	LD$_{50}$* mmol/kg
Na[Gd(DOTA)]	3.4	~10
Na$_2$[Gd(DTPA)]	3.7	~10
Na$_2$[Mn(EDTA)]	2.2	7†
Na[Fe(EDTA)]	1.6	3.4
Nitroxides	≤0.7‡	≤25§

* Dose causing 50 percent mortality.
† Reference 2.
‡ Highest from Reference 15.
§ Highest from Reference 16.

metabolites generally do not have strong relaxivity. Diamagnetic compounds Fe(II) and Mn(III) have very low relaxivity. Some Mn(III) porphyrins appear to be exceptions.[21]

The Fe(III) agents are intuitively appealing because iron is so plentiful in the body. This is not, however, necessarily an advantage, since the mammalian body maintains avid mechanisms for sequestering and retaining excess iron.[24] This is also true to some extent for manganese.[24] In addition, Fe(III) chelates can catalyze very powerful radical reactions.[25] These can be minimized by saturating all the available coordination positions on the iron atom, as has been done for Fe(EHPG)$^-$,[8] but the relaxivity is greatly diminished when water molecules cannot coordinate the metal ($^{20}k_1$ = 0.9 mM^{-1}s^{-1} for Fe(EHPG)$^-$), as will be demonstrated in the following discussion.

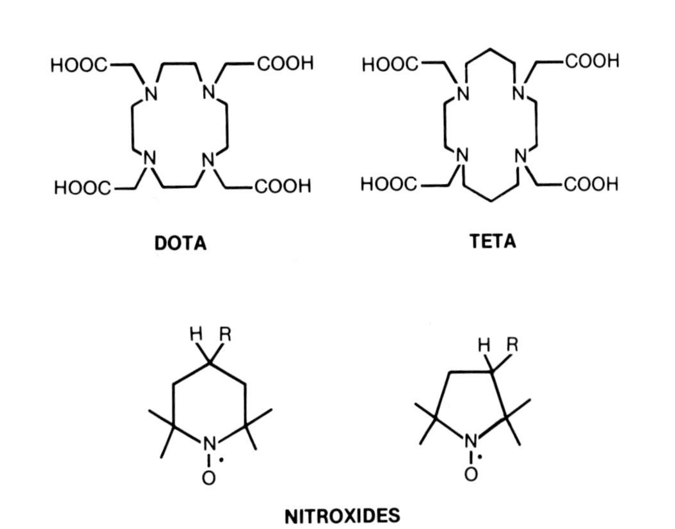

EDTA   DTPA

Figure 46–3. Structures of nitroxides and of the chelating ligands: EDTA, ethylenediaminetetraacetic acid; DTPA, diethylenetriamine-pentaacetic acid; DOTA, 1,4,7,10-tetraazacyclododecane-1,4,7,10-tetraacetic acid; TETA, 1,4,8,11-tetraazacyclotetradecane-1,4,8,11-tetraacetic acid.

DOTA   TETA

NITROXIDES

CHARACTERIZATION OF PARAMAGNETIC METAL COMPLEXES

The relaxivity of a paramagnetic compound, in this case a metal complex, depends on the magnitude of the dipole-dipole (through space) interaction between the electron spin (on the metal) and the proton spin (on the water). The interaction is described by the Solomon-Bloembergen-Morgan (SBM) equations (Ref. 1, p. 26; Refs. 26–28), a simplified form of which follows as Equation (5).

$$k_1 = \frac{q\mu_{eff}^2 t_c}{r^6} \tag{5}$$

$$t_c^{-1} = t_r^{-1} + t_S^{-1} + t_M^{-1} \tag{6}$$

Constant terms and the frequency and temperature dependence of t_c have been omitted. A similar equation can be written for k_2, but we will restrict our discussions to k_1. k_1 is the longitudinal relaxivity in $M^{-1}s^{-1}$ from Equation (3); q represents the number of water molecules involved per paramagnetic metal. μ_{eff} is the effective magnetic moment of the paramagnetic metal in units of Bohr magnetons. The effective magnetic moment for the metals we will discuss is equal to $n(n + 2)^{1/2}$, where n is the number of unpaired electrons. r is the distance between the protons on the water molecules and the paramagnetic center. t_c is called the correlation time, and its components, t_r, t_S, and t_M, refer to contributions to the correlation time from brownian molecular rotation of the metal-water complex, the relaxation time of the paramagnetic moment, and the lifetime of the water proton in the complex, respectively.

Efficient catalysis by a dilute (e.g., millimolar) metal complex in 55.5 M water requires that a water molecule reside at the metal no longer than necessary to be relaxed. The change observed in $T1$ of bulk water protons when a dilute paramagnetic metal complex, P, is dissolved has been described[29] by

$$\Delta T1^{-1} = [P](n/55.5)(T_{1p} + t_M)^{-1} \tag{7}$$

where $\Delta T1^{-1}$ is the difference in the reciprocal of the relaxation times measured in the presence and absence of P, n is the number of water molecules associated with (usually coordinated to) the metal, and T_{1p} is the relaxation time (catalyzed) of the protons on the coordinated water. From equations (3) and (7)

$$k_1 = n/55.5(T1_p + t_M)^{-1} \tag{8}$$

$T1_p$ for water coordinated to a paramagnetic metal is on the order of microseconds. To the extent t_M is long relative to $T1_p$, "slow exchange" conditions will exist, and no communication between the metal and the bulk water will occur. "Fast exchange" conditions will exist when $t_M \ll T1_p$, and it is these conditions that will generally lead to high relaxivities. Thus, t_M plays a dual role. It first establishes the exchange conditions and then acts as a contributor to t_c.

Magnetic Moment and k_{ex}

Table 46–2 lists the $^{20}k_1$ relaxivities ($^f k_1$ where $f = 20$ MHz) for several chelate complexes. The complexes are chosen so that q is well defined, r is similar (the metal-OH$_2$ bond distances are 2.1 to 2.5 A), and t_c is dominated by t_r, which is $\sim 10^{-11}$ s for small molecules. Gd(III) has the largest magnetic moment, $\mu_{eff}^2 = 63$ BM^2 for Gd(III), compared with $\mu_{eff} = 35$ BM^2 for Mn(II) and Fe(III), and $\mu_{eff} = 15$ BM^2 for Cr(III) and so, with other variables equal, the Gd(III) complexes have the largest $^{20}k_1$ values.

Although these complexes show the order of relaxivities expected based on their

Table 46–2. RELAXIVITIES (39°C) OF METAL
COMPLEXES

Complex	$^{20}k_1$ (mM^{-1}s^{-1})
[Gd(DTPA)(H$_2$O)]$^{2-}$	3.7
[Gd(DOTA)(H$_2$O)]$^-$	3.4
[Mn(EDTA)(H$_2$O)]$^{2-}$	2.0
[Fe(EDTA)(H$_2$O)]$^-$	1.6
[Cr(EDTA)(H$_2$O)]$^-$	0.2

magnetic moments, the relaxivity for the Cr(III) complex is lower than would be expected based only on the magnetic moment. The reason for its inefficient relaxation is probably to be found in the water exchange rates typical of Cr(III). The rate at which coordinated water exchanges with bulk water is governed by the rate constant k_{ex} (equivalent to t_M^{-1}).

$$Cr(EDTA)(H_2O^*)^- + H_2O \rightleftharpoons Cr(EDTA)(H_2O)^- + H_2O^* \quad k_{ex}$$

Cr^{3+} compounds generally have very poor relaxivities because $k_{ex} = t_M^{-1} \sim 10^{-6}$ s^{-1} [29] leads to $t_M \sim 10^6$, and the "slow exchange" condition. Note that it is not meaningful to calculate the contribution of t_M to t_c under conditions of "slow exchange."

The k_{ex} values for Mn^{2+} and Fe^{3+} aqua ions are $k_{ex} = t_M^{-1} = 10^{7.5}$, and 10^3 s^{-1} [30] respectively, and would lead one to predict that [Mn(EDTA)(H$_2$O)]$^{2-}$ would be a far better relaxation catalyst than [Fe(EDTA)(H$_2$O)]$^-$. However, for the 3d metals, as the waters on the free ion are replaced with other ligands, k_{ex} for the remaining coordinated waters increases, sometimes by orders of magnitude. This effect is particularly strong for [Cr(EDTA)(H$_2$O)]$^-$, which has $k_{ex} = t_M^{-1} \sim 1$ s^{-1} [31] or about six orders of magnitude higher than the Cr^{3+} aqua ion, although the exchange conditions are still "slow" for [Cr(EDTA)(H$_2$O)]$^-$. A similar enhancement going from the Fe^{3+} aqua ion to the [Fe(EDTA)(H$_2$O)]$^-$ probably increases k_{ex} from 10^3 s^{-1} (slow exchange) to $\geq 10^6$ s^{-1} (fast exchange), leading to the relatively high $^{20}k_1$ value observed for [Fe(EDTA)(H$_2$O)]$^-$. Mn(II) and Gd(III) aqua ions and complexes are generally very labile and fall into the fast exchange regime; for example, [Mn(EDTA)(H$_2$O)]$^-$ has $k_{ex} \simeq 7 \times 10^8$ s^{-1} [30] and [Gd(PDTA)(H$_2$O)$_n$]$^-$ has $k_{ex} \sim 3.3 \times 10^8$ s^{-1} [32].

The Hydration Number, q

For the preceding discussion we chose complexes with similar hydration shells in order that we could isolate the effects of magnetic moment and water exchange. In this section we will concentrate on hydration numbers, represented by q, and will use complexes similar in other respects as examples. The relaxivity of a paramagnetic metal complex is more precisely described as the sum of two components designated inner sphere and outer sphere relaxivities.[29,33]

$$k_1 = k_{1\ outer} + k_{1\ inner} \tag{9}$$

Inner and outer sphere refer to the position of the water molecule relative to the metal. An inner sphere water is coordinated through a chemical bond to the paramagnetic metal. Outer sphere water is associated with the metal, but not through a bond to the metal (for example, a water molecule hydrogen bonded to a portion of the ligand). The outer sphere waters have greater values for r, and so lower relaxivity on a per water basis. However, there are more water molecules in the outer than in the inner sphere, so the outer sphere contribution to the relaxivity can be appreciable.

One way to estimate the outer sphere relaxivity is to measure relaxivity for molecules whose inner coordination spheres are saturated with ligands other than water. Note the relaxivities of some presumably outer sphere Mn(II) and Fe(III) compounds (Table 46–3).

The Mn(II) and Fe(III) complexes of the octadentate ligands, DOTA and DTPA, are presumed to have no coordinated water molecules. These metal ions are normally six coordinate, seven coordinate at most, and it is unlikely that water would find a coordination position permanently available. It is possible, though, that some intermittent hydration occurs owing to lability of the acetate groups. The lower relaxivity of the Fe(III) complexes may arise, in part, from lability differences and also from a contribution of t_s to t_c that does not exist for Mn(II). Assuming that the relaxivities in Table 46–3 represent mostly outer sphere relaxivity, and assuming, based on the known solid state structures, that one water is coordinated to the metal when the ligand is EDTA, $^{20}k_1$ outer $\simeq$ $^{20}k_1$ inner $\simeq 1$ mM^{-1}s^{-1} for Mn(EDTA)(H$_2$O)$^{2-}$. Averaging the Fe data in Table 46–3 and subtracting that from the relaxivity of Fe(EDTA)(H$_2$O)$^-$ (1.6 mM^{-1}s^{-1} from Table 46–2) gives 0.55 and 1.05 mM^{-1}s^{-1} for the outer sphere and inner sphere contribution to the relaxivity of Fe(EDTA)(H$_2$O)$^-$. Note that the outer sphere contribution can be expected to give "fast exchange" conditions.

It is more difficult to be sure of having a fully outer sphere complex of Gd^{3+} owing to its extreme lability and its ability to bind up to 12 donor atoms. As an alternative, one can determine the inner sphere hydration number, q_{IS}.[34] By measuring the relaxivities of a series of similar Gd(III) complexes and experimentally determining the hydration numbers, the relative contributions of inner and outer sphere relaxation to the relaxivity can be estimated for the series. Estimates for outer and inner sphere contributions to the relaxivity of some Gd polyaminecarboxylates can be made using this approach. The $^{20}k_1$ and q_{IS} values for [Gd(L)(H$_2$O)$_q$], where L = EDTA, DOTA, or TETA, are shown in Table 46–4. $^{20}k_1$ was experimentally determined by the authors. q_{IS} values were determined[35] for the europium(III), Eu(III), complexes by the Horrocks method.[36] Eu is adjacent to Gd on the periodic table, and its chemistry is very similar. $^{20}k_1$'s ranged from 2.1 to 5.4 mM^{-1}s^{-1}, but the three $^{20}k_1$ values correlated linearly with the measured q_{IS}; that is, a plot of q_{IS} versus $^{20}k_1$ was linear with slope = 1.66 $\pm$ 0.23 mM^{-1}s^{-1}; intercept = 1.36 $\pm$ 0.32 mM^{-1}s^{-1}, $r = 0.97$. The slope and intercept of the relaxivity versus hydration number data are taken to be reasonable estimates of, respectively, the inner sphere relaxivity contribution per coordinated water and the outer sphere relaxivity contribution for all waters in the outer sphere. We can assume that the number of waters contributing substantially to the outer sphere relaxivity is constant through this series of similar complexes. If we assume that one water is hydrogen bound to each coordinated carboxylate oxygen,[29] we have $q_{outer sphere}$ = 4 for each complex. Considering the experimental errors, the outer sphere contribution may be as high as 1.68 mM^{-1}s^{-1}, or 0.42 mM^{-1}s^{-1} per water. The inner sphere contribution to the relaxivity is larger on a per water basis, as would be expected from the theoretical r^{-6} dependence.

Table 46–3. RELAXIVITIES (39°C) OF OUTER SPHERE COMPOUNDS

Complex	$^{20}k_1$ (mM^{-1}s^{-1})
[Mn(DOTA)]$^{2-}$	1.1
[Mn(DTPA)]$^{3-}$	1.1
[Fe(DTPA)]$^{2-}$	0.7
[Fe(DOTA)]$^-$	0.4

Table 46–4. RELAXIVITIES (39°C) AND
COORDINATED WATERS FOR COMPLEXES

Complex	q	$^{20}k_1$ mM^{-1}s^{-1}
[Gd(EDTA)(H$_2$O)$_q$]$^-$	2.5	5.4
[Gd(DOTA)(H$_2$O)$_q$]$^-$	1.2	3.4
[Gd(TETA)(H$_2$O)$_q$]$^-$	0.6	2.1

The Rotational Correlation Time, t_r

Paramagnetic Mn(II) and Gd(III) complexes bound to protein and macromolecules have relaxivity enhanced over that of the unbound complexes owing to increased t_c. The correlation time, t_c, is dominated by the rotational correlation time, $t_r \sim 10^{-11}$ s, for small (<1000 amu) molecules. t_r increases as a function of molecular size and leads to increased relaxivity. This proton relaxation enhancement (PRE) effect increases with increasing molecular weight up the point at which one of the other correlation times, usually t_s for Gd(III) and Mn(II), becomes dominant. Studies of the frequency dependence of the relaxivities of protein-bound ions have long been used to probe these correlation time effects, but there are usually more variables than there are independent ways to relate them. As a result, q, and perhaps some of the other parameters, have been rather poorly determined by this method.[28]

It would be useful to know the limits to the PRE effect in terms of relaxivity per coordinated water because increased relaxivity translates, other things being equal, into lower dose. For example, measuring both the relaxivity and the hydration number of Gd^{3+} bound to large macromolecules and proteins, trial and error has led us to a tentative lower limit for the effect for Gd at 20 MHz and 39°C. The highest $^{20}k_1$ per coordinated water determined was $^{20}k_1 = 29$ mM^{-1}s^{-1} for Gd(rabbit IgG antibody). Compared with the data in Table 46–2, it seems safe to assume that at least one order of magnitude of PRE is available. More systematic studies in this area are needed, particularly with emphasis on independent determinations or control of the contributing chemical factors, combined with measurements of the frequency dependence of the relaxivity.

Since relaxivity is strongly affected by correlation phenomena, relaxivity of new chelates should be measured in biologic fluids of interest, ideally using variable frequency data, and in tissues from animals that have been injected with the solutions of the complex. Table 46–5 shows examples of ex vivo 20 MHz relaxivity data for [Gd(DTPA)]$^{2-}$ and [Gd(DOTA)]$^-$ in water, dog serum, and a mouse tumor. These tissues were chosen to model the extracellular fluid space in a brain tumor. ^{153}Gd was used to determine tissue concentrations in molal. Control $T1$'s for the tumor study were obtained from tissues of animals having tumors of the same age and size. The errors

Table 46–5. $^{20}k_1$ VALUES OF GADOLINIUM CHELATES 39°C

Complex	(mM^{-1}s^{-1}) Water*	(mM^{-1}s^{-1}) Dog Serum*	(mM^{-1}s^{-1}) Mouse Tumor†
[Gd(DTPA)]$^{2-}$	3.7 ± 0.1	4.1 ± 0.4	5.6 ± 1.9
[Gd(DOTA)]$^-$	3.4 ± 0.2	3.8 ± 0.5	4.8 ± 1.3

* ±97.5 percent confidence limits.
† In mM^{-1}s^{-1}, 5 min post 0.4 mmol/kg, i.v., in 25 gm MRL +/+ mice (N = 3) 8 days post implantation of mammary adenoacanthomas. [Gd] = 2.2 ± 0.2 molal in 300 mg tumors (± standard deviation).

in the tumor relaxivities are large because even with tumors of the same age and size, the *Tl* values of the control tumors were the largest source of error.

Little proton relaxation enhancement is evident for these chelates (at least no substantial progress has been made toward the figure of 29 mM^{-1}s^{-1} per water determined for the Gd-[rabbit IgG]). This was not unexpected since these chelates are highly hydrophilic, and protein binding is usually low when hydrophilicity is high. The small increases in the mean (the units are in millimolal^{-1} rather than millimolar^{-1}) seen in tumors are within the range expected based on the reduced water content of tumor tissue relative to serum or water. Although not observed in this study, nonlinear Tl^{-1}–Gd concentration curves have been observed in some compartmentalized tissues. Biexponential water relaxation behavior has been reported in rabbit kidney.[13] It will be important to understand these effects, as they could complicate (or enhance) kinetic studies using NMR imaging to follow paramagnetic agents in vivo.

Complex Stability and Biologic Studies

In studies with animals, it is common to see a great deal of effort put into multiple determinations in order to obtain meaningful statistics. The efforts are wasted, however, if the compound being tested is inconsistently prepared, or worse, consistently prepared containing high levels of impurities.[37] Radiochemical techniques can be used to great advantage in this area. Radiodetection of TLC and HPLC of radiolabeled complexes is particularly useful.[35] The technique can be used to monitor reactions of metal chelates, determine compound purity, and monitor reactions of the chelates with endogenously available ions. Some examples of our results using ^{153}Gd-labeled chelates will be reported.

In chelate formation reactions, it is necessary to determine that a complete reaction of metal with ligand has occurred, or that a recrystallization or chromatographic purification has succeeded. Ligands and metal sources are generally hydrated to uncertain degrees, and formation reactions are pH dependent and can be exceedingly slow, despite high formation constants. For example, to prepare ^{153}Gd-Gd(DOTA)$^{-}$, ^{153}Gd-Gd(acetate)$_3$ is first made by dissolving the Gd(acetate)$_3$(H$_2$O)$_4$ reagent in water at about 50 mM and adding ^{153}Gd (97.4, 103.2 keV, half-life 242 days) as the nitrate or chloride (from Oak Ridge or New England Nuclear) to make a specific activity of 1 mCi/mmol. The free acid form of DOTA is added in slightly less than one molar equivalent, the pH adjusted to 4 with HCl or NaOH, and the solution heated at 88°C for 15 minutes. An aliquot of the solution is then adjusted to pH 7 and mixed with a solution of the HPLC mobile phase, which contains EDTA (Fig. 46–4). An HPLC radiochromatogram is then taken using the conditions outlined in Figure 46–4. The excess (weakly chelated) Gd in the reaction solution appears as ^{153}Gd(EDTA) in the HPLC. If no ^{153}Gd(EDTA) is detected, additional Gd(acetate)$_3$(H$_2$O)$_4$ is added to the reaction mixture and the heating procedure repeated. Once ^{153}Gd(EDTA) is detected, the reaction can be titrated by adding small aliquots of free acid DOTA (adjusted to pH 4) until the ^{153}Gd(EDTA) peak disappears. This procedure yields a solution that is free of unreacted gadolinium and DOTA.

This procedure works for other ligands, such as DTPA, as long as they have higher affinity for Gd than EDTA, and rapid kinetics. The free ^{153}Gd^{3+} can be determined by ITLC-SG (instant thin layer chromatography with silica gel impregnated in glass fibers) using the conditions shown in Figure 46–5. The ITLC-SG (Fig. 46–5) is of the completed reaction. For this assay an aliquot of the reaction mixture is adjusted to pH 7 with NaOH and mixed with 0.067 M Na$_3$PO$_4$ at pH 7. After 15 minutes, five ITLC-SG strips are spotted at 1 cm and eluted to 11 cm with 10 percent NH$_4$OAc, 50 percent H$_2$O/

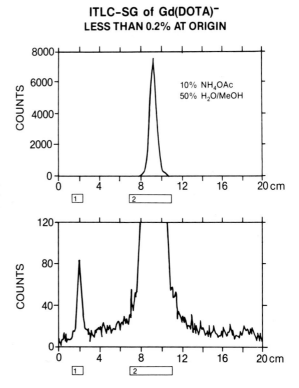

Figure 46–4. HPLC chromatograms of completed reaction (left) and after adding ^{153}Gd(acetate) to the completed reaction (right). Incomplete reactions appear as on the right, with the area under the Gd(EDTA)$^-$ peak proportional to the uncomplexed gadolinium in the reaction mixture. Mobile phase: 50 mM tris acetate, 2 1mM EDTA, 2 % CH$_3$CN, pH 7.3. Flow: 1 ml/min. Column: Nucleosil C18.

MeOH. The strips are scanned on a Bioscan System 200 Imaging Scanner. The strips can also be cut into segments and counted in a well counter. Uncomplexed and weakly chelated Gd remains at the origin. The ITLC-SG method is used on the final solutions to provide accuracy at very low levels of uncomplexed ^{153}Gd. The HPLC is more convenient to use during the titration. The ITLC-SG technique works as long as the 0.067 M phosphate ($K_{sp} = 10^{-22}$ for GdPO$_4$[39]) is unable to compete with the ligand of interest for binding Gd. Measured origin counts changing with phosphate mixing

Figure 46–5. ITLC-SG radiochromatogram of final reaction solution of ^{153}Gd(DOTA)$^-$ after 0.067 M phosphate was added to an aliquot of reaction solution. The bottom trace is the same data as the top trace with the ordinate expanded ($< 0.2\%$ free ^{153}Gd^{3+} was detected at the origin).

time is an indication that phosphate is slowly removing Gd from the chelate. This suggests special caution in interpretation of subsequent biologic results, since mammalian blood contains mM phosphate and other Gd-avid anions such as CO_3^{2-}, K_{sp} = 10^{-32} for $Gd_2(CO_3)_3$[39] and OH^-, K_{sp} = 10^{-26} for $Gd(OH)_3$.[39]

If possible, unchelated ligand should also be determined. Ligands that bind to Gd^{3+} will also generally bind avidly to Ca^{2+} and could affect biologic results. Unchelated ligands of the polyaminecarboxylate variety are often difficult to detect directly at mM concentrations. In some cases a transition metal can be added to a solution of the Gd-chelate, and the visible spectrum of the transition-metal-ligand monitored, but in many cases the transition metal has a higher affinity for the chelating ligand than for Gd, and the transition metal then replaces ^{153}Gd in the chelate, leaving free $^{153}Gd^{3+}$ in the solution (see below).

Many polydentate ligands bind Ca^{2+}, and these can be highly toxic when injected intravenously as the free ligand. Injecting the Ca^{2+} complexes should raise the LD_{50} when hypocalcemia is the toxic mechanism. This appears to be the major mechanism for the toxicity of the ligand DTPA (Table 46–6).

Determining LD_{50} values for new materials requires that the solutions injected be scrupulously pure. When the drug is a metal chelate, the problem of impurities is magnified by the fact that the starting materials are the main source of toxic impurity. The magnitude of the problem is illustrated by the data in Table 46–6, which show, from the LD_{50} values for the free DTPA ligand and free Gd^{3+}, that they are 25 to 100 times more toxic than the complex. Obviously, an error of a few percent excess free ligand or free metal in chelating in any preparation could control the determined LD_{50}.

Unchelated metal can also be a crucial factor in biodistribution studies because it is often much slower to be excreted than metal complexes.[37] The data in Table 46–7 illustrate the problem. $[Gd(DTPA)]^{2-}$ and $[Gd(DOTA)]^-$ are quantitatively excreted, mainly into urine, while unchelated $^{153}Gd^{3+}$ is retained, with liver being the main repository. Chromatographic analyses are needed to determine with confidence whether or not retained ^{153}Gd for a new chelate was injected as unchelated $^{153}Gd^{3+}$. In this case, ≤0.3 percent (to 95 percent confidence) of the injected dose was in the form of free $^{153}Gd^{3+}$ by ITLC, and HPLC of the injected dose showed one peak, with 100 ± 1 percent recovery of activity from the column. Using the chromatography data along with the known distribution of aqueous gadolinium, we can conclude that the activity retained at seven days could have come from free $^{153}Gd^{3+}$ injected with the chelate. For example, if ≤ 0.3 percent of the injected dose were unchelated Gd, 41 percent of it, or ≤ 0.12 percent of the injected dose, would be expected in the liver, and 86 percent, or ≤0.26 percent of the injected dose, would be expected in the whole animal. Knowing the amount of uncomplexed Gd in the injected solutions allows us to conclude that all of the Gd remaining at seven days in the whole animal and in the liver for $Gd(DTPA)^{2-}$ and $Gd(DOTA)^-$ could have originated as uncomplexed Gd in the injected solution. There is, therefore, in these data no evidence that either complex is metabolized in such a way that free Gd is produced.

Table 46–6. INTRAVENOUS ACUTE TOXICITY IN MICE

Compound	LD_{50} (mmol/kg)
$Na_2[Gd(DTPA)]$	~10
$GdCl_3$	0.4
$Gd(OH)_3$	0.1
$Na_3[Ca(DTPA)]$	3.5
Na_2H_3DTPA	0.1

Table 46–7. URINARY EXCRETION AND WHOLE BODY RETENTION IN MICE FOLLOWING INTRAVENOUS INJECTIONS

	% ID ± 95% Confidence Limits			
	$GdCl_3$	Gd(acetate)	$Gd(DTPA)^{2-}$	$Gd(DOTA)^-$
Urine				
5 min	0.92 ± 1.72	2.11 ± 2.32	44.9 ± 14.4	20.6 ± 21.7
60 min	1.38 ± 1.14	4.45 ± 1.14	95.4 ± 12.0	89.5 ± 23.1
Whole Animal				
1 day	93.6 ± 2.13	93.7 ± 8.08	1.26 ± 0.10	1.83 ± 1.60
7 day	72.2 ± 10.7	86.1 ± 14.2	0.35 ± 0.13	0.18 ± 0.06
Liver				
7 days	40.3 ± 12.1	41.0 ± 7.25	0.022 ± 0.004	0.008 ± 0.008

Pharmacokinetic studies can also be affected by injected free metal or free metal formed as a result of reaction of the complex in vivo. For example, Figures 46–6 and 46–7 show blood clearance curves in rats as semilog plots of percent injected dose in blood versus time for ^{153}Gd-labeled $Gd(DOTA)^-$ and for unchelated ^{153}Gd (as the acetate) in the presence of unlabeled $Gd(DOTA)^-$. These data were obtained by a dual isotope method using coinjected ^{99m}Tc(DTPA) as a standard. Data for $Gd(DOTA)^-$ are similar in all respects to those for ^{99m}Tc(DTPA). Uncomplexed, or very weakly complexed, Gd shows markedly different behavior, being an order of magnitude more slowly eliminated. The elimination rate constants, k_{el}, calculated from the curves assuming a two-compartment open model,[40] are $9.9 \pm 1.2 \times 10^{-2}$ min^{-1} for $Gd(DOTA)^-$ and $3.9 \pm 4.3 \times 10^{-2}$ min^{-1} for free $Gd(acetate)_n$; the corresponding rate constants for the coinjected ^{99m}Tc(DTPA) are $11.0 \pm 0.8 \times 10^{-2}$ min^{-1} and $11.1 \pm 0.1 \times 10^{-2}$ min^{-1}, respectively.[41]

In addition to being a by-product of an incomplete reaction, free metal can arise as a product of the reaction of endogenous elements with the metal complex. Table 46–8 shows data for Gd^{3+} released from complexes in the presence of ions available in vivo. Chelates and ions were mixed at 25 mM in tris-acetate-buffered water, and precipitated Gd^{3+} was determined after 30 minutes of reaction.

$[Gd(TETA)]^-$ reacts with all of the agents (it continues to produce free Gd with

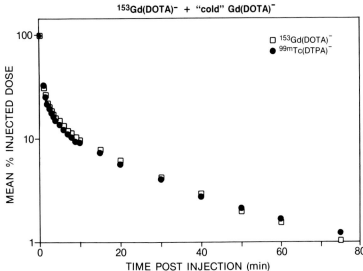

Figure 46–6. Mean % injected dose in blood (n = 6 rats) for coinjected ^{99m}Tc(DTPA) and ^{153}Gd-Gd(DOTA)$^-$ (0.1 mmol/kg).

BLOOD CLEARANCE IN RATS (N = 6)

^{153}Gd(DOTA)$^-$ + "cold" Gd(DOTA)$^-$

□ ^{153}Gd(DOTA)$^-$
● ^{99m}Tc(DTPA)$^-$

MEAN % INJECTED DOSE

TIME POST INJECTION (min)

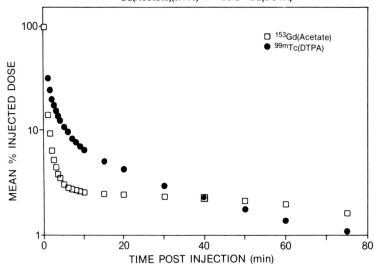

Figure 46–7. Mean % injected dose in blood (n = 6 rats) for coinjected $^{99m}Tc(DTPA)$, ^{153}Gd-Gd(acetate)$_n$ (0.1 μmol/kg), and unlabeled Gd(DOTA)$^-$ (0.1 mmol/kg).

longer reaction times). [Gd(EDTA)]$^-$ also readily reacts with Fe^{3+} and Cu^{2+}. Interestingly, [Gd(DTPA)]$^{2-}$, a drug undergoing clinical trials in humans, reacts rapidly with Cu^{2+}; after one day and one week reaction intervals, the free Gd^{3+} released from Gd(DTPA)$^{2-}$ was 47.1 and 48.7 percent, respectively, indicating that one Gd^{3+} was released for every two Cu^{2+} present in solution. DTPA is known to form a very stable [Cu$_2$(DTPA)]$^-$ complex (K_{eq} = 10^{28} M^{-2}),[42] which accounts for the 2 Cu:1 Gd stoichiometry. The rigid macrocyclic structure of DOTA does not allow it to incorporate two Cu^{2+} ions in the interior binding cavity, so DOTA prefers Gd^{3+} to two Cu^{2+} ions. DTPA, owing to its flexibility, is able to accommodate and prefers coordination with two Cu^{2+} ions over one Gd^{3+}.

About 55 μmol of copper are found in the human plasma.[43] The human dose for Gd(DTPA)$^{2-}$ is about 7 mmol, so a complete 2 Cu:1 Gd reaction could liberate 0.4 percent of the injected gadolinium dose at equilibrium. This kind of problem could become more important in renally impaired patients, in whom, presumably, the drug would be more slowly excreted by the kidneys with more of the drug excreted through the liver. That organ has 189 μmol of copper localized in only 1.8 kg.[43] Other endogenous ions, Zn^{2+}, for example, have not yet been investigated and may also compete with Gd^{3+} for its ligands. These, along with biochemical decomposition mechanisms, must ultimately be overcome, presumably by optimizing the structure of the ligand, to produce an ideal agent.

Table 46–8. PERCENT Gd^{3+} RELEASED (95% CL) FROM CHELATES AT pH 7.0

Complex	Na$^+$	PO$_4^3$	Fe^{3+}	Cu^{2+}
Gd(OAc)$_3$	—	99(1)	—	—
[Gd(TETA)]$^-$	22(3)	37(2)	28(3)	24(1)
[Gd(EDTA)]$^-$	3(3)	1(1)	21(12)	60(1)
[Gd(DTPA)]$^{2-}$	0.3(0.1)	0.2(0.2)	1.4(0.4)	34(4)
[Gd(DOTA)]$^-$	0.0(0.1)	0.2(0.1)	0.3(0.8)	0.2(0.0)

SUMMARY AND OVERVIEW

Initial evaluations of paramagnetic materials known to influence NMR relaxation kinetics have led most researchers to the same few metal ions and to one class of organic radical, the nitroxides. For a variety of reasons, the free metal ions are considered by most investigators to be too toxic for use as contrast agents, and only the strongest known chelating agents are able to sufficiently stabilize them in the biologic milieu. So far, physical chemical and in vivo results support the use of strongly chelated gadolinium compounds as NMR contrast agents but also suggest that existing complexes can be improved. For example, reactivity with endogenously available ions can be reduced. With a longer view, relaxivities can be increased by at least an order of magnitude, although not without substantial research involving the synthesis of new molecules. New structures are also likely to improve other pharmaceutically important properties such as water solubility and osmolality.

Engineering generally moves faster than synthetic chemistry, so improvements in the instrumentation can be expected to change in ways that will find new uses for the agents we have faster than new agents can be created and tested. Fortunately, several candidates from the chemical literature qualify as first-generation NMR agents, and these will provide us with a base of physical and clinical data upon which to build better agents. The first generation of paramagnetic MRI contrast agents will have in vivo distribution, kinetics, and excretion similar to iodinated x-ray agents. They will probably be used initially in MR imaging for the same indications that iodinated x-ray contrast media (e.g., diatrizoic acid, Renografin; iopamidol, Isovue) are currently used, e.g., as intravenous agents in cerebral imaging to observe the absence of a completely intact blood-brain barrier.

It is very likely that the current MR imaging agents will see improvements in tolerance, but the acute toxicity to dose ratio is already as high as for the safest x-ray media with the same indication. This is because MRI is more sensitive to Gd than x-ray is to iodine. From direct quantitative comparisons,[44,45] there seems to be about one order of magnitude difference in molar detectability favoring Gd/MRI over iodine x-ray. The clinical trial dose of $NMG_2[Gd(DTPA)]$ is 0.1 mmol Gd per kg, and the highest dose so far needed in our own animal studies of brain lesions was 0.25 mmol per kg. A dose of 4.5 mmol I per kg is used in cerebral CT scans. This difference in sensitivity to the agents compensates for the relatively crude state of the chemical art in MRI agents, as regards their acute toxicity. Iopamidol has an acute intravenous LD_{50} in mice of 172 mmol I per kg compared with 10 to 20 mmol Gd per kg for $Na_2[Gd(DTPA)]$, but the toxicity to dose ratios are about 40 in each case. Table 46–9 shows how the tolerance of iodinated x-ray media has increased with time.

If similar improvements can be made in the MRI agents and if they are shown to be equally safe in long-term studies, it seems natural that contrast-enhanced MRI should

Table 46–9. IMPROVEMENT OF ACUTE TOXICITY
OF X-RAY AGENTS WITH TIME*

Agent	Year Introduced	LD_{50}(mmol I/kg) IV in Mice
Diodone	1931	21
Acetrizoate	1952	52
Diatrizoate	1954	71
Iopamidol	1985	172

* Adapted from Grainger RG: Br J Radiol 55:1, 1982.

at least replace competitive x-ray procedures when other factors are equal. Eventually, we could even see tissue- or metabolism-specific agents of the kind routinely used as radiopharmaceuticals.

References

1. Wolf GL, Popp C: NMR, a Primer for Medical Imaging. Thorofare, New Jersey, SLACK, 1984.
2. Wolf GL, Burnett KR, Goldstein EJ, Joseph PM: Contrast agents for magnetic resonance imaging. *In* Magnetic Resonance Annual. New York, Raven Press, 1985.
3. Runge VM, Clanton JA, Lukehart CM, Partain CL, James AE: Paramagnetic agents for contrast-enhanced NMR imaging: A review. AJR, *141*:1209, 1983.
4. Brasch RC: Inherent contrast in magnetic resonance imaging and the potential for contrast enhancement. West J Med, *142*:847, 1985.
5. Sovak M (ed.): Radiocontrast Agents. Handbook of Experimental Pharmacology. New York, Springer-Verlag, 1984, p 73.
6. Chilton HM, Jackels SC, Hinson WH, Ekstrand KE: Use of a paramagnetic substance, colloidal manganese sulfide, as an NMR contrast material in rats. J Nucl Med *25*:604, 1984.
7. Eisenberg AD, Conturo TE, Mitchell MR, Schwartzberg MS, Price RR, Rich MF, Partain CL, James AE: Enhancement of red blood cell proton relaxation with chromium labeling. Invest Radiol *21*:137, 1986.
8. Lauffer RB, Grief LW, Stark DD, Vincent AC, Saini S, Weden VJ, Brady TJ: Iron-EHPG as an hepatobiliary MR contrast agent: initial imaging and biodistribution studies. J Comput Assist Tomogr *9*:431, 1985.
9. Canby RC, Elgavish GA, Reeves RC, Pohost GM: Biodistribution of the paramagnetic contrast agent Gd(BDP)₃ as measured by NMR relaxation rate enhancement of tissue water. Abstracts of the Fourth Annual Meeting of the Society of Magnetic Resonance in Medicine, 1985, p 842.
10. Burnett KR, Wolf GL, Shumacher HR, Goldstein EJ: Gadolinium oxide: a prototype agent for contrast enhanced imaging of the liver and spleen with magnetic resonance. Magn Reson Imag *3*:65, 1985.
11. Wolf GL: Vitalism and proton relaxation. Invest Radiol *21*:427, 1986.
12. Bloch F: Nuclear induction. Phys Rev *70*:460, 1946.
13. Spiller M, Koenig SH, Wolf GL, Brown RD: Compartmentalization of water and distribution of injected Gd-DTPA in the rabbit kidney medulla, investigated through the magnetic field dependence of 1/$T1$. Abstracts of the Fourth Annual Society of Magnetic Resonance in Medicine, 1985, p 904.
14. Laniado M, Weinmann HJ, Schorner W, Felix R, Speck U: First use of GdDTPA/dimeglumine in man. Physiol Chem Phys Med NMR, *16*:157, 1984.
15. Ehman RL, Brasch RC, McNamara MT, Erikkson U, Sosnovsky G, Lukszo J, Li SW: Diradical nitroxyl spin label contrast agents for magnetic resonance imaging, A comparison of relaxation effectiveness. Invest Radiol *21*:125, 1986.
16. Gries H, Niedballa U, Weinmann HJ: Patent Application. Derwente Number AN 85-051054/09.
17. Lauterbur PC, Mendonca-Dias MH, Rudin AM: Augmentation of tissue water proton spin-lattice relaxation rates by in vivo addition of paramagnetic ions. Front Biol Energ *1*:752, 1978.
18. Brown MA, Johnson GA: Transition metal-chelate complexes as modifiers in nuclear magnetic resonance. Med Phys *11*:67, 1984.
19. Weinmann HJ, Brasch RC, Press WR, Wesby GE: Characteristics of gadolinium-DTPA complex: a potential NMR contrast agent. AJR *142*:619, 1984.
20. Runge VM, Clanton JA, Herzer WA, Gibbs SJ, Price AC, Partain CL, James AE: Intravascular contrast agents suitable for magnetic resonance imaging. Radiology *153*:171, 1984.
21. Chen CW, Cohen JS, Myers CE, Sohn M: Paramagnetic metalloporphyrins as potential contrast agents in NMR imaging. FEBS Lett *168*:70, 1984.
22. Carr DH, Brown J, Leung AWL, Pennock JM: Iron and gadolinium chelates as contrast agents in NMR imaging: preliminary studies. J Comput Assist Tomogr *8*:385, 1984.
23. Tweedle MF, Brittain HG, Desreux JF, Gaughan GT: Gadolinium complexes as NMR contrast agents. J Nucl Med *27*:915, 1986.
24. Ochai E-I: Bioinorganic Chemistry, An Introduction. Boston, Allyn and Bacon, 1977, p 168. Fe; p 436, Mn.
25. Barb WG, Baxendale JH, George P, Hargrave KR: Reactions of ferrous and ferric ions with hydrogen peroxide. Trans Faraday Soc., *47*:462, 1951.
26. Bloembergen N, Purcell EM, Pound RV: Relaxation effects in nuclear magnetic resonance absorption. Phys Rev *73*:679, 1948.
27. Solomon I: Relaxation processes in a system of two spins. Phys Rev *99*:559, 1955.
28. Koenig SH, Brown RD: *In* Bertini I, Drago RS (eds): ESR and NMR of Paramagnetic Species in Biological and Related Systems. Dordrect, Reidel, 1979, p 89.
29. Oakes J, Smith E: Structure of Mn-EDTA²⁻ complex in aqueous solution by relaxation nuclear magnetic resonance. J Chem Soc Faraday 77:299, 1981.
30. Burgess J: Metal Ions in Solution. Chapter 11. Chichester, New York, Ellis Horwood, 1978.

31. Ogino H, Watanabe T, Tanaka N: Equilibrium and kinetic studies of the reactions of *N*-substituted ethylenediamine-N,N',N''-triacetatoaquochromium(III) with acetate ions. Inorg Chem *14*:2093, 1975.
32. Southwood-Jones RV, Earl WL, Newman KE, Merbach AE: Oxygen-17 NMR and EPR studies of water exchange from the first coordination sphere of gadolinium(III) propylenediamine-tetraacetate. J Phys Chem *73*:5909, 1980.
33. Alsaadi BM, Rossotti FJC, Williams RJ: Studies of lanthanide(III) dipicolinate complexes in aqueous solution. Part 2. Hydration. J Chem Soc 813, 1980.
34. Tweedle MF, Brittain HG, Krumwiede AL, Wedeking PW: Solution and tissue relaxivities of some paramagnetic complexes. Abstract 143. Int Soc Radiopharm Chem, 1986, p 325.
35. Bryden CC, Reilley CN: Europium luminescence lifetimes and spectra for evaluation of 11 europium complexes as aqueous shift reagents for nuclear magnetic resonance. Anal Chem *54*:610, 1982.
36. Horrocks W De W, Sudnick DR: Lanthanide ion probes of structure in biology. Laser induced luminescence decay constants provide a direct measure of the number of metal coordinated water molecules. J Am Chem Soc *101*:334, 1979.
37. Wedeking PW, Tweedle MF: Comparison of the biodistribution of 153-gadolinium–labeled Gd (DTPA)$^{-2}$, Gd (DOTA)$^{-1}$ and Gd (acetate) in mice. Int J Nucl Med Biol. In press.
38. Wieland DM, Tobes MC, Mangner TJ (eds): Analytical and Chromatographic Techniques in Radiopharmaceutical Chemistry. New York, Springer-Verlag, 1986.
39. Martell AE, Smith RM: Critical Stability Constants. Vol I. New York, Plenum Press, 1974.
40. Wagner JC: Fundamentals of Clinical Pharmacokinetics. Drug Intelligence Publications. Hamilton, Illinois, Hamilton Press, 1975.
41. Tweedle MF, Eckelman WC, Wedeking PW, Yost FJ: Pharmacokinetics and metabolism of 153-Gadolinium complexes. Abstract 142. Boston, Int Soc Radiopharm Chem, 1986, p 323.
42. Martell AE, Smith RM: Critical Stability Constants. Vol III. New York, Plenum Press, 1974.
43. Report of the Task Group on Reference Man. ICRP Publication 23. New York, Pergamon Press, 1984, p 290.
44. Price AC, Runge VM, Allen G, James AE: MR imaging contrast enhancement with Gd-DTPA: imaging experience with 30 intracranial neoplasms at 0.5 T. Radiology *157(P)*:37, 1985.
45. Runge VM, Price AC, Allen G, James AE: Sequence optimization for visualization of Gd-DTPA in human intracranial neoplastic disease. Radiology *157(P)*:37, 1985.
46. Grainger RG: Intravascular contrast media—the past, the present and the future. Br J Radiol *55*:1, 1982.

47

Intravenous Contrast Media

VAL M. RUNGE

HISTORICAL PERSPECTIVE

Since its introduction in the late 1970s, magnetic resonance imaging has rapidly evolved from an experimental technique to a significant clinical tool. Signal intensity in proton MRI depends upon at least four parameters: proton density, *T1, T2,* and flow. The advent of chemical-shift imaging adds an additional dimension, with the ability to discriminate between signals originating from water and fat (hydrocarbon chains). The clinical potential of MR was apparent very early owing to the high intrinsic tissue contrast and its noninvasive nature. Despite rapid clinical acceptance, investigators in 1982 continued to cite the need for intravenous contrast media.[1]

The use of paramagnetic metal ion chelates in MRI was first advocated by Runge et al. at the 1982 RSNA. This work led to the first published article in the field in mid-1983.[2] Chromium EDTA was identified as a prototype agent for this chemical group, from which gadolinium (Gd) DTPA has emerged as a likely compound for clinical application. Work with this agent (Berlex Laboratories, New Jersey, and Schering AG, West Berlin) has rapidly proceeded to Phase III clinical trials in both the United States and Europe.

Work with Cr-EDTA in vitro (Figs. 47–1 and 47–2) rapidly led to experimental animal work in late 1982 (Fig. 47–3) at 0.3 tesla.[3] At that point, cooperative work began with the University of Aberdeen, in Scotland. Having already confirmed the feasibility of intravenous contrast media application in animals, research was pursued with chromium EDTA in rabbits. The ability of contrast-enhanced MR to assess renal function (Figs. 47–4 and 47–5) was thus demonstrated in early 1983.[4]

Work continued at Vanderbilt University in mid-1983 upon delivery of one of the early Technicare 0.5 tesla instruments. High-resolution spin-echo images (in contrast to the spin-warp technique employed in Aberdeen) were thus obtained, with comparison studies of Cr-EDTA and Gd-DTPA and early pulse technique optimization pursued (Figs. 47–6 to 47–8).[5]

This work led to further animal experimentation elucidating other potential roles for intravenous contrast media, comparative studies with newer agents (including Gd-DOTA and non-ionic compounds), and clinical trials (see below). Parallel work with potential oral contrast agents, in particular the particulate compounds, has also been pursued and will be briefly summarized under New Contrast Media.

An alternative class of intravenous MR contrast agents was initially advocated by Brasch et al.[6]—the nitroxide spin labels. Although this chemical group has received much attention, no example has yet to reach clinical trials and is unlikely to do so in the future. This is primarily because of concerns about carcinogenesis and poor effectiveness of these agents when compared with paramagnetic metal ion chelates.

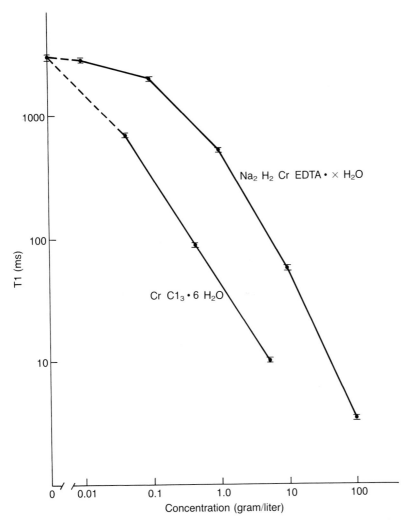

Figure 47–1. The paramagnetic effect of Cr-EDTA on $T1$, compared with that of free Cr 3^+ ion. In vitro, 90 MHz. (From Runge VM, et al: Invest Radiol *19*:408, 1984. Used by permission.)

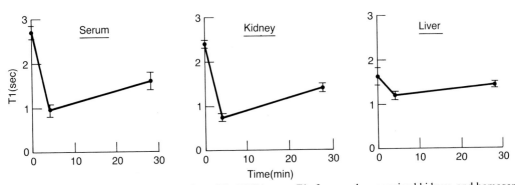

Figure 47–2. The effect of intravenous injection of Cr-EDTA upon $T1$ of serum, homogenized kidney, and homogenized liver (in mice). Each data point represents three animals, mean ± SEM. (From Runge VM, et al: Invest Radiol *19*:408, 1984. Used by permission.)

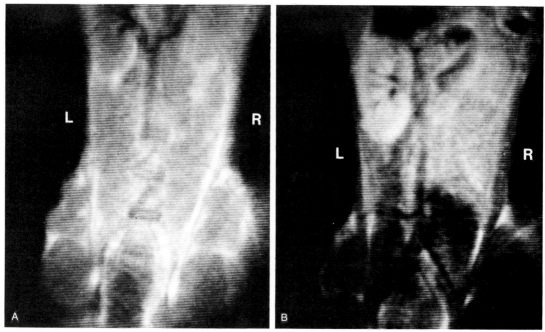

Figure 47–3. SE 500/30 coronal images of a canine at 0.3 tesla prior to (A) and following (B) IV administration of 0.1 gm/kg Cr-EDTA. Enhancement of the left kidney (cortex and medulla) is noted following contrast medium injection. (From Runge VM, et al: Invest Radiol *19*:408, 1984. Used by permission.)

RESEARCH

Relaxation agents such as Gd-DTPA (supplied as the meglumine salt by Berlex Laboratories and Schering AG) affect primarily $T1$ and $T2$ (Fig. 47–9). If the effect upon relaxation rate ($1/T1$ or $1/T2$) is plotted versus agent concentration, the resultant graph will be linear. The slope of the graph relates to the relative effectiveness of the agent. Referring to Figure 47–9, one will observe that Gd-DTPA has a much greater effect upon $T1$ than does Cr-EDTA, given equal concentrations. In this case, the disparity between agents is primarily a result of the difference in number of free electrons for Gd^{3+} versus Cr^{3+} (7 versus 3).

It is the $T1$ effect of the relaxation agents (in general) and not their $T2$ effect that is of interest. On spin-echo images, a decrease in $T1$, caused, for example, by the presence of Gd-DTPA, leads to an increase in signal intensity—thus "positive" contrast enhancement. Because of the complicated relationship of signal intensity in MR to $T1$, $T2$, and proton density, a decrease in $T2$ (which paramagnetic agents such as Gd-DTPA cause in addition to their $T1$ effect) leads to a reduction in SI. High contrast agent concentration thus appears as black on $T2$ weighted scans. Considering the effects upon $T1$ and $T2$ together, $T1$ weighted scans and contrast media with a relatively greater effect on $T1$ (versus $T2$) are desired to achieve "positive" enhancement. If one considers the actual curves of SI versus contrast agent concentration (Fig. 47–10), SI increases to a peak with increasing paramagnetic concentration, after which SI decreases. The upslope can be principally related to $T1$ effects, while the decrease in signal intensity with further increases in contrast agent concentration is caused by progressively more $T2$ shortening. With $T2$ weighted techniques, the upslope becomes less prominent, with negative enhancement becoming the dominant characteristic.

Early work (discussed previously) defined the ability of contrast-enhanced MRI to assess renal function. Experimental work in animals included models of normal renal

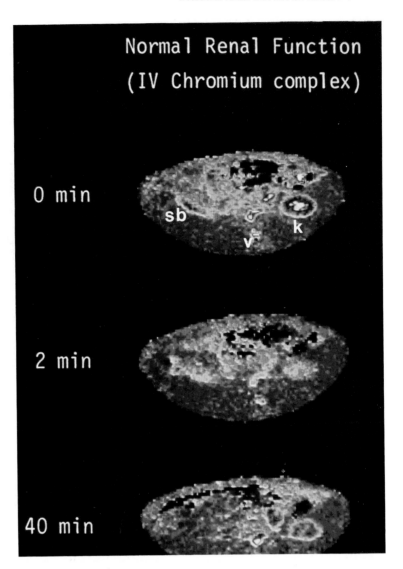

Figure 47–4. Axial calculated *T1* images of a rabbit at 0.04 tesla prior to and immediately following IV bolus injection of 0.07 gm/kg Cr-EDTA. *T1*'s of the kidney (k) are decreased by approximately 100 ms following paramagnetic chelate injection, as evidenced by the change in signal intensity in the kidney in the 2-minute image. In the 40-minute image, the kinetics of contrast enhancement are illustrated by the fact that the signal intensity in the kidney has returned toward the precontrast level owing to an increase in *T1* of the kidney (sb = small bowel; v = vertebral column). (From Runge VM, et al: Radiology *152*:123, 1984. Used by permission.)

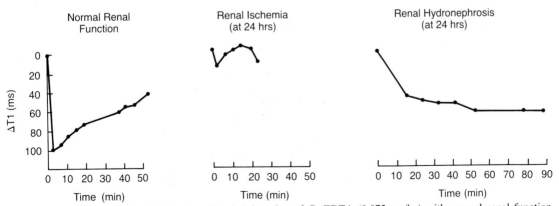

Figure 47–5. The change in *T1* following IV administration of Cr-EDTA (0.075 gm/kg) with normal renal function, ischemia, and hydronephrosis. (From Runge VM, et al: Radiology *152*:123, 1984. Used by permission.)

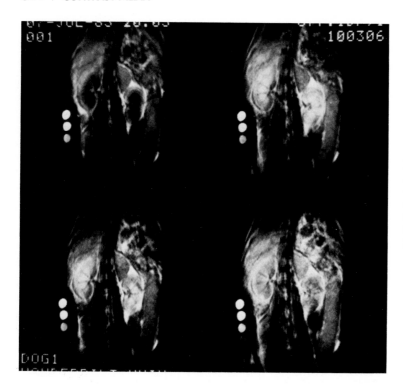

Figure 47–6. Coronal sections through the kidneys in a canine (0.5 tesla, SE 500/30 technique) prior to and following IV 0.25 mmol/kg Cr-EDTA administration. Normal renal function. (From Runge VM, et al: AJR *141*:1209, 1983. Used by permission.)

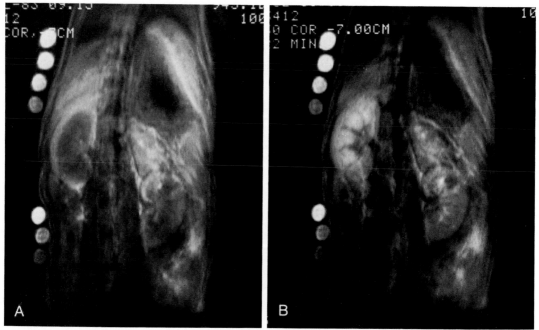

Figure 47–7. Acute right renal hydronephrosis in the canine, prior to (A) and 21 minutes following (B) IV injection of 0.25 mmol/kg Gd-DTPA. Retention of agent in the hydronephrotic right kidney, with prolonged enhancement, is noted. (From Runge VM, et al: AJR *141*:1209, 1983. Used by permission.)

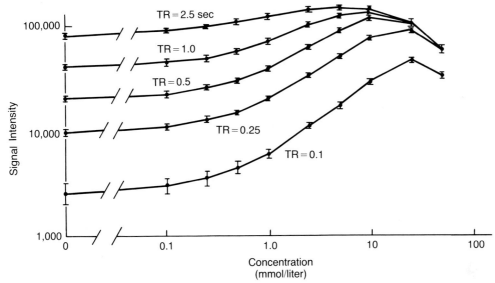

Figure 47–8. The dependence of signal intensity on both contrast agent concentration (in this instance, Cr-EDTA) and pulse technique at 0.5 tesla. TE = 30 ms. (From Runge VM, et al: AJR 141:1209, 1983. Used by permission.)

function, partial and total obstruction (hydronephrosis), and renal ischemia (ligation of renal artery and vein). With normal renal function, maximum enhancement of renal cortex and medulla is seen rapidly (within minutes) following intravenous injection. From this point, clearance of the agent is confirmed by a gradual reduction in SI of renal tissue with time over the next hour. These results have been confirmed with Gd-DTPA dosages of 0.1 to 0.25 mmol per kg. Higher dosages could potentially modify this effect if sufficiently high renal concentrations were achieved to manifest a "$T2$ effect" and thereby decrease SI.

Chromium-EDTA and gadolinium-DTPA[7] were compared in ten canines with normal renal function (Figs. 47–11 and 47–12). Excellent renal enhancement was achieved with each agent utilizing a dose of 0.25 mmol/kg IV. Enhancement was significantly greater and more prolonged with Gd-DTPA, primarily owing to its greater relaxivity

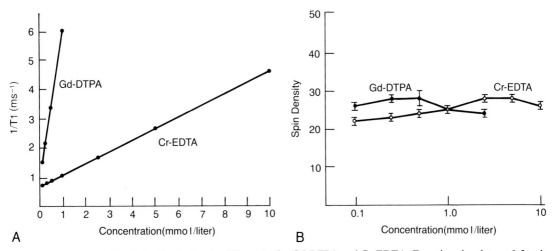

Figure 47–9. Calculated $T1$ (*A*) and spin-density (*B*) graphs for Gd-DTPA and Cr-EDTA. From imaging data at 0.5 tesla. (From Runge VM, et al: Radiology 153:171, 1984. Used by permission.)

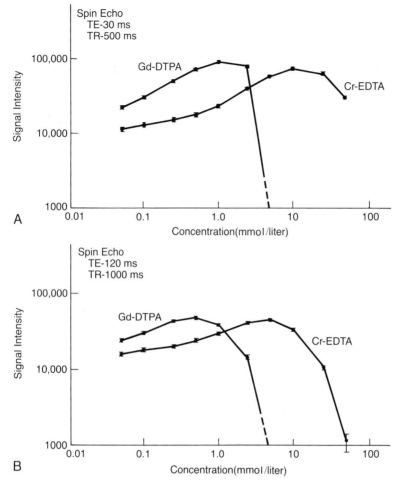

Figure 47–10. Signal intensity versus contrast agent concentration (data from a 0.5 tesla imager) for two pulse techniques: *TR/TE* 500/30 (*A*) and 1000/120 (*B*). The more *T1* weighted technique (500/30) emphasizes positive contrast enhancement to a greater extent than the more *T2* weighted sequence. With the *T2* weighted technique, negative enhancement (a decrease in signal intensity following contrast agent injection) is possible even at relatively low concentrations. (From Runge VM, et al: Radiology *153*:171, 1984. Used by permission.)

(relative effectiveness as a *T1* relaxation agent). Given this greater effectiveness at equal dosages and the known higher LD_{50} for Gd-DTPA, further experimental work concentrated on applications for Gd-DTPA.

In five canines a portion of the spleen and kidney was infarcted by surgical ligation of feeding arterial vessels.[7] MR examination was performed at 0.5 tesla approximately 24 hours following surgical intervention. These partial infarcts were confirmed by radionuclide and x-ray CT studies. Both *T1* weighted (IR 1500/450/30) and *T2* weighted images (SE 1000/120) were utilized in an attempt to visualize ischemic tissue prior to contrast agent injection. The splenic infarcts could be seen only in retrospect on heavily *T1* weighted images, and the renal infarcts were not visualized at all on precontrast images. These partial infarcts were well seen in all cases following injection of Gd-DTPA (Figs. 47–13 and 47–14). Some caution should be exercised in interpretation of these results, however, since the data presented may reflect, in part, the relatively primitive state of MRI development in 1983.

Following initial abdominal work, the application of Gd-DTPA to MRI of the central nervous system was rapidly investigated.[8] Using a canine alpha-streptococcus brain abscess model, seven animals were studied by both contrast-enhanced x-ray CT (GE 8800) and contrast-enhanced MRI (0.5 tesla Technicare). Each animal was studied at two time points during evolution of the abscess: early cerebritis (day 1) and late cerebritis (days 6 to 8). The abscess was created by surgical implantation of 10^8 colony-forming units of bacteria in 0.1 ml sterile 1 percent agarose.

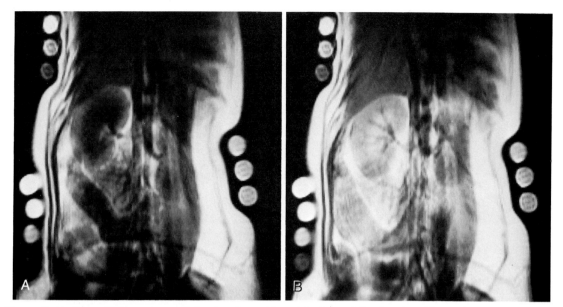

Figure 47–11. Coronal MR sections at 0.5 tesla prior to (*A*) and 6 minutes following (*B*) 0.25 mmol/kg Cr-EDTA (given as an IV bolus). The normal right kidney in this canine is displayed in cross section and is seen to enhance following IV injection of this paramagnetic metal ion chelate. (From Runge VM, et al: Radiology *153*:171, 1984. Used by permission.)

Contrast-enhanced MR proved to be more sensitive than either unenhanced MR or iodinated CT for the detection of early inflammatory changes. This was due to enhancement on MR of areas of blood-brain barrier (BBB) disruption following injection of Gd-DTPA. At the late cerebritis stage (Figs. 47–15 and 47–16), ring enhancement of the lesion was also noted, corresponding to the region of BBB breakdown. This permitted better differentiation of the central necrotic portion of the lesion from surrounding cerebral edema. As had been previously noted in CT studies, with time fol-

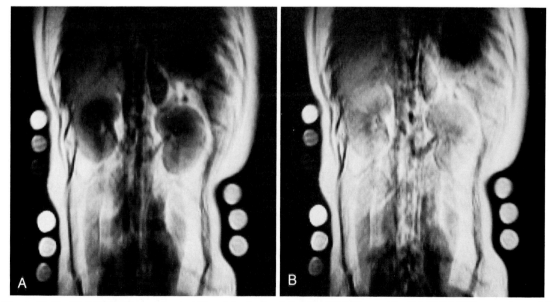

Figure 47–12. SE 500/30 images prior to (*A*) and 6 minutes following (*B*) 0.25 mmol/kg Gd-DTPA IV in a canine at 0.5 tesla. Uniform enhancement of both kidneys (seen in cross section) following contrast agent injection is noted. (From Runge VM, et al: Radiology *153*:171, 1984. Used by permission.)

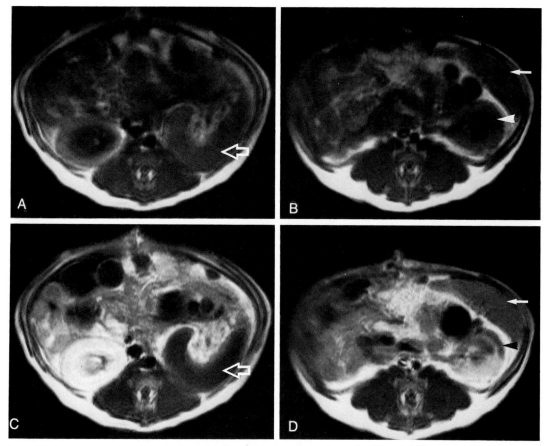

Figure 47–13. Acute partial splenic and renal infarction in a canine prior to (*A–B*) and following (*C–D*) 0.25 mmol/kg Gd-DTPA IV. Normal splenic tissue (small white arrow) enhances following contrast agent injection, unlike infarcted spleen (open arrow), which does not increase in SI post contrast. The right kidney and dorsal half of the left kidney enhance normally. The ventral portion of the left kidney is markedly abnormal on postcontrast images (arrowheads), owing to ischemia (acute ligation of arterial blood supply). (From Runge VM, et al: Radiology *153*:171, 1984. Used by permission.)

lowing injection of Gd-DTPA the ring of enhancement thickened and the central portion of the lesion filled in. Further studies with this model demonstrated the efficacy of Gd-DTPA as a contrast-enhancing agent at very low field strengths (0.15 tesla) and high fields (1.5 tesla). However, *T1* is prolonged with increasing field strength. Thus the effect of Gd-DTPA does change somewhat with the magnetic field, a finding that was confirmed by in vitro studies (Fig. 47–17).

Following this work, a canine model of BBB disruption using intra-arterial injection of hyperosmolar mannitol was investigated.[9] This model was used because of the large, uniform BBB lesion created and the time course of contrast enhancement. Following the initial increase in *SI*, enhancement is relatively stable 10 to 30 minutes post injection. Contrast enhancement using this model is illustrated in Figures 47–18 and 47–19.

This lesion proved to be difficult to detect on unenhanced MR (the lesion was identified in only one of five control animals), whereas it was readily recognized following Gd-DTPA administration (five of five animals). This finding again demonstrates the improved sensitivity of contrast-enhanced MR when compared with unenhanced studies. In a study of pulse technique efficacy, short spin-echo sequences and inversion-recovery techniques proved best for detection of Gd-DTPA. Specifically, the use of *TE*'s as short as 18 ms improved the contrast-to-noise ratio change from pre- to post-

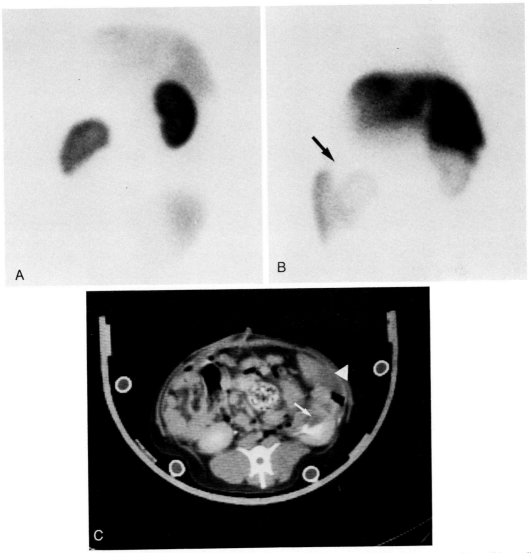

Figure 47–14. Confirmation of the partial renal and splenic infarcts illustrated in Figure 47–13 by radionuclide studies (*A–B*) and x-ray CT (*C*). *A*, Absence of activity in the infarcted portion of the left kidney in a posterior Tc-99m DMSA study. *B*, The upper pole of the spleen (arrow) is not visualized (owing to infarction) in a Tc-99m sulfur colloid examination. *C*, Lack of enhancement of a portion of both the spleen (arrowhead) and the left kidney (arrow) on x-ray CT following iodinated contrast injection. (From Runge VM, et al: Radiology *153*:171, 1984. Used by permission.)

contrast scans. Contrast enhancement is at times detected on *T2* weighted techniques, this being due to residual *T1* sensitivity with such sequences.

In vivo gadolinium concentrations were measured, allowing the first calculation of *T1* relaxivity due to Gd-DTPA in an experimental CNS lesion. In the area of BBB disruption, *T1* decreased typically by 300 ms following Gd-DTPA injection—with Gd concentration in the lesion being 0.12 mmol per kg (results determined by ion coupled plasma measurement). Relaxivity in vivo for Gd-DTPA was thus calculated to be 7.8 (inverse mmolar, inverse seconds), significantly higher than that (4.5) in aqueous solution.

Work has also proceeded with canine and rat glioma models (Figs. 47–20 and 47–21). Specialized receiver coils and pulse techniques are necessary to achieve high-resolution rat brain images (1.0 tesla unit, Siemens Medical Systems) such as those

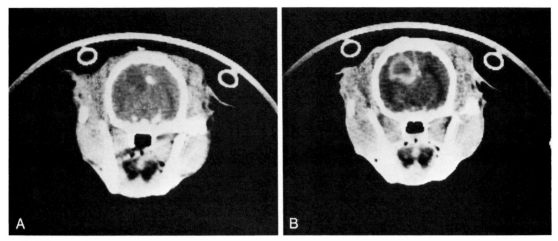

Figure 47–15. Precontrast (*A*) and postcontrast (*B*) x-ray CT of a canine α-streptococcus brain abscess. These examinations were made in correlation with Gd-DTPA contrast-enhanced MR. (From Runge VM, et al: Am J Neuroradiol 6:139, 1985. Used by permission.)

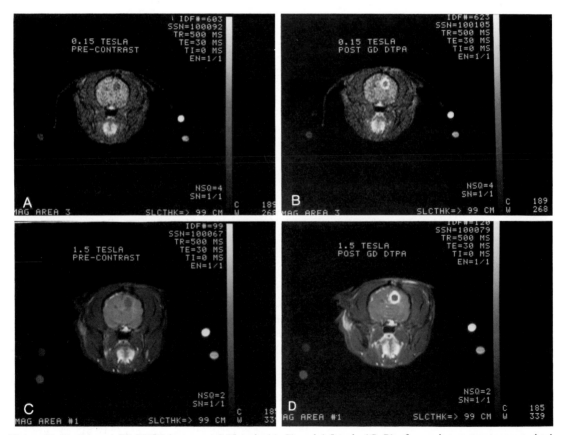

Figure 47–16. Coronal SE 250/30 images at 0.15 tesla (*A–B*) and 1.5 tesla (*C–D*) of a canine α-streptococcus brain abscess. Scans were obtained prior to and 10 minutes following 0.25 mmol/kg Gd-DTPA IV. Ring enhancement is noted in the region of blood-brain barrier disruption following contrast medium injection. The appearance correlates well with the CT scan in Figure 47–15. (From Runge VM, et al: Am J Neuroradiol 6:139, 1985. Used by permission.)

Gd-DTPA—T1
Change with Magnetic Field

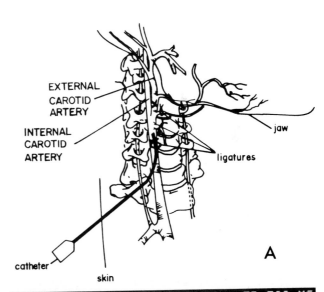

Figure 47-17. The effectiveness of a paramagnetic contrast agent, such as Gd-DTPA, is influenced by field strength. *T1* is prolonged with increasing field, and relaxivity (an expression of the general effectiveness of the agent) is lower.

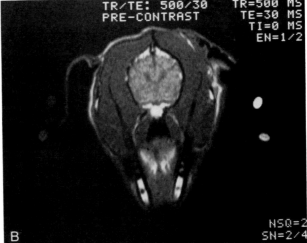

Figure 47-18. Disruption of the blood-brain barrier (BBB) induced by intra-arterial injection of hyperosmolar mannitol. *A*, Surgical placement of the arterial line.

Illustration continued on following page

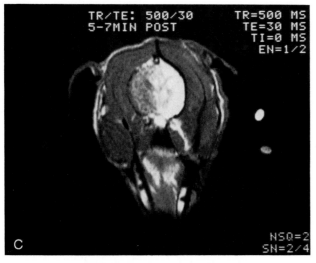

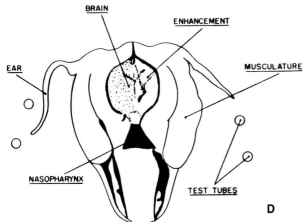

Figure 47–18 *Continued* Precontrast (*B*) and postcontrast (*C*) coronal images (SE 500/30) illustrating contrast enhancement in the left cerebral hemisphere following disruption of the BBB; 0.25 mMol/kg Gd-DTPA was injected intravenously. *D*, Diagram of *C* presented for orientation. (From Runge VM, et al: Invest Radiol *20*:830, 1985. Used by permission.)

shown in Figure 47–21. However, the development of a rat glioma model is highly desirable. Use of such a model would allow a statistical comparison of different contrast media, which might be available in only limited doses owing to their experimental nature.

In the heart, Gd-DTPA may provide for enhancement of ischemic myocardium, owing to its delayed washout (Fig. 47–22). Although this application has been demonstrated in experimental models,[10,11] the utility of Gd-DTPA contrast-enhanced MR in the detection and quantitation of human myocardial ischemia and infarction is as yet unknown.

NEW CONTRAST MEDIA

Following the advent of Gd-DTPA, alternative contrast media with potential for human application, such as Gd-DOTA and Gd-DO3A, have been suggested.[12] Gd-DOTA has imaging characteristics and pharmacokinetics quite similar to those of Gd-DTPA (Fig. 47–23). Synthetically this agent is, however, more difficult and costly to prepare in pure form. It offers no known advantages over Gd-DTPA. The development of stable non-ionic paramagnetic metal ion chelates, such as Gd-DO3A, should have a significant impact upon MRI. Toxicity theoretically could be substantially lower,

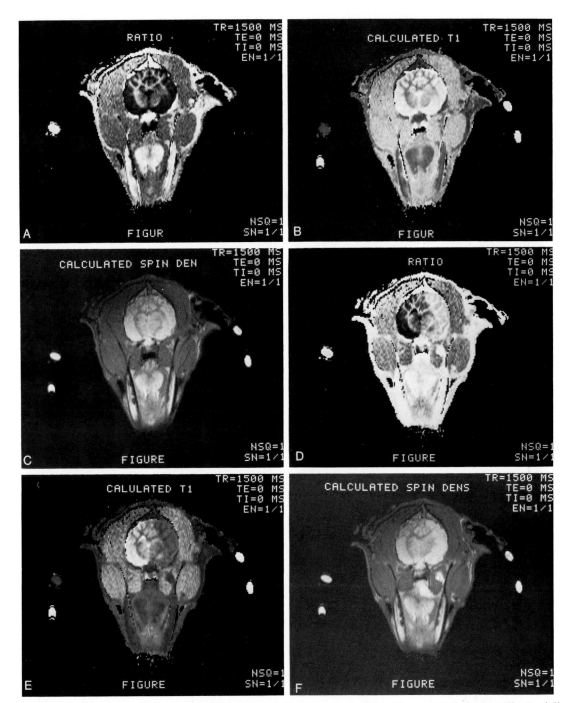

Figure 47–19. Pre–mannitol infusion ratio (*A*), calculated *T1* (*B*), and calculated spin-density (*C*) images. The "ratio" image is obtained by dividing the SI of an IR 1500/450/30 scan by that of a SE 1500/30 sequence. *D–F*, The same set of images is presented at 51 minutes following barrier disruption and IV injection of 0.25 mMol/kg Gd-DTPA. Contrast enhancement is noted as an increase in signal intensity on the ratio images (heavily *T1* weighted) and a decrease in SI on the calculated *T1* images (corresponding to a numerical decrease in *T1*). The spin-density image is relatively unaffected by contrast injection. (From Runge VM, et al: Invest Radiol *20*:830, 1985. Used by permission.)

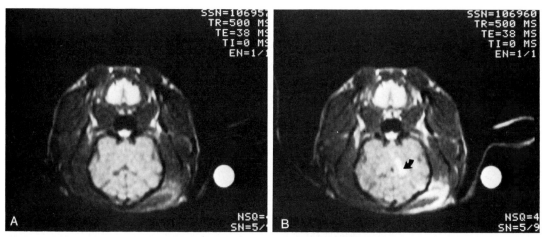

Figure 47–20. A canine gliosarcoma approximately two weeks following surgical implantation. Images are presented prior to (*A*) and following (*B*) IV Gd-DTPA administration. Enhancement is noted in the intracerebral and extracerebral components of the lesion.

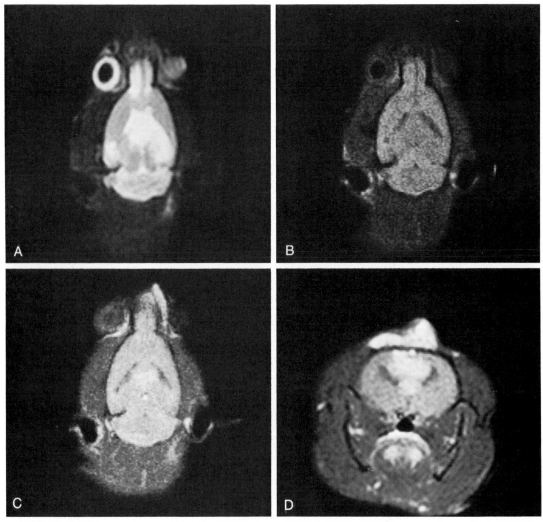

Figure 47–21. An implanted rat glioma on *T2* weighted (*A*) and *T1* weighted (*B–C*) SE technique. *C*, Following 0.25 mMol/kg Gd-DTPA injection IV. The lesion was initiated by stereotactic implantation of approximately 1 million live tumor cells. Growth of the tumor has caused hydrocephalus (seen on *A*). The lesion is best seen on the postcontrast scans (*C–D*, coronal image). A preacquisition magnification factor of 6 was utilized with 3 mm slice thickness (multislice acquisition). Results at 1.0 tesla.

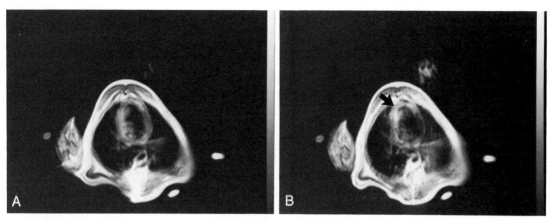

Figure 47–22. Enhancement of a region of myocardial ischemia in the canine. Images are prior to (*A*) and 20 minutes following (*B*) 0.25 mmol/kg Gd-DTPA IV. *TE* = 30 ms, data acquisition ECG-gated to every heartbeat. *B* is approximately 70 minutes following ligation of the distal LAD. (From Runge VM, et al: Physiol Chem Physics Med NMR *16*:113, 1984. Used by permission.)

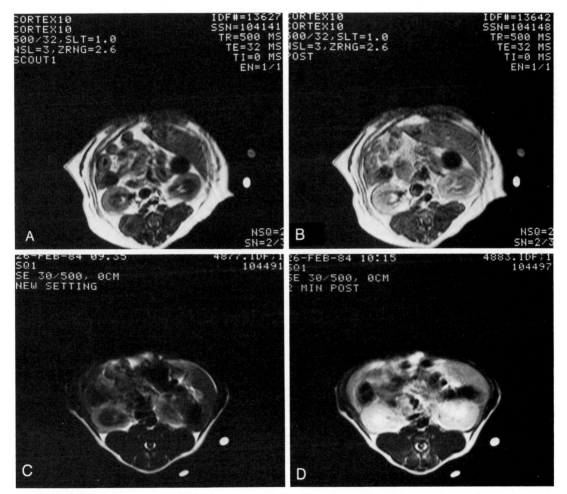

Figure 47–23. Comparison of renal enhancement with Gd-DTPA (*A–B*) and Gd-DOTA (*C–D*). Images are prior to and following IV administration of 0.1 mmol/kg of the respective gadolinium compound in a canine. Spin-echo 500/30 technique at 0.5 tesla.

allowing use of "megadoses"—at least an order of magnitude higher dosage than that currently permitted with Gd-DTPA. This could open up the detection of brain perfusion by use of contrast-enhanced MRI.

Development of intravenous contrast media with improved stability in vivo and enhanced relaxivity is also likely in the next few years.

Gd-DTPA and other intravenous contrast media of the paramagnetic metal ion chelate group can be formulated for oral administration and utilized for opacification of the gastrointestinal tract. Such oral contrast media are needed in MRI, particularly for improved imaging of the pancreas (by opacification of the C-loop of the duodenum) and for the differentiation of intra-abdominal mass lesions from fluid-filled bowel loops. Of particular interest are the particulate contrast media (see Chapter 48). These agents affect primarily $T2$, not $T1$, and result in a decrease in SI. Thus they are visualized as "black", although certain formulations may allow use as "positive" or "white" contrast media. These agents are insoluble. Therefore, the entire dosage is passed through the gastrointestinal tract without absorption, resulting in very low toxicity.[13]

CLINICAL APPLICATION

Animal investigation with Gd-DTPA has demonstrated the potential application of this agent for improved lesion visualization, improved sensitivity, and improved differentiation of central neoplastic tissue from surrounding cerebral edema. These projec-

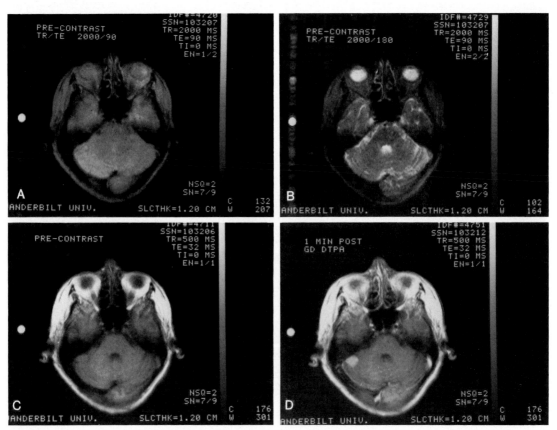

Figure 47–24. A small meningioma of the petrous ridge. This lesion is poorly identified on the precontrast images: SE 2000/90 (*A*), SE 2000/180 (*B*), and SE 500/32 (*C*). Following IV administration of 0.1 mmol/kg Gd-DTPA (*D*, SE 500/32), the lesion enhances strongly, making diagnosis possible. Images at 0.5 tesla.

tions have been confirmed in Phases II and III clinical studies in the United States with meglumine Gd-DTPA (Figs. 47–23 and 47–24). The detection of both intra- and extra-axial lesions (such as metastatic disease and meningiomas) is improved with Gd-DTPA. Small metastatic deposits and meningiomas may both exhibit $T1$'s and $T2$'s similar to normal brain tissue. Other such "isointense" CNS lesions may occur, in which case the use of an agent that identifies areas of BBB disruption will improve lesion detection (technique sensitivity). The use of a contrast agent such as Gd-DTPA also improves specificity to some degree, owing to the enhancement characteristics of a lesion. Meningiomas and glioblastomas are two such lesions in which a typical pattern of contrast enhancement adds some tissue specificity to the diagnostic interpretation. Gd-DTPA also improves the ability to differentiate between a central lesion and surrounding cerebral edema (Fig. 47–25).

MR continues to undergo rapid technological advances, with fast gradient echo techniques (Figs. 47–26 and 47–27) and half Fourier imaging being two significant recent developments. Angiography-like contrast-enhanced CNS studies (with single slice scan times <5 seconds) are thus feasible, opening yet another avenue for research and clinical application. Much, however, remains to be done in optimization of these techniques for both signal-to-noise (S/N) and tissue (or contrast agent) contrast. Single breath–hold imaging of the body is, however, possible (Fig. 47–27), perhaps conquering

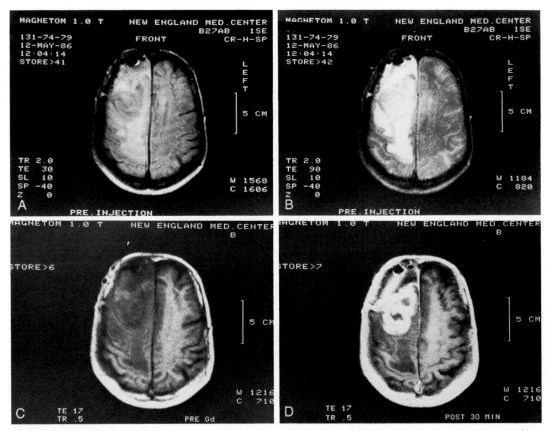

Figure 47–25. On precontrast images (*A–C*), neoplastic tissue cannot be differentiated with certainty from surrounding cerebral edema and postoperative change. *A*, SE 2000/30. *B*, SE 2000/90. *C*, SE 500/17. Clinical history: recurrent glioblastoma. Contrast enhancement with 0.1 mmol/kg Gd-DTPA enables identification of blood-brain barrier disruption, providing the best available marker of viable tumor tissue (*D*, SE 500/17). The pattern of enhancement (frondlike) also lends specificity in diagnosis.

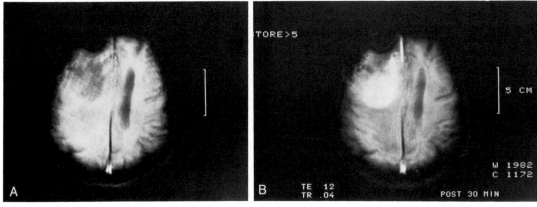

Figure 47–26. Precontrast (*A*) and 30 minutes postcontrast (*B*) 10-second FLASH technique images of the patient in Figure 47–25. Gradient echo technique with *TE* = 12 ms, *TR* = 40 ms, and a 40 degree tip angle; 128 × 256 image matrix, two acquisitions, 1.0 tesla field strength.

the one remaining stumbling block to successful application of MRI in the upper abdomen.

Gd-DTPA has emerged as the first agent likely to be approved for widespread use as a contrast agent for MRI. This paramagnetic metal ion chelate serves as a prototype for a large class of chemical compounds from which agents with improved relaxation properties and substantially lowered toxicity are likely to emerge in the next few years. This may include specifically the development of non-ionic paramagnetic metal ion chelates.

Gd-DTPA improves both the sensitivity and the specificity of MRI in the study of CNS disease (the latter because of the pattern of contrast enhancement observed). It also allows for improved lesion definition. The primary initial application of this agent will be in the study of intracranial neoplastic and inflammatory disease. The assessment of disease activity, for example, with multiple sclerosis, may be a secondary use.[14] Its application in body MRI is still under investigation, although animal studies and initial clinical trials indicate possible utility in multiple areas.

Paramagnetic metal ion chelates act as indirect contrast agents. The presence of these compounds causes a decrease in the *T1* and *T2* of surrounding protons (thus enhancing proton relaxation). This effect is quite different from the direct action of iodinated agents in conventional radiology.

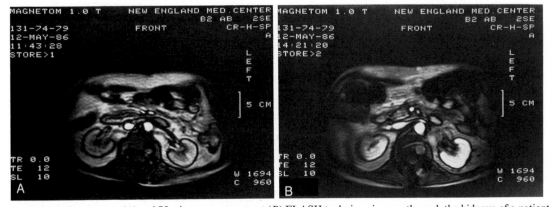

Figure 47–27. Precontrast (*A*) and 75 minutes postcontrast (*B*) FLASH technique images through the kidneys of a patient with normal renal function. Gradient echo 40/12, 40 degree tip angle, 128 phase-encoding steps, 10 second scan time, image acquisition performed during breath holding. Marked enhancement is seen in both kidneys owing to renal excretion of the intravenously administered Gd-DTPA.

It is the *T1* effect that is responsible for the increase in *SI* observed post contrast. Thus short spin-echo sequences, with high *T1* sensitivity, are utilized for contrast agent detection. Our own experimental work has included experimentation with *TE*'s as low as 12 ms (performed by Hahn spin-echo technique).

Perhaps the greatest advantage of MR contrast media, and specifically Gd-DTPA, (when compared with iodinated agents) is the absence of patient morbidity. Owing to the lower dosage (less than 1/20th that of an iodinated agent on a per gram basis), there has been no significant patient morbidity in the first 4000 examinations. Specifically, nausea, vomiting, and allergic reactions have not been observed. At present the only side effect noted is a transient increase in serum iron following intravenous administration.

Contrast enhancement with Gd-DTPA on MRI is generally superior to that observed on x-ray CT. Owing to this factor, the improved diagnostic quality of the examination (following contrast administration), and the low patient morbidity, paramagnetic metal ion chelates are likely to have a great impact upon MRI and thus even on the practice of radiology. Furthermore, this field is still in its infancy, with development of superior agents, additional applications, and differential targeting of compounds anticipated in the near future.

ACKNOWLEDGMENTS

This research was supported by both Berlex Laboratories (New Jersey), which supplied the meglumine salt of Gd-DTPA, and the Squibb Institute for Medical Research (New Jersey), which supplied the sodium salts of both Gd-DTPA and Gd-DOTA.

With many thanks to the researchers whose efforts made this work possible, including Dean Kaufmann, Mark Osborne, Michael Wood, John Kirsch, Samuel Wolpert, Jan Breslin, Joanne Incerpi, Jeff Clanton, Leon Partain, and A. Everette James, Jr.

With special thanks to Siemens Medical Systems for their technical assistance.

References

1. Young IR, Bailes DR, Burl M, et al: Initial clinical evaluation of a whole body nuclear magnetic resonance tomography. J Comput Assist Tomogr *6*:1, 1982.
2. Runge VM, Stewart RG, Clanton JA, et al: Potential oral and intravenous paramagnetic NMR contrast agents. Radiology *147*:789, 1983.
3. Runge VM, Clanton JA, Foster MA, et al: Paramagnetic NMR contrast agents: Development and evaluation. Invest Radiol *19*:408, 1984.
4. Runge VM, Foster MA, Clanton JA, et al: Contrast enhancement of magnetic resonance images by chromium EDTA: An experimental study. Radiology *152*:123, 1984.
5. Runge VM, Clanton JA, Lukehart CM, et al: Paramagnetic agents for contrast-enhanced NMR imaging: A review. AJR *141*:1209, 1983.
6. Brasch RC, London DA, Wesbey GE, et al: Work in progress: Nuclear magnetic resonance study of a paramagnetic nitroxide contrast agent for enhancement of renal structures in experimental animals. Radiology *147*:773, 1983.
7. Runge VM, Clanton JA, Herzer WA, et al: Intravascular contrast agents suitable for magnetic resonance imaging. Radiology *153*:171, 1984.
8. Runge VM, Clanton JA, Price AC, et al: Contrast enhanced magnetic resonance evaluation of a brain abscess model. Am J Neuroradiol *6*:139, 1985.
9. Runge VM, Price AC, Wehr CJ, et al: Contrast enhanced MRI: Evaluation of a canine model of osmotic blood-brain barrier disruption. Invest Radiol *20*(6):830, 1985.
10. Runge VM, Clanton JA, Price AC, et al: Paramagnetic contrast agents in magnetic resonance imaging: Research at Vanderbilt University. Physiol Chem Phys Med NMR *16*:113, 1984.
11. Runge VM, Clanton JA, Wehr CJ, et al: Gated magnetic resonance imaging of acute myocardial ischemia in dogs. Magn Reson Imag *3*:255, 1985.
12. Runge VM: Gd-DTPA: Experimental studies in animals—cardiac/blood-brain barrier. *In* Runge VM (ed): Contrast Agents in Magnetic Resonance Imaging. New York, Excerpta Medica, 1986.
13. Runge VM, Foster MA, Clanton JA, et al: Particulate oral NMR contrast agents. Int J Nucl Med Biol *12*(1):37, 1985.
14. Runge VM, Price AC, Kirshner HS, et al: The evaluation of multiple sclerosis by magnetic resonance imaging. RadioGraphics *6*(2):203, 1986.

48

Oral Contrast Agents

JEFFREY A. CLANTON

There has been periodic controversy regarding the need for contrast agents in conjunction with magnetic resonance imaging (MRI). This relatively new modality has an extensive number of pulse sequences that theoretically could provide adequate, natural contrast between normal and diseased tissues. Of the pulse sequences used today clinically, *T2* weighted images have demonstrated the greatest promise for soft tissue contrast differentiation, but *T2* weighting alone is not a practical technique because it has too many limitations associated with diagnostic accuracy, anatomic resolution, patient comfort, long collection times, susceptibility to motion artifacts, and economics. The concomitant use of contrast agents with *T1* weighted MR images helps to resolve these limitations. Thus, it is necessary to research the feasible development of oral contrast agents and explain what pharmaceutical considerations should be taken into account in the process of this development.

Numerous studies have been performed using various paramagnetic compounds for intravenous systemic contrast.[1-5] Initial human studies indicate that intravenous contrast will assist in the diagnosis of several types of brain lesions.[6,7] Unfortunately, only a limited number of studies have been performed using orally administered contrast agents for MRI.[8-11] Comparable to the development of computerized tomography (CT), MRI examinations of the abdomen and gastrointestinal tract have not been as effective as had been hoped. This lack of effectiveness is the primary result of technical problems, such as long acquisition times, which contribute to motion artifacts and the lack of appropriate contrast necessary to differentiate with certainty bowel from other abdominal structures.

PHARMACEUTICAL CONSIDERATIONS

The most important pharmaceutical considerations in developing and using any new drug—including oral contrast agents—are, of course, patient safety and effectiveness. There are, however, other requirements that are somewhat different for agents taken by mouth than for their intravenous counterparts, and these requirements vary (slightly) depending on the rate of absorption of the agent from the gastrointestinal tract.

Absorbed Agents

If a soluble contrast agent is to be used, several factors must be evaluated. First, the concentration and volume of the proposed agent for effective contrast of the gastrointestinal tract will have to be determined by experimentation with phantoms or animal models. Next, the amount of drug absorbed systemically will have to be determined at that dose level and compared with LD_{50} data. A safety level of 100:1 (lethal dose/absorbed dose) is considered practical in animal models. Once the initial safety and effectiveness of a contemplated oral agent has been established in animals, chemical evaluations should be performed.

Since the pH of the stomach and intestine varies substantially (1.2 versus 7.5), the new agent should be tested in simulated gastric fluid and simulated intestinal fluid[1] for chemical interaction and alteration. The absorption of an agent chemically transformed in the gastrointestinal tract could have disastrous effects on true toxicity. Finally, the agent should be tested in simulated gastrointestinal fluids with suspect orally administered therapeutic drugs (e.g., cholestyramine) for possible chemical effects.

Nonabsorbed Agents

The essential nature of nonabsorbed agents makes the toxicity of such compounds almost irrelevant. Similar to the absorbed agents, the concentration and volume must be determined for effectiveness. Next, strenuous testing of the compound in simulated gastrointestinal fluids should be performed and the results analyzed for any soluble species that would contribute to toxicity. Provided that the agent is found to be truly insoluble and its suspending agent is innocuous, possible drug interactions should be tested, as with the absorbed agents.

After the proposed agent has passed the in vitro and animal studies, the next required procedure is submitting a physician-sponsored Investigational New Drug Application (IND) with the Food and Drug Administration (FDA).

INVESTIGATIONAL NEW DRUGS

The first phase of studies involving an investigational drug requires that form 1571 be filed with the US FDA. Although the form itself is easy to address (Fig. 48–1), the material that must accompany this form, unfortunately, is rather voluminous. Among other items, the accompanying material must contain the name of the drug; the components used to prepare the drug and its final composition; the source and preparation of components; data obtained from animal studies regarding biodistribution, toxicity, proposed dose, and proposed use; and, finally, the methods of record-keeping as well as the qualifications of the investigators. After approval by the FDA and the investigator's institutional review committee, the Phase I trials can proceed.

Phase I investigations are designed to perform safety and biodistribution studies on a limited number of normal volunteers. They should be designed to foresee future problems (e.g., elevated liver enzymes) that might occur during the clinical trials and clinical use of the drug. Determination of biodistribution is also an important portion of Phase I studies owing to changes (sometimes alarming) attributed to species variation. Once Phase I studies are complete with no adverse findings, Phase II may begin.

Phase II studies are initiated by filing FDA form 1572. This form contains information similar to form 1571. In addition, it contains any changes in components or protocol made as a result of findings in the Phase I investigation as well as the results of the safety and biodistribution data in human volunteers. Phase II studies should be designed to study safety and effectiveness in a small group of patients and normal volunteers. Once the drug is deemed worthy after review of results in Phase II, it should be advanced to Phase III.

Phase III studies begin with the filing of FDA form 1573. This form contains all

---

DEPARTMENT OF HEALTH AND HUMAN SERVICES PUBLIC HEALTH SERVICE FOOD AND DRUG ADMINISTRATION	*Form Approved; OMB No. 0910-0014* *Expiration Date: December 31, 1984*
NOTICE OF CLAIMED INVESTIGATIONAL EXEMPTION FOR A NEW DRUG	**NOTE:** No drug may be shipped or study initiated unless a complete statement has been received. *(21 CFR 312.1(a)(2)).*

Name of Sponsor _____ Date _____

Address _____ Telephone ( )

Name of Investigational Drug _____

FOR A DRUG:

Food And Drug Administration
Office of New Drug Evaluation *(HFN-106)*
5600 Fishers Lane
Rockville, Maryland 20857

FOR A BIOLOGIC:

Food and Drug Administration
Office of Biologics *(HFN-823)*
8800 Rockville Pike
Bethesda, Maryland 20205

Dear Sir:

    The sponsor, _____ , submits
this notice of claimed investigational exemption for a new drug under the provisions of section 505(i) of the Federal Food, Drug, and Cosmetic Act and § 312.1 of Title 21 of the Code of Federal Regulations.

    Attached hereto in triplicate are:

Figure 48–1. Front page of US FDA form 1571.

the information from the previous two phases. The Phase III studies are designed primarily to determine effectiveness in a diverse group of patients, with an emphasis on the agent's safety. Normally, several hundred patients are enrolled in a closely controlled study designed to determine the performance of the new drug with differing individuals and varied levels of disease. Following the analysis and summation of this data, a New Drug Application (NDA) can be filed with the FDA. The typical time for approval of a NDA is 18 to 24 months.

ORAL CONTRAST AGENTS

    Oral contrast agents for MRI described to date can be divided into three classes: (1) soluble ionic agents, (2) soluble chelates, and (3) insoluble particulate paramagnetic and ferromagnetic preparations. For clarity, the various oral agents will be discussed as individual classes.

Soluble Ionic Agents

    This class of oral agents consists of ionic components such as ferric ammonium citrate, ferrous gluconate, and ferrous sulfate heptahydrate.[8,9] Since these components are the active ingredients of common NDA approved over-the-counter iron supplements (Geritol, Fergon, and Fer-In-Sol) and the amount of drug required to obtain adequate contrast in MRI does not exceed the recommended daily dose, a physician may use these as contrast agents without filing INDs or NDAs.

    Ferrous gluconate is easily utilized in the clinic by adding 20 ml of Fergon to 480 ml of water (5 mM) for patient administration. After oral ingestion, the stomach and C-loop of the duodenum are easily distinguished from other abdominal structures (Fig.

48–2). As with other images of the abdomen when MRI is used, respiratory motion as well as peristalsis creates artifacts. Therefore, for optimal studies, techniques such as respiratory gating and the administration of glucagon can be utilized to reduce motion artifacts (Fig. 48–2*B*). As with other soluble oral contrast agents, the soluble ionic preparations have some limitations.

Because of absorption and slow clearance of the paramagnetic iron, obtaining good resolution of the stomach and intestinal walls is difficult, if not impossible, with this class of agent. In addition, dilution with intestinal fluids combined with absorption makes it difficult to acquire images with good definition in regions beyond the duodenal C-loop.

Soluble Chelates

This class of compounds includes agents such as Gd-DTPA, Cr-EDTA, and Mn-EDTA. These agents are all investigational for human application and require appropriate documentation and approval if human use is anticipated. Of the aforementioned media, the only one with the appropriate stability and characteristics for use in humans appears to be Gd-DTPA. The oral administration of the soluble paramagnetic chelates provides good contrast of the stomach and intestine (Fig. 48–3). As previously described for soluble ionic agents, the stomach and intestinal walls are not easily distinguished (Fig. 48–4) owing to absorption of the agent. To date, no published data are available on the oral administration of soluble chelates in humans.

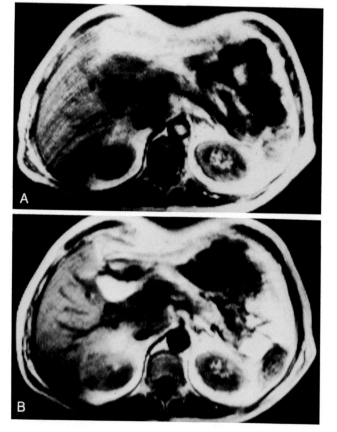

Figure 48–2. *T1* weighted (32/500 *TE/TR*) transverse image through the pancreatic region of a patient before (*A*) and after (*B*) the oral administration of 500 ml of 5 mM ferrous gluconate and application of respiratory gating during image acquisition.

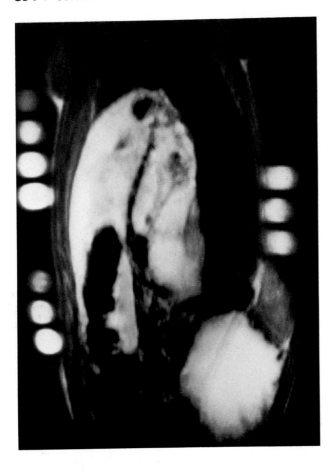

Figure 48–3. Coronal *T1* weighted image of a dog after the oral administration of Cr-EDTA via nasogastric tube. Seen faintly is the stomach, demonstrating enhancement of the stomach (increased intensity). Rectal addition of Cr-EDTA demonstrates contrast enhancement of intraluminal fluid in large bowel adjacent to fecal material.

Insoluble Particulates

Initial studies with insoluble particulate compounds for oral MRI contrast included agents such as gadolinium oxalate and insoluble forms of chromium.[12] More recent studies with this class of agent have centered on insoluble salts of paramagnetic iron.[13] These agents provide excellent definition of the stomach and intestinal walls as well as differentiation of the bowel from other abdominal anatomy (Fig. 48–5). The major advantage of this class of compound is that there is no absorption, which eliminates

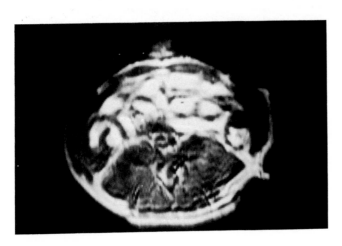

Figure 48–4. Transverse *T1* weighted image through the intestinal region of a dog following oral administration of Cr-EDTA. The differentiation provided by oral contrast agents between bowel and normal abdominal tissues is illustrated.

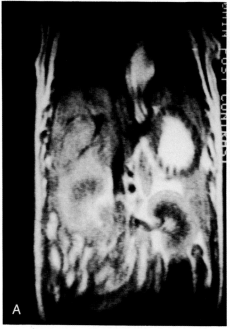

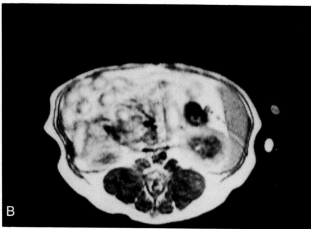

Figure 48–5. *T1* weighted image through the abdomen of a dog following oral administration of a paramagnetic insoluble iron compound. *A*, Coronal image through the region of the stomach. *B*, Transverse image of small intestine. Note the definition of gastric folds and bowel wall in comparison with the soluble oral agents.

toxicity problems and permits superb definition of the gastrointestinal tract. In addition, agents can be designed to provide "negative" gastrointestinal contrast similar to the use of air-contrast enhancement in CT (Fig. 48–6).

The particulate oral contrast agents are investigational, and no use in humans has been published to date.

Miscellaneous

Other agents proposed for oral use include ferromagnetic, albumin-coated magnetite[14] as well as Fluosol-DA for ^{19}F MRI.[15] The albumin-coated magnetite should correspond to negative insoluble particulate agents; however, no data on the solubility of this agent have been published.

The successful application of a promising agent such as Fluosol-DA will depend on the development and utilization of ^{19}F MRI. When utilized for this purpose, Fluosol-DA should correspond functionally to soluble chelated compounds.

Figure 48–6. *T1* weighted transverse image through the region of the stomach of a dog following oral administration of an insoluble compound that affects *T2* to a greater extent than *T1*, providing a "negative" (decreased intensity) gastrointestinal tract contrast agent.

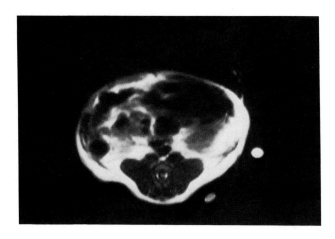

FUTURE DIRECTIONS

As previously discussed, motion artifacts that seriously degrade images in the abdomen have decreased the utility of MR in this region. Respiratory gating[16] used in conjunction with antiperistaltic drugs is a successful means of decreasing motion artifacts. Unfortunately, not all patients gate successfully and examination time is generally increased two to three times normal, limiting clinical usefulness. However, recent technical developments have demonstrated promise for the clinical application of abdominal imaging.

Of the methods recently described, low flip-angle imaging[16] as well as the respiratory compensating pulse sequences (e.g., ROPE, COPE, MAST, Exorcist) show excellent potential for abdominal MRI.

Fast-gradient echo, low flip-angle, and other fast-scanning techniques that provide abdominal data collections in less than 10 seconds are being evaluated. Fast acquisition of this type would allow data collection during a single breath-hold, thus eliminating detrimental motion artifacts. One sacrifice made by using these pulse techniques is low contrast, especially in the *T1* weighted pulse sequences.[18,19] Therefore, as these sequences become more prevalent in the clinical environment, paramagnetic oral contrast agents will be utilized more extensively to provide contrast lost in the utilization of fast scanning, in addition to providing increased lesion/bowel differentiation.

The respiratory compensating techniques use more standard pulse sequences and are fairly effective at eliminating artifacts due to respiratory motion. With these techniques, the problem of differentiating abdominal structures and bowel loops that simulate lesions still exists. Therefore, the use of oral MR contrast, both positive and negative, will increase diagnostic sensitivity and specificity.

References

1. Runge VM, Clanton JA, Lukehart CM, et al: Paramagnetic agents for contrast enhanced NMR imaging: A review. AJR *141*:1209, 1983.
2. Weinmann HJ, Brasch RC, Press WR, Wesbey GE. Characteristics of gadolinium-DTPA complex: A potential NMR contrast agent. AJR *142*:619, 1984.
3. Young IR, Clarke GJ, Bailes DR, et al: Enhancement of relaxation rate with paramagnetic contrast agents in NMR imaging. CT *5*:543, 1981.
4. Runge VM, Foster MA, Clanton JA, et al: Contrast enhancement of magnetic resonance images by chromium EDTA: An experimental study. Radiology *152*:123, 1984.
5. Brasch RC: Work in progress: Methods of contrast enhancement for NMR imaging and potential applications. Radiology *147*:781, 1983.
6. Carr DH, Brown J, Bydder GM, et al: Gadolinium-DTPA as a contrast agent in MRI: Initial clinical experience in 20 patients. AJR *143*:215, 1984.
7. Schörner W, Felix R, Laniado M, et al: Human testing of the nuclear spin tomographic contrast medium gadolinium-DTPA. Tolerance, contrast affect, and the 1st clinical results. ROFO *140*(5):493, 1984.
8. Runge VM, Stewart RG, Clanton JA, et al: Potential oral and intravenous paramagnetic NMR contrast agents. Radiology *147*:789, 1983.
9. Wesbey GE, Brasch RC, Engelstad BL, et al: Nuclear magnetic resonance contrast enhancement study of the gastrointestinal tract of rats and a human volunteer using nontoxic oral iron solutions. Radiology *149*:175, 1983.
10. Wesby GE, Brasch RC, Goldberg HI, et al: Dilute oral iron solutions as gastrointestinal contrast agents for magnetic resonance imaging: initial clinical experience. Magn Reson Imag *3*(1):57, 1985.
11. Runge VM, Clanton JA, Price AC, et al: Paramagnetic contrast agents in magnetic resonance imaging: research at Vanderbilt University. Physiol Chem Phys Med NMR *16*(2):113, 1984.
12. Runge VM, Foster MA, Clanton JA, et al: Particulate oral NMR contrast agents. Int J Nucl Med Biol *12*(1):37, 1985.
13. Unpublished data obtained at Vanderbilt University, 1986.
14. Renshaw PF, Owen CS, McLaughlin AC, et al: Ferromagnetic contrast agents: A new approach. Magn Reson Med *3*(2):217, 1986.
15. McFarlan E, Koutcher JA, Rosen BR, et al: In vivo ^{19}F NMR Imaging. J Comput Assist Tomogr *9*(1):8, 1985.

16. Haase A, Frahm J, Matthaei D, et al: FLASH imaging: Rapid NMR imaging using low flip angle pulses. J Magn Reson *67*:258, 1986.
17. Runge VM, Clanton JA, Partain CL, James AE Jr: Respiratory gating in magnetic resonance imaging at 0.5 tesla. Radiology *151*:521, 1984.
18. Osborne MA, Runge VM, Wood M, Kirsch J: Clinical applications of FLASH and FISP. (Abstr. Tam-A3). Society for Magnetic Resonance Imaging, 5th Annual Meeting, San Antonio, February 28–March 4, 1987.
19. Hahn D, Nägele M, Seelos K, Lissner J: Gd-DTPA contrast enhancement in conventional and fast MR-imaging of mediastinal masses. (Abstr. Wam-B1). Society for Magnetic Resonance Imaging, 5th Annual Meeting, San Antonio, February 28–March 4, 1987.

49

Free Radical Contrast Agents for MRI

EDWARD J. GOLDSTEIN
GERALD L. WOLF
ROBERT C. BRASCH

Contrast agents for use in MRI must have the property of localizing in a tissue zone, either normal or pathologic, and altering the MRI signal intensity arising from that zone such that the region of contrast localization becomes more readily distinguished from surrounding areas. Materials that are paramagnetic as a consequence of having unpaired electrons in outer orbitals have the ability to alter signal intensity by causing significant changes in tissue proton relaxation times, $T1$ and $T2$. These concepts have been discussed elsewhere in this text and extensively in the literature and will not be presented in this chapter.[1,2]

Free radicals are substances with unpaired electrons that endow them with paramagnetic properties. These compounds are currently under investigation for application as MRI contrast agents. Most free radicals that have been produced in the chemistry laboratory or that occur in nature are short-lived intermediates in a chemical reaction with half-lives in the range of thousandths to millionths of a second. Examples of two free radical intermediates are seen in the following structures.

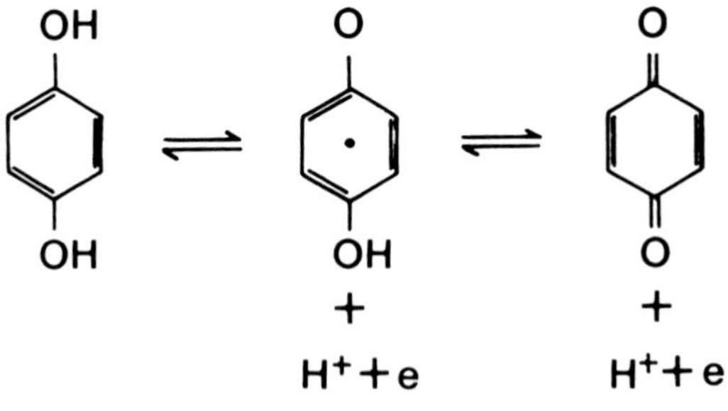

Hydroquinone   Semiquinone   Quinone

The free radical species semiquinone and methyl radical are at an excited state relative to the ground-state hydroquinone and azomethane. These are highly reactive species and have short half-lives. The $T_{1/2}$ for semiquinone is far greater than for methyl radical, since its unpaired electron can be incorporated in a large electron cloud distributed over the entire molecule in a form of resonance stabilization. A second mech-

$$CH_3-N=N-CH_3 \xrightarrow{h\gamma} 2CH_3\cdot + N_2$$

Azomethane   Methyl radical

anism whereby free radicals may acquire stability results from steric hindrances at the free radical reaction site. This means that there are structural components at or near the reactive site that block a second atom or molecule from easily reaching this area. A reaction is thus less likely to occur. When a free radical undergoes a reaction at the unpaired electron site, the molecule loses its paramagnetic property.

Because free radicals are so reactive as electron donors, they may react indiscriminately in an inappropriate manner in naturally occurring biologic systems. To curb this process, naturally occurring compounds are present in biologic systems, such as reduced glutathione, that act as antioxidants by reacting with the active radicals to eliminate them in a benign reaction pathway.

For a free radical to be effective as an MRI contrast agent it must be stable, in order to retain in vivo its paramagnetic property. The compound must also be safe, such that no significant adverse effect or abnormal biochemical process occurs either directly or indirectly from metabolites. Certain nitroxyl compounds appear to fulfill these criteria. The nitroxyl group may be represented in Lewis resonance structures: The unpaired electron is delocalized in the molecular orbitals between nitrogen and oxygen, which aids in stabilization of the free radical moiety. The formal charge on

Nitroxyl Resonance Structures

the resonance structure at the left is zero on both O and N. The structure on the right has a formal charge of $+1$ on N and -1 on O for a net charge of zero. The formal charge on an atom is estimated by subtracting the sum of half the shared electrons plus all the unshared electrons around the atom from its valence electrons. Nitrogen has five valence electrons, oxygen six. We can see that in both resonance structures an unpaired electron exists, rendering the molecule paramagnetic.

Brasch and coworkers[4,6,7,11] have studied two such nitroxyl compounds, PCA 3-carboxy-2,2,5,5-tetramethyl-1-pyrrolidinyloxy and TES 4-[(3-carboxy-1-oxopropyl) amino]-2,2,6,6-tetramethyl-1-piperidinyloxy for use as MRI contrast agents. Nitroxyl

compounds undergo degrees of reduction to the nonparamagnetic hydroxyamine and are partially devitalized in vivo as MRI contrast agents. In the compounds PCA and TES, the methyl groups flanking the nitroxyl group sterically hinder the approach of potential reducing agents (e.g., ascorbic acid) and to some degree prolong the half-life of these reagents in vivo and in vitro.

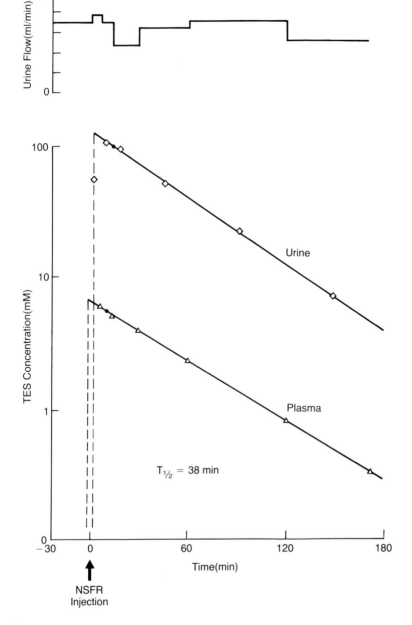

Paramagnetic   Non-paramagnetic

After intravenous administration these reagents are primarily eliminated via the urinary tract (over 80 percent) in either the nitroxyl or the reduced hydroxylamine form. The five-membered ring structure (PCA) is more resistant to reduction than the

Figure 49–1. Graph demonstrating TES concentrations in the urine and plasma of a cat following intravenous administration of TES, 1.0 gm/kg, indicates a biologic half-life (T½) of 38 minutes. Urine flow demonstrates a relatively uniform rate (top curve). The clearance rate suggests that TES is excreted by glomerular filtration (lower two curves). (From Brasch RC, et al: Radiology *147*:775, 1983. Used by permission.)

six-membered ring. Following the intravenous introduction of TES in cats the renal clearance of TES was observed to be 9.8 ml/min, a value approximating the GFR. The biologic $T_{1/2}$ was determined to be approximately 38 minutes (Fig. 49–1).[3] Only trace levels of TES, <0.005 mmol/L, were detected in CSF. This reagent does not appear to significantly cross the intact blood-brain barrier. Curves for the elimination of TES in low and high doses from the blood stream in rats are depicted in Figure 49–2.[4]

Griffith and coworkers have demonstrated that the strongly charged forms of nitroxyl compounds, such as quaternary salts, are less fat-soluble and have a different tissue distribution than the less ionic, more lipophilic compounds.[4] Tissue distributions from rat experiments are shown in Figure 49–3. These data were obtained via EPR spectra of tissue homogenates after intravenous introduction of nitroxyl compounds. The ability to alter the lipid solubility of nitroxyl compounds by altering structure may lead to a method of controlling the target organs or target tissue zones of these MRI contrast agents.

In rats the LD_{50} of PCA was determined to be 15.1 mmol/kg and that of TES between 15.1 and 25.2 mmol/kg.[5] For comparison, the meglumine diatrizoate salt demonstrated an LD_{50} of up to 37 mmol/kg. The more ionic salt may be less toxic owing to decreased tissue concentration as a consequence of decreased lipophilic property and more rapid urinary clearance. These LD_{50} values are more than 100 times the least effective contrast-enhancing dose. No genotoxic effects of PCA and TES, or their reduced metabolites, have been observed in cell cultures. In vitro MRI imaging of TES solutions using spin-echo technique demonstrated increasing signal intensity with increasing TES concentrations up to 10 mmol/L followed by a decrease in signal intensity with further increases in TES concentration (Fig. 49–4).[3]

At the operating parameters (*TR, TE*) used in this study, the phenomenon observed

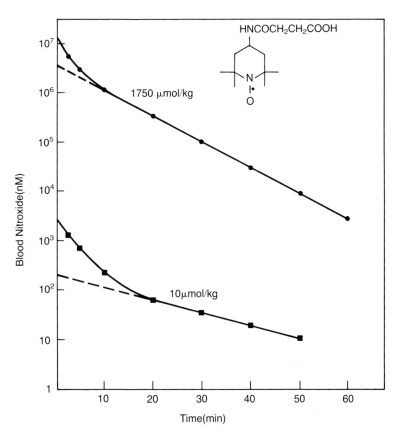

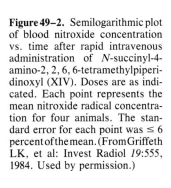

Figure 49–2. Semilogarithmic plot of blood nitroxide concentration vs. time after rapid intravenous administration of *N*-succinyl-4-amino-2, 2, 6, 6-tetramethylpiperidinoxyl (XIV). Doses are as indicated. Each point represents the mean nitroxide radical concentration for four animals. The standard error for each point was ≤ 6 percent of the mean. (From Griffeth LK, et al: Invest Radiol *19*:555, 1984. Used by permission.)

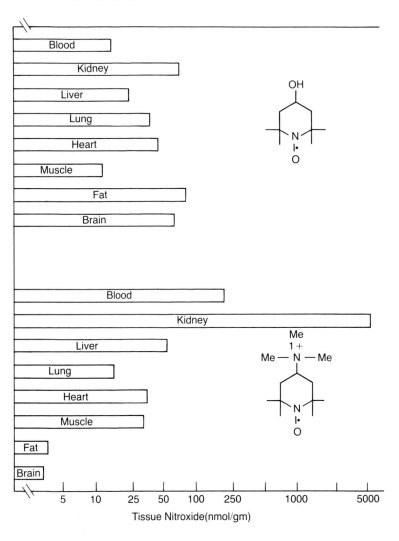

Figure 49–3. Tissue distribution of two nitroxides 60 minutes after high-dose (1.75 mmol/kg) administration is depicted. Each value represents the mean nitroxide radical concentration for four animals. The standard error for each value was ≤10 percent of the mean. A simple non-ionized nitroxide (III) was found to be almost equally distributed among the various tissues examined. In contrast, a completely ionized quaternary ammonium nitroxide (VII) was excluded from lipophilic tissues (e.g., fat and brain) and is roughly 100 times more concentrated in the kidney than in the remaining tissues investigated. (From Griffeth LK, et al: Invest Radiol *19*:561, 1984. Used by permission.)

occurs, since *T1* and *T2* affect signal intensity in opposite ways. As *T1* decreases, signal intensity increases; when *T2* decreases, however, signal intensity decreases. The paramagnetic nitroxyl compound reduces both *T1* and *T2*. Initially the *T1* effect dominates the signal intensity up to 10 mmol/L. Beyond this concentration, the *T2* shortening effect begins to dominate and reverses the signal intensity profile.

Canine renal imaging with PCA is demonstrated in Figure 49–5.[6] Intravenous administration of PCA at 1.0 mmol/kg was used for these images, which were obtained on a 0.35 tesla superconducting facility with spin-echo technique (*TE* at 28 ms and *TR* at 1000 ms). Significant contrast enhancement is observed in the kidney at 12 minutes post injection. No adverse effects in the dogs were observed. Using a rat model with unilateral hydronephrosis, the change in signal intensity arising from the remaining functioning kidney after intravenous administration of TES at 0.5gm/kg is seen (Fig. 49–6).[3]

Magnetic resonance imaging of acute canine myocardial infarcts was conducted with and without the use of PCA.[7] Infarcts in adult mongrel dogs were created by ligation of the left anterior descending coronary artery distal to the first septal branch. Dog hearts were imaged in vitro 24 hours post ligation. Dogs with hearts to be imaged after use of contrast received 3.0 mmol/kg of PCA intravenously, 5 or 15 minutes prior to sacrifice. Imaging was carried out within two hours post sacrifice with a 0.35 tesla

Figure 49–4. Graph of changes in spin-echo intensity signals from test tubes containing increasing concentrations of TES. The intensity change is nonlinear with respect to NSFR concentration, which can be attributed to the differential effects of NSFR on *T1* and *T2* relaxation enhancement at various concentrations. The maximum intensity, observed at 10.0 mmol/L for two echo delays (28 and 56 ms), is approximately 300 percent higher than the intensity signal of water. (From Brasch RC, et al: Radiology *147*:775, 1983. Used by permission.)

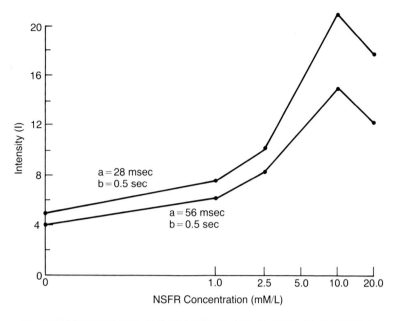

Figure 49–5. Enhancement of canine kidney with PCA (arrowhead). (From Ehman RL, et al: Magn Reson Imag *3*:96, 1985. Used by permission.)

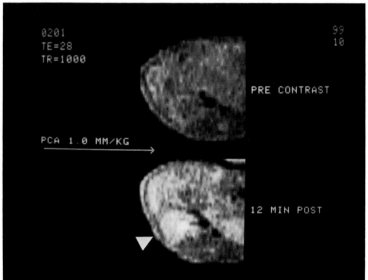

Figure 49–6. Enhancement of normal kidney (arrow) with IV TES in rat with unilateral hydronephrosis. (From Brasch RC, et al: Radiology *147*:778, 1983. Used by permission.)

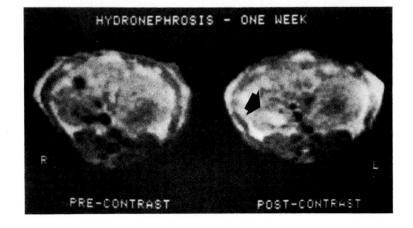

Table 49–1. IMAGE INTENSITY AND RELAXATION TIMES FOR CONTROL GROUP: NO PCA

Dog	T1 (ms) Normal Myocardium	Infarct	% Difference T1	T2 (ms) Normal Myocardium	Infarct	% Difference T2	% Difference Intensity (N vs. I)*
1	516	567	10	38	47	24	33
2	662	793	20	39	50	38	42
3	599	618	3	43	53	23	14
Mean	592.3	659.3	11.0	43.3	46.7	25.0	30
SD	73.2	118.5	4.0	8.4	3.5	2.6	14

* = SE 2000/56.
SD = standard deviation; N = normal myocardium. I = infarcted myocardium; ms = milliseconds.
From McNamara ML, et al: Invest Radiol 20:592; 1985. Used by permission.

superconducting facility using spin-echo technique. With T2 weighted precontrast images, increased signal intensity was observed at the site of infarction owing to increased T2 values (Table 49–1). The T1 values were also prolonged in the infarct. This increase in relaxation time at the infarct site is partially due to increased water content arising from edema.[8–10] Following the use of contrast media, T1 and T2 values at the infarct site were shortened; however, the effect was greater on T1 such that the T1 values were lower at the infarct relative to normal myocardium, whereas the T2 values remained higher (Table 49–2). These results suggest that PCA localized in five minutes at the infarct site to a greater degree than in normal myocardium, resulting in significant focal T1 shortening. Proton relaxation times were calculated from the images. A calculated T1 image of a myocardial infarct heart is seen in Figure 49–7. The infarct appears as a low signal intensity zone in the T1 weighted image.

Cerebritis secondary to experimentally produced abscesses in dogs was studied with MRI in conjunction with the intravenous use of TES.[11] Contrast enhancement is observed at the abscess site in postcontrast views (Fig. 49–8). These images were obtained on a 0.35 tesla superconducting facility at TR = 0.5 sec and TE = 28 ms using spin-echo technique. Greatest enhancement is seen 10 minutes post injection.

PCA has been used to improve tumor soft tissue contrast in xenograft implants of human breast carcinoma in athymic mice.[6] After intravenous administration of PCA at 3 mmol/kg, significant contrast enhancement of the subcutaneous tumor is observed at 4 minutes post injection (Fig. 49–9).

The investigation of stable paramagnetic free radicals for use as MRI contrast agents is at a very early stage. Nitroxyl-containing compounds have drawn particular attention as potential MRI contrast agents because of their chemical versatility; they

Table 49–2. IMAGE INTENSITY AND RELAXATION TIMES FOR PCA GROUP: 5 MINUTES POSTINJECTION

Dog	T1 (ms) Normal Myocardium	Infarct	% Difference T1	T2 (ms) Normal Myocardium	Infarct	% Difference T2
4	659	339	−39	33	43	12
5	632	463	−27	40	43	8
6	673	484	−28	39	42	7
Mean	645.7	448.7	−31.3	39.0	42.7	9.0
SD	20.8	44.3	6.7	1.0	0.6	4.0

SE 500/56.
SD = standard deviation; ms = milliseconds.
From McNamara ML, et al: Invest Radiol 20(6):592, 1985. Used by permission.

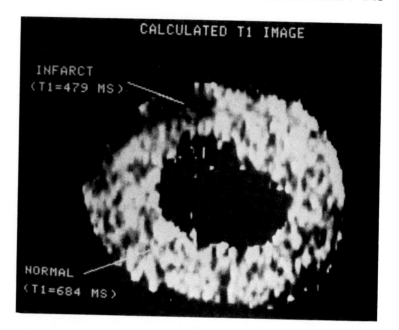

Figure 49–7. Calculated *T1* image of canine myocardial infarct following IV PCA. (From McNamara ML, et al: Invest Radiol *20*:594, 1985. Used by permission.)

can be synthesized with widely varying properties of size, lipophilicity, and charge. Nitroxyls can also be readily conjugated to carrier molecules. Furthermore, these compounds, by virtue of their small molecular weight, are capable of penetrating into cells and thus potentially probing the intracellular environment. These favorable properties must, however, be weighed against their lack of complete in vivo stability and the

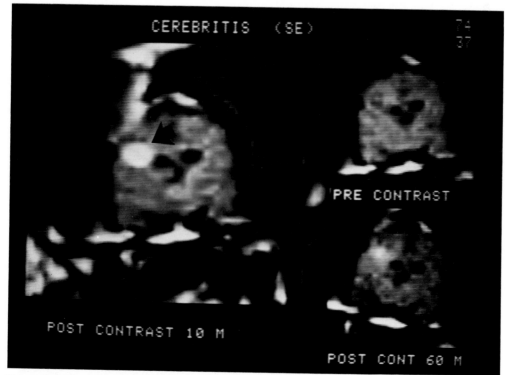

Figure 49–8. Contrast enhancement of cerebritis following use of IV TES (arrow). (From Brasch RC, et al: AJNR *4*:1037, 1983. Used by permission.)

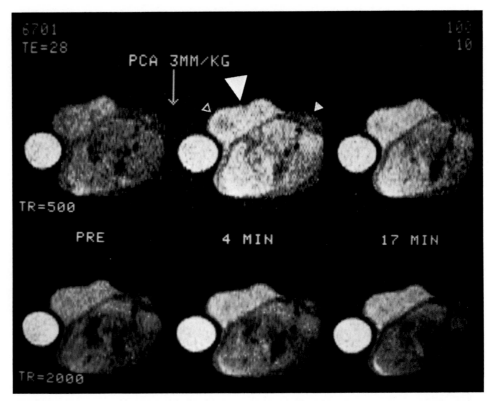

Figure 49–9. Enhancement of breast carcinoma xenograft (arrowhead) in an athymic mouse using IV PCA as the contrast agent. (From Ehman RL, et al: Magn Reson Imag *3*:91, 1985. Used by permission.)

relatively weak proton relaxation effects of nitroxyls. Early results, however, are encouraging.

References

1. Wolf GL: Contrast enhancement in biomedical NMR: A symposium. Physiol Chem Phys *16*:(2):1, 1984.
2. Wolf GL, Burnett KR, Goldstein EJ, Joseph PM: Contrast agents for magnetic resonance imaging. *In* Kressel HY (ed): Magnetic Resonance Annual. New York, Raven Press, 1985.
3. Brasch RC, et al: Nuclear magnetic resonance study of a paramagnetic nitroxide contrast agent for enhancement of renal structures in experimental animals. Radiology *19*:559, 1984.
4. Griffeth LK, et al: Pharmacokinetics of nitroxide NMR contrast agents. Invest Radiol *19*:559, 1984.
5. Afzal V, Brasch RC, Nitecki DE, Wolff S: Nitroxyl spin label contrast enhancers for magnetic resonance imaging: studies of acute toxicity and mutagenesis. Invest Radiol *19*:549, 1984.
6. Ehman RL, et al: Enhanced MRI tumors utilizing a new nitroxyl spin label contrast agent. Magn Reson Imag *3*:89, 1985.
7. McNamara ML, et al: Magnetic resonance imaging of acute myocardial infarction using a nitroxyl spin label (PCA). Invest Radiol *20*:591, 1985.
8. Hazlewood CF, Cleveland G, Medina D: Relationship between hydration of proton nuclear magnetic resonance relaxation times in tissues of tumor bearing and non-tumor bearing mice. J Natl Cancer Inst *52*:1848, 1974.
9. Brown J, Slutsky R: Proton nuclear magnetic resonance tissue analysis of normal, volume overloaded and dehydrated rabbit myocardium. Am Heart J *108*:159, 1984.
10. Higgins CB, et al: Nuclear magnetic resonance imaging of acute myocardial infarction in dogs. Am J Cardiol *52*:184, 1983.
11. Brasch RC, et al: Brain nuclear magnetic resonance imaging enhanced by a paramagnetic nitroxide contrast agent. AJNR *4*:1035, 1983.

50

Iron Ethylene bis (2-Hydroxyphenylglycine) as a Hepatobiliary MRI Contrast Agent

RANDALL B. LAUFFER
THOMAS J. BRADY

The superiority of proton (^{1}H) magnetic resonance (MR) imaging for lesion detection is apparent in certain anatomic regions such as the central nervous system and is explained by exogenous differences in proton relaxation behavior in normal and pathologic tissue.[1-3] The initial experience of MR imaging of the liver does not reflect the same high level of sensitivity. If only a single pulse sequence is employed, lesions can be missed. Thus, multiple spin-echo (SE) and inversion-recovery (IR) pulse sequences are often necessary to confidently exclude liver disease. In addition, if the relaxation times of the specific pathology overlap normal values, the sensitivity is reduced irrespective of the pulse sequence utilized. Current MR imaging techniques employed to screen the liver for focal lesions are therefore time-consuming and no more sensitive than computed tomography (CT).[4]

To improve the sensitivity and clinical efficacy of MR imaging of the liver, suitably designed paramagnetic contrast agents may offer great potential. These agents are usually complexes of transition or lanthanide metal ions, the unpaired electrons of which give rise to a large magnetic moment that efficiently relaxes the protons of coordinated or solvated water molecules. The predominant effect of such substances in MR imaging is to increase signal intensity owing to decreases in the longitudinal relaxation time (TI).[5-12] To date, the development of MR contrast agents has emphasized derivatives such as Gd(DTPA)$^{-2}$, which have a nonspecific distribution in the extracellular space.[9-13] While offering great potential for evaluating the integrity of the blood-brain barrier,[9-11] this agent holds less promise in hepatic imaging. Extracellular agents localize in lesions as well as normal liver and thus can reduce inherent tissue contrast and even obscure lesions.[12] Clearly, an agent whose distribution reflects organ function, as opposed to passive distribution in the extracellular space, would be preferable for detection of liver lesions.

TARGETING STRATEGIES FOR LIVER ENHANCEMENT

Of the two major cell types present in the liver, the Kupffer cells and hepatocytes, the former are more often the targets of imaging agents in nuclear medicine. These reticuloendothelial (RE) cells, along with those in the spleen and bone marrow, avidly scavenge particulate substances from the blood. This uptake mechanism forms the basis of the widely employed ^{99m}Tc sulfur colloid scan for detection of focal liver disease.[14]

An alternative RE-targeting strategy is to enclose the imaging agent within liposomes, which are cleared in a similar fashion.

Preliminary investigations reveal that both particulate and liposomal preparations can be utilized to direct paramagnetic Mn^{+2} to the liver, yielding significant changes in the liver relaxation times.[15,16] Nevertheless, the Kupffer cells may not be the optimal target for a hepatic MR contrast agent. These cells constitute approximately 2 percent of the liver volume,[17] and thus a paramagnetic agent contained within them may enhance the relaxation rates of only a portion of the total water protons that give rise to the observed signal. The dominant signal arises from water in the hepatocytes, which constitute 78 percent of the liver volume.[17] The relaxation rates of the water molecules in these cells will be affected by an RE-targeted relaxation agent only if the rates of water exchange between the two populations of cells is very fast or if the agent is transferred into the hepatocytes. The formulation and stability of pharmacologically acceptable suspensions or liposomes also represent a major problem for the clinical use of these agents. In addition, an RE-avid agent can have extensive residence times in the body, which may increase its long-term toxicity. This is a major concern for the recently investigated ferromagnetic iron particles.[18] These substances are very effective in reducing the $T2$ (and therefore signal intensity) of liver and spleen but are retained indefinitely in these tissues as well as in the lungs, creating the potential for eventual carcinogenic response (via free radical generation, for example) or other toxic effects.

A more attractive target for a hepatic MR contrast agent are the polygonal cells of the liver, which are particularly adept in the extraction, metabolism, and biliary excretion of a wide variety of endogenous and exogenous compounds. The ^{99m}Tc-iminodiacetic (^{99m}Tc-IDA) complexes currently used in nuclear medicine exploit this biliary excretion pathway, allowing sequential visualization of hepatic parenchyma, bile ducts, and gallbladder in normal individuals as well as in the detection of pathologic states.[19] The uptake of a suitable paramagnetic agent would reflect hepatocellular function, and the efficient clearance of the substance would minimize toxicity and provide enhanced high-resolution images of biliary structures. In addition, such an agent would presumably have direct contact with most of the liver water and thus might be more effective than RE agents (on a mole-to-mole basis) in altering the tissue relaxation times.

REQUIREMENTS FOR A HEPATOBILIARY MR CONTRAST AGENT

General requirements in the design and use of a clinically applicable hepatobiliary MR agent include the following:
1. Sufficient hepatocellular uptake and biliary excretion of the compound.
2. Sufficient paramagnetism to alter the relaxation times of the liver parenchyma.
3. Stability of the compound in vivo, both before and after biliary excretion.
4. Low toxicity or high margin of safety for the effective dose.

CHOICE OF FE(EHPG)⁻ AS A PROTOTYPE HEPATOBILIARY AGENT

In consideration of the foregoing requirements, we selected the high-spin iron(III) complex of ethylene bis(2-hydroxyphenylglycine) [Fe(EHPG⁻)] for initial evaluation.[20] A major reason for selecting this complex, besides its paramagnetic properties, is the structural requirement for biliary excretion rather than renal excretion. While almost any small molecular weight and hydrophilic complex will be nonspecifically filtered into the urine, biliary excretion appears to be more selective. Properties such as polarity, molecular weight, and chemical structure determine what percentage of an administered compound is excreted in the bile. Although the exact details of the hepatic uptake and transport of compounds to the bile are not known, the overall requirements for biliary excretion include a molecular weight greater than 300 and a balance between lipophilic and hydrophilic characteristics.[21,22]

The structure of Fe(EHPG)$^-$ is shown in Figure 50–1. The EHPG ligand is a hexadentate chelating agent that wraps tightly around the ferric ion, coordinating in an octahedral manner with two nitrogens, two carboxylate oxygens, and two phenolic oxygens.[23] The overall structure is similar to that of the ^{99m}Tc-IDA complexes used in cholescintigraphy.[19] The common features include molecular weights greater than 400 [412 for Fe(EHPG)$^-$ and greater than 600 for the ^{99m}Tc-IDA derivatives], octahedral coordination of the metal ion, a single negative charge, and two phenyl rings.

The chemical properties of Fe(EHPG)$^-$ are favorable for in vivo applications. Most importantly, the stability afforded by a hexadentate ligand is superior to, for example, the use of two tridentate ligands, such as the IDA derivatives. The metal-ligand formation constant of Fe(EHPG)$^-$ is 10^{34} M^{-1}, which makes it one of the most stable metal complexes ever characterized.[24] Transferrin, a circulating iron transport protein, has a formation constant for iron of only 10^{22} M^{-1} [25] and has been shown to be unable to remove iron from Fe(EHPG)$^-$.[26] In addition, Fe (EHPG)$^-$ is stable over a pH range of 3.6 to 10[26] and undoubtedly has a very low reduction potential arising from the metal-phenol interaction, which stabilizes the trivalent state.[27] This latter property will prevent conversion to the highly labile ferrous complex by in vivo reductants such as ascorbate. The total enclosure of the metal ion by the hexadentate chelate also prevents the formation of the cytotoxic hydroxyl radical, which can be generated by the Fenton reaction in the presence of superoxide and iron complexes with open coordination sites.[28]

The water relaxation ability, or relaxivity, of Fe(EHPG)$^-$ appears adequate despite the fact that the six-coordinate EHPG ligand, while providing for the stability of the complex, simultaneously prevents direct water coordination to the iron center. It is generally thought that one or more open coordination sites on a paramagnetic complex are required for a close approach of the water protons to the metal ion and thus appre-

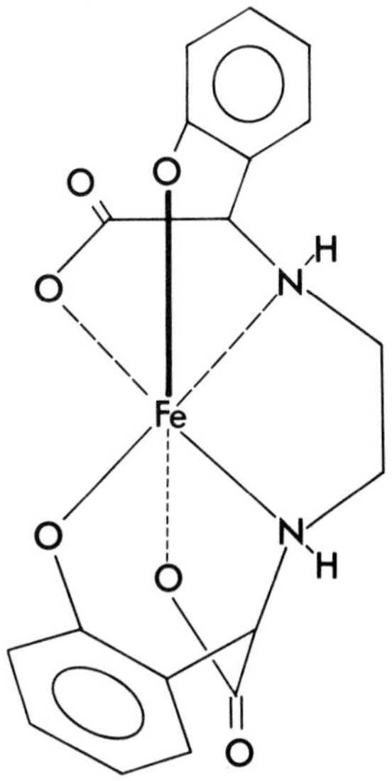

Figure 50–1. Structure of Fe(EHPG)$^-$. Other isomers exist owing to the chirality of EHPG. (From Lauffer RB, et al: J Comput Assist Tomogr 9:431, 1985. Used by permission.)

ciable relaxivity. However, waters of solvation that form hydrogen bonds to coordinating heteroatoms can bring a number of solvent protons sufficiently close. The cumulative effect of these "outer sphere" waters yields appreciable relaxivity. The measured longitudinal relaxivity for Fe(EHPG)$^-$ (change in $1/T1$ of water protons per mM of complex), $R_1 \sim 1$ s^{-1}mM^{-1} (20 MHz and 37°) is not that much lower than that for Gd(DTPA)$^{-2}$ (~ 4 s^{-1}mM^{-1}) when the higher magnetic moment of Gd^{3+} and single water coordination site of the latter is taken into account.[20]

Interestingly, the relaxivity in vivo may be somewhat higher than in solution. Any binding of the complex to serum albumin, intracellular proteins, or membrane structures will hinder the molecular motion and may lead to some enhancement in relaxivity.[29] Indeed, in the case of human serum albumin, we have recently shown that substantial binding of Fe(EHPG)$^-$ derivatives to this plasma protein can occur and that the binding enhances the relaxivity roughly twofold.[30]

INITIAL EVALUATION OF FE(EHPG)$^-$

We found that the intravenous administration of 0.2 mmol/kg Fe(EHPG)$^{-1}$ to fasted rats produced a rapid increase in the signal intensity of the liver with the use of the IR 1460/400/15 pulse sequence on a 1.4 tesla imaging system.[20] Figure 50–2 shows the preinjection and various postinjection images of the rat liver in one experiment. With our experimental parameters, the liver intensity increases approximately 200 percent in the first few postinjection images and then decreases over time. The average liver intensities observed in three animals after administration of Fe(EHPG)$^-$ are plotted in Figure 50–3. These values are background-subtracted and normalized to any changes in phantom intensities.

The clearance of the agent is observed over a three-hour period, with an apparent $t_{1/2}$ (time between maximum and half-maximum intensities) of approximately 80 minutes. These image changes are consistent with significant uptake of Fe(EHPG)$^-$ by

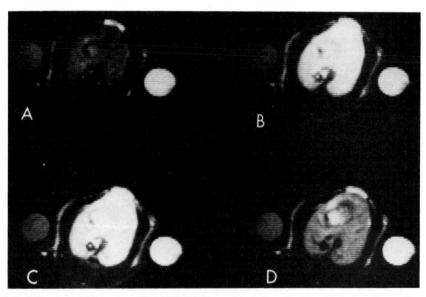

Figure 50–2. Transverse MR images (IR 1460/400/15) at a level through the midportion of a rat liver before (*A*) and 16, 56, and 182 minutes after intravenous administration of 0.2 mmol/kg Fe(EHPG)$^-$ (*B–D*, respectively). The images depict the animal on its back with the bright phantom on the left side. (From Lauffer RB, et al: J Comput Assist Tomogr 9:431, 1985. Used by permission.)

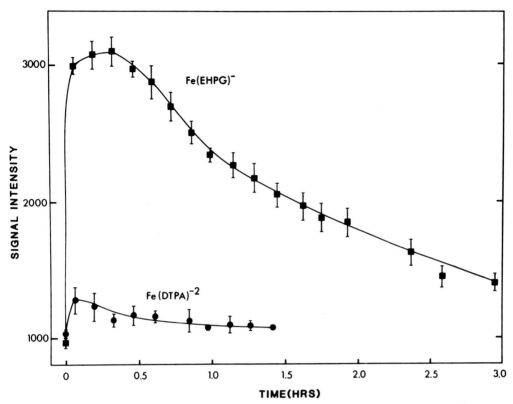

Figure 50–3. Average signal intensities (mean ± s.d.) of the liver on IR 1400/400/15 MR images of rats over time after intravenous administration of $Fe(EHPG)^-$ or $Fe(DTPA)^{-2}$. The intensity values were background subtracted and normalized for any changes in phantom intensities. Values shown are averages of three animals in each group. (From Lauffer RB, et al: J Comput Assist Tomogr 9:431, 1985. Used by permission.)

the liver and slow but efficient excretion into the bile, in good agreement with a previous report.[31]

Imaging studies conducted with equivalent doses of a different iron chelate, $Fe(DTPA)^{-2}$, revealed only small and transient increases in liver intensity. The average intensities observed over 90 minutes (n = 3) are compared with those seen with $Fe(EHPG)^-$ (Fig. 50–3). Administration of $Fe(DTPA)^{-2}$ increases the liver intensity only ~30 percent in the first postinjection image, and the clearance of the agent follows at $t_{1/2}$ of ~30 minutes. These observations reflect the known extracellular distribution of $Fe(DTPA)^{-2}$, which results in relatively low liver uptake and rapid renal excretion.[32]

The imaging characteristics of $Fe(EHPG)^-$ in rats compared well with rat bio-distribution behavior. We found that 20 percent of the injected dose of the ^{59}Fe-labeled complex (0.2 mmol/kg, n = 6) was present in the liver 10 minutes after intravenous administration. This uptake caused a substantial increase in the $1/T1$ of the liver, from 3.2 to 4.3 s^{-1} (20 MHz, n = 3), leading to the image-enhancement effects observed. No significant alterations of $1/T2$ outside of the error in these measurements were found.

Other experiments demonstrate conclusively that $Fe(EHPG)^-$ is excreted into the bile. Figure 50–4 displays pre- and postinjection abdominal images of a dog obtained on a 0.6 tesla imaging system using an IR 1500/200/20 pulse sequence. The agent increases the liver intensity approximately 70 percent (seen better on other slices directly through the liver) and causes an intense signal from newly formed bile in the gallbladder that layers on top of the denser, previously concentrated bile with low signal intensity. Direct evidence for biliary excretion of $Fe(EHPG)^-$ was obtained in a rabbit experiment

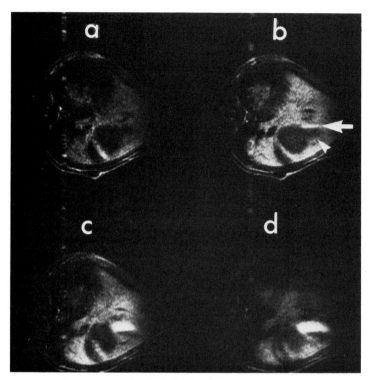

Figure 50–4. Transverse MR images (IR 1500/200/20) at the level of the gallbladder in a dog positioned on its right side before (*a*) and 14, 50, and 60 minutes after intravenous administration of 0.2 mmol/kg Fe(EHPG)⁻ (*b–d*, respectively). Bile in the gallbladder prior to injection appears dark (arrowhead), whereas newly formed bile appears bright (arrow) and layers on top. (From Lauffer RB, et al: J Comput Assist Tomogr 9:431, 1985. Used by permission.)

in which bile was collected by bile duct cannulation post injection. Visible spectra and *T1* measurements confirmed the presence of high concentrations of the intact metal complex.

The successful results with Fe(EHPG)⁻ in three species of animals ensure that this and similar complexes will have considerable hepatocellular affinity in humans as well. The use of several species (especially rabbits) in screening hepatobiliary agents for human use is important, since there can exist a marked variation among species as to the percentage of a substance that will be excreted into bile.[21,22]

Nevertheless, we expect that improvements over Fe(EHPG)⁻ both in relaxation efficiency and in liver targeting can be achieved. Certainly, a suitable Gd^{3+} hepatobiliary agent would be preferable on the basis of higher relaxivity and hence lower effective dose; such agents are currently under development in our laboratory. Toward the improvement of Fe(EHPG)⁻, the ligand itself can be modified to achieve higher liver uptake with its Fe^{3+} complexes. Substituted EHPG complexes of $^{99m}Tc^{3+}$ or ^{68}Ga, particularly the 5-chloro and 5-bromo derivatives, have been reported to have much higher biliary excretion ratios, and therefore doses much lower than 0.2 mmol/kg may be effective using the iron complexes of these ligands.[33,34]

The acute intravenous toxicity of Fe(EHPG)⁻ is unknown at present, but evidence suggests that the 0.2 mmol/kg dose used in the present study for contrast enhancement is well tolerated. No ill effects over a two to three month period were observed at this or at a tenfold higher dose. Furthermore, the free ligand EHPG has been administered to human patients at comparable dose levels in early studies on iron metabolism, with no untoward effects.[35] It should be noted that, while the clinical use of analogous hepatobiliary media for CT (e.g., isoefamate[36]) has been limited by toxicity considerations,[37] the margin of safety for MR agents most likely will be higher owing to the smaller doses necessary for contrast enhancement.

THE IMPORTANCE OF PULSE SEQUENCE SELECTION

The reproducibility of Fe(EHPG)$^-$ uptake and clearance in the rat as well as the large homogeneous sampling area of the liver prompted a systematic study of pulse sequence selection in contrast-enhanced MR imaging with this agent.[38] We compared the enhancement of the liver [16 minutes after injection of 0.2 mmol/kg Fe(EHPG)$^-$] divided by background noise, E_L/N, for several IR and spin-echo (SE) pulse sequences. Figure 50–5 displays pre- and postinjection images of the rat abdomen using two different IR sequences with *TE*'s of 30 and 15 ms. The greater enhancement and signal-to-noise observed for the 15 ms *TE* sequence illustrates the major conclusion of our study: that the minimum *TE* available must be used to obtain the maximum contrast enhancement with agents that predominantly reduce *T1*. The proper selection of pulse sequence parameters will allow the use of minimum doses of contrast media, resulting in the highest margin of safety for the patient.

CLINICAL RELEVANCE

The liver represents an important area of diagnostic imaging. Assessment of both structural and functional problems currently requires at least two imaging modalities,

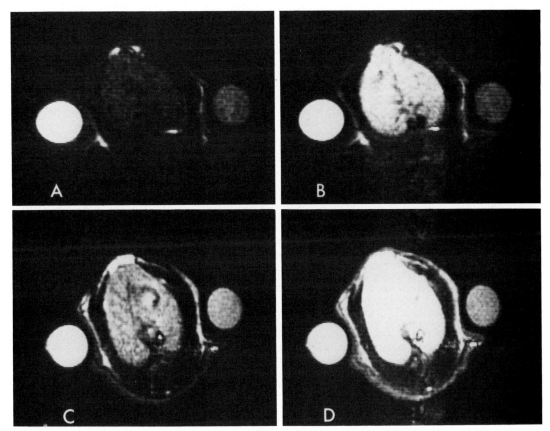

Figure 50–5. Representative images of the rat liver before (*A*) and 16 minutes after administration of Fe(EHPG)$^-$ using an IR 1484/400/30 pulse sequence (*B*). Similar pre- and postimages (*C* and *D*, respectively) are shown using the IR 1462/400/15 sequence. (From Greif WL, et al: Radiology *157*:461, 1985.)

such as x-ray CT and radionuclide scintigraphy. The availability of a safe and effective paramagnetic hepatobiliary contrast agent in concert with high-resolution MR tomography may provide a powerful tool for the assessment of both space-occupying lesions and hepatocellular disease as well as structural and functional assessment of the biliary system. Preclinical (and eventual clinical) studies are required to determine the ultimate utility of this class of agents.

References

1. Bydder GM, Steiner RE, Young IR, et al: Clinical NMR imaging of the brain: 140 cases. AJNR *3*:459, 1982.
2. McGinnis BD, Brady TJ, New PFJ, et al: Nuclear magnetic resonance (NMR) imaging of tumors in the posterior fossa. J Comput Assist Tomogr *7*:575, 1983.
3. Brant-Zawadzki M, Badami JP, Mills CM, et al: Primary intracranial tumor imaging: a comparison of magnetic resonance and CT. Radiology *150*:435, 1984.
4. Moss AA, Goldberg HI, Stark DD, et al: Hepatic tumors: magnetic resonance and CT appearance. Radiology *150*:141, 1984.
5. Brady TJ, Goldman MR, Pykett IL, et al: Proton nuclear magnetic resonance imaging of regionally ischemic canine hearts: effect of paramagnetic proton signal enhancement. Radiology *144*:343, 1982.
6. Goldman MR, Brady TJ, Pykett IL, et al: Quantification of experimental myocardial infarction using nuclear magnetic resonance imaging and paramagnetic ion contrast enhancement in excised canine hearts. Circulation *66*:1012, 1982.
7. Brasch RC, London DA, Wesbey GE, et al: Nuclear magnetic resonance study of a paramagnetic nitroxide contrast agent for enhancement of renal structures in experimental animals. Radiology *147*:773, 1983.
8. Wesbey GE, Brasch RC, Engelstad BL, Moss AA, Crooks LE, Brito AC: Nuclear magnetic resonance contrast enhancement study of the gastrointestinal tract of rats and a human volunteer using nontoxic oral iron solutions. Radiology *149*:175, 1983.
9. Brasch RC, Weinmann HJ, Wesbey GE: Contrast-enhanced NMR imaging: animal studies using gadolinium-DTPA complex. AJR *142*:625, 1984.
10. Carr DH, Brown J, Bydder GM, et al: Intravenous chelated gadolinium as a contrast agent in NMR imaging of cerebral tumours. Lancet *1*:484, 1984.
11. Grossman RI, Wolf G, Biery D, et al: Gadolinium enhanced nuclear magnetic resonance images of experimental brain abscess. J Comput Assist Tomogr *8*:204, 1984.
12. Carr DH, Brown J, Bydder GM, et al: Gadolinium-DTPA as a contrast agent in MRI: initial clinical experience in 20 patients. AJR *143*:215, 1984.
13. Weinmann HJ, Brasch RC, Press WR, Wesbey GE: Characteristics of gadolinium-DTPA complex: a potential NMR contrast agent. AJR *142*:619, 1984.
14. Larson SM, Nelp WB: Radiopharmacy of a simplified technetium-99m-colloid preparation for photoscanning. J Nucl Med *7*:817, 1966.
15. Caride VJ, Sostman HD, Winchell RJ, Gore JC: Relaxation enhancement using liposomes carrying paramagnetic species. Magn Reson Imag *2*:107, 1984.
16. Chilton HM, Jackels SC, Hinson WH, Ekstrand KE: Use of a paramagnetic substance, colloidal manganese sulfide, as an NMR contrast material in rats. J Nucl Med *25*:604, 1984.
17. Jones AL: Anatomy of the normal liver. *In* Zakim D, Boyer TD (eds): Hepatology: A Textbook of Liver Disease. Philadelphia, WB Saunders, 1982, pp 3–31.
18. Mendonca-Dias MH, Bernardo ML Jr, Muller RN, Acuff V, Lauterbur PC: Ferromagnetic particles as contrast agents for magnetic resonance imaging. Abstract presented at the Fourth Annual Meeting of the Society of Magnetic Resonance in Medicine, London, August 1985.
19. Chervu LR, Nunn AD, Loberg MD: Radiopharmaceuticals for hepatobiliary imaging. Semin Nucl Med *12*:5, 1984.
20. Lauffer RB, Greif L, Stark D, Vincent AC, Wedeen V, Brady TJ: Iron-EHPG as an hepatobiliary NMR contrast agent: Initial imaging and biodistribution studies. J Comput Assist Tomogr *9*:431, 1985.
21. Milburn PM: Factors in the biliary excretion of organic compounds. *In* Fishman WH (ed): Metabolic Conjugation and Metabolic Hydrolysis. New York, Academic Press, 1970, pp 1–74.
22. Klaassen CD, Walkins JB III: Mechanisms of bile formation, hepatic uptake, and biliary excretion. Pharmacol Rev *36*:1, 1984.
23. Bailey NA, Cummins D, McKenzie ED, Worthington JM: Iron(III) compounds of phenolic ligands. The crystal and molecular structure of iron(III) compounds of the sexadentate ligand N,N'-ethylene-bis-(o-hydroxyphenylglycine). Inorg Chim Acta *50*:111, 1981.
24. Frost AE, Freedman HH, Westerback SJ, Martell AE: Chelating tendencies of N,N'-ethylenebis-[2-(o-hydroxyphenyl)]-glycine. J Am Chem Soc *80*:530, 1958.
25. Aisen P, Listowsky I: Iron transport and storage proteins. Ann Rev Biochem *49*:357, 1980.
26. Korman S: Iron metabolism in man. Ann NY Acad Sci *88*:460, 1960.
27. Patch MG, Simolo KP, Carrano CJ: The cobalt(III), chromium(III), copper(II), and manganese(III) com-

plexes of ethylenebis [(o-hydroxyphenyl)glycine]: models for metallotransferrins. Inorg Chem *21*:2972, 1982.

28. Graf E, Mahoney JR, Bryant RG, Eaton JW: Iron-catalyzed hydroxyl radical formation. Stringent requirement for free iron coordination site. J Biol Chem *259*:3620, 1984.
29. Lauffer RB, Brady TJ: Preparation and water relaxation properties of proteins labeled with paramagnetic metal chelates. Magn Reson Imag *3*:11, 1985.
30. Lauffer RB, Betteridge DR, Padmanabhan S, Brady TJ: Albumin binding of paramagnetic hepatobiliary contrast agents: enhancement of outer sphere relaxivity. Abstract presented at the Fourth Annual Meeting of the Society of Magnetic Resonance in Medicine, London, August 1985.
31. Haddock EP, Zapolski EJ, Rubin M, Princiotto JV: Biliary excretion of chelated iron. Proc Soc Exp Biol Med *120*:663, 1965.
32. Rubin M, Pachtman E, Aldridge M, Zapolski EJ, Bagley DA Jr, Princiotto JV: The metabolism of parenteral iron chelates. Biochem Med *3*:271, 1970.
33. Theodorakis MC, Groutas WC, Bermudez AJ, Magnin D, Stefanakow SS: Localization of technetium 99m-ethylene-diamine-N,N′-bis-(α-2-hydroxy-5-bromophenyl)acetic acid and technetium 99m-N-(2-mercapto-1-oxopropyl)glycine in hepatobiliary system. J Pharm Sci *69*:581, 1980.
34. Hunt FC: Phenolic aminocarboxylic acids as gallium-binding radiopharmaceuticals. Nuklearmedizin *23*:123, 1984.
35. Cleton F, Turnbull A, Finch CA, Thompson L, Martin J: Synthetic chelating agents in iron metabolism. J Clin Invest *42*:327, 1963.
36. Koehler RE, Stanley RJ, Evans RG: Iosefamate meglumine: an iodinated contrast agent for hepatic computed tomography scanning. Radiology *132*:115, 1979.
37. Moss AA: Computed tomography of the hepatobiliary system. *In* Moss AA, Gamsu G, Genant HK (eds): Computed Tomography of the Body. Philadelphia, W.B. Saunders, 1983, pp 615–619.
38. Greif WL, Buxton RB, Lauffer RB, Saini S, Stark DD, Wedeen VJ, Rosen BR, Brady TJ: Pulse sequence optimization for MR imaging using a paramagnetic hepatobiliary contrast agent. Radiology *157*:461, 1985.

51

Hepatobiliary Contrast Agents

EDWARD J. GOLDSTEIN
GERALD L. WOLF

Concepts and theory regarding proton relaxation and its relationship to MRI contrast agents are discussed in great detail in Chapters 46 to 50 and 52. The reader may also refer to the literature for similar information.[1-3] We will provide a brief introduction pertinent to contrast agents and jump right into a discussion of specific substances under investigation with examples of laboratory data and imaging results.

THEORY

The signal generated in proton magnetic resonance imaging arises primarily from tissue water protons. Most human tissues are 75 to 80 percent water by weight. The MRI signal intensity is governed by a host of factors, these being as follows: (1) tissue proton density; (2) the velocity of moving protons; (3) imaging techniques and operating parameters (*TR, TE, TI,* number of excitations, slice thickness) in conjunction with different pulsing sequences (e.g., inversion recovery, spin echo, gradient echo); and (4) intrinsic tissue longitudinal proton relaxation time, *T1*, and transverse proton relaxation time, *T2*.

Frequently, in magnetic resonance imaging of two distinct tissue zones, all parameters may be similar. These zones will not be well distinguished with MRI. Under these circumstances, contrast agents have great utility. Ideally, a contrast agent should have the ability to selectively localize in either normal or abnormal tissue, altering *T1* and *T2*, thereby changing the signal intensity arising from one tissue zone relative to surrounding contiguous tissue. This results in better visual distinction of the two regions. An alteration of approximately 25 percent in relaxation time is required.

With the selection of appropriate imaging techniques in conjunction with contrast agents, patient throughput should be increased in two ways: (1) as a consequence of eliminating the necessity to carry out screening imaging with several imaging techniques to optimize visualization of the lesion; and (2) by utilizing the faster pulsing sequences that are applicable with the use of contrast agents. An effective MRI contrast agent must be tissue- or lesion-specific, nontoxic, effective in altering proton relaxation time, and chemically stable.

Contrast agents useful for hepatic imaging localize in any of three areas: hepatocytes, Kupffer cells (RE cells), and extracellular sinusoidal or vascular spaces. The reagents may be introduced intravenously or orally. Localization is a dynamic process in which the contrast agents move from one zone to another in a predominantly nonreversible manner until excretion occurs. This process may last from minutes to many hours and, in some cases, days to years. Most blood-pool agents that remain extracellular are rapidly eliminated by the urinary tract. The reagents that are in the form of particle suspensions or colloids are trapped by Kupffer cells and are slower to be excreted. Reagents that enter hepatocytes have an intermediate lifetime prior to excretion in bile. Various paramagnetic and ferromagnetic substances fulfill all the requirements for use as MRI hepatic contrast agents.

Ferromagnetic substances such as iron oxide particles, Fe_2O_3, have intrinsic magnetic properties and, when distributed in tissue that is placed in a magnetic field, disrupt the homogeneity of the external flux surrounding tissue protons. This local inhomogeneity of field causes rapid dephasing of proton spin with a preferential effect on *T2*. Ferromagnetic materials have large magnetic moments and may retain their magnetic properties after the external field is no longer present, whereas paramagnetic substances exhibit their magnetic properties only in the presence of an external magnetic field and develop smaller magnetic moments. The paramagnetic materials have unpaired outer orbital electrons, endowing them with electron spin magnetic moments. Certain metal ions have this property (Table 51–1) and are also able to decrease proton relaxation times of both *T1* and *T2*. The paramagnetic metal ions are usually chelated or complexed to large organic molecules to reduce toxicity and produce tissue specificity. Chelation, unfortunately, reduces paramagnetic efficacy owing to the formation of coordinated covalent bonds between metal ion and ligand, resulting in partial shielding of coordination sites previously available for metal ion–water molecule encounters. The water molecule need not contact the metal ion but must reach a critical distance to undergo proton relaxation.

The concentration of paramagnetic substances per unit volume of tissue also affects the degree of proton relaxation: the greater the concentrations, the greater the reduction of *T1* and *T2*.

Paramagnetic ions need not be chelated to localize in hepatocytes. Free manganese II ion is excreted by the hepatobiliary system and during its transit from blood to hepatocyte to bile serves as a contrast agent.

Insoluble paramagnetic particles such as gadolinium oxide (Gd_2O_3), iron oxide (Fe_2O_3), and liposomes containing gadolinium or manganese chelates may also serve as hepatic contrast agents. A list of substances that have demonstrated promise for use as liver MRI contrast agents is found in Table 51–2.

Table 51–1. PARAMAGNETIC CATION ELECTRON DISTRIBUTION

Transition Series Cations		Electron Distribution in Third Orbitals							Spin Quantum Number
Vo^{+2}	$3d^1$	↑	_	_	_	_			1/2
Ti^{+2}	$3d^2$	↑	↑	_	_	_			2/2
Cr^{+3}	$3d^3$	↑	↑	↑	_	_			3/2
Cr^{+2}, Mn^{+3}	$3d^4$	↑	↑	↑	↑	_			4/2
Mn^{+2}, Fe^{+3}	$3d^5$	↑	↑	↑	↑	↑			5/2
Fe^{+2}, Co^{+3}	$3d^6$	↑↓	↑	↑	↑	↑			4/2
Co^{+2}, Ni^{+3}	$3d^7$	↑↓	↑↓	↑	↑	↑			3/2
Ni^{+2}, Cu^{+3}	$3d^8$	↑↓	↑↓	↑↓	↑	↑			2/2
Cu^{+2}	$3d^9$	↑↓	↑↓	↑↓	↑↓	↑			1/2
Cu^{+1}	$3d^{10}$	↑↓	↑↓	↑↓	↑↓	↑↓			0
Gd^{+3}	$4f^7$	↑	↑	↑	↑	↑	↑	↑	7/2

Table 51–2. LIVER MRI CONTRAST AGENTS

Paramagnetic Metal Chelates
MnPDTA
MnEGTA
MnPP
GdDTPA
GdHIDA
FeEHPG
Paramagnetic Particles
Gd_2O_3
Liposomes = GdDTPA
Liposomes = MnDTPA
MnS
Ferromagnetic Particles
Fe_2O_3
Paramagnetic Metal Ions
$MnCl_2$ I.V.
$Mn(oAC)_2$ I.V.
$MnCl_2$ oral

DISCUSSION

Paramagnetic Metal Chelates

MnPDTA, MnEGTA. Manganese propanoldiaminotetracetate (MnPDTA) is a hexadentate chelate that forms six coordination bonds with bivalent manganese ion through four carboxylate groups and two nitrogen atoms having lone pairs of electrons as bonding sites. Its paramagnetic properties arise as a consequence of its five unpaired 3D outer orbital electrons, resulting in a spin quantum number of 5/2 with an effective electron spin magnetic moment. This endows MnII with great efficacy in reducing the relaxation time of water protons in tissue. The chelate of MnII, MnPDTA, is depicted in Figure 51–1. We envision tissue water molecules rapidly migrating in and out of an inner relaxation zone surrounding the chelated manganese ion. Manganese ethyleneglycol-bis(B-aminoethylether) tetraacetate, MnEGTA, has paramagnetic properties and tissue specificity similar to MnPDTA. It is also a hexadentate chelate (Fig. 51–2).

Mn PDTA

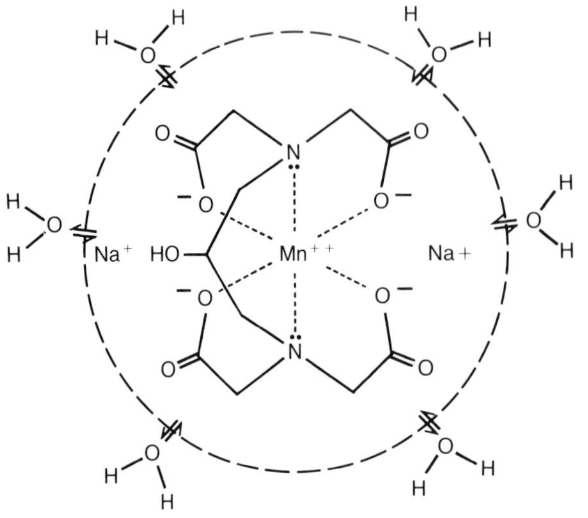

Figure 51–1. Hexadentate chelate, Mn PDTA.

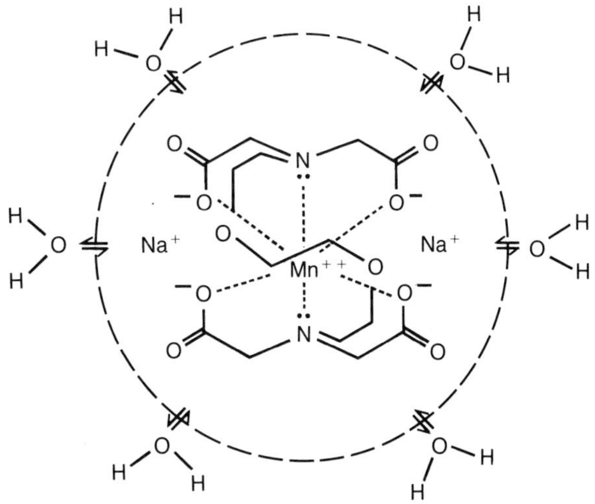

Figure 51-2. Hexadentate chelate, Mn EGTA.

Tissue studies carried out on rabbits, using intravenous doses of these two chelates, have demonstrated them to be effective in reducing liver proton relaxation times by 90 percent within 15 minutes after the administration of manganese chelate at doses between 15 and 50 μmol/kg. Tissue proton relaxation times were measured on a RADX proton spectrometer at 5 and 10 MHz at 37° C.[4] Chelation of manganese II significantly reduces toxicity relative to the free ion and reduces its paramagnetic efficacy to a lesser degree (Table 51-3). The chelate has more utility as a contrast agent than the free ion, as evidenced by its larger, more favorable therapeutic safety index.

Examples of the use of MnPDTA and MnEGTA for imaging are seen in Figures 51-3 to 51-5. There is considerable increase in signal intensity arising from normal rabbit liver following intravenous administration of MnEGTA. The use of MnEGTA to contrast-enhance normal rabbit liver is demonstrated (Fig. 51-3). MnPDTA is injected into a rabbit with a liver abscess (Fig. 51-4). A larger gradient of signal intensity between normal liver and abscess is obtained after the use of contrast. The gallbladder is also enhanced. The two round areas within the liver at its posterior aspect represent stomach. The increased signal arising from the dependent segment of the stomach is due to manganese in rabbit chow. Intravenous use of MnPDTA in a rabbit with a VX2 carcinoma introduced into the liver is demonstrated in Figure 51-5. This temporal study shows significant liver enhancement in a matter of minutes post injection. The VX2 carcinoma does not sequester the compound as do the normal hepatocytes, but there is a definite ring sign around tumor nodules at 54 minutes. The images in Figures 51-3 to 51-5 were obtained on a 1.4 tesla superconducting small-bore MR unit constructed by Peter Joseph at the University of Pennsylvania Pendergrass Research Laboratory.

MnPPIX. Manganese protoporphyrin IX (MnPPIX) is a chelate of manganese III

Table 51-3. RELATIVE RELAXATION EFFICACY AND TOXICITY OF FREE AND CHELATED MANGANESE II

Compound	$T1$ (ms)*	LD_{50} (μmol/kg)	Liver ED_{50} (μmol/kg)†	Therapeutic Safety Index LD_{50}/ED_{50}
MnCl$_2$	92	220	8.0	27.5
MnEGTA	435	750	7.2	104
MnPDTA	298	2500	6.8	368

* Proton relaxation time measured on a RADX spectrometer at 5MHz for a 10^{-3} aqueous solution.
† ED_{50} defined as dose required to reduce $T1$ by 50%.

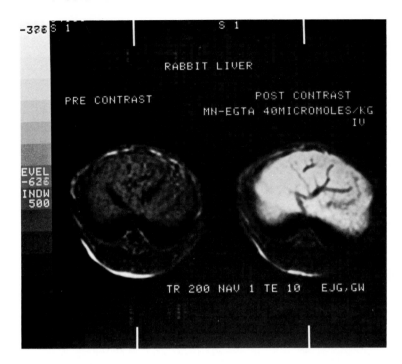

Figure 51–3. Contrast enhancement of normal rabbit liver after IV administration of Mn EGTA at a dose of 40 μmol/kg. Image obtained on 1.4 tesla superconducting facility with partial saturation spin-echo technique; *TR* 200, *TE* 10, number acquisitions = 1.

in which the metal ion retains its paramagnetic properties. The protoporphyrins are large molecules containing four pyrrole type five-membered rings linked by four methane bridges. A series of side chains on the five-membered rings occur in nature and give rise to a large number of structures—hence the Roman numeral designation. At the center of each protoporphyrin molecule are four nitrogen molecules capable of chelating to a metal ion (Fig. 51–6). In hemoglobin the metal ion is iron II. MnPPIX has been studied by Jackson and coworkers.[5] It is a water-soluble material that, when injected intravenously in rats, reduces liver *T1* values up to 70 percent at a dose of 2.5 mg Mn/kg. These data were obtained on liver tissue samples in a proton spectrometer

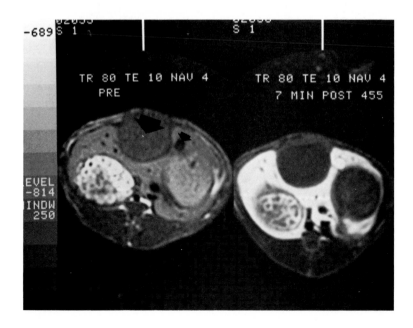

Figure 51–4. Contrast enhancement of rabbit liver with abscess present (large arrow) after IV administration of 33 μmol/kg of Mn PDTA. The gallbladder is also enhanced (small arrow). Image obtained on 1.4 tesla superconducting facility with partial saturation spin-echo technique; *TR* 80, *TE* 10, number acquisitions = 4.

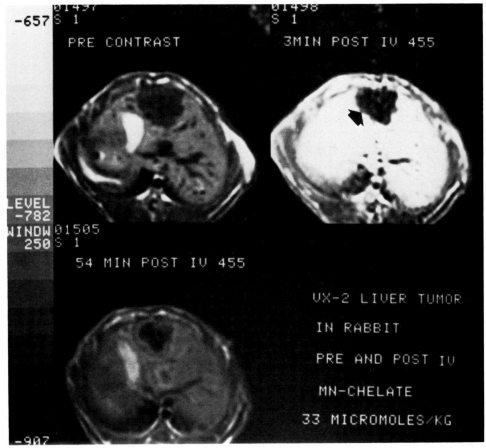

Figure 51–5. Contrast enhancement of rabbit liver with VX2 carcinoma present (arrow) after IV administration of 33 μmol/kg of Mn PDTA. Image obtained on 1.4 tesla superconducting facility with partial saturation spin-echo technique; *TR* 80, *TE* 10, number acquisitions = 2.

operating at 20 MHz. Liver MRI studies obtained on a Varian 12 inch, 2.4 tesla unit operating at 1 tesla confirmed increased signal intensity from liver 30 minutes after injection of MnPP. The effect is lost by 53 hours, which suggests effective elimination of the reagent from the liver, either in an intact form or through a metabolic breakdown process.

Of note is a preliminary report discussing manganese chelates of other porphyrins that have shown promise in contrast enhancement of colon tumors as a consequence of selective uptake by the neoplasm.[6]

Figure 51–6. Porphyrin ring structure with potential chelation site at center, Mn PPIX.

GdDTPA. Gadolinium diethylenetriaminepentaacetate (GdDTPA) is a stable non-toxic octadentate chelate with great potential as an MRI contrast agent because of its strong paramagnetic properties in an external magnetic field. This metal ion has seven unpaired electrons in its 4F orbitals endowing it with this property.[7] Five carboxylate groups and three nitrogen atoms with lone pairs of electrons on each serve as chelation sites. The coordinate number of gadolinium III is believed to be 10. This number reflects the number of possible hydration sites surrounding the metal ion in solution. The coordination number is usually twice the valence charge but may, and usually does, exceed this value in the lanthanide series of metals. Recent x-ray crystallography data suggest that the molecule is dimeric (Fig. 51–7). The stability constant of GdDTPA in solution is 10^{23}, which implies that there is very little free Gd III ion in solution. This reagent is cleared by the urinary tract and has been demonstrated to enhance CNS tumors. It is primarily a blood-pool agent but has been included for hepatobiliary imaging since it has been shown to be effective as a contrast agent for liver metastasis.[8] Using intravenous doses of 100 μmol/kg in humans, Carr[8] found significant enhancement of metastatic carcinoma of the colon to liver. Pre- and post-MRI images using spin-echo techniques at *TR* 540 ms and *TE* 40 ms are shown in Figure 51–8. Increased signal intensity arises from the kidney in the postcontrast image, in which GdDTPA is excreted. This indicates that the signal is not purely a *T2* weighted image, since this would result in decreased signal intensity arising from kidney. The increased signal arising from the liver metastasis must therefore represent significant *T1* shortening in tumor as a consequence of greater concentration of GdDTPA at these sites compared with normal hepatic parenchyma. This postcontrast image was obtained 20 minutes post injection. A delayed image should demonstrate eventual decrease in tumor enhancement as the GdDTPA is eliminated from the tumor. More vascular tumors might be expected to enhance earlier and wash out sooner.

GdHIDA. Gadolinium dimethylacetanilideiminodiacetic acid (GdHIDA) is a paramagnetic chelate that is an analogue of the well-known hepatobiliary nuclear medicine imaging agent technetium 99M HIDA. The latter reagent is 85 percent excreted by the

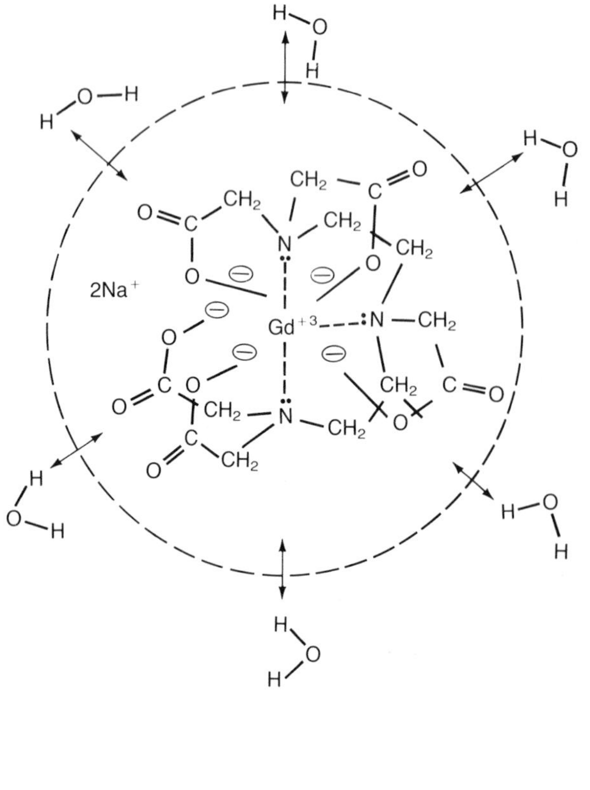

Figure 51–7. Octadentate chelate, Gd DTPA.

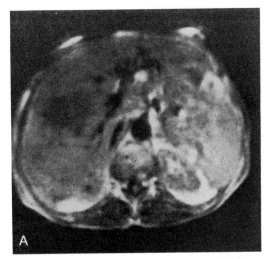 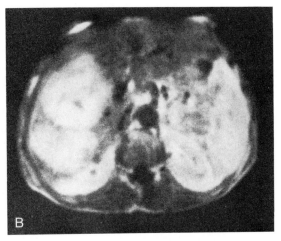

Figure 51–8. Precontrast (*A*) and postcontrast (*B*) images of human liver following IV administration of 100 μmol/kg of Gd DTPA. The liver metastases from colon are enhanced in the postcontrast image. (From Carr DH: Magn Reson Imag *3*:17, 1985. Used by permission.)

hepatobiliary system and 15 percent excreted by the urinary tract.[9] Uptake by the liver occurs within 5 to 10 minutes post injection and is visualized in the gallbladder and duodenum 15 to 30 minutes post injection. GdHIDA is also rapidly sequestered by the liver. MRI studies on rabbit liver infiltrated with VX2 carcinoma demonstrated significant contrast enhancement 10 minutes after intravenous administration of 30 μmol/kg GdHIDA (Fig. 51–9). Images were obtained on a 1.4 tesla small-bore superconducting unit with partial saturation spin-echo technique. The *T1* weighted image demonstrated increased gradient between the normal liver parenchyma and tumor following

Figure 51–9. Contrast enhancement of rabbit liver with VX2 carcinoma present (mottled rounded black areas) after IV administration of 30 μmol/kg of Gd HIDA. Image obtained on a 1.4 tesla superconducting facility with partial saturation spin-echo technique; *TR* 400, *TE* 10, number acquisitions = 4.

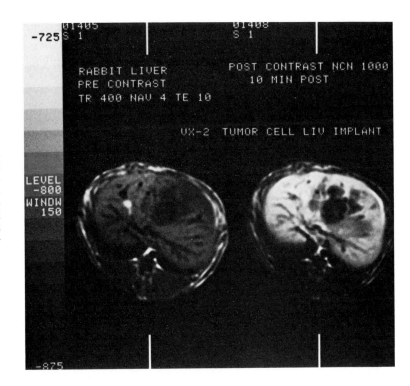

the use of contrast. The ligand for this water-soluble contrast agent is shown in Figure 51–10. The ratio of metal to ligand is in question.

FeEHPG. Iron ethylenebis(2-hydroxyphenylglycine) (FeEHPG) is a hexadentate chelate with FeIII as the paramagnetic center surrounded by the large EHPG ligand.[10] Iron III has a coordinate number of six and forms coordination bonds with two carboxylate groups, two hydroxy groups, and two nitrogen atoms with lone pairs of electrons. After chelation the molecule is likely to assume an octahedral configuration (Fig. 51–11). The formation constant of 10^{34} M^{-1} implies a very tightly bound metal chelate with little free iron III in solution. Extensive studies by Lauffer[10] demonstrated that this reagent is excreted by both hepatobiliary and urinary routes in intact form. The heptatobiliary route accounts for 6 percent of the injected dose. Imaging studies were carried out on a 1.4 tesla 8 cm bore superconducting unit (Technicare Corporation). Using inversion recovery with $T1$ weighted imaging, IR 1460/400/15, increases of 200 percent in signal intensity are observed in rat liver following intravenous injection of 200 μmol/kg of FeEHPG (Fig. 51–12). The increase in signal intensity occurs rapidly, within 10 minutes post injection, and slowly decreases over several hours. The toxicity of this reagent has not yet been assessed.

Paramagnetic Particles

Gd₂O₃. Gadolinium oxide (Gd_2O_3) has been studied in the form of a finely divided suspension for use as a paramagnetic MRI contrast agent.[11] Following intravenous introduction in laboratory rabbits, this material preferentially localized in lung, liver, and spleen. At a dose of 120 μmol/kg, lung, spleen, and liver $T1$ values are reduced by 74 percent, 63 percent, and 58 percent, respectively, at 30 minutes post injection. Peak reduction of $T1$ for liver occurs at one hour post injection. Some effect persists at 48 hours. The site of localization of the particle is in dispute. Some researchers have observed the presence of the oxide in liver and spleen sinusoids, whereas others report its presence in RE cells.[11,12] Differing results may be related to the size of the particle being used. Toxicity results also differ, ranging from nontoxic to moderately toxic. Pre- and postcontrast MRI images obtained on a rabbit liver containing VX2 carcinoma are seen in Figure 51–13. These images were obtained on a 1.4 tesla superconducting unit using partial saturation spin-echo technique TR 100 ms, TE 10 ms. The tumor is the dark area in a midline location at the anterior aspect of the liver, and the rounded gray area at the lateral aspect of the abdomen that does not contrast-enhance is stomach. At a dose of 50 μmol there is significant liver contrast enhancement at 10 minutes after intravenous injection, which increases at 39 minutes. An obvious increase in the gradient of signal intensity post contrast is observed when tumor and normal liver are compared. Gadolinium oxide should have potential for liver imaging if it does not prove too toxic.

Liposomes. Liposomes are lipid spheres that are composed of single or multiple lipid layers separated by a water zone.[13] Each lipid lamella consists of phospholipid bilayers reminiscent of the structure of cell membrane. The size of the spheres can be

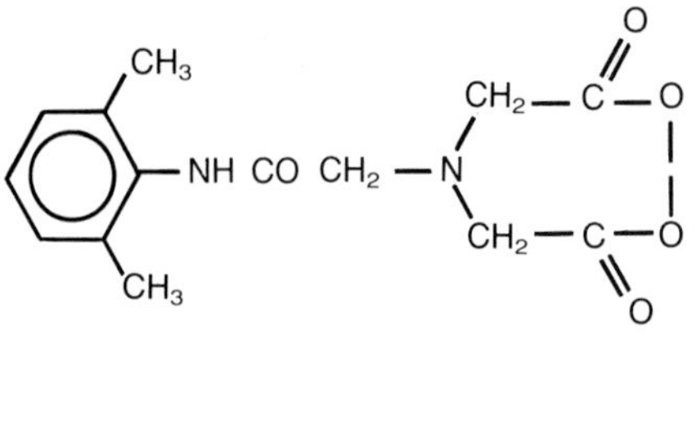

Figure 51–10. Dimethylacetanilideiminodiacetic acid, HIDA.

Figure 51–11. Fe EHPG: a hexadentate chelate of ferric ion. (From Lauffer RB, et al: J Comput Assist Tomogr 9:431, 1985. Used by permission.)

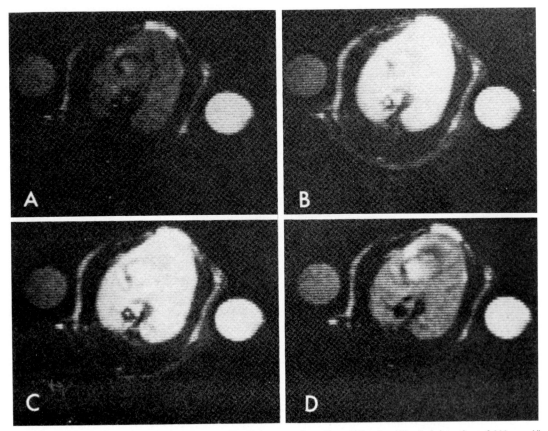

Figure 51–12. Precontrast (*A*) and postcontrast (*B–D*) images of rat liver following IV administration of 200 μmol/kg of Fe EHPG. The liver is seen to contrast-enhance (*B–D*). Images obtained on a 1.4 tesla superconducting unit with IR 1460/400/15. (From Lauffer RB, et al: J Comput Assist Tomogr 9:431, 1985. Used by permission.)

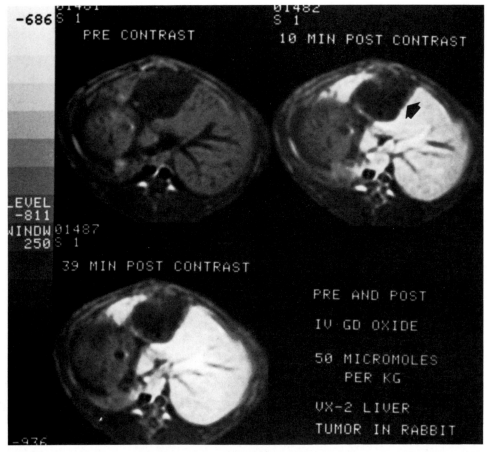

Figure 51–13. Contrast enhancement of rabbit liver with VX2 carcinoma present (arrow) following IV administration of 50 μmol/kg of Gd$_2$O$_3$ particles. Image obtained on a 1.4 tesla superconducting facility with partial saturation spin-echo technique; *TR* 100, *TE* 10, number acquisitions = 2.

controlled as well as the lipid composition. Phosphatidylcholine and cholesterol are commonly used in their preparation. These spheres are nontoxic and are trapped by the RE cells in the liver. The particles are also trapped in lung and spleen. The size of the spheres governs the location of their deposition: Large liposomes are trapped by lung; very small liposomes may remain in the blood pool. Fortunately, homogeneity in the size of the spheres can be achieved during their preparation.

Liposomes have been prepared with paramagnetic chelates incorporated into their structure. This is achieved by incorporating into the liposome a fatty acid amine, such as stearylamine, which can then bind the chelate. Liposomes containing MnDTPA and GdDTPA have been prepared in this manner. The MnDTPA liposomes, when injected intravenously into laboratory mice, result in significant reduction in longitudinal proton relaxation time, *T1*, of liver and spleen, amounting to 59 percent and 30 percent, respectively. These results were obtained one hour after injection of liposomes. The delivery of the chelate to the liver is increased by 207 percent compared with the use of MnDTPA alone. Similarly, an increase of spleen uptake of 1444 percent is observed. In similar experiments Buonocore et al.[14] reported a 25 to 35 percent reduction in intensity of mouse liver and spleen after intravenous introduction of GdDTPA liposomes. Approximately 50 percent of these liposomes accumulate in the liver 30 minutes post injection. The percent reduction in liver intensity, and spleen proton relaxation time after the use of these paramagnetic liposomes, indicate that these substances have great promise as MRI contrast agents.

MnS. Manganese sulfide in colloid form has been studied by Chilton et al.[15] for use as a liver MRI contrast agent. MnS has been prepared in particle sizes ranging from 0.1 to 10 μ. Following intravenous introduction of this nontoxic paramagnetic substance as a colloid at dose levels of 0.7 to 2.0 mg/kg into laboratory rats, $T1$ values of liver at 30 minutes were reduced significantly. Typical results of these experiments are listed in Table 51–4. It is likely that this material is sequestered by the RE cells in the liver similarly to technetium sulfur colloid. The significant reduction of liver $T1$ achieved following the use of MnS suggests that it should be effective as an MRI contrast agent.

Ferromagnetic Particles

Fe_2O_3. Magnetite particles (Fe_2O_3) are ferromagnetic and develop intrinsic magnetic fields when placed in an extrinsic magnetic flux. The Fe_2O_3 particle magnetic moment is far greater than that of a paramagnetic substance or tissue proton owing to its large positive magnetic susceptibility. The effect of the Fe_2O_3 micromagnetic fields in an external flux is to preferentially shorten transverse relaxation times, $T2$, of protons encountering the particle's field. This may be related to the creation of small zones of field heterogeneity in close proximity to the proton, resulting in an increased rate of loss of coherence.

Magnetite particles of appropriate size are sequestered by the RE cells of the liver after their intravenous introduction. The $T2$ effect of these particles is demonstrated in Table 51–5, which contains data obtained by injecting 0.3 μ magnetite particles into rabbits. $T2$ values of tissue were measured on a RADX proton spectrometer at 10 MHz. The rabbits were sacrificed 30 minutes post injection. A Carr-Purcell-Meiboom-Gill pulse sequence is used. A train of 64 echoes and best-fit curve processing of the data is used to arrive at a $T2$ value.

Pre- and postcontrast magnetic resonance images of rabbit liver invaded with VX2 carcinoma are shown in Figure 51–14. The instrument used is a 1.4 tesla superconducting unit with partial saturation spin-echo technique. Weighting for $T2$ is obtained with a TR of 500 ms and TE of 100 ms. In the precontrast image, tumor is not distinguished from normal liver. Postcontrast images represent the normal liver as dark areas of decreased signal intensity, the tumor appearing white. The ferromagnetic particles reside in normal liver, reduce $T2$ in this zone, and decrease signal intensity relative to the magnetite-free tumor. The results yield a negative contrast effect. These preliminary results are indeed promising.

Table 51–4. EFFECT OF INTRAVENOUS MnS ON RAT LIVER $T1$

Mn Dose (mg/kg)	$T1$ (ms)	Reduction in $T1$ (%)
(control)	275	—
0.7	227	17
1.0	175	36
1.5	159	42
2.0	128	53

The $T1$ values were obtained on a proton spectrometer at 24 MHz.
From Chilton HM, et al: Magn Reson Imag *1*:238, 1982. Used by permission.

Table 51–5. EFFECTS OF MAGNETITE PARTICLES
ON TISSUE PROTON RELAXATION TIME

Organ	Normal $T2$ (ms)*	$T2$ Post I.V. Magnetite Particles (10 mg/kg)
Heart	57	35
Lung	91	55
Liver	52	8
Spleen	74	8
Pancreas	70	53
Renal cortex	69	57

* Measured on a RADX proton spectrometer at 10 MHz. Animals studied were New Zealand white rabbits.

Paramagnetic Metal Ions

MnII. Although unchelated metal ions will generally have greater toxicity than their chelated counterparts, a great deal of investigative work has been directed toward their use as MRI contrast agents for hepatobiliary imaging. Manganese II in particular has been studied extensively for both intravenous and oral use. Schuhmacher et al.[16] studied the effect of intravenous manganese II on the longitudinal relaxation time, $T1$, of rat liver. Liver manganese II concentration was increased with intravenous doses of aqueous manganous acetate. The results are shown in Table 51–6. It is clear from these data that increasing concentration of liver manganese II significantly reduces proton relaxation time. The manganese II is transported from blood in liver sinusoids to hepatocytes to bile canaliculi. The significant reduction in liver $T1$ would indeed manifest a visible change on liver signal intensity in magnetic resonance images.

The effect of protein binding to manganese II has been studied by Brown and Koenig.[17] Once bound, manganese II has greater efficacy per molecule in reducing proton relaxation. The efficacy of the protein-metal complex is field-dependent (Fig.

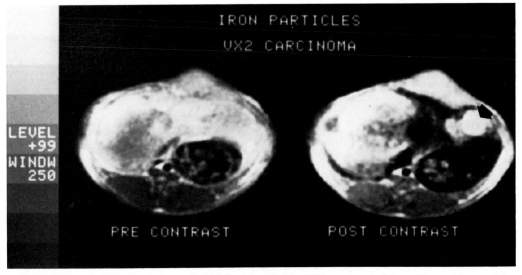

Figure 51–14. Pre- and postcontrast views of rabbit liver invaded by VX2 carcinoma. Magnetite particles are injected, IV, at a dose of 10 mg/kg. Normal liver becomes darker, revealing tumor as white island (arrow). Image obtained on 1.4 tesla superconducting facility with partial saturation spin-echo technique; *TR* 500, *TE* 100, number acquisitions = 2.

Table 51–6. EFFECT OF MANGANESE
ON RAT LIVER *T1*

MnII Injected	*T1* (ms)	Mn (mg/gm liver)
None	262	2.32
30 mg	238	2.94
80 mg	209	3.79
120 mg	177	5.34
300 mg	135	7.76

T1 measured on Bruker NMR spectrometer operating at 20
MHz at 22°C. All rats were of similar weight and were sacrificed one hour after administration of MnII. Liver manganese concentration was determined with neutron activation
analysis.
From Schuhmacher JH, et al: Invest Radiol *20*:601, 1985.
Used by permission.

51–15). The complex of manganese II with the protein ConA has greatest efficacy at
between 3 and 60 MHz. It is also noted that manganese II in water, MnII aquoion, is,
in general, less affected than the protein complex. Proton relaxivity is proportional to
the reciprocal of *T1*, or 1/*T1*. The graph (Fig. 51–15) is called an NMRD curve, or
nuclear magnetic resonance dispersion curve.

The enhancement effect on manganese II of protein binding has been examined
by Kang and Gore.[18] These studies demonstrated significant increase in relaxation rate
of liver after intravenous use of $MnCl_2$ solutions in mice. Measurements were made
at 20 MHz at 37° C. A proton relaxation enhancement ratio, E*, is defined and used
to measure the Mn-protein binding enhancement effect on relaxation rates:

$$E^*_1 = \frac{\Delta R_1 \text{ tissue}}{\Delta R_1 \text{ water}}$$

Figure 51–15. Koenig-Brown NMRD
curve demonstrating field strength
and protein-binding effects on Mn II
proton relaxivity. (Modified from
Koenig SH, et al: Magn Reson
Med *1*(4):498, 1984.)

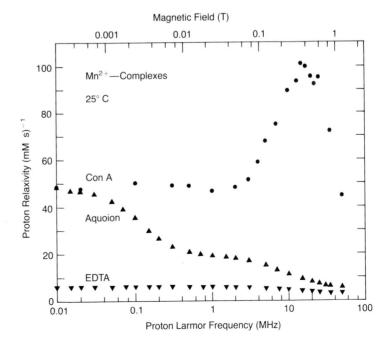

where $R = 1/TI$; ΔR tissue = increase in relaxation rate of the tissue after addition of manganese II; and ΔR water = increase in relaxation rate of pure water for the same concentration of manganese II.

If $E^*_1 > 1$, there is an enhancement effect by tissue protein. A value of 5.2 was observed for mouse liver. This can be interpreted at the molecular level as being due to binding of MnII to a cellular component that produces a manganese ion–ligand complex resulting in an increased rotational correlation time. The manganese II is thus endowed with greater proton relaxation efficacy in its bound form. Since not all paramagnetic ions have increased efficacy when bound to tissue components, manganese may prove the reagent of choice for future practical application. The field strength of imaging is also critical, since the enhancement effect is maximized at a specific flux range.

Manganese II has also been studied as a hepatic MRI contrast agent via oral administration.[19] Experiments were conducted by tube-feeding rats with $MnCl_2$ solution. A sample of these results is seen in Figure 51–16. After an oral dose of 500 mg/kg, a significant reduction in liver TI is observed within 15 minutes of oral intake. Liver relaxation times were measured on a RADX proton spectrometer operating at 5 and 10 MhZ at 37° C. The effect persists for several hours. A 90 percent reduction in liver TI is obtained in this manner. The significant reduction of TI at low doses of $MnCl_2$ suggests presystemic elimination or extraction of manganese II by the liver via the portal system. This happens at doses below 125 mg/kg. The oral route of $MnCl_2$ administration, which permits presystemic elimination, adds to the potential of $MnCl_2$ as a contrast agent, since its toxicity is reduced by nearly 50 percent.[20]

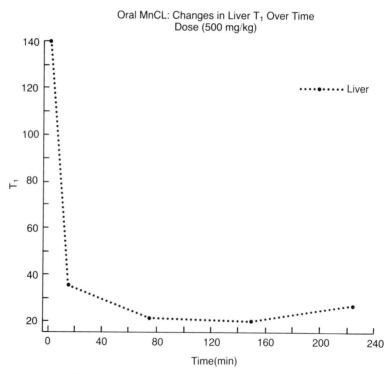

Figure 51–16. Rabbit liver TI values versus time, measured on proton spectrometer operating at 10 MHz and 37°C, following oral administration of $MnCl_2$.

References

1. Axel L: Relaxation times and NMR signals. Magn Reson Imag 2:121, 1984.
2. Brown MA: Effects of the operating magnetic field on potential NMR contrast agents. Magn Reson Imag 3:3, 1985.
3. Wolf GL, Burnett KR, Goldstein EJ, Joseph RM: Contrast agents for magnetic resonance imaging. *In* Magnetic Resonance Annual. New York, Raven Press, 1985, pp 231–266.
4. Wolf GL, Burnett KR, Goldstein EJ: NMR In vitro measurements: a quality control study of the RADX tabletop spectrometer. Physiol Chem Med NMR 16:6, 1985.
5. Jackson LS, Nelson JA, Case TA, Burnham BF: Manganese protoporphyrin IX: a potential intravenous paramagnetic NMR contrast agent. Invest Radiol 20:226, 1985.
6. Lyon R, et al: Tissue distribution and stability of metalloporphyrin MRI contrast agents. Scientific Program Society of Magnetic Resonance Imaging, London, August 1985, pp 885–886.
7. Goldstein EJ, Burnett KR, Wolf GL, et al: Gadolinium DTPA (an NMR proton imaging contrast agent): chemical structure, paramagnetic properties and pharmacokinetics. Physiol Chem Phys Med NMR 16:97, 1984.
8. Carr DH: The use of proton relaxation enhancers in magnetic resonance imaging. Magn Reson Imag 3:17, 1985.
9. Weissman HS, Frank MS, Berstein LH, Freeman LM: Rapid and accurate diagnosis of acute cholecystitis with TcHIDA cholescintigraphy. AJR 132:523, 1979.
10. Lauffer RB, et al: Iron-EHPG as an hepatobiliary MR contrast agent: initial imaging and biodistribution studies. J Comput Assist Tomogr 9(3):431, 1985.
11. Burnett KR, Wolf GL, Schumacher RH, Goldstein EJ: Gadolinium oxide: a prototype agent for contrast enhanced imaging of the liver and spleen with magnetic resonance. Magn Reson Imag 3:65, 1985.
12. Seltzer SE, et al: Hepatic contrast agents for CT: High atomic number particulate material. J Comput Assist Tomogr 5:370, 1981.
13. Caride VJ, Sostman HD, Winchell RJ, Gore JC: Relaxation enhancement using liposomes carrying paramagnetic species. Magn Reson Imag 2:102, 1984.
14. Buonocore E, et al: Potential organ specific MRI contrast agents for liver and spleen: gadolinium labeled liposomes. Program of Society of Magnetic Resonance Imaging, London, August 1985, pp 838–839.
15. Chilton HM, et al: Contrast enhancement of *T1* signal in rat liver tissues using manganese sulfide colloid. Magn Reson Imag 1:238, 1982.
16. Schuhmacher JH, et al: Contribution of paramagnetic trace elements to the spin-lattice relaxation time in the liver. Invest Radiol 20:601, 1985.
17. Brown RD III, Brewer CF, Koenig SH: Conformation states of concanavalin A: kinetics of transitions induced by interactions with MnII and CaII ion. Biochemistry 16:3883, 1977.
18. Kang YS, Gore JC: Studies of tissue NMR relaxation enhancement by manganese. Invest Radiol 19:399, 1984.
19. Mamourian AC, et al: Proton relaxation enhancement in tissue due to injected manganese chloride. Physiol Chem Phys Med NMR 16:123, 1984.
20. Thompson TM, Klaassen CD: Presystemic elimination of manganese in rats. Toxicol Appl Pharmacol 64:236, 1983.

52

Dynamic Contrast-Enhanced MRI and Mathematical Modeling

C. LEON PARTAIN
JEFFREY A. CLANTON
MYRON HOLSCHER
TIMOTHY ASHBAUGH
MICHAEL McCURDY
B. G. TWEEDY

Twenty years of experience in radiopharmaceutical development and nuclear medicine kinetic techniques have preceded the initial consideration of dynamic contrast-enhanced magnetic resonance imaging. It is most interesting to note the exact parallel between radioisotope labeled pharmaceuticals for specific metabolic medical imaging and the opportunity that we now have to develop a completely new range of magnetically labeled pharmaceuticals for organ function. This circumstance combines the significant anatomic resolution of magnetic resonance imaging and the detailed functional information of contrast-enhanced kinetic studies. The resulting data may serve as the basis to develop more accurate diagnostic criteria for multiple organ systems and multiple pathophysiologic processes. Recent investigators have reported the utilization of paramagnetic labeled MRI contrast agents.[1-4]

The excretory route of gadolinium-DTPA is by renal excretion using 100 percent glomerular filtration. This is the same route as for the nuclear medicine agent technetium-DTPA and the conventional hydrophilic iodinated contrast media used in angiography and computed tomography.[5] It is understood that gadolinium-DTPA diffuses to extracellular fluid soon after it is injected. Dynamic studies with 0.5 tesla MRI, using short *TE* and *TR* values and spin-echo sequences, can obtain dynamic data on its distribution in normal and abnormal tissues. Illustrated in this chapter are dynamic contrast-enhanced MR images in the liver and kidneys of rats using injected concentration of 0.1 mmol/kg to assess the feasibility of dynamic time-intensity curves in the liver and kidney for distinguishing normal and abnormal hepatic-renal function on a quantitative and possibly metabolic basis.[6-10]

MATERIALS AND METHODS

Eighty Fischer 344 rats, each approximately 80 gm, were imaged in this study. Forty normal controls were used and 40 received three concentrations of oral azo dye, 0.06 percent *N,N*-dimethyl-*p* (m-tolylazoaniline) with 100 percent corn oil, mixed with laboratory rat chow. This chapter illustrates normal and toxic liver time-intensity curves and differential renal curves. Liver toxicity resulted from the oral injection of azo dye. Differential renal function apparently was not related to the azo dye injection. The injected dose of 0.1 mmol/kg (in 1 to 2 ml) of gadolinium-DTPA was administered over a ten-second period using a 23-gauge needle into the tail vein of the rat. Injection was followed by a flush of 1 ml of sterile saline.

Contrast enhancement was demonstrated with serial images in the transverse plane using a specially designed surface coil, with images taken every minute for 30 minutes after injection following a precontrast image. Data were acquired using a Technicare 0.5 tesla superconducting MR system and a spin-echo imaging technique with *TR* 500 ms and *TE* 32 ms. Imaging time was approximately four minutes for a multislice collection, each slice being 0.5 cm thick. Data were collected on a 128 × 256 matrix and interpolated for 256 × 256 display. Signal intensities were normalized to maximum intensity for analysis. Time-intensity curves were generated, yielding the functional dependence of relative intensity versus time as the independent variable. Since the 50 cm bore total-body human MRI system was utilized, a special surface coil was designed for the rat in order to facilitate the magnified anatomic imaging. The coil is illustrated in Figure 52–1 with the subject in place in the coil.

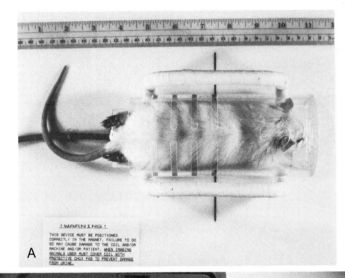

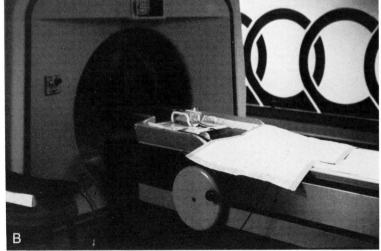

Figure 52–1. Fischer 344 rat (100 gm) in surface coil specially designed for liver and kidney imaging. *A*, Four-inch rectangular surface with anesthetized animal in place. *B*, Surface coil and animal during imaging in total-body 0.5 tesla MRI system.

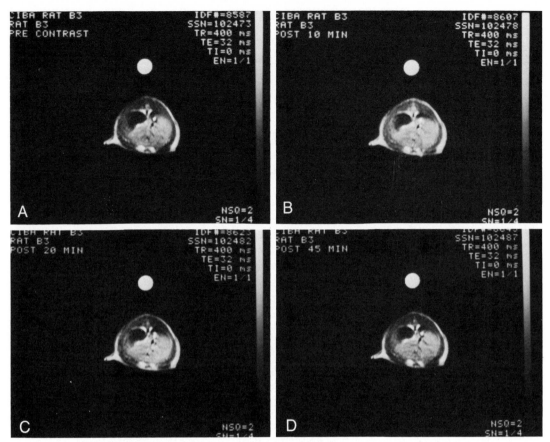

Figure 52–2. Normal liver MRI kinetic study, 0.5 tesla, SE 500/32, before and after the intravenous injection of 0.1 mmol/kg of Gd-DTPA. *A*, Precontrast. *B*, Ten min post contrast. *C*, Twenty min post contrast. *D*, Forty-five min post contrast.

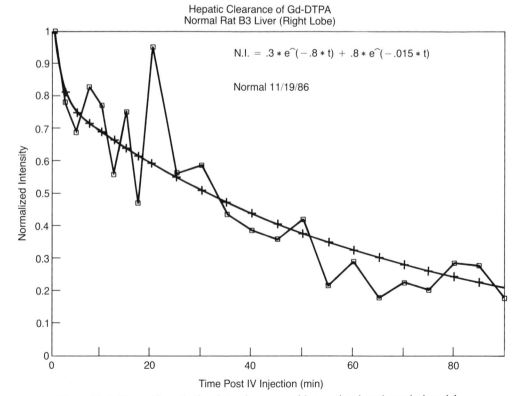

Hepatic Clearance of Gd-DTPA
Normal Rat B3 Liver (Right Lobe)

$N.I. = .3 * e\hat{\ }(-.8 * t) + .8 * e\hat{\ }(-.015 * t)$

Normal 11/19/86

Figure 52–3. Normal hepatic time-intensity curve with associated mathematical model.

RESULTS

Serial images are illustrated in Figure 52–2 before and after intravenous injection of gadolinium-DTPA. The normal liver contrast-enhanced MRI kinetic curve is illustrated in Figure 52–3. Mathematical modeling was performed using an equation of the form

$$I(t) = Ae^{-\lambda 1t} + Be^{-\lambda 2t}$$

where the parameters are defined as

I(t) = intensity as a function of time

A = a constant

B = a constant

λ1 = first rate constant

λ2 = second rate constant.

These parameters were fit to the experimental data using a modified least-squares fitting algorithm. Notice that the data are well behaved, that the time to peak in this study is approximately two minutes, and that the longer rate constant for removal of contrast from the kidney is equal to 0.015 sec^{-1}.

Abnormal liver serial contrast-enhanced dynamic studies, abnormal hepatic time-

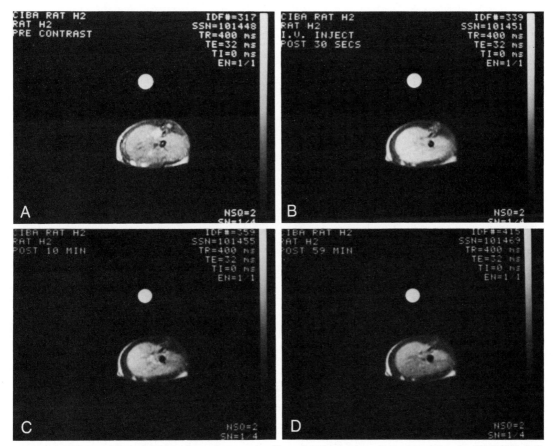

Figure 52–4. Abnormal liver MRI kinetic study: a toxic effect of oral injection of azo dye, 0.5 tesla, SE 500/32, before and after the intravenous injection of 0.1 mmol/kg of Gd-DTPA. *A*, Precontrast. *B*, Thirty sec post contrast. *C*, Ten min post contrast. *D*, Fifty-nine min post contrast.

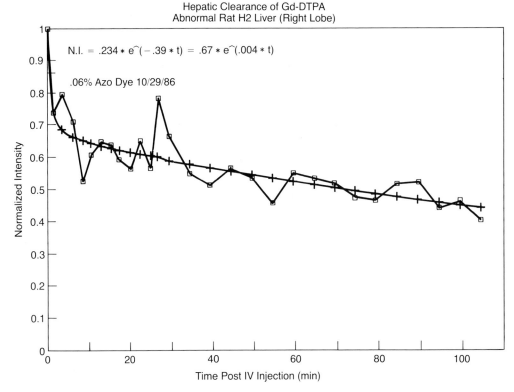

Hepatic Clearance of Gd-DTPA
Abnormal Rat H2 Liver (Right Lobe)

N.I. $= .234 * e\hat{}(-.39 * t) = .67 * e\hat{}(.004 * t)$

.06% Azo Dye 10/29/86

Normalized Intensity

Time Post IV Injection (min)

Figure 52–5. Abnormal hepatic time-intensity curve with associated mathematical model.

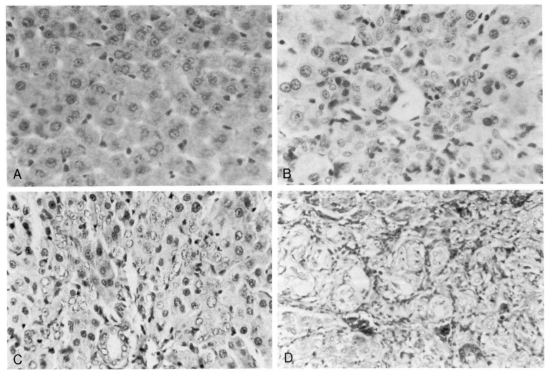

Figure 52–6. Histology of hepatic toxicity with periportal round cell proliferation. *A*, Normal liver. *B*, Mild toxicity. *C*, Moderate toxicity. *D*, Marked toxicity with tumor nodules.

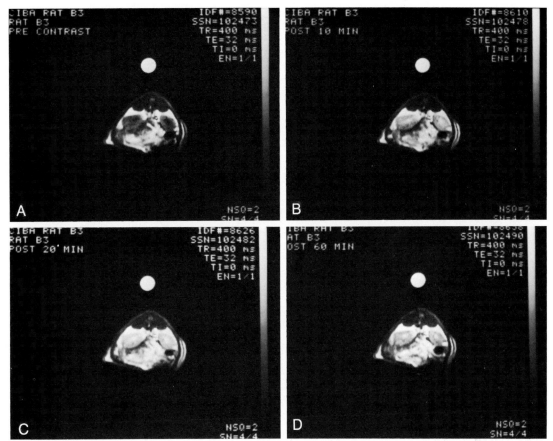

Figure 52–7. Bilateral renal MRI dynamic study, 0.5 tesla, SE 500/32, before and after the intravenous injection of 0.1 mmol/kg of Gd-DTPA. *A*, Precontrast. *B*, Ten min post contrast. *C*, Twenty min post contrast. *D*, Sixty min post contrast.

intensity curves with corresponding mathematical model, and supporting histologic evaluation are illustrated in Figures 52–4 to 52–6.

Typical bilateral renal MRI dynamic studies are illustrated in Figure 52–7 after intravenous injection of 0.1 mmol/kg gadolinium-DTPA. Corresponding differential dynamic MR renograms are shown in Figure 52–8 and illustrate differential renal function with no known cause for abnormal function in the left kidney of this animal.

DISCUSSION

Dynamic MRI, contrast-enhanced, time-intensity curves are comparable in shape and form to similar curves using radiopharmaceuticals in nuclear medicine[11,12] and iodinated contrast agents in contrast-enhanced x-ray CT in angiography and digital radiography.[5] The technique of dynamic imaging using gadolinium-DTPA allows the evaluation of diffusion to the kidney and liver and allows differences in normal and abnormal hepatic and renal function to be quantitatively observed.

It is obvious that while reproducible time-intensity curves are available in the liver, DTPA is not an ideal hepatic MR contrast pharmaceutical because it is a blood-pool agent cleared by the kidney. Two improved pharmaceuticals are available for hepatic MR contrast. One is a labeled aminodiacetic acid cleared physiologically by the hepatocyte, an analogue to the hepatobiliary nuclear medical agents. A second example,

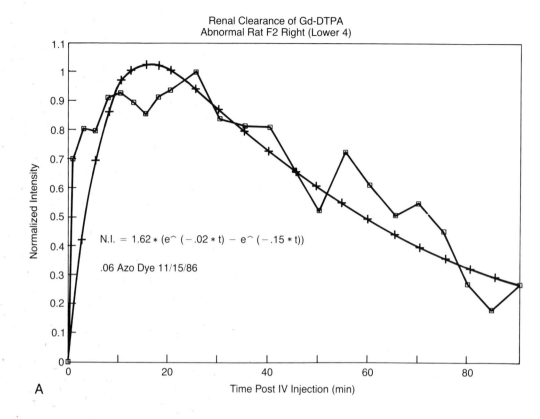

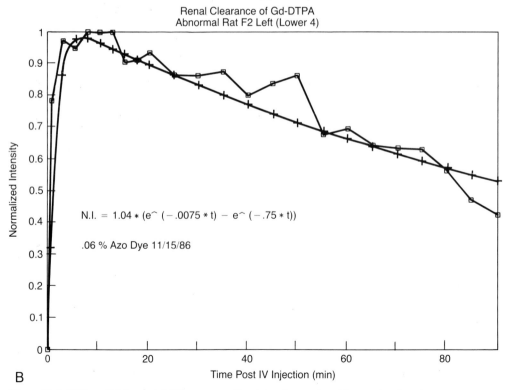

Figure 52–8. Differential dynamic MRI renogram time intensity curves with associated mathematical models. *A*, Normal right renogram ($\lambda_2 = 0.15 \text{ sec}^{-1}$). *B*, Abnormal left renogram ($\lambda_2 = 0.75 \text{ sec}^{-1}$).

ferrite, as recently reported, is an agent handled by the Kupffer cell and reticuloendothelial system of the liver.[7,8]

It is anticipated that a wide range of contrast pharmaceuticals will be developed for study of the brain, heart, liver, kidney, endocrine organs, and reproductive organs. These will include paramagnetically labeled monoclonal antibodies, which will provide added sensitivity and specificity and, hence, increase the diagnostic accuracy of a multitude of lesions that are amenable to magnetic resonance imaging. The future offers a most interesting comparison of pulse sequence optimization, contrast-enhanced dynamic magnetic resonance imaging, and in vivo NMR spectroscopy as these new additions are made to the diagnostic armamentarium of the clinician.

References

1. Weinmann HJ, Brasch RC, Press WR, Wesbey GE: Characteristics of gadolinium-DTPA complex: A potential NMR contrast agent. AJR *142*:619, 1984.
2. Runge VM, Clanton JA, Lukehart CM, Partain CL, James AE: Paramagnetic agents for contrast-enhanced NMR imaging: A review. AJR *141*:1209, 1983.
3. Runge VM, Clanton JA, Foster MA, Smith FW, Jones MM, Lukehart CM, Price RR, Partain CL, James AE: Paramagnetic NMR contrast agents: Development and evaluation. Invest Radiol *19*:408, 1984.
4. Brasch RC, Weinmann HJ, Wesbey GE: Contrast-enhanced NMR imaging: Animal studies using gadolinium-DTPA complex. Am J Roentgenol *142*:625, 1984.
5. Kormano M, Dean PB: Extravascular contrast material: The major component of contrast enhancement. Radiology *121*:379, 1979.
6. Iio M, Yoshikawa K, Ohotomo K, Yashiro N, Okada Y, Ito M, Nishikawa J: Dynamic magnetic resonance imaging with Gd-DTPA. *In* Runge VM, Clausson C, Felix R, James AE (eds): Contrast Agents in MRI. Amsterdam, Excerpta Medica, 1987, pp 183–185.
7. Saini S, Stark DD, Hahn PF, Wittenberg J, Brady TJ, Ferrucci, JT: Ferrite particles: A superparamagnetic MR contrast agent for the reticuloendothelial system. Radiology *162*:211, 1987.
8. Saini S, Stark DD, Hahn PF, Bousquet JC, Introcasso J, Wittenberg J, Brady TJ, Ferrucci, JT: Ferrite particles: A superparamagnetic MR contrast agent for enhanced detection of liver carcinoma. Radiology *162*:217, 1987.
9. Partain CL, Clanton JA, McCurdy M, Ashbaugh T, Holburn G: Dynamic contrast enhanced MRI: a sensitive measure of hepatic toxicity to azo dye. Radiology *161*(P):315, 1986.
10. Pettigrew RI, Avruch L, Dannels W, Coumans J, Bernardino ME: Fast-field-echo MR imaging with GD-DTPA: physiologic evaluation of the kidney and liver. Radiology *160*:561, 1986.
11. Cohen M: Radionuclide clearance techniques. Semin Nucl Med *4*:23, 1975.
12. Sarper R, Fajman WA, Rypins EB, et al: Non-invasive method for measuring portal venous/total hepatic blood flow by hepatosplenic radionuclide angiography. Radiology *141*:179, 1981.
13. Chervu LR, Blaufox MD: Renal radiopharmaceuticals: an update. Semin Nucl Med *12*:224, 1982.

XI

CONCLUSIONS

53

Clinical Efficacy: 5000 MRI Cases Between 0.15 and 0.6 Tesla

MARK A. LUTHE
HARVEY V. FINEBERG

As the first medical imaging modality subject to the full impact of broad legislation guiding the development, marketing, purchase, and reimbursement of medical imaging devices, magnetic resonance imaging has faced a most rigorous challenge in its attempt to achieve acceptance as a standard clinical test. The enactment of the Medical Device Amendments Act, on May 28, 1976, broadened the federal government's authority to oversee the safety of medical devices and was given substance by the FDA's published regulations for premarket applications in December 1980.[1] While these laws were passed to increase the responsibilities of device manufacturers, independent actions were taken to ensure hospitals' financial restraint in the use of the new technology.[2] Section 1122 of the Social Security Act was passed in 1972, requiring prior approval by local and state planning agencies for capital expenditures that would seek reimbursement under Medicare and/or Medicaid, and, most recently, the Health Care Financing Administration, in 1983, issued the list of diagnosis-related groups (DRGs) for Medicare prospective payment of health care costs.[3]

The technical nature of MR imaging requires the consideration of more interdependent parameters (*TE, TR, TI,* and so forth) than were previously encountered in other imaging modalities, necessitating an even larger number of studies to standardize its clinical use. While anecdotal reports and specific applications of MR imaging have clearly made a weighty (if inconclusive) contribution to a host of medical journals, it should be recognized that the largest repositories of clinical data on magnetic resonance imaging systems reside with the device manufacturers themselves. In order to meet compliance with the aforementioned laws, MRI manufacturers have found themselves involved in increasingly detailed studies to prove the clinical effectiveness, safety, and, recently, cost-effectiveness of their products. As the worldwide leader in MRI installations, Technicare Corporation has the largest source for its database of clinical MRI studies. This and the following chapter are attempts to aid the radiologic community by sharing the compiled results from these wide-ranging investigations. The current study reviews the findings from a large pool of early results. As will become apparent, the constantly changing nature of the technology involved in MR imaging has had an impact on every attempt to obtain an accurate assessment of its abilities. Nevertheless, the enormity of the data pool here presented allows for a reasonable review of the modality's strengths and weaknesses.

BACKGROUND

Initiation of the Technicare protocol for a multi-institutional evaluation of its Teslacon Magnetic Resonance Imaging system against established diagnostic modalities occurred during late 1981; it involved Massachusetts General Hospital, University Hospitals of Cleveland, and The Cleveland Clinic Foundation. As part of the premarket approval process, a two-page, open-ended questionnaire was developed with these institutions in March 1982 to ascertain subject history, final diagnoses, and etiology as well as the comparative detection rates of standard imaging modalities. During this initial phase, Technicare monitored the study progress and reviewed the questionnaires for completeness and accuracy prior to their inclusion in the study. In addition, an independent monitoring firm randomly reviewed approved records at the participating institutions, rechecking results against the patients' medical records.

Investigators were required to maintain files on all normal volunteers and patients entering the imaging device. No criteria for subject selection were specified, other than exclusion of populations who at that time were considered potentially at risk: patients having metal prostheses and/or surgical clips, pregnant females, and infants. All subjects were required to sign a letter indicating consent to the procedure, and all patients were to have undergone or been scheduled for comparative diagnostic imaging tests. Although not required, pathologic confirmation of disease was requested when available.

Because a secondary aspect to the study was definition of appropriate imaging techniques, investigators were permitted and encouraged to develop and use imaging parameters that they deemed appropriate to the condition under study. Subject files therefore contained the aforementioned questionnaire, informed consent, patient medical records (including reports of all relevant diagnostic tests), a written summary of MRI techniques and findings, and sample MRI images. Each file was reviewed jointly by the monitor and a Technicare staff physician before data were entered into the main subject pool. Discrepancies between these recorded summaries and the questionnaire synopses were resolved through consultation between the study monitors and the clinical investigators and their associates. As the number of completed studies neared 300 in September 1982, and the FDA requirements for marketing applications became known, the questionnaire results were organized into a computer database.

Between the deadline for the initial marketing application (November 1982) and May 1983, eight additional institutions became participants in the study. In order to better quantify the results from this expanding subject base, new questionnaires (compatible with the earlier version) were designed and distributed. In addition to the questions previously asked, assessment of MRI pulse techniques, anatomy localization, and a four-point scale of detection confidence were introduced. Corresponding changes were incorporated into the database.

Following the establishment of routine procedures for the review, collection, and entry of data by the MRI Clinical Program in July 1983, the duplicate monitoring efforts of the independent firm were discontinued. Simultaneously, patient exclusion criteria were eased, allowing infants and those with prosthetic devices to be imaged upon approval by the presiding Institutional Review Boards. The study continued similarly with few changes, other than the number of participating institutions: 22 as of May 1984, and represented herein. The dates of inclusion for the participating institutions and the corresponding number of submitted studies are presented in Figure 53–1.

Data analysis for this review was accomplished with sorting and record-selection methods inherent in the VAX-11 Datatrieve system, in conjunction with custom-designed statistical programs based on standard analysis procedures. Tests of each analysis procedure were performed on subsets of the data and verified against independent calculations.

Summaries of subsets of this study have been submitted to the Food and Drug Administration in support of marketing approval for the Teslacon, and to state and local health care agencies requesting data for technology assessment and reimburse-

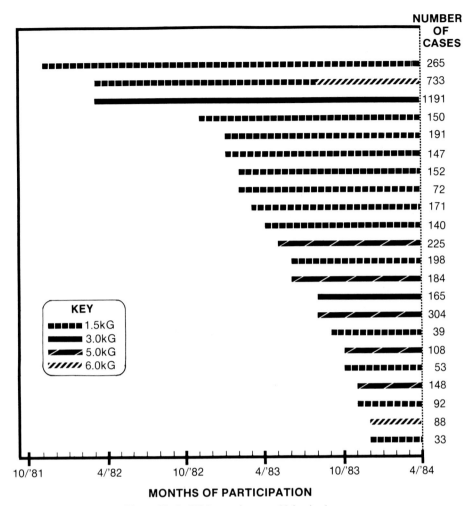

Figure 53–1. MRI experience at 22 institutions.

ment decisions. The full set of data was organized into a menu-driven system displayed at RSNA 1984 in Washington, D.C., and at the Third Annual Meeting of the Society of Magnetic Resonance in Medicine in New York City. This report on the findings constitutes the first published summary of the complete results.

OBJECTIVES

The primary goal of the multi-institutional study was to define those areas of medical imaging where MRI could surpass existing modalities through increased sensitivity and specificity to disease identification, lower risk, and/or decreased cost. From a manufacturer's viewpoint, it was also intended to direct improvements in design and, thus, clinical utility.

Among variables available for analysis were field strength, MRI concurrence with diagnosis (and other modalities), type of scan (*T1* weighted, *T2* weighted, IR, and so forth), anatomic location, etiologic category, final diagnosis, and degree of experience. The second generation of forms furthermore asked for observations of abnormalities to be recorded using a four-point ranking order ("Definitely normal" to "Definitely abnormal") in order that Receiver Operating Characteristic (ROC) curves might be constructed from the data. To provide a comprehensive look at the results of the study, two approaches will be taken. The first will examine all results for such variables as lesion location, etiology, and final diagnosis. The second is an ROC analysis based only on those cases confirmed by biopsy or surgery.

METHODS

The preliminary nature of this study has potentially subjected it to several forms of bias, most notably (1) selection bias of the subject population, (2) recall bias when reporting the results, and (3) information bias due to prior knowledge of the results of comparison modalities.

Selection of patients generally followed two criteria; either investigators wished to determine MRI's ability to depict lesions previously noted on standard imaging modalities, or they sought aid in diagnoses that had confounded other available means. In the first case, MRI results are negatively skewed in relation to other modalities by virtue of the fact that other studies were known to be positive prior to the decision to compare their results with those obtained by MRI. In the second case, unusually difficult cases were selected; these results, however, negatively skew the results for both MRI and the comparison modality. Thus, it should be noted that if selection bias has affected the results reported herein, it has probably done so in such a manner as to cause MRI to appear less accurate than is likely to be the case in a purely random population. Limitations to classes of diseases studied are, in themselves, significant and will be addressed.

The potential problem of recall bias has been addressed by the careful scrutiny of all supporting documents for the data considered. That is, the reports of all modalities compared against MRI were carefully reviewed to assure that the reports were an accurate representation of all the findings.

The problem of prior knowledge from results of competing modalities is not resolvable except for the document review noted previously. The extent of bias can be inferred from Table 53–1. The only means to eradicate the effects of prior knowledge would be to conduct blinded studies, such as those presented in Chapter 54. An attempt to correct for this potential bias is provided later, when ROC curves are presented for the subset of studies verified by pathologic confirmation.

Before the results are reported, it will benefit the reader to briefly capsulize the numbers and subsets of data, so that the specific discussions can be easily followed. This is especially important because the use of two data forms allows different subsets of results to be included for specific purposes (e.g., lesion etiology was always a re-

Table 53–1. SEQUENCE OF IMAGING EXAMINATIONS

Other Study	MRI Prior to Other Study (%)	Other Study Prior to MRI (%)	Studies Performed on Same Day (%)
CT	18	68	19
Radiography	15	79	6
Angiography	12	75	13
Ultrasound	8	85	7
Nuclear medicine	24	57	19
Mammography	11	84	5
Myelography	3	90	7

Percentages based on random sampling of 100 lesions per modality; each institution represented proportionately to comparisons provided.

quired parameter, whereas specific lesion location was not requested until the latter form version).

For the purposes of this investigation, a study was defined as all sets of MR images obtained during a single imaging session. However, many subjects had complaints referable to different areas of anatomy, on which individual comparisons were drawn. When determined to be normal, these areas have been referred to as regions of interest ("regions," henceforth identified as N_N); when abnormal, as "lesions" (identified as N_D). Figure 53–2 reflects the relationship between "studies," "lesions," and "regions." For patients with disease, the average number of lesions per subject was 1.19; certain subsets of patients averaged more lesions per patient, specifically those with multiple sclerosis (2.69), cerebral infarction (1.75), and metastatic disease (1.90).

The 5781 studies represented herein were obtained over a period of 29 months (between October 1981 and April 1984) from 22 institutions. Cases were deemed ac-

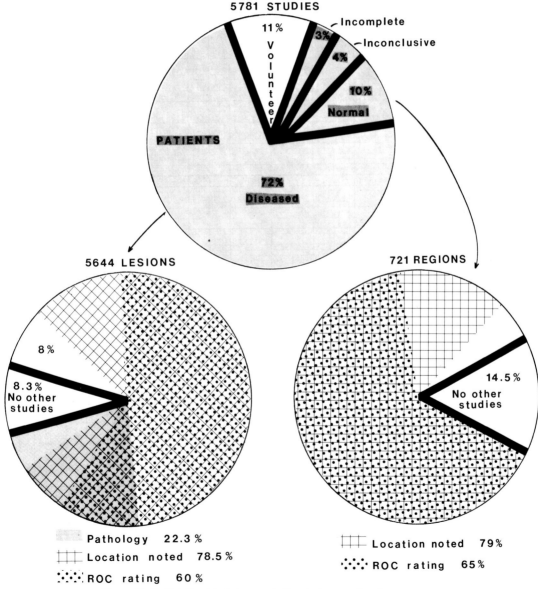

Figure 53–2. Relationship between studies, lesions, and region.

ceptable and entered into the study when evidence was available that alternative imaging results had been accurately reported and that a final decision regarding the subject's condition had been reached (even though this decision was "Inconclusive" in about 5 percent of the patients studied). It is important to note the dates of inclusion for these studies, as they represent early (and technically simplistic) results. For example, multislice and multiecho capabilities—now industry standards—were not available during this period of investigation. Similarly, cardiac-gated studies compose a small percentage (28 percent) of the reported thoracic cases, and the only surface coils used were prototype breast coils—both were under preliminary development during that time. Nevertheless, this "historic" summary offers preliminary suggestions for the clinical use of MRI, borne out by subsequent studies, as well as several insights into the seeming shortcomings of the new modality.

RESULTS

The most reliable part of this study involves those cases that are incontestably supported by pathologic proof (i.e., biopsy). To limit discussion to these cases, however, necessarily excludes the vast majority of studies for which pathologic proof was not obtained. While there is a rationale for one to discount these "uncontrolled" cases as anecdotal, it is felt that their inclusion in the initial survey is warranted. All patients were discharged or treated as though the reported diagnosis had been confirmed. Realistically, the opportunity to obtain pathologic proof is not always consistent with the patient's well-being; for patients with multiple sclerosis or certain CNS tumors, laboratory and neurologic examination are frequently sufficiently specific to convince the physician of the type and region of pathology. The purpose of this study was to determine if MRI could detect a wide variety of disease—limiting the investigation to those pathologies that are routinely pursued by surgery seemed incomplete. Great care has been taken since the initiation of this study to ensure that subjects with inconclusive findings do not contaminate the general results. Thus, the pool of patients without pathologic proof maintains its integrity through the exclusion of lesions whenever discrepancies among the varying clinical results were unresolvable. These "inconclusive" cases are therefore excluded from all analyses.

In order to maximize the report's completeness and validity, results with both standards of "proof" will be reviewed, clearly identified, and directly compared when possible. Results are therefore subdivided into six sections: four utilizing the full study results and prefaced by the heading "Modality Concordance," and two restricted to pathology-confirmed lesions and assessed through ROC methods entitled "ROC Evaluation."

Modality Concordance: Sensitivity and Specificity

The primary question asked when a new imaging modality enters into competition with standard methods of imaging is, "How does it compare?" In the course of the present study, every imaging modality that had been used to locate abnormalities sought by MRI was directly compared in its ability to identify the cause of the patient's symptoms. The complete results are reported in Table 53–2; MRI was shown to be at least as sensitive to disease as all tests other than myelography and mammography, and at least as specific as all except myelography and plain film radiography. Subsets of these data were also compared using the methods of ROC analysis for pathology-proven lesions only (see ROC Evaluation: Modality Comparison).

Table 53–2. CONCORDANCE BETWEEN MRI AND OTHER MODALITIES: ALL LESIONS

Modality	N_D	Sensitivity	N_N	Specificity
MRI		0.87		0.95
vs. CT	4462	0.72	433	0.90
MRI		0.86		0.94
vs. Angiography	731	0.74	48	0.94
MRI		0.83		0.79
vs. Ultrasound	448	0.82	34	0.68
MRI		0.87		0.87
vs. Nuclear medicine	513	0.70	52	0.75
MRI		0.79		0.90
vs. Myelography	418	0.81	39	0.92
MRI		0.81		0.86
vs. Mammography	112	0.92	14	0.71
MRI		0.85		0.86
vs. Radiography	1118	0.74	81	0.90

Modality Concordance: Anatomic Regions

A second method of organizing the results involved an analysis of MRI's accuracy within specific anatomic regions. The data forms allowed for 100 different locations to be specifically identified; 34 of these, however, were fine gradations between areas of the brain. In reviewing the results, it became apparent that such fine gradations limited useful conclusions. Results are therefore presented as conglomerates of the 100 categories, based on anatomic similarity and proximity (Table 53–3).

Findings support the generally widespread belief that MRI is highly sensitive to lesions in the CNS (including the spinal cord), and of equal or less value than existing modalities elsewhere in the body. This indication probably reflects more than simple discrepancies between head and body imaging, however. Body examinations by MRI are significantly fewer in number, owing not only to discouragement over previous failure but also to the lack of research expended on areas of uncertainty. This perception

Table 53–3. ALL RESULTS BY ANATOMIC SITE

Anatomic Site	Other Study	Sensitivity			Specificity		
		MRI	N_D	*Other*	*MRI*	N_D	*Other*
CNS							
Cerebrum	CT	0.95	787	0.69	0.94	16	0.62
Cerebellum	CT	0.93	151	0.68	0.80	5	0.80
Brainstem	CT	0.88	211	0.58	1.00	20	0.85
Sinuses	CT	0.93	78	0.80	1.00	1	0.00
Ventricles	CT	0.96	140	0.81	1.00	7	0.86
Pituitary and sella	CT	0.89	144	0.83	1.00	13	0.77
Spine and spinal cord	CT	0.84	438	0.82	0.93	54	0.94
Neck—soft tissues	CT	0.75	47	0.87	0.89	9	1.00
Lungs	CT	0.91	66	0.96	1.00	1	1.00
Breast	MAM	0.80	91	0.96	0.88	16	0.75
Heart/great vessels	ANG	0.78	128	0.88	1.00	2	1.00
Thorax	CT	0.93	57	0.90	0.86	7	0.57
Liver	CT	0.77	186	0.88	0.95	20	0.95
Pancreas	CT	0.80	30	0.87	1.00	2	1.00
Urinary tract	CT	0.86	167	0.93	0.67	6	0.67
Reproductive system	CT	0.86	44	0.84	0.75	4	0.75
Lymph nodes	CT	0.92	118	0.86	0.80	10	0.60
Bone and soft tissue	CT	0.87	99	0.91	0.67	3	0.33

is borne out by reviewing the reported results of specific institutions for which concentrated research efforts on these areas of generally low results had been developed. For one institution that had an early interest in developing spinal and hepatic applications, the reported results were 94 percent positive in spine cases ($N_D = 114$) and 83 percent in liver studies ($N_D = 63$); as opposed to 84 percent and 77 percent, respectively, for the general population. Another institution's interests in pituitary and breast imaging placed the accuracy at 92 percent for the pituitary ($N_D = 52$) and 82 percent for the breast ($N_D = 68$)—several percentage points higher than the average. What must be recognized is that the results tell average performance over a wide spectrum of clinical settings. The effects of concentrated research can alter, and have already improved, some of these results, but only when used consistently by all involved investigators.

Modality Concordance: Lesion Etiology

Similarly, results have been classified and analyzed according to type of disease process involved (Table 53–4). As might be expected from the previous discussion, the prevalence of specific categories of disease within the study tends toward higher samples of the most successful categories. Neoplastic disease alone accounts for 40 percent of all lesions examined by both MRI and CT. This does not reflect disease incidence, for neoplasm accounts for only 12 percent of confirmed diseases in the general population,[4] and cerebrovascular disease is diagnosed as the cause of 85 percent of intracranial pathologies.[5]

One further point to be made is in regard to MRI's only apparent area of inadequacy: metabolic lesions. The superiority of CT in this category was almost exclusively due to its inclusion of calcific plaques, accounting for 15 of 18 lesions observed by CT but missed by MRI. Moreover, early studies involving such plaques frequently considered them nondetectable by MRI because of their absence of signal; later experience

Table 53–4. COMPARISON BETWEEN MRI AND CT FOR LESIONS OF KNOWN ETIOLOGY

Etiology		All Lesions		Pathology-Proven Lesions	
		N_D	Sensitivity	N_D	Sensitivity
Neoplastic	MRI	1601	0.93	690	0.93
	vs. CT		0.90		0.93
Traumatic	MRI	205	0.89	16	0.81
	vs. CT		0.84		0.88
Vascular	MRI	451	0.87	13	0.92
	vs. CT		0.71		0.92
Congenital	MRI	189	0.93	27	0.93
	vs. CT		0.83		0.89
Hydrocephalic	MRI	76	0.99	0	
	vs. CT		0.91		
Inflammatory	MRI	299	0.81	48	0.79
	vs. CT		0.64		0.81
Degenerative	MRI	1027	0.91	30	0.77
	vs. CT		0.52		0.93
Metabolic	MRI	87	0.45	13	0.39
	vs. CT		0.81		0.69
Cystic	MRI	81	0.90	11	0.73
	vs. CT		0.85		0.73

increased the rate of detection for these plaques when investigators learned to recognize their "negative" contrast appearance.

A feature of Table 53–4 to be noted is its direct comparison between the total pool of lesions and those conclusively proven by pathologic confirmation. While some samples contained in this latter group are admittedly small, the concurrence between the lesions with different levels of "proof" supports MRI's wide range of applications. The greatest disparities, those for "degenerative" and "cystic" lesions, are probably reflected more accurately by the totality of studies than by those restricted to pathologic proof, since surgical intervention in the majority of these cases is an infrequently chosen option.

Modality Concordance: Selected Diagnoses

One of the customized capabilities of the database is a hierarchical listing of final diagnoses as indexed by the *International Classification of Diseases, Ninth Revision* (ICD-9-CM).[6] By cataloguing several thousand diagnoses for which medical imaging might be of value, a decimal-based organization of diseases was developed, whereby subsets of studies could be examined along multiple levels of complexity (superset: neoplasm; set: malignant neoplasm of cerebrum; subset: frontal astrocytoma) insofar as the diagnoses were reported in equally specific terms. By updating the directory to include unforeseen types of cases, a powerful reference to over 5000 cases has been developed. Besides being a means of analysis for various classes of disease, the index has been of use in identifying both patterns of experience among the 22 institutions and previous examples of rare imaging situations (lightning injury, decompression illness, and so forth). Among the diagnoses with sufficient sample sizes (greater than 25), MRI results were particularly high for multiple sclerosis, Chiari malformation, acute cerebrovascular disease, and closed head injury with hemorrhage. Disappointing results were obtained on patients with liver metastases, intervertebral disc degeneration, and cystic kidney disease.

A comparison of matched samples between MRI and CT is presented in Table 53–5. The results are inclusive of patients both with and without pathologic confirmation. Although it would be preferable to have pathologic confirmation on all lesions, the variety and number of cases investigated have made this an unobtainable goal. Therefore, rather than ignore a magnitude of studies that are regularly treated without obtaining pathologic confirmation (e.g., multiple sclerosis, stroke), all cases are presented in this part of the evaluation, using the clinically accepted criteria. While similar to the type of information presented in Table 53–4, evaluation according to specific diagnosis allows for finer direction of research interests.

ROC Evaluation: Modality Comparison

Owing to the inclusion of the ranking method for lesion discernibility, the ability to construct ROC curves was planned into the second version of data forms. An essential characteristic of ROC curves is that bivalent situations are presented (e.g., presence or absence of disease), and multivariate responses are reported indicating certainty in one of the two possibilities.[7] By analyzing the number of correct and incorrect responses, the reader's discrimination abilities can be tested. In such a test, readers rate the presence or absence of a given lesion with an incremental scale ranging from "definitely present" to "definitely absent." By systematically raising the threshold of detection, a graph can be constructed that relates the trade-off of fewer detections

Table 53–5. COMPARISON OF MRI AND CT: MATCHED SAMPLES

Final Diagnosis	ICD-9	N_D	MRI Sensitivity	CT Sensitivity
Cysticercosis	123.1	27	0.96	0.70
Malignant neoplasm of				
Oropharynx	146	29	1.00	0.97
Bones and articular cartilage	170	58	0.95	0.93
Ovary and uterine adnexa	183	27	0.85	0.82
Bladder	188	28	0.71	0.68
Kidney and urinary organs	189	43	0.98	1.00
Brain	191	363	0.97	0.88
Cerebellum	191.6	38	0.94	0.79
Adrenal gland	194	44	0.96	0.98
Pituitary	194.3	85	0.92	0.88
Lymph nodes (metastatic)	196	68	0.90	0.90
Liver (metastatic)	197.7	124	0.85	0.89
Meningitis	322	39	0.72	0.67
Childhood CNS degeneration	330	59	0.88	0.51
Multiple sclerosis	340	570	0.92	0.28
Acute cerebrovascular disease	436	53	0.91	0.70
Intervertebral disc disorders	722	89	0.92	0.88
Intervertebral disc degeneration	722.6	44	0.75	0.96
Chiari malformation	742.4	51	1.00	0.63
Congenital cardiac anomalies	746	30	0.87	0.87
Cystic kidney disease	753.1	39	0.90	0.97
Closed head injury with hemorrhage	852	51	0.98	0.77

to the increase in certainty of those correctly identified.[8] As the threshold is lowered, a reverse situation occurs, in that more occurrences are identified but with an accompanying decrease in certainty. In diagnostic practice, the first situation (high specificity, low sensitivity) is analogous to "under-reading," or "false negative" results. The second (high sensitivity, low specificity) results in "over-reading," or "false positive" results. Since ROC analysis presents the functional relationship between these two types of errors, it allows the physician to better gauge the consequences of various confidence levels in his tests. Because the graph is based on percentages, its total area can equal no more than 1; thus, the "perfect test" (100 percent sensitive and 100 percent specific) would have an area equal to 1. This estimate of the area is often called the performance of the test (designated "W," the Wilcoxon statistic) and is the single parameter by which ROC curves are most frequently compared. For ROC data generated under similar conditions, the test with the greater "W" (area beneath the curve) is deemed the superior test. Areas beneath two curves are compared as a function of the standard deviation of each in a statistical test called the critical ratio ("z").[9] Critical ratios must be of significant magnitude (usually greater or equal to 1.96) to assure that a level of certainty exists (usually 90 to 99 percent) and that the differences in the curves are not due to sampling error.

    The subset of data used for the ROC analysis of MRI versus comparative imaging modalities consists of 614 lesions confirmed by pathology and rated on a four-point scale by investigators, in addition to 470 regions determined to be normal and rated similarly. For each of the seven modalities, all common examinations by MRI and the comparison modality were evaluated. Because each set of data constituted a matched pair between MRI and the other study, the statistical significance was calculated using a method specifically appropriate to matched samples. This method, developed by Hanley and McNeil,[10] adjusts the standard error between two ROC curves by correcting for the degree of inherent correlation due to the matching process. They have calculated a table of correlation coefficients that provide the correct coefficient when the average areas and average Kendall tau are known. This coefficient (r) is then used to calculate the standard error between the areas via the formula

$$SE(A_1 - A_2) = [(SE_1)^2 + (SE_2)^2 - 2r(SE_1)(SE_2)]^{.5}.$$

As in the general formula, this allows calculation of the critical ratio (Z) by:

$$Z = (A_1 - A_2)/[SE(A_1 - A_2)].$$

Subscripts in the prior formulae refer to the first or second comparative imaging test, whereas "A" represents the area of the curve, "SE" the standard error, and "Z" the critical ratio.

Results of the seven comparisons with MRI are graphically displayed in Figures 53–3 to 53–9. Values on each table indicate the number of lesions compared (N_D), the normal subjects examined (N_N), and the calculated critical ratio (Z). Of all the modalities, the comparison with radiography has the greatest statistical significance—MRI is superior at the 99 percent level of significance.[11] The comparisons with CT, angiography, nuclear medicine, and mammography do not fall far behind, however, and have statistical significance at the 90 percent confidence level. Thus, the lowest common level of statistical confidence (90 percent) supports the conclusion that MRI is performed accurately 2 percent more frequently than CT, 5 percent more frequently than angiography, 10 percent less frequently than mammography, 9 percent more frequently than radiography, and 10 percent more frequently than nuclear medicine. Comparisons with ultrasound and myelography did not support the existence of real differences between these modalities and MRI.

ROC Evaluation: MRI Field Strength

The final evaluation involved a comparison of MRI's performance at different field strengths (0.15, 0.3, 0.5, and 0.6 tesla) for those cases constituting the MRI versus CT (ROC) comparison reviewed previously. The results of this comparison are presented in Figure 53–10.

The comparison and methods of evaluation are identical to those noted above, with one exception. Because the studies are not matched samples, the standard error is calculated using

$$SE(A_1 - A_2) = [(SE_1)^2 + (SE_2)^2]^{.5}$$

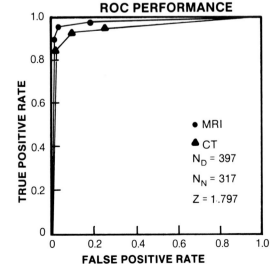

Figure 53–3. Matched ROC analysis between MRI and CT resulted in an area for MRI equal to 0.969 ($SE^2 = 0.000051$) and for CT, 0.949 ($SE^2 = 0.000082$).

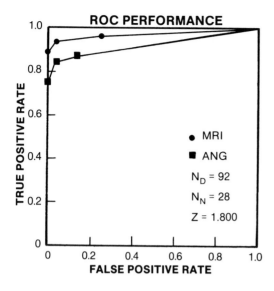

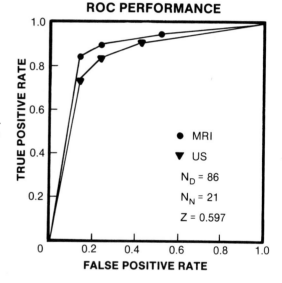

Figure 53–4. Matched ROC analysis between MRI and angiography resulted in an area for MRI equal to 0.969 (SE^2 = 0.000222) and for angiography, 0.919 (SE^2 = 0.000594).

Figure 53–5. Matched ROC analysis between MRI and ultrasound resulted in an area for MRI equal to 0.876 (SE^2 = 0.002437) and for ultrasound, 0.836 (SE^2 = 0.002735).

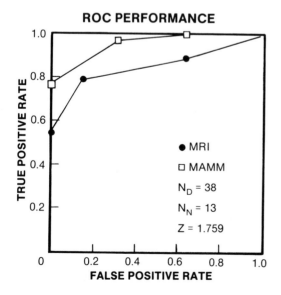

Figure 53–6. Matched ROC analysis between MRI and mammography resulted in an area for MRI equal to 0.856 (SE^2 = 0.002670) and for mammography, 0.955 (SE^2 = 0.000681).

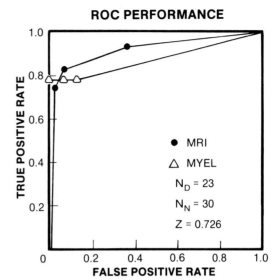

Figure 53–7. Matched ROC analysis between MRI and myelography resulted in an area for MRI equal to 0.925 ($SE^2 = 0.001583$) and for myelography, 0.877 ($SE^2 = 0.003177$).

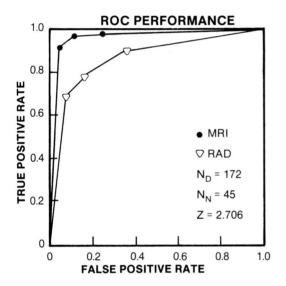

Figure 53–8. Matched ROC analysis between MRI and radiography resulted in an area for MRI equal to 0.961 ($SE^2 = 0.000387$) and for radiography, 0.870 ($SE^2 = 0.000865$).

Figure 53–9. Matched ROC analysis between MRI and nuclear medicine resulted in an area for MRI equal to 0.884 ($SE^2 = 0.001589$), and for nuclear medicine, 0.781 ($SE^2 = 0.002317$).

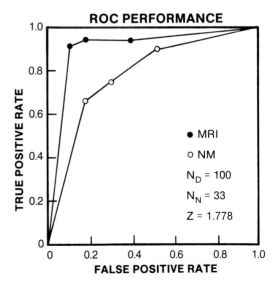

**ROC PERFORMANCE OF MRI
AT DIFFERENT FIELD STRENGTHS**

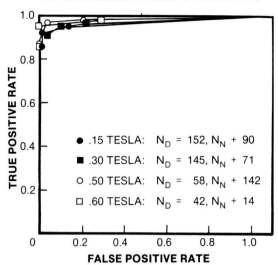

Figure 53–10. Unmatched ROC analysis for MRI at varying field strengths resulted in the following areas and SE^2: 0.15 T (0.963, 0.000285), 0.3 T (0.958, 0.00028), 0.5 T (0.963, 0.001717).

rather than the modified version noted above. Calculation of the critical ratios between each pair of curves indicates that differences in MRI results between field strengths are not statistically significant; the calculated critical ratios are given in Table 53–6.

Despite its limitations, several basic conclusions can be drawn from the current study. MRI performs at least as well, and very likely better, than established modalities (other than mammography) in regard to detection of disease. This assertion is supported both by an examination of the extraordinarily large number of studies reported generally in this report and by ROC analysis of a smaller subset of matched samples proven by pathology. MRI's inferiority to mammography supports the necessity of application-specific techniques and accessories for MRI to become a serious replacement for current highly specialized devices. One would be hesitant to extrapolate the reported differences in a predictive fashion because of several important considerations. In MRI's favor would be the fact that the technology here represented has already been surpassed; it might be expected that the intervening research and development of surface coils for the spine, for example, has significantly increased MRI's performance when compared with myelography for a variety of spinal pathologies. On the negative side, there remains a potentially great bias in the results that is due to prior knowledge of the other examinations; this bias can be resolved only through blinded readings of each modality's images. Furthermore, it has yet to be determined that the population evaluated reflects the usual patient pool referred for imaging tests. The comparisons with angiography, for example, reflect a subpopulation of angiography studies most suitable to MR imaging. Aortic aneurysms, myocardial infarcts, and congenital ab-

Table 53–6. CRITICAL RATIO COMPARISONS AMONG MRI FIELDS

Field Strength	0.30 t	0.50 t	0.60 t
0.15 t	0.251	1.306	0.016
0.30 t	—	1.384	0.104
0.50 t	1.384	—	0.543

Comparisons among each possible combination of the tested MRI field strengths resulted in performance differences that were insignificant at the 90% confidence interval.

normalities are heavily represented, whereas studies of vessel patency—a highly effective use of angiography—have been infrequently compared.

When the results of the current study are considered for knowledge regarding MRI's abilities to detect lesions within certain anatomic regions, the results are not surprising. MRI appears superior to CT in the brain and is equally, or less, effective elsewhere. Motion has been a particular problem in the short history of MRI, and the relative lack of gating and surface coils available during this investigation is readily apparent.

The current report indicates that MRI is highly sensitive to a wide variety of disease pathologies. There are, however, two disclaimers to this statement. First, it is assumed that the physician has in mind some specific diagnosis for confirmation. Second, he must have the knowledge to choose parameters that differentiate between diagnostic alternatives. At this stage, both these prerequisites (especially the latter) may hinder the use of MRI as a screening tool. It is not surprising that diseases of greatest severity and cost have been explored earliest, particularly when the imminent goal of reimbursement for such uses is considered. Because this stage of investigation is potentially the most liberal in its research opportunities, the concentration of efforts on limited applications is disappointing. As reimbursement for MRI procedures is approved for specific conditions, fiscal responsibilities will tend to allow less experimentation with unproven techniques and conditions in all but heavily endowed research institutions.

Finally, the question of the relative effectiveness of varying field strengths was examined through the use of ROC curves. The current evaluation does not conclusively support any differences attributable to this variable. In order to provide a more definitive analysis, those institutions with the resources to do imaging at multiple fields might attempt blinded readings of subjects imaged on devices at different field strengths. Until that time, it appears to be an unresolvable issue.

A clinical efficacy study of 300 MRI cases at 1.5 tesla is presented in Chapter 54.

ACKNOWLEDGMENTS

The authors wish to extend their gratitude to the following investigators, their colleagues, and their institutions for the diligent efforts and wholehearted cooperation in compiling the studies of which this report is composed.

AMC Cancer Institute (Denver, Colorado): Lewis Schiffer, M.D.
Baylor University Medical Center (Dallas, Texas): Steven Harms, M.D.
The Cleveland Clinic Foundation (Cleveland, Ohio): Thomas Meaney, M.D.
Charlotte Memorial Hospital (Charlotte, North Carolina): Edward Easton, M.D.
Dent Neurologic Institute (Buffalo, New York): William Kinkel, M.D.
Greenberg Radiology Clinic (Deerfield Park, Illinois): Irving Greenberg, M.D.
Houston Imaging Center (Houston, Texas): Marcos Calderon, M.D.
Hershey Medical Center (Hershey, Pennsylvania): William Weidner, M.D.
Massachusetts General Hospital (Boston, Massachusetts): Thomas Brady, M.D.
Messina & Liebeskind Associates (New York, New York): Arie Liebeskind, M.D.
North Shore University Hospital (Manhasset, New York): Harry Stein, M.D.
New York Hospital (New York, New York): Joseph Whalen, M.D.
Ontario Cancer Institute (Toronto, Ontario): Marc Henkelman, M.D.
Rush Presbyterian–St. Luke's Medical Center (Chicago, Illinois): David Turner, M.D.
St. Joseph's Hospital (London, Ontario): Lionel Reese, M.D.
St. Luke's Hospital (Jacksonville, Florida): Harry McEuen, M.D.
Scottsdale Memorial Hospital (Scottsdale, Arizona): Samuel Hessel, M.D.
Shands Teaching Hospital (Gainesville, Florida): Clyde Williams, M.D.
University Hospitals of Cleveland (Cleveland, Ohio): Ralph Alfidi, M.D.
University Hospital of Indianapolis (Indianapolis, Indiana): Eugene Klatte, M.D.
University Hospital of Kentucky Medical Center (Lexington, Kentucky): Harold Rosenbaum, M.D.
Vanderbilt University Medical Center (Nashville, Tennessee): C. Leon Partain, M.D., Ph.D.

References

1. Swets JA, Pickett RM, et al: Assessment of diagnostic techniques. Science *205*(4407):753, 1979.
2. Evens RG: National Guidelines and Standards for Health Planning—Their Relationship to Radiology. St. Louis, Washington University School of Medicine, Dept. of Radiology, 1985.
3. The states and health care: Girding for DRGs, budget cuts and rate control fights. FAH Review, September/October 1983, pp 16–36.
4. National Cancer Institute (NCI) 1977 Fact Book Estimate of New Cases.
5. National Center for Health Statistics (NCHS) 1977 Hospital Discharge Survey (HDS) Estimates.
6. International Classification of Diseases, 9th Revision: Clinical Modification (ICD-9-CM), Vols 1 & 2: Commission on Professional and Health Activities. Ann Arbor, Edwards Brothers Inc., 1980.
7. Metz CE: Basic principles of ROC analysis. Semin Nucl Med *8*:283, 1978.
8. Hanley JA, McNeil BJ: The meaning and use of the area under a receiver operating characteristic (ROC) curve. Radiology *143*:29, 1982.
9. Hogg RV, Tanis EA: Probability and Statistical Inference. Macmillan Publishing Co, New York, 1977.
10. Hanley JA, McNeil BJ: A method of comparing the areas under receiver operating characteristic curves derived from the same cases. Radiology *148*:839, 1983.
11. Korin BP: Introduction to Statistical Methods. Cambridge, Winthrop Publishers, 1977.

54

Clinical Efficacy: Analysis of 300 MRI Cases at 1.5 Tesla

MARK A. LUTHE
ALAN A. STEIN

As part of its continuing investigations of the Teslacon, Technicare Corporation has completed two evaluations using clinical images collected on a 1.5 tesla MRI device. The first involved unblinded clinical evaluations, as an extension of studies done earlier with systems operating from 0.15 to 0.6 T (see Chapter 53).[1] The results of 298 subjects imaged between 3 April 1984 and 29 July 1985 are presented and compared with findings reported for the lower field systems.

The second study sought to define the effectiveness of MRI when unaided by any outside information or when supplemented only by clinical history. This blinded study, employing 150 cases and 1200 separate readings, was organized concurrently with the first study, utilizing the same cases in a blinded fashion, and completed on 10 August 1985.

PROSPECTIVE STUDY

Objectives

The purpose of the prospective study was to measure the ability of the 1.5 T Teslacon to determine the presence or absence of disease as determined by accepted medical diagnostic criteria. Clinical investigators from three institutions accepted referrals of patients with proven or expected abnormalities for MR imaging. After a conclusion was reached regarding the subject's condition, a data form was completed listing that decision as well as the success of comparison modalities in relation to MRI. Because each investigator has at his disposal the results of all tests, the prospective study simulated actual clinical conditions but did not attempt to blind investigators from any relevant clinical or diagnostic information.

Methods

Potential subjects for the prospective investigation included all patients for whom an imaging procedure had been prescribed. Results of the MRI examination were evaluated for their consistency with other imaging modalities and the final diagnosis, as determined by accepted clinical criteria.

The protocol for the prospective study was in most details unchanged from that of previous investigations: Investigators were unrestricted in their choice of patients

Table 54–1. COMPARISON BETWEEN MRI AND FINAL DIAGNOSIS

	MRI +	MRI −	
Final diagnosis +	201	25	Of 226 patients examined by MRI: success of MRI = 201/226 = 89%
Final diagnosis −	2	57	Of 59 normal subjects examined by MRI: success of MRI = 57/59 = 97%

"MRI +" denotes true positive when "Final Diagnosis +", and false positive when "Final Diagnosis −".
"MRI −" denotes true negative when "Final Diagnosis −", and false negative when "Final Diagnosis +".

and imaging parameters appropriate to the expected pathology. Investigators responsible for providing the prospective study population were directed only in regard to the case mix needed for fulfillment of the blinded protocol. Any remaining investigator bias is a reflection of differences in patient referrals. The inclusion of radiologists with differing backgrounds (i.e., a community hospital, consulting practice, and specialty center) should compensate for these referral variations. Patients were excluded from the study only if the presence of pacemakers, ferromagnetic clips, or prostheses was thought to harbor potential danger to the individual.

A detailed explanation of the study design is presented in Chapter 53 under Methods.[1] The only variation from those earlier studies involved format changes to the questionnaire used for data collection. A revision, made to the forms on 3 October 1984, affected the investigator's responses in the following manner: (1) The numerical rating scale for comparing imaging tests was replaced by a symbolic system $(0, >, <, =)$; (2) a method for identifying useful MRI pulse sequences was added; (3) the 99 anatomic codes were collapsed to a 9-region system; and (4) the previous 10 etiologic categories were reorganized to a 14-category system.

Results

The prospective study evaluated MRI results for consistency with the final diagnosis as well as with other imaging modalities. Of the 298 studies reported, 13 had been deemed technically inadequate. Eight were inadequate because of patient motion, three because of operator error, and two because of technical problems. The 285 satisfactory studies consisted of 226 patients diagnosed as abnormal and 59 patients diagnosed as normal. The results of the comparisons between MRI and the final diagnoses for these 285 cases are presented in Table 54–1.

Table 54–2. CONCORDANCE BETWEEN MRI AND OTHER MODALITIES

	MRI +	MRI −	
CT +	157	6	Of 189 patients examined by MRI and CT:
CT −	13	13	success of MRI = 170/189 = 90%
			success of CT = 163/189 = 86%
Ultrasound +	10	0	Of 11 patients examined by MRI and US:
Ultrasound −	0	1	success of MRI = 10/11 = 91%
			success of US = 10/11 = 91%
Angiography +	4	2	Of 11 patients examined by MRI and ANG:
Angiography −	2	3	success of MRI = 6/11 = 55%
			success of ANG = 6/11 = 55%
Radiography +	23	0	Of 31 patients examined by MRI and RAD:
Radiography −	4	4	success of MRI = 27/31 = 87%
			success of RAD = 23/31 = 73%

Patients represented are a subset of those in Table 54–1; patients for whom multiple imaging tests were done appear separately under each category.

Table 54–3. COMPARISON OF MRI RESULTS VERSUS FINAL DIAGNOSIS AT VARIOUS FIELD
STRENGTHS

	MRI Results								
	1.5 T			*0.5–0.6 T*			*0.15–0.3 T*		
Final Diagnosis	MRI+	MRI−		MRI+	MRI−		MRI+	MRI−	
Pathology present	89%	11%	[226]	89%	11%	[767]	89%	11%	[308]
Pathology absent	3%	97%	[59]	1%	99%	[168]	4%	96%	[54]

Numbers in brackets represent the number of abnormalities studied (for the row labeled "Pathology present"), or the number of normal subjects (for the row labeled "Pathology absent") at each field strength. "MRI +" denotes true positive when "Pathology present" and false positive when "Pathology absent."

Evidence of MRI's concordance with other imaging modalities is presented in Table 54–2. Each column shows the number of patients imaged by both MR and the comparison modality. Within each column, a plus (+) indicates detection of an abnormality, whereas the minus (−) indicates nondetection.

The results of comparisons between MRI and computerized tomography, angiography, ultrasonography, and radiography indicate that for the population studied, the 1.5 T Teslacon was highly effective in its ability to identify abnormalities of the head and body. The similarity of the findings to results reported for lower field Teslacon systems is illustrated for the comparison between MRI and the final diagnosis in Table 54–3, and between MRI and CT in Table 54–4. In order that similar levels of system development and physician experience be compared, results in Tables 54–3 and 54–4 are abstracted from Technicare's FDA premarketing applications as they were prepared for each range of systems.[2,3]

The section of Table 54–3 labeled "1.5 T" summarizes the results of the 285 studies completed on the 1.5 T Teslacon and compares the findings with initial experiences at lower field systems. Despite differences in the number of patients studied, the detection of lesions defined by the final diagnosis has remained constant at 89 percent. Although the percentage of correctly diagnosed normal subjects has fluctuated slightly, consistently there has been over-reading of less than 5 percent of the cases.

Historically, the concordance rate between CT and MR has been of interest as one of the best tests of MR performance. Table 54–4 presents a synopsis of this comparison as documented by Technicare through its investigations of low- , mid- , and high-field systems. Each column lists the earliest cases imaged by both MR and CT, respectively, at each field strength.

Although the concordance rate has varied among the populations studied (e.g., a high percentage of multiple sclerosis patients in the 0.5 to 0.6 T group), MR has consistently detected abnormalities at a rate higher than that of CT. Similar comparisons between the 1.5 T Teslacon and angiography, ultrasonography, radiography, and nu-

Table 54–4. CONCORDANCE OF LESION DETECTION FOR MRI AND CT
AT VARIOUS FIELD STRENGTHS

	MRI Results					
	1.5 T		*0.5–0.6 T*		*0.15–0.3 T*	
Final Diagnosis	MRI+	MRI−	MRI+	MRI−	MRI+	MRI−
CT+	83%	3%	55%	5%	74%	3%
		[189]		[598]		[263]
CT−	7%	7%	34%	6%	16%	7%

Numbers in brackets represent the number of lesions examined by both MRI and CT at each field strength. In each panel, " + " indicates detection of a lesion, while " − " indicates nondetection.

clear medicine have shown MRI to be comparable to each in detecting lesions among these specific populations.

BLINDED INVESTIGATION

Objectives

In view of concerns regarding prospective payment and cost-containment of health care, it becomes a necessity that unbiased scientific studies be conducted to determine the risks and benefits associated with the various medical technologies. While previous Technicare studies have concentrated on the concordance of lesions in diverse anatomic areas and disease states with established imaging modalities, no study has yet examined the inherent performance of MRI. As MRI continues to be disseminated throughout the medical community, the need arises for an accurate assessment of its ability to detect and differentiate various disease states. This necessity arises not only from the physician specialists involved in interpretation of this new technology but also from the primary care physicians who must decide when its use is to be prescribed.

The goal of the blinded study was to determine the extent to which a physician, highly trained in the reading of MR images, could distinguish pathologic from normal tissue based solely on the appearance of the images or, at most, supplemented by a minimum of relevant clinical history. Furthermore, it was the objective of the investigation to determine the accuracy with which a diagnosis could be made under those conditions.

Methods

From the prospective studies, 150 cases (49 abnormal heads, 26 normal heads, 51 abnormal bodies, 24 normal bodies) were selected for inclusion in a blinded reading study. Since the aim of this study was to determine the effects of clinical history on the accuracy of MRI interpretation, selection took into account the availability of a final diagnosis, relevant patient history, and consistent numbers and types of images. The final determination could include the results of the MRI examination but only when verified by other means (laboratory results, other imaging tests, pathology). Because of the inherent difficulty in verifying the absence of pathology in clinically normal subjects (those presenting with symptoms, though deemed to be free of disease), consenting Technicare employees were used to supplement the clinically normal group in order to achieve the required case mix. The number of subjects per etiologic category as used in the blinded study is included in Table 54–5. Other than the 19 normal studies of Technicare employee volunteers, Table 54–5 is a direct subset of the studies performed under the prospective study.

The sample population comprised 75 head and 75 body studies per the planned ratio of 1:1. Likewise, the intended ratio of abnormal to normal subjects was met at 2:1. The final anatomic distribution of cases included in the blind readings is provided in Table 54–6.

This study was conducted by Technicare with assistance from eight Teslacon users currently working at field strengths lower than 1.5 tesla: Four specialists in cranial imaging read the 75 head cases, and four specialists in extracranial imaging read the 75 body cases. Readers were selected from among Technicare's experienced pool of clinical MRI investigators, excluding those previously familiar with the cases to be read.

Table 54–5. SUBJECT DISTRIBUTION PER ETIOLOGIC CATEGORY

Etiology of Diagnoses	Total
Normal	50
Tumor	44
Hemorrhage/hematoma	2
Infarct/ischemia	10
Inflammation/edema	5
Aneurysm	4
Obstructive	0
Traumatic	5
Degenerative	16
Metabolic	2
Atrophic	0
Cystic	5
Abscess	2
Congenital	5
Uncertain	0
Total	150

Prior to the actual examination, readers were instructed in the mechanics of the test through a standard script read by the test administrator, and all questions asked of the administrator and clarification given were noted. During the readings, cases were identified by unique case identification numbers appearing on each sheet of images, clinical history summary, and data acquisition sheet. Owing to the expected length of the test, presentation order was a potential source of bias. In order to assure that cases were not consistently misread because of reader fatigue, each series of readings was presented in a unique randomly selected order.

Each reader had two occasions to read 75 sets of films from either head or body data. During the first reading, each case was presented by the test administrator with a copy of the questionnaire. During the second series, the cases were reordered and reread with the inclusion of a summary of limited clinical symptoms and history. During this trial, normal cases were accompanied by appropriate contrived histories, readers having been forewarned of the ruse (an example is shown in Figure 54–1). For control purposes, five randomly selected cases were never accompanied by clinical information. Sample cases, including images and patient histories, are provided as Figures 54–1, 54–2, and 54–6 to 54–9. Included with these samples, though they were not available to the readers, are the subjects' final diagnoses.

The questionnaires required the readers to rate the quality of the scan, assign a confidence value to the probability of disease ("Definitely normal" to "Definitely abnormal"), record the number of lesions observed, and divide 100 points among a variety of pathologies. Several types of protocol deviations were encountered during the course

Table 54–6. ANATOMIC DISTRIBUTION OF PATHOLOGIC AND NORMAL CASES IN 1.5 T BLINDED STUDY

Anatomic Region	Normal (No.)	Abnormal (No.)	Total
Head	26	49	75
Body	24	51	75
Spine	6	13	19
Thorax	7	9	16
Abdomen	3	10	13
Pelvis	6	13	19
Extremities	2	6	8
Total	50	100	150

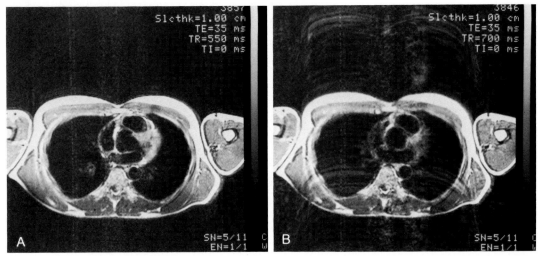

Figure 54–1. *A–B*, A 27-year-old male with history of pneumococcal pneumonia two years earlier. Patient complained of fatigue and was found on physical examination to have faint heart murmur and borderline splenomegaly. Diagnosis: Normal (example of fictitious history).

of the 1.5 T blinded study. In order of discussion, they are as follows: test administration errors, changes in the protocol, and failure to foresee a consistent reading aberration.

In the reporting of the ROC data, it will be noted that the number of readings for the extracranial data totals 297 (rather than 300, the correct number for four readers × 75 cases). Likewise, the composite total for the head and body data is three less than the expected total of 600. The source of the discrepancy was a test administration error; during the production of the randomization lists for the four body case readings, three erroneous case identification numbers were entered into the randomization program. The result was that the administrator of the first trial found himself with three cases listed for which he had no films or history. The substitution error was corrected prior to the remaining readings.

The sole protocol change involved modification of the instructions presented to readers of the extracranial studies. Prior to administration of these four reading tests, it was recognized that the expanse of anatomy that readers would be required to wade through undirected made for both an impossible task and a clinically unrealistic one. Additionally, the possibility of distraction by nonclinical findings could dramatically shadow the true sensitivity of the reading test. For example, the frequent MRI depiction of degenerated discs might readily be noted as an abnormality in lieu of more subtle changes (Fig. 54–2). Because correlation is seldom warranted for these findings, and because the spine is apt to appear in most body images, it was decided that readers would be directed to examine a single organ system for each case. Therefore, each of the extracranial cases (both normal and abnormal) was identified as belonging to one of the following groups: cardiothoracic, musculoskeletal, hepatic, gastrointestinal, and urogenital. Readers were informed during the initial instructions that abnormalities outside the identified category were to be ignored. Identification of groups became part of the case identification number, which was permanently affixed to each MR film; thus, it was available for both the pre- and posthistory readings.

A similar problem to that requiring the protocol change was uncovered in the data from the head cases during the course of the studies. As early as the first reading, the test administrators were asked by the readers whether sinusitis should be considered an abnormality. Uncertain as to whether sinusitis cases had been part of the protocol, and not wishing to unduly bias the data, the administrators responded that *all* abnor-

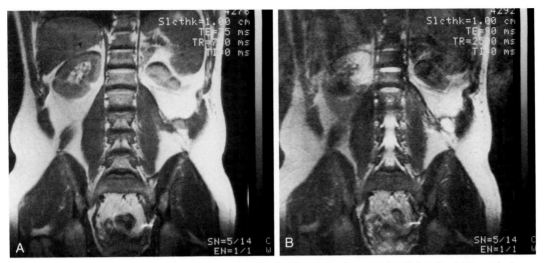

Figure 54–2. *A–B,* A 45-year-old male with a complaint of left side pain for three weeks. Patient has history of sebaceous cyst removal 15 years ago and left nephrectomy for tumor three years ago. Diagnosis: Left flank abscess.

malities were to be included. Readers were asked, thenceforth, to make notations on any data questionnaires for which their responses were based solely on the presence of sinusitis. Upon analysis of the data, it became obvious that several of the normal subjects received "definitely abnormal" ratings as the result of the presence of sinusitis. As with the case of degenerative discs noted earlier, MR tends to show maxillary sinusitis and cysts with greater sensitivity than other imaging modalities, yet the findings are frequently ignored unless clinically warranted. In order to correct this aberration of the data, it was decided that there was justification to reassign the ratings given to these cases. Specifically, for six cases during the prehistory series and five cases during the posthistory series the readers had marked the questionnaires as 100 percent inflammation, in addition to explicitly noting that sinusitis was the cause. For all cases with those two conditions, the 100 percent certainty rating was reallocated from "Inflammation" to "Normal" and the case rating from "Definitely abnormal" to "Definitely normal." All of the cases marked in said manner were, in fact, clinically normal.

Results

Results of this study are presented as Figures 54–3 to 54–5 in the form of receiver operating characteristic (ROC) curves, a recognized method of measuring subject discrimination.[3–6] In such a test, readers rate the presence or absence of a given lesion with a five-step incremental scale ranging from "definitely present" to "definitely absent." By systematically raising the threshold of detection, a graph can be constructed that relates the trade-off of fewer detections to the increase in certainty of those correctly identified. The estimate of the area beneath the curve is called the performance of the test (designated as "W") and is the single parameter by which ROC curves are most frequently compared.

The ROC curve in Figure 54–3 plots the points obtained as a composite of all head and body cases read at 1.5 T; the graphs shown represent a comparison of the pre- and posthistory test conditions. Computation of the critical ratio (z) gives a z-value of 0.6744, indicating that the difference between the areas underlying the curves (0.81 prehistory, 0.83 posthistory) is not statistically significant with 95 percent certainty (p = 0.05).[7,8] Only one pair of ROC curves proved to have statistically significant

COMPOSITE RECEIVER OPERATING CHARACTERISTIC (ROC) CURVES FOR BLIND READINGS OF 1.5 TESLA MR IMAGING CASES

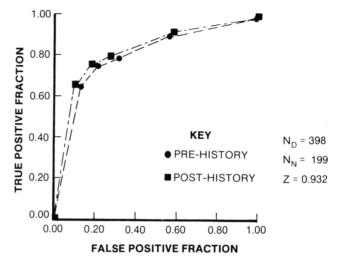

Figure 54–3. ROC curves for blind readings of 1.5 tesla MR imaging cases.

differences at this level; with the inclusion of clinical history, head cases were read more accurately than body cases (critical ratio was 2.568). Other pairs of ROC curves are included as Figures 54–4 and 54–5, with tables of the data points from which they were constructed.

The ROC performance (W, the Wilcoxon statistic) of individual readers varied considerably, and the range and mean for each subgroup of readings is provided in Table 54–7. Considering the strict nature of the reading test, the results (Table 54–7) indicate a high degree of sensitivity (ability to detect disease) and specificity (ability to recognize normality) when the 1.5 T Teslacon is used alone or in conjunction with limited clinical history.

The final task put to the readers was one of discriminating among a wide variety of clinical pathologies with the limited knowledge obtainable from the MR images (or the images in conjunction with clinical history). In order to examine diagnostic specificity, readers were required to divide 100 points among the listed categories during each viewing. By totaling the results of all readers for patients with a specific etiology, it is possible to gather some impressions about the rates of correct and incorrect pathology discrimination. Concordance between the final etiology and the readers' opinions were calculated for each of six situations: prehistory studies, posthistory studies, prehistory head studies, posthistory head studies, prehistory body studies, and posthistory body studies. In Tables 54–8 to 54–10, each row represents all subjects having a primary discharge diagnosis of the designated category, and the columns represent the readers' attempts at correctly identifying them. Thus, the point of cross section gives the percentage at which a certain category of disease was correctly identified

Table 54–7. READERS' PERFORMANCE (W) FOR 1.5 T READINGS

	Head Studies		Body Studies	
	Images Alone	*Images + History*	*Images Alone*	*Images + History*
Range	0.731–0.900	0.804–0.904	0.772–0.831	0.727–0.827
Mean	0.828	0.873	0.796	0.780

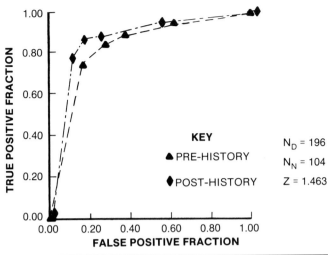

RECEIVER OPERATING CHARACTERISTIC (ROC) CURVES FOR BLIND READINGS OF 1.5 TESLA HEAD CASES

KEY

▲ PRE-HISTORY

◆ POST-HISTORY

$N_D = 196$

$N_N = 104$

$Z = 1.463$

IMAGES ONLY

	DEFINITELY NORMAL x = 1	PROBABLY NORMAL x = 2	POSSIBLY ABNORMAL x = 3	PROBABLY ABNORMAL x = 4	DEFINITELY ABNORMAL x = 5	N
1) Normals = x	39	26	10	11	18	104
2) Abnormals > x	187	174	164	146	0	
3) Abnormals = x	9	13	10	18	146	196
4) Normals < x	0	39	65	75	86	

W(area) = .82763   SE = 2.6704E-02 $SE^2 = 0.000713$

IMAGE + HISTORY

	DEFINITELY NORMAL x = 1	PROBABLY NORMAL x = 2	POSSIBLY ABNORMAL x = 3	PROBABLY ABNORMAL x = 4	DEFINITELY ABNORMAL x = 5	N
1) Normals = x	46	31	8	7	12	104
2) Abnormals > x	187	174	168	150	0	
3) Abnormals = x	9	13	6	18	150	196
4) Normals < x	0	46	77	85	92	

W(area) = .87252   SE = 2.3194E-02 $SE^2 = 0.000538$

Each column denotes the number of cases rated at a particular value (rows 1 and 3), or relative to a particular rating (rows 2 and 4). In the final row, "W" denotes the Wilcoxon statistic, "SE" the standard error of the graph values, and "SE^2" the standard error squared.

Figure 54–4. ROC curves for blind readings of 1.5 tesla head cases (z = 1.2693).

Table 54–8. CLINICAL DIFFERENTIATION: FINAL DETERMINATION VERSUS BLIND READER RESPONSE*

Actual Etiology	Sample Size	Percentage Response (Pre/Post)								
		NEO	CVA	INF	FLU	DEG	CON	TRM	HYP	NML
Neoplastic (NEO)	44	57/65	11/2	3/3	5/2	8/6	2/3	0/1	3/3	11/15
Infarction (CVA)	10	6/6	39/56	5/3	4/2	26/18	5/1	NA	NA	16/14
Inflammation (INF)	7	11/7	4/0	33/31	0/0	1/0	0/13	13/0	0/0	38/49
Fluid (FLU)	8	1/0	4/5	5/8	25/36	8/0	42/28	0/0	0/0	15/24
Degeneration (DEG)	19	2/2	18/8	1/1	0/0	62/75	5/5	0/0	0/0	11/8
Congenital (CON)	5	11/7	17/17	11/3	0/0	27/49	4/1	0/0	0/0	29/23
Trauma (TRM)	5	2/0	NA	0/0	0/0	0/0	18/1	2/16	0/0	78/83
Hypertrophy (HYP)	2	2/0	NA	0/0	0/0	0/0	18/1	2/16	0/0	78/83
Normal (NML)	50	4/4	4/6	2/3	5/0	7/5	4/2	1/0	3/0	70/80

* Composite results of all readers for both head and body cases.

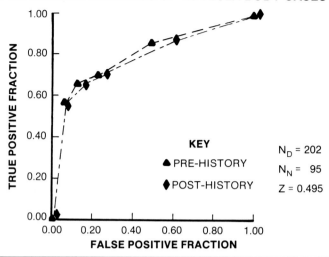

RECEIVER OPERATING CHARACTERISTIC (ROC) CURVES FOR BLINDED READINGS OF 1.5 TESLA BODY CASES

KEY

▲ PRE-HISTORY

◆ POST-HISTORY

$N_D = 202$
$N_N = 95$
$Z = 0.495$

IMAGES ONLY

	DEFINITELY NORMAL x = 1	PROBABLY NORMAL x = 2	POSSIBLY ABNORMAL x = 3	PROBABLY ABNORMAL x = 4	DEFINITELY ABNORMAL x = 5	N
1) Normals = x	48	25	10	4	8	95
2) Abnormals > x	173	142	134	114	0	
3) Abnormals = x	29	31	8	20	114	202
4) Normals < x	0	48	73	83	87	
W(area) = .79570		SE = 2.6959E-02		SE² = 0.000727		

IMAGES + HISTORY

	DEFINITELY NORMAL x = 1	PROBABLY NORMAL x = 2	POSSIBLY ABNORMAL x = 3	PROBABLY ABNORMAL x = 4	DEFINITELY ABNORMAL x = 5	N
1) Normals = x	37	32	10	8	8	95
2) Abnormals > x	178	143	133	111	0	
3) Abnormals = x	24	35	20	22	111	202
4) Normals < x	0	37	69	79	87	
W(area) = .77989		SE = 2.7627E-02		SE² = 0.000763		

Each column denotes the number of cases rated at a particular value (rows 1 and 3), or relative to a particular rates (rows 2 and 4). In the final row, "W" denotes the Wilcoxon statistic, "SE" the standard error of the graph values, and "SE²" the standard error squared.

Figure 54–5. ROC curves for blinded readings of 1.5 tesla body studies (z = .40955).

Table 54–9. CLINICAL DIFFERENTIATION: HEAD STUDIES

Actual Etiology	Sample Size	Percentage Response (Pre/Post)						
		NEO	*CVA*	*INF*	*FLU*	*DEG*	*CON*	*NML*
Neoplastic (NEO)	20	57/68	16/3	4/4	5/2	11/8	1/1	7/14
Infarction (CVA)	10	6/6	40/58	5/3	4/2	27/19	2/0	16/12
Inflammation (INF)	1	24/17	10/0	30/17	0/0	3/0	0/0	33/67
Fluid (FLU)	4	0/0	8/9	0/11	33/44	13/0	36/24	10/11
Degeneration (DEG)	9	3/3	25/11	1/1	0/0	59/77	4/4	9/4
Congenital (CON)	5	9/6	14/14	9/2	0/0	23/41	17/7	27/29
Normal (NML)	26	5/4	5/8	2/3	7/1	7/4	3/2	71/79

Table 54–10. CLINICAL DIFFERENTIATION: BODY STUDIES

Actual Etiology	Sample Size	Percentage Response (Pre/Post)							
		NEO	*HYP*	*INF*	*FLU*	*DEG*	*CON*	*TRM*	*NML*
Neoplastic (NEO)	24	58/60	9/9	3/0	3/0	0/0	5/8	0/4	23/18
Hypertrophy (HYP)	2	25/10	25/40	0/0	0/0	0/0	0/0	0/0	50/50
Inflammation (INF)	6	6/1	0/0	34/40	0/0	0/0	0/20	20/0	40/39
Fluid (FLU)	4	5/3	0/0	19/5	26/43	0/0	25/25	0/0	25/25
Degeneration (DEG)	10	1/0	0/0	0/0	0/0	70/70	10/10	0/0	20/20
Congenital (CON)	0	0/0	0/0	0/0	0/0	0/0	0/0	0/0	0/0
Trauma (TRM)	5	2/0	0/0	0/0	0/0	0/0	18/1	2/16	78/83
Normal (NML)	24	2/1	12/0	0/2	0/0	8/6	8/2	4/2	66/86

(e.g., Neoplastic (NEO) × NEO), or incorrectly identified as one of the alternatives (e.g., Neoplastic (NEO) × INF). The preliminary look at MRI's diagnostic specificity led to the composite head and body results (Table 54–8), head results (Table 54–9), and body results (Table 54–10). Each column contrasts the responses for identical cases both before and after the clinical history was presented (Pre/Post); percentages preceding each slash reflect prehistory confidence in the column category as the primary process, while numbers following the slash indicate the same for posthistory readings. Rows identify the etiology and number of cases composing the test.

Besides providing an initial look at MRI's ability to correctly differentiate disease, Tables 54–8 to 54–10 are of greater benefit when used to determine the causes of the most significant incorrect responses. As should be expected, correct differentiation generally increased upon inclusion of clinical history. Since this is more akin to the actual clinical setting, discussion will focus on the misclassifications that occurred during this trial. Particular attention is given to misreadings that help to define the criteria necessary for appropriate MRI examinations.

One of the most unexpected findings was a 7 percent higher rate of false positive responses for normal head studies than for normal body cases. That 12 percent of these misreadings were assigned to the degenerative/demyelination and infarction categories seems to support an observation by Dr. Meredith Weinstein of The Cleveland Clinic Foundation. Dr. Weinstein has noted a frequent occurrence of subclinical UBO's (unidentified bright objects), which can be easily confused with multiple sclerosis plaques or multiple infarcts. In this respect, then, there appears to be at least a minimal learning curve followed for high-field imaging, above that required with lower field systems.

Blinding readers to the results of other imaging tests dramatically decreased their ability to discriminate pathologic from nonpathologic images. Whereas the sensitivity was 89 percent and the specificity 97 percent for unblinded readings, these values dropped to 81 percent and 70 percent, respectively, during the fully blinded readings. Implications of this finding are unclear. While MRI sensitivity and specificity have probably been exaggerated in the medical literature, it must be acknowledged that the restrictiveness of the current study does not accurately reflect the clinical use of any imaging test.

Among the more disappointing findings are the reported results of the five traumatic lesions. Three of these cases were universally missed by the readers and involved ligamentous injury or bone trauma to the extremities; a fourth was an example of spinal fracture. Because surface coils and thin-slice imaging were not included in the protocol, these changes went unnoticed. More than one of the readers commented, "I keep seeing these extremity cases, and I know there must be something wrong in some of them, but I'll be darned if I can see it." Thus, the axiom to be learned is that sensitive applications often require specialized tools and techniques for proper imaging. An example of one of these extremity cases is provided in Figure 54–6.

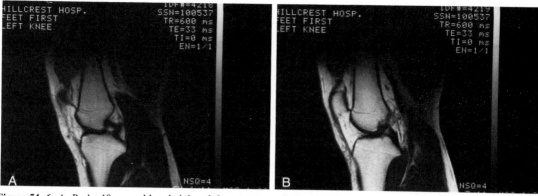

Figure 54–6. *A–B,* An 18-year-old male injured three years earlier in skiing accident. Patient complained of pain in right knee, swelling, and difficulty walking. Diagnosis: Torn cruciate ligament.

The inflammatory/infectious category is a third example of misclassification, arising in large part from one cranial study (Fig. 54–7). That study involved a patient with AIDS who had developed diffuse cerebral cryptococcosis. Owing to the clinical history, virtually all readers correctly identified the fact that the patient suffered from AIDS, yet most assumed the mottled appearance of the MR images to be due to system noise rather than widespread infection. Familiarity with the MRI characteristics of specific disease traits is another factor that must be considered when assessing a new modality— a factor that strongly requires exceptional training and continual accommodation to an ever-changing art. Lesion differentiation during this stage of development depends primarily on anatomic location and pattern recognition of lesion shape and size. Only for a few well-researched disease processes is differentiation based upon MR image contrast currently possible.

Other specific cases that were frequently misread included a left ovarian abscess (inflammatory category) called normal by three readers (Fig. 54–8) and several patients with Huntington's disease (congenital category), in which changes in the basal ganglion were overlooked by the majority of readers (Fig. 54–9).

Unblinded readings of 1.5 tesla MR images were shown to have nearly identical sensitivity and specificity to reports at similar stages of development for lower field strength MR systems. While no attempts were made to match data from the various

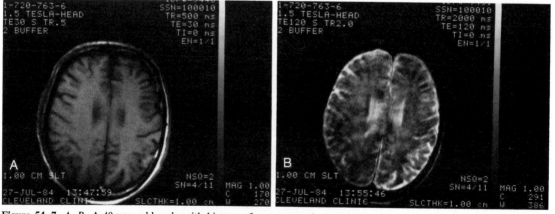

Figure 54–7. *A–B,* A 40-year-old male with history of pneumocystis pneumonia four months earlier, readmitted with severe leg weakness, foot numbness, dysuria, and rectal discharge. Physical examination revealed generally wasted appearance and wide-eyed stare, cervical adenopathy, diminished lower extremity strength, and decreased sensation to soft touch. Diagnosis: Cerebral cryptococcosis (secondary to AIDS).

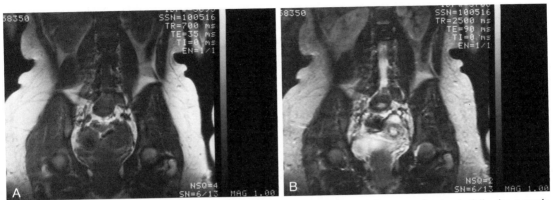

Figure 54–8. *A–B*, A 30-year-old female with six-month history of persistent left lower quadrant pain following a staphylococcal infection. Patient complained of constant painful abdominal cramps. Diagnosis: Left ovarian abscess.

populations, the variable of field strength has shown no influence on MRI's ability to discriminate between pathologic and normal tissue.

These previously reported results of MR sensitivity and specificity have been frequently criticized for failing to exert proper controls (i.e., blinding) to assure the integrity of the results. The current blinded study reports results supportive of the notion that MRI is an effective tool for differentiating diseased from normal anatomy. Statistical tests did not support the hypothesis that clinical history made a significant difference in the detection of lesions. Regardless of the inclusion of clinical history, blinding readers to the results of other imaging tests led to a significant drop in the sensitivity and specificity of MR imaging.

An initial examination of diagnostic specificity showed MRI to be unable to accurately discriminate among disease processes. The most positive findings showed MRI able to differentiate neoplasm and degenerative disease 65 percent and 75 percent of the time, respectively, from other disease processes when the study was accompanied by clinical history. These values were slightly higher when confined to cranial examinations and slightly lower when restricted to extracranial studies. Overall disease differentiation was greater with the inclusion of relevant clinical history. Poor discrimination was shown for a number of other etiologic processes, specifically trauma, inflammation/infection, and congenital lesions. Possible implications of, and reasons for, these findings have been discussed.

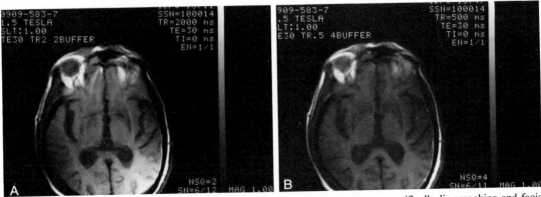

Figure 54–9. *A–B*, A 66-year-old male with a history of involuntary movements, specifically lip-smacking and facial grimacing. Physical examination revealed irregular speech cadence, irregular respiration, lurching, ataxic gait, involuntary head-turning and oral-facial movements, and hyperactive deep tendon reflexes. Diagnosis: Huntington's disease.

Regardless of the method by which it is evaluated, MRI has consistently proved itself to be a highly effective imaging tool. Its reported level of accuracy has varied somewhat, depending on the stringency of the evaluation as well as the extent of pathology and anatomy researched. Nevertheless, when an appropriate comparison with established modalities is agreed upon, and when all the assorted specialized MRI accessories have been identified and developed, MRI is certain to be acknowledged among the battery of standard radiologic tests.

ACKNOWLEDGMENTS

The authors wish to extend their gratitude to the following investigators, their colleagues, and their institutions for the diligent efforts and wholehearted cooperation in collecting the case studies from which this study was generated:

The Cleveland Clinic Foundation (Cleveland, Ohio): Thomas Meaney, M.D.
Hillcrest Hospital (Mayfield Heights, Ohio): James Zelch, M.D.
Hill & Thomas Associates (Cleveland, Ohio): Glenn Sykora, M.D.

The following physicians are also gratefully acknowledged for having donated their time to participate in the blind readings of the clinical cases:

AMC Cancer Institute (Denver, Colorado): Chris Morgan, M.D.
Baylor University Medical Center (Dallas, Texas): Steven Harms, M.D.
Massachusetts General Hospital (Boston, Massachusetts): Ken Davis, M.D., Robert Edelman, M.D.
Rush Presbyterian–St. Luke's Medical Center (Chicago, Illinois): David Turner, M.D., Eric Russell, M.D.
University of Texas Medical Branch (Galveston, Texas): Eugene Amparo, M.D.
Vanderbilt University Medical Center (Nashville, Tennessee): Madan Kulkarni, M.D.

References

1. Luthe MA, Fineberg HV: Clinical efficacy: 5000 MRI cases between 0.15 and 0.6 tesla, *In* Partain CL, Price RR, Patton JA, et al (eds): Magnetic Resonance Imaging, 2nd ed., Philadelphia, W. B. Saunders, 1988.
2. Technicare Pre-Market Approval Application for Teslacon™, FDA Docket No. P830051. Solon, Ohio, Technicare Corporation, 28 January 1983.
3. Technicare Pre-Market Approval Supplement for Teslacon™: Clinical Data for 0.5- and 0.6-Tesla Teslacons™, FDA Docket No. P830051. Solon, Ohio, Technicare Corporation, 27 January 1984. MRI Imaging Devices operating at .5–.6 T.
4. Swets JA, Pickett RM, et al: Assessment of diagnostic techniques. Science 205(4407):753, 1979.
5. Hanley JA, McNeil BJ: The meaning and use of the area under a receiver operating characteristic (ROC) curve. Radiology 143:29, 1982.
6. Hanley JA, McNeil BJ: A method of comparing the areas under receiver operating characteristic curves derived from the same cases. Radiology 148:839, 1983.
7. Metz CE: Basic principles of ROC analysis. Semin Nucl Med 8:283, 1978.
8. Hogg RV, Tanis EA: Probability and Statistical Inference. New York, Macmillan Publishing Co, 1977.
9. Korin BP: Introduction to Statistical Methods. Cambridge, Winthrop Publishers, 1977.

55

Legal Aspects of MRI

A. EVERETTE JAMES, JR.
JOHN GORE
A. EVERETTE JAMES III
JEANNETTE CROSS JAMES
C. LEON PARTAIN
F. DAVID ROLLO
TIMOTHY DEVINNEY
TOM GREESON

The societal, ethical, and legal considerations of magnetic resonance provide a window at the pinnacle to view the multiple changes, movements, and challenges that affect medicine today. Magnetic resonance imaging (MRI), as stated on many occasions throughout this text, represents a significant advance in our ability to differentiate health and disease, even suggesting a redefinition of our concepts of illness from histopathologic to chemical-physiologic terms. This technology will foster new issues of standards and credentials as well as a possible redefinition of "standard of care." The fascination with technology will result in a multitude of demands from both providers and consumers. These will generate challenges in the area of distribution and access, leading to litigation under the aegis of antitrust. Financial implications due to the initial costs involved, and the profit potential coupled with policy enactments such as TEFrA, DRGs, RAPs and vestiges of CON, will require accommodations of an unprecedented nature. One of those, the so-called free-standing medical imaging center, will be considered in detail in this chapter as will the implications of a retrospective system of compensation for services provided while medical care is administered.

Magnetic resonance imaging also presents challenges to certain more classic areas of medical law, such as agency relationships and informed consent. Because the technology is unique and the settings wherein this technology is performed may be quite different, the legal implications may differ from conventional radiography and the other new modalities of ultrasound, x-ray computed tomography, digital radiography, single photon emission computed tomography (SPECT), and positron-emission tomography (PET).

Recognizing that a single chapter on the legal aspects of MRI will not be encyclopedic, we will comment on those general aspects that will apply to all of medical imaging and elaborate on those that seem to be most applicable.

THE LAW OF AGENCY

Agency law is particularly important to magnetic resonance imaging. An agency relationship enables physicians to utilize the services of others and thus to accomplish what they could not achieve alone. Today, many aspects of the practice of medicine as well as nearly all forms of business and professional activity are conducted by agents.[1,2] Because of this widespread use of agents, the courts have formulated rules dealing with the agency relationship and its impact upon third parties.

The law of agency has been almost the exclusive province of the courts rather than legislatures.[3] As a result, it has not achieved the same degree of uniformity as other areas of law. The varied use of terms and concepts by the courts in dealing with agency problems has created confusion. However, certain general propositions that can offer substantial guidance to physicians may be stated. We will review some of the basic concepts of agency and study their relationship to MRI.

An agency relationship involves at least two parties,[3,4] principal and agent, in situations in which the issue is contractual in nature; that is, the agent enters into a contract on behalf of the principal. As for a tortious act or omission, when the agent has injured another person or property while acting on behalf of the principal, the law refers to the relationship as "master and servant." More recently, the terms "employer" and "employee" have been used. These terms, while encompassing the traditional view of the employment relationship, may include other persons who are not commonly viewed as employees but who meet the legal definition of the term.[3]

Formation of an Agency Relationship

An agency relationship has been said to exist when two parties consent to enter into a relationship whereby one party acts for the benefit of and under the direction or control of the other. Depending upon the circumstances, the controlling party may be termed the principal, master, or employer, and the party controlled is referred to as the agent, servant, or employee. Agency is in this instance consensual rather than contractual.[4] There need not be a contract between the two parties nor need the agent be compensated for his service; it is not uncommon to see a gratuitous agency relationship.

If consent is present, the next requirement for the formulation of an agency relationship is that the agent must be acting on behalf of the other party. This is often phrased in terms of benefit; that is, the agent's actions operate to benefit the principal.[4] This benefit element is not difficult to locate or identify and rarely causes any interpretive problems when there is a question of an agency relationship.

The third element in an agency relationship is that of control by the principal over the agent. This does not mean absolute physical control over all acts performed by the agent, nor does it imply that the agent must constantly look to the principal for direction. Instead, it means that the principal has a general power to control the agent's actions. The courts often phrase it as a right to control.[3] Thus, since a physician has the administrative control to order a technologist to discontinue or to alter a procedure, the right to control may be said to exist even though the MRI physician may not be present when the technologist is performing his duties.

Because an agency relationship can be found to exist when there is consent, benefit and control parties may create an agency relationship without realizing that they have done so. As a practical matter, agency relationships are created constantly, and the law is clear that the intent of the parties is not relevant in determining whether or not one exists. Physicians often specifically request the performance of acts of potential injury (and benefit) to patients to be executed by technologists, assistants, nurses, and attendants. In this informal manner and without formal disclosure, agency relationships may be created.

An unwitting agency relationship can also occur when an agent creates a subagency. For example, a technologist acting clearly as an agent may, in turn, request an assistant or attendant to perform certain actions that ultimately are for the benefit of the MRI physician. This act on the part of the technologist may constitute the creation of a subagency, although the physician has not interacted directly with the subagent. The only requirement is that a subagency be implicitly or expressly authorized or that it be reasonably foreseeable that a subagency may be necessary in order to carry out the requests of the MRI physician. In the event that a court finds a subagency to exist, the physician may be held responsible for the actions of the subagent.[4]

It is not difficult to find an unwitting agency relationship between two physicians. An example is the case of *Rockwell v. Kaplan*, 404 Pa. 574, 173 A2d 54 (1961). The plaintiff submitted to surgery for removal of a bursa from his right elbow by Dr. Kaplan. The anesthesiologist selected by Dr. Kaplan, who was chief of the hospital's anesthesiology department, administered Pentothal anesthesia by injection to Rockwell's left arm in such a manner as to obstruct blood flow to the extremity. The surgeon, Dr. Kaplan, did not discover the error until the arm had been so damaged that amputation was required. In this litigation the issue involved only the extent of the surgeon's liability. The court found that Dr. Kaplan had not been negligent but that the anesthesiologist had, and the court held that the anesthesiologist had been acting, during the course of the operation, as the "employee" or agent of the surgeon. Thus, Dr. Kaplan was held liable for the error of his "employee."

These physicians believed that they had not created an agency relationship but were acting as independent professionals. The court found the requisite elements of agency: consent, benefit, and the potential right to control. The court stated that the necessary right to control existed; although the surgeon would not tell the anesthesiologist how to perform the anesthesia, he could have discontinued the operation at any time. This control over the procedure for which the faulty injection was administered was held to be adequate evidence of control by the surgeon over the anesthesiologist. The foregoing decision, while not stating the universal rule, does indicate how some courts may be persuaded to find an agency relationship. This "master of the ship" logic for surgeons in operating theaters may also apply to specialists in magnetic resonance.

The Question of Vicarious Liability

Once an agency relationship has been found to exist, the question becomes to what extent and under what circumstances the principal shall be held responsible for the conduct of the agent. The characteristic result of an agency relationship is the ability of the agent (1) to create contractual rights in favor of the principal, and (2) to subject the principal to personal liability. The significant question for the physician is the power of the agent to make the principal responsible for the acts or omissions of the former. The law generally refers to this as "respondeat superior" ("let the master respond") or "vicarious liability," and this doctrine was applied by the court in *Rockwell v. Kaplan* (supra). Whatever the term employed, the law contemplates that the principal shall be held liable regardless of any fault of his own.

This doctrine of liability without fault is a significant exception to most of Anglo-American jurisprudence, which generally tends to equate legal responsibility with fault. Perhaps the primary reason to create liability without fault in the agency situation is that the principal enjoys benefits conferred upon him by the agent. The law has determined that in return for the privilege of employing agents, the principal should be prepared to take responsibility for any harm suffered by others as a result of the agent's actions.[4]

However, the imposition of vicarious liability is not an automatic and inevitable consequence of an agency relationship. Indeed, many relationships will permit the agent to bind the principal to a contractual obligation but do not contain the two elements necessary to create vicarious liability for the agent's wrongful conduct. Assuming the existence of an agency relationship, the first additional element that must exist is the principal's right to control the *details* of the agent's work. If this right to control is found, the courts will term the relationship to be one of "employer-employee" or "master-servant." The second element that affects the imposition of vicarious liability is the determination that the employee's actionable conduct took place "within the scope of employment." Both these factors must exist before a court will find the "employer" liable.[4] Scope of employment for an MRI technologist may be difficult to determine at present.

The right to control should be specific and direct. The issue of whether this right to control exists is an elusive one and depends upon the facts and circumstances of each case in terms of the employment relationship in each instance. Courts have looked to certain factors that are outward manifestations of a right to control the details of an employee's activities.

Even though a court may find an agency relationship, and more than that, an employment relationship, the employer will not be held liable for the acts of his employee unless it is also determined that the employee caused the injury complained of while acting within the "scope of his employment." Whether or not a person is acting within the scope of his employment is also a question of fact and is perhaps as difficult to answer in a particular case as is the question of whether or not a right to control exists. As a general proposition, to be within the scope of employment, conduct by an employee must be of the same general nature as that authorized by the employer, or it must be incidental to, or a reasonable and foreseeable consequence of, the conduct authorized.[4] Stated and "working" policies here may differ in MRI facilities, but it is generally the routine conduct of the department that is considered policy. An example is intravenous injection of contrast media for MRI studies. If it is the general conduct of the department to allow technologists or nurses to perform these injections, then it is considered within the scope of their employment to do so despite disclaimers to that effect in the formal instrument of their contract. Thus, the MRI physician is liable for the untoward results of such an injection. It is important to note that the courts are willing to interpret scope of employment quite liberally, thus including a broad range of activities that arguably would fall outside the normal duties of an employee.

Other Consequences of an Agency Relationship

In addition to vicarious liability for the wrongful acts of an employee, the formation of an agency relationship may have other implications. For example, if an agent or employee becomes aware of certain facts or, by virtue of his position, should be aware of certain facts, that knowledge or notice may be imputed to the physician. Liability may occur even though the physician does not presumably have any knowledge or reason to know of the facts in question. Agency law holds that agents have a duty to disclose relevant information acquired within the scope of their employment to their employer.[3] Thus, the responsibility for disclosure by a patient to a nurse, assistant, or technologist of certain information important in making a diagnosis may be imputed to the physician although the physician may never have received that information from the nurse or technician or from the patient. As a result, an incorrect diagnosis may lead to liability, since the physician would be on notice of the information given to an employee.

In complex MRI facilities a patient may have great difficulty identifying the professional staff from the technological or nonprofessional staff. Disclosure of a significant medical fact to an employee that should be transmitted to the professional person in charge can result in vicarious liability for the employer physician. This obtains if it can be shown that the assumption made by the patient was a reasonable and logical one and that the employee should have been expected to transmit the information to the physician because of the nature of the employment relationship.

With the extension of MRI practices and the formation of partnerships, the law of agency increases in complexity. Generally, a medical partnership will be treated by the courts just as any other business partnership. Partnership law declares that each partner shall be held responsible for the acts or omissions of the other partners. In effect, partners are mutual agents. Thus, if a patient enters a radiology office or department in which he may be seen by different radiologists who are members of that partnership, each physician may be jointly and severally liable for the improper treatment of the patient by an employee of the partnership. Such vicarious liability cannot be contracted away, although the law does provide that any judgment against the partnership be collected from the partnership assets first and subsequently from the assets of the individual partners. Certainly, each partner has a right of reimbursement from a partner whose wrongful conduct caused the injury, but this right will not be available if all the partners are blameless and the injury was due to the negligence of an employee.[5]

When a physician acts as a consultant, he will generally be considered to be an "independent contractor." The finding of independent contractor status is the converse of finding an employee relationship. An independent contractor may and, in most cases will, be considered an agent. However, under agency law an independent contractor, by definition, is not an employee because he is not subject to a right to control over the details of his work by the contracting party. Note, however, that the court in *Rockwell v. Kaplan*, discussed previously, found that the anesthesiologist was subject to a right of control by the surgeon and thus could not be considered an independent contractor but was, in fact, an employee. This decision does not conform to the general rule. To the extent that any injury to the patient can be attributed to the other physician or his agents, the physician would not be held responsible. There may, however, be cases in which the injurious result to the patient can be attributed both to the primary care physician and to the MRI specialist. In such a case, both parties would be held jointly and severally liable. Yet a third situation would occur, in which the primary care physician acts upon the performance and interpretation of study by the MRI physician, such interpretation having been negligently made, thus causing harm to the patient. In such situations the MRI physician will be held responsible, since his acts caused the injury in question. Under a *Rockwell v. Kaplan* rationale, the primary care physician may also be held responsible despite no fault on his part. When the *Rockwell v. Kaplan* rationale is not recognized, the radiologist would be deemed an independent contractor rather than an agent of the primary care physician. Therefore, the primary care physician would not be subjected to vicarious liability for any wrongful conduct by the MRI physician. Since the level of expertise would not be equal, it is generally held that the MRI physician is liable, as the physician ordering the study is in a secondary and dependent role.

An area of concern is often encountered in the consultative process when the conclusions of the MRI physician are at variance with those of his clinical colleague who is primarily responsible for the patient's care as to the most appropriate next study in the diagnostic evaluation. At times, the primary care physician can object to the recommendations of the radiologist and continue to request the study not recommended by the MRI physician. Because the MRI specialist is an independent physician he is at liberty to refuse to perform a study requested when his judgment so dictates. The

MRI physician understandably could be held responsible for any damages to the patient because of a study's not being performed. It is a good practice for a physician to document his basis for refusal to perform a certain study on a patient at the time such a refusal occurs.[6] The professional obligation to a patient for appropriate services is that of the physician. The legal obligation will be based upon the issue of causation: Did the acts or omissions of the radiologist or his employees cause the injury in question? The liability, however, will be based upon the determination of negligence by the MRI physician in refusing the study.

With the increased demands upon the health care delivery system, it is inevitable that MRI will continue to depend upon large numbers of persons to perform many significant functions in the care of patients. Therefore, vicarious liability will continue to exist and grow. Certain basic aspects must be appreciated by the physician. It is important to understand under what circumstances individuals will be acting as employees and in what situations MRI specialists may have liability for their actions.

INFORMED CONSENT

The legal considerations of informed consent principally involve the elementary tort doctrines of battery, negligence, and interference with peace of mind. An example of the last is failure to disclose a risk or collateral hazard associated with a certain procedure or treatment.[10] These are fundamentally different types of wrongs (for which the legal redresses are not equal), involve separate and distinct treatments by the courts, and require different reasonable self-protective steps.

The basic theory of a battery action is a physical touching that is not consented to by the patient. Negligence is behavior that does not conform to the standard of care exercised by a prudent MRI physician. The guidelines and understanding of the issues involved in battery cases are much more familiar than the disclosure required and what circumstances require that disclosure, according to the tenets of informed consent.

A landmark informed consent case in which a number of important considerations were articulated is *Salgo v. Leland Stanford, Jr., Board of Trustees*, 154 Cal. App. 2d 560, 317 P.2d 170 (1957).[2] An angiographic procedure performed upon the plaintiff resulted in paralysis. A critical issue involved the content of the preangiographic instructions by the physician: Did the physician properly disclose the dangers attendant to angiography? It was pointed out that the physician subjects himself to liability if he withholds facts necessary to form the basis of an intelligent (informed) consent. However, it was also recognized that placing the welfare of the patient foremost means that the physician must sometimes choose between two alternative positions. One is to explain every attendant risk, no matter how remote, in explicit detail. This mode of action may make a patient unduly apprehensive, especially with a new technology such as MRI, which could in itself increase the risk of an untoward event.[8,9] The other mode of action is to recognize the importance of the individual's perception of the associated risk and to exercise discretion consistent with full disclosure of the facts necessary for an informed consent.[10]

Another important case is *Bang v. Charles T. Miller Hospital*, 251 Minn. 42, 88 N.W. 2d 186 (1958), in which the court did not appear to have a very clear understanding of the nature of the disclosure required to avoid liability for malpractice when seeking informed consent. The court suggested that "substantial disclosure" was needed, but at another point said that "reasonable disclosure" or "full disclosure of the facts necessary to ensure an informed consent" were necessary. A landmark opinion in this case was that the decision of how a physician should most appropriately discharge his or her obligation to the patient in a difficult situation of informed consent is primarily a question of medical judgment. The court ruled that the physician would not be medically negligent and would not be liable for malpractice so long as his disclosures and actions were such that his motivation appeared to be in the best interests of the patient. It was insisted that the physician conducted himself in such a manner as a competent medical man would have in a similar situation.

These examples point to two substantial conditions that must be established in informed consent cases and reveal two excellent methods of legal defense. It must be shown that the physician was motivated by some desire not in the best interest of his patient for him to be liable. Additionally, the physician must have deviated from the standard of practice either in failing to obtain a truly informed consent or in choosing not to disclose a particular fact or collateral risk to the patient. This permits or even suggests the necessity for expert medical testimony as to what constitutes acceptable standards, and also allows specialty organizations to establish a "standard of care" by official policy statements.[11]

In the practice of medicine, certain procedures have well-established significant inherent risks.[9,12] Other procedures also have associated known risks wherein these untoward events are much less common. An important consideration for diagnostic procedures such as magnetic resonance imaging is to know exactly what it is that constitutes "adequate" disclosure to provide an informed consent, or what set of circumstances of performance constitutes an implied consent (interaction of the physician and patient to indicate consent).

Physicians often adopt two types of rationalization for not establishing formalized informed consent. Little sympathy is evoked by the assertion that the nature and character of an MRI study cannot be explained without use of complex technical language that would prove confusing and anxiety-provoking to the layman.[8,13] The validity of the second argument, however, appears to have much greater general acceptance. This is the assertion that the risk involved is exceedingly uncommon; choosing not to inform the patient of the collateral or associated risk is within the physician's prerogative and within the scope of his best medical judgment as to what is most desirable for his patient.[11,14] In other words, the physician believes that the hazards of informing the patient of the risk are greater than the risk of the study itself.

In cases involving plaintiff claims of not being fully or correctly informed as to collateral hazards attendant on the medical procedure, the judicial approach is different from that of battery cases. The defendant's obligation is more flexible in character and subject to great variation, whereas the plaintiff's rights are less certain. The physician's obligation is an elastic concept in this instance; it cannot be prescribed with specificity.

In the case of *Nathan v. Kline*, 187 Kan. 186,354 P 2d 670 (1960) the court recognized that a circumstance might exist in which the duty to refer to collateral hazards would be minimal. In the case of *Roberts v. Wood*, 206 F. Supp. 579, 583 (D.C. Ala. 1962) it was agreed that "the anxiety, apprehension, and fear generated by a full disclosure of the risks may have a detrimental effect on some patients." However, with a discipline as new as MRI, the database to determine the hazards and risk is still being developed.

One does not wish to dismiss the importance of emotional stress.[8] In the latter circumstance, failure to disclose by the physician should not be defended on the grounds that the patient's knowledge of collateral risks increases the chance of an untoward event, but rather upon sound medical judgment and the reasonable standard of practice. Again, a very important factor that influences court decisions as to whether or not there is a duty to disclose collateral dangers for a procedure is the likelihood that the risk will materialize. A general rule is that the greater the incidence of an untoward event, the greater obligation a physician has to patients to warn them of this specific risk. In the case of *Roberts v. Young*, 369 Mich. 133, 139–40, 119 N.W. 2d 627, 630

(1963) regarding postoperative infection, the court recognized that they were dealing with the "mere possibility" of an untoward event. It ruled in this instance that what should be done was whatever the general practice customarily followed by the medical profession in the locality. The apparent logic was that many complications may occur following a procedure. Some appear fairly likely because of the nature of the procedure and may even be expected to some degree. Others are possible but highly unlikely. The former collateral risks should probably be disclosed to the patient, whereas the latter are not necessarily disclosed.

In the case of *Ball v. Mallinckrodt Chem. Works*, 53 Tenn. App. 218, 381 S.W. 2d 563 (1964) the court approved an instruction that gave the physician great latitude in determining the extent to which he was obligated to disclose the potentially dangerous results of a translumbar aortogram. Again, it was recognized that the physician's knowledge was so much greater than the patient's that the amount of disclosure was to be left to the discretion of the physician.

In *Fischer v. Wilmington General Hospital*, 51 Del. 554, 149 A 2d 749 (Sup. Ct. 1959) the relatively low incidence (less than 1 percent) of the collateral hazard (hepatitis from a transfusion) was relied upon to warrant a finding of no duty to disclose this hazard to the patient. Again, the thesis was that many collateral risks are possible, but those only remotely possible need not be detailed to a patient prior to a procedure. The court also recognized that whether or not a physician should warn a patient of collateral hazards associated with a medical procedure is essentially a medical question, one upon which judges or juries are not competent to make a decision. This thesis, however, has not always been universally accepted. Courts and juries can decide whether the physician deviated from a standard of care. With a recognized discipline the standard of care would be that practiced by other members of the specialty, the recommendations in scientific publications, and that which is recommended by statements and position papers of the appropriate societies. However, with MRI the standard of care is being established on a continual basis.

Courts have attempted to recognize the impracticality of disclosing to each patient all the collateral risks of a procedure. In *Williams v. Menehan*, 191 Kan. 6, 379 P 2d 292, 295 (1963) the court stated that it specifically did not wish to adopt the posture that a physician is under legal obligation to disclose hazards that might possibly follow a procedure. It was recognized that there may well be circumstances under which such disclosure would constitute poor medical practice. Another important legal principle in this case was that the physician could utilize expert testimony to establish that voluntary lack of disclosure complied with standards of good practice in a particular instance. From the viewpoint of physicians, this seems a logical extension of the fiduciary or dependent relationship that characterizes the physician-patient status. In recent years, the constraints on this type of relationship have been much more severe. In a review of a number of cases that apply to this general issue, the courts seemed to be approaching unanimity in the view that in a cause of action based upon medical negligence because of failure to disclose a collateral hazard, expert testimony is necessary to establish a standard against which one can measure the defendant physician's conduct.

Two significant cases seem to support a collateral or even deviant trend in the nature of informed consent. Because of the current implications, these two cases will be considered in detail. The first case is *Canterbury v. Spence*, 464 F 2d 772 (D.C. Cir. 1972), which takes into account the specific needs of an individual patient and places upon the physician additional responsibilities of judgment. The patient tolerated an operation well and was recuperating normally when he fell during urinary voiding in his room while unattended. After this time, despite emergency surgery, the patient had a permanent disability of lower extremity paralysis and urinary and bowel incontinence.

The court discussed criteria by which failure to disclose a risk should be interpreted as negligence. It was felt that the patient's right of self-decision shapes the boundaries of the duty to reveal a particular hazard. The scope of the physician's communications to the patient should be measured by the patient's needs or by the materiality of the information to an informed decision. The court further recognized that a very small chance of death or serious disability may well be significant. Some dangers, however, are inherent in any procedure, and there is not an obligation to communicate those of which patients of average sophistication are aware. A physician's privilege to withhold information does not allow him to remain silent because divulgence might prompt the patient to forgo a procedure the physician believes the patient needs.

Two other considerations regarding the physician's obligation are discussed in the appeal. Certain aspects place an undue burden upon the physician. If the patient can retrospectively claim that, had the risk at question been known prior to the procedure, the patient would have refused the procedure, it would seem to obligate the physician to predict every particular patient response. A more reasonable criterion would seem to resolve the causality issue in terms of what a prudent person in the patient's position would have decided if suitably informed of all perils bearing significance.

Regarding the importance of risk, it has been historically followed that medical expert testimony was necessary. However, this court and others have recently felt that nonmedical persons are competent to determine the value of a disclosure in having a patient render an informed consent. The physician's duty to disclose is governed by the same legal principles applicable to others in comparable situations. Is the treatment worth the risk? This type of consideration would require the physician to weigh the different lifestyles and circumstances of patients. In this area, a physician may not be any more competent than the average lay person. Again, it would appear that the physician should elect to disclose those risks that have some reasonable likelihood of occurring.

If one examines the closing statements at the end of the appeal, it seems that the issue of informed consent is not a central one. Rather, the court felt that Mr. Canterbury was deprived of compensation for his disability because he could never establish whether the primary causation was his surgery or his original physical condition, or whether the disability resulted from the accident in the hospital. The element of negligence appears to surround whatever circumstances resulted in his serious physical limitation, and he was thus compensated. After view of the considerations of this case, it does not seem to mean that lack of total disclosure is negligence, as it is often presented.

In *Cobbs v. Grant*, 8 Cal. 3d 229, 502 P 2d 1 (1972), it was determined that information should be given by the physician such that a prudent person could make a reasoned decision. This is a very interesting example of a case that is viewed with great concern by physicians.

In this medical malpractice case, a verdict was rendered against the surgeon, who appealed. The plaintiff underwent an operation for an "active duodenal ulcer." His primary physician advised the plaintiff in general terms of the risks of undergoing a general anesthetic, and the surgeon explained the nature of the operation to the patient—but did not discuss any of the inherent risks. Eight days following the surgery and an uneventful postoperative course the patient was discharged. The following day, the plaintiff experienced abdominal pain and returned to the hospital. He went into shock, and emergency surgery was performed because of suspected internal hemorrhage. At surgery a severed splenic artery was found and splenectomy performed. Again, his postoperative course was satisfactory and he was discharged two weeks after splenectomy. A month following discharge the patient was found to have a gastric ulcer, which subsequently led to a gastrectomy.

In the initial trial, expert medical testimony established that the first operation was within good medical practice and that the subsequent untoward results, while unfortunate, did not constitute malpractice. The central point at issue was the surgeon's decision not to disclose these risks to the plaintiff. The court relied upon *Berkey v. Anderson*, 1 Cal. App. 3d 790, 803, 82 Cal. Rptr. 67 (1969), a case in which it was held that if the defendant failed to make a sufficient disclosure of the risks inherent in the operation, he was guilty of "technical battery." The appeals court disagreed and characterized failure to obtain informed consent as negligence.

In the very exhaustive discussion of both the patient's right of self-determination and the physician's obligation to assure that the consent is an informed one, the court appeared to find the incidence and likelihood of risk as fundamentally important. It was stated that during a common procedure the physician must make such inquiries to determine if the procedure is contraindicated for that particular patient. Beyond those inquiries, however, no warning is required as to the remote possibility of death or serious bodily harm. If the procedure is simple and the danger remote, the physician is not under legal obligation to disclose the danger. The judgment was reversed for this reason.

A central issue in the question of informed consent is the frequency of adverse outcomes. Extrapolating from the legal decisions regarding "reasonable likelihood," it would appear that a patient should be informed of minor risks because they are sufficiently common. It seems that the primary consideration is not the seriousness of the reaction provided that it is sufficiently rare. The *Wilkinson v. Vesey*, 295 A.2d 676 (Sup. Ct. R.I. 1972), case is at variance with the trend in what is generally regarded by both medical and legal experts as an appropriate direction. In this case, the logic of the award was to seek compensation for the dramatic event from the "deepest pocket" without proof of malpractice, negligence, or battery. Further examination of the judgment in this case should establish that it has not been supported by similar future judgments.[2,11,15]

When general medical conditions suggest to the physician that a full disclosure of attendant hazard and collateral is preferred, but specific patient circumstance makes it not in the patient's best interest to do so, two options are available to the clinician. It is acceptable for the physician to tell patients only as much as they desire to know, as long as the physician makes them aware that they have the option to obtain additional information.[15] A second technique is for the physician to explain to a responsible family member or appropriate representative the nature and reasons for the lack of disclosure to the patient. Additionally, this should be documented in detail in the patient's medical record. The evidentiary nature of this type of medical record makes this mandatory. Not only should the failure of disclosure be recorded, but also the considerations and intent with regard to the patient's general welfare. The physician should place the decision of disclosure on a medical basis and so state it within that frame of reference.

It is a principle in law that "the courts will decide." Physicians have often adopted the attitude that they are in a completely passive role and dependent upon the intentions of their legal colleagues. Certainly, informed consent decisions to date have allowed, during trial, the medical profession an opportunity to influence future decisions regarding this issue. If the courts are to rely upon medical judgment and standard of practice to determine whether or not negligence or malpractice occurred in informed consent cases, it would seem that physicians have an opportunity to create criteria for these legal judgments. Pronouncements by organized medical groups or societies supported by appropriate available data can be introduced into court to significantly influence these considerations.

Physicians, by documenting the collateral risks attendant on any diagnostic procedure, and by translating these into the context of expected medical benefit, can create the guidelines for informed consent. Not to do so will force the courts to decide on the basis of incomplete data, which could result in legal precedents that encourage poor medical practice. The initial responsibility to establish these precedents and guidelines lies in the hands of the physician. It would seem appropriate for clinicians to formulate guidelines based on the accumulation of well-documented data and to utilize these guidelines to assist the individual specialists in the conduct of their practices. The American legal system is a common law system, in which each case is decided on its own merits guided by rulings in similar prior cases. Legal precedent is the basis on which these decisions are made. Countersuits, while dramatic, will not be as effective as an effort to establish precedent for specific diagnostic procedures such as MRI studies. MRI precedent cases do not currently exist in any great number. One would believe that certain principles applied in cases involving x-ray computed tomography would also apply to cases involving MRI.

PROSPECTIVE PAYMENT

Public and industry investment in medical imaging research has indeed produced an array of expensive and sophisticated diagnostic modalities.[16-21] In the past decade, we have experienced the introduction of x-ray computed tomography,[22] gray-scale real-time and pulsed Doppler ultrasound,[23,24] digital radiology,[25] positron-emission tomography (PET), and magnetic resonance imaging. These technologies have traditionally been hospital-based. Since 1970, hospital costs have increased more than 450 percent with a dramatic rise since 1983. Expenditures for Medicare doubled in the five-year period between 1974 and 1979. They have again doubled in the past five years. Many have predicted that, given present trends, the Medicare fund will be bankrupt by the last decade of this century. Health care costs are over 340 billion dollars annually at present.

One recognizes that technology is not entirely responsible for spiraling health care costs. Changes in demography and increased cost of labor and supplies have contributed substantially to this phenomenon. The expansion of government regulation and the rising incidence of large malpractice awards have created a climate that also contributes to a substantial increase in health costs.

In the past four decades, America developed a complex system of financing hospital care and developing programs for the provision of care for selected groups, such as veterans and the poor. This system essentially protected patients from the cost of care and assured provider compensation. In doing so, the public health care provision system created obvious adverse incentives for cost containment. Providers received little or no benefit from cost reductions, while the primary consumers had no reason to make price comparisons or quality trade-offs. The ultimate effect was an escalation in health care costs along with what were taken as dramatic improvements in quality, especially in the area of high-technology medicine.

Our health care financing system, until recent times, encouraged the provision of complete care with minimum regard for expense; it provided all benefits, although the gain at the margin might be quite small. With proliferation of the expensive imaging technologies, the cost-inflating effects of the health care payment system were magnified.[26-28] The retrospective payment system largely obviated the need to weight benefits of certain physician-controlled activities or to stimulate physicians to undertake a true cost-benefit analysis. Under the retrospective system, physicians were allowed to provide almost any diagnostic service that appeared to have potential benefit to the patient. Ultrasound and x-ray computed tomography certainly experienced geometric growth in this environment.

The retrospective system largely ignored the policing activities that are natural phenomena in business markets. From the supply side, the scheme of cost plus nature of reimbursement makes efforts at cost control of little value. Also, with no price advertising in medicine and with consumer search for the most efficient, effective, and inexpensive provider being very costly, the least-cost provider cannot be ensured of greater volume as a result of a lower price. On the demand side, consumers have little incentive to search for lower-priced providers, since they are generally not paying for the services rendered; and search provides little ultimate benefit, since providers have no incentive to reduce prices.

Recent changes in the nature of health care compensation schemes have partially recognized these weaknesses. The source of these changes is in the increasing burden and the ever-larger expected burden being assumed by the paying parties, the government, and the employers. Just as institutional investors were largely responsible for the dramatic decline in brokerage fees, the budget pressures on the government and the profit motive of businesses have been the primary motivation behind recent economic developments in the health care system.[28] Obviously, deficit reductions such as the DRG measures will be a major factor in the future of health care.

Efforts have recently been instituted to dramatically change provider practices, to relate consumer choices to recognition of costs, and to decrease the upward trend in expenditures for health care. Implicit in these efforts is the recognition that "quality at any price" is no longer a realistic aim. There also appears to be growing consensus that consumer sovereignty, once thought valueless in the medical market, has no less valuable a role than in any other financial market. The growth in the influence of PPOs, HMOs, and the like is an example of this. The federal government has instituted the prospective payment system based upon diagnosis-related groups (DRGs) as a part of this phenomenon.[29] The prospective payment system is designed to force the alteration of physicians' practices and to stem the rising tide of Medicare costs. In what is actually a form of price forecasting, states are also in the process of imposing budget limits on medicine, especially hospital care. Many large businesses are moving from a fee-for-service health care provider arrangement to health maintenance organizations (HMOs) and preferred provider organizations (PPOs). With these types of arrangements, consumer and, primarily, payer bargaining power will provide the potential to decrease costs for a unit service rendered. In a field such as magnetic resonance imaging, in which the individual unit charge is quite high, decisions about these costs will become even more crucial.

An assumption underlying these and other initiatives in the health care field is that medical charges contain much waste, inappropriate use of resources, and significant inefficiencies in the delivery of a given service. Assuming this to be correct, it would logically follow that health care costs can be reduced painlessly and without compromise of quality. Those proponents of cost containment and prospective payment believe that we can maintain present standards, experience our historical medical advances, such as MRI, in the future, and curtail the present growth of health care costs.

We would contend for MRI that it is naive to assume that medical advances will occur without the prerequisite basic research. In the overall strategy to balance the budget and reduce the nation's deficit, across-the-board reductions that are currently planned will affect magnetic resonance research to a profound degree. We will comment on this later.

We have come increasingly to depend upon private resources through industry to fund our imaging research. With an increase in corporate taxes, there is less incentive for private industry to fill in where public funds have decreased in this area, following the reduction in government funding. We believe that to significantly decrease the growth of health care costs, certain benefits that accrue from the use of medical services, including magnetic resonance imaging technology, will have to be compromised.

We may need to discontinue the uniform provision of high-technology medicine. There is public recognition of this choice, one that is difficult for patients to participate in. From a societal standpoint, there is no indication that the discontinuation of the uniform provision of certain medical services is per se wrong. In a society with heterogeneous preferences there is no way to quantitate the value of uniform provision of services. Provided that consumers are reasonably informed about available choices there is little reason to expect them to choose identical houses or identical medical services or to make any less "efficient" a decision. Certainly, the lay literature is replete with articles extolling the virtues of magnetic resonance, but analyses of its relative efficacy have not been widely published.

One might consider the questions that are actually being addressed by these measures to decrease health care costs. Do we have useless and unnecessary medical imaging technology? Is the technology inefficiently employed, maldistributed, and improperly funded? Both health care policy makers and significant sectors of the American public have proposed that redundant and duplicated medical imaging facilities exist to the degree that they contribute significantly to the rise in health care costs. In response to these assumptions, such measures as distribution limitation and certificates-of-need legislation[30] as well as legislation such as the Tax Equity Federal Act (TEFRA) of 1982 have been enacted. Agencies such as the Health Resources Administration (HRA) have recommended guidelines for distribution and use of high-technology medical imaging equipment (National Guideline for Health Planning, 1978). As a more recent example, the Health Care Financing Administration (HCFA) and the Food and Drug Administration (FDA) have insisted that the subject of this text, magnetic resonance imaging, demonstrate a certain level of efficacy before they will recommend third-party compensation for these procedures.[31] We have yet to determine who will pay to research and develop modalities such as MRI and to perform the clinical trials on this very expensive equipment if these costs are no longer to be indirectly passed on to patients. This will probably affect the middle-class taxpayer, who normally pays medical bills even if not covered by insurance. Will this be a case of whether the patient pays now or pays later? We will subsequently consider the societal aspects.

One should obviously consider those possible gains afforded by the elimination of inappropriate use of sophisticated medical imaging technology, such as MRI. Recent studies have demonstrated that if present policy goals are achieved, the effects on hospital costs will not be significant.[32,33] Furthermore, if one limits the distribution of certain facilities of medical imaging technologies such as MRI, many patients may be forced to travel great distances for diagnostic evaluation and might incur significant expense, discomfort, and possibly increased medical risk. We will return to this consideration later. By eliminating nonefficacious application of medical imaging technology some savings could be achieved, but studies have shown that the impact on overall hospital costs would be relatively small. Additionally, the application of antitrust legislation will stimulate suits from both consumers and providers in this type of environment.

The rationale for limited distribution of medical imaging facilities, like that of certificate-of-need legislation, can be argued on public utility grounds. Dramatic economic savings may be possible given the presence of only one facility in a specified region because it could operate more efficiently. However, as in the case of classic public utilities, the validity of this argument in the case of medical imaging technology, including magnetic resonance imaging, is not a strong one. If such economies did exist, regardless of government involvement, the providers would have the incentive to merge since cost per unit would be reduced. Government involvement would be superfluous in this instance, which leads one to question the role of involvement. In addition, the marginal cost of the majority of medical imaging procedures appears to be low. Calculations have shown that, if the equipment is already in place, reduction of studies by 33 percent would lower hospital expenditures by only 2 to 3 percent.[34-36] Evidence of decreased volume leading to decreased cost is evidence against economies in imaging technology. Thus, little validity can be found for the public utility– wasteful competition rationale in imaging technology. The major reason is the fixed overhead that exists in the operation and maintenance of the type of equipment represented by MRI. Additionally, patient and referral physician demand makes this type of response problematic.

Biomedical advances in recent years have made it possible to replace an invasive diagnostic imaging examination with a noninvasive one[37] or a study employing ionizing radiation with one using a non-ionizing energy form, such as MRI.[38] Although the initial capital expense for this sophisticated technology may appear formidable, the instrumentation could allow one to perform an imaging procedure on an outpatient rather than an inpatient basis. This could effect considerable savings in many types of health care resources, including financial and legal ones. Obviously, proponents of this line of reasoning must take a long view of health care economic theory.

We believe it to be doubtful that any new modality, including MRI, would be readily accepted regardless of cost if the sole difference between the new modality and more standard imaging procedures was the utilization of non-ionizing radiation versus ionizing radiation. For example, if all that magnetic resonance imaging offered was the substitution of non-ionizing radiation for computerized tomography, which utilizes x-rays, it would be very difficult to justify the cost to the consumer of adding another layer of expensive technology to that which already existed. If the MRI procedure simply replaced the x-ray CT study, however, this might be favorably received.

HMOs have been proposed by the enthusiasts as a panacea for reduction of health care costs. However, their effect upon medical imaging technology may not reflect the positive effects predicted. HMOs appear to be less expensive than the fee-for-service sector, but this is mainly because they experience 30 percent less hospital admissions. The nonadmissions are, by definition, in this framework "unnecessary" and are said to be accompanied by no loss of potential medical benefits. HMOs propose to reduce baseline costs and growth rates of medical expenditures. Baseline costs are to be reduced by eliminating zero-benefit care and decreasing waste in the health care delivery system. However, per capita, the number of overall diagnostic imaging studies is not growing at a very rapid rate[35,36] and the 30 percent admission rate difference has remained constant for a number of years. This latter fact implies that the rate of useless admissions in relation to HMOs has not grown in the general health care delivery area.

It has been said that DRGs are designed to provide an incentive for parsimony.[34] This prospective compensation system may create an entirely new environment for health care providers. They may be forced to establish rigid priorities to purchase only the most cost-effective (in dollar terms) medical imaging equipment and to decide what new modalities they can afford under the DRG guidelines of fixed, limited resources. Physicians may be placed in the role of deciding which patients to admit for the medical imaging study and determine which patients to reject based upon criteria to be developed. They may have to engage frequently in the now uncommon practice of deciding which methods of diagnostic imaging are too costly to provide. MRI may then flourish in the central nervous system and spine and not fare so well in the abdomen, where its value is not as well established. Physicians may have to estimate the relative value added by a medical imaging study and to then decide if the expenditure of resources is appropriate. Balancing costs and medical benefits is anathema to some physicians; yet with the proposed regulatory systems this activity appears both implicitly and explicitly unavoidable. Notwithstanding is the legal responsibility as a concomitant to this type of activity. In the United States, our traditional attitudes of the "best" (often equivalent to the most technical) medical care to all citizens and our previous system of compensation will make these transitions difficult. Reducing hospital revenues could have a profound effect upon which medical imaging procedures can be undertaken in a particular institution. The task of ensuring optimal use of magnetic resonance equipment could be characterized by confrontations between the medical imager and physician colleagues as well as hospital administrators. DRGs will eventually come to affect physicians in addition to those considered under present RAPs (radiologists, anesthesiologists, and pathologists), eventually affecting all physicians.

The best and most efficient hospitals may suffer along with the worst in global efforts at reductions. The better quality tertiary care facility will certainly have more complicated cases destined to be outliers, yet will suffer with many hospitals that are much less efficient in their prior and present operations. Might these be the criteria upon which MRI facilities are placed? Studies have shown that services can be more easily reduced if patients are unaware of the benefits they are forgoing. In Great Britain, there are approximately 35 x-ray computed tomographic (CAT) scanners in the entire country, whereas in the United States there are several thousand. The British decision makers (presumably the National Health Service Administration) reasoned that their patients were sufficiently uninformed that few would ever realize that this sophisticated medical imaging technology was being denied them. In the United States, physicians, news media, and personal interchange have made consumers quite aware of the medical advantages of this modality, not to mention the present high public and professional expectations for magnetic resonance imaging.

If physicians and health policy decision makers accept rationing of highly technical medical imaging devices such as MRI, consumers could offer resistance even in the form of litigation.[23,39,40] This will be discussed in more detail when we consider medical imaging centers for MRI. This form of rationing of technology in medicine may require a redefinition of the legal concept of "standard of care." If resource constraints change the alternative diagnostic studies available to patients, the legal system (courts) may be the vehicle whereby the consumer's right to access and entitlement of service is sought. However, will the consumer consider the responsibility to be that of the physician or the government in such litigation? Also, in a modality with unique characteristics such as MRI, what level of expertise represents competency, how much training is involved, what is the prerequisite professional background? Additionally, who should be the accrediting body? Historically, demands from the health policy sector upon the legal system have resulted in turmoil and chaos.[41,42] Applications of legislative activity, precedent rulings, and laws intended for other sectors of our society have encountered significant difficulty when applied to the health care system.[41,43–47] Physicians, often acting upon a real or perceived mandate from patients, have traditionally adopted measures to obviate many forms of health care regulation and have adopted policies to circumvent the system. To escape certain of the constraints of certificates of need, physicians placed CT scanners in private offices and clinics when medically they might have been more appropriately located in hospitals.[30] At present, the corollary phenomenon of free-standing diagnostic imaging centers is experiencing geometric growth; this subject will be considered in detail later.

EXCLUSIVE CONTRACTS IN MEDICINE: POST-HYDE

Exclusive contracts will become much more commonplace in the future. The provision of MRI services by exclusive contracts will predictably be the norm. An exclusive contract is an arrangement whereby one party arranges to deal exclusively with another party. Two types of exclusive contracts may exist. Two (or more) parties may sign a contract, willingly, in which they agree to deal only with the other party for a particular set of transactions. Alternatively, a seller may find that a manufacturer requires any dealer selling its product to handle only its product. In the first case, both contractors desire the exclusive arrangement. In the second case, one party may desire a nonexclusive arrangement but is not given a choice.

Many feel the issues of exclusive contracts between hospitals and physicians have been resolved by the U.S. Supreme Court decision in *Hyde v. Jefferson Parish Hospital District No. 2*, 686 F. 2d 286 [5th Cir. 1982], cert granted 51 U.S. U.S.L.W. 3649 [1983]. Under both *per se* and "rule of reason" logic, the Supreme Court concluded unanimously that the anesthesiology contract in this case did not violate Section One of the Sherman Antitrust Act.

We believe that although some of the issues regarding exclusive contracts have been more appropriately defined, many are yet to be resolved and that other areas in our society related to medicine will raise new and different concerns. In this chapter, we will analyze the *Hyde* case and then suggest areas of potential future conflict and legal activity.

In the United States there is considerable case law regarding exclusive contracts. Specifically, the *Hyde* case provided an opportunity to establish under what antitrust analysis exclusive physician contracts might be considered appropriate arrangements. Defendant hospitals and plaintiff physicians are not in agreement regarding their attitude toward what are proper economic arrangements between physicians and their institutions. Defendant hospitals most commonly view an exclusive physician contract as a method by which the hospital can secure the medical services necessary to discharge the service aspect of health care responsibility. Hospitals often regard themselves, and not the physicians, as the providers of medical services. They produce health care by contracting with physicians, paramedics, and others acting as agents for these physicians.[48] Hospitals contend that hospital-based physicians compete with other groups to acquire privileges in any particular medical institution. Hospitals would contend, for instance, that they survey a national market in order to secure these qualified professionals for magnetic resonance and enter into an exclusive contract with them. Thus, the hospital's search is a national one, and competition for the contract is at this level. In an antitrust context, the market to provide these magnetic imaging services would also be a national one. A contracting MRI group or a particular medical institution, therefore, should not have the potential to capture a substantial market share. Contracts between one hospital and a service provider group would be viewed as affecting an insignificant part of the national marketplace and would not be considered as a restraint of trade. The exclusive contract is an arrangement that allows the hospital to meet competition for health care services.

Central to this consideration is the antitrust query of whether an exclusive contract of this type creates a tying arrangement. Certain tying arrangements are *per se* illegal, while others may unreasonably restrain competition. An invalid tying arrangement occurs when a seller has a resource or ability (market power) to force a purchaser (physician) or consumer (patient) to do something they would not do in a competitive market. If patients are forced to purchase the services of an exclusive contractor because of the hospital's market power, the contractual arrangement may have anticompetitive consequences.

Physicians generally do not view exclusive contracts in the same manner as do hospital administrators. Physicians usually contend that the relevant market is the specific hospital where that purveyor of health care wishes to compete for patients and privileges to perform MRI. Hospital privileges viewed in this manner would then be the important issue in terms of which group will provide the MRI service.[38] A contract may give a certain group virtually a tacit monopoly to provide MRI services in any individual hospital or, if it is the only hospital in that vicinity to provide services, then in that particular geographic area.

Competition is not present in an exclusively contracted medical imaging service because other physicians do not have the opportunity to compete for the privilege of providing MRI service in that hospital. If the particular medical service is unique to that community (for instance, magnetic resonance imaging), then a "tying arrangement" could be claimed. From the point of view of physicians, competition for patients could be eliminated by an exclusive contract that allowed only one group access to some unique resource, such as MRI. From the hospital's position, the competition is for the contract, and this is secured and maintained based upon continuous performance by the provider group.

These two interpretations of exclusive contracts make analysis altogether different. In the *Hyde* case, the U.S. Supreme Court agreed with the position taken by the hospital. Because of the *Hyde* decision, the status of antitrust law in the area of exclusive physician service contracts is better defined. The majority opinion of the Supreme Court severely constrained *per se* logic. The minority opinion believed that this analysis should not be applied in the health care field. Exclusive contracts could become equivalent to ordinary employment contracts, and antitrust challenges of the type considered in *Hyde* could be dismissed upon pleading.

In the *Hyde* case, the Fifth Circuit Court of Appeals characterized the exclusive contract of an anesthesiology group as an unlawful tying arrangement and a *per se* violation of antitrust law. They reasoned that the surgery for which the anesthesiology was administered represented a "tied product." The appeals court decision in *Hyde* declared as *per se* unlawful the "common practice in the health care industry of hospitals to enter into exclusive contracts with physicians." (*Dos Santos v. Columbus-Cuneo-Cabrini Medical Center*, 684 F 2d 1346, 1351 (7th Cir. 1982).

Before the court of appeals decision in *Hyde*, every state and federal court in the United States had upheld the traditional position and rationale that the exclusive contract provided a public benefit under Judge Brandeis's "rule of reason." Courts have traditionally rejected the argument that exclusive medical contracts amount to a group boycott or that they represent any other *per se* violation of antitrust law. A historical example in the medical imaging field is that of *Harron*.[49]

In *Harron v. United Hospital Center, Inc.*, an antitrust challenge to an exclusive medical contract was deemed so "frivolous" that the suit was dismissed because of lack of federal jurisdiction. In another important case, *Capili v. Schott*,[50] the court ruled that an exclusive arrangement was "reasonable." They also determined that the challenge failed to show that the exclusive contract had any effect on interstate commerce, which would make antitrust challenges more logical. The issue that medicine does involve interstate commerce has been previously commented upon in the U.S. courts. Analysis of the cases *Datillo v. Tucson General Hospital*,[51] *Blank v. Palo Alto–Stanford Hospital Center*,[52] and *Robinson v. Magovern*[53] will demonstrate the logic that courts have used to reject a great number of different antitrust claims other than that of tying arrangements. U.S. courts have adopted the attitude that the health care system in America is so complex and multifaceted that it may represent a unique industry. Additionally, significant costs related to certain activities of this industry (such as magnetic resonance imaging) involve choices that are not subject to typical business analysis. These considerations have created a favorable and understanding climate for the arguments that hospitals may employ exclusive contracts to protect their investment, to maintain quality of service, and to contain costs. Technologies such as MRI are particularly relevant to these considerations.

That patients as consumers should have their welfare protected is viewed by many as a primary reason for the application of antitrust legislation to the health care delivery industry.[41] The general facts regarding the cases cited, such as *Datillo v. Tucson General Hospital*, are those of placing sophisticated medical technology in specific locations and then limiting hospital privileges. These combined effects can create a number of tying arrangement issues that relate directly to not only the structure of hospitals but also the structure of exclusive contracts. In *Harron v. United Hospital Center, Inc.*, the issues arose when two hospitals in a single community were merged. The major issues in this case were determination of what represented the marketplace and whether the plaintiff was denied entry into the marketplace by not having a contract with the only existing hospital in that particular community. This type of case will be very important from the standpoint of "market penetration" analysis, especially if this involves a single hospital with a unique facility or a medical instrument such as an MRI scanner. The *Hyde* case involved an anesthesiology group without unique characteristics practicing in an urban community with many hospitals. For this reason, subsequent cases involving MRI may be decided with an entirely different outcome.

The law of exclusive dealing contracts under the provisions of the Clayton Act in the United States apply only to arrangements that involve goods, wares, merchandise, machinery, and supplies. Thus, one of the fundamental issues in medical antitrust cases is whether or not the delivery of health care can be considered under one of these categories. The Sherman Act, which does not contain such limitations, is applicable when the delivery of a particular type of service is involved. If this service is tied to yet another service (for example, MRI to neurosurgery), the analysis becomes more complex. For a tying arrangement to have an undesirable effect under antitrust reasoning, it must preclude freedom of choice or obviate true freedom of choice about the related service.

Under the Sherman Act, exclusive dealing contracts had not, until the Hyde case in the Fifth Circuit U.S. Court of Appeals, been deemed *per se* violations. As noted, "rule of reason" analysis had been applied to all preceding similar cases. Market foreclosure because of an exclusive medical contract for MRI will predictably be a subject of great importance in medicine. Crucial to the argument of market foreclosure seems to be the effect upon alternatives for obtaining the MRI studies and treatment by the physicians and patients involved. Excluded physicians may act as advocates for the consumer/patient.

Under the "quantitative substantiality test," the relative market must be defined and the degree of foreclosure by the contract from any particular activity determined. If the market for the MRI service is believed to be a national one, then the degree of market foreclosure represented by an MRI instrument or contract should be considered insignificant. An exclusive contract in this instance would neither pose general antitrust issues nor sustain an action in antitrust by an individual plaintiff. If a local market definition is assumed, then market foreclosure by the granting of exclusive contracts or hospital privileges may be viewed to be significant or fundamentally important.

The U.S. courts have generally based their decisions regarding exclusive contracts and denial of hospital privileges upon the testimony of physicians, hospital administrators, and policymakers. It has been generally contended that closed staff policies are desirable and necessary in certain health care provider circumstances. The usual benefits cited are operating and utilization efficiency, protection from duplication of costly and sophisticated instrumentation (such as MRI instruments), standardization of credentials and practice patterns, and financial savings. It has also been claimed that these benefits are transferred to the patient and eventually to the consumer public. The desirability of exclusive contracts and the high standards that allegedly result from these arrangements have been considered by the courts to be of greater merit than the negative effects of the monopolistic elements that might be present.

An additional antitrust theory is that exclusive medical contracts constitute an illegal group boycott. Antitrust causes will be sustained when plaintiffs establish that their competitors have precluded them from the marketplace. In such cases, it may be shown that the defendant controls a unique resource (such as a magnetic resonance imaging device) that is necessary for the particular trade or business of the plaintiff. In a more general context, one might claim that access to this resource is essential to protect public welfare. Accessibility to a scarce and important resource (such as MRI) may be an antitrust issue. A number of correlative and precedent cases can be found in other segments of business and industry.[41]

One of the important distinctions between group boycott and the general logic applied to exclusive medical contracts is in their antitrust analysis in the United States. Exclusive contracts have been treated under "the rule of reason," but group boycotts are considered *per se* violations of the U.S. Sherman Antitrust Act. Therefore, notwithstanding any redeeming virtue, an activity deemed to represent a group boycott would be deemed *per se* illegal. This distinction is an important one from the perspective of the *Hyde* case.

Viewed from the perspective of a single medical group, an exclusive contract can serve to eliminate rivalry for each hospital patient, allowing one firm of physicians to efficiently organize and deliver their service. In *United States v. Addyston Pipe & Steel Co.*,[54] and *Broadcast Music, Inc., v. Columbia Broadcasting System, Inc.*,[55] a number of legal principles were articulated and antitrust legislation interpreted. In the latter case it was found that elimination of a rival ancillary to a collaborative productive economic endeavor is not necessarily an unlawful violation of antitrust. This form of reasoning has also been applied to health care. If a medical service is delivered more efficiently under contract by a single group of physicians, all parties appear to benefit. In the course of exclusive hospital contract litigation, defendants have produced evidence of a number of efficiencies intrinsic to exclusive arrangements.

One benefit for an exclusive contract often cited is that of economic integration. A contract, like the internal arrangement of any firm, has the potential to organize, coordinate, and secure the efficient use of medical services. In many of the cases involving the legality of exclusive contracts, this has been termed a "scheduling" benefit. Hospital-based specialties in the United States have generally recognized scheduling problems because they operate in a response mode. Elimination or amelioration of these difficulties would be accepted as a desirable feature of any medical activity.

Regarding exclusive contracts, physicians in the United States have adopted a sequence of positions over a period of time. As practitioners, they must exercise their independent medical judgment as freely as possible. However, patients rely upon hospitals to procure certain services, many of which are termed hospital-based. In the precedent case, *Capili v. Schott*, a federal court ruled that hospital-based ancillary services are defined as radiology, pathology, anesthesiology, and emergency services. These are the services a hospital must guarantee as available to all their patients. Because patients do not select the individual physicians rendering these services, hospitals have a greater burden of responsibility in assuring the proper quality and quantity of these services.[50]

However, the New York Court of Appeals has ruled that a medical facility has no responsibility to supervise or intervene in the course of treatment recommended by the personal physician of a patient.[56,57] These factors support the concept that a general contract, which may be exclusive in nature, must be present to guarantee the availability of certain medical services for patient benefit and protection.

Whenever a hospital contracts for a medical service to the exclusion of noncontracting groups, certain activities can be organized and consolidated in a ready fashion. For example, the contracting group might better coordinate its activities, train the technological and support staff, and provide continuous clinical coverage. Additionally, the consulting group will attempt to maintain the contract by performing certain services that may be costly in terms of resources of the group, yet are essential to patient welfare and the general hospital mission. A noncontracting physician or group could acquire an arrangement by selecting the more lucrative aspects of a particular service, while leaving the contracting group with the costly obligations. In this instance, the result could be that the contracted services could deteriorate in overall quality.

In *Continental T.V., Inc., v. GTE Sylvania, Inc.*,[58] the United States Supreme Court recognized that when one party supplies services, and another selects only a part of that responsibility, the contracting firm, industry, and public could suffer from the decline in quality of service. Present "turf" issues in MRI may well be resolved on the same logic. A medical group under exclusive contract could come under intense pressure to maintain a contract in the national market, where competition may be vigorous and ongoing. If contracting physicians lose their administrative contract, they may also lose permission to practice in that particular hospital. Therefore, physicians should understand how "permission to practice" rights might be affected by other contracts that they might negotiate. These interrelationships can be complex in a free enterprise country.[39] Owning the contract for the MRI scanner may not be enough.

As noted in the United States, hospitals are entering increasingly into contractual relationships with medical groups to provide professional services. Hospitals form these contracts to ensure the continuous availability of certain services, to allocate equitably the responsibility for coverage, and to guarantee the performance of necessary administrative functions. These issues of antitrust and conflicts regarding hospital privileges will become increasingly important in the future.[38,59] The triers of fact have a very different problem. The level of expertise required to formulate policy regarding the distribution of sophisticated technology will necessitate requests for information and testimony from vested-interest groups who often are the only available experts.[30] Bias, influence, and self-serving activities by the groups will be difficult to detect and to minimize.[41,60]

In many countries, policymakers will receive a much stronger mandate to regulate the health care industry in the future.[21] Regulations will assume a more legal character, and many fundamental issues of medical practice will be resolved by court decisions.[61] High technology such as MRI in some countries will drive many of these issues to the forefront of public attention.[40,46] The patients' advocate in the legal arena and the patients' provider in the health care area should each attempt to understand the limits and constraints under which the other must function. Although we have seen this activity greatly increased in the past decade, this circumstance will be increasingly experienced in the future.

MAGNETIC RESONANCE IMAGING CENTERS

The decrease in funding sources from DRGs and the decline in capitalization grants, investment tax credits, charges in amortization, and traditional extramural funding have resulted in a search for new capital sources. These changes created a growing legion of physician entrepreneurs. In some states, physicians have been able to provide high technology access by circumventing the regulatory system. These activities have to date been accepted by the public because expectations of patients regarding technology are largely determined by the wishes of their physicians and rarely by the informed consent and desires of the consumers as patients. Our present environment has often placed MRI physicians in the position of competing financially with established medical institutions, even at times their own parent medical facility. Medical imaging physicians might well have instrumentation in their imaging centers that they could not acquire by traditional methods of funding in their parent institutions.

As noted earlier, the cost of health care delivery in the United States has achieved remarkable numbers in the past decade (10 percent GNP and over $340 billion per annum). At this level it has become apparent that broad public policy measures will be required to address issues of cost containment in medicine. In partial response to this challenge have come the Tax Equity Finance Reform Act (TEFRA) of 1982 and the enactment and implementation of a prospective payment system (DRGs) to compensate medical service.[29]

One of the short-term changes that will result from implementation of DRGs will be a shift of pretreatment diagnostic evaluation from an inpatient to an outpatient setting. This will favor the initiation and maintenance of magnetic resonance imaging centers. Our present mix of regulatory mechanisms (including the application of CON to control the distribution of costly instrumentation such as MRI machines), policies that make hospital privileges more difficult to obtain, and increased cost-consciousness of the American public will work in a complementary fashion to favor the placement of magnetic resonance imaging centers outside traditional institutional setting. These phenomena will be examined in some depth, possibly with some overlap with earlier considerations.

Financial analysis of medical costs has repeatedly demonstrated that outpatient diagnostic imaging studies can be performed less expensively than those performed in an inpatient setting.[27,28,62] Present policies of reimbursement make outpatient studies more profitable owing to the rapidity and efficiency by which they can be performed and the comparative decrease in overhead costs.[21,28,29,62]

This disparity between the outpatient and inpatient settings may become even greater in the future. Hospital overhead, personnel requirements, and equipment costs will probably remain relatively fixed. If fewer procedures are performed in hospitals in the future, this will necessitate higher charge per inpatient MRI procedure or unit of medical service.

Historically, refusal of third-party payers to provide compensation for certain diagnostic studies performed on an outpatient basis forced admissions of "nonsick" individuals or ambulatory patients for inpatient evaluation to ensure collections. But we believe that this will no longer be the circumstance. Under DRGs, a fixed amount of money will be allocated for diagnosis and treatment of certain symptom complexes. Thus, the physician's choice regarding whether to choose an outpatient or inpatient diagnostic evaluation will be driven by a different set of circumstances. Freestanding magnetic resonance imaging centers should become relatively more profitable in this environment.

From other chapters, one can see that the efficacy of MRI in certain areas remains to be established. Large institutions, already encumbered with a substantial debt service, may be unwilling to incur the financial risk of acquiring or upgrading and expanding this capability. However, there are individual investors, financial institutions, and entrepreneurial groups who appear very willing to undertake the business risk of a magnetic resonance imaging center. No matter how attractive any of these schemes may appear, each may be characterized by an associated risk.

Outpatient evaluation by MRI of individuals with serious illnesses may result in their being maintained outside of hospitals for more extended periods for preadmission tests than they would have before DRGs. This may not represent the best interests of the patient. As more and more complex MRI procedures are performed on individuals in the outpatient setting, complications from these procedures could occur more often in areas without ready access to fully trained advanced life-support teams, emergency rooms, or intensive care units. Care of patients might be compromised in transporting them to the outpatient setting, even from the hospital.

A full complement of alternative imaging procedures may not be present at an MRI facility or in the immediate vicinity; this might preclude the use of ultrasound, x-ray computed tomography, and angiography when one of these, rather than MRI, is the appropriate imaging study. Additionally, if the MRI center is located at a remote site, students, residents, fellows, and clinical colleagues may not be able to utilize the learning experience of the facility.

We have previously alluded to possible antitrust issues raised by MRI centers. A discussion of the granting of hospital privileges should be helpful. Following the *Darling v. Charleston Medical Center* case, more stringent JCAH requirements and increased awareness of hospital liability for physicians have resulted in greater difficulty in acquiring hospital privileges.[63] Because it has been established that the ultimate responsibility for the quality and expertise of the professional staff in any given medical institution rests in its board of trust, procedures to grant hospital privileges have become more standardized and increasingly problematical. These combined effects may well exclude certain physicians, and subsequently their patients, from access to the inpatient magnetic resonance imaging facilities placed in specific hospitals. Freestanding MRI centers in this instance would offer an alternative means of access to this expensive, state-of-the-art imaging modality.

We have noted that MRI centers provide certain opportunities to imaging physicians; however, they are not without potential risks. Increased profitability of imaging centers will predictably lead to greater competition for ownership and governance. Hospitals, attorneys, venture capitalists, and other physicians as well as imaging physicians may wish to benefit from the independence, flexibility, and potential financial profit. These inducements may lead to the formation of a variety of ownership–service provision arrangements. The owners of imaging centers may choose to contract physicians to interpret the diagnostic studies on a fee-for-service basis, as a share of the revenue of the center, or on a straight salary basis. The financial arrangements for compensation and reimbursement as well as return on investment in some of the MRI centers will predictably create antitrust issues.

To finance the initiation of these magnetic resonance imaging centers, certain physicians and/or other investors may become general partners, while other participants will enter into the arrangement as limited partners. Each will incur financial risks in exchange for the opportunity to share in the subsequent profits. The limited partners may be and often are the referring physicians who will utilize the center by sending their patients to be studied in their facility. These limited partners have the potential to control a large segment, or all, of the patients who could be referred to the MRI facility for diagnostic studies.

By preselecting certain subspecialty categories or the parent specialty disciplines of limited partners, the general partners could choose the most "profitable" equipment (including the MRI) based upon the diagnostic studies that they know would be obtained in their MRI center. Selection of the most appropriate and profitable equipment is possible owing to prior knowledge of those studies to be ordered by the carefully chosen limited partners.[64–66] Some element of "free choice" of patients and physicians might be eliminated by this arrangement.

It might further be contended that the effort to serve the acquisition and operational debt of the center may significantly bias the owner-physician's choices. A number of queries as to the propriety of the potential responses may be considered. For those who believe that the patient's interests are paramount and that the welfare of the patient supersedes that of the physician, the investor–limited partner arrangement will be viewed with some skepticism.

Other ethical issues also arise from these arrangements. Is it legal or ethical to have as limited partners physicians who will financially profit from the MRI study they order in their MRI center? Is this not a rather complex form of "fee-splitting" or, at best, self-referral? These activities are judged to be unlawful in a few states. More importantly, they have traditionally been considered unethical by organized medicine. At present, certain states require disclosure of a financial interest in centers by physicians to patients. But others are considering more stringent measures to limit ownership.

In consideration of the *Hyde* case, could a single magnetic resonance imaging center in a certain geographic location represent capture of the marketplace? Also, does the imaging physician have corporate responsibility to the parent medical specialty group? The answers to these concerns are not readily apparent, because precedents for MRI centers have not been established and extrapolations from other areas of medical activity are sometimes difficult. Regarding antitrust concerns and "tying arrangements" for the MRI venture arrangements, certain concepts seem to be applicable. As long as the referring physician-partner in the MRI facility financially benefits as a result of return upon investment and not relative to the numbers or types of patients referred or by some scale or weighting factor for the examinations requested, the arrangement will be deemed legal.[24] A legal arrangement, however, is not by definition necessarily a moral or an ethical one.

Many long-existing referral patterns in medicine present mutually beneficial financial incentives among physicians. Would the organization, purpose, and incentives for the magnetic resonance imaging center have these traditional characteristics? We should apply the same stringent ethical guidelines of conduct in these arrangements to the MRI centers. Before we can form meaningful conclusions about these fundamental moral issues, we might return for reconsideration of the fundamental premises of antitrust theory and relate them to these activities. Challenges on moral and ethical grounds, if they are appropriate, would be valid only after a considered analysis of the multiple factors involved in these issues.

In any antitrust analysis of medical practice, the characterization of "marketplace" is of fundamental importance.[39] A magnetic resonance imaging center in a small community may represent the only facility that has the ability to provide this unique mode of diagnostic inquiry. In larger communities, because of the unique nature of this technology, an MRI center may still represent significant market "capture" or "penetration." Penetration would be viewed from the aspect of instrument distribution and capture from consideration of physician and patient choices and access.

The existence of a magnetic resonance imaging center could, thus, be challenged on several antitrust bases, especially that of capture by control of a resource of a unique and essential nature. Might the ownership of the MRI center by the referring physicians constitute a unique "tying arrangement"[39] in the tradition of the *U.S. v. Terminal R.R. Assn., Tampa Electric Co. v. Nashville Coal Co.*, and *Associated Press v. United States* cases?[48,67,68] The ownership of the MRI center by a certain physician group may constitute control of a vital resource for the conduct of a particular business, the practice of medicine. Limited ownership in an MRI center could also adversely affect a physician's, and ultimately the patient's, choice of whether to utilize a particular resource and which resource to utilize. Other physicians might claim exclusion from the marketplace by a competing provider, the MRI center. The challenge would be directed at the physicians with a financial partnership in the competing MRI center.

The probability of a court case developing on the antitrust basis of a "tying arrangement" or self-referral is moderate. Challenges posed to regulatory agencies by competing groups or businesses and professional codes enacted by state legislatures, however, are to be expected.

Many communities or geographic areas may have the patient demand or resource capacity for only a single magnetic resonance imager. Should not all physicians in that community have equal access to this unique medical resource? On the "quantitative substantiality" theory of antitrust analysis, does single ownership of an MRI unit for an isolated area constitute sufficient market capture that the questions of antitrust become valid concerns?[69,70] We would suggest that it does and that a general moral and social responsibility regarding access for physicians and patients exists.

DRGs may in the future affect outpatient or freestanding facilities, as may application of CON legislation and the limitations upon technology proliferation that these impose. At present the magnetic resonance imaging centers are clearly separate and independent of an inpatient facility, although they may be geographically adjacent, and thereby will escape these constraints. These nonregulated MRI facilities may represent momentary "windfall" profit centers.

Hospitalized patients in many instances could be relegated to a second-class status owing to lack of physician or patient access to the separate MRI center or potential third-party reduction in fees for services in inpatient facilities and possible disallowance of charges. Hospital governance bodies will prove increasingly reluctant to invest in costly technology if return on equity falls below a certain level of expectation. Over a period of time the medical instrumentation in insititutions and hospitals might become "dated" in relation to these diagnostic imaging centers. More general social trends may also result in lower technology hospital-based medicine owing to a multitude of factors, some of which have been discussed.

The current structuring of MRI centers could reduce access to this high technology for the low-income population. Because of their "for profit" structure, MRI centers are likely to demonstrate a corporate attitude of reduced care for patients who are covered by Medicare or who have limited insurance, or whose personal financial resources are inadequate to compensate for service rendered.[31] Such policies to ensure profitability might also include active solicitation of those patients with well-identified means to pay for the magnetic resonance imaging studies. These types of activities might alter the health care delivery system, especially in attempts to provide adequate care to the financially underprivileged.

Certain ethical issues that result from these financial arrangements are dependent upon the societal interpretation and concept of the medical system. If health care is viewed as a basic social right, rationing of care based upon financial grounds would be deemed inappropriate. If medical care is believed to be a purchasable commodity available in the marketplace, magnetic resonance imaging centers would represent a response to a consumer and marketplace need as well as an investment opportunity. Traditionally, substantial emphasis has been placed on the health care professional's responsibility to serve as an advocate for patients and society, while recognizing the appropriateness of payment for services rendered.

Ethical responsibility and obligation are clearly relevant to all manners of medical practice, including MRI centers. Physicians also have an affirmative ethical obligation to disclose their ownership in MRI centers to patients. Given these principles, magnetic resonance imaging centers will remain an ethical and moral concern for many physicians. A number of centers will be initiated, for the most part to avoid the constraints of currently enacted distribution and compensation arrangements (especially DRGs). Others will be formed because capital expenditure budgets in traditional health care facilities will not permit the acquisition of the MRI equipment desired by physicians.[71,72] These acquisitions can now be financed under the venture capital and limited partnership structure, providing a definite advantage over other more traditional methods.

Some facilities in magnetic resonance imaging centers may be overutilized because of the ownership by referring physicians. Facility selection and choice of diagnostic studies will be biased to some degree in certain of these centers owing to the organizational arrangement and financial profitability of the participants. Would the potential for this bias be in the best interests of the image of the medical profession? We believe that this will at least represent a considerable change in the traditional fiduciary posture relative to patients.

Imaging centers of all types have the real potential to capture a substantial part of the patient population, alter referral patterns, and essentially redefine the "marketplace." These centers also have the potential to exclude physicians from a segment of the health care delivery system.[36,73,74] Given the alternatives, a solution has been offered for physicians to become active participants in the planning of centers to positively influence these arrangements and protect patient welfare by maintaining the quality of health care delivery.

Another option available to the MRI physician is to become part of the policy-making process and remove certain of the financial incentives to these types of organization by making them subject to similar arrangements as inpatient-, and hospital-, or institution-based facilities.[75] Might another position be taken that the policies be changed or reoriented to equally affect all segments of the health care delivery system? Freestanding imaging centers are a phenomenon of present health care policies.[76–78] They represent challenges and risks to all components of the system.

In this chapter we have discussed selected legal topics that we felt had both current interest and application to the discipline of magnetic resonance imaging as a form of diagnostic inquiry. Many of the societal concerns and ethical principles are, in our opinion, timeless. Since we live in an environment of precedent and case-made law, the legal principles are much more subject to change.

It is our hope that these considerations will assist in providing the reader some perspective regarding magnetic resonance imaging that could not be gained elsewhere.

ACKNOWLEDGMENTS

The authors are indebted to Steven Hirschtick, J.D., Paul G. Gebhard, L.L.B., Otha Linton, M.S.J., Gerald Freedman, M.D., Henry S. Allen, J.D., Richard Sanders, J.D., Barbara Chick, M.D., Richard Robinson, J.D., Frank Sloan, Ph.D., Tom Reed, J.D., Stanley Baum, M.D., Martin Silbiger, M.D., Henry Pendergrass, M.D., Jim Blumstein, J.D., Terry Calvani, J.D., Ron Evens, M.D., and W. Hoyt Stephens, M.S., for thoughts and advice. The resources of the Schools of Law and Medicine and Institute for Public Policy Studies at Vanderbilt University were utilized in this communication.

References

1. Holder AR: Medical Malpractice Law. New York, John H Wiley & Sons, 1975.
2. Curran WJ, Shapiro ED: Law, Medicine, and Forensic Science, 3rd ed. Boston, Little, Brown, and Co, 1982.
3. American Law Institute: Restatement (2nd) of the Law of Agency. American Law Institute Publishers, 1959.
4. Seavey WA: The Law of Agency. St Paul, West Publishing Co, 1964.
5. Crane JA, Bromberg AR: Law of Partnership. St Paul, West Publishing Co, 1968.
6. James AE Jr, Hall DJ, Johnson BA: Some applications of the law of evidence to the specialty of radiology. Radiology *124*:845, 1977.
7. Plante ML: An analysis of informed consent. Fordham Law Review *36*:639, 1968.
8. Lalli AF: Urographic contrast media reactions and anxiety. Radiology *112*:267, 1974.
9. Witten DM, Hirsch FD, Hartman GW: Acute reactions to urographic contrast medium. Incidence, clinical characteristics, and relationships to history of hypersensitivity status. AJR *119*:832, 1973.
10. Coleman LL: Terrified consent. Physicians World *1*(5):5, 1974.
11. Allen R: Informed consent: a medical decision. Radiology *119*:233, 1976.
12. Ansul GM: Adverse reactions to contrast agents. Invest Radiol *5*:374, 1970.
13. Alfidi R: Controversy, alternatives, and decisions in complying with the legal doctrine of informed consent. Radiology *114*:231, 1975.

14. Bucklin R: Informed Consent: Past, Present, and Future Legal Medicine Annual 1975. New York, Appleton-Century-Crofts, 1976.
15. Rubasem DS: What every doctor should know about changes in informed consent. Med World News *14*(6):66, 1973.
16. James AE Jr, Anderson JH, Higgins CB: Digital Image Processing in Radiology. Baltimore, Williams & Wilkins, 1985.
17. Partain CL, James AE Jr, Rollo FD, Price RR (eds): Nuclear Magnetic Resonance (NMR) Imaging, 1st ed. Philadelphia, WB Saunders, 1983.
18. Coulam CM, Erickson JJ, Rollo FD, James AE Jr (eds): The Physical Basis of Medical Imaging. New York, Appleton-Century-Crofts, 1981, pp 1–4.
19. James AE Jr: Ethical choices in high technology medicine: current dilemmas in diagnostic imaging. Health Care Instrumentation *1* (5):158, 1986.
20. James AE Jr, Partain CL, Patton JA, et al: The Marshal Eskridge Lecture: Current status of magnetic resonance imaging. South Med J *78*(5):580, 1985.
21. James AE Jr: The Walter Herbert Memorial Lecture: Certain legal aspects of medical imaging. *In* Margulis AR, Gooding CA (eds): Diagnostic Radiology. San Francisco, University of California Press, 1985, pp 309–315.
22. James AE Jr: The newer imaging procedures in radiological sciences: choices of informational content and imaging quality. *In* Proceedings of the 18th Annual Meeting of the National Council on Radiation Protection and Measurements. Washington DC, April 1982.
23. James AE Jr, Fleischer AC, Thieme GA, Bundy AL, Sanders RC, Johnson B, Boehm FH: Diagnostic ultrasonography: certain legal considerations. J Ultrasound Med *4*:427, 1985.
24. Fleischer AC, James AE Jr: Real-time sonography. Norwalk, Connecticut, Appleton-Century-Crofts, 1984.
25. Price RR, Rollo FD, Monahan WG, James AE Jr: Digital Radiography: A Focus on Clinical Utility. New York, Grune & Stratton, 1982.
26. Stephens WH, James AE Jr, Winfield AC, Pendergrass HP: Financial implications of NMR imaging. *In* Partain CL, James AE Jr, Rollo RD, Price RR: Nuclear Magnetic Resonance (NMR) Imaging, 1st ed. Philadelphia, WB Saunders, 1983.
27. Freedman GS, Stephens WH, Fisher B: Economic considerations in MRI. Appl Radiol *13*(3):55, 1984.
28. Freedman GS, James AE Jr: Comparison of outpatient digital angiography and inpatient arteriography: some financial implications. *In* Price RR, Rollo FD, Monahan WG, James AE Jr (eds). Digital Radiography: A Focus on Clinical Utility. New York, Grune & Stratton, 1982.
29. James AE Jr, Sloan FA, Carroll FE, Pendergrass HP, Winfield AC, Blumstein J, Hamilton RJ, Chapman JC: Hospital cost regulation: some cumulative effects from certificate of need and diagnosis related groups. Noninvas Med Imag *1*(4):259, 1984.
30. James AE Jr, Hickey Lecture: Medical imaging technology in a societal context. AJR *144*:1109, 1985.
31. James AE Jr, Pendergrass HP, Partain CL, Rollo FD, Quimby C, Johnson B, Price RR: Legal considerations of NMR imaging. *In* Partain CL, James AE Jr, Rollo FD, Price FF (eds): Nuclear Magnetic Resonance (NMR) Imaging, 1st ed. Philadelphia, WB Saunders, 1983.
32. Schwartz WB, Joskow PL: Duplicated hospital facilities: how much can we save by consolidating them? N Engl J Med *303*:1449, 1980.
33. Aaron JH, Schwartz WB: The Painful Prescription: Rationing Health Care. Washington, DC, The Brookings Institute, 1984.
34. Schwartz WB, Aaron HJ: Health care costs: the social tradeoffs. Issues in Sci Technology. Winter: 39–46, 1985.
35. Griner PF: Use of laboratory tests in a teaching hospital: long-term trends, reduction in use and relative costs. Ann Intern Med *90*:243, 1979.
36. Showstack JA, Schroeder SA, Matsumoto MF: Changes in the use of medical technologies, 1971–1977: a study of 10 inpatient diagnoses. N Engl J Med *306*:706, 1982.
37. James AE Jr, Price RR, Erickson JJ, et al: Advances in digital imaging: experience at Vanderbilt University. Contrast Media in Digital Radiography, International Workshop, Berlin. Amsterdam, Excerpta Medica, 1983.
38. James AE Jr, Winfield AC, Rollo FD, et al: An analysis of the combined effects of certificate of need legislation and changes in the granting of hospital privileges. Radiology *145*(1):229, 1982.
39. James AE Jr, et al: Legal and ethical issues in a technologic discipline: New times, new choices. Invest Radiol *21*(8):673, 1986.
40. James AE Jr: Antitrust law and the practice of radiology. Radiology *132*:233, 1979.
41. Calvani T, James AE Jr: Antitrust law and the practice of medicine. *In* James AE Jr (ed). Legal Medicine with Special Reference to Diagnostic Imaging. Baltimore, Urban & Schwartzenberg, 1980.
42. Covington RN: Medical malpractice insurance: what went wrong? *In* James AE Jr (ed): Legal Medicine with Special Reference to Diagnostic Imaging. Baltimore, Urban & Schwartzenberg, 1980.
43. James AE Jr, Sherrard TJ: The law of agency as applied to radiology. Radiology *128*:257, 1978.
44. James AE Jr: Law and medicine: Can antitrust legislation secure better health care? The Vanderbilt Lawyer *13*(2):20, 1983.
45. James AE Jr, Waddill WB III, Feazell GL, et al: The new medical imaging technologies as evidence. J Contemp Law *11*(1):105, 1984.
46. James AE Jr, Sloan FA, Hamilton RH, et al: Antitrust aspects of exclusive contracts in medical imaging. Radiology *156*:237, 1985.

47. James AE Jr, Partain, CL, et al: A critique of the concept of MRI centers. Magn Reson Imag *5*:71, 1987.
48. *Hyde* v. *Jefferson Parish Hospital District No. 2*, 686 F. 2d 286 (5th Cir. 1982), cert. granted 51 U.S.L.W. 3649 (1983).
49. *Harron* v. *United Hospital Center, Inc.* 522 F. 2d 1133 (4th Cir. 1975), cert. denied, 424 U.S. Hospital Center, Inc., 916 (1976).
50. *Capili* v. *Schott* 487 F. Supp. 710, 711–12 aff'd 620 F. 2d 438 (4th Cir. 1980).
51. *Datillo* v. *Tucson General Hospital* 23 Ariz. App. 392, 533 P. 2d 700, 1975.
52. *Blank* v. *Palo Alto–Stanford Hospital Center* 234 Cal. App. 2d 377, 44 Cal. Rptr 572, 1965.
53. *Robinson* v. *Magovern* 521 F. Supp. 842 (W.D.Pa 1981) aff'd mem., 688 F. 2d 824 (d Cir. 1982), cert. denied, 1982.
54. *United States* v. *Addyston Pipe & Steel Co.*, 85 Fed. 271 (6th Cir. 1898) (Taft J), 175 U.S. 211, 1899.
55. *Broadcast Music, Inc.* v. *Columbia Broadcasting System, Inc.*, 441 U.S. 1, 60 L.Ed. 2d 1, 99 S.Ct. 1551, 1557 (1979) ("ASCAP").
56. *Fiorentino* v. *Wenger* 19 NY 2d 407 (1967).
57. *Matter of Storar* 52 NY 2d 363 (1981).
58. *Continental T.V., Inc.* v. *G.T.E. Sylvania, Inc.* 433 U.S. 36 (1977).
59. *National Gerimedical Hospital and Gerontology Center* v. *Blue Cross of Kansas City* 101 S.Ct. 2415 (1981).
60. James AE Jr, Sloan FA, Blumstein JF, et al: Certificate-of-need in an antitrust context. J Health Polit Policy Law *8*(2):314, 1983.
61. Sanders R, James AE Jr (eds): The Principles and Practice of Ultrasonography in Obstetrics and Gynecology, 3rd ed. Norwalk, Connecticut, Appleton-Century-Crofts, 1984.
62. Stephens WH, Patton JA, Lagan JE, et al: Certain economic considerations in NMR imaging. *In* Partain CL (ed): Nuclear Magnetic Resonance and Correlative Imaging Modalities. New York, Society of Nuclear Medicine, 1983, pp 263–269.
63. *Darling* v. *Charleston Community Memorial Hospital*, 33 Ill. 2d 326, 211 N.E. 2d 253 (1965), cert. denied 282 U.S. 946 (1966).
64. Evens R, Jost RG, Evens R Jr: Economic and utilization analysis of magnetic resonance imaging units in the United States in 1985. AJR *145*:393, 1985.
65. Partain CL (ed): Nuclear Magnetic Resonance and Correlative Imaging Modalities. New York, Society of Nuclear Medicine, 1983.
66. Price RR, Rollo FD, Monahan WG, James AE Jr (eds): Digital Radiography: A Focus on Clinical Utility. New York, Grune & Stratton, 1982.
67. *U.S.* v. *Terminal Railroad Association*. 224 U.S. 383 (1912).
68. *Tampa Electric Co.* v. *Nashville Coal Co.*, 365 U.S. 320, 329 (1961).
69. *Associated press* v. *United States*, 326 U.S. 1, 17 (1945).
70. James AE Jr, Partain CL, Rollo FD, et al: Nuclear magnetic resonance: certain legal and proprietary questions. *In* Partain CL (ed): Nuclear Magnetic Resonance and Correlative Imaging Modalities. New York, Society of Nuclear Medicine, 1983, pp 271–298.
71. Nutler DO: Access to care and the evaluation of corporate for-profit medicine. N Engl J Med *311*:917, 1984.
72. Fineberg H, Wittenberg J, Ferrucci J, et al: The clinical value of body computed tomography over time and technologic change. AJR *141*:1067, 1983.
73. Evens R, Siegel B, Welch M, Ter-Pogossian M: Cost analysis of positron emission tomography for clinical use. AJR *141*:1073, 1983.
74. Freeland M, Schendler C: Health spending in the 1980s: Integration of clinical practice patterns with management. Health Care Financing Review *5*(3):1, 1984.
75. Ginzberg E: The monetarization of medical care. N Engl J Med *310*(18):1162, 1984.
76. Relman AS: Who will pay for medical education in our teaching hospitals? Science *26*:20, 1984.
77. Relman AS: Dealing with conflicts of interest. N Engl J Med *313*:749, 1985.
78. Silbiger ML: Innovations to assure the future of academic radiology. Appl Radiol Sept/Oct, 1985.

56

The Economics and Regulation of MRI

EARL P. STEINBERG
OTHA W. LINTON
JANE E. ERICKSON

In today's health care environment, the cost of new technologies, the availability of third-party payment for them, and the strength of state and federal regulations governing their use are as important determinants of their adoption by the medical profession as is their clinical efficacy.[1] This is particularly true in the case of high-cost medical technologies, such as magnetic resonance (MR) imagers.

The purpose of this chapter, therefore, is to examine a number of the most important issues related to the economics and regulation of magnetic resonance imaging (MRI). We begin with a discussion of the current and expected diffusion of MR imagers, both in the United States and worldwide. We then analyze the costs of several types of MR imagers and compare those costs with those of state-of-the art x-ray CT scanners. We also discuss the impact of MRI on overall health care costs and describe a newly developed computer model that estimates the volume of MRI and x-ray CT scans likely to be generated by an individual hospital's inpatient case mix. The current status of third-party payment for MRI is reviewed and a number of payment issues identified. These include variation in payment rates for MRI scans performed on different types of MRI systems and how Medicare is likely to pay for capital costs in the future—issues that are likely to attract increasing attention. We discuss the status and impact of certificate-of-need (CON) and Food and Drug Administration (FDA) regulation of MRI and present a number of conclusions.

DIFFUSION OF MRI

In the United States

Despite the high costs of MRI and the increased cost consciousness of the health care industry, the cumulative number of MR imagers installed in the United States more than tripled in 1985.[2] By the end of 1985, more than 360 MR imagers had been installed,[2] compared with 108 at the end of 1984.[3] Recent estimates from industry analysts suggest that an additional 300[4] MRI units were shipped to United States installations in 1986, and that as many as 1400 MRI units will have been shipped to sites nationwide by the end of 1988.[5] Even if these industry sales estimates are correct, the installed base of MRI units in the United States by the end of this decade will probably fall short of the more than 2000 CT scanners that are currently operating.[6] Nonetheless, with the current exponential rate of installation of MR imagers, it is clear that MR imaging will account for a substantial proportion of radiology capital costs in this country by the end of this decade.

Outside the United States

Although worldwide MRI diffusion data have not recently been published, our own data obtained from manufacturers suggest that approximately 140 MRI units had been installed outside the United States by the end of 1985.[2] Thus, more than 70 percent of all MRI units installed worldwide by the end of 1985 were in the United States. Despite recent efforts to control health care costs in the United States, and recent concerns about the effect of those efforts on the adoption of new technologies, it seems clear that MRI is being adopted more widely and rapidly in the United States than in the rest of the world.

Siting Patterns

Based on reports from manufacturers, nearly half the MRI units that have been installed in the United States have been located outside of acute care hospitals.[1,2] Many of these MR imagers were purchased to form the core of a freestanding diagnostic imaging center that also commonly includes a CT scanner and other imaging devices. These centers frequently have been established as for-profit enterprises with quite varied patterns of ownership.

Developers of outpatient imaging centers have included single hospitals, groups of hospitals, hospitals joining with members of their medical staff, groups of radiologists, radiologists joined with other physicians, and venture capitalists having no other involvement with health care. In some instances, freestanding imaging centers have been developed to avoid health care planning restrictions that apply only to hospitals or to increase revenues or earn investment profits in an era of prospective payment.

The involvement of clinicians as investors in these imaging centers has raised issues about medical ethics and propriety. Several states have considered, but none has enacted, legislation that would restrict the participation of physicians as investors in imaging centers. The American Medical Association in 1984 asserted that physicians should acknowledge their ownership of an imaging facility at the time they refer a patient to it.[27] The American College of Radiology, a year later, urged radiologists to avoid participation in centers where clinicians received a direct financial return on each patient referred for an examination.[28] Despite these cautions and concerns, there continues to be considerable interest among physicians in investing in imaging centers that include MRI.

ECONOMICS OF MRI

Considerable experience with MRI has now been amassed, and several estimates of the annual operating costs have been published.[7-10] Certain conclusions can be drawn from these analyses. First, the annualized cost of an MRI scanner varies with the type of magnet employed. Second, the break-even cost per MRI scan is largely dependent on the specific assumptions regarding depreciation of equipment and facilities, cost of capital, rates of partial pay/bad debt, and, most important, patient throughput (number of patients scanned per year). Third, even when an MR imager is operated efficiently with maximum patient throughput, the cost of an MRI scan is greater than the cost of a CT scan. Fourth, with efficient operation and reasonable patient throughput, the cost of an MRI scan is not prohibitively high. Finally, few data are available regarding the marginal impact of MRI on the cost of patient care, particularly on the per-hospitalization costs of patients admitted in specific DRGs.

Tables 56–1 to 56–3 present data from the literature that we believe reflect the costs of purchasing and operating various types of MRI scanners. The annualized cost data (Table 56–2) and the break-even cost per scan data (Table 56–3) assume that 1500 MRI scans will be done annually with one shift (6 scans per day, 5 days per week, 50 weeks per year) and that 3000 scans will be done annually with two shifts (12 scans per day, 5 days per week, 50 weeks per year). Although few sites are currently achieving this level of throughput,[9] it seems clear from information reported in the literature[9] as well as information informally provided by manufacturers and several MRI sites that an average throughput of one patient per hour is achievable. The per-scan cost estimates (Table 56–3) do not include either professional fees or allowance for partial pay/bad debt.

The data reported in Tables 56–1 to 56–3, based in large part on estimates made by the U.S. Congressional Office of Technology Assessment, provide cost estimates that are similar to those developed by Evens et al.[9] Based on a 1985 survey of 77 MRI sites operating in the United States, these investigators projected that the "typical" MRI unit in the United States cost $1,360,000 to purchase and $378,000 to install and had an annualized operating cost of $841,500. Based on these estimates, Evens et al. determined that the break-even cost of an MRI scan varies from $501 to $702 (assuming 16 percent and 40 percent partial pay/bad debt, respectively) when only eight patients are scanned per day; the break-even cost of an MRI scan varies from $350 to $490 (assuming 16 percent and 40 percent partial pay/bad debt, respectively) if 12 patients are scanned per day.

To put these MRI cost estimates into perspective, data are presented in Tables 56–4 and 56–5 for the costs of purchasing and operating a high-quality CT scanner in 1985. Based on these cost estimates and an assumption of a patient throughput of 5000 CT scans per year (the average annual throughput per CT machine at Johns Hopkins Hospital[26]), the per-scan cost of a CT scan, exclusive of bad debt and professional

Table 56–1. ESTIMATED COSTS OF MRI IMAGING SYSTEMS BY TYPE OF MAGNET

	Resistive (0.15T)	Permanent (0.3T)	Superconductive (0.5T)	Superconductive (1.5T)
Capital Costs				
Purchase	$800,000*	1.5m*	1.5m*	2.0m*
Site Renovation	150,000–510,000*	75,000–250,000*	350,000–1.3m†	600,000‡–1.3m†
Annual Operating Costs				
Cryogens and/or electricity	20,000*	8,200* 6,000–11,000†	20,000–40,000*	30,000–50,000* 21,000–82,000†
Personnel	70,000–140,000§ 85,000–138,000‖	70,000–140,000§ 85,000–138,000‖	70,000–140,000§ 85,000–138,000‖	70,000–140,000§ 85,000–138,000‖
Supplies	30,000¶ 60,000**	30,000¶ 60,000**	30,000¶ 60,000**	30,000¶ 60,000**
Maintenance contract	40,000–60,000*	40,000–75,000†	119,000*	140,000*
Overhead	40,000–82,000*	46,000–82,000*	51,000–98,000*	59,000–104,000*

* Source: Reference 7.
† Source: Reference 8.
‡ Source: Reference 11.
§ Source: Reference 7 for one shift and two shifts, respectively.
‖ Source: Reference 8 for one shift and two shifts, respectively.
¶ Assumes 1500 scans per year (6 scans/day), $20 per scan.
** Assumes 3000 scans per year (12 scans/day), $20 per scan.

Table 56–2. ESTIMATED ANNUALIZED COSTS OF MRI IMAGING SYSTEMS BY TYPE OF MAGNET

	Resistive (0.15T)	Permanent (0.3T)	Superconductive (0.5T)	Superconductive (1.5T)
Capital				
Equipment	$204,000*	382,000*	382,000*	510,000*
Site	24,000*	12,000*	103,000*	111,000*
Total	228,000	394,000	485,000	621,000
Operating	180,000†–280,000‡	183,200†–283,200‡	249,000†–349,000‡	290,000†–390,000‡
Overhead	82,000*	82,000*	98,000*	104,000*
TOTAL				
1 shift	490,000	659,200	832,000	1,015,000
2 shifts	590,000	792,200	932,000	1,115,000

* Source: Reference 7.
† Assumes 1 shift, 1500 scans annually.
‡ Assumes 2 shifts, 3000 scans annually.

fees, is approximately $159 to $171. At a less busy community hospital, where the annual CT throughput may be only 4000 scans, the break-even cost per CT scan, exclusive of professional fees and bad debt, would range from $177 to $192. Thus, with high patient throughput, the cost of an MRI scan on a resistive magnet system might be similar to the cost of a CT scan, whereas the cost of an MRI scan on a high-field unit could be two to three times that of a CT scan, depending on patient throughput.

Comparison of the costs of MRI scanning to those of CT scanning, though useful, does not address several other fundamental issues pertinent to an analysis of the cost impacts of MRI. These include the *marginal* impact of MRI on the frequency of use of other diagnostic modalities, such as CT, myelography, angiography, ultrasonography, nuclear imaging, and biopsy and surgery; and the impact of MRI on therapeutic practices, lengths of hospital stay, frequency of outpatient versus inpatient evaluations, and the ultimate quality of patient care. Until further experience with, and insight into, these issues are gained, the economic component of decisions regarding acquisition of MRI units will be based largely on assessments such as those in Tables 56–1 to 56–5 and estimates of the probable volume of utilization of MRI at individual sites.

With regard to the latter point, a computer model has been developed by one of us (EPS) that utilizes historical DRG-specific patterns of use of x-ray CT scanning, as well as expert opinion regarding rates of substitution of MRI for CT, to estimate the number of inpatient MRI scans that would be generated by an individual hospital's or area's case mix.[12] DRG-specific patterns of CT use were derived by linking Johns Hopkins Hospital's Inpatient Management Detail File, which includes billing codes for 22 different clinical categories of CT scans and documentation of CT utilization for all inpatients, with the Johns Hopkins Hospital Casemix Discharge Data Base, which includes information on the DRG in which each inpatient is discharged. Analysis of

Table 56–3. ESTIMATED BREAK-EVEN COST PER MRI SCAN BY TYPE OF MAGNET*

	Resistive (0.15T)	Permanent (0.3T)	Superconductive (0.5T)	Superconductive (1.5T)
Cost per Scan				
1 shift	$327	$439	$555	$677
(1500 scans/year)				
2 shifts	$197	$253	$311	$372
(3000 scans/year)				

* Excluding professional fees and allowances for partial pay/bad debt.

Table 56–4. ESTIMATED COST OF HIGH-QUALITY X-RAY CT SYSTEM

Capital Costs	
Purchase	$900,000*
Site Renovation	100,000*–200,000†
Annual Operating Costs	
Electricity	20,000†
Personnel	85,000‡
	133,333§
Supplies	180,000‖
	235,000¶
Maintenance	80,000*–94,000†
Overhead	70,000*

* Source: Reference 11.
† Source: Reference 26.
‡ Source: Reference 11 for 1.5 shifts.
§ Source: Reference 11 for 2 shifts.
‖ Assumes 4000 scans per year, $35 per scan including contrast, and $40,000 per year for tubes.
¶ Assumes 5000 scans per year, $35 per scan including contrast, and $60,000 per year for tubes.

CT utilization during 19,000 hospitalizations at Johns Hopkins in fiscal year 1984 was used to develop the DRG-specific profile of CT use. This profile was then linked to the results of a survey of eight nationally recognized MRI experts, who provided estimates of expected rates of substitution of MRI for CT in 1986 and in 1990 in each of the 22 clinical categories of CT use. In the final model, adjustments are made for differences in case mix and patterns of CT use between Johns Hopkins and other hospitals. The model, which provides an estimate of a hospital's CT and MRI use in 1986 and 1990 if the number of CT scanners and MR imagers were not constrained, is currently being field-tested in several hospitals across the country.

In its current form, the model suggests that, were there to be an unlimited supply of MRI and CT scanners in the United States, aggregate MRI and CT scanning would increase between 1984 and 1986, but would decrease between 1986 and 1990 as MRI more fully substituted for CT in many clinical applications.[13] The model also suggests that in 1986 two thirds of aggregate CT and MR scanning would be accounted for by CT, whereas in 1990 two thirds of aggregate CT and MR scanning would be accounted for by MRI.[12,13] Models of this sort, though useful in estimating likely volumes of use, cannot substitute for clinical trials designed to define the efficacy of MRI compared with other diagnostic modalities and the actual volume of scans or scanners needed to serve a particular population.

Table 56–5. ESTIMATED ANNUALIZED COST OF HIGH-QUALITY X-RAY CT SYSTEM

Capital	
Equipment	$229,500*
Site	45,500–91,000†
Total	$275,000–320,500
Operating	
4000 scans/year	$365,000–379,000‡
5000 scans/year	$468,333–482,333§
Overhead	$ 70,000
TOTAL	
4000 scans/year	$710,000–769,5000‡
5000 scans/year	$793,333–852,833

* Assumes useful life for equipment of 5 years, and 10% interest rate.
† Assumes useful life for site of 5 years and 10% interest rate.
‡ Assumes that personnel work 1.5 shifts.
§ Assumes that personnel work two shifts.

THIRD-PARTY PAYMENT ISSUES

As with any technology, considerations related to the availability of third-party payment are integral to any assessment of the economics of MRI. We will therefore briefly review the status of payment for MRI from various third-party payers.

By June 1984, at least ten commercial insurers were paying for MRI as "generally accepted practice" and at least three Blue Cross plans had approved payment for MRI.[14] In May 1985, the American College of Radiology (ACR) reported that 11 commercial insurers had approved unrestricted coverage of MRI, 14 others had agreed to review claims for MRI on a case-by-case basis, and 5 others had their MRI coverage determination policy under consideration.[15] The ACR also reported that by May 1985 more than a dozen Blue Cross/Blue Shield plans had agreed to provide coverage for designated MRI procedures.[15] By October 1985, 67 private carriers, including several local BC/BS plans, had approved at least some type of coverage for MRI.[16]

Because approximately 40 percent of a hospital's revenues are attributable to Medicare beneficiaries,[17] coverage of MRI by Medicare is critical to the economic viability of almost any hospital's MRI program. As is now well known, in November 1985 the Health Care Financing Administration (HCFA) approved coverage for MRI scans performed on Medicare beneficiaries on or after November 22, 1985. Coverage was limited to MRI units that had received premarket approval by the FDA and to scans that were "reasonable and necessary for the diagnosis or treatment" of specific patients. Coverage was not approved for MRI scans performed on patients with cardiac pacemakers or metallic clips on vascular aneurysms, or for women with a viable pregnancy. Coverage was also not provided for MRI scans that employ gating devices or surface coils, or for paramagnetic contrast materials, although this will probably change when these techniques receive premarket approval from the FDA. MRI scans for measurement of blood flow or spectroscopic analysis were deemed investigational and thus not eligible for coverage.[18]

Overall, the coverage provided by Medicare appears to be quite broad and includes head, thoracic, abdominal, pelvic, and many types of bone studies. Until more is known about how intermediaries will interpret and apply HCFA's guidelines, however, little can be said about specific clinical applications of MRI that are or are not covered by Medicare.

When it approved coverage for MRI, HCFA did not specify an amount that should be paid by intermediaries for an MRI scan. Instead, HCFA advised carriers "to apply their own judgments when making individual reasonable charge determinations for MRI."[18] Although HCFA did provide an estimate of the cost of an MRI scan ($474), which assumed an annual operating cost of $947,000 and a throughput of 2000 scans per year, carriers were instructed not to be bound by HCFA's cost estimates or methodology.[18]

HCFA's coverage approval for MRI is important for several reasons. First, it means that payment will now be made for outpatient MRI scans performed on Medicare beneficiaries. Second, it means that capital costs for MRI scanners now qualify for payment under the current "capital passthrough" mechanism. Third, it means that MRI use and costs will now be considered whenever DRG payment rates are recalibrated. Finally, it provides a strong precedent for coverage of MRI by other insurers.

Under Medicare's DRG-based prospective payment system, hospitals will not receive specially designated payments for the operating costs related to MRI scans performed on Medicare inpatients. Rather, hospitals will receive a predetermined DRG payment rate for each patient regardless of whether an MRI scan (or any other procedure) is performed. During its 1985 and early 1986 meetings, the Prospective Payment Assessment Commission (ProPAC) considered whether to recommend that Medicare make a special payment in addition to the regular DRG payment rate for MRI scans performed on inpatients. Concerned that MRI scanners would increase the cost of patient care (at least in the short run) and that as a result hospitals would be slow to adopt MRI scanning, ProPAC recommended that for a period of three years Medicare should pay a "DRG add-on" for each covered MRI scan performed on an inpatient Medicare beneficiary.[19] ProPAC recommended that in fiscal year 1987 the add-on be set at $124 for each scan performed by the hospital caring for the beneficiary and at $282 for each scan performed at a facility other than that in which the beneficiary is hospitalized.[19] (The latter add-on is set at a higher level to take account of the fact that the capital costs of the latter scan are not paid for in the usual passthrough manner.[19]) Despite ProPAC's recommendation, HCFA officials have predicted that it is unlikely that HCFA will approve such an add-on for MRI, since such a policy would violate many of the cost-containment incentives incorporated into the prospective payment system (PPS).

Two final issues of considerable importance related to Medicare payment for MRI should be mentioned. The first is that, at present, despite the variation in cost of MRI scans performed with different types of magnets, there is no indication that Medicare will vary the amount it pays to providers as a function of the type of scanner (i.e., type of magnet and field strength) used to perform the study. Rather, in an effort to provide an incentive to contain costs, Medicare may set its payment level for MRI scans in a middle range of possible costs, or at a level that reflects the number and cost of the particular MRI scanners that have been installed across the country. Such a policy has incited considerable criticism, particularly from manufacturers of higher-priced systems.

The second issue relates to how Medicare intends to pay for capital costs in the future. Currently, Medicare continues to pay for capital expenses separately from operating costs. The legislation mandating the adoption of PPS by Medicare permitted, for the short term, payment of capital expenses on a cost basis. Thus, even under PPS, hospitals receive reimbursement on a cost basis for equipment and facilities depreciation and interest expenses that are attributable to Medicare patients. This "passthrough" of capital expenses was intended to continue only until a system for incorporating funding for capital expenses into the DRG payment system could be devised.

The Department of Health and Human Services was expected to propose such a system for consideration by the United States Congress by October 1986 but has not yet done so. Several options are being considered. One alternative is to make an additional payment to each hospital equal to 7 percent of its total DRG payment rate. This approach is predicated on the fact that, historically, capital expenses have constituted approximately 7 percent of hospitals' budgets.

A major advantage of this option is that capital payments would be set prospectively, offering predictability to both the payer and the hospital. In addition, it provides hospitals with an incentive to economize in their purchasing and financing decisions, an incentive that was not present under cost-based reimbursement. In addition, a 7 percent capital payment would treat all hospitals equally, reimbursing them for their caseload of Medicare patients rather than their ability to raise capital.

A 7 percent payment, however, is based on the average proportion of hospitals' costs attributable to capital. Thus, hospitals whose capital costs are lower than the average would be overpaid and those whose capital costs are higher than the average would be underpaid under this plan. This option also may be insensitive to hospital-specific factors, such as construction costs and the phase of individual hospitals' capital-acquisition cycles.

A second option being considered is the incorporation into DRG payments of an amount equivalent to the average capital cost per case for a Medicare patient. This amount would be determined using previous years' Medicare data and would be adjusted for inflation and other factors. Debate on this proposal has included discussion of which base year to use in determining the average capital cost per case; which inflation index to use in updating costs; how to define capital; how to structure a "transition period" during which Medicare would gradually adopt this prospective approach and discard use of cost-based reimbursement; and whether or how any adjustments might be made for hospitals' teaching status, geographic location, or area construction costs.

This option, like the one discussed previously, offers predictability to hospitals and to Medicare. In addition, it encourages prudent investment of hospital resources, eliminates the incentive established by cost-based reimbursement to finance capital through debt, and may discourage overinvestment. Also like the option discussed previously, it relies on the use of averages to determine payment rates and may result in overpayment of some providers and underpayment of others.

Another suggested method that could be used to pay for new technologies is a lump-sum capital payment approach. With this approach, a hospital that acquires MRI would receive a payment for the proportion of the cost of the purchase that is attributable to Medicare beneficiaries. This differs from current cost-based reimbursement in that the lump-sum payment would be drawn from a pool of funds set aside for acquisition of technologies. This lump-sum option would be used in conjunction with another method of payment for types of capital other than that for simply new technologies.

One unresolved issue in this method relates to whether funds from the pool will be available to purchase any technologies or only specially designated technologies. The latter would require a determination of which technologies are to be financed through lump-sum payments by Medicare as well as the time period during which lump-sum payments would be available. If funds were available for only a limited period, erratic diffusion patterns could result.

The method that is ultimately adopted could greatly affect hospitals' purchasing decisions. Whatever the outcome of these deliberations, including the possibility that Congress will take no definitive action regarding Medicare payments for hospital capital costs during the 1980s, it is likely that MRI will be competing against other equipment for scarce capital dollars. The effect of this competition on the diffusion of MRI may be offset in part by competition among hospitals for patients. To the extent that owning a magnetic resonance imager enhances an institution's reputation, acquisition of an MR imager may offer a competitive advantage in the local hospital market.

REGULATION

Health Planning

National and state health planning, as it applies to MRI, generally involves regulatory decision-making regarding (1) the overall number of MRI units that are necessary, appropriate, or desirable in a particular geographic area; and (2) the equitable or efficient distribution of these units among individual health care providers. Advocates of health planning bemoan the proclivity of providers to adopt new technology before its efficacy or role in clinical medicine is well defined.[20] Opponents of health planning, on the other hand, complain about the undue restraints and costs imposed by the health planning process, and the general historical failure of health planning programs to assure the equitable distribution of equipment across providers in the United States.[21]

Early on, state health planning agencies adopted one of four strategies with regard to the introduction of MRI: (1) pro forma denial of applications; (2) a formalized strategy of delay in approval of applications; (3) predetermined limits on diffusion; or (4) uncontested approval of applications.[7] In many instances, CON applications for MRI units were denied in an effort to restrain investment in this high-cost technology until more was known about optimal magnet design and strength, and to help health planners learn more about the clinical efficacy of MR imaging from the experiences of early MRI installations. As of April 1984, the last date for which national data were collected, at least 30 CON applications for MR imagers had been denied or deferred in the United States.[22] Nonetheless, hundreds of MRI units had been installed in the United States by the end of 1985 compared with only 140 in the rest of the world. This pattern of diffusion, which is common in the case of high-cost technology, is probably in part a reflection of stronger health planning controls in European and other countries than in the United States.[23]

One effect of health planning in the United States has been an increased tendency to install MRI units in nonregulated outpatient facilities. By the end of 1984, approximately 39 percent of the 108 MRI scanners installed in the United States were located in outpatient facilities—roughly twice the percentage of CT scanners that had been similarly situated at a comparable point in CT's diffusion history.[3] This increased tendency to install MRI units in outpatient settings is undoubtedly due partly to the fact that certificate-of-need laws in the United States tend more to apply to hospital facilities than to physicians' offices or outpatient diagnostic imaging centers.[3] Whether this increased tendency to install MRI units in outpatient facilities will lead to a reduction or an increase in health care costs, or to an increase or decrease in access to and quality of care, remains to be seen.

An increasingly common pattern of distribution and ownership of MRI units, as well as the impact of health planning on that pattern, is well illustrated by the experience with MRI in the Washington, D.C., metropolitan area. This region is commonly defined as the District of Columbia, the Maryland counties of Montgomery and Prince George, and the Virginia counties of Arlington and Fairfax. The area, which has a population of approximately 3.4 million, is served by 37 acute-care hospitals, including five major facilities operated by the federal government. The four military hospitals, Walter Reed Army Medical Center, the National Naval Medical Center, DeWitt Army Hospital, and the Air Force's Malcolm Grow, serve active-duty and retired military personnel and their dependents. The fifth government facility, the Clinical Center of the National Institutes of Health, is a research institution caring exclusively for patients accepted for research protocols.

By the spring of 1986, nine MRI units were operating in the Washington, D.C., area and six others were in some stage of planning or installation (Table 56–6). The location of these units reflects the strength of CON regulation in the relevant areas. The District of Columbia has a relatively strong CON program, which applies both to hospitals and to physicians' offices. The D.C. health planning agency approved three of five CON applications that were submitted by hospitals. (Although Walter Reed is located in the District, it is not subject to CON regulation.) No office-based MRI units have been installed in the District. Only two MRI units, both hospital-based, are located in the Virginia suburbs. Like the District, Virginia has a strong health planning program.

In Maryland, by contrast, CON regulations have never applied to outpatient facilities. Until the spring of 1985, Maryland did have a CON regulatory program that applied to hospitals. Prior to the Maryland legislature's elimination of CON regulation in 1985, the state's health planning commission had approved MRI units only for the two major teaching hospitals in Baltimore (Johns Hopkins and the University of Maryland). While hospital installations were restrained, office-based units proliferated, par-

Table 56—6. MRI INSTALLATIONS IN THE WASHINGTON, D.C., METROPOLITAN AREA: APRIL 1986

Location	Operational	Type of Site
District of Columbia		
Walter Reed Army Medical Center	Yes	Hospital*
Washington Hospital Center/Children's Hospital	No	Hospital
Howard University Hospital	No	Hospital
Georgetown University Hospital	No	Hospital
Montgomery County, Maryland		
NIH Clinical Center	Yes	Hospital*
NIH Clinical Center	No	Hospital*
MRI of Washington	Yes	Office
Grover, Christie and Merritt, P.C.	Yes	Office
Georgetown/Montrose	Yes	Office
Holy Cross/George Washington University	Yes	Mobile (Office/Hospital)
Shady Grove	Yes	Office
Prince Georges County, Maryland		
MRI of P.G. County	Yes	Office
Wener, Boyle & Associates	Yes	Office
Fairfax County, Virginia		
Fairfax Hospital	No	Hospital
Arlington/Alexandria Hospital	No	Hospital

* Exempt from CON regulation.

ticularly in the Maryland suburbs adjacent to Washington, D.C. The first MRI unit to operate in Maryland was located in a freestanding facility operated by the same group of neurologists and neurosurgeons who introduced CT scanning to the D.C. area a decade ago. A second MRI unit in Maryland is owned and operated by a group of radiologists based in the Washington area. Two other Maryland units involve venture capitalists as major partners, with radiologists and clinicians as minor shareholders, while two others are owned by consortia of physicians with radiologists as managing partners. The radiology groups serving George Washington University Hospital in the District and Holy Cross Hospital in suburban Maryland have jointly leased a mobile MRI unit located on the grounds of Holy Cross Hospital. Of further interest is the fact that since CON regulation in Maryland was eliminated in early 1985, six MRI units have been installed in the Baltimore area, in addition to the two at the University of Maryland and Johns Hopkins, and a seventh is operating in Frederick, Maryland, within 30 miles of both Washington, D.C., and Baltimore.

Overall, health planning efforts in the case of MRI have suffered from the absence of well-defined criteria or techniques for estimating either "need" or demand for MRI scans,[24] the rapid rate of change in the quality and number of clinical applications of MRI scanning, and the resourcefulness of providers in installing units in nonregulated settings.

FDA Premarket Approval

Beginning in 1976, the FDA assumed responsibility for ensuring that medical devices are safe and effective before they are marketed. MR imagers are the first imaging devices to have been subjected to the FDA premarket approval (PMA) process. By the end of 1985, 6 of 15 manufacturers worldwide had been granted premarket approval for at least one MRI model (Table 56–7).[25] Although early analyses suggested that the PMA process was not substantially limiting the number of MRI units that were being installed,[7] it seems likely that the FDA PMA process is now having a more substantial

Table 56–7. MRI MANUFACTURERS GRANTED PREMARKET APPROVAL BY FDA:
November 1985

Manufacturer	Type of Unit	Field Strength (Tesla)	Date PMA Granted
Technicare*	Whole body	0.15, 0.3, 0.6	3/29/84
Diasonics	Whole body	0.35	3/29/84
Picker	Head	0.15, 0.26	5/10/84
Fonar	Whole body	0.3	9/26/84
Siemens	Whole body	0.35, 0.5, 0.10	12/14/84
General Electric	Whole body	0.5, 1.0, 1.5	4/25/85

* Now owned by General Electric.
Source: Reference 25.

impact, particularly on individual manufacturers, now that system development and production capabilities are at a more advanced stage. Possession of FDA PMA became even more important in November 1985, when the Health Care Financing Administration approved coverage for MR imaging provided to Medicare beneficiaries only on those machines that had been granted PMA.[18]

Two issues related to the FDA PMA process are likely to receive increasing attention. The first relates to how much information manufacturers must provide to establish the safety and effectiveness of their devices now that over 600 MRI scanners are operating in the United States, and Medicare and other insurers have determined that MRI has advanced to the point where it is worthy of payment on a routine basis. Manufacturers who already have PMA are likely to argue that those who do not yet have such approval should be forced to meet the same standards of proof as had been expected of early PMA recipients. Current and future applicants, on the other hand, are likely to argue that demonstration of certain standards of performance should be sufficient for FDA approval now that the safety and effectiveness of MRI is generally accepted.

The second PMA issue likely to receive increasing attention relates to the type of FDA approval that will be required (and the type of approval process that will be applied) for software improvements and hardware innovations (e.g., surface-coil design and use) by manufacturers who have already been granted PMA. It is unclear whether the FDA has the manpower or inclination to review the large number of MRI innovations that are certain to be made in the coming years.

In an economic and political sense, the introduction of MRI has presented a reprise of the issues that arose a decade ago when CT scanners were introduced. The environment in which MRI has arrived, however, is different in several important respects from that in which CT was introduced. Many forces working to curb health care cost increases have coalesced; Medicare now pays for inpatient care on a prospective rather than cost-based reimbursement basis; there is now an FDA premarket approval process for technologies; and for-profit medical care and physician entrepreneurialism have increased markedly.

Within this new environment, MRI has diffused widely and relatively rapidly, although not as quickly as CT scanners did a decade ago. As was the case with CT, there are many more MRI scanners being installed in the United States than in the rest of the world. Many more of these scanners are being installed outside of hospitals than was the case for CT, however, and increasing numbers of MR imagers are owned by physician investors and entrepreneurs.

The break-even cost of an MRI scan depends on the type of magnet employed and on annual patient throughput. Although the cost of an MRI scan can be two to three times that of a CT scan, an MRI scan is not prohibitively expensive. With reasonable patient throughput, for instance, MRI scans cost less than many types of nuclear scans.

Third-party payment for MRI is becoming more common. This trend will undoubtedly continue. Still unknown is the impact that MRI will have on health care costs, either in aggregate or per hospitalization. It is hoped that, as experience is gained and progress is made in software and surface coils, MRI increasingly will substitute for more invasive technologies and decrease the need for many types of inpatient evaluations.

With regard to health care regulation, MRI presents a formidable challenge to state and local health planners, who still suffer from a poor image gained from their attempts to regulate CT scanners. Whether there is still a role for CON applied to high capital cost medical equipment in the new era of prospective payment may be clarified by the experience with MRI.

Finally, MRI is the first imaging device to be subject to the FDA premarket approval (PMA) process. Acquisition of PMA has become increasingly important to manufacturers now that Medicare has begun paying for MRI scans performed on scanners that have received PMA. Whether PMA will continue to be required for MR imagers or whether it will be replaced by performance standards is unclear. The FDA will undoubtedly take up this issue again, in addition to considering the process through which approval will be provided for software and hardware innovations.

ACKNOWLEDGMENTS

We are grateful to Charlotte Chalmers for technical preparation of the manuscript.

References

1. Steinberg EP: The impact of regulation and payment innovations on acquisition of new imaging technologies. Radiol Clin North Am 23(3):381, 1985.
2. Steinberg EP: Johns Hopkins Hospital. Unpublished data.
3. Steinberg EP, Sisk JE, Locke KE: X-ray CT and magnetic resonance imagers: diffusion patterns and policy issues. N Engl J Med 313(14):859, 1985.
4. Hess TP: MR vendors surrender discounts in battle for market supremacy. Diagn Imag, 9:61, 1987.
5. Biomedical Business International 9(3):23–24, February 11, 1986.
6. Schroeder SA: Magnetic resonance imaging: present costs and potential gains. Ann Intern Med 102:551, 1985.
7. Steinberg EP, Cohen AB: Health Technology Case Study 27: Nuclear Magnetic Resonance Imaging Technology: A Clinical, Industrial, and Policy Analysis. Washington, DC, US Congress, Office of Technology Assessment, OTA-HCS-27, September 1984.
8. American Hospital Association: Hospital Technology Series Guideline Report. NMR-Issues for 1985 and Beyond 4(3/4):1985.
9. Evens RJ, Jost RG, Evens RJ Jr: Economic and utilization analysis of magnetic imaging units in the United States in 1985: AJR 145:393, 1985.
10. Is it now time to acquire magnetic resonance imaging? J Health Care Technol 2(1):23, 1985.
11. Linda Lillybeck, Manager of MR Market Development, General Electric Company: Personal communication, January 1986.
12. Steinberg EP, diMonda R: Projecting MRI utilization: Two new approaches. Hospital Technology Series Guideline Report, Vol. 6, No. 13. Chicago, American Hospital Association, March 1987.
13. Steinberg EP, Anderson GF, Steinwachs D, et al: Financing Magnetic Resonance Imaging in an Era of Prospective Payment: Issues and Options. Report submitted to the Health Industry Manufacturers Association, February 1986.
14. Mobile Technology, Inc: Unpublished data, Los Angeles, June 16, 1984.
15. American College of Radiology: Report of the ACR Commission on MRI. Reston, Virginia, May 1985.
16. Biomedical Business International 8(19/20):191–194, October 10, 1985.
17. Gibson RM, Levit KR, Lazenby H, Waldo DR: National health expenditures, 1983. *In* Health Care Financing Review 6(2):1–29, Winter 1984.
18. Department of Health and Human Services, Health Care Financing Administration, Transmittal No. 1134, November 1985.

19. Technical Appendices to the Report and Recommendations to the Secretary, Department of Health and Human Services (Washington DC, Prospective Payment Assessment Commission, April 1, 1986).

20. Schersten T, Sisk JE: An international view of magnetic resonance imaging and spectroscopy. Introduction. Int J Tech Assess Health Care *1*(3):479, 1985.

21. Pardini AP, Cohodes DR, Cohen AC: Certificate of Need and High Capital Cost Technology: The Case of Computerized Axial Tomographic Scanners, contract No. 231-77-1004. Submitted to the U.S. Department of Health and Human Services, HRA Bureau of Health Planning, Cambridge, MA, 1980.

22. Office of Health Planning: 1984 Summary of nuclear magnetic resonance (NMR) regulations/guidelines/standards and criteria/program positions by states within regions (Program information letter). Washington, DC, Department of Health and Human Services, August 24, 1984.

23. Steinberg EP, Sisk JE, Locke KE: The diffusion of magnetic resonance imagers in the United States and worldwide. An international view of magnetic resonance imaging and spectroscopy. Int J Technol Assess Health Care *1*(3):499, 1985.

24. Steinberg EP: Expert witness providing testimony regarding magnetic resonance imaging utilization projection methodologies before the Maryland Health Resources Planning Commission. Baltimore, December 5, 1984.

25. FDA Announcement: Status of magnetic resonance imaging devices. Food and Drug Administration Center for Devices and Radiologic Health. Silver Spring, Maryland, November 15, 1985.

26. Gaylor R, M.D., Associate Director, Department of Radiology, Johns Hopkins Hospital: Personal communication, 1986.

27. Report of the Council on Medical Services of the American Medical Association: Accepted at the Annual Session of the American Medical Association House of Delegates, Chicago, June 1984.

28. ACR Bulletin, October 1985, p 1.

57

Role and Scope of MRI in Diagnostic Medicine

R. E. STEINER

Worldwide clinical experience with magnetic resonance imaging is now sufficiently advanced to provide adequate data for a critical look at its present impact on diagnostic radiology and also to look at its future potential. Our own clinical experience in the NMR Unit at Hammersmith Hospital started in March 1981, when a prototype Picker cryogenic 0.15 tesla scanner operating at 6.4 MHz was installed; its technical performance has been described previously.[1]

Before MRI can be accepted as an established imaging modality, some definitive criteria must be laid down and some important questions answered. Firstly, is the information provided by MRI already so incisive that the technique can be used as a primary method of investigation? Secondly, is the technique better than other noninvasive well-established imaging methods? Thirdly, has MRI already influenced patient management and care to a significant degree? In the investigation of some neurologic disorders MRI has already fulfilled some of these criteria, a comment supported in a number of other chapters.

IMAGE QUALITY AND INTERPRETATION

It is already established that contrast resolution of MRI is superior to that of CT. On the other hand, spatial resolution with modern CT equipment still appears to be better in some parts of the body than that obtained by MRI. In the central nervous system, however, contrast and spatial resolution has already achieved a high level and in some areas surpasses that of CT.[2-4] The absence of motion and bone artifacts together with the small imaging volume is partly responsible for this. In the thorax and abdomen these facts do not apply; in the pelvis[5-8] and the limbs,[9,10] however, cardiac and respiratory motion artifacts present no problems, so that MRI is already approaching the diagnostic capability of CT. As far as specificity is concerned, both MRI and CT are equally disappointing. There are many areas of general pathology where the diagnosis is still unsatisfactory, as for example in liver[11-13] and renal disorders,[14,15] such as the various types of cirrhosis or nephritis.

Absolute numbers of $T1$ and $T2$ relaxation times can be obtained from normal and abnormal tissues, but the variability of these numbers among medical centers is still considerable. These differences depend on many factors[16]—the type of scanner, the sequences used, repeatability of measurements, and sampling errors. To this one must add a significant overlap of the $T1$ and $T2$ values between some normal and pathologic tissues in various organs; good examples are, again, diffuse liver and kidney diseases.[11,14] The final choice of optimum sequences has not yet been established; those used for the central nervous system are not necessarily ideal for body imaging in view of their sensitivity to motion artifacts. For this reason alternative sequences, which will be discussed later, will have to be considered.

Imaging in different planes is more readily achieved with MRI than with CT, which is a further great advantage in midline structures of the brain, brainstem, craniocervical junction, and neural canal.[17-19] In imaging of the mediastinum,[20,21] the heart,[22] and some abdominal and pelvic organs,[5-8] the multiplanar capability can also have some advantages. The availability of multiple sequences that are capable of demonstrating different types of pathology makes MRI more flexible and sensitive than CT. It is fully appreciated that the selection of these sequences is very much a problem and is dependent on the underlying pathology as well as on the type of scanner. Sufficient experience now has been acquired in many centers to develop definitive imaging strategies for specific disease processes, taking account of all the points raised.

MRI OF THE CENTRAL NERVOUS SYSTEM

Compared with CT the important advantages of MRI are (1) high level of gray–white matter contrast; (2) absence of bone artifact; (3) variety of sequences that are sensitive to pathologic change; and (4) absence of known hazard.

In some types of neurologic disease MRI has definitely established its diagnostic capability, as, for example, in the demonstration of white matter disorders and lesions in the posterior fossa, the craniocervical junction, and the spinal cord, where intra-axial and extra-axial lesions are well visualized. The application of surface coils has contributed considerably to the image quality of the neural canal and its contents.[23] In the investigation of pathology in the posterior fossa[24,25] and the spinal cord,[19,26] the absence of bone artifact gives MRI a significant advantage over CT. By contrast, the inability to demonstrate calcification or cortical bone directly by MRI is a definite disadvantage compared with CT.

The absence of known hazards has made MRI particularly suitable for the investigation of neurologic disorders in pediatrics,[27] quite apart from its ability to demonstrate progressive myelination as well as gray and white matter pathology very clearly. One would not hesitate to repeat examinations with MRI for follow-up purposes to monitor treatment and disease progress.

In other areas of pathology the efficacy of MRI is still not fully established, as, for instance, in cerebral vascular disease, infarction, and hemorrhage. The same applies in cerebral tumors when MRI is used without paramagnetic contrast medium, where separation of a mass lesion from surrounding edema may be very difficult.[28]

PARAMAGNETIC CONTRAST MEDIA

Although the value of intravenous or oral paramagnetic contrast media in MRI has not been fully established, one fact has definitely emerged. When gadolinium-DTPA is administered intravenously, it selectively crosses the diseased blood-brain barrier. By reducing the relaxation time of the tumor and highlighting it, the unaffected surrounding edema is clearly separated.[28,29] In gliomas of the brain the reduction of relaxation time by paramagnetic contrast, such as Gd-DTPA, is greater with IR than with SE sequences[28]; the same has been observed in meningiomas.[30] Although experience with paramagnetic contrast media in neurologic disorders is still limited, results so far suggest a place for its use in the future. A great deal more experimental and clinical work will have to be done before definitive answers become available.

There are a number of disadvantages of MRI compared with CT in imaging some neurologic disorders. There is the inability to demonstrate calcification. Patient throughput is slower than with CT. There still remains the problem of investigating the very sick patient on a life-support system. Finally, the higher cost of MRI equipment is a significant disadvantage in the general hospital setting. This, together with some of the other points mentioned, makes MRI not yet really suitable as a screening technique.

MRI OF THE BODY

The indications for MRI as a primary imaging technique for the body are still limited for a number of reasons. To be acceptable as an established clinical and universal imaging technique, magnetic resonance must be at least as good as, or even better than, the other well-established noninvasive techniques, such as ultrasound and CT. Only then can one truly justify the high initial costs of equipment, installation, and operation.

Experience to date is adequate to suggest, however, that in some areas of body imaging the results are more than encouraging. For example, images of the pelvis and limbs can be of excellent quality owing to the absence of motion artifacts[5,6]; in the thorax, good images of the heart, mediastinum, and pulmonary hila can be obtained; and adequate images of the liver, kidney, and retroperitoneal space can be produced. The important questions still remain unanswered, however. Are these images providing better and new information that is unobtainable by the established techniques, which at present are faster and cheaper from a patient management point of view? There is a further question that must be asked: Is there any additional information magnetic resonance can provide that is not obtainable by other techniques? Some progress has been made in combining in vivo spectroscopy and imaging.[31,32] It is also possible to image sodium,[33] and some advances have been made in quantifying blood flow.[34–37]

Paramagnetic Contrast Studies

The use of contrast media in abdominal organs in man is still limited. Some experience has been gained at Hammersmith Hospital in a number of patients with primary and secondary mass lesions of the liver. In our experience so far, hepatic masses in most instances become isodense with surrounding normal liver tissue following the administration of Gd-DTPA (Fig. 57–1). Subtraction of pre- and postcontrast images

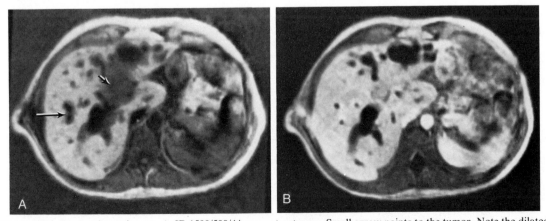

Figure 57–1. Cholangiocarcinoma. *A*, IR 1500/500/44 precontrast scan. Small arrow points to the tumor. Note the dilated bile ducts in portal veins (large arrow). *B*, Following the administration of gadolinium-DTPA the tumor appears isointense with the normal liver. Some of the dilated vascular structures are no longer visible (note the one indicated by the large arrow in *A*). Portal venous branches are now isointense with the liver, and only the dilated bile ducts are still visible in black. Note signal from the aorta and vena cava and the differences in signal from the spleen and left kidney due to contrast.

can overcome this problem by highlighting the contrast-enhanced pathologic areas within the liver.

It is also possible following contrast injection to separate the bile ducts from portal veins. The bile ducts do not emit a signal and remain black, whereas the portal veins do emit a signal and in most instances become isodense with normal liver tissue (Fig. 57–1). Gadolinium-DTPA has also been used in other types of pathology in the abdomen and retroperitoneal space, but experience is too limited to draw any definite conclusions as yet.

POSSIBLE FUTURE DEVELOPMENTS

Contrast and spatial resolution for inversion-recovery and spin-echo sequences can be improved with high-resolution scans. Furthermore, the development of a 512 × 512 matrix may provide some additional improvement, and so will a reduction in slice thickness, preferably down to 2 to 3 mm. This will be of particular advantage in the head for midline lesions or very small structures, such as the pituitary fossa, cranial nerves, and spinal outlet foramina.

Motion artifacts are important problems when imaging the thorax or the abdomen. ECG gating has already been established and taken care of cardiac motion, of considerable help when imaging the heart and mediastinum[38–40] The problem of respiratory motion artifact has not yet been solved. The standard technique of respiratory gating imposes a major time penalty.[40] However, an alternative method of respiratory ordered phase encoding (ROPE) overcomes the problem by controlling the respiratory artifact

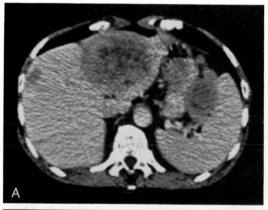

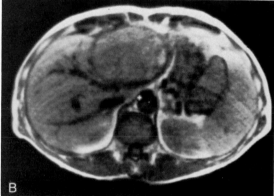

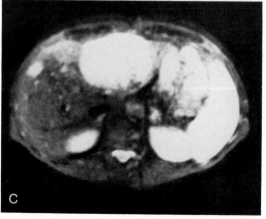

Figure 57–2. Metastases from a primary carcinoma of the colon. *A*, CT scan demonstrating two areas of abnormal attenuation, one involving the greater part of the left lobe, and the other the margin of the right lobe. *B*, Spin-echo scan 544/44. Only the large metastatic deposit is outlined, the smaller marginal one being invisible. Note respiratory motion artifacts (small central white cross is a central artifact). *C*, STIR sequence 1500/100/44. The metastatic deposits are now highlighted. There are also some parenchymal changes visible in the right and the remaining left lobe of the liver. Fluid in the gut is highlighted as well as the spleen and the kidneys.

to some extent.[41] Once motion artifacts have been eliminated, image quality of the chest and abdomen will improve significantly.

New Sequences

The application of new sequences that are less motion-dependent and also highlight specific pathology will represent a further advance in imaging technique. A good example is the short $T1$ inversion-recovery (STIR) sequence (TR 1500/100/44), which suppresses fat.[42] In fat-containing organs such as the liver, where there are significant imaging problems, this sequence can be of considerable value. For instance, ghost artifacts from anterior abdominal wall fat are frequently present in the phase-encoded direction (Fig. 57–2). The short $T2$ of the liver means that medium $T1$ inversion-recovery sequences become relatively more $T2$ dependent and therefore suffer a loss of contrast. Intra-abdominal fat has a long $T2$ and may therefore simulate long $T2$ lesions when spin-echo sequences are used. Furthermore, respiratory motion produces a loss of contrast with long TE, long TR sequences. The STIR sequence to some extent overcomes these problems by suppressing the signal from fat. After the 90 degree pulse it makes the $T1$ and $T2$ dependent contrast additive. When combined with ROPE it also provides a reasonable control of respiratory artifacts (Figs. 57–3 and 57–4).

The use of the STIR sequence also can be of help when imaging other regions of the body containing a great deal of fat, such as the orbit, bone marrow, the retroperitoneum, and the pelvis, where tumor spread may be difficult to detect and where the STIR sequence will highlight pathology (Figs. 57–5 and 57–6). Similarly, chemical-shift

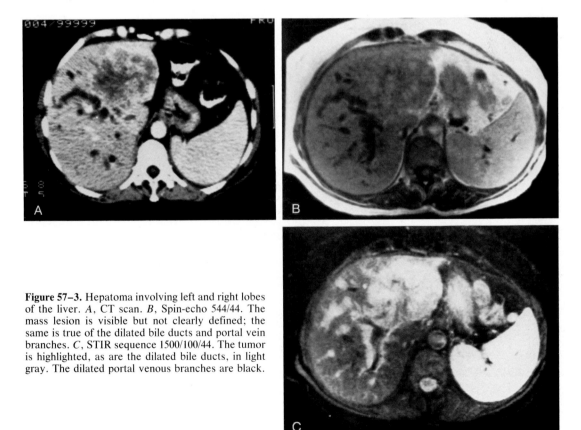

Figure 57–3. Hepatoma involving left and right lobes of the liver. *A*, CT scan. *B*, Spin-echo 544/44. The mass lesion is visible but not clearly defined; the same is true of the dilated bile ducts and portal vein branches. *C*, STIR sequence 1500/100/44. The tumor is highlighted, as are the dilated bile ducts, in light gray. The dilated portal venous branches are black.

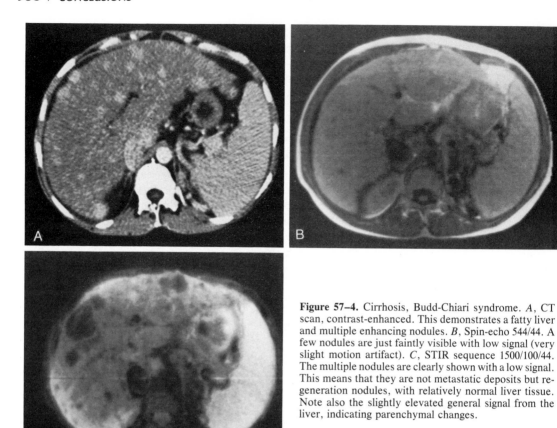

Figure 57–4. Cirrhosis, Budd-Chiari syndrome. *A*, CT scan, contrast-enhanced. This demonstrates a fatty liver and multiple enhancing nodules. *B*, Spin-echo 544/44. A few nodules are just faintly visible with low signal (very slight motion artifact). *C*, STIR sequence 1500/100/44. The multiple nodules are clearly shown with a low signal. This means that they are not metastatic deposits but regeneration nodules, with relatively normal liver tissue. Note also the slightly elevated general signal from the liver, indicating parenchymal changes.

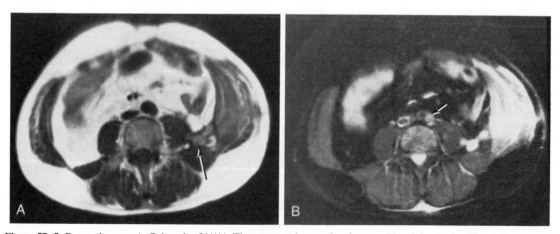

Figure 57–5. Psoas abscess. *A*, Spin-echo 544/44. The arrow points to the abscess. The abdominal wall and iliac muscle adjacent to the abscess are swollen; some of the muscle groups are separated by fluid. *B*, STIR sequence 1500/100/44. The psoas abscess is highlighted and so is the fluid in the region of the swollen abdominal muscle. Some fluid can also be seen subcutaneously posteriorly with a high signal. Slow-flowing blood in some of the lumbar veins gives a signal. Small arrow points to a small swollen para-aortic lymph node (not seen on *A*).

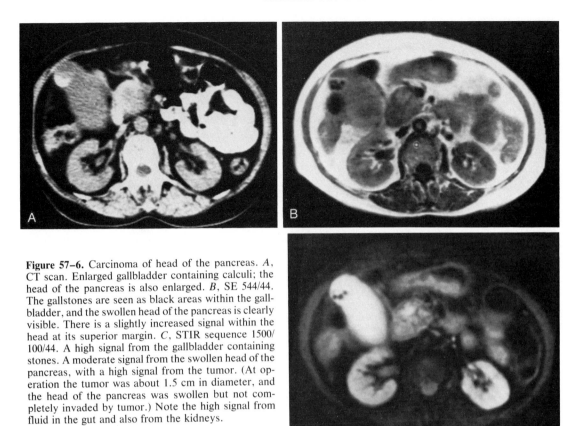

Figure 57–6. Carcinoma of head of the pancreas. *A,* CT scan. Enlarged gallbladder containing calculi; the head of the pancreas is also enlarged. *B,* SE 544/44. The gallstones are seen as black areas within the gallbladder, and the swollen head of the pancreas is clearly visible. There is a slightly increased signal within the head at its superior margin. *C,* STIR sequence 1500/100/44. A high signal from the gallbladder containing stones. A moderate signal from the swollen head of the pancreas, with a high signal from the tumor. (At operation the tumor was about 1.5 cm in diameter, and the head of the pancreas was swollen but not completely invaded by tumor.) Note the high signal from fluid in the gut and also from the kidneys.

imaging can be used to separate lipid and water or to cancel the signal from both. Using this approach a qualitative estimate of the lipid or water content of the tissue can be achieved (Figs. 57–7 to 57–10).[42–44]

An improvement of spatial resolution can also be obtained by specially designed rf coils helping to collect more signal.[4] Surface coils have already been developed and are used widely for imaging of the orbit, the petrous bone, the neural canal, and the breast. Close coupled body receiver coils for head, thorax, abdomen, and limb imaging are also already well advanced in their development.[23]

The further question that will be resolved in time is the choice of an optimum field strength for MRI.[45] There is no doubt that satisfactory images can be obtained at low magnetic fields of 0.08 to 0.5 tesla and similarly with high fields of 1.0 to 1.5 tesla. Therefore, if imaging is the primary clinical indication, a low field will be satisfactory, thus reducing the price of the scanner as well as installation and running costs. If, on the other hand, spectroscopy is the main clinical requirement, a high-field scanner of 1.5 to 2.0 tesla is necessary. There is not yet sufficient worldwide experience to decide whether a multipurpose scanner for imaging and spectroscopy is the ideal solution. This is an important question, since the answer will affect patient throughput, staffing requirements, and, above all, costs. Ultimately, two systems, one for imaging and one for spectroscopy, may be the optimum solution. There is also a considerable difference in the type of equipment required for routine clinical work in the general hospital and for research purposes.

Once all the technical advances discussed have been achieved, MRI will become fully competitive with CT as a whole-body imaging technique. But one must not forget

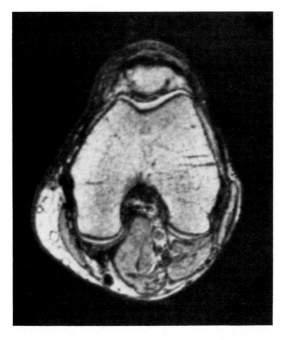

Figure 57–7. Normal lower end of the femur, including the knee joint. Chemical-shift image, partial saturation recovery 500/22. Cartilage is clearly demonstrated, separated from bone by a black line representing cortical bone. Some of the wider trabeculae in the lower end of the femur are highlighted against the high signal from fatty marrow. Note the cancellation lines between muscle groups in the posterior aspects of the knee joint and the different flow effects in the different vascular structures.

other noninvasive imaging modalities such as real-time ultrasound, which is still the primary method of investigation in obstetrics, in some areas of cardiology, and in liver and kidney diseases. Since it is the quickest and cheapest method of study, it can also be used as a simple screening technique. The same applies to dynamic and metabolic studies using isotope techniques, although spectroscopy may supersede this method in some areas once its clinical application has been established. In vivo spectroscopy in man is still in an experimental stage. This no longer applies to magnetic resonance imaging.

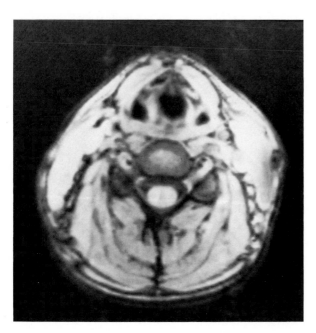

Figure 57–8. Transverse section of the neck at C3 level. Chemical-shift image, partial saturation recovery 500/22. The nucleus and anulus have different densities. Anterior and posterior nerve roots arising from the cord are displayed. Note the cancellation lines between the different structures in the laryngeal region and muscle groups of the neck.

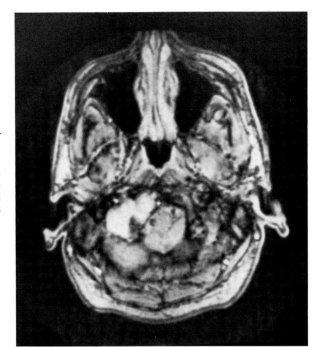

Figure 57–9. Glomus jugulare tumor at the base of the skull. Chemical-shift image, partial saturation recovery 500/22. The tumor is clearly demonstrated, with a high signal displacing the medulla and also the cerebellum. Note the cancellation lines between the various anatomic structures in the facial region and posteriorly in the neck. Note also the varying signals from blood vessels.

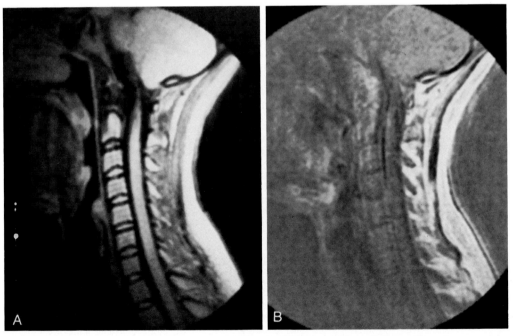

Figure 57–10. Chronic myeloid leukemia. Chemical shift imaging. Dixon technique.[44] Symmetric and asymmetric spin-echo scans 1044/44. *A,* The water component image shows no significant change in signals. *B,* The lipid component image shows no signal from the cervical vertebrae, which are now virtually isointense with brain structures and therefore indicate a low lipid content. This is compatible with the more cellular leukemic marrow.

References

1. Young IR, Burl M, Clarke GJ, et al: Magnetic resonance properties of H_2: imaging the posterior fossa. AJR 137:895, 1981; AJNR 2:487, 1981.
2. Bydder GM: Nuclear magnetic resonance imaging of the brain. Br Med Bull 40(2):170, 1984.
3. Young IR: Considerations affecting signal and contrast in NMR imaging. Br Med Bull 40(2):139, 1984.
4. Curati WL, Graif M, Kingsley DPE, Niendorf HP, Young IR: Acoustic neuromas: Gd-DTPA enhancement in MR imaging, Radiology 158:447, 1986.
5. Hricak H, Williams RD, Spring JB, et al: Anatomy and pathology of the male pelvis as imaged by magnetic resonance. AJR 141:1101, 1983.
6. Hricak H, Alpers C, Crooks LE, Sheldon PE: Magnetic resonance imaging of the female pelvis: initial experience. AJR 141:1119, 1983.
7. Bryan PJ, Butler HE, LiPuma JP: Magnetic resonance imaging of the pelvis. Radiol Clin North Am 22(4):897, 1984.
8. Hricak H: NMR imaging of the retroperitoneum and pelvis. Br Med Bull 40(2):197, 1984.
9. Brady TJ, Rosen BM, Pykett IL, McGuire MH, Makin HG, Rosenthal DI: NMR imaging of leg tumors. Radiology 149:181, 1983.
10. Scott JA, Rosenthal DI, Brady TJ: The evaluation of muscular skeletal disease with magnetic resonance imaging. Radiol Clin North Am 22(4):917, 1984.
11. Doyle FH, Pennock JM, Banks LM, et al: Nuclear magnetic resonance imaging of the liver. AJR 138:193, 1982.
12. Stark DD, Goldberg HI, Moss AA, Bass NM: Chronic liver disease: evaluation by magnetic resonance. Radiology 150:149, 1984.
13. Haaga JR: Magnetic resonance imaging of the liver. Radiol Clin North Am 22:879, 1984.
14. Leung AW, Bydder GM, Steiner RE, Bryant DJ, Young IR: NMR of the kidney. AJR 143:1215, 1984.
15. LiPuma JP: Magnetic resonance imaging of the kidney. Radiol Clin North Am 22(4):925, 1984.
16. Bradley WJ Jr: Notes and impressions from meetings. Third annual meeting of Society of Magnetic Resonance in Medicine. J Comput Assist Tomogr 9(1):220, 1985.
17. Flannigan RB, Bradley WG, Mazziotta JC, et al: MRI of internal brain stem anatomy with clinical correlation. In Scientific Program, Society of Magnetic Resonance in Medicine. Abstracts, 1984, pp 231–232.
18. Han JS, Bonstelle TE, Kaufman B, et al: Magnetic resonance imaging in the evaluation of the brainstem. Radiology 150:705, 1984.
19. Han JS, Benson JE, Yoon YS: Magnetic resonance imaging in the spinal column and craniovertebral junction. Radiol Clin North Am 22(4):805, 1984.
20. Gamsu G, Webb RW, Sheldon P, et al: Nuclear magnetic resonance imaging of the thorax. Radiology 147:473, 1983.
21. Cohen AM: Magnetic resonance imaging of the thorax. Radiol Clin North Am 22(4):829, 1984.
22. Dinsmore RE, Wisman GL, Levine RA, Obada RD, Brady TJ: Magnetic resonance imaging of the heart: positioning and gradient angle selection for optimal imaging places. AJR 143:1142, 1984.
23. Bydder GM, Curati WL, Gadian DG, et al: Use of closely coupled receiver coils in MR imaging. Practical aspects. J Comput Assist Tomogr 9:987, 1985.
24. Bydder GM, Steiner RE, Thomas DJ, Marshall J, Gilderdale DY, Young IR: NMR imaging of the posterior fossa: 50 cases. Clin Radiol 34:173, 1983.
25. Randell CP, Collins AG, Young IR, et al: Nuclear magnetic resonance (NMR) imaging of posterior fossa tumours. AJR 141(3):489, 1983.
26. Modic MT, Weinstein MA, Pavlicek W, et al: Nuclear magnetic resonance imaging of the spine. Radiology 148:757, 1983.
27. Johnson MA, Bydder GM: NMR imaging of the brain in children. Br Med Bull 40(2):175, 1984.
28. Graif M, Bydder GM, Steiner RE, et al: Contrast enhanced MRI of malignant brain tumours. AJNR. 6:855, 1985.
29. Carr DH, Brown J, Bydder GM, et al: Intravenous chelated gadolinium as a contrast agent in NMR imaging of cerebral tumours. Lancet 1:484, 1984.
30. Bydder GM, Kingsley DPE, Brown J, Niendorf HP, Young IR: MR Imaging of meningiomas including studies with and without gadolinium DTPA. J Comput Assist Tomogr 9(4):690, 1985.
31. Radda GR, Bore PJ, Rajagopalan B: Clinical aspects of 31P NMR spectroscopy. Br Med Bull 40(2):155, 1984.
32. Bottomley PA, Hart HR Jr, Edelstein WA, et al: Anatomy and metabolism of the normal human brain studied by magnetic resonance at 1.5T. Radiology 150:441, 1984.
33. Hilal SK, Maudsley AA, Simon HE, et al: In vivo NMR imaging of the tissue sodium in the intact cat before and after acute cerebral stroke. AJNR 4:245, 1983.
34. Crooks LE, Kaufman L: NMR imaging of blood flow. Br Med Bull 40(2):167, 1984.
35. Bryant DJ, Payne JA, Firmin D, Longmore DM: Measurement of flow with NMR imaging using a gradient pulse and phase difference technique. J Comput Assist Tomogr 8(4):588, 1984.
36. Bradley WG, Waluch V, Lai KS, Fernandez EJ, Spalter C: Magnetic resonance appearances of rapidly flowing blood. AJR 143:1167, 1984.
37. Bradley WG, Waluch V: Blood flow: magnetic resonance imaging. Radiology 154:443, 1985.
38. Lanzer P, Botvinik EH, Schiller NB, et al: Cardiac imaging using gated magnetic resonance. Radiology 150:121, 1984.

39. Fletcher BD, Jacobstein MD, Melrose AD, Riemeschneider TA, Alfidi RJ: Gated magnetic resonance imaging of congenital cardiac malformations. Radiology *1150*:137, 1984.
40. Lieberman JM, Alfidi RJ, Nelson AD, et al: Gated magnetic resonance imaging of the normal and diseased heart. Radiology 152:465, 1984.
41. Bailes DR, Gilderdale DJ, Bydder GM, Collins AG, Firmin DN: Respiratory ordered phase encoding (ROPE) a method of reducing respiratory motion artefact in magnetic resonance imaging. J Comput Assist Tomogr 9(4):435, 1985.
42. Bydder GM, Young IR: MR Imaging: Clinical use of the inversion recovery sequence. J Comput Assist Tomogr 9(4):659, 1985.
43. Pykett IL, Rosen BR: Nuclear magnetic resonance: in vivo proton chemical shift imaging. Radiology *149*:197, 1983.
44. Dixon WT: Simple proton spectroscopy imaging. Radiology *153*:189, 1984.
45. Chen CN, Sark VJ, Hoult DI: Probing image frequency dependence. *In* Program and Abstracts, Society of Magnetic Resonance in Medicine. Third Annual Meeting, August 1984, pp 148–152.

58

Future Directions

C. LEON PARTAIN
WILLIAM G. BRADLEY
LEON AXEL
JAMES A. PATTON

In the early years of MRI, many investigators felt that new developments probably would come more slowly and be less dramatic than the rapid acceleration of generations 1 through 4 in x-ray computed tomography. However, the opposite seems to be true. New developments and advances seem to be announced almost monthly. The purpose of the final chapter of Volume I is to summarize the more significant of those technical innovations that, at the time of publication, are in various stages of development.

MRI "Fluoroscopy." The concept of fluoroscopic imaging was recently illustrated[1] utilizing the kinetic display of the temporomandibular joint (TMJ) in multiple graduated positions from opened to closed. The technique utilizes a variable position mouthpiece that can be advanced by the patient at the proper timing sequence for each data collection period. The results may be viewed in a cine-format demonstrating the movement of the TMJ articular surfaces and facilitating assessment of the condylar disc. Logical extensions of this technique soon will include sagittal images of the cervical spine in varying positions from flexion to extension, coronally viewed shoulder images in varying positions from internal to external rotations, coronal views of the hip in anterior and frog-leg positions, and multiplanar dynamic images of the knee in positions varying from flexion to extension. See TMJ MRI illustrated in Chapter 19.

MRI Angiography. Very recent developments taking advantage of flow-related enhancement phenomena[2,3] and fast scan techniques (see Chapters 36 and 96) now allow the three-dimensional and rotational imaging of vascular branches, either arterial or venous. Impressive examples include the carotid and vertebral arteries,[4] the intracerebral arteries,[5] the mediastinal vessels,[6] the abdominal and pelvic vessels,[7] and the popliteal artery together with its distal branches.[8] MRI coronary artery visualization presents a special challenge owing to the multiple axes of rotation and movement. Currently, only visualization of the more proximal coronary arteries is possible with MRI angiography.[9] Further creative development is required in order for MRI angiography to have a significant impact in coronary arteriography.

MRI Flow and Perfusion Measurement. Numerous centers currently are applying MRI techniques to the noninvasive measurement of intravascular flow.[9,10] This capability for in vivo flow measurement in large and moderate-sized vessels is anticipated to be a routine capability within the next year (see Chapters 36 and 98). In addition to intravascular flow measurement, the phenomenon of organ and tissue perfusion may be observed and quantitated using MRI techniques.[11]

MRI Dynamic Cardiac Cine. Cine-mode, thin-section, multiplanar, tomographic imaging allows kinetic, quantitative visualization of cardiac pathophysiology, including congenital and developmental cardiac defects.[12] Included are the measurement of functional indices, such as ejection fraction and wall-motion,[13] and assessment of the functional results of myocardial ischemia and infarction[14] (see also Chapters 23 to 25). Further developments are likely to combine MRI cardiac cine with MRI angiography of the coronary arteries in order to assess myocardial function noninvasively.

MRI Contrast Development and New Applications. Intravenous and oral contrast agents are under development in numerous laboratories (see Chapters 46 to 52). The hope of increased diagnostic sensitivity and specificity using these agents seems realized to some extent in work accomplished to date.[15] Further development in the area of dynamic contrast-enhanced MRI is expected to provide a mechanism to evaluate a growing list of MRI contrast pharmaceuticals, which may allow organ-specific and pathology-specific enhancement for MRI investigations[16,17] (see Chapter 52).

MRI Fast Scan, Under 1 Minute. Various approaches to fast scan techniques using gradient echoes and partial flip-angle techniques[18-20] allow 3D data collection in a reasonable time period. There also is the capability for dynamic, very thin sections (under 2 mm) and adequate signal-to-noise for high-quality anatomic evaluation. In addition, breath-holding techniques[21] provide improved (CT quality) imaging of most of the abdomen without the time-consuming necessity of respiratory gating.

MRI Ultrafast Scan, Under 1 Second. MRI scans in the millisecond range have been demonstrated in laboratory animals and in a few pediatric applications in vivo.[22,23] Image quality currently remains very limited.

In Vivo Multinuclear NMR Spectroscopy. Practical, clinically useful NMR spectroscopy will offer the capability of quantitative substrate metabolism studies by allowing evaluation, for multiple nuclei, of the distribution and pharmacokinetics of numerous compounds that contain, or may be labeled with, the magnetically and biomedically interesting isotopes of H-1, C-13, F-19, Na-23, and P-31 (see Chapters 88 to 95). Several nontrivial challenges currently need engineering solutions. Not the least of these are precise localization of NMR spectra, magnetic field uniformity, and anatomic registration and correlation with H-1 MRI imaging.[24,25]

MRI Guided/Assisted Interventional Diagnosis and Therapy. The potential exists for MRI to be utilized in interventional procedures in a fashion parallel to CT and ultrasound-guided biopsies, drainage, and retrieval procedures. This assumes that adequate nonmagnetic needles and surgical tools are available. The capability must be balanced against the time required for these procedures, since in most medical centers there is an increasing demand for MR scanning for diagnostic purposes. One apparent alternative is to provide stereotactic data automatically in the operating room in a form that is accurate, reliable, and compatible with correlative studies from CT, PET, ultrasound, and DSA. All these forms of computer-based, digital data are, in principle, compatible, archivable, and retrievable[26] (see Chapter 79).

MRI, One Node of a Comprehensive Picture Archiving and Communication System (PACS). Medical centers all over the world are becoming acutely aware of the need for automatic transmission and storage of medical imaging data. The problems inherent in reporting and filing this type of data are exacerbated by volume and demand. On the one hand, there are increasing numbers and varieties of "high-technology" imaging modalities. On the other hand, the quantity of imaging procedures per unit time is accelerating. The amount of resultant data places maximum stress upon postprocessing and storage requirements at most medical centers. Timely and high-quality transmission may become problematic. The possibility of collecting, transmitting, archiving, and retrieving these data is available through the technology of a PAC system. However, there is significant cost associated with PACS. Unfortunately, funding mechanisms are difficult to develop because of the typical absence of incremental income to pay the bill for these needed systems (see Chapter 79).

Conclusion. Although many MRI practitioners predicted a slower pace, as compared with x-ray CT, in the realization of new generations of MRI and NMR-S, the opposite has occurred. This explosion of technological innovation has further complicated the attempts to identify and interpret the proper role and scope of MRI applications and correlative imaging. Our social system is increasingly complex. Those who help define high-quality and affordable health care include interested parties beyond the patient and the physician. The "best available technology" must stand the scrutiny of government regulations, economic constraints, medicolegal concerns, and the distribution of biotechnology. Third-party payers are interested in alternative procedures—those that are equivalent and those that are adequate. Decisions about the mode or timing of health care delivery, specifically with regard to imaging procedures, are constrained by the limited knowledge and sometimes competing objectives of those who are part of the process. Therefore, it is essential that medical imaging professionals (basic scientists and clinicians) adequately evaluate the capability, limitations, and clinical role of each technical development. These evaluations then may be used to educate the referring physicians, the lay public, and the health care system of management in the successful utilization of these diagnostic modalities (see Chapters 53 to 57).

References

1. Anderson QN, Katzberg RW, Helms CA: Current developments in imaging of the temporomandibular joint. Radiology *161*(P):172, 1986.
2. Fellmeth BD, Price RR, Ertzner TW, Stein S, Sandler MP: Peripheral Vascular Imaging. *In* Sandler MP, Patton JA, Shaff MI, Powers TA, and Partain CL (eds): Nuclear Medicine, Magnetic Resonance and Correlative Imaging Modalities. Baltimore, Williams & Wilkins, 1988.
3. Axel L: Review: Blood flow effects in magnetic resonance imaging. Am J Roentgenol *143*:1157, 1984.
4. Dumouliu CL, Hart JR Jr.: MR angiography. Society of Magnetic Resonance in Medicine. Montreal Book of Abstracts, August 1986, pp 1095–1096.
5. Dumouliu CL, Souza SP, Feng H: Multi-echo magnetic resonance angiography. Magn Reson Med *5*:147, 1987.
6. Sommerhoff BA, Sechtem UP, Schiller NB, Higgins CB: MR imaging of the thoracic aorta in patients with Marfan syndrome. Radiology *161*(P):137, 1986.
7. Karstaedt N, Markisz JA: MR imaging of the abdomen and pelvis. Radiology *161*(P):260, 1986.
8. Jaffe RB, Soulen RL: Advances in noninvasive evaluation of congenital heart and great vessel disease: roles of Doppler echocardiography and MR imaging. Radiology *161*(P):171, 1986.
9. Price RR, Pickens DR, Smith G, Patton JA, Wolfe O, Partain CL, James AE: Blood flow effects in MR imaging. Radiology *161*(P):374, 1986.
10. Axel L, Morton D: MR imaging of arterial blood flow by saturation washout. Radiology *161*(P):152, 1986.
11. Feinberg DA, Mark AS: Tissue blood perfusion measurements by two-dimensional Fourier transform velocity MR imaging. Radiology *161*(P):152, 1986.
12. Feiglin DHI, Moodie DS, Gill CC, Sterba R, O'Donnell JK, Go RT, MacIntyre WJ: Cine-MR imaging in the evaluation of preoperative and postoperative patients with congenital heart disease. Radiology *161*(P):198, 1986.
13. Utz JA, Herfkens R, Glover GH, Pelc NJ: Dynamic MR imaging of the heart. Radiology *161*(P):185, 1986.
14. Pflugfelder P, White RD, Sechtem U, Gould RG, Higgins CB: Cine MR imaging assessment of regional left ventricular systolic wall thickening in patients with remote myocardial infarction. Radiology *161*(P):338, 1986.
15. Runge VM, Clausson C, Felix R, James AE: Contrast Agents in MRI. Amsterdam, Excerpta Medica, 1986.
16. Iio M, Yoshikawa K, Ohotomo K, Uashiro N, Okada Y, Ito M, Nishikawa J: Dynamic magnetic resonance imaging with Gd-DTPA. *In* Runge VM, Clausson C, Felix R, James AE (eds). Contrast Agents in MRI. Amsterdam, Excerpta Medica, 1986, pp 183–185.
17. Partain CL, Clanton JA, McCurdy MW, Ashbaugh TJ, Holburn GE: Dynamic, contrast-enhanced MR imaging: A sensitive measure of liver toxicity to azo dye. Radiology *161*(P):315, 1986.
18. Runge VM, Kirsch JE, Wood ML: "FAST" imaging techniques and other motion reduction schemes. Radiology *161*(P):375, 1986.
19. Zeitler E, Barfuss H: Functional analysis of the heart with fast imaging with steady precession (FISP) in patients with congenital and acquired heart disease. Radiology *161*(P):400, 1986.

20. Hanicke W, Merboldt, KD, Frahm J: Rapid T1 imaging using FLASH MR images. Radiology *161*(P):333, 1986.
21. Glazer HS, Cohen AM: MR imaging of the chest. Radiology *161*(P):53, 1986.
22. Worthington BS, Doyle M, Chapman B, Turner R, Ordidge RJ, Cawley M, et al: Real-time, cardiac imaging of adults using variations of the echo-planar imaging. Radiology *161*(P):338, 1986.
23. Rzedzian RR, Pykett IL: Instant scan technique for real-time MR imaging. Radiology *161*(P):333, 1986.
24. Brittoun J, Aubert B, Leroy-Willig A, Ricard M, Idy I, Aubert N: Feasibility of routine in-vivo spectroscopy using a clinical MR imager. Radiology *161*(P):148, 1986.
25. Semmler W, Gademann G, van Kaick G, Zabel J, Lorenz WJ: In vivo P31 spectroscopy in humans with a 1.5 T whole body scanner: therapy response of tumors. Radiology *161*(P):92, 1986.
26. van Sonnenberg E, Hajek PC, Baker LL, Casola G, Gylys-Morin V, Mattrey RF, et al: Materials for MR-guided interventional radiologic procedures: laboratory and clinical experience. Radiology *161*(P):121, 1986.

GLOSSARY OF MRI TERMS

ABSORPTION LINE: Peak in NMR spectrum indicating absorption of radio frequency (rf) power by a spin system at a particular frequency.

ADIABATIC FAST PASSAGE: A technique that produces reorientation of the magnetization by sweeping either the external magnetic field or the applied frequency of an rf field through resonance (the Larmor frequency) in a time that is short compared with the relaxation times. Often used for the inversion of spins.

ALIASING: Also called wrap-around artifact, a phenomenon resulting from digitizing fewer than two samples per period in a periodic function. Can occur in MRI when object extends beyond field of view. Portions of object extending beyond field of view boundaries are aliased back to appear at artifactual locations. *See also* Nyquist limit.

ANALOG TO DIGITAL CONVERTER (ADC): Part of the electronic interface that produces a number, in digital, computer-readable form, that is proportional to a (analog) voltage, such as the detected MR signals.

ANGULAR FREQUENCY (ω): Frequency of oscillation or rotation expressed in radians, rather than revolutions or cycles, per second. There are 2π radians in a circle; therefore, $\omega = 2\pi f$, where f is the frequency in terms of cycles or revolutions per second, usually called Hertz (Hz).

ANGULAR MOMENTUM: A measure of rotational or spinning motion. Individual atomic nuclei possess an intrinsic angular momentum, i.e., they rotate about their axes. This intrinsic angular momentum is referred to as spin, or spin moment, and is measured in multiples of Planck's constant divided by 2π. In the absence of external torques, angular momentum remains constant. Generally, a nuclear magnetic dipole moment is associated with a nuclear spin. The ratio of the magnetic to spin moments is called the gyromagnetic ratio, or *g*-value, and may be positive or negative. A torque applied to a gyromagnetic body, such as that produced by a magnetic field acting on a spinning magnetic moment, induces a steady precession of the spin, at constant angle, about the magnetic field direction. This is known as Larmor precession or frequency.

ARTIFACTS: False features in the image produced either by the imaging processor or by the experimental methodology.

Aliasing artifact: In MRI, this artifact occurs when the diameter of the imaged object exceeds the field of view. It is due to low sampling rates in the frequency-encoded direction. It has a more complex cause in the phase-encoded direction. The

---

* Compiled in part with the aid of the ACR Glossary of MRI Terms, 2nd ed., by S. Koenig, R. Brown, R. Price, and R. Tarr with permission of the American College of Radiology and Dr. Leon Axel, Chairman of the Subcommittee on MR nomenclature.

artifact appears as a series of ghost images along the frequency-encoded axis of the imaged object.

Asymmetric brightness: Uniform decrease in signal intensity along the frequency-encoded axis as a result of filters that are too narrow compared with the signal bandwidth. A similar artifact may be caused by nonuniformity in slice thickness, or by nonuniform receiver-coil sensitivity.

Chemical-shift artifact: Chemical shifts in tissue result from the difference in the Larmor frequency of hydrogen molecules in fat and in water. The chemical-shift artifact occurs only along the frequency-encoded axis as a low- or high-intensity band at one side of a structure with high fat content.

Bounce-point artifact: This artifact may occur when magnitude reconstruction is used with an inversion-recovery pulse sequence. The artifact occurs when $TI = 0.693 \times T1$ for any tissue, and $TR \geqslant T1$, and results in an absent signal.

Metallic artifacts: These artifacts are due to distortions of the main magnetic field caused by ferromagnetic materials. The spectrum of appearances includes spatial distortions, a region of signal void, a region of signal void surrounded by a zone of high intensity, or multiple high-intensity rings.

Motion artifact: Ghost images are due to the failure of compensatory gradients to completely eliminate the phase contribution of either the slice-select or the frequency-encoding gradient, when motion occurs in these planes. They may appear along the encoded axis or as blurring in the direction of motion. Temporal lag between phase encoding and signal read-out may cause ghost images along the phase-encoded axis.

Power gradient drop-off: This artifact is seen as a compression of the image along the faulty gradient axis and is due to power drop-off in the frequency- or phase-encoding gradient amplifiers causing the gradient to be less than that assumed by the computer software.

RF tip angle inhomogeneity: Produced by variation in rf energy required to tip protons 90 or 180 degrees within the selected slice volume. Presents as patchy areas of increased or decreased signal intensity.

Truncation artifact: Due to the inability of a truncated Fourier series or finite number of sine waves to perfectly describe abrupt changes in signal intensity. The artifact consists of multiple high- and low-intensity bands that parallel zones of such abrupt changes. This artifact may cause difficulty in the evaluation of complex anatomic areas, such as the larynx, and in the evaluation of small structures, such as the menisci of the knee. Also called Gibbs phenomenon.

Zeroline or star artifacts: Due to system noise or radio frequency interference; appear as a bright linear signal in a dashed pattern that decreases in intensity across the screen, either as a line or as a star pattern.

ATTENUATION: Reduction of power. Attenuation in electrical systems is commonly expressed in dB. (*See also* Decibel.)

ATTENUATOR: A device that reduces signal power by a specific fraction or ratio, commonly given in dB.

BANDWIDTH: In the case of pulsed radio frequency (rf) radiation, it is the range of frequencies present that combine to create a pulse. Also, it is the range of frequencies over which an amplifier or filter is effective.

BLOCH EQUATIONS: Phenomenological equations, proposed by the late Felix Bloch of Stanford University, that describe the motion of the macroscopic magnetization vector. The equations include the effects of external magnetic fields, both static and rf, and of longitudinal ($T1$) and transverse ($T2$) relaxation. They have been generalized by Torrey to include particle diffusion.

BOLTZMAN DISTRIBUTION: Energy distribution of a system of particles at thermal equilibrium. The relative number of particles N_1 and N_2 in two particular energy states with energies E_1 and E_2 is given by

$$\frac{N_1}{N_2} = \exp\left[-(E_1 - E_2)/kT\right]$$

where k is Boltzman's constant and T is the absolute temperature. In the case of a large ensemble of nuclear spins with moment μ in field B, the number of magnetic moments N_p (parallel) and N_a (antiparallel) alignment will be such that there will be a small majority of nuclear moments in the lower energy (parallel alignment) state.

CARR-PURCELL (CP) SEQUENCE: A sequence consisting of an initial 90 degree, followed by a series of equally spaced 180 degree, radio frequency (rf) pulses, often used to measure transverse relaxation ($T2$). This approach can minimize effects of molecular diffusion in a gradient, which often predominates in simpler spin-echo experiments.

CARR-PURCELL-MEIBOOM-GILL (CPMG) sequence: A modification of the Carr-Purcell rf pulse sequence, which uses a 90 degree phase shift between the initial 90 degree pulse and the subsequent series of 180 degree pulses. This reduces the cumulative effects of variations in the 180 degree pulses over the sample volume. (Alternatively, suppression of the effects of pulse error accumulation can be achieved by switching phases of the 180 degree pulses by 180 degrees.)

CHEMICAL SHIFT (σ): The difference in the Larmor frequency of a given nucleus when bound in different sites of a molecule, due to diamagnetic screening effects of the electron orbitals. Chemical shifts provide information about chemical structure and are usually expressed in parts per million (ppm) shift relative to some reference standard.

CHEMICAL-SHIFT IMAGING: A magnetic resonance imaging technique that provides mapping of the spatial distribution of a restricted range of chemical shifts corresponding to individual spectral lines or groups of lines.

CHEMICAL-SHIFT REFERENCE: A compound with which the chemical shifts of other compounds are compared. The reference standard can be used internally (i.e., dissolved in the sample) or can be external, either in a separate sample compartment or set by the software. Because of the need for possible corrections due to differential magnetic susceptibility between an external standard and the sample being measured, and which depend on the shape of the sample, the use of internal standards is generally preferred.

COHERENCE: A constant phase relationship between components of a rotating or oscillating system, or between the system and a reference signal.

COIL: Single or multiple loops of wire designed either to produce a magnetic field from a current flowing through the wire, or to detect a changing magnetic flux by the voltage it induces in the wire.

CONTINUOUS WAVE (Cw): A NMR spectroscopic technique that utilizes continuous rather than pulsed radio frequency irradiation, more common before the development of present-day Fourier technique.

CONTRAST: The relative difference of signal intensities in two adjacent regions of an image.

CONTRAST AGENT: A substance administered to a subject that selectively alters the image intensity of a particular anatomic or functional region. In MRI, this is usually accomplished by altering the relaxation times. *See also* Paramagnetic.

CONTRAST-TO-NOISE RATIO: The ratio of the absolute difference in intensities between two regions of an image to the level of random fluctuations in intensity due to noise.

CORRELATION FREQUENCY; CORRELATION TIME: The correlation frequency characterizes the high frequency limit of fluctuations in the local magnetic field experienced by a spin, often due to motion of that spin relative to others nearby. The correlation time is the reciprocal of the correlation frequency. Transverse and longitudinal relaxation times at a given field are functions of the correlation time and vary significantly with field whenever the Larmor frequency becomes comparable with the correlation frequency.

CPMG: Carr-Purcell-Meiboom-Gill sequence.

CROSSED COIL: Pair of rf coils arranged such that their magnetic fields are at right angles, to minimize their mutual magnetic interaction.

CRYOSTAT: Apparatus for maintaining a constant low temperature (often by means of liquid helium).

CT: X-ray computed tomography.

dB/dt: The rate of change of the magnetic flux density with time. Its magnitude is a potential concern for safety limits, since changing magnetic fields induce electrical voltages.

DECIBEL (dB): A measure of relative power. It is defined as 20 $\log_{10}$ of the amplitude of the voltage in an electrical circuit relative to some standard, or 10 $\log_{10}$ of the relative power.

DECOUPLING: Specific rf irradiation technique designed to remove multiple structure in a particular resonance due to spin-spin coupling with other nuclei. Also, a technique used to avoid interactions between coils, such as occur with separate rf transmitting and receiving coils.

DETECTOR: Portion of the rf receiver that demodulates an rf signal to recover the information contained in the frequency signal. Coherent detection involves a comparison with a reference oscillator.

DIAMAGNETIC: Property of a substance that tends to reduce the penetration of the substance by an external magnetic field. Diamagnetic effects are typically minute (ppm) unless the substance is superconducting, in which case the exclusion of field can be total.

DIFFUSION: The process by which molecules and other particles mix and migrate owing to thermal motion.

DIPOLE-DIPOLE INTERACTION: The interaction of two magnetic dipole moments due to the magnetic field that one generates at the location of the other. Fluctuation in this interaction due to random thermal motion is responsible for magnetic relaxation of both nuclear and atomic moments. In liquids and tissues, protons are generally relaxed by fluctuations in the dipole-dipole interaction with neighboring protons or paramagnetic ions.

DISPERSION: Variation of a quantity with energy in frequency. In NMR, variation of relaxation rates *R1* and *R2* with Larmor frequency (or magnetic field).

DRESS: Depth Resolved Surface Coil Spectroscopy. A method in which spectroscopic data are depth resolved by special applications of shaped rf pulses and gradients.

ECHO: *See* Spin echo.

ECHO PLANAR IMAGING: A technique of planar imaging in which a complete planar image is obtained from one selective excitation pulse. The FID is observed while periodically switching the *y*-magnetic field gradient in the presence of a static *x*-magnetic field gradient. The Fourier transform of the resulting spin-echo train can be used to produce an image of the excited plane.

ECHO TIME: See *TE*.

EDDY CURRENTS: Electrical currents induced in a conductor by a changing magnetic flux, produced either by motion of the conductor through a magnetic field or by a time dependence of the field. Eddy currents are a potential hazard to subjects in very high magnetic fields or rapidly varying gradients. They can also be a practical problem for superconducting magnets, or when induced in shim coils during gradient switching.

EXCITATION: Increasing the energy of a spin system above its Boltzman equilibrium value. If a net transverse magnetization is produced, an MR signal can be observed.

FARADAY SHIELD: Electrical conductor interposed between transmitter and/or receiver coil and patient to block out external electrical fields.

FAST FOURIER TRANSFORM (FFT): An efficient algorithm for calculating Fourier transforms of a given set of data.

FID: Free induction decay.

FIELD GRADIENT: In MRI, a spatial variation of the external magnetic field along a specific direction, e.g., a linear gradient has a constant variation with distance (*see* Gradient).

FIELD-FREQUENCY LOCK: A feedback control used to maintain resonance conditions in the presence of drift of the external field, usually done by monitoring the resonance frequency of a reference sample or line in a spectrum and adjusting the rf transmitter frequency accordingly.

FILLING FACTOR: A measure of the geometrical relationship of the rf coil and the object being studied. It affects the efficiency of irradiating the object and detecting MR signals, thereby affecting the signal-to-noise ratio and, ultimately, image quality.

FILTERING; FILTER: Filtering is a process that alters the relative frequency composition of a signal. A filter is a hardware or software implementation of filtering.

FILTERED BACK PROJECTION: An algorithm used in many technologies to reconstruct an image from a set of projection data (used in CT, MRI, PET, and SPECT).

FISP: Fast Imaging With Steady State Free Precession. Similar to FLASH, which uses small flip angles and gradient echoes, but in which the phase encoding is reversed after data collection. Image intensities are dependent on the ratio $T1/T2$.

FLASH: Fast Low Angle Shot. A fast scanning technique utilizing small flip angles and gradient echoes. Image intensities can be made to have $T1$ and $T2$ dependence.

FLIP ANGLE: The amount of rotation of the macroscopic magnetization vector produced by an rf pulse, measured with respect to the direction of the static magnetic field.

FLOW-RELATED ENHANCEMENT: The increase in image intensity that may be seen for flowing blood or other liquids using appropriate MR imaging techniques; due to the flux of equilibrium spins into the imaging region.

FOURIER-ACQUIRED STEADY-STATE (FAST): MR technique that utilizes variable tip angles in combination with short repetition times in order to allow decreased acquisition times with preserved image contrast.

FOURIER TRANSFORMATION: In MRI, a technique for resolving a complex waveform into the sum of its many frequency components. Fourier transformation of the FID signal gives the NMR spectrum of the sample. In the case of a single spin component resonant system, the spectrum full width at half height is inversely proportional to the time constant of the exponentially decaying FID signal, which by definition, is $1/T2$.

FREE INDUCTION DECAY (FID): The MR signal that follows a radio frequency (rf) pulse, usually 90 degrees. In practice, the initial part of the FID is not observable, owing to the electronics of the receiver (the receiver dead time) by the rf excitation.

FREQUENCY ENCODING: Encoding the distribution of sources of MR signals along a direction in space by generating the signal in the presence of a magnetic field gradient along that direction so that there is a corresponding gradient of resonance frequencies along that direction.

GAUSS (G): Unit of magnetic induction or flux, no longer standard. 1 tesla = 10^4 gauss. (Earth's magnetic field is 0.6 G.)

GIBBS PHENOMENON: A truncation artifact consisting of multiple bands of high and low-intensity bands that parallel zones of abrupt changes in signal intensity. *See also* Truncation artifact.

GOLAY COIL: Term for a particular kind of gradient coil commonly used to create magnetic field gradients perpendicular to the main magnetic field.

GRADIENT: The change in the value of a quantity with location in space; specifically, its first derivative. For example, a magnetic field that is not uniform, but is continuously changing in the x direction, has a magnetic field gradient in the x direction.

GRADIENT COILS: Current-carrying coils designed to produce a desired magnetic field gradient.

GRADIENT ECHO: A spin echo produced by reversing the direction of a magnetic field gradient or by applying balanced pulses of magnetic field gradient before and after a refocusing rf pulse so as to cancel out the position-dependent phase shifts that have accumulated because of the gradient.

GRASS: Gradient Recalled Acquisition in Steady State. A fast scan technique, similar to FLASH, that uses small flip angles and gradient echoes.

GYROMAGNETIC RATIO (γ): Ratio of the magnetic moment of a particle to its spin moment, usually expressed in dimensionless units. (*See* Angular momentum.)

HELMHOLTZ COIL: A pair of current-carrying coils, with well-defined geometries, designed to optimize the uniformity of the magnetic field near the center of Helmholtz pair. The distance between the two single wire loops is set equal to their radius.

HERTZ (Hz): The standard (SI) unit of frequency; the same as cycles per second.

HOMOGENEITY: Uniformity in space. In MR, the homogeneity of the magnetic field is an important criterion of the quality of the magnet.

HYBRID TECHNIQUE: MR fast scanning technique in which the phase-encoding gradient oscillates, allowing multiple views to be obtained with a single repetition, thereby smoothing motion-induced noise while retaining a relatively high signal-to-noise ratio.

INVERSION: A nonequilibrium state in which the macroscopic magnetization vector is oriented opposite to its equilibrium direction; produced either by adiabatic fast passage or by a 180 degree rf pulse. The rate of recovery of the magnetization to its equilibrium value is governed by the longitudinal relaxation time (*T1*).

INVERSION-RECOVERY PULSE SEQUENCE (IR): A pulse sequence that inverts the nuclear magnetization at a time of the order of *T1*; applied before the regular imaging pulse-gradient sequences. The subsequent partial relaxation of the magnetizations being imaged can be used to produce an image that is strongly weighted by *T1*.

INVERSION SPIN-ECHO PULSE SEQUENCE (ISE): A form of inversion recovery in which an initial 180 degree (inverting) pulse is followed in time *T1s* by a 90 degree measuring pulse. A subsequent 180 degree refocusing pulse creates a spin echo for read-out. The sequence can provide images with either *T2* weighting or almost pure *T1* weighting.

INVERSION TIME (*T1S*): In inversion recovery, the time between the middle of the 180 degree inverting rf pulse and the middle of the subsequent 90 degree measuring pulse; the latter is used to detect the amount of residual longitudinal relaxation.

ISOTOPE: Any of one or more species of atoms (elements) with the same atomic number but different atomic mass. Isotopes have different physical properties but nearly identical chemical properties.

LARMOR EQUATION: Relation between the Larmor precession frequency, the gyromagnetic ratio, and the magnetic field H_0.

$$\omega = H \text{ (radians/second)}$$

or

$$f_0 = \gamma H_0 / 2\pi \text{ (Hertz)}$$

where ω_0 or f_0 is the frequency, γ is the gyromagnetic ratio, and H_0 is the magnetic field strength. *See also* Angular momentum.

LARMOR FREQUENCY: The frequency of precession given by the Larmor equation. *See also* Angular momentum.

LATTICE: The thermal environment with which nuclei exchange magnetic energy.

LINE SCANNING: Class of MR imaging methods in which spin density distribution is determined along one line in space at a time. The line is scanned sequentially through a sample to obtain the total image.

LONGITUDINAL MAGNETIZATION (Mz): Component of the macroscopic magnetization vector along the static magnetic field. Following excitation by an rf pulse, Mz will return to its thermal equilibrium value Mo with a characteristic time constant $T1$, the longitudinal relaxation time. In solids, this time is often called the spin-lattice relaxation time.

LONGITUDINAL RELAXATION: Return of nonequilibrium longitudinal magnetization to its equilibrium value. Longitudinal relaxation involves exchange of energy between the magnetized nuclear spin system and the lattice.

LONGITUDINAL RELAXATION TIME $T1$ (SPIN-LATTICE RELAXATION TIME): *See* Longitudinal magnetization.

MACROSCOPIC MAGNETIZATION VECTOR M: The net magnetic moment per unit volume of a sample, the vector sum of all the nuclear magnetic moments.

MAGNETIC DIPOLAR MOMENT: The equivalent of a small bar magnet or current loop, characterized by the geometry of the magnetic field it produces.

MAGNETIC FIELD STRENGTH (H): Magnetic field is a vector quantity that produces torques on magnetic moments. It also induces the macroscopic magnetization M. Its SI unit is amperes/meter; an older unit is Oersted.

MAGNETIC INDUCTION OR FLUX DENSITY (B): A vector quantity related to H that exerts forces on wires carrying current. Often not distinguishable from H, the fundamental difference becomes important in strongly magnetized materials. There are no sources of B other than H. The SI unit is tesla.

MAGNETIC MOMENT, NUCLEAR: The magnetic moment associated a given nucleus. Nuclei with zero spin have zero magnetic moment, but not conversely. The relationship between nuclear spin and magnetic moments is complex.

MAGNETIC MOMENT, PARAMAGNETIC: The magnetic moment associated with a given electronic distribution of an ion or atom; also called "electronic moment." Electron spin resonance (ESR), also electron paramagnetic resonance (EPR), is the analog for the electronic moment of NMR for nuclear moments.

MAGNETIC RESONANCE (MR): The resonant absorption of electromagnetic energy by an ensemble of atomic nuclei or electrons situated in a magnetic field. The frequency of the magnetic resonance coincides with the frequency of the Larmor precession of the magnetic moments in the magnetic field.

MAGNETIC RESONANCE IMAGING (MRI): The use of magnetic resonance phenomena to create images of objects. Currently, this primarily involves imaging the distribution of water and aliphatic protons in the body. The signal intensity of a pixel, and the contrast between pixels, depends on the spin density $[N(H)]$ and the relaxation times $T1$ and $T2$, their relative importance depending on the pulse sequence used. The relaxation times, and therefore the appearance of the image, can be altered by paramagnetic contrast-enhancing agents.

MAGNETIC SHIELDING: A method of restricting the range of the strong magnetic field that surrounds a magnet. This is most commonly done with the use of material with high permeability.

MAGNETIC SUSCEPTIBILITY χ: Measure of the extent to which a substance becomes magnetized in the presence of H. The magnetization is given by $M = 4\pi\chi H$. For diamagnetic materials, $\chi \leq 1$; for paramagnetic materials, $\chi \geq 1$.

MAST: Motion artifact suppression technique. A software technique to correct for motion occuring during data collection.

MAXWELL COIL: A particular type of gradient coil commonly used to create magnetic field gradients along the direction of the main magnetic field.

MEIBOOM-GILL SEQUENCE: A modification of the Carr-Purcell sequence intended to minimize effects resulting from inaccuracies in the 180 degree pulse lengths. (*See* CPMG.)

MULTIECHO IMAGING (ME): Spin-echo imaging using spin echoes acquired in series. A separate image is produced from each echo of the series.

MULTIPLE LINE-SCAN IMAGING (MLSI): Variation of sequential line-scan imaging techniques that can be used if selective excitation methods that do not affect adjacent lines are employed. Adjacent lines are imaged while waiting for relaxation of the first line toward equilibrium. This process can result in decreased image-acquisition time.

MULTIPLE SENSITIVE POINT: Sequential line-imaging technique utilizing two orthogonal oscillating magnetic field gradients, a steady-state free precession pulse sequence, and signal averaging to restrict the NMR spectrometer sensitivity to a desired line in the body.

MULTIPLE-SLICE IMAGING: Adjacent slices are imaged while waiting for relaxation of the first slice toward equilibrium, resulting in a decreased image-acquisition time for the set of slices.

NMR SIGNAL: Electromagnetic signal in the radio frequency range produced by Larmor precession of the transverse magnetization of the sample. Rotation of the transverse magnetization induces a signal voltage in a coil, which is amplified and demodulated by the receiver.

NOISE: That component of the reconstructed image due to random and unpredictable processes.

NUCLEAR MAGNETIC RELAXATION DISPERSION (NMRD): The magnetic field dependence (dispersion) of nuclear relaxation rates, also referred to as NMRD profiles.

NUCLEAR MAGNETIC RESONANCE (NMR): *See* MR.

NUCLEAR OVERHAUSER EFFECT (NOE): A change in the steady-state magnetization of a particular nucleus due to irradiation of a neighboring nucleus of a different isotope or element with which it is magnetically coupled. Such an effect can occur during decoupling and must be taken into account for accurate intensity determinations during such procedures.

NUCLEAR SPIN QUANTUM NUMBER (I): The angular momentum of a nucleus in units of $h/2\pi$. The number of possible quantitized orientations, and thus energy levels, for a given nucleus in a fixed magnetic field is equal to $2I + 1$.

NUCLEON: A proton or a neutron.

NUCLEUS: The positively charged central core of an atom composing nearly all its mass and consisting of protons and neutrons.

NUTATION: A slow, periodic variation of the angle of Larmor precession, generally produced by a resonant rf field.

NYQUIST LIMIT: Frequency of a signal beyond which aliasing will occur in the sampling process. This frequency is equal to one half of the sampling rate.

OERSTED: An old unit for H. It has the convenience that B in gauss, and H in Oersteds, have essentially the same numerical value in air.

PARAMAGNETIC: A substance with the property of becoming magnetized in the direction of an applied field, but not retaining this directional magnetization when the field is removed. The addition of a small amount of paramagnetic substance may greatly reduce the relaxation time of water. Most common paramagnetic substances contain transition metal ions or lanthanides: Gd^{+3}, Dy^{+3}, Ho^{+3}, Fe^{+3}, Fe^{+2}, Ni^{+2},

Cr^{+3}, and Mn^{+2}. O_2 is an exception. Substances with complexes of these ions with paramagnetic properties are being investigated for use as MRI contrast agents. *See* Magnetic susceptibility.

PARTIAL SATURATION (PS): Pulse sequence technique of applying repeated rf pulses in times on the order of or shorter than *T1*. Although this pulse sequence technique results in decreased signal amplitude, there is a possibility of generating images of increased contrast between regions with different relaxation times.

PARTIAL SATURATION SPIN ECHO (PSSE): Pulse sequence technique that utilizes partial saturation, but for which the signal is detected as a spin echo. Even though a spin echo is used, there will not necessarily be significant *T2* weighting unless the echo time (*TE*) is on the order of or longer than *T2*.

PASSIVE SHIMMING: Shimming by adjusting the position of suitable pieces of ferromagnetic metal within or around the main magnet of an MR system. This is in contrast to active shimming, which is achieved by adding extra gradient coils.

PERMANENT MAGNET: A magnet whose magnetic field originates from permanently magnetized material.

PERMEABILITY: Permeability equals $1 + 4\pi\chi$ for diamagnetic and paramagnetic substances, and more generally is given by the ratio B/H, an expression that holds for ferromagnetic substances.

PET: Positron emission tomography.

PHASE CYCLING: Techniques of excitation in which the phases of the exciting or refocusing rf pulses are systematically varied, and the resulting signals are then suitably combined in order to reduce or eliminate certain artifacts.

PHASE ENCODING: Process of encoding the distribution of sources of MR signals along a direction in space with different phases by applying a pulsed magnetic field gradient along that direction prior to detection of the signal.

PLANAR IMAGING: A type of MR imaging in which the information is gathered from an entire plane simultaneously.

POINT SCANNING: A type of MR imaging in which information is integrated one point at a time. A complete image is obtained by sequentially scanning throughout the sample. (Also called "sensitive point" imaging.)

PRECESSION: Rotation of the spin axis produced by a torque applied about an axis mutually perpendicular to the spin and the axis of the resulting rotation.

PROBE: The part of an NMR spectrometer that contains the sample and radio frequency (rf) coils.

PROJECTION PROFILE: A one-dimensional projection of nuclear spin density on the frequency axis.

PROJECTION-RECONSTRUCTION IMAGING: MR imaging technique in which a set of projection profiles of the body is obtained by observing MR signals in the presence of a suitable corresponding set of magnetic field gradients.

PULSE–90 DEGREES: RF pulse that rotates (nutates) the macroscopic magnetization vector 90 degrees in space about an axis at right angles to the main magnetic field and the applied rf field. This pulse will produce transverse magnetization from an initial longitudinal component, and conversely.

PULSE–180 DEGREES: RF pulse designed to rotate the macroscopic magnetization vector 180 degrees in space about an axis at right angles to the main magnetic field and RF field. Inversion of longitudinal magnetization is produced by these pulses.

PULSE LENGTH (WIDTH): Time duration of an rf pulse.

Q FACTOR: Most often, the coil quality factor. A measure of energy loss described as a ratio of energy in the system to energy that is lost in one oscillating radian. The Q factor affects the signal-to-noise ratio, since the detected signal increases proportionally to Q while the noise is proportional to the square root of Q.

QUENCHING: The sudden loss of superconductivity of a current-carrying coil.

RADIO FREQUENCY (rf): The part of the electromagnetic energy spectrum associated with radio waves. The approximate wavelengths involved range from 10^1 to 10^3 meters, with corresponding frequencies being 10^5 to 10^9 Hz.

RADIO FREQUENCY (rf) PULSE: A shaped burst of radio frequency radiation.

RARE: Rapid Acquisition with Relaxation Enhancement. A rapid scan technique that uses multiple spin echoes to produce separate phase-encoding projections.

RECEIVER COIL: Portion of the MR apparatus that picks up the NMR signal, for subsequent amplification and detection.

RELAXATION RATES: Inverse of the relaxation times. Longitudinal relaxation rate $R_1 = 1/T1$. Transverse relaxation rate $R_2 = 1/T2$.

RELAXATION TIMES: Characteristic NMR parameters of magnetized materials, particularly $T1$ and $T2$. $T1$ (longitudinal) is a measure of the time required for the longitudinal magnetization to return to thermal equilibrium with its surroundings. $T2$ (transverse) is a measure of the decay time of the transverse (x,y) component of magnetization, when it is not due to loss of phase due to gradients of the magnetic field. In liquids and in tissue, both R_1 and R_2 of water protons and aliphatic protons arise from spin-spin interactions of a given proton with either its neighboring protons or a nearby paramagnetic ion.

RELAXOMETER, RELAXOMETRY: The measurement of relaxation rates, with length precision, over a range of magnetic field values and temperature requires a specialized instrument called a relaxometer. Relaxometry is the name for the discipline that involves all aspects of relaxation rate measurements and their interpretation. Relaxometry and relaxometer are analogs to, but quite distinct from, spectroscopy and spectrometer.

RESOLUTION: The limit set by noise, hardware, or software to the ability to perceive differences in neighboring parts of a spectrum in spectroscopy or regions of an image in MRI.

RESONANCE: A specific and large response of a physical system to excitation at a specific frequency near an absorption peak. In NMR experiments and MR imaging, the excitation is generated by rf energy.

ROPE: Respiratory Ordered Phase Encoding. A motion suppression technique that reorders the phase-encoding steps of the acquired image data according to the respiratory cycle.

ROTATING FRAME OF REFERENCE: A frame of reference that rotates at the Larmor frequency with respect to the laboratory frame. In this reference frame, the motion of the net magnetization describes a much simpler path than in the laboratory frame.

SADDLE COIL: Coil design that is commonly used when the static magnetic field is coaxial with the axis of the coil along the long axis of the body.

SAMPLING: The process of converting an analog signal into a series of digital values by measurement at a set of particular times. Aliasing will occur if the rate of sampling is less than twice the highest frequency.

SATURATION; PARTIAL SATURATION: After exposure to a single 90 degree rf pulse, if $T2$ is much shorter than $T1$, the net transverse magnetization will disappear before significant repolarization of the spin occurs. The sample is said to be saturated during this time. If the pulse is less than 90 degrees, so that only a part of the signal disappears, the sample is said to be partially saturated.

SATURATION RECOVERY: A type of partial saturation in which the preceding pulses leave the spins in a state of saturation. In this condition, recovery at the time of the next pulse will have taken place from the initial condition of no magnetization.

SELECTIVE EXCITATION: Modulated rf exciting radiation designed to excite only a limited spatial region of the sample, defined by the field gradient.

SHIFT REAGENTS: Paramagnetic compounds designed to induce a shift in the resonance Larmor frequency of nuclei with which they interact.

SHIM COILS: Shaped coils used to produce small field gradients of an NMR magnet to reduce field inhomogeneities needed for NMR spectroscopic analysis.

SHIMMING: Correction of magnetic field inhomogeneity either by changing the configuration of coils or adding shim coils (active shimming) or by adding small pieces of metal (passive shimming).

SIGNAL AVERAGING: A process of averaging repeated signals acquired under similar conditions in a manner that suppresses the effects of noise.

SIGNAL-TO-NOISE RATIO: Term used to describe the relative contributions to a signal of the true signal and random superimposed noise signals.

SPECT: Single photon emission computer tomography.

SPECTRUM: The display of absorption peaks in the frequency domain of the MR signal.

SPIN: The intrinsic angular momentum of an electron or nucleus, usually given in units of $h/2\pi$, and called I. For electrons and protons, $I = 1/2$.

SPIN DENSITY (N): The number of resonating nuclei per unit volume of sample. The true spin density is generally not imaged directly, but can be calculated from signals derived using different interpulse times.

SPIN ECHO (SE): A phenomenon discovered by Erwin Hahn. The reappearance of an NMR signal arising from refocusing or rephasing of the various components of magnetization in the x,y plane. This usually results from the application of a 180 degree pulse (90 degree in the first experiments) after an initial 90 degree pulse and the decay of the initial FID. Measurement of $T2$ values by the Hahn method is complicated by effects of the magnetic field inhomogeneities. The Carr-Purcell and CPMG sequences, which apply a series of 180 degree pulses, can be used for more accurate measurements of $T2$.

SPIN-ECHO PULSE SEQUENCE: In MRI, a pulse sequence utilizing a 90 degree rf pulse followed in time ($TE/2$) by a 180 degree rf pulse that produces a spin echo at time TE. This can be used to produce images with strong $T2$ weighting if TE is approximately equal to the $T2$ of the tissues of interest. Some $T1$ weighting can be gained if the repetition time (TR) is approximately equal to the $T1$ value of the tissues of interest and if TE is much less than the $T2$ value of the tissues of interest.

SPIN TAGGING: Since nuclear magnetization retains its orientation for a time approximately equal to $T1$, this property can be used to trace spatial motion, such as flow, in a region for a time of the order of $T1$, by "tagging" the spins at the start and following the magnetization in space by imaging.

SPIN-WARP IMAGING: Fourier transform imaging in which the phase-encoding gradient pulses are applied for a constant duration but with varying amplitude. This method, as with other Fourier imaging techniques, is relatively tolerant of inhomogeneities in the magnetic field. Also called two-dimensional Fourier transformation (2-DFT) imaging.

STEADY-STATE FREE PRECESSION (SSFP): An MR pulse sequence technique in which a series of rf pulses are used with interpulse spacings that are short compared with $T1$ and $T2$.

STIR (SHORT *TI* INVERSION RECOVERY): Variation of the inversion spin-echo (ISE) pulse sequence using short inversion times (TI). This pulse sequence allows increased image contrast, owing to synergism of $T1$ and $T2$ effects.

STEAM: Stimulated Echo Acquisition Mode. A fast scan technique that produces multiple $T1$ weighted images in the same scan.

SUPERCONDUCTING MAGNET: A magnet whose magnetic field originates from current flowing through a superconductor. Such a magnet must be enclosed in a cryostat.

SUPERCONDUCTOR: A substance whose electrical resistance disappears at temperatures near absolute zero, and below some critical maximum magnetic field. A commonly used superconductor is a niobium-titanium alloy embedded in a copper matrix.

SURFACE COIL: An rf sample coil that does not surround the body, but is placed close to the body surface to limit the region of the body contributing to the detected signal.

T1: *See* Longitudinal relaxation time.

T2: *See* Transverse relaxation time.

TE (ECHO TIME): Time between the center of an initial 90 degree pulse and the center of a subsequent spin echo.

TESLA (T): A unit of magnetic induction: 1 tesla = 10^4 gauss.

THERMAL EQUILIBRIUM: A state in which all parts of a system are at the same time-independent state, characterized by a temperature.

TI (INVERSION TIME): The time between the middle of the inverting (180 degree) rf pulse and the middle of the subsequent exciting (90 degree) pulse, used to measure the longitudinal magnetization in inversion recovery or inversion spin-echo pulse sequences.

TORQUE: A twisting moment, which produces or tends to produce rotation.

TR (REPETITION TIME): The time between the beginning of a pulse sequence and the beginning of the succeeding (essentially identical) pulse sequence.

TRANSVERSE MAGNETIZATION (Mxy): Component of the macroscopic magnetization at right angles to the static magnetic field. Precession of the transverse magnetization at the Larmor frequency gives rise to the detectable NMR signal. In liquids, the transverse magnetization will relax toward zero, its equilibrium value, with the characteristic time constant *T2*.

TRANSVERSE RELAXATION TIME (*T2*; SPIN-SPIN RELAXATION TIME): A measure of the decay time to lose transverse magnetization. *See* Relaxation times.

ZEUGMATOGRAPHY: The name given by Lauterbur to what has now become MRI. Taken from the Greek *zeugma* (to join together); referring to the combining of the static *B* field and its gradient with the NMR signal from tissue nuclei to produce a graphic image.

Appendix Tables

PROPERTIES OF BIOLOGICALLY SIGNIFICANT MAGNETIC NUCLEI

Isotope	Atomic Number	Atomic Weight	NMR Frequency MHz (at 1 tesla)	Spin	Natural Abundance (%)	Relative Sensitivity (Constant field)
H	1	1	42.5759	$\frac{1}{2}$	99.985	1.00
C	6	13	10.7054	$\frac{1}{2}$	1.108	1.59×10^{-2}
N	7	14	3.0756	1	99.63	1.01×10^{-3}
N	7	15	4.3142	$\frac{1}{2}$	0.37	1.04×10^{-3}
O	8	17	5.772	$\frac{5}{2}$	3.7×10^{-2}	2.91×10^{-2}
F	9	19	40.0541	$\frac{1}{2}$	100.0	0.833
Na	11	23	11.262	$\frac{3}{2}$	100.0	9.25×10^{-2}
P	15	31	17.235	$\frac{1}{2}$	100.0	6.63×10^{-2}
K	19	39	1.9868	$\frac{3}{2}$	93.1	5.08×10^{-4}
Ca	20	43	2.8646	$\frac{7}{2}$	0.145	6.40×10^{-3}
Fe	26	57	1.3758	$\frac{1}{2}$	2.19	3.37×10^{-5}

From CRC Handbook of Chemistry and Physics, 49th ed., Cleveland, The Chemical Rubber Co., 1968–69. Used by permission.

PHYSICAL CONSTANTS

Physical Quantity	Symbol	Value
Avogadro constant	N_A	6.0225×10^{26}/kmol
Boltzmann constant	k	1.38042×10^{-16} erg/degree
Bohr magneton	M_B	9.2732×10^{-21} erg/gauss
Electron rest mass	m_e	9.1085×10^{-28} gm
Electronic charge	e	1.602×10^{-19} coulomb
Permeability of free space	μ_0	$4\pi \times 10^{-7}$ henry/meter
Planck's constant	h	6.625×10^{-27} erg sec
Speed of light	c	2.998×10^{10} cm/sec

SELECTED ELECTRICAL AND MAGNETIC QUANTITIES

Physical Quantity	Defined Units	Fundamental Units
Force	newton (N)	kg m/s^2
Energy	joule (J)	N m = kg m^2/s^2
Power	watt (W)	J/S = kg m^2/s^3
Electric charge	coulomb (C)	C
Electric current	ampere (A)	C/s
Magnetic inductance (L)	henry (H)	J/A^2 = kg m^2/s^2 A^2
Magnetic flux (ϕ)	weber (W)	J/A = kg m^2/s^2 A
Magnetic intensity (B)	tesla (T)	Wb/m^2 = kg/s^2 A
Magnetizing force (H)	oersted (O)	A/m
	($B = \mu H$ where μ is permeability)	
Magnetization (M)	oersted (O)	A/m
	($M = \chi H$ where χ is susceptibility)	

Permeability: (μ) of a material is the ratio of the magnetic intensities from a current-carrying coil of wire with and without the material present.

Susceptibility: (χ) of a material is related to the ability of a material to become magnetized when subjected to a magnetizing force, H.

APPROXIMATE RELAXATION TIMES OF SELECTED TISSUES

	T2*\nmsec	T1 (0.5 T)\nmsec	T1 (1.5 T)\nmsec
Adipose	80	210	260
Liver	42	350	500
Muscle	45	550	870
White matter	90	500	780
Gray matter	100	650	920
CSF	160	1800	2400

* *T2* values are approximately field-strength independent.
From Sprawls P Jr: Physical Principles of Medical Imaging. Rockville, MD, Aspen Publishers, 1987. Used by permission.

INDEX

Numbers in *italics* refer to illustrations; numbers followed by t refer to tables.

Abdomen. *See also* Pelvis.
  hematomas in, 499–500
  in pediatric patients, 677–679
    alimentary canal and, 677–678, *678*
    solid organs and, 678, *678, 679*
    urinary tract and, 678–679, *679*
  low field strength and, 701, *703,* 711–714, *712–714*
  MRI applications, in Germany, *772,* 772–773, *773*
Abscesses, hepatic, in pediatric patients, 678, *678*
  of brain, 189–191, *190–192*
    epidural, frontal, in pediatric patients, 662, *664*
  of musculoskeletal system, 623, *624*
    iliacus muscle and, 499, *499*
  ovarian, 910, *911*
  renal, 514
Absolute signal difference (ASD), *1779,* 1779–1781
  noise and, 1780–1781, *1781*
Acquisition node, throughputs for, 1392–1394, 1393t
ACR. *See* American College of Radiology.
Active shielding, 1442
  gradient coils and, 1413
ADC. *See* Analog-to-digital converter.
Adenocarcinomas, low field strength and, 712, *712, 713*
  mammary, hyperthermia and, tumor metabolism and, 1598
  of paranasal sinuses, 311
Adenomas, chromophobe, 235, *235, 236,* 237
  Cushing's, *239,* 239–240, *530,* 530–531, *531*
  follicular, 337, *338*
  in hyperaldosteronism, primary, *532, 533, 533*
  nonhyperfunctioning, adrenal pathology in, 534–535, *535–537*
  parathyroid, 341–344, *342, 343, 365, 365,* 366, *366*
  thyroid, 337, 356
Adenosine diphosphate (ADP), phosphorus-31 studies and, 1504–1508, 1512–1514
Adenosine triphosphate (ATP), creatine kinase flux and, *1751,* 1751–1752
  in ischemic cerebrovascular disease, 198
  phosphorus-31 studies and, 1502–1504, 1506–1508, 1511–1514
  synthesis of, rate of, 1753
Adhesions, of temporomandibular joint, 294, *294*
Adiabatic fast passage, radiofrequency amplitude artifacts and, 1325
ADP. *See* Adenosine diphosphate.
Adrenal glands, 65, 524–543
  anatomy of, 525–526
    left adrenal and, 526, *528*

Adrenal glands *(Continued)*
  anatomy of, right adrenal and, 525–526, *526, 527*
  image optimization and, *526,* 528, *528, 529*
  imaging technique and, 524–525, 525t
  pathology of, 530–543
    adenoma and, nonhyperfunctioning, 534–535, *535–537*
    carcinoma and, 530, 536–537
    Cushing's syndrome and, *530,* 530–531, *531*
    cysts and, 537–538, *539, 540*
    hyperaldosteronism and, primary, *529,* 531, *532, 533, 533*
    metastases and, 536, *536–538*
    myelolipoma and, 538
    neuroblastoma and, *542,* 542–543
    pheochromocytoma and, *538,* 539–540, *541*
    virilizing states and, 534, *534*
  radiofrequency magnetic fields and, low intensity, 1477
  signal intensity and, *526,* 527–528
Agency law, 913–918
  relationship and, consequences of, 916–918
    formation of, 914–915
  vicarious liability and, 915–916
Airway, 436–440, *437*
Aldosteronomas, *532, 533, 533*
Aliasing, 79–80, *79–81*
Alimentary canal. *See* Gastrointestinal tract.
Aluminum, resistive magnets and, 1134
Alveoli, filling of, *437,* 437–438
Alzheimer's disease, 212, 213
Ameloblastoma, of paranasal sinuses, 313, *313*
American College of Radiology (ACR), 941
  third-party payment and, 945
American Conference of Governmental Industrial Hygienists, 1474
American Medical Association, 941
American National Standards Institute (ANSI), 1473
Amniotic fluid, 596–599, *598*
Amplitude modulation, 1417–1418
Anal atresia, in pediatric patients, 677, *678*
Analog-to-digital converter (ADC), 1353–1355, *1354*
Anatomic regions, efficacy and, 889t, 889–890
Anencephaly, 590, *591*
Anesthetics, biodistribution, retention, and perfusion studies of, 1547–1548, *1548*
Aneurysm(s), 63
  aortic, 518, *518,* 521, 773, *773*
    abdominal, combined sonography and MRI and, 764

xv